Clinical Neuroscience *for* Rehabilitation

Margaret L. Schenkman
University of Colorado

James P. Bowman
Retired, PhD

Robyn L. Gisbert
University of Colorado

Russell B. Butler
Emerson Hospital

Dennis Giddings
Giddings Studios, Illustrator

Steven Sawyer
Consulting Editor, Texas Tech University

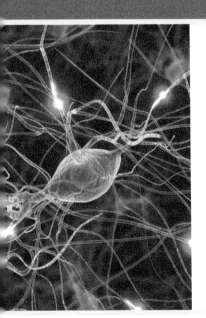
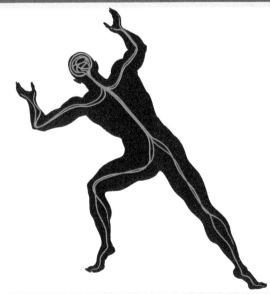
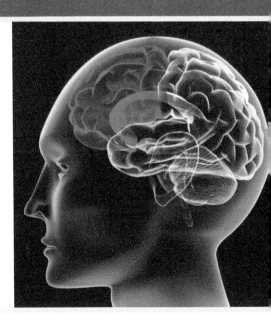

PEARSON

Boston Columbus Indianapolis New York San Francisco Upper Saddle River
Amsterdam Cape Town Dubai London Madrid Milan Munich Paris Montréal Toronto
Delhi Mexico City São Paulo Sydney Hong Kong Seoul Singapore Taipei Tokyo

Publisher: Julie Levin Alexander
Publisher's Assistant: Regina Bruno
Executive Editor: John Goucher
Editorial Project Manager: Melissa Kerian
Editorial Assistant: Erica Viviani
Development Editor: Barbara Price
Director of Marketing: David Gesell
Executive Marketing Manager: Katrin Beacom
Marketing Coordinator: Alicia Wozniak
Senior Managing Editor: Patrick Walsh
Project Manager: Patricia Gutierrez
Senior Operations Supervisor: Ilene Sanford
Operations Specialist: Lisa McDowell
Art Director: Jayne Conte
Text Designer: Ilze Lemesis

Cover Designer: Suzanne Behnke
Cover Art and Chapter Openers: (L) Active nerve
    cell—Sebastian Kaulitzik/Shutterstock Images
    (R) Human Brain scan by X-ray—
    Yakobchuk vasyl/Shutterstock.com
    (C) Illustration—Giddings Studios
Media Editor: Amy Peltier
Lead Media Project Manager: Lorena Cerisano
Full-Service Project Management: Integra Software
    Services
Composition: Integra Software Services
Printer/Binder: R.R. Donnelley
Cover Printer: Lehigh-Phoenix
    Color/Hagerstown
Text Font: 10/12, Times Ten LT Std

Credits and acknowledgments for content borrowed from other sources and reproduced, with permission, in this textbook appear on appropriate page within text.

Notice: The authors and the publisher of this volume have taken care that the information and technical recommendations contained herein are based on research and expert consultation, and are accurate and compatible with the standards generally accepted at the time of publication. Nevertheless, as new information becomes available, changes in clinical and technical practices become necessary. The reader is advised to carefully consult manufacturers' instructions and information material for all supplies and equipment before use, and to consult with a health care professional as necessary. This advice is especially important when using new supplies or equipment for clinical purposes. The authors and publisher disclaim all responsibility for any liability, loss, injury, or damage incurred as a consequence, directly or indirectly, of the use and application of any of the contents of this volume.

Library of Congress Cataloging-in-Publication Data
    Clinical neuroscience for rehabilitation/Margaret L. Schenkman...[et al.].
        p. ; cm.
    Includes bibliographical references and index.
    ISBN 978-0-13-302469-2
    I. Schenkman, Margaret L.
    [DNLM: 1. Nervous System Physiological Phenomena.   2. Rehabilitation.
WL 102]
    LC Classification not assigned
    616.8'04651—dc23

                                2012008761

Printed in the Unites States of America

12 2023

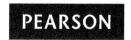

ISBN 10:   0-13-302469-5
ISBN 13: 978-0-13-302469-2

Dedication

For Parthasarthi Rajagopalachari

— Margaret Schenkman

Preface

The nervous system provides an elegant, dynamic, and highly organized mechanism by which humans appreciate, interact with, and navigate the world. An appreciation for neuroscience is foundational for understanding how we feel, perceive, and interpret the world around us; similarly, it is foundational for understanding how we organize movements from relatively simple tasks such as rising from sitting to standing to the execution of highly complex routines, as performed by a professional athlete. When the nervous system operates effectively, an individual can function without ever realizing the complex processes that are ongoing. When the nervous system malfunctions due to injury or disease, the impact on a person's life can be substantial, sometimes even devastating. As such, neuroscience provides a foundational basis for many approaches to rehabilitation.

The nervous system is highly complex and can be studied from many different perspectives. In this text, we present principles of neuroscience in a manner that is intended to make concepts comprehensible for the learner. Thus, we introduce information in a logical and accessible manner, while providing sufficient depth and challenge for the reader to build an appreciation for the intricacies and elegance of this system that underlies so much of our lives. Throughout the text, emphasis is on content of greatest applicability for clinical practice.

Learning and applying this critical content, much of which is abstract, can be anything but simple. For example, pathways of the nervous system cannot be seen in dissection as readily as can the muscles, nerves, and ligaments that form a basis for human anatomy. Mastering an understanding of the nervous system requires a new vocabulary with specialized terms along with a three-dimensional appreciation of complex integrated structures.

We organized this text into seven parts that are designed to facilitate learning, beginning with broad concepts and becoming systematically more detailed as readers progress through the content. The first four parts of the text lay the groundwork for understanding how the nervous system is constructed and how it operates. The final three parts of the text apply this content, first to understanding how the nervous system organizes functionally important information and then to understanding the impact of disease and injury. The sections of this text are outlined in detail in the Introduction.

To assist readers in mastering neuroscience, we employed several specific strategies. First, we present the material in the way that many instructors teach this content. That is, we begin with an overview of the nervous system, with some of the basic definitions that are necessary to learning this content, and with a basic appreciation for the organization of the nervous system from cells to tracts. We then build on that content, introducing increasing layers of complexity. Thus, the reader has many opportunities to revisit content in a format specifically designed to enhance the ability to learn. Second, we emphasize those concepts and constructs of greatest importance to rehabilitation. The role of the motor and sensory systems in control of movement and function is emphasized. Cognitive functions, emotion, and language also are considered in context of rehabilitation. Third, clinical examples are provided throughout the text to illustrate the application of neuroscience across systems (e.g., musculoskeletal as well as neurological) and across the lifespan. Each chapter includes clinical previews, designed to engage readers in thinking about the clinical relevance of the material on which they are about to embark. Throughout each chapter are thought questions, many of which are designed to further assist readers to appreciate the clinical relevance of neuroscience. Each chapter ends with applications in which readers apply material that they learned to clinical problems.

About the Authors

Margaret L Schenkman, PT, PhD, FAPTA, received her PhD from Yale University in microbiology in 1974. In 1980, she received a master's degree in physical therapy from Boston University. Currently, she is a professor, the Associate Dean for Physical Therapy Education, and Director of the Physical Therapy Program, School of 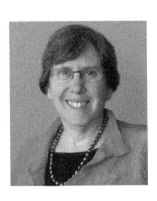 Medicine, at the University of Colorado. Her clinical practice is with individuals who have neurological disorders. Over the past 20 years, she has published numerous clinical papers and research studies. Much of her work has focused on issues faced by people who have Parkinson's disease. She has taught neuroanatomy at Northeastern University, MGH Institute of Health Professions, and the University of Colorado Physical Therapy Program and was a member of the team that taught neuroscience at Duke University.

James P. Bowman, PhD, received his PhD from Northwestern University. Dr. Bowman conducted research in and taught neurobiology to medical, undergraduate, and graduate students for 33 years. He is now retired and is a professional sculptor.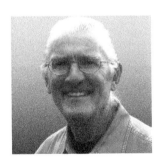

Robyn L. Gisbert, PT, DPT, received her MS in physical therapy in 1994 and her DPT in 2009, both from the University of Colorado, Physical Therapy Program. Currently, she is a senior instructor at the University of Colorado Physical Therapy Program, where she has taught neuroscience and neurological physical therapy since 2007. 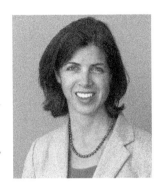 Much of her clinical work has focused on older adults and individuals who have neurological disorders.

Russell B. Butler, MD, is a graduate of Cornell University and received his Doctor of Medicine Degree from the University of Chicago. He trained at the University of Minnesota in neurology and had a fellowship in aphasia and neurobehavior at Boston University. He has taught medical students and residents at Boston University and has taught students in al- 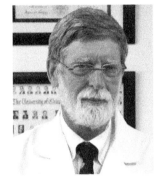 lied health sciences at Boston University, Northeastern University, Tufts University and the MGH Institute of Health Professions. He was a commissioner and chairman of the Commission for Accreditation of Physical Therapy Education. He has been a practicing neurologist and on the staff of Emerson Hospital in Concord, Massachusetts, for 35 years.

Dennis Giddings, medical illustrator, brings 51 years of medical illustration, graphic artistry, and anatomical study to the digital age. Giddings has illustrated and published numerous books and lecture presentations, including *Atlas of Surgical Approaches to the Bones and Joints of the Dog and Cat, Handbook of Small Animal Orthopedics and Fracture Repair, the Virtual Edge Human Prosection Guide, and Pocket Manual of Basic Surgical Skills.* His latest contribution is the complete, illustrated/animated online course offered by the University of New England School of Osteopathic Medicine: "Human Anatomy for the Health Professions." He directed the medical graphics section at the Colorado State University, School of Veterinary Medicine and Biomedical Sciences, and contributed to publications and presentations of that school for 29 years.

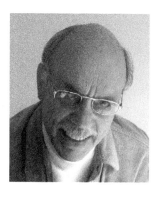

Steven Sawyer, PT, PhD, consulting editor, received a PhD in neuroscience from the University of California at San Diego in 1988, and a master's degree in physical therapy in 1997 from Texas Tech University Health Sciences Center (TTUHSC). He has been on the faculty of the physical therapy program at TTUHSC since 1996 and is currently professor and chair of the Department of Rehabilitation Sciences within the School of Allied Health Sciences. Over the course of his scientific and clinical career, he has 20 years of experience in teaching neuroscience to medical students and physical therapy students.

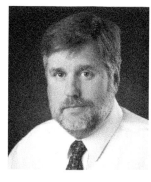

Acknowledgments

We express our tremendous gratitude to Steven Sawyer, PT, PhD, Professor and Chair of Rehabilitation Sciences at Texas Tech University Health Sciences. Dr. Sawyer read each chapter of the text as it was finalized. He made outstanding and valuable recommendations regarding content, organization, and clarity.

Dennis Giddings, who illustrated the text, was an exceptional collaborator and an incomparable illustrator. We thank him for his patience and dedication to excellence.

We express our appreciation to all of the team at Pearson Health Science who shepherded this text through publication. In particular, we thank Barbara Price, who worked with us through the copyedit and page proof processes with patience and dedication to the quality of this text. And we thank Mark Cohen, who was Editor in Chief of Pearson Health Professions; he helped us to navigate the shoals from the beginning and provided support and guidance over many years.

A number of colleagues reviewed chapters in the final stages of preparation of the text and provided invaluable insight. We thank each of them. Kenda Fuller, PT, NCS, and Susan Whitney, PT, PhD, FAPTA, reviewed Chapter 17; Michelle Woodbury, PhD, OTR/L, reviewed Chapter 21;

Sandra Brotherton, PT, PhD, reviewed Chapter 23; Terry Ellis, PT, PhD, reviewed Chapters 24 and 26; Karen McCulloch, PT, PhD, reviewed Chapter 25, and Kathleen Gill-Body, PT, DPT, NCS, reviewed Chapters 22 and 25. Jennifer Stevens-Lapsley, PT, PhD, provided an example of central activation for Chapter 10.

The many professionals listed in the Reviewers section reviewed specific chapters (sometimes through multiple revisions) and provided recommendations that greatly enhanced this book.

We thank our students, who have taught us over many years both through their questions about the content and their curiosity and insights. One of our students, Kyle Ridgway, PT, DPT, reviewed earlier chapters of the text and provided useful comments.

Richard Krugman, MD, Dean of the School of Medicine, and Dennis Matthews, MD, Chair of Physical Medicine and Rehabilitation, created an environment conducive to this project. Finally, we gratefully acknowledge the faculty and staff at the University of Colorado, who graciously gave us space and good humor throughout the task—especially as the task drew to a close.

Reviewers

Roy Lee Aldridge, PT, EdD
Arkansas State University
Jonesboro, Arkansas

Kristine Beekhuizen, PT, PhD, OGCS
Nova Southeastern University
Fort Lauderdale, Florida

Sandra Brotherton, PT, PhD
Medical University of South Carolina
Charleston, South Carolina

John Buford, PT, PhD
The Ohio State University
Dublin, Ohio

Jennifer Christy, PT, PhD
University of Alabama at Birmingham
Birmingham, Alabama

Jamie Duley, MSPT, NCS
Delta College
University Center, Michigan

Gammon Earhart, PT, PhD
Washington University
St. Louis, Missouri

Terry Ellis, PT, PhD, NCS
Boston University
Boston, Massachusetts

Steve Fehrer, PT, PhD
University of Montana
Missoula, Montana

Kathleen M. Gill-Body, DPT, MS, NCS
Newton-Wellesley Hospital
Newton, Massachusetts

Richard Johnson, PT, MA
Stony Brook University
Stony Brook, New York

James Karnes, PT, PhD
D'Youville College
Buffalo, New York

Valerie Kelly, PT, PhD
University of Washington
Seattle, Washington

Gary Krasilovski, PT, PhD
Hunter College
New York, New York

Wen Ling, PT, PhD
New York University
New York, New York

Scott Livingston, PT, PhD, ATC, SCS
University of Kentucky
Lexington, Kentucky

Roberto López Rosado, MSPT, DPT, MA
Florida Gulf Coast University
Fort Myers, Florida

Marybeth Mandich, PT, PhD
West Virginia University
Morgantown, West Virgina

Gary Mattingly, PT, PhD
University of Scranton
Scranton, Pennsylvania

Michael McKeough, PT, EdD
California State University at Sacramento
Sacramento, California

Jim McPherson, PhD, OTR/L, FAOTA
Shawnee State University
Portsmouth, Ohio

Gabriele Moriello, PT, MS, GCS
Sage Colleges
Troy, New York

Lawrence Pan, PT, PhD
Marquette University
Milwaukee, Wisconsin

Robert Ragusa, PT, PhD
University of Cincinnati
Cincinnati, Ohio

Rose Rine, PT, PhD
University of North Florida
Jacksonville, Florida

Clare E. Safran-Norton, PT, PhD, MS, OCS
Boston University
Boston, Massachusetts

Contents

Introduction to the Text

The nervous system provides the means by which humans explore and interpret their environment and determine when, where, and how to move, think, feel, remember, and imagine. The nervous system also processes information about the person's internal state and controls autonomic functions such as heart rate, blood pressure, and homeostasis. When the nervous system functions well, the individual can function efficiently and often with grace. When the system is damaged through injury, disease, or congenital disorders, the individual may have difficulty in any or all of his or her functions. The specific difficulties that a person encounters (e.g., trouble learning, communicating, moving) depend on the cause, extent, and location of the damage, as well as the time in the lifespan at which damage occurred.

This text provides readers with a basis from which to appreciate the nervous system structures and their functions that allow for complex neurophysiological processing subserving human functions. Clinical connections are provided in each chapter to reinforce learning and to illustrate how information is used by the rehabilitation professional. The reader begins to develop the ability to predict neurological problems that will occur with specific diseases or injury and can use this information to understand how interventions might assist individuals to recover function.

To understand the complex functions of the nervous system and the behavioral manifestations that occur when its specific parts malfunction, one must learn a vocabulary, develop an appreciation of the three-dimensional structural organization of the nervous system, learn the basic mechanisms by which information is communicated throughout the system, and learn how given sets of structures are linked anatomically and functionally to mediate specific behaviors. To truly understand the nervous system and its disorders, one must be able to draw *concurrently* from each of these areas of knowledge. The overarching goal of this text is to help the reader attain this understanding. Reaching this goal can prove challenging in the beginning for two reasons: (1) the vocabulary of the nervous system is extensive and unfamiliar, and (2) the vocabulary makes the most sense once one has an appreciation of the three-dimensional structure and the function of the nervous system. Hence, as the reader begins to learn about the nervous system, he or she often is faced with learning terms and constructs out of a context of full understanding. While this can pose challenges, the outcome is well worthwhile.

To facilitate this learning process, basic information is introduced early in the text, and then more detailed information is provided systematically with additional structures and terms added as new functional aspects are considered. Definitions are carefully provided as we proceed; however, it can be difficult to retain all of the definitions initially. For this reason, a glossary of terms is provided on the Companion Website to this text. Important acronyms are provided in a box at the beginning of the chapter.

Information about structure and function of different parts of the nervous system is revisited throughout the text, with more detailed and complex information progressively added to the initial basic content. In addition, in each of the chapters, functional and clinical correlates are introduced. The text is organized in the following fashion:

Part I of the text introduces the fundamental organizational principles of the nervous system. Chapter 1 provides a preliminary three-dimensional overview of nervous system structure and discusses specific aspects of development that are important for understanding the overall structure of the adult nervous system. Chapter 2 then builds on the basic structure, providing more of the detailed naming of parts and relationships. Chapters 3 and 4 focus on the cellular organization of the nervous system. Chapter 3 details the types of cells that make up the nervous system and the functional specializations that equip them to perform unique tasks in brain function. Chapter 4 addresses the neurophysiological processes that underlie all aspects of brain function, allowing neurons to communicate with one another.

With this overall appreciation of the nervous system, it is possible to learn the names and basic external and internal features of the nervous system in more detail. Hence, Part II, including Chapters 5, 6, and 7, provides a more in-depth introduction to the spinal cord and brainstem, diencephalon and cerebellum, and cerebral hemispheres, respectively. The blood supply of each of these five major subdivisions of the central nervous system (CNS) is addressed.

Part III of the text represents a transition from the introduction of structure and terminology to the introduction of systems. This part of the text introduces the somatosensory and motor systems innervating the extremities and trunk, as well as the autonomic nervous system. In these chapters, the overall components of these systems are built anatomically. In the case of the somatosensory system, we begin with the spinal cord and progress to the cerebral cortex; in the case of the motor system, we begin with the cerebral cortex and proceed to the spinal cord. Chapter 8 provides us with our first look at the organizational principles that apply to all somatosensory and motor systems and delineates principles of functional organization as well. Chapter 9 then describes the somatosensory system of the extremities and trunk, including the specific tracts involved in several of the major systems. Chapters 10 and 11 focus on the somatic motor system innervating the extremities and trunk, again focusing on several systems of particular importance for rehabilitation. Chapter 12 builds the autonomic system. Included in each of these chapters are some of the major nuclei, location of major tracts, and blood supply that are most relevant to rehabilitation sciences. In these chapters, cross-sectional representations of the spinal cord are presented, with an emphasis on the relationship of one cross section to the next and to the entire three-dimensional structure of the nervous system.

Part IV presents the sensory and motor systems that innervate structures of the head and neck. In certain respects, this innervation parallels the innervation of the extremities and trunk; in other respects, this innervation is unique because the head contains systems not found in the extremities and trunk. Therefore, Part IV begins with a presentation of the cranial nerves innervating structures of the head and neck (Chapter 13). The functional components contained in each of the 12 pairs of cranial nerves are detailed, along with the clinical methods used to test the integrity of each cranial nerve. Additionally, Chapter 13 discusses common disorders that affect each nerve and the symptoms such disorders produce. Chapter 14 then details the somatosensory and motor innervation of the head and neck. The somatosensory innervation parallels the organization of the somatosensory innervation of the extremities and trunk and is largely confined to just one cranial nerve, the trigeminal (CN V). The somatic motor innervation supplying striated muscle of the head and neck is also presented. The clinical manifestation is discussed for disorders of the somatosensory and motor innervations. Part IV concludes with Chapter 15, which presents an overall review of brainstem structure. The blood supply of the brainstem is detailed, and common clinical syndromes resulting from the disruption of specific arteries are described. With an appreciation of basic neurophysiology and neuroanatomy, including tracts and blood supply associated with basic systems, it is possible to begin to appreciate special functional systems of the nervous system.

Part V of the text addresses what the authors define as *special functional systems* of the CNS. These are systems designed to subserve unique and specific functions in the CNS. Such special functional systems fall into three categories: sensory, motor, and cognitive. Part V addresses the first two: sensory and motor. Included in the sensory systems are pain (Chapter 16), the auditory and vestibular systems (Chapter 17), and vision (Chapter 18). As in other chapters about sensory systems, these special systems are discussed from receptors in the periphery to the cerebral cortex, and clinical conditions resulting from damage to each system are considered. The motor system includes three systems that have specialized functions in mediating motor behavior: the cerebellum, basal ganglia, and motor areas of the cerebral cortex. The cerebellum and basal ganglia are the topics of Chapter 19. When either of these structures is damaged from trauma

or disease, specific and distinctive clinical syndromes result. The control of voluntary movement is detailed in Chapter 20. Although planned and initiated by motor areas of the cerebral cortex, the cerebellum, and basal ganglia each make important contributions to the final, goal-directed voluntary movement.

Part VI continues with a discussion of special functional systems of the CNS, focusing on those of importance for cognition. Chapter 21 focuses on association areas of the cerebral cortex. Such cortical areas subserve specific cognitive functions such as spatial cognition and facial recognition. Association cortices are involved in a host of identifiable cognitive functions (e.g., spatial perception, contingency planning). Not all cognitive function resides just in the cerebral cortex. Both the cerebellum and parts of the basal ganglia are reciprocally linked to cortical association areas, and this linkage means that they, too, participate in cognition. Some of these functions have been identified and are discussed. Chapter 22 addresses systems subserving three other cognitive functions: emotion, memory, and language. Divisions between the systems subserving emotion, memory, and language have dissolved, reflecting the fact that they were arbitrary in the first place. For example, the limbic system is considered to subserve emotion, but it is also intimately involved in memory, and there is a limbic substrate subserving language. Disorders of emotion, memory, and language (aphasias) are discussed in detail. The last chapter in this part, Chapter 23, introduces concepts related to the influence of aging and Alzheimer's disease, with particular emphasis on alterations to cognitive systems.

Finally, Part VII focuses on some of the neurophysiological and neuroanatomical processes associated with injury, disease, and recovery. Chapter 24 focuses on stroke, the resulting cortical lesions, their combined deficits (affecting sensory, motor, and cognitive/perceptual systems), and language. Chapter 25 explores traumatic brain injury and its impact on bony, membranous, and fluid environments in which the brain resides, as well as the clinical consequences of these types of injury. The final chapter, Chapter 26, synthesizes some of the evidence for brain plasticity and its role in recovery following nervous system injury. Neuroplasticity is an area of neuroscience that is just beginning to emerge and that has the potential to radically alter approaches to rehabilitation.

The information in this text, taken together, provides a basis for understanding control of normal movement and perception of the environment, both within and around us. Examples are provided throughout, illustrating the clinical relevance of the material in each chapter. In addition, each chapter ends with applications designed to assist the reader to integrate and absorb some of the critical content as well as to further explore the clinical relevance of the material.

PART I

Fundamentals: The Relationships and Development of Structures and the Basis of Their Communication

The nervous system has a unique and complex structure; each part is exquisitely designed so that it can fulfill its responsibilities. We begin the journey of exploration of the structures and functions of the nervous system by learning the names, shapes, and roles of some of the major features. This includes both the gross, three-dimensional overall structure of the nervous system and its fundamental building blocks—the cells.

With regard to the gross overall structure of the nervous system, it is necessary to learn and recall a myriad of names and shapes of the nervous system. To begin our journey, we introduce some of the major structural components. Only selected components are introduced at this time; we will continue to build on these components throughout the remainder of the text, allowing you to develop a working understanding of the nervous system in a systematic manner, but taking small pieces at a time. Major divisions are introduced first, including distinctions among three functional and structural components of the system (i.e., the peripheral, central, and autonomic nervous systems). Later in Chapter 1, we explore development of the nervous system. An appreciation of some of the fundamental aspects of development will greatly enhance your ability to understand and learn components of the adult nervous system. First, the events that occur during development explain why certain structures are geographically related to others in the adult nervous system. This will be particularly evident in structures such as the brainstem that take on complex structural relationships. Secondly, developmental terminology is carried forward into the adult nervous system. Hence, learning the language of development can assist you in learning the names of adult structures. For these reasons, development is introduced early in this text so that we can draw on names, geographic relationships, and functional relationships from the beginning of our exploration of the nervous system.

In Chapter 2, more structural details are provided (e.g., lobes or divisions of the cortex are differentiated). We also introduce the concept of identifying nervous system structures in two-dimensional sections through the spinal cord and brain, focusing on some of the key areas that will form a basis of all of our future work. This introduction allows you to begin learning how to translate three-dimensional structures into series of thin slices in which structures appear in only two dimensions. The skill of translating information from two dimensions to three dimensions is critical as you proceed through the nervous system—linking different structural components to more and more refined appreciations of functional roles.

All of the three-dimensional structures of the nervous system are constructed out of cells. Cells of the nervous system are particularly intriguing from a functional point of view. They have the unique ability to translate signals from specific modalities (e.g., a sharp object underfoot; colors and shapes associated with visual images) into meaningful constructs that the nervous system can codify, interpret, and act upon. To process all types of information, cells of the nervous system transmit information across great distances.

To appreciate how this happens, it is necessary to appreciate the unique structural elements of cells of the nervous system. Cellular structures and their communication are introduced in Chapters 3 and 4. Included are those elements that transmit information across distances and those that provide support to these communicating cells. Cellular structure is introduced, differentiating the neuron, which transmits information, from other cellular structures that provide support to the nervous system. Finally, the mechanisms are introduced by which cells signal one another and communicate across distances to near and far locations.

Basic Design and Development of the Nervous System

LEARNING OUTCOMES

This chapter prepares the reader to:

1. Recall the meaning of the following terms and any alternate names: nuclei, tracts, column, fasciculus, capsule, commissure, decussation, presynaptic neuron, postsynaptic neuron, afferent, and efferent.

2. Differentiate neurons from neuroglia according to their structure and function.

3. Explain the role of each of the following with respect to communication between cells: presynaptic cell, postsynaptic cell, neurotransmitter, and synaptic vesicle.

4. Differentiate the peripheral nervous system (PNS) from the central nervous system (CNS), describing the locations and major components of each.

5. Differentiate the function of the somatic nervous system from the autonomic nervous system (ANS).

6. Identify five major regions of the central nervous system.

7. Name the portions of the ventricular system and identify the role of this system.

8. Differentiate gray from white matter and explain the major components that comprise each.

9. Explain the importance of apoptosis and name the proteins that are involved.

10. Recall the major events that occur during gastrulation, neurulation, and vesicle development and the terms associated with each.

11. Relate the alar and basal plates to the relative position of motor and sensory nuclei in the brainstem.

12. Identify the brain flexures.

13. Relate the following developmental conditions to the specific structures that fail to develop appropriately: spina bifida, Arnold-Chiari malformation, and anencephaly.

ACRONYMS

AFP Alpha fetal protein
ANS Autonomic nervous system
CNS Central nervous system
CSF Cerebrospinal fluid
PNS Peripheral nervous system

Introduction

The first section of this chapter presents the basic structural organization of the adult nervous system and the terminology applied to it. Two types of cells—neurons and neuroglia—make up the solid tissue structure of the nervous system, which is subdivided into peripheral and central nervous systems (PNS and CNS, respectively). The PNS is subdivided into two major divisions—the somatic and autonomic nervous systems—which have markedly different functions. The CNS essentially is a system of fluid-filled cavities, called the ventricular system, surrounded by neurons and neuroglia that have organized themselves into gray matter and white matter. Note that gray matter consists of the cell bodies of neurons as well as neuroglia and that white matter consists of the axons of neurons as well as neuroglial cells. The CNS consists of five major subdivisions: the spinal cord, brainstem, cerebellum, diencephalon, and cerebral hemispheres. With the exception of the spinal cord and cerebellum, each of these subdivisions is composed of additional named parts. The brainstem (consisting of a medulla, pons, and midbrain); the diencephalon, consisting of a thalamus, hypothalamus, epithalamus, and subthalamus; and the cerebrum (including the cerebral cortex and subcortical nuclei such as the basal ganglia). Information travels between different parts of the CNS—for example, between the spinal cord and cerebral cortex—via tracts and pathways, and these are defined structurally. The entire nervous system is surrounded by a series of three connective tissue coverings. In the case of the CNS, these are called the meninges.

The second major section of this chapter discusses how this adult configuration is attained by considering the embryonic and fetal development of the nervous system. During these developmental periods, the brain progressively differentiates from a single hollow neural tube surrounded by progenitor cells that will become neurons and neuroglia into the definitive five major subdivisions of the adult nervous system with their additional named components. The names in the adult nervous system are derived from those applied during development. Thus, each named subdivision is traced from its origin in development to its adult configuration, which retains its embryonic nomenclature. But as noted earlier, the CNS retains its essential embryonic organization of a fluid-filled ventricular system surrounded by gray and white matter. Structural changes that occur during development result in a dramatic shift in the axes of orientation of CNS structures. Thus, rather than the single longitudinal axis that characterizes early development, the adult CNS has two longitudinal axes: one that applies to the spinal cord and brainstem and a second that applies to the diencephalon and cerebral hemisphere. These two axes meet at an angle, resulting in different orientation terminology being applied along the two axes. This section ends by linking development to important clinical conditions such as defective closure of the neural tube and the bony structures that surround the CNS.

BASIC DESIGN OF THE ADULT NERVOUS SYSTEM

Cells of the Nervous System

The nervous system is made up of two types of cells: **neurons** (nerve cells) and **neuroglial** (glial) cells (Figure 1-1a ■). Both cell types are enclosed by a continuous **plasma membrane**. There are about 100 billion (give or take a few billion) neurons and 5 to 10 times as many neuroglial cells. Neuroglial cells form about half the total volume of the brain. There are different types of cells within both groups that vary from one another in terms of their structure, chemistry, and function. A typical neuron consists of different parts: a **cell body** and two different types of processes extending from the cell body, a single **axon**, and numerous **dendrites**. Neurons sense changes in the environment, communicate these changes to other neurons, and control the body's response to these sensations. Glial cells contribute to nervous system function by insulating, supporting, and nourishing adjacent neurons. The axons of neurons, also called fibers, anatomically connect different parts of the nervous system with one another.

Axons connect the cell body of one neuron with other neurons located in a different part of the nervous system. They are the basis of communication of one part of the nervous system with another. Axons do this by conducting **nerve impulses**, or **action potentials**, along their length.

The main function of neurons is to process information and communicate with other neurons. Communication between neurons occurs at a specialized site of apposition between two neurons called a **synapse** (Figure 1-1b). The first neuron, the one containing the information to be communicated, is called the **presynaptic neuron**; the second, the neuron to receive the information, is called the **postsynaptic neuron**. When nerve impulses arrive at the end of the presynaptic neuron's axon, they cause the release of a chemical, called a **neurotransmitter**, which is packaged and stored in the presynaptic terminal in specialized structures called **synaptic vesicles**. The molecules of released neurotransmitter then diffuse across the fluid-filled cleft separating the two neurons and form transient chemical bonds with receptors located on the membrane of the postsynaptic neuron. The neurotransmitter and

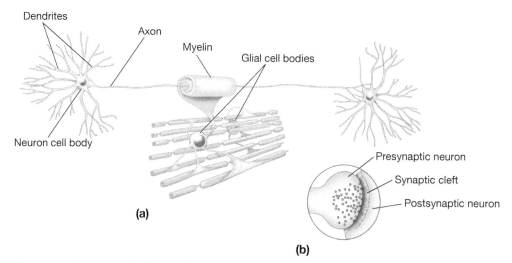

(a)

(b)

FIGURE 1-1 (a) Neurons and neuroglia (glia) are the two types of cells that make up nervous tissue. Neurons consist of a cell body and two types of processes extending from it: a single axon and multiple dendrites, although neuronal morphology is quite variable. Various different types of neuroglial cells exist (see Chapter 3), only one of which is shown in this illustration. Note that this particular glial cell (an oligodendrocyte) has an intimate structural (and functional) relationship with the neuron's axon, called the myelin sheath. (b) A chemical synapse represents a site of structural apposition, not contact, between two neurons because there is a gap, the synaptic cleft, between them. It is the specialized site at which a presynaptic neuron communicates information to a postsynaptic neuron. The information exchange is mediated by a chemical called a neurotransmitter.

> **Thought Question**
>
> The function of synapses will be discussed in detail in Chapter 4. In preparation for understanding that information, it is necessary to recognize the structures related to synapses. What is the convention for naming neurons on either side of the synapse?

its specialized receptor then interact with one another to cause a response in the postsynaptic neuron. Thus, information has been conveyed from the presynaptic to postsynaptic neuron via a chemical mediator, the neurotransmitter. One of the many possible responses of the postsynaptic neuron may be to generate another set of action potentials that then will carry the message on to yet another nerve cell.

Divisions of the Nervous System

Central and Peripheral Nervous System

Neurons are organized into specific nervous system structures that have distinct names. The two principal divisions of the nervous system are the **central nervous system (CNS)** and the **peripheral nervous system (PNS)**. The CNS is encased within the skull and vertebral column. It consists of the **brain**, located within the skull, and the **spinal cord**, located within the vertebral column (Figure 1-2 ■).

The PNS emerges from this bony vault by way of numerous foramina. The PNS is composed of 31 pairs

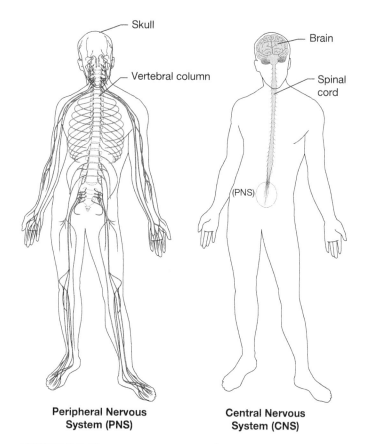

Peripheral Nervous System (PNS)

Central Nervous System (CNS)

FIGURE 1-2 The nervous system consists of two principal divisions. A peripheral nervous system (PNS), made up of spinal and cranial nerves (left), and a central nervous system (CNS), made up of the brain and spinal cord (right).

of **spinal nerves** that attach to the spinal cord, and 12 pairs of **cranial nerves**, 10 of which attach to the brainstem (Figure 1-3 ■). The spinal and cranial nerves are composed of the axons of neurons as well as specific neuroglial cells.

Somatic and Autonomic Nervous System

The PNS is divided into two major divisions: the **somatic nervous system**, which innervates structures of the body wall such as voluntary muscle, and the **autonomic nervous system (ANS)**, which innervates smooth muscle, cardiac muscle, and glands (Figure 1-4 ■). The ANS, in turn, is divided into two divisions: a **sympathetic division** and a **parasympathetic division**, often innervating the same organs but differing from one another both structurally and functionally. In general, the sympathetic division mobilizes body systems during, for example, emergency situations and, in so doing, expends energy, while the parasympathetic division promotes nonemergency functions and restores energy. Thus, a spinal or cranial nerve potentially can contain somatic, sympathetic, and parasympathetic (i.e., autonomic) peripheral nerve fibers, as well as fibers related to the special senses like vision and hearing in the case of cranial nerves.

Organizing Principles

Regions

The brain is further subdivided into four major regions: the **cerebral hemispheres**, **diencephalon**, **cerebellum**, and **brainstem**. Together with the spinal cord, the CNS thus consists of five major regions (Figure 1-5 ■). The term **cerebrum** encompasses the cerebral hemispheres, which include the **basal ganglia**, and diencephalon. Most of these regions are made up of additional named anatomical components. The diencephalon consists primarily of a **thalamus** and **hypothalamus**. The brainstem consists of three parts: the **midbrain**, **pons**, and **medulla**.

The entire central nervous system is surrounded by three connective tissue membranes collectively called the **meninges** (Figure 1-6 ■). These membranous coverings provide important supportive and protective functions to the easily damaged neural tissue of the brain and spinal cord. From outer to inner, these continuous connective sheets are the **dura mater**, the **arachnoid**, and the **pia mater**. Between the arachnoid and pia mater is the **subarachnoid space**, which is traversed by delicate **arachnoid trabeculae**. The subarachnoid space is filled with a fluid called **cerebrospinal fluid (CSF)** and numerous blood vessels.

Directions and Planes

The subdivisions of the CNS differ markedly from one another in terms of their specific anatomical organizations. To understand this variation, it is necessary to have a set of terms that allows us to navigate through the CNS in known directions. This set of directional terms is based on the long axis of the structure being studied. Because of a flexure of the CNS that occurs during development (the cephalic flexure, see section on Development, brain flexures) the longitudinal axis of the cerebrum and diencephalon is bent about 80 degrees in relation to the longitudinal axis of the brainstem and spinal cord. The directional terms applied to the CNS are referenced to these longitudinal axes (Figure 1-7 ■). Because some of these axes differ along the neuroaxis, certain of the directional terms have different meanings, depending on the structure being described. As illustrated, a structure located *anterior* to a reference point in the cerebral hemisphere or diencephalon may also be referred to as *rostral* in position. However, a structure located *anterior* to a reference point in the brainstem or spinal cord cannot be referred to as rostral. Rather, the term *ventral* is used as a synonym for anterior.

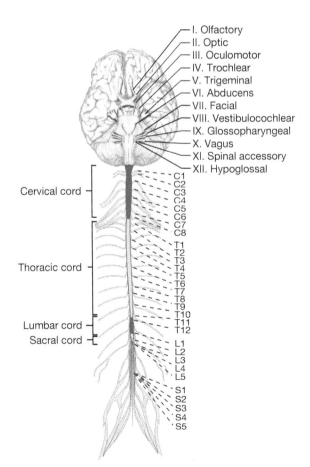

I. Olfactory
II. Optic
III. Oculomotor
IV. Trochlear
V. Trigeminal
VI. Abducens
VII. Facial
VIII. Vestibulocochlear
IX. Glossopharyngeal
X. Vagus
XI. Spinal accessory
XII. Hypoglossal

Cervical cord
C1
C2
C3
C4
C5
C6
C7
C8

Thoracic cord
T1
T2
T3
T4
T5
T6
T7
T8
T9
T10
T11
T12

Lumbar cord
Sacral cord
L1
L2
L3
L4
L5
S1
S2
S3
S4
S5

FIGURE 1-3 Pairs of cranial and spinal nerves.

Thought Question

The central nervous system can be differentiated into five major regions. What are their names? Which major region is not part of the brain?

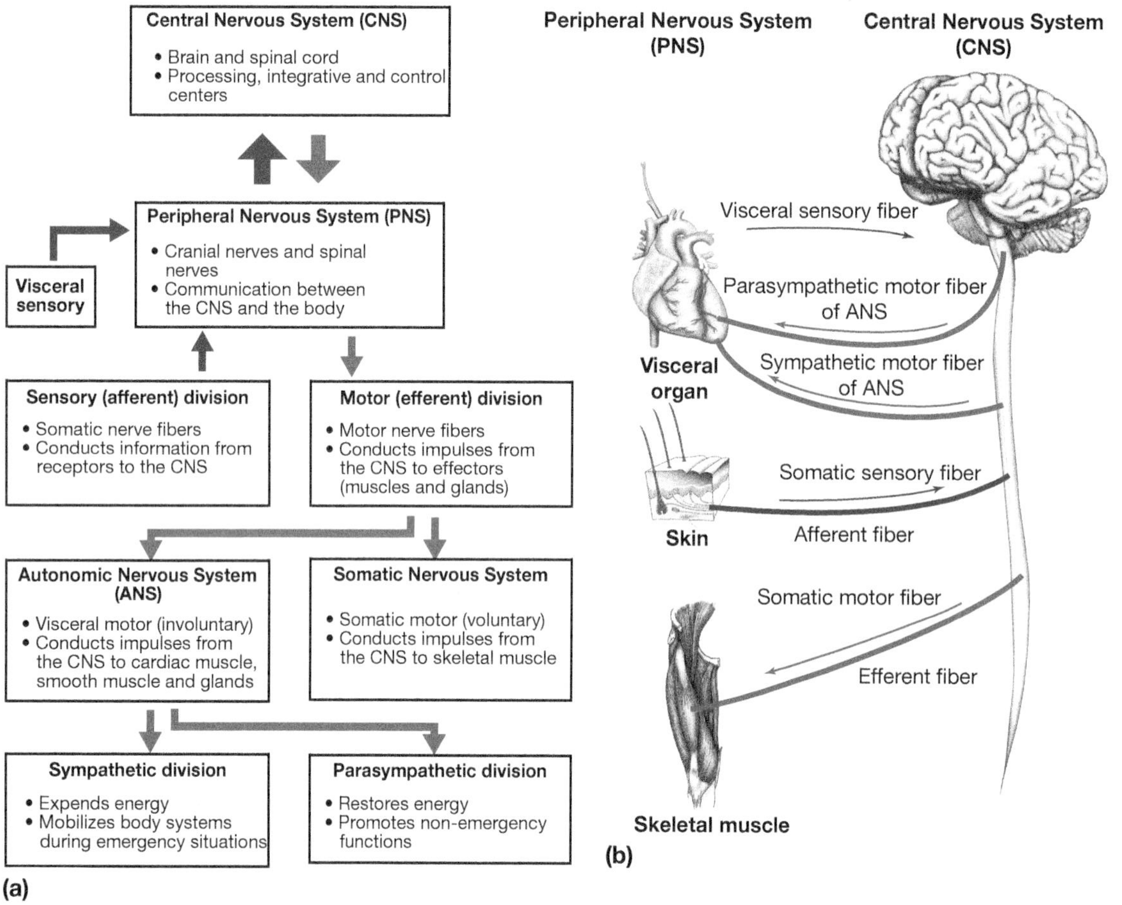

Central Nervous System (CNS)
• Brain and spinal cord
• Processing, integrative and control centers

Peripheral Nervous System (PNS)
• Cranial nerves and spinal nerves
• Communication between the CNS and the body

Visceral sensory

Sensory (afferent) division
• Somatic nerve fibers
• Conducts information from receptors to the CNS

Motor (efferent) division
• Motor nerve fibers
• Conducts impulses from the CNS to effectors (muscles and glands)

Autonomic Nervous System (ANS)
• Visceral motor (involuntary)
• Conducts impulses from the CNS to cardiac muscle, smooth muscle and glands

Somatic Nervous System
• Somatic motor (voluntary)
• Conducts impulses from the CNS to skeletal muscle

Sympathetic division
• Expends energy
• Mobilizes body systems during emergency situations

Parasympathetic division
• Restores energy
• Promotes non-emergency functions

(a)

Peripheral Nervous System (PNS)   **Central Nervous System (CNS)**

Visceral sensory fiber

Parasympathetic motor fiber of ANS

Visceral organ

Sympathetic motor fiber of ANS

Somatic sensory fiber

Skin   Afferent fiber

Somatic motor fiber

Efferent fiber

Skeletal muscle

(b)

FIGURE 1-4 Functional overview of the nervous system. The organizational chart (a) indicates the sensory and motor functional divisions of the CNS. Arrows (b) indicate the direction of nerve impulses of somatic and autonomic fibers.

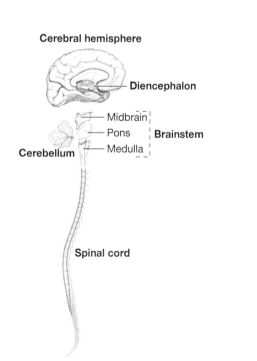

Cerebral hemisphere

Diencephalon

Midbrain
Pons   **Brainstem**
Medulla

Cerebellum

Spinal cord

FIGURE 1-5 The five major subdivisions of the central nervous system include the cerebral hemispheres (telencephalon), diencephalon, cerebellum, brainstem, and spinal cord.

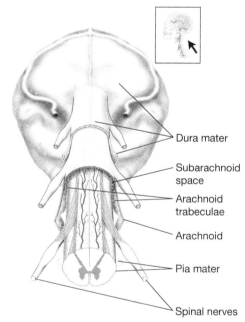

Dura mater

Subarachnoid space

Arachnoid trabeculae

Arachnoid

Pia mater

Spinal nerves

FIGURE 1-6 The entire central nervous system is surrounded by three layers of connective tissue meninges. From outer to inner these are the dura mater, the arachnoid, and the pia mater. Note that there is a space—the subarachnoid space—between the arachnoid and pia mater that is traversed by delicate arachnoid trabeculae that anchor the arachnoid to the pia. The subarachnoid space is filled with cerebrospinal fluid.

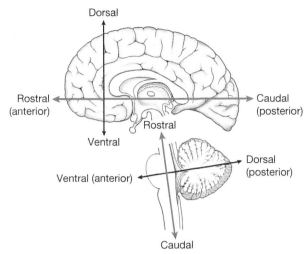

FIGURE 1-7 All directional terms in the CNS are referenced to the long axis (red arrows) of the structure being talked about. Note that the orientation of the long axis of the cerebrum is different than that of the long axis of the brainstem and spinal cord due to the cephalic flexure at the level of the midbrain. This means that some directional terms have different meanings, depending on the structure being discussed.

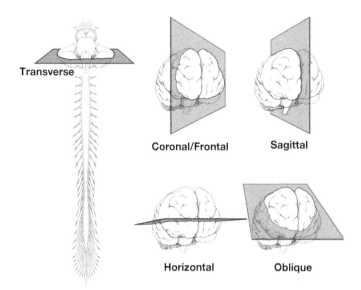

FIGURE 1-8 Planes of section used to study the interior structures of the CNS.

The structures making up the interior of the CNS are studied by examing sections (or slices) at representative levels in each of the five major regions. A **transverse section** is taken at right angles to the longitudinal axis of a structure (Figure 1-8 ■). In the brain, but not in the spinal cord, a transverse section is equivalent to a **frontal** or **coronal**, section dividing the CNS into rostral and caudal components. The **sagittal plane** runs in an anterior–posterior direction, dividing the CNS into right and left components. A **midsagittal plane** divides the brain into two symmetrical halves. **Parasagittal planes** are parallel to the midsagittal plane but do not divide the brain into symmetrical halves. The **horizontal plane** is parallel to the line of the horizon and perpendicular to the sagittal plane dividing the CNS into dorsal and ventral components. An oblique section through the brain also is illustrated.

Ventricles, Gray Matter, and White Matter

The basic design of the brain is a system of cavities, called **ventricles**, surrounded by collections of neuronal cell bodies, called **gray matter**, and collections of neuronal axons, called **white matter** (Figure 1-9 ■). The basic design of the spinal cord is a narrow cavity, called the **central canal**, surrounded by gray matter and white matter.

VENTRICLES There are four ventricles within the brain with three interconnections between them (Figure 1-10 ■). The four ventricles are the left and right **lateral ventricles**, the **third ventricle**, and the **fourth ventricle**. The interconnections are the two **interventricular foramina**, which connect the two lateral ventricles with the third ventricle, and the **cerebral aqueduct**, which connects the third and fourth ventricles. The central canal may be partially

or completely obliterated in the spinal cord of normal adults, serving only as a landmark. The ventricles, like the subarachnoid space, are filled with cerebrospinal fluid (CSF). CSF structurally supports and protects the CNS and also participates in the metabolic activity of neurons. The CSF of the ventricles and that of the subarachnoid space communicate with one another through specific openings as described in Chapter 2.

GRAY MATTER NAMES Gray matter refers to areas of the CNS where there is a preponderance of neuronal cell bodies and dendrites (Figure 1-11 ■). In reality, gray matter is actually a pinkish-gray color because of its abundant blood supply. White matter refers to areas of the CNS where there is a preponderance of neuronal axons. Many axons are invested with an insulating myelin sheath that is mostly lipid and, therefore, has a fatty, white appearance. When a cross section of white matter is stained with a myelin staining technique and the section is examined under high enough magnification, the myelinated axons will appear as circular spaces surrounded by myelin. When the section is examined under low magnification, the white matter appears black after myelin staining and the gray matter a light brown because the neuronal cell bodies are unstained by the myelin staining technique. Neuroglial cells are present in both gray and white matter.

Areas of gray matter in the CNS may be referred to by a variety of terms such as **nucleus**, **cortex**, and **cell column** (Figure 1-12 ■). The term **nucleus** as used here refers to a

---

Thought Question

Nervous system tissue can be differentiated into white and gray matter. What parts of the neuron comprise each?

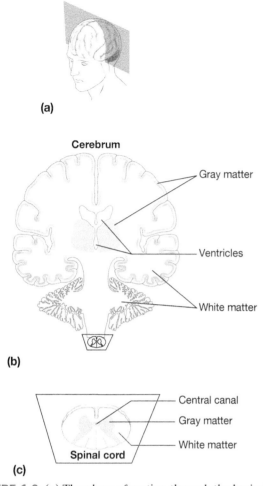

(a)

(b)

Cerebrum

Gray matter

Ventricles

White matter

Central canal

Gray matter

White matter

Spinal cord

(c)

FIGURE 1-9 (a) The plane of section through the brain is frontal. (b) The basic design of the brain and spinal cord is a centrally located cavity surrounded by gray matter and white matter. The brain contains a system of cavities called ventricles, whereas the spinal cord contains only a single cavity called the central canal. (c) The plane of section through the spinal cord is transverse.

more or less discrete collection of neuronal cell bodies within the CNS, and not to the nucleus that occurs within the cell body of a single neuron. The term **ganglion** (pl. *ganglia*) also refers to certain collections of cell bodies or nuclei, specifically those located in the peripheral nervous system. For example, the dorsal root ganglion refers to the cell bodies of peripheral nerves, which are located just outside the spinal cord in the PNS. (Note that the term *basal ganglia* is also used to describe one group of cell bodies in the central nervous system). The term *cortex* (L., *rind*) refers to the layer of nerve cell bodies that covers the cerebral hemispheres and cerebellum. The term *cell column* is applied to nerve cell bodies in the spinal cord that extend over multiple levels of the spinal cord.

WHITE MATTER NAMES In all parts of the CNS, the white matter organizes itself into anatomically distinct collections of axons. Such organizations are described by a variety of terms such as **peduncle** (L., a little foot), **pyramid** (G., a pyramid), **tract**, **fasciculus** (L., a little bundle), **funiculus** (L., a little cord), **column**, **bundle**, **brachium** (L., arm), **lemniscus** (G., a fillet, a group of threads), and **capsule** (Figure 1-13 ■). Some such terms are applied to different subdivisions of the CNS. For example, fasciculus, funiculus, and column are used for structures in the spinal cord, whereas lemniscus, peduncle, and pyramid are applied to structures in the brainstem. Note that the term *column* can be used with both gray and white matter.

Many portions of the white matter are composed of tracts. A **tract** represents a collection of many axons, gathered together in a discrete portion of the white matter, that have the same origin, termination, and function (Figure 1-14 ■). The illustrated tract has its origin in an elongated nucleus (cell column) located in the spinal cord. The tract's termination is in a nucleus located in the brain. The specific name of a tract often is derived from the name of the structure in which its axons originate (e.g., the spinal cord) and the structure in which its axons terminate (e.g., a nucleus of the thalamus). The specific name of this tract would then be the **spinothalamic tract**. Note that the spinothalamic tract extends through the spinal cord and all three subdivisions of the brainstem

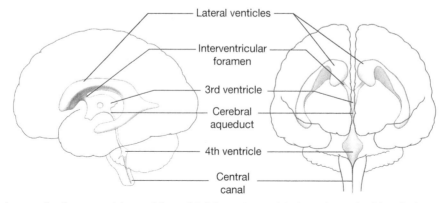

Lateral ventricles

Interventricular foramen

3rd ventricle

Cerebral aqueduct

4th ventricle

Central canal

FIGURE 1-10 The brain contains four ventricles: a right and left lateral ventricle in each cerebral hemisphere, an unpaired third ventricle in the diencephalon, and an unpaired fourth ventricle in the pons and medulla of the brainstem. Each lateral ventricle is connected to the third ventricle by an interventricular foramen, and the third ventricle is connected to the fourth ventricle by the cerebral aqueduct located in the midbrain. The fourth ventricle of the brainstem is continuous with the central canal of the spinal cord.

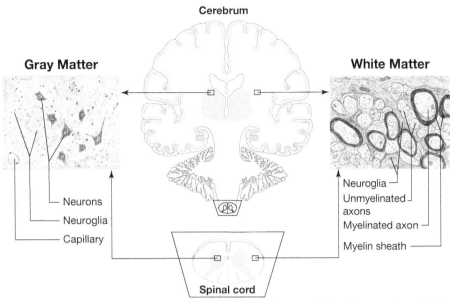

FIGURE 1-11 Gray matter and white matter each have distinctive structural compositions irrespective of their locations in the CNS. The panel on the left shows cells a Nissl stain, while the panel on the right is a myelin stain.

before it terminates in the thalamus. Such tracts are referred to as **long tracts** (or **through tracts**).

A **pathway** is the route nerve impulses (action potentials) travel between two given points in the CNS (Figure 1-15 ■). With this definition, the term *pathway* is interchangeable with the term *tract*. In many instances, a pathway involves more than just a single tract. In this illustration, the pathway is one that carries pain and temperature information from one side of the body to the opposite side of the brain. The information is carried in the form of nerve impulses from the right body wall to the left cerebral cortex. Note that this pathway has crossed from one side of the spinal cord to reach the opposite thalamus

and cerebral cortex. The pathway is composed of three components: peripheral nerve fibers, the spinothalamic tract (which crosses), and **thalamocortical fibers**. Note that the latter two components are named according to the origin and termination of their fibers.

The CNS is divided into symmetrical halves by a midline sagittal plane. In specific locations, axons (fibers) cross this median plane from one side of the CNS to the other. The terms applied to the structures in which this crossing occurs are **commissure** and **decussation** (Figure 1-16 ■). Both halves of the CNS contribute equal numbers of axons to a commissure or decussation. The term *commissure* is used when the origin and termination of the crossing axons are in

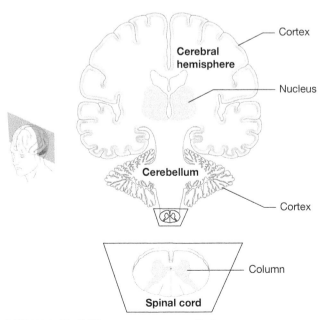

FIGURE 1-12 Different terms are applied to gray matter depending on its location in the CNS.

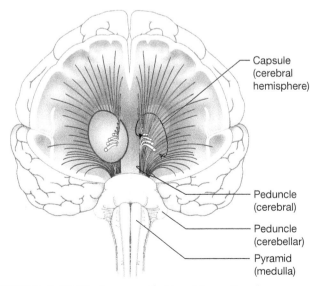

FIGURE 1-13 The terms applied to white matter also vary depending on its location in the CNS and are more varied than those applied to gray matter. Not all terms applied to white matter are illustrated.

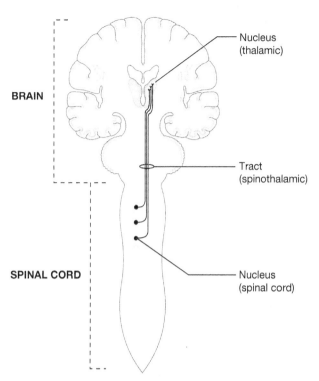

FIGURE 1-14 A tract represents a more or less discrete collection of axons (white matter) in the CNS that have the same origin, termination, and function(s).

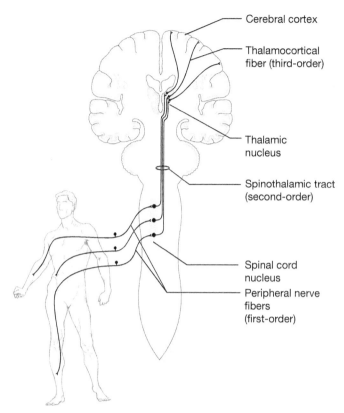

FIGURE 1-15 This is an example of a pathway with one of its components in the PNS (first order) and two components in the CNS (second order and third order).

equivalent areas on the opposite sides of the midline plane. The term *decussation* is used when the axons that cross the midline plane have an origin on one side of the CNS that is different from its termination on the opposite side.

The term **afferent** means *toward* a center, while the term **efferent** means the opposite, or *outward* from a center (Figure 1-17 ■). In discussing nerve fibers of the PNS, the terms *afferent* and *efferent* have constant meanings because the point of reference always is the CNS. An afferent (sensory) fiber always refers to a nerve fiber that conducts information from the body periphery toward the CNS, while an efferent (motor) fiber refers to one that conducts information outward from the CNS to the body periphery (see Figure 1-4). In contrast, when discussing fibers in the CNS, the terms *afferent* and *efferent* are relative. Each usage must be defined with reference to a specific anatomical structure (i.e., the center). Figures 1-14 and 1-15 show the spinothalamic tract that originates in the spinal cord and terminates in the thalamus. When the point of reference is the spinal cord, these axons are *efferents* from the spinal cord. However, when the point of reference is the thalamus, these same axons are *afferents* to the thalamus.

DEVELOPMENT

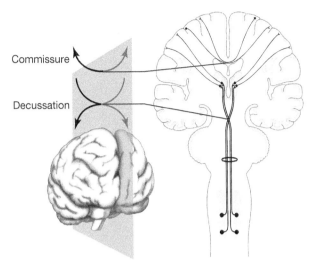

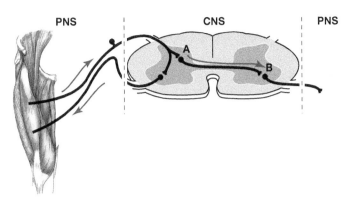

FIGURE 1-16 Fibers (axons) that cross from one side of the CNS to the opposite (contralateral) side are said to decussate or to be commissural fibers. The structures in which this crossing occurs are called either a decussation or commissure. The term *commissure* is used when the origin and termination of the crossing axons are in equivalent areas on the opposite sides of the midline plane. The term *decussation* is used when the axons that cross the midline plane have an origin on one side of the CNS that is different from its termination on the opposite side.

FIGURE 1-17 The terms *afferent* (traveling to the CNS) and *efferent* (traveling from the CNS) have consistent meanings when applied to fibers in the PNS because the point of reference always is the body periphery. However, there is no consistent structural point of reference in the CNS. Thus, in the CNS, a given fiber can be *either* afferent or efferent, depending on the structure selected as the point of reference.

Development of the nervous system involves two simultaneous processes: morphogenesis and histogenesis. **Morphogenesis** focuses on the processes that lead to the normal shape of the adult nervous system. **Histogenesis** concerns the processes by which nervous tissue cells proliferate and develop their form, chemical composition, arrangement (migration), and connections. This chapter focuses on morphogenesis, histogenesis being beyond the scope of the book. One process involving neurons that looms large in development is apoptosis. Apoptosis also is important following damage to the adult brain.

It may seem counterintuitive to state that the development of the nervous system depends not just on the proliferation of neurons and their establishment of appropriate synaptic connections (synaptogenesis) but also on the death of neurons. However, an excess number of neurons are produced by the embryonic nervous system, and their axons establish an overabundance of synaptic connections. In addition, a process of competition for synaptic contact also influences which synapses and neurons survive during development. Thus, during development this surplus must be eliminated and the excess synaptic connections they establish retracted. This normal winnowing process is called **apoptosis**, and its purpose is to establish an appropriate match between the number of presynaptic neurons and their postsynaptic target cells (e.g., other neurons, muscle cells, glandular cells). Apoptosis is in part genetically determined. Therefore, the process is referred to as "programmed cell death" and the genes that mediate it as "death genes." Note that apoptosis also occurs in diseases such as Parkinson's disease (see Chapters 19 and 23).

The number of embryologically generated neurons that survive into adulthood depends on the target cells with which they interact during development. The target cells of developing neurons produce limited quantities of chemical factors that are taken up by nerve terminals and transported in a retrograde direction to the neuronal cell body. These factors were named **neurotrophins** because they originally were thought to promote the survival of neurons by stimulating their metabolism in life-promoting ways. Today, it is known that such factors act predominantly by suppressing a latent biochemical pathway that is present in all cells of the body—a pathway that is, in effect, a suicide program. The neurotrophins are a family of small proteins that include **nerve growth factor (NGF)**, **brain-derived neurotrophic factor (BDNF)**, **neurotrophic factor-3**, and **neurotrophic factor-4/5**. Different types of neurons in the nervous system depend on different neurotrophins or different combinations of factors. But because they are produced in limited quantities, neurons must compete for them. Those that capture sufficient quantities survive.

Neurotrophins bind to specific cell surface receptors, called trk receptors, which they then phosphorylate. Phosphorylation stimulates a second-messenger cascade that ultimately alters gene expression in the cell's nucleus. The key gene is Bcl-2, which is the anti-apoptotic gene that suppresses the latent genetic program for the cell to self-destruct. In the face of neurotrophin deprivation, the actions of the Bcl-2 gene are antagonized, which allows the enzyme caspase-3 to be activated. Caspase-3 activation commits the neuron to an apoptotic death and thus is the executor of cell death. The neuron is systematically disassembled: the neuron shrinks, nuclear DNA fragments, and membrane and cytoskeletal components disintegrate.

While knowing how the nervous system develops clearly assists our understanding of the shape and components of the adult nervous system, it must be recognized that the development of nervous tissue is not isolated from the development of other body tissues (e.g., connective tissue).

> **Thought Question**
>
> Apoptosis is a *destructive process* that goes hand-in-hand with the proliferation of neurons that occurs during development. Explain what apoptosis is and why this process is necessary during embryonic development.

The concurrent development of multiple body tissues is key to understanding malformations of the CNS, in particular a frequently debilitating form of the most common developmental disorder, spina bifida (see Clinical Connections). Development of the nervous system involves several stages: gastrulation, neurulation, and vesicle formation.

Morphogenesis

Gastrulation and Neurulation

The first stage of embryonic development is **gastrulation**, an event that occurs during the third week following conception and involves formation of the three germ layers and notochord. In addition, it defines the midline and anterior–posterior axis of the embryo. During gastrulation the two-layered embryonic disc is converted into a three-layered embryonic disc consisting of **ectoderm**, **mesoderm**, and **endoderm**. Each of these layers gives rise to specific tissues and organs. Ectoderm is our primary concern because it is the origin of nervous tissue and its associated structures. However, a type of cell called **mesenchyme** arises from the mesoderm and is of vital importance in development. Mesenchymal cells are migratory (ameboid) and become distributed singly and in groups to lodge eventually in the spaces between the three germ layers. Additionally, they are pluripotential in that they possess the capacity to develop into a variety of cell types that give rise to the various connective tissues of the body (connective tissue, cartilage, and bone). Of special importance to development is the fact that some mesenchymal cells migrate cranially from their origin to form a median cellular cord, the **notochord** (Figure 1-18 ■).

Interaction between the notochord and its overlying ectoderm is critical because the notochord will induce the process of **neurulation** in the overlying ectoderm. Neurulation, which results in the formation of the **neural tube**, begins during the early part of the fourth week of fetal life. Induction is a general phenomenon by which cell-to-cell signaling (via a variety of signaling proteins such as growth factors) from one group of cells to an adjacent group causes the latter to proliferate, differentiate, and develop into a specific set(s) of cells with irreversibly determined form and function. (Induction is a process that continues throughout embryogenesis, but the specific signaling cells, their proteins, and particular influence on given cellular developments vary as a function of time.)

During the process of neurulation, the notochord and midline mesoderm first induce a longitudinal band of ectoderm to form the **neural plate**, a thickened slipper-shaped region of ectoderm (now referred to as neuroectoderm).

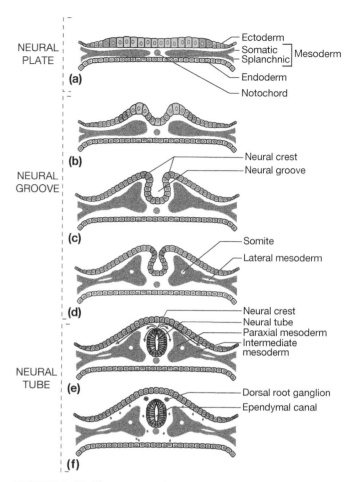

FIGURE 1-18 The process of neurulation. The neural plate (a) thickens during the third week of embryonic development. The neural plate folds inwards to form the neural groove (b), (c) and (d). By week four, the neural tube is formed (e) and (f).

The proliferation of cells at the lateral margins of the neural plate exceeds that of the midline so that the neural plate folds inward at the midline forming a longitudinal **neural groove** flanked on either side by parallel elevated **neural folds** (see Figure 1-18). Appearance of the neural folds coincides with the thickening and segmentation of paraxial mesoderm into discrete **somites**, the precursors of the axial skeleton and skeletal muscle. As the neural folds approach one another in the midline, the neural groove deepens. The folds then fuse in the midline to form the hollow neural tube with a central lumen, the **neural canal**. The walls of the neural tube thicken to form the brain and spinal cord, while the neural canal is converted into the ventricular system of the brain and the central canal of the spinal cord.

Fusion of the neural tube is a critical event. It occurs at multiple sites along the tube, and a failure of closure at these different sites results in specific neural tube defects (see Clinical Connections). For example, anencephaly results from a failure of closure of the rostral neural tube such that there is an absence of the cerebral hemispheres along with an absence of the bones of the cranial vault. Failure of closure at a different site in the more caudal neural tube results in spina bifida cystica.

Fusion progresses in both cranial and caudal directions until only small areas remain open at both ends of the neural tube. There is thus an **anterior (rostral) neuropore** and a **posterior (caudal) neuropore**, where the neural canal communicates freely with the amniotic cavity (Figure 1-19 ■). The anterior neuropore closes on about the 25th day and the zone of closure becomes the **lamina terminalis**. The posterior neuropore closes some two days later. By the time the neural tube is completely closed, the rostral portions of the neural tube have enlarged, and three primary brain vesicles are apparent (see "Vesiculation").

As the neural folds meet and fuse, the thin lateral margins of the neural plate approximate one another, and their cells separate from the neuroectoderm to form the **neural crest** (see Figure 1-18). Initially, neural crest cells form a layer continuous across the midline interposed between the surface ectoderm and neural tube. They then migrate laterally and are segregated into cell clusters. The clusters move to different locations and develop into a variety of cell types within the PNS. These include sensory neurons of the dorsal root ganglia of spinal nerves and sensory ganglia of cranial nerves, postganglionic neurons housed in the ganglia of the autonomic nervous system, Schwann cells of the peripheral nervous system, pigment cells (melanocytes) of the skin (epidermis), and others.

Vesiculation

The process of **vesiculation** begins with the formation of three primary brain vesicles: a **prosencephalon** (forebrain), **mesencephalon** (midbrain), and **rhombencephalon** (hindbrain) (Figure 1-20a, b ■). The prosencephalon and rhombencephalon each subdivide further into two parts at

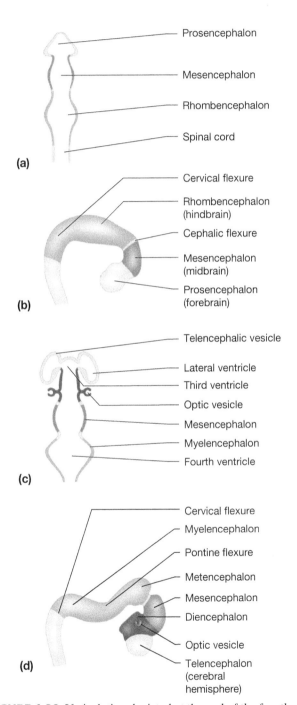

FIGURE 1-20 Vesiculation depicted at the end of the fourth week. (a) A schematic of the three primary vesicles: prosencephalon, mesencephalon, and rhombencephalon. (b) A lateral view of the neural tube illustrating the bends/flexures. Vesiculation is depicted at the end of the sixth week. (c) A schematic of the secondary vesicles and optic vesicles. (d) Lateral view of the neural tube.

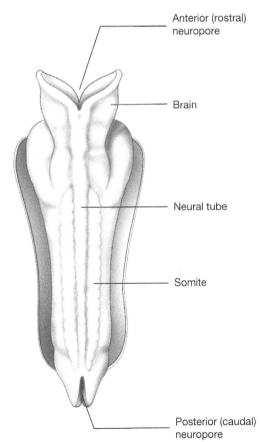

FIGURE 1-19 The anterior and posterior neuropore close by week four of embryonic life. Somites indicate the location of the developing spinal cord.

about the 32nd day of intrauterine life. These subdivisions are referred to as secondary vesicles (Figure 1-20c, d). The prosencephalon becomes the telecephalon and diencephalon. Two evaginations from the telencephalon extend beyond the limit of the lamina terminalis (where the anterior neuropore fused) to form the **telencephalic vesicles** that eventually differentiate into the cerebral hemispheres. On each side of the diencephalon, bulges develop, thus forming the **optic vesicles**.

The five secondary vesicles that differentiate from the rostral part of the neural tube give rise to the entire brain. The diencephalon eventually differentiates into the thalamus, hypothalamus, epithalamus, and subthalamus. The mesencephalon remains undivided. The rhombencephalon subdivides into the **metencephalon** and **myelencephalon**. The metencephalon develops into the pons and cerebellum of the adult, while the myelencephalon differentiates into the medulla oblongata. The optic vesicles eventually differentiate into the optic nerves and retina. It is important to know these names because they are used in describing the adult brain. These developmental events are summarized in Table 1-1 ∎.

Brain Flexures

The different parts of the developing brain undergo different growth rates. As a result, three flexures appear so that the five brain vesicles are not arranged in a straight line (Figure 1-21 ∎; see also Figure 1-20d). Beginning caudally, the **cervical flexure** develops at the junction of the spinal cord and rhombencephalon, but it gradually disappears as the body posture changes and the head becomes erect. The cervical flexure does not persist in the adult. The **pontine flexure** develops in the rhombencephalon and divides it into two portions—the metencephalon and myelencephalon. The **cephalic (or mesencephalic) flexure** develops in proximity to the junction of the metencephalon and mesencephalon. The myelencephalon extends from the level of the first spinal nerve of the cervical cord to the beginning of the pontine flexure, while metencephalon

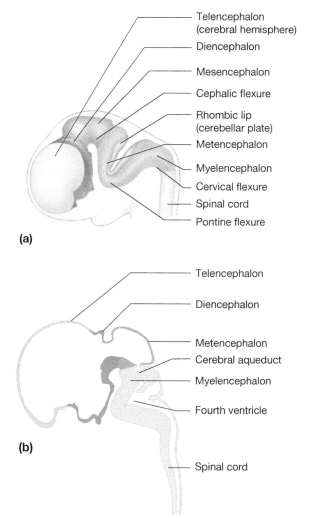

(a)

Telencephalon (cerebral hemisphere)
Diencephalon
Mesencephalon
Cephalic flexure
Rhombic lip (cerebellar plate)
Metencephalon
Myelencephalon
Cervical flexure
Spinal cord
Pontine flexure

(b)

Telencephalon
Diencephalon
Metencephalon
Cerebral aqueduct
Myelencephalon
Fourth ventricle
Spinal cord

FIGURE 1-21 Development at 12 weeks. (a) The cerebral vesicles and (b) brainstem flexures. Depicts the ventricular system.

extends from the pontine flexure to the rhombencephalic isthmus. This prominent flexure creates the deep **transverse rhombencephalic sulcus** on the dorsal surface of the brainstem (Figure 1-21). Although the pontine flexure does not persist in the adult as a bend in the axis of the brainstem, it is

Table 1-1 Vesicles of the Neural Tube and Their Derivatives

PRIMARY VESICLE	SECONDARY VESICLE	ADULT DERIVATIVES	VENTRICULAR CAVITY
Prosencephalon	Telencephalon	Cerebral hemispheres	Lateral ventricles
	Diencephalon	Parts of the basal ganglia	Third ventricle
		Thalamus	
		Hypothalamus	
		Parts of the basal ganglia	
Mesencephalon	Mesencephalon	Midbrain	Cerebral aqueduct
Rhombencephalon	Metencephalon	Pons	Rostral fourth ventricle
	Myelencephalon	Cerebellum	Caudal fourth ventricle
		Medulla	

important in understanding adult brain configuration. This deep flexure has an effect similar to that of flexing a thick rubber hose. That is, the rhombencephalon flattens and widens (producing a diamond, or rhomboid, shape—hence the name *rhombencephalon*) so that only a thin membranous roof unites the two sides. The lateral walls of the resulting rhomboid fossa enclose what will become the fourth ventricle covered only by this thin membranous roof.

Ventricular System

The ventricular system, derived from the lumen of the neural tube, comprises a continuous, fluid-filled series of cavities, components of which are present in all the major subdivisions of the CNS. The general pattern of its adult configuration is clearly apparent in a 12-week fetus. The cavity of the rhombencephalon is the fourth ventricle (see Figure 1-20). As noted earlier, the fourth ventricle consists of a diamond-shaped depression, the rhomboid fossa, covered by a thin membranous roof. As the walls of the midbrain expand, the cavity of the mesencephalon shrinks markedly to eventually form the narrow tube-like cerebral aqueduct. The cavity of the diencephalon is the third ventricle. It, too, shrinks markedly because of the pronounced medial growth of the diencephalon, ultimately becoming a narrow, midline, slit-like cavity. Each of the two telencephalic vesicles contains a lateral ventricle. As the cerebral hemispheres expand and reconfigure themselves dramatically, the shape of each lateral ventricle is correspondingly altered (see Figure 1-10). Communication between each lateral ventricle and the unpaired midline third ventricle is via large openings behind the lamina terminalis called the interventricular foramina.

Regional Development of the Nervous System

The major subdivisions of the CNS are the spinal cord and the subdivisions of the brain: the myelencephalon, metencephalon, mesencephalon, diencephalon, and telencephalon. In the following, each of these subdivisions will be considered separately, although it is to be understood that the described embryologic events unfold simultaneously.

Alar and Basal Plates

Initially, the walls of the neural tube consist of neural epithelial cells arranged as a pseudostratified epithelium. Further development of the neural tube occurs by mitotic division in this zone of germinal cells lining the neural canal. All of the structural components of the CNS except

microglia, blood vessels, and meninges develop from this source. The cells of this innermost germinal zone divide, with most migrating to a new layer where they differentiate into neuroblasts (proliferating further and giving rise to neurons of the gray matter) and glioblasts (that develop into specific types of supporting neuroglial cells).

The wall of the developing spinal cord consists of three layers (zones). The innermost layer is called the ependymal layer because its cells become the ependyma that line the central canal. The bulky intermediate mantle layer becomes butterfly-shaped gray matter of the spinal cord, while the outermost marginal layer develops into the white matter that contains the ascending and descending fiber tracts (Figure 1-22 ■).

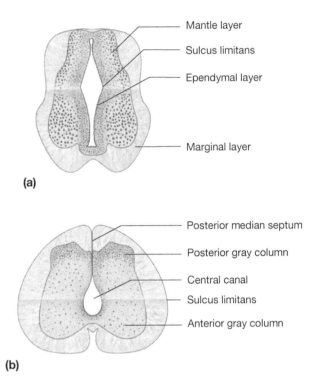

(a)

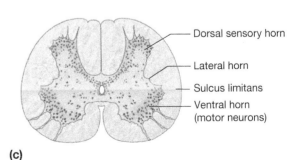

(b)

(c)

FIGURE 1-22 Spinal cord development. (a) At week 5, note the inner ependymal layer, intermediate mantle layer, and outermost marginal layer. (b) At week 8, the central canal is forming. (c) At week 10, the presence of the dorsal, intermediate, and ventral horns is observed. The alar plate is shaded yellow, the basal plate shaded green. The sulcus limitans is not apparent in the mature cord.

Differential thickening of the walls of the neural tube as a result of continued cell proliferation in the mantle layer produces a longitudinal groove, the **sulcus limitans**, on each side of its lumen. The sulcus limitans separates a dorsal bulge, the **alar plate**, from a ventral bulge, the **basal plate**, joined together by thinner roof and floor plates. This separation is important because in subsequent development of the spinal cord and brainstem, the alar plate is associated with sensory (afferent) functions while the basal plate is associated with motor (efferent) functions. Within both the alar and basal plates, neurons associated with visceral (autonomic) functions are located nearest the sulcus limitans.

The sulcus limitans is clearly distinguishable, extending through the hindbrain and midbrain, but its termination in the forebrain is not known. Regions of the brain rostral to the mesencephalon (the diencephalon and telencephalon) develop from the alar plate as does the cerebellum. However, the diencephalon and telencephalon both have sensory as well as motor functions.

Development of the alar and basal plates is a generalized process underlying the development of a number of components of the adult nervous system. We next consider the development of specific subdivisions of the nervous system, important parts of which are known derivatives of the alar and basal plates.

Spinal Cord

The embryonic pattern of the neural tube is maintained in the adult spinal cord, wherein a central cavity (the central canal) is surrounded by a core of gray matter that is surrounded by a peripheral mantle of white matter. The portions of the neural tube that develop into the spinal cord have—in addition to cellular ependymal and mantle layers—a clearly distinguishable outer third layer: the marginal layer that is cell-sparse.

Although the sulcus limitans cannot be distinguished in the adult spinal cord, proliferation of cell bodies in the alar plates gives rise to dorsal gray columns that extend the entire length of the spinal cord. These appear as the **dorsal**

(sensory) horns of the spinal cord in transverse sections (see Figure 1-22c). Dorsal root ganglion cells of the PNS, derived from the neural crest, extend their central processes into the spinal cord to terminate primarily on neurons of the dorsal horn. Their peripheral processes form the sensory component of spinal nerves. Cell bodies of the basal plate give rise to a ventral gray column that also extends the entire length of the spinal cord, as well as to a lateral gray column that is present only over thoracic and upper lumbar levels of the adult spinal cord. In transverse sections, these columns appear as the **ventral (motor)** and **lateral (autonomic) horns**. In the fourth week, axons of the motor neurons exit the neural tube to form the ventral root. The peripheral processes of dorsal root ganglion cells join axons of the ventral roots to form the spinal nerves. As the ventral horns of the two sides continue to expand (along with the ventral funiculus), they bulge out beyond the floor plate to form a deep midline groove—the **ventral (anterior) median sulcus** of the adult spinal cord.

The axons of neuroblasts in the mantle layer grow out into the cell-sparse marginal layer beginning in the fourth week. These axons help form the peripherally located white matter of the adult spinal cord. Some interconnect different levels of the spinal cord (intersegmental axons), while others—specifically axons from neuroblasts in the alar plate—develop into long, ascending sensory tracts of the spinal white matter. Descending (motor) tracts of the spinal cord white matter derive from cells located rostral to the spinal cord (i.e., in the brainstem and telencephalon).

The ectoderm as well as the mesenchyme immediately surrounding the neural tube condense to form the primordium of the meninges. The ectoderm gives rise to the pia mater and arachnoid while the mesoderm gives rise to the dura mater. The origin of the pia and arachnoid from a single layer is indicated in the adult by the presence of the arachnoid trabeculae. The trabeculae are strands of connective tissue that anchor the overlying arachnoid to the pia, an arrangement necessitated by the fact that the space between these two meninges (the subarachnoid space) is filled by a fluid (the cerebrospinal fluid) that begins to form during the fifth week of intrauterine life.

Medulla

The medulla, the most caudal subdivision of the brain, is derived from the myelencephalon and is continuous with the spinal cord. However, the organizational pattern in the spinal cord of a centrally placed core of gray matter surrounded by a mantle of white matter is not present in the medulla. The walls of the neural tube in the developing medulla are spread apart by the pontine flexure. This affects the positions of the alar and basal plates and the configuration of, in particular, the roof plate. The expansion of the rhomboid fossa (fourth ventricle) stretches out the roof plate into a thin single layer of ependymal cells covered by pia mater (Figure 1-23 ■). But the floor plate holds the sidewalls of the neural tube together ventrally

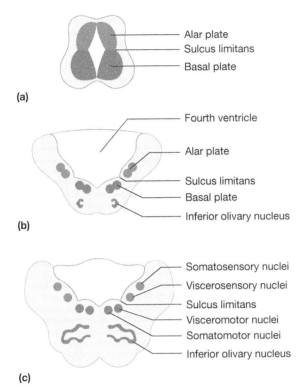

(a)

(b)

(c)

FIGURE 1-23 The medulla is derived from myelencephalon. (a) At week 5, the sulcus limitans divides the dorsal alar plate and ventral basal plate. (b) At week 8, cranial nerve nuclei and other brainstem nuclei begin to differentiate, including the inferior olivary nucleus. (c) At week 10, there are distinct nuclei. Due to the expansion of the rhomboid fossa, the cranial nerve sensory nuclei (derived from the alar plate) are now lateral to the sulcus limitans, and the cranial nerve motor nuclei (derived from the basal plate) are medial. The sulcus limitans is apparent in the mature medulla as two longitudinal indentations in the floor of the fourth ventricle.

so that the sidewalls flatten out into a plate-like structure. The result is that the alar plates come to be located lateral to the basal plates on each side of the medulla. The sulcus limitans, no longer discernable in the adult spinal cord, remains distinct in the adult medulla and separates alar plate derivatives with sensory functions from the more medially placed basal plate derivatives that have motor functions. However, rather than forming longitudinally continuous sensory and motor cell columns as in the spinal cord, the alar and basal plate derivatives in the medulla (and pons and midbrain as well) consist of separate and distinct aggregations of neuronal cell bodies called **nuclei**.

Many, but not all, of these adult brainstem nuclei are associated with cranial nerves. The **motor cranial nerve nuclei** are more medially placed in the floor of the fourth ventricle; their axons innervate somatic and autonomic structures via cranial motor nerves. The **sensory cranial nerve nuclei** are more laterally placed in the floor of the fourth ventricle and receive axons from sensory ganglia associated with sensory cranial nerves innervating somatic and visceral structures.

Thought Question

Compare and contrast the location of the motor and sensory nuclei in the spinal cord and brainstem. Provide several reasons that explain why the locations differ in these two regions of the CNS.

Pons

The pons is derived from the ventral part of the metencephalon. Its configuration is in many respects like that of the medulla (Figure 1-24 ■). The floor of the tapering fourth ventricle is occupied by alar and basal plate derivatives separated by the sulcus limitans. These cranial nerve motor and sensory nuclei reside in a dorsal portion of the pons referred to as the **tegmentum** (L., covering) (see Chapter 2). A larger ventral portion of the pons is referred to as the **basilar portion**. The terms *tegmentum* and *basilar* are commonly used terminology in describing the adult brainstem. Among other structures, the basilar portion contains massive collections of cell bodies that have migrated ventrally from the alar plates. These are the **pontine nuclei**, and they are related to the overlying cerebellum.

Cerebellum

The most pronounced changes that occur in the metencephalon involve development of the cerebellum. The dorsolateral portions of the alar plates in rostral metencephalon thicken markedly to form the **rhombic lips** (Figure 1-25 ■). Each lip projects partly into the fourth ventricle (intraventricular) and partly on the surface of the metencephalon above the roof plate (extraventricular). At first, the rhombic lips of each side are widely separated from one another. But as the lips thicken and the transverse rhomencephalic sulcus at the pontine flexure deepens, the lips approach one another to fuse in the midline caudal to the roof of the mesencephalon. After this midline fusion, the developing

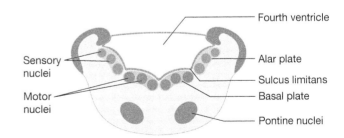

FIGURE 1-24 The pons is derived from the metencephalon, depicted here at approximately week 10. As with the medulla and due to the expansion of the rhomboid fossa, the cranial nerve sensory nuclei (derived from the alar plate) are now lateral to the sulcus limitans, and the cranial nerve motor nuclei (derived from the basal plate) are medial. The sulcus limitans is apparent in the mature pons as indentations in the floor of the fourth ventricle. Note the wide fourth ventricle and presence of the pontine nuclei.

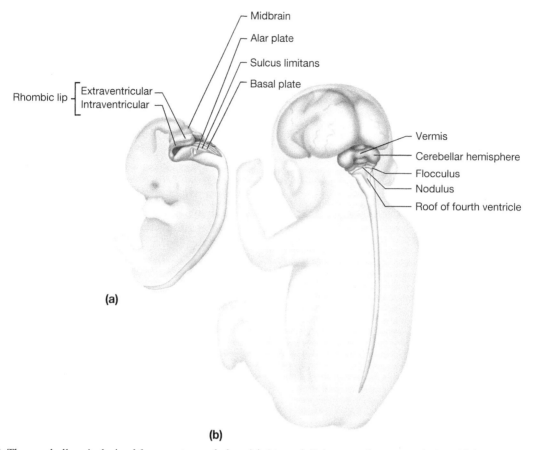

FIGURE 1-25 The cerebellum is derived from metencephalon. (a) At week 7, the rostral metencephalon thickens to form the rhombic lips. (b) By week 16, the rhombic lips are fused, and the midline vermis and hemispheres are apparent in the developing cerebellum.

cerebellum at about three months has a dumbbell shape. The unpaired central part represents the **vermis** of the adult cerebellum, while the lateral expansions develop into the **cerebellar hemispheres**.

Fissures begin to develop in the primordial cerebellum in the fourth month. These are important because they serve to subdivide the adult cerebellum into more or less functionally specific lobes (see Chapter 6).

Mesencephalon

The mesencephalon, smallest of the primary brain vesicles, is also the smallest component of the adult brainstem. Its walls thicken markedly such that its ventricular cavity is narrowed to a small tube, the cerebral aqueduct. An imaginary horizontal line drawn through the cerebral aqueduct serves to subdivide the midbrain into a dorsal part, the **tectum** (L., roof), and a ventral part (Figure 1-26 ■). The dorsal part, or tectum, is derived from the alar plates. It develops longitudinal and transverse depressions that subdivide the tectum into four elevations (the corpora quadrigemina): a rostral pair, or the **superior colliculi**, and a caudal pair, or the **inferior colliculi**. The ventral part consists of the **midbrain tegmentum** dorsally and the **cerebral peduncle (crus cerebri)** ventrally. The alar plate also gives rise to the **periaqueductal (central) gray matter** that surrounds the cerebral aqueduct. Basal plate derivatives give rise to the cranial nerve motor

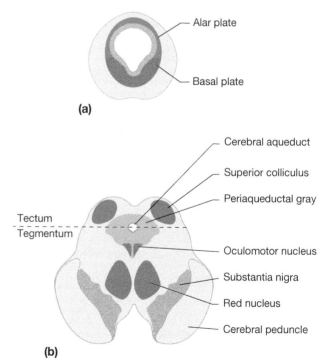

FIGURE 1-26 The midbrain is derived from mesencephalon. (a) The neural depicted at approximately five weeks. (b) A mature midbrain several important structures are observable.

nuclei of the midbrain that includes both somatic and visceral motor nuclei. There are no sensory cranial nerve nuclei that belong exclusively to the midbrain.

Diencephalon

The diencephalon develops from the thickened lateral walls of the caudal part of the prosencephalic vesicle. It usually is considered to arise solely from the alar plate. Three swellings in the lateral wall of the third ventricle give rise to the main subdivisions of the diencephalon: the **epithalamus, thalamus, hypothalamus, and subthalamus** (Figure 1-27 ■). The **hypothalamic sulcus** appears as a longitudinal groove in the lateral wall of the third ventricle and separates the dorsal thalamus, the largest subdivision of the diencephalon, from the ventral hypothalamus. The thalamus forms the lateral aspect of the third ventricle. In many brains, the two sides join across the midline within the third ventricle in a junction of gray matter called the **massa intermedia**. Development of the thalamus is closely related to the development of the cerebral cortex, and the two structures are intimately related in the adult brain. The hypothalamus is a horseshoe-shaped structure consisting of two sides joined by a floor extending across the midline. In the adult, the floor includes the **tuber cinereum**, **infundibulum**, and **mammillary bodies**. This horseshoe configuration has led to the belief that the floor plate and ventral part of the basal plate of the diencephalon may be involved in the formation of the hypothalamus.

A major part of the epithalamus is the **epiphysis** or **pineal gland**. It arises as an evagination of the roof plate between the thalamus and corpora quadrigemina. (These structures are discussed in detail in Chapter 6.) Rostral to the pineal gland, the roof plate remains as a single layer of ependymal cells covered by a highly vascular mesenchyme. The mesenchyme coalesces into pia mater.

Telencephalon

The most dramatic developmental changes are seen in the tremendous growth of the two telencephalic vesicles that are joined across the midline by the thin lamina terminalis (the site at which the anterior neuropore fused). The lamina terminalis provides the only bridge between the two developing cerebral hemispheres (Figure 1-28 ■ ; see also Figure 1-20). Because it is the only site where bundles of nerve fibers can pass from one hemisphere to the other, it is the region where commissural (crossing) fibers begin to grow. By far, the largest bundle of commissural fibers in the adult is the massive **corpus callosum**, while the **anterior commissure** is much smaller. However, both commissures remain attached to the thin lamina terminalis.

Soon after the telencephalic vesicles have formed the basal wall of each vesicle immediately adjacent to the diencephalon, the telencephalon thickens to form the primordia of the basal ganglia, several more or less distinct masses of gray matter buried deep in each cerebral hemisphere of the adult. As the more dorsal parts of the telencephalic vesicle expand tremendously, the primordia of the basal ganglia fold down alongside the diencephalon and become overgrown by the rapidly developing cerebral cortex. The cerebral cortex overlying the developing basal ganglia becomes the **insula** of the adult.

The fibers that connect the telencephalic vesicle with the diencephalon and rest of the brain pass through the developing gray matter of the basal ganglia. As a result, these masses of gray matter acquire a striped appearance—hence the name **corpus striatum** that is applied to the basal ganglia. As the cerebral hemispheres expand rapidly, there is an associated increase in the number of fibers connecting each hemisphere with the rest of the brain. These fibers coalesce into the internal capsule that incompletely

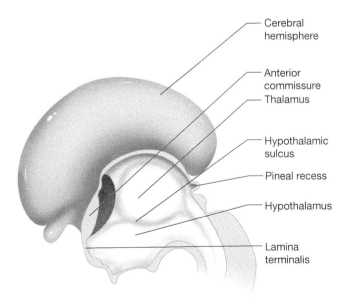

FIGURE 1-27 Lateral view of the developing cerebral hemispheres (telencephalon), with a cutaway midline view of the developing diencephalon.

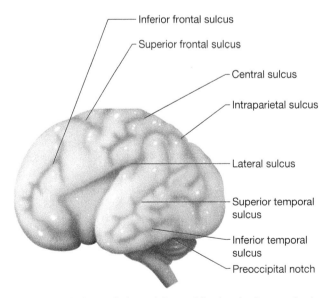

FIGURE 1-28 Lateral view of the rapidly developing cerebral cortex. Sulci are apparent in a fetus at seven months of intrauterine development.

separates the corpus striatum into a **caudate nucleus** and a **lentiform nucleus**. The internal capsule also passes lateral to the diencephalon.

The cortex above the primordial insula expands tremendously during the second through fourth months so as to push the posteroventral part of the telencephalic vesicle downwards and forwards in the shape of a large arc. This portion becomes the future **temporal lobe** (see Figure 1-28). Ultimately, the size and shape of the cerebral hemispheres overlap the structures of the mid- and hindbrains. Because the ventricular cavity of the telencephalic vesicle follows these changes in the shape of the developing hemisphere, the lateral ventricles, too, acquire a C shape (see Figure 1-10). Other structural components of the telencephalon also acquire C shapes; these include the caudate nucleus, the hippocampus and fornix, and the limbic lobe. Continued growth of the cerebral cortex eventually covers the cortex of the insula.

The bony cranial vault limits continued expansion of the hemisphere as a result of ongoing rapid cell proliferation. Thus, to accommodate continued expansion, the initially smooth (lissencephalic) cortex of each hemisphere becomes folded. This infolding results in the formation of grooves, called **sulci**, that demarcate elevations (convolutions) in the cortex called **gyri**. In the adult, fully two-thirds of the cerebral cortex is hidden from view, lying buried in the walls and floor of the sulci.

Sulci appear in an orderly sequence in the developing fetus. In a seven-month fetus, the major sulci of the adult brain can be identified. These are shown in Figure 1-28.

Somites: Development of Vertebrae

The vertebrae and cranium that surround and protect the CNS develop simultaneously with the neural tube. Formation of the notochord and neural tube is accompanied by a thickening of the paraxial mesoderm into two longitudinal columns. During the third week of intrauterine life, these columns become divided into blocks of mesoderm called **somites**. Each somite differentiates into three regions that form different parts of the embryo (Figure 1-29 ■). The outermost layer of a somite is the **dermatome** (Gr. skin slice) that develops into the dermis of the skin. The middle layer of a somite is the **myotome** (Gr. muscle slice), whose myoblasts develop into striated muscle. The innermost layer of a somite is the **sclerotome** (Gr. hard slice), whose cells give rise to bone (vertebrae and ribs).

During the fourth week, cells of the sclerotome surround the neural tube and the notochord. The mesoderm

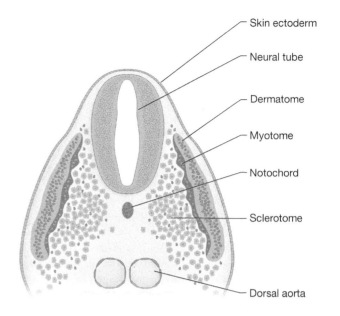

FIGURE 1-29 The development of the tissues surrounding and protecting the neural tube during the third week of intrauterine life. The mesoderm divides into three layers of somites: sclerotome, myotome, and dermatome.

(mesenchymal) cells that surround the notochord develop into the bodies of the vertebrae. As the bodies of the vertebrae develop, the notochord degenerates, but it persists as the nucleus pulposus of each intervertebral disc (Chapter 5). The mesenchymal cells that surround the neural tube form the vertebral arches or laminae, lying dorsal to the developing spinal cord. After formation of the cartilaginous model of a vertebra, including the fusion of the vertebral arches, ossification is evident in the vertebral arches at the end of the eighth week. The cranium develops from mesenchyme (mesoderm) surrounding the developing brain, derived from both somites and neural crest cells.

CLINICAL CONNECTIONS
Neural Tube Defects

A number of congenital disorders occur that result from defective closure of the neural tube. These disorders result when the neural tube fails to close during the third to fourth weeks of development. Neural developmental tube defects are associated with inadequate folic acid consumption, especially during early development. These disorders differ because of the location within the neural tube where the defect occurs; such abnormalities can affect the spinal cord or brain either singly or in combination. However, they are not confined just to neural tissue but may involve associated bony structures as well. The incidence of severe neural tube defects such as anencephaly has been declining because of early prenatal detection as well as dietary supplementation of folic acid. Defective neurulation can be detected through the determination of alpha-fetoprotein (AFP) and acetylcholinesterase levels in the amniotic fluid. AFP increases in amount in the amniotic fluid as well as in the maternal blood serum. Pregnant women with elevated blood serum levels of AFP undergo *amniocentesis* to determine the level of AFP in amniotic fluid, which is a more reliable indicator of a neural tube defect than blood serum level. Acetylcholinesterase is produced by nervous tissue and is excreted in cerebrospinal fluid. It passes into the amniotic fluid when there is a neural tube defect. Ultrasound scans are also used in the prenatal detection of neural tube defects.

Spina Bifida

The term **spina bifida** refers to a failure of the primordial halves of the vertebral arches to fuse in the midline. In severe cases, the contents of the vertebral canal (the meninges and spinal cord) gain access to the body surface. **Spina bifida occulta** is the least severe form of the disorder (Figure 1-30 ■),

typically occurring in the L5 or S1 vertebrae. In spina bifida occulta, the defect is confined to the vertebral arches. The meninges do not extend through the defect such that there is no protrusion of the overlying skin. This condition usually produces no clinical symptoms, but the presence of the defect may be marked by a tuft of hair on the overlying skin.

Several more severe types of spina bifida are referred to as **spina bifida cystica** because the meninges—with or without the spinal cord—protrude (herniate) through the vertebral arch defect to form a translucent cyst-like sac filled with cerebrospinal fluid on the surface of the back. In spinal bifida cystica, which occurs in about 1 of every 1,000 births, the neural tube closes normally. Although spina bifida cystica can occur anywhere along the vertebral column, it is most common in the lumbar region. When just the dura and arachnoid herniate dorsally, the disorder is called **spina bifida with myelomeningocele** (see Figure 1-30). The spinal

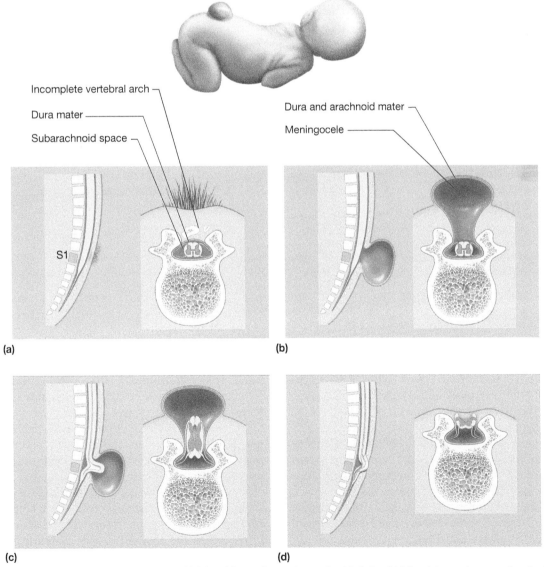

FIGURE 1-30 (a) Spina bifida cystica. (b) Spina bifida with myelomeningocele. (c) Spina bifida with meningomyelocele. (d) Spina bifida with myeloschisis.

cord and spinal nerve roots remain in their normal position, but there still may be abnormalities in the spinal cord. When the spinal cord and nerve roots herniate into the CSF-filled cyst, the condition is called spina bifida with meningomyelocele (see Figure 1-30c). The incidence of meningomyelocele is 2 to 3 per 1,000 births, and approximately 80 percent occur in the lumbar region. The condition is about 10 times more common than spina bifida with meningocele; the clinical consequences also are much more severe.

The marked neurological deficits in meningomyelocele manifest themselves inferior to the level of the protruding cyst. With lumbosacral involvement, a saddle anesthesia is almost always present in which the area of skin without sensation is in the region of the body that would rest on a saddle during riding. Paralysis of the bladder and anal sphincters is common, along with partial or complete paralysis of skeletal muscle of the legs. Because nerve fibers do not develop normally in this disorder, even successful surgical treatment of the meningomyelocele does not usually eliminate the neurological symptoms.

The most severe type of spina bifida is spina bifida with myeloschisis in which there is no meningeal cyst (see Figure 1-30d). In this disorder, the neural folds of the caudal neuropore fail to fuse (Gr. *schisis*, cleavage). The open spinal cord is exposed on the surface of the back, and the neural epithelium is continuous with adjacent skin (surface epithelium). Spinal nerve roots are attached to the ventral surface of the exposed neural tissue. The neurological deficits are severe because neurons in the region of myeloschisis fail to differentiate normally.

Arnold-Chiari Malformation

Most meningomyeloceles (more than half) in the lumbosacral region are associated with another congenital defect called the **Arnold-Chiari malformation**, or cerebellomedullary defect. This is a congenital anomaly in which the medulla and posterior cerebellum are elongated and extend into the foramen magnum, with displacement of the medulla into the inferior part of the fourth ventricle and cervical spinal canal. In many individuals, there are no clinical symptoms. However, if the malformation is severe enough, there can be obliteration of the ventricular drainage system resulting in hydrocephalus. Symptoms typically result from involvement of the medulla and its associated cranial nerves such as respiratory problems, difficulty in swallowing, diminished gag reflex and noisy breathing or laryngeal stridor, resulting from vocal cord paralysis. In addition to spina bifida, syringomyelia of the cervical spinal cord and hydrocephalus are commonly associated with this congenital anomaly. These conditions are discussed in Chapters 9 and 25.

Anencephaly

Anencephaly, in which the rostral neuropore fails to close, is one of the more common and dismaying congenital malformations of the brain. Its incidence varies from 0.5 to 2.0 per 1,000 live births, with females significantly predominating. Northern Ireland and South Wales are the areas with the highest incidence. Large portions of the scalp, cranial bones, and cerebral hemispheres (both cortex and white matter) are absent, and the brain appears as a small, vascularized mass lacking structure. A brainstem, spinal cord, and cerebellum are present, but they, too, usually are malformed. Most anencephalic fetuses (65 percent) die in utero and virtually all by the end of the first postnatal week.

Thought Question

Defective neurulation results in developmental defects. As a rehabilitation professional, you may treat children or adults with such deficits. What are the common malformations, which structures failed to develop properly, and how do you expect these malformations to affect the individual's physical abilities?

Summary

The nervous system is composed of two types of cells: neurons and neuroglia. The parts of a typical neuron are the cell body and the processes extending from it: a single axon and multiple dendrites. The main function of neurons is to process information and communicate with other neurons, while the main function of neuroglial cells is to support the activities of neurons. Neurons communicate with one another via a chemical neurotransmitter that is released at a specialized structure—the synapse—which occurs between two neurons. The nervous system consists of two major divisions: the CNS and PNS, each of which is further subdivided into different components. The basic design of the CNS is a system of cavities surrounded by gray and white matter, each of which is defined in terms of its major structural components. A variety of terms applied to the nervous system were defined including tract, pathway, decussation, commissure, afferent, efferent, and others.

The development of the nervous system was described in order to better understand the configuration and subdivisions of the adult nervous system. Morphogenesis of the nervous system involves three stages: gastrulation, during which three cellular layers are differentiated with the ectoderm, giving rise to the nervous system; neurulation, during which the neural tube is formed; and vesicle formation, during which the rostral portion of neural tube expands into five vesicles from which the subdivisions of the adult brain develop, including the telencephalon, diencephalon, mesencephalon, metencephalon, and myelencephalon. The caudal portion of the neural tube gives rise to the spinal cord. The ventricular system develops from the lumen of the neural tube and thus has a component in each of the subdivisions of the adult brain. Development of the alar and basal plates of the neural tube is a key event because the alar plate gives rise to neurons with sensory functions and the basal plate to neurons with motor functions not only in the spinal cord but also in the brainstem. In terms of structural reorganization, that occurring in the telencephalon is the most dramatic. The cerebral hemispheres expand to overlie the diencephalon and hide most of the midbrain from view. A variety of developmental defects can occur—the most common being those involving neurulation, in particular, spina bifida.

Applications

1. Diagram a cross-sectional representation of the neural tube during the fourth week of development. Identify the sulcus limitans, alar plate, basal plate, and neural crest cells.

2. Diagram a cross-sectional representation of the embryonic spinal cord during the sixth week of development. Identify the sulcus limitans, alar plate, and basal plate. Draw a dorsal root ganglion cell sending its central process into the alar plate via the dorsal root. Draw a motor neuron with its cell body in the basal plate and axon exiting via the ventral root.

3. Diagram a cross-sectional representation of the adult spinal cord. Draw a dorsal root ganglion cell sending its central process into the dorsal gray via the dorsal root. Draw a motor neuron with its cell body in the ventral gray and axon exiting via the ventral root. Although the sulcus limitans cannot be distinguished in the adult spinal cord, note the relationship of sensory and motor information.

4. Diagram a cross-sectional representation of the adult medulla. Identify the sulcus limitans. Identify the location of the sensory and motor cranial nerve nuclei in relationship to the sulcus limitans.

References

Edwards, A. *Vocabulary Guide to Neuroanatomy*. East Bay Publishing Co., Berkeley, CA, 1967.

Moore, K. L., and Persaud, T. V. N. *The Developing Human: Clinically Oriented Embryology*, 7th ed. W. B. Saunders, Philadelphia, 2003.

Nolte, J. *The Human Brain: An Introduction to Its Functional Anatomy*. Mosby Elsevier, Philadelphia, 2009.

Parent, A. Ch. 3. Development of the nervous system. In: *Carpenter's Human Neuroanatomy*, 9th ed. Williams & Wilkins, Baltimore, 1996.

Ropper, A. H., and Brown, R. H. Ch. 38. Developmental diseases of the nervous system. In: *Adams and Victor's Principles of Neurology*. 8th ed. McGraw-Hill, New York, 2005.

Van Allen, M. I., et al. Evidence for multi-site closure of the neural tube in humans. *Am J Med Genet* 47:723, 1993.

PEARSON
myhealthprofessionskit™

Use this address to access the Companion Website created for this textbook. Simply select "Physical Therapy" from the choice of disciplines. Find this book and log in using your username and password to access self-assessment questions, a glossary, and more.

Regional Anatomy and Blood Supply

LEARNING OUTCOMES

This chapter prepares the reader to:

1 Recall the meaning of the following terms: ganglion, peduncle, colliculus, dermatome, and myotome.

2 Name five regions of the spinal cord and identify their relative locations.

3 Explain why the cervical and lumbar levels of the spinal cord are large (bulge) in comparison to the thoracic and sacral levels.

4 Explain why an injury to neurons in the cervical spinal cord could affect sensory and motor function for both the arms and legs, whereas an injury to neurons in the lumbar spinal cord could only affect sensory and motor function of the legs, but not the arms.

5 Relate spinal nerve roots to the mucsle groups that they innervate.

6 Recognize major structures on the surface of the brainstem, including the following: cerebellar peduncles, pyramids, olives, basilar sulcus, cerebral peduncles, and corpora quadrigemina.

7 Name the nerve roots for cranial nerves 3 through 12 and identify them on the surface of the brainstem.

8 Name the portions of the corpus callosum and identify the importance of this structure.

9 Identify the major lobes, gyri, and sulci of the cerebral hemispheres.

10 Name the components of the diencephalon.

11 Identify the components of the ventricular system and discuss where each is located in relationship to the cerebral hemispheres, brainstem, and spinal cord.

12 Differentiate the function of commissural, projection, and association fibers of the cerebral hemispheres.

13 Recall the major arteries and the vascular territories of the CNS.

ACRONYMS

ACA Anterior cerebral artery

CSF Cerebrospinal fluid

CNS Central nervous system

MCA Middle cerebral artery

PCA Posterior cerebral artery

PNS Peripheral nervous system

Introduction

As outlined in Chapter 1, the human CNS consists of five major subdivisions: the spinal cord, brainstem, cerebellum, diencephalon, and cerebral hemispheres. The term *cerebrum* includes the cerebral hemispheres and diencephalon as well as the basal ganglia. This chapter provides an overview of each of these subdivisions in a separate section. With the exception of the section on the cerebellum, all are organized such that major surface features are discussed first, followed by a consideration of the general internal organization of that subdivision. The interior of each subdivision is made up of specific arrangements of gray and white matter. Recall that a fundamental feature in the basic design of the brain and spinal cord is the division into areas of gray and white matter and that the white matter consists of the axons of neurons that structurally join one part of the nervous system with another. Importantly, axons (nerve fibers) are the basis of communication between different parts of the nervous system by virtue of their capacity to conduct nerve impulses. This chapter's overview of CNS structure establishes the framework within which the cells of the nervous system—the neurons and neuroglia—function. An understanding of the anatomical layout of the CNS helps us appreciate the demands placed on neurons with respect to their routing of information between, for example, the spinal cord and brain and between the various components of the brain. This communication occurs over identifiable tracts and pathways that reside in the white matter of the interior of the CNS. The overview of regional anatomy of the CNS provided in this chapter provides a foundation for a more detailed consideration of each of these major structures that will be presented in Parts II and III of this text.

SPINAL CORD

Clinical Preview

Maria Rodriguez is a 14-year-old girl who was in a skiing accident that left her with a complete transaction of the spinal cord at the thoracic level. She was admitted to the rehabilitation facility where you work.

Jonathan Perry is an 18-year-old boy who was also admitted to your facility. He has a tumor in his spinal cord that resulted in only sensory loss.

As you read through this chapter, consider the following:

- What types of loss would Maria likely sustain (motor, sensory, or both)?
- For Maria, given that the injury is to the thoracic cord, consider what muscle groups would likely still be innervated and which would not. (Note that we will revisit this issue in Chapters 9, 10, and 11.)
- For Jonathan, what part of the cord (anterior, posterior, or both) is most likely affected, given that he only sustained a sensory loss?

Thought Question

Does the dorsal horn arise from the basal or alar plate?

Surface Features

Spinal Cord Segments and Enlargements

Thirty-one pairs of spinal nerves attach to the cord, giving the spinal cord an appearance of external segmentation. Thus, a *spinal cord segment* is defined as the region of the cord occupied by the nerve roots of a single (pair) spinal nerve (Figure 2-1 ■). As each spinal nerve approaches the cord, it bifurcates into a **dorsal root**, whose filaments attach to the dorsolateral surface of the cord, and a **ventral root**, whose filaments attach to the ventrolateral surface of the spinal cord. The dorsal root contains afferent (sensory) axons whose cell bodies are located in a **dorsal root ganglion**, a swelling along the distal part of a dorsal root. These afferent axons are also called **first-order fibers** because they represent the initial fiber in a chain of synaptically linked neurons that carry information to a particular site in the CNS. First-order fibers are components of a spinal nerve belonging to the PNS. The ventral root is composed of efferent (motor) axons whose cell bodies are located in the spinal cord gray matter of the CNS but whose axons continue into the PNS as a component of a spinal nerve.

Corresponding to the 31 pairs of spinal nerves, there are 31 spinal cord segments: 8 **cervical**, 12 **thoracic**, 5 **lumbar**, 5 **sacral**, and 1 **coccygeal**. Although used to specify the location of spinal cord lesions, the spinal cord segment is purely a product of superficial anatomy, because there is little in the internal structure of the cord

Thought Question

Name the five regions of the spinal cord. How many segments are associated with each region? What is a nerve root, and how many are associated with each segment?

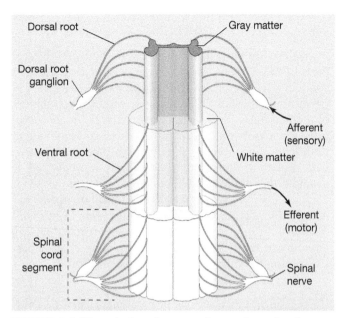

FIGURE 2-1 The spinal cord segment is a product of surface anatomy and is defined as that portion of the spinal cord occupied by one pair of spinal nerve roots belonging to one pair of corresponding spinal nerves. Afferent fibers of the dorsal root of a spinal nerve have cell bodies in the dorsal horn of the spinal gray, while efferent fibers of a ventral root of a spinal nerve have their cell bodies in the ventral horn of the spinal gray. For segments with preganglionic nuclei (T1–L2, S2–S4), autonomic efferent fibers travel in the ventral roots and their cell bodies are in the intermediate zone, not ventral horn.

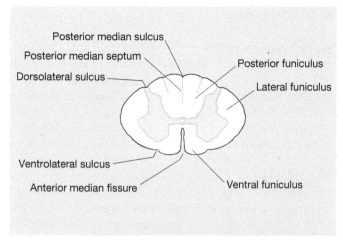

FIGURE 2-2 A cross section of the spinal cord showing the locations of the longitudinally running sulci and fissures observable on the surface of the spinal cord.

to justify its division into segments. Many of its axons both originate and terminate in the spinal cord and serve to bilaterally interconnect its segments in some cases throughout its length (see the spinospinal, or propriospinal system, Chapter 5).

Because of its segments, the spinal cord is referred to as the **segmental level** of the nervous system. The term *suprasegmental* refers to the brain—that is, all parts of the CNS that are superior to the (segmentally organized) spinal cord. For example, the brainstem, cerebellum, and cerebral cortex all represent suprasegmental structures.

The spinal cord extends from the foramen magnum, where it is continuous with the brainstem, to the level of the junction of the L1 through L2 vertebra (see Figure 5-3). It is approximately cylindrical in shape but somewhat flattened anteroposteriorly. A number of longitudinal furrows can be distinguished on the surface of the spinal cord (Figure 2-2 ■). On its posterior surface the **posterior**, or **dorsal**, **median sulcus** is evident as a shallow groove running the entire length of the cord. A partition, the **posterior median septum**, extends ventrally from the sulcus and passes deeply into the substance of the cord. The **anterior**, or **ventral**, **median fissure** is a considerably more prominent external landmark, penetrating deeply into the cord on its ventral surface. The

fissure also runs the entire length of the cord. Two less distinct sulci, the **dorsolateral** and **ventrolateral**, are present on the lateral aspect of the cord and divide each lateral half into approximate thirds. Fibers making up the dorsal (posterior) root of each spinal nerve attach to the dorsolateral sulcus. Similarly, ventral (anterior) root fibers emerge from the ventrolateral sulcus.

Two grossly visible enlargements occur along the length of the spinal cord: the **cervical** and **lumbosacral enlargements**. The cervical (**brachial**) enlargement extends over spinal cord segments C4 through T1, while the lumbosacral enlargement occupies segments L2 through S3 (Figure 2-3 ■). The enlargements represent, respectively, the regions of the spinal cord supplying the upper and lower extremities. In evaluating the integrity of spinal cord function, the extremities are used for assessing somatosensation, testing various spinal reflexes, and determining the person's capacity for voluntary movement. Thus, it is important to the clinician to know which segments of the spinal cord innervate the upper and lower limbs.

Enlargements provide excellent examples of the correlation of structure with function. Spinal nerves derived from cord segments C4 through T1 unite to form the **brachial plexus** from which the nerves innervating the arm and hand originate. In addition to being capable of executing delicate, skilled movements, the hand is highly sensitive to tactile stimulation. These motor and sensory

Thought Question

The spinal cord is partitioned throughout its length by distinct fissures or grooves. Name them.

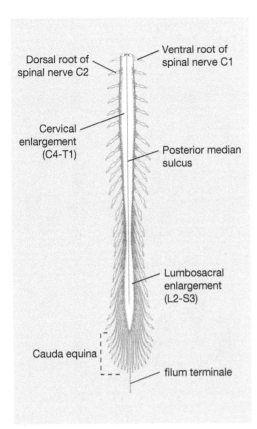

Dorsal root of spinal nerve C2

Ventral root of spinal nerve C1

Cervical enlargement (C4-T1)

Posterior median sulcus

Lumbosacral enlargement (L2-S3)

Cauda equina

filum terminale

FIGURE 2-3 Posterior view of the spinal cord showing its focal enlargements and other surface features. The cervical enlargement corresponds to spinal nerves that form the brachial plexus whose nerves innervate the upper extremity, while the lumbosacral enlargement corresponds to spinal nerves that form the lumbosacral plexus whose nerves innervate the lower extremity. Because the thoracic region does not have as much muscle or sensory innervation, it will be smaller. Note that for most people, there is no C1 dorsal root.

functions both require large numbers of individual nerve fibers. The CNS's capacity to finely grade movements of the fingers is dependent upon its ability to control small groups of muscle fibers. This requires that there be a large number of motor nerve fibers relative to the number of muscle fibers in the fingers (Figure 2-4 ■). That is, there must be a **high innervation density** of the upper extremity, especially the hand.

Likewise, the capacity of the fingertips to accurately discriminate the properties of tactile stimuli requires large numbers of receptors per unit of skin area. This means that large numbers of afferent nerve fibers must be available to transmit the message from peripheral receptors to the spinal cord. The spinal cord, in turn, must contain a large number of neurons to receive and process this afferent information. Therefore, the region of the spinal cord innervating the upper extremities sends, relative to the mass of the structure, a disproportionately large number of motor fibers to the extremity and,

likewise, receives a large number of sensory fibers from it. The higher innervation density of the upper extremity is reflected in spinal cord segments C4 through T1 as the cervical enlargement.

The lumbosacral enlargement extends over spinal cord segments L2 through S3. Spinal nerves from these segments contribute to the **lumbosacral plexus** that innervates the lower extremity. The innervation density of the lower extremity is not as high as that of the upper limb. Although the same factors that produce the cervical enlargement contribute to the lumbosacral enlargement, the latter would appear to be relatively related more to the mass of the structure innervated (leg vs. arm). In contrast to both enlargements, thoracic segments of the spinal cord are small. This is because of the relatively low somatosensory and motor innervation densities of the trunk.

Caudal to the lumbosacral enlargement, the spinal cord tapers rapidly in diameter and forms a cone-shaped termination known as the **conus medullaris** (Figure 2-5 ■). Because disproportionate growth rates result in a spinal cord that is much shorter than the vertebral column, the more caudally placed nerve roots must descend in progressively more oblique directions before reaching their foramina of entry or exit. Lumbar and sacral nerve roots descend almost vertically for a considerable distance (e.g., the S1 root has a six-inch course) and, beyond the conus medullaris, form a collection of rootlets and nerves called the **cauda equina**, from its fancied resemblance to a horse's tail.

The fact that the spinal cord ends at the lower border of the L1 vertebra means that herniations of the lumbar intervertebral discs below spinal level L1 or trauma below spinal level L1 can only compress the nerve roots of the cauda equina and do not damage the spinal cord itself. As a result, symptoms referable to spinal cord damage do not occur.

Segmental Innervation: Dermatomes and Myotomes

A **dermatome** is the area of skin supplied by the somatosensory fibers via the dorsal roots of one segment of the spinal cord. In humans, dermatomes were first determined by mapping the areas of cutaneous rash and pain in herpes zoster (shingles), wherein the virus often affects a single dorsal root ganglion. In the trunk, the dermatomes follow one another consecutively, each dermatome forming a band that encircles the trunk from the midposterior to midanterior line. However, in both the upper and lower extremities, the dermatomes do not *all* follow one another consecutively because of the manner in which the extremities develop embryologically. The dermatomes of the limbs from the fifth cervical to the first thoracic in the upper extremity, and from the third lumbar to the second sacral in the lower extremity, extend as a series of bands from the mid-dorsal line of the trunk into the limbs as illustrated in Figure 2-6 ■ . Each dermatome is also partially innervated by the dorsal roots

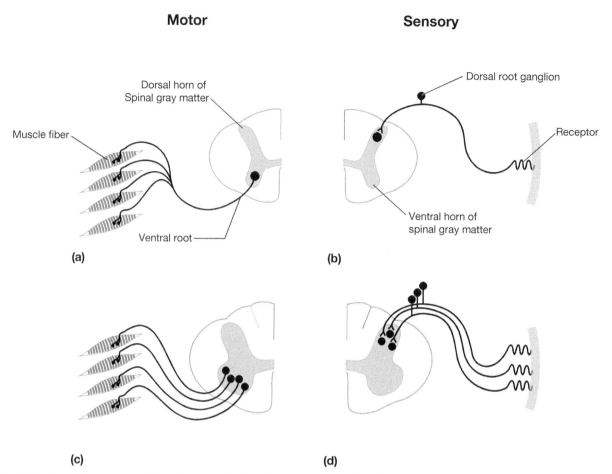

FIGURE 2-4 Schematic representations of motor (a, c) and somatosensory (b, d) innervation densities. Panel (a) illustrates a low motor innervation density, while (c) illustrates a high motor innervation density such that the spinal cord gray matter in (c) must expand to accommodate a large number of motor neurons. Panel (b) illustrates a low somatosensory innervation density, while (d) illustrates a high somatosensory innervation density such that the spinal cord gray matter in (d) must expand to accommodate the large number of cells required to receive and process the information.

above and below the dermatome. Because of this overlap, cutting just one spinal dorsal root results in virtually no loss in cutaneous sensibility. The best method to detect and plot an area of diminished cutaneous sensibility is by the use of light pin scratch for pain sensation.

It is important to differentiate a *spinal root* lesion from *spinal nerve* damage such as occurs in a peripheral neuropathy. Thus, the cutaneous distribution of the various peripheral nerves must be known in addition to the dermatomal map. These two maps are compared in Figure 2-6. This distinction is important clinically because while damage to a single dorsal root may result in little or no detectable loss of cutaneous sensation due to the partial overlapping of adjacent dermatomes, damage to a single cutaneous nerve may cause a profound loss of cutaneous sensibility.

Myotomes are groups of muscles innervated via the ventral roots by a segment of the spinal cord. The segmental organization of myotomes is less obvious than that of dermatomes. Most muscles, in particular those of the limbs,

> **Thought Question**
>
> As a rehabilitation professional, you may be called upon to use information from dermatomes to interpret the location of your patient's lesion. Explain why damage to a *single dorsal* nerve root may not cause a sensory loss, whereas damage to the dorsal spinal cord at that level will certainly cause a sensory loss. Use terms such as *peripheral* and *central* in your explanation. How will the pattern of loss be similar and how will it be different when a *single ventral* root is damaged?

are innervated by motor axons that arise from multiple adjacent segments of the spinal cord. Because the different axons arise from different spinal segments, the myotome is formed from several adjacent spinal roots. Thus, damage to a single ventral root may only weaken a muscle or have little discernable effect. There are, however, certain

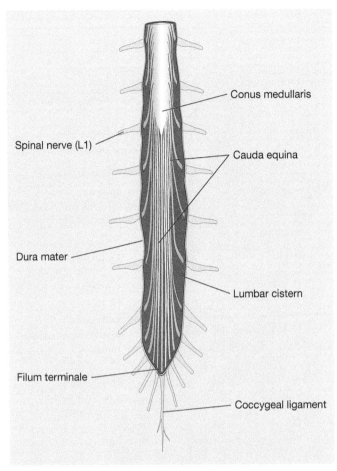

FIGURE 2-5 The spinal cord ends in a cone-shaped configuration called the conus medullaris, but the spinal nerve roots derived from caudal spinal cord segments continue to descend caudal to the conus medullaris to form a structure called the cauda equina. The nerve roots of the cauda equina lie in a cul-de-sac formed by the dura mater and arachnoid mater called the lumbar cistern.

muscles whose weakness or atrophy suggests damage to a single ventral root or adjacent roots, and these are summarized in Table 2-1 ■.

Internal Organization

It can be seen in cross section that the posterior median sulcus and anterior median fissure virtually split the spinal cord into symmetrical halves (Figure 2-7 ■). Throughout its length, the spinal cord consists of a centrally situated core of gray matter surrounded by a mantle of white matter of varying thickness. These have an obvious demarcation from one another.

Gray Matter

The spinal gray matter is composed primarily of neuronal cell bodies embedded in a rich capillary network. The gray matter appears in cross section as a deeply notched column in the shape of a butterfly or the letter H (see Figure 2-7). The vertical bars of the H form the dorsal and ventral horns, while the cross bar forms the **gray commissure** within which the central canal is situated. The central canal is so small as to be barely visible to the naked eye. The dorsal and ventral horns extend the entire length of the spinal cord, although each exhibits regional variations in size, depending on the number of neuron cell bodies making up the horn.

> ### Thought Question
>
> In future chapters, we will find that neurons can be differentiated into first-, second-, and third-order neurons (and sometimes a fourth order). Where do the first-order sensory (afferent) neurons always originate? Where is the cell body for the first-order neuron located?

Each dorsal horn is that portion of the gray matter extending posteriorly from the gray commissure. Dorsal horn neurons receive many of the terminations of first-order neurons. These sensory fibers originate in peripheral receptors and reach the cord via dorsal roots. Dorsal horn neurons function in a sensory capacity.

The ventral horns extend anteriorly from the gray commissure. These contain the large motor neurons innervating skeletal muscle as well as other types of cells. The cell bodies of motor neurons are within the CNS but their axons emerge from the spinal cord through the ventral roots to terminate in the body periphery. Motor neurons appear as pale spots in myelin-stained sections and as dark spots in Nissl-stained sections.

The **intermediate gray** is located between the dorsal and ventral horns. Most neurons of this region are interneurons and function in an integrative capacity. At its simplest level, interneurons link sensory with motor neurons thereby integrating their activity.

White Matter

Spinal cord white matter is composed of densely packed, long, myelinated fibers running in a longitudinal direction. The entering dorsal roots and the exiting ventral roots divide the white matter of each half of the cord into three zones known as **funiculi**, or **columns** (see Figure 2-2). The **dorsal funiculus** is situated between the posterior median sulcus and the dorsolateral sulcus where the dorsal roots attach to the spinal cord. The **lateral funiculus** is located between the dorsolateral sulcus and the ventrolateral sulcus where the ventral root attaches to the spinal cord, while the **ventral funiculus** lies between the ventral root and the anterior median fissure. Because the dorsal horn extends almost to the surface of the cord, the dorsal funiculus is sharply demarcated from the remaining white matter. However, the ventral horn ends at some distance from the cord surface so that the lateral and ventral funiculi are not sharply delimited from one another. Indeed, some authors consider them to comprise a single funiculus, the ventrolateral or

PERIPHERAL NERVES   **DERMATOMES**   **PERIPHERAL NERVES**

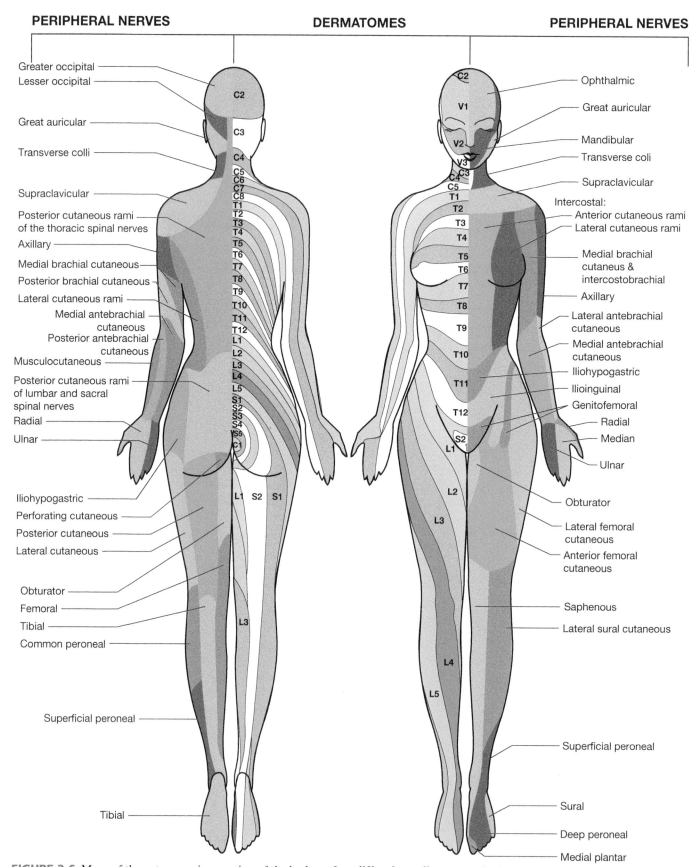

FIGURE 2-6 Maps of the cutaneous innervation of the body surface differ, depending upon whether one is looking at the areas of the skin innervated by a single pair of spinal dorsal roots (center) or peripheral nerves (left and right). The area of skin innervated by a single pair of dorsal roots is referred to as a dermatome. Note that the spinal cord segment C1 has no dorsal roots and therefore does not innervate the skin. The difference between a dermatome and innervation by a peripheral nerve is clinically important.

Table 2-1 Myotome Chart Relating Muscles, Their Function, and the Related Nerve Roots

MUSCLE	PRIMARY FUNCTION	ROOT
Diaphragm	Respiration	C3, C4, C5
Deltoid	Abduction of arm	C5
Biceps	Flexion of forearm	C5
Brachioradialis	Flexion of forearm	C6
Triceps	Extension of forearm	C7
Quadriceps femoris	Extension of knee	L3, L4
Extensor hallucis longus	Dorsiflexion of great toe	L5
Gastrocnemius	Plantar flexion	S1

Thought Question

Think about the anatomy of axons versus dendrites. Why do axons make up columns in the spinal cord but dendrites do not? What is the role of dendrites?

anterolateral. Specific ascending and descending tracts (collections of axons) run in the three funiculi. These tracts will be presented in subsequent chapters.

Commissures

In addition to the gray commissure, two white commissures are recognized, the most significant of which is the ventral (anterior) white commissure. The ventral white commissure is positioned between the gray commissure and anterior median fissure and contains the axons of neurons that decussate from one side of the spinal cord to the other (see Figure 2-7). The ventral white commissure is a structure of unquestionable clinical significance. It is the location where the spinothalamic tract (which carries information about pain and temperature) crosses and will be discussed in Chapters 5 and 9. This structure must always be taken into account when determining the location of a lesion based on the sensory symptoms displayed by an individual.

Level Variation in Cord Structure

Both the internal and external (size and shape) structures of the spinal cord vary at different levels. Several primary trends characterize this variation (Figure 2-8 ■ and Figure 2-9 ■). First, the amount of gray matter at a given level of the spinal cord varies locally, depending on the size of the spinal nerve roots at different levels. This is because the amount of gray matter at any spinal level is related primarily to the richness of peripheral innervation

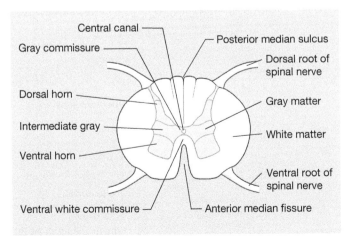

FIGURE 2-7 Cross section of the spinal cord showing the configuration of its gray matter and its subdivision into dorsal and ventral horns and the intermediate gray matter.

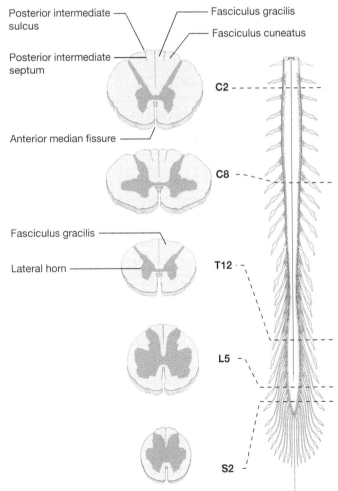

FIGURE 2-8 The configuration of the spinal cord and the amount of gray and white matter vary at different levels.

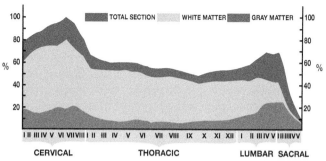

FIGURE 2-9 Curves showing the variation in cross-sectional area of the gray matter, white matter, and entire cord in the different segments of the human spinal cord.

(i.e., to the size of the dorsal and ventral roots) as was discussed earlier. Thus, the brachial and lumbosacral enlargements are characterized by large gray columns, especially the ventral horn. Conversely, thoracic levels contain small amounts of gray matter because of the low peripheral innervation density of the trunk.

The second factor is this: all levels of the spinal cord are connected to the brain by bundles of long fibers. Thus, more rostral levels of the spinal cord contain more white matter because they contain (1) all of the ascending fibers that have originated from more caudal segments of the cord and (2) all of the descending fibers that have not yet terminated in more caudal segments. From a clinical standpoint this is very important: given that ascending fibers from more caudal levels accumulate progressively in moving rostrally, the more rostrally situated a spinal cord lesion, the greater the region of the body displaying a sensory alteration. For example, damage

to upper cervical segments results in somatosensory deficits in both the lower and upper extremities, whereas damage to thoracic segments results in somatosensory alterations only in the lower extremities. Likewise, the more rostral a cord lesion, the greater the portion of the body displaying a motor alteration because not as many descending fibers have terminated. Damage to upper cervical segments produces motor deficits in both the upper and lower extremities, whereas thoracic damage causes deficits in the lower extremity.

But still, these variations are trends in terms of their anatomy. Both gray and white matter vary locally and govern the configuration of the spinal cord in specific segments.

Table 2-2 ■ and Figure 2-9 summarize the characteristic features of transverse sections through different levels of the spinal cord. The changing shapes are determined by the size of the cell columns at the different levels. Recall that a cell column refers to the neuronal cell bodies that extend over several levels of the cord.

CLINICAL CONNECTIONS
Relationship of Symptoms to Lesions within the Pyramidal Tract

The side on which symptoms occur following spinal cord and brainstem injury depends on whether the injury is above or below the decussation of the pyramids. When injury occurs in the spinal cord, the pyramidal tract (carrying motor fibers) already has decussated. Therefore, the pyramidal tract acts on motor neurons that are on the same side as the muscles that will eventually be innervated. This means that a lesion to the pyramidal tract in the spinal

Table 2-2 Characteristic Features of Transverse Sections through the Spinal Cord at Different Levels

FEATURE	CERVICAL	THORACIC	LUMBAR	SACRAL
Outline	Oval, greatest diameter is transverse	Oval to circular	Nearly circular	Circular to quadrilateral
Volume of gray matter	Large	Small	Large	Relatively large
Anterior gray column	Massive	Slender	Massive	Massive
Posterior gray column	Relatively slender, but extends far posteriorly	Slender	Massive	Massive
Lateral gray column	Absent	Well demarcated	Demarcated to L3	Demarcated to S4
White matter	In large amount	Less than in the cervical region; relatively large amount in comparison to the gray matter	Slightly less than in the thoracic region; very little in comparison to the large volume of the gray matter	Very little
Dorsal intermediate sulcus	Present throughout	Present in upper six thoracic segments	Absent	Absent

cord will produce symptoms on the same side as the lesion. In contrast, when a lesion occurs in the brainstem above the decussation of the pyramids (e.g., in the pons or midbrain), the symptoms will be contralateral to the lesion (on the opposite side). This is because those fibers would have crossed over on the way to the motor neurons that innervate muscles on the opposite side.

Furthermore, the regions of the body that are affected are determined by whether the lesion is above or below the decussation. Above the decussation, both body and face may be affected, whereas below the decussation, only the body will be affected. This is because cranial nerves exit the brainstem to go to the head, neck and face.

Putting these two factors together, a pyramidal tract lesion in the brainstem and *above* the decussation of the pyramids causes symptoms contralateral to the extremities and torso as well as symptoms in the head, neck and face. Some of these symptoms will be contralateral and some ipsilateral, as will be seen in later chapters. In contrast, a pyramidal tract lesion *below* the decussation can only affect the extremities and torso. Therefore, if a lesion causes symptoms in muscles of the extremities, head, neck, and face, the lesion is almost certainly above the pyramidal decussation, whereas if a lesion causes symptoms of the extremities and torso, typically it is below the pyramidal decussation.

BRAINSTEM

Clinical Preview

Gordon Wagner, a 55-year-old gentleman, sustained a traumatic brain injury that mainly affected his brainstem. He was admitted to the rehabilitation unit where you work. As a rehabilitation professional, you will need to predict signs and symptoms of his injury, based on the location of his lesion. As you read through this chapter, begin to consider how knowledge of the location of cranial nerves will assist you. Note that we will continue to build on this information in Chapters 13, 14, and 15; this is just the beginning!

Surface Features

The surface features of the brainstem differ markedly from those of the spinal cord. This is due to a number of factors. First, the uniform appearance of external segmentation imparted to the spinal cord by the dorsal and ventral roots of spinal nerves stops abruptly at the spinomedullary junction. Nerve roots attaching to the brainstem comprise the cranial nerves, of which 10 pairs are irregularly distributed over the brainstem subdivisions. Whereas each spinal nerve has a dorsal root ganglion (belonging to the PNS), only four of the cranial nerves have an equivalent **sensory**

ganglion (cranial nerves V, VII, IX, and X). Second, in general, the circumference of the brainstem is larger than that of the spinal cord. There are several reasons. For one thing, there are sensory systems in the head subserved by cranial nerves that have no counterparts in the body served by spinal nerves. Thus, hearing, balance, vision, and taste require the presence of special sensory cranial nerve nuclei that are in addition to the general sensory cranial nerve nuclei that serve general somatic sensation in the head. For another thing, the brainstem governs functions such as respiration and cardiovascular function, as well as others, and this requires the elaboration of neural networks not found in the spinal cord. These factors and others contribute to an enlargement of the brainstem that occurs during development.

In a whole brain, much of the brainstem is hidden from view by the cerebellum. In order to view the dorsal surface of the brainstem, it is necessary to remove the cerebellum. This is accomplished by transecting the three cerebellar peduncles that attach the cerebellum to the brainstem. The **inferior cerebellar peduncle** attaches the cerebellum to the medulla, the **middle cerebellar peduncle** attaches the cerebellum to the pons, while the **superior cerebellar peduncle** attaches the cerebellum to the midbrain (Figure 2-10 ■). Recall that the term *peduncle* refers to white matter.

The three components of the brainstem were identified previously. The pons is the most readily identified subdivision. Its caudal and rostral borders are delimited by the **inferior** and **superior pontine sulci**, respectively (see Figures 2-10 and 2-11). The most outstanding surface

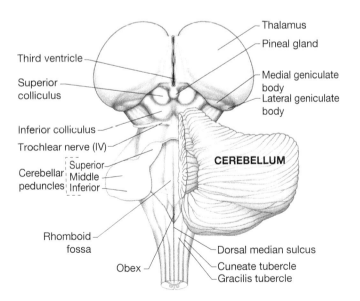

FIGURE 2-10 The dorsal surface of the brainstem is fully visualized when the overlying telencephalon is removed and the cerebellum has been removed by transecting the three cerebellar peduncles that attach the cerebellum to the brainstem. The floor of the rhomboid fossa is made up of the dorsal surfaces of the medulla and pons. Note that components of the diencephalon (thalamus, pineal gland, third ventricle) also are illustrated.

feature of the pons is the bulging, massive band of transversely running fibers making up its ventral surface. These are the **transverse fibers of the pons**. The medulla, the most caudal brainstem subdivision in structural continuity with the spinal cord, extends from the inferior pontine sulcus to approximately the caudal border of the cerebellum. Extending cranially from the pons is the midbrain. This is the least differentiated and smallest brainstem component; it extends from the superior pontine sulcus to a region just caudal to the **mammillary bodies**. The mammillary bodies are located on the ventral brainstem surface and belong to the hypothalamus; each is a small, round structure just lateral to the midline.

Medulla and Pons: Anterior Aspect

The anterior median fissure of the spinal cord continues rostrally into the medulla, but at the spinomedullary junction it sometimes is obliterated by the crossing fibers of the **pyramidal decussation** (Figure 2-11 ■). The term *decussation* was defined in Chapter 1. Rostral to the decussation, the anterior median fissure deepens and is flanked on either side by prominent longitudinal ridges known as the **pyramids**. Each pyramid is composed of descending motor fibers that cross in the pyramidal decussation. They then enter the contralateral lateral funiculus of the spinal cord, where they descend as the lateral corticospinal tracts.

> **Thought Question**
>
> Here is a critical concept related to the pyramids. What tract makes up the pyramids? Where does this tract decussate, and where does it terminate? Why is the location of this decussation of clinical importance to the rehabilitation professional?

Ultimately, many of these descending motor fibers synapse on motor neurons that innervate striated muscle.

Lateral to each pyramid is the **olivary eminence**, or **olive**, produced by cells of the large underlying **inferior olivary nucleus** of the medulla. The olive is an important landmark, especially with respect to identifying cranial nerves. The olive is demarcated from adjacent structures by the **preolivary** and **postolivary sulci**. The four pairs of cranial nerves attaching to the medulla do so in relation to the olive (see Figure 2-11). The **hypoglossal nerve** (cranial nerve XII) exits as a series of rootlets along the preolivary sulcus, between the olive and pyramid. The remaining three cranial nerves form a nearly continuous line of rootlets attaching at the postolivary sulcus, immediately lateral to the olive. The most caudal of these rootlets, at about the inferior border of the olive, form the **accessory nerve** (XI). The largest contingent of rootlets unites to form the **vagus**

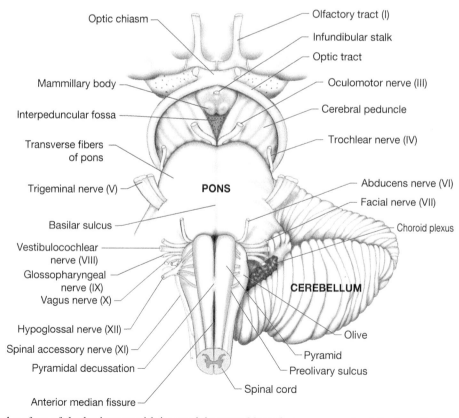

FIGURE 2-11 Ventral surface of the brainstem with its cranial nerves. Note that components of the hypothalamus (mammillary body and tuber cinereum) also are shown.

nerve (X), the longest and functionally most complex of the cranial nerves. The most rostral contingent of rootlets belong to the **glossopharyngeal nerve** (IX). A more detailed anatomy as well as the functions of all cranial nerves is provided in Chapter 13.

A number of structurally obvious changes are evident in progressing superiorly from the medulla to the pons. First, as already mentioned, the most conspicuous feature of the pons is the bulging band of fibers on its ventral surface composed of the transverse fibers of the pons. These fibers appear as a sling that anchors the cerebellum to the pons. As the transverse fibers of the pons are traced laterally, they become more compact and form the middle cerebellar peduncle (**brachium pontis**). The name *pons* (L., bridge) comes from the fact that its superficial transverse fibers look like a bridge between the cerebellar hemispheres, strapping the cerebellum to the pons. In fact, fibers of the middle cerebellar peduncle directly connect the pons with the overlying cerebellum. A shallow midline depression can be identified on the ventral pontine surface. This is the **basilar sulcus**, within which lies the **basilar artery** (see Figure 2-10).

Four pairs of cranial nerves attach to the ventral or ventrolateral aspect of the pons (see Figure 2-11). The **abducens nerve** (VI) is most medial, emerging from the inferior pontine sulcus in line with hypoglossal rootlets. The **facial nerve** (VII), also attaching at the pontomedullary junction, is situated lateral to the abducens nerve. The **vestibulo-cochlear nerve** (VIII) is immediately lateral to VII and much larger. As the name states, cranial nerve VIII consists of two functional components, a larger and more medial **vestibular division** and a smaller **cochlear division**. The **trigeminal nerve** (V) is the largest of the cranial nerves. It attaches to the ventrolateral aspect of the middle cerebellar peduncle.

Medulla and Pons: Posterior Aspect

The dorsal aspect of the medulla and pons can be viewed only after the three cerebellar peduncles (reciprocally connecting the cerebellum and brainstem) have been transected and the cerebellum removed (see Figure 2-10). This exposes the floor of the fourth ventricle, the caudal portion of which is formed by the dorsal surface of the medulla, the rostral portion by the dorsal surface of the pons. The floor of the fourth ventricle is approximately diamond shaped and is called the **rhomboid fossa**. The point at which the lateral walls of the fourth ventricle begin to diverge is known as the **obex**. The obex demarcates the point at which the central canal in the caudal medulla expands into the fourth ventricle and forms the ventricle's caudal boundary.

In looking at the dorsal medullary surface, it appears as though the lateral walls of the ventricle are formed by diverging dorsal column fibers that ascend from the spinal cord. This actually is not the case because a number of structures form these walls. One of the visible features is the inferior cerebellar peduncle (**restiform body**), most of whose

Thought Question

The cerebellum is connected to the brainstem through peduncles. Name the three cerebellar peduncles and the part of the brainstem with which each is connected.

fibers originate in the medulla (from the inferior olivary nucleus) and serve to connect the medulla with the cerebellum (see Figure 2-10). The walls of the rostral, pontine portion of the fourth ventricle are formed by the superior cerebellar peduncles. These stout bundles of fibers originate in the cerebellum and project to the midbrain and thalamus. A number of eminences and sulci can be identified in the rhomboid fossa. The dorsal median sulcus of the spinal cord continues rostral through the medulla and pons. The eminences flanking the dorsomedial sulcus are produced largely by dorsally positioned cranial nerve nuclei of the brainstem.

Midbrain: Anterior and Posterior Aspects

Two massive, longitudinally running fiber bundles comprise most of the anterolateral surface of the midbrain (see Figure 2-11). They are called the cerebral peduncles and were defined in Chapter 1 (see Figure 1-13). (Note that some authors use the term *cerebral peduncle* to refer to all of the midbrain except the tectum, whereas other authors use the term to refer to the massive bundle of corticospinal, corticobulbar, and corticopontine fibers located in the ventral aspect of the midbrain. We use the latter definition in this text.) The cerebral peduncles extend from the superior pontine sulcus to a transversely running discrete band of fibers called the optic tracts, where they disappear into the substance of the brain. The longitudinally running, descending fibers of the cerebral peduncles originate in the cerebral cortex and terminate in a number of structures: cranial nerve motor nuclei of the brainstem, brainstem reticular formation, pons, and the spinal cord. Corticospinal fibers coursing within the cerebral peduncles continue their descent toward the spinal cord in the pyramids of the medulla; these fibers thus are referred to as the pyramidal tract. The cerebral peduncles are separated by a deep, triangular-shaped depression, widest rostrally, called the **interpeduncular fossa** (see Figure 2-11). The fossa extends from the mammillary bodies to the superior pontine sulcus. Emerging from the midportion of the fossa are fibers of the large **oculomotor nerve** (III). This motor nerve innervates all of the extraocular musculature, save the two muscles supplied by the abducens and trochlear nerves

Four large eminences, the **corpora quadrigemina**, can be observed on the dorsal aspect of the midbrain (see Figure 2-10). The corpora quadrigemini also are called colliculi (singular colliculus) from the Latin *colliculi*, meaning small mounds or hills. The rostral pair comprises the superior colliculi and the caudal pair, the inferior colliculi. Recall that the superior and inferior colliculi on one side are referred to as the tectum. Immediately caudal to the inferior colliculi are exiting fibers of the **trochlear nerve** (IV). This is the only cranial nerve to attach to the dorsal brainstem surface. The nerve of each side travels laterally and anteriorly around the lateral surface of the cerebral peduncle to emerge on the ventral surface of the midbrain.

Immediately inferior and lateral to the superior colliculus is a prominent band of fibers. This is the **brachium of the inferior colliculus** (L., *brachium*, arm). It can be traced from the inferior colliculus rostrolaterally to another eminence, the **medial geniculate body**, which is part of the diencephalon. The brachium of the inferior colliculus contains axons connecting the inferior colliculus with the medial geniculate body. All three of these structures (the inferior colliculus, its brachium, and the medial geniculate body) are parts of the auditory system. There also is a **brachium of the superior colliculus**, but it is difficult to identify on the surface of the brainstem. This brachium connects the superior colliculus with the **lateral geniculate body**. The lateral geniculate body, also part of the diencephalon, can be identified as a small swelling on the distal end of the optic tract. The superior colliculus, its brachium, and the lateral geniculate body are parts of the visual system.

Table 2-3 ■ summarizes the cranial nerves that attach to each of the three brainstem subdivisions.

Internal Organization

A core of tissue extends through all three subdivisions of the brainstem and is referred to as the **tegmentum** (Figure 2-12a ■). The term *tegmentum* is commonly used with the pons and midbrain because both of these structures contain parts in addition to the tegmentum. However, the tegmentum makes up virtually the entire medulla, so the term *tegmentum* is usually not applied to the medulla. The term *medulla* alone suffices. Many nuclei and tracts are found within the tegmentum of the brainstem, just as in the spinal cord.

Table 2-3 Cranial Nerves of the Brainstem

DIVISION	CRANIAL NERVES
Medulla	Hypoglossal (XII)
	Accessory (XI)
	Vagus (X)
	Glossopharyngeal (IX)
Pons	Vestibulo-cochlear (VIII)
	Facial (VII)
	Abducens (VI)
	Trigeminal (V)
Midbrain	Trochlear (IV)
	Oculomotor (III)

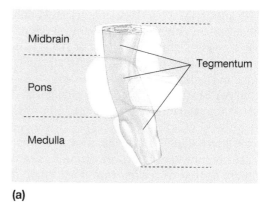

(a)

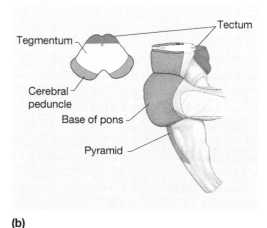

(b)

FIGURE 2-12 (a) The interior of the brainstem is characterized by a core, called the tegmentum, that extends uninterrupted through all three of its subdivisions. (b) Added to the tegmental core are ventral components in all three brainstem subdivisions and a dorsal component in the case of the midbrain. The added components are visible both in cross section and on the brainstem surface.

> **Thought Question**
>
> The brainstem has two *cerebral* and three *cerebellar* peduncles. What is the anatomical difference between these types of peduncles? Contrast the location and destination of each.

Ventral to the tegmentum of the midbrain, pons, and medulla is a **basilar portion** that has a different name for each brainstem subdivision (Figure 2-12b). In the midbrain, the basilar portion is referred to as the cerebral peduncle. In the pons, it is referred to as the basal pons, and in the medulla as the pyramid. The cerebral peduncle of the midbrain and pyramids of the medulla are composed of fiber tracts, while the basilar portion of the pons consists of both fiber tracts and nuclei. Dorsal to the tegmentum and cerebral aqueduct of the midbrain is a structure called the **tectum** (L., roof). Dorsal to the tegmentum of the pons and rostral half of the medulla is the floor of the fourth ventricle.

The transition from the spinal cord to the brainstem is characterized by a complete reorganization of the internal pattern of gray and white matter (Figure 2-13 ■). In the spinal cord, sensory neurons in the dorsal horn form what amounts to a general somatic sensory column. Somatic motor neurons in the ventral horn form a somatic motor column. Both columns extend as uninterrupted aggregations of gray matter over the entire length of the spinal cord. In contrast, there are no uninterrupted sensory or motor columns of gray matter that extend throughout the length of the brainstem. Rather, the cell bodies of brainstem neurons aggregate themselves into anatomically isolated and identifiable nuclei. However, the functional specificity of the dorsal, ventral, and lateral horns is retained in many brainstem nuclei so that we identify **sensory nuclei**, **motor nuclei**, and **visceral nuclei**, whose axons form sensory, motor, or mixed cranial nerves. Moreover, the positions of sensory and motor nuclei relative to one another are in a mediolateral sequence in the brainstem rather than a dorsal ventral sequence as in the spinal cord. This is because the pontine flexure in embryonic development opens the part of the neural tube that develops into the hindbrain (medulla and pons). Thus, rather than a somatic sensory column being located dorsal to the somatic motor column as in the spinal cord, in the brainstem the general somatic sensory nuclei (alar plate derivatives) are lateral to the medially located somatic motor nuclei (basal plate derivatives) (see Figure 1-22). As in the spinal cord, visceral motor nuclei occupy an intermediate position between the motor and sensory nuclei.

Another notable difference between the brainstem and spinal cord is that many tracts of the brainstem segregate themselves into identifiably separate bundles of axons, as opposed to the homogeneous appearance of the white funiculi of the spinal cord. These discrete bundles of axons contain various ascending (sensory) or descending (motor) tracts. Thus, for example, there is no line of demarcation separating the spinothalamic tracts from the corticospinal tracts in the lateral funiculi of the spinal cord, whereas the two tracts are anatomically more distinguishable in their trajectory through the brainstem. A third difference is that the brainstem subserves many functions not subserved by the spinal cord (such obvious functions as vision, balance, hearing, sleep, and many others as noted before). Thus, the brainstem contains nuclei and tracts having *no counterparts* in the spinal cord. A fourth conspicuous difference is that the distinct internal gray matter–external white matter pattern of the spinal cord is not preserved in the brainstem where nuclei and tracts are intermingled. Lastly, the brainstem homologue of the spinal cord intermediate gray matter, the **reticular formation** of the brainstem, is larger and functionally far more diversified than the spinal intermediate gray.

> **Thought Question**
>
> Compare the location of the somatic motor and sensory nuclei in the brainstem and spinal cord.

CEREBELLUM

The cerebellum, positioned dorsal to the medulla and pons but partially separated from them by the fourth ventricle (see Figure 2-10), is made up of three major regions: a small, unpaired midline band called the **vermis** (from its fancied resemblance to a worm) and large, lateral regions on either side of the vermis, the **cerebellar hemispheres** (Figure 2-14 ■). The cerebellum is further subdivided into a number of lobes and lobules, each of which consists of a vermal and hemispheral portion. The vermis is largely hidden from view in a whole brain, while in the hemisected brain, the cut passes through the vermis (see Figure 2-10).

> ## Clinical Preview ··················
>
> When working on a rehabilitation unit where you treat many patients post-stroke, you will find that you need to be able to differentiate the signs and symptoms and their implications for physical function, based on location of the patients' lesions. As a first step in this process, consider four patients with whom you are working. One had a stroke that affected her frontal cortex, another had a stroke that affected the parietal cortex, a third had involvement of his temporal cortex, and the fourth had damage to her occipital cortex. In reading through this chapter, begin to consider the location of these four different areas in preparation for understanding the signs and symptoms you will encounter later.

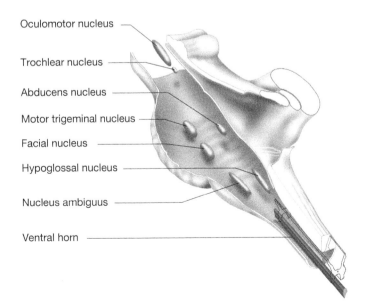

Oculomotor nucleus
Trochlear nucleus
Abducens nucleus
Motor trigeminal nucleus
Facial nucleus
Hypoglossal nucleus
Nucleus ambiguus
Ventral horn

FIGURE 2-13 Reorganization of the brainstem gray matter relative to that in the spinal cord. Note that there is a longitudinal distribution of discrete cranial nerve motor (and sensory, not shown) nuclei in the three subdivisions of the brainstem, in contrast to the continuous column of motor neurons in the spinal cord.

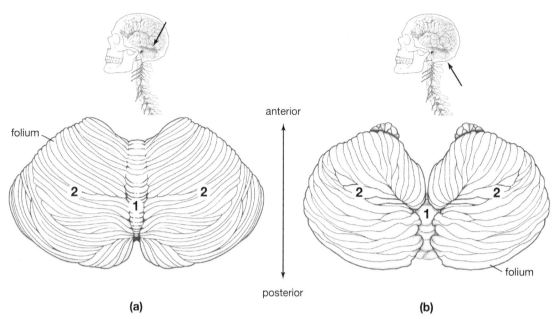

FIGURE 2-14 Superior (a) and inferior (b) views of the cerebellar surface. Note the largely transversely oriented ridges characterizing the surface, each of which is called a folium. Abbreviations: 1. vermis; 2. cerebellar hemisphere.

CEREBRUM

Surface Features

The right and left **cerebral hemispheres** make up the bulk of the cerebrum and are separated from one another by the deep **longitudinal fissure** (Figure 2-15 ■). If you were to look down at the superior surface of the cerebrum and gently separate right and left hemispheres, you would see the superior surface of the **corpus callosum**, a massive bundle of commissural (L., *commissura*, joining together connection) fibers interconnecting the two hemispheres. The corpus callosum provides the only connection between the two hemispheres. If you examine a hemisected brain, you can see that the medial hemispheral surface is not cut except at the commissures. You also can see the configuration of the corpus callosum as a shallow, inverted C. The corpus callosum is divided into four major regions (Figure 2-16 ■): an anterior portion known as the **genu** tapers into the ventrally directed **rostrum**, a middle portion dorsal to the thalamus is termed the **body**, and the enlarged caudal part is called the **splenium**. In rare cases, a neurosurgeon will cut the corpus callosum to relieve incapacitating epilepsy that is unresponsive to conventional medication (referred to as intractable epilepsy). This somewhat controversial operation is termed a **commissurotomy** and has yielded a small population of exceptionally interesting patients whose intensive study has revealed fascinating insights into cognitive functions and their localization in a given hemisphere.

From a structural standpoint, the right and left cerebral hemispheres appear to be essentially symmetrical. Both contain the same named lobes and the same named gyri, sulci, and fissures (also see Chapter 7). But there are subtle discernable differences in the structure of the right and left

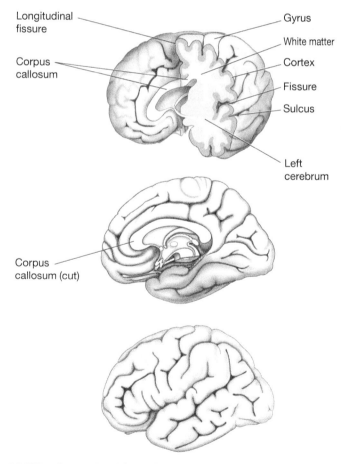

FIGURE 2-15 The right and left cerebral hemispheres are separated by the deep longitudinal fissure. The massive band of fibers joining the two hemispheres, the corpus callosum, has been cut by the midsagittal section, but the medial surfaces of the hemispheres have not.

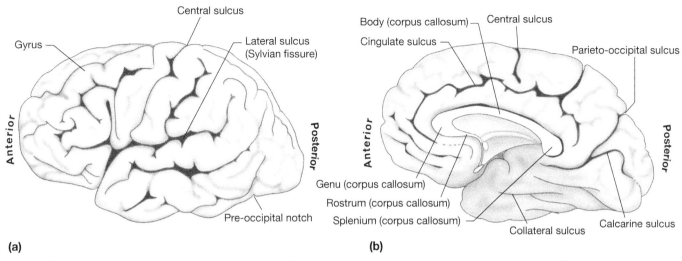

FIGURE 2-16 Major sulci on the lateral (a) and medial (b) hemispheral surfaces used to delineate the lobes of the hemisphere. The subdivisions of the corpus callosum also are shown.

Thought Question

Why is the corpus callosum important? What kind of fibers make up this structure? Name the four major portions of this structure.

hemispheres. These differences relate to the documented functions of the right and left hemispheres as determined by the clinical deficits resulting from lesions confined to just one hemisphere. Language was the first and best documented example. Damage to the left cerebral hemisphere results, in the vast majority of people, in deficits in the expression or comprehension, or both, of language. The deficits are called aphasias and are discussed in Chapter 22. Thus, the left hemisphere was designated the **dominant hemisphere**. Today, when one speaks of a dominant hemisphere, it is almost universally assumed that one is speaking of the left hemisphere. However, it subsequently was documented that the right cerebral hemisphere is dominant for its own, but different, functions. For example, the right hemisphere is dominant for visuospatial functions such as drawing correct three-dimensional spatial representations (e.g., a cube) or constructing three-dimensional block designs (see Chapter 21).

Lobes of the Cerebral Hemisphere

Each hemisphere is divided into four major lobes: the **frontal**, **parietal**, **temporal**, and **occipital lobes**. In addition, there is a functionally defined region, comprised of parts of the frontal, parietal, and temporal lobes and referred to as the limbic system, or sometimes as the limbic lobe. Although based in part on definite anatomical landmarks, this lobular subdivision is arbitrary, as will become even more obvious once we begin to consider the functions of the cerebral hemispheres. But this is not to dismiss the necessity of subdivision: we must have a common language by which to refer to

different hemispheral parts, and some primary hemispheral functions are, in fact, differentially located in the four lobes.

Each hemisphere is composed of an inner core of white matter surrounded by a superficial layer of gray matter, the **cerebral cortex**. In viewing the intact cerebrum, what one is looking at is the cortical surface. It is highly folded in curves and tortuous windings (convoluted). The ridges are known as gyri (singular, gyrus), the grooves as sulci (singular, sulcus). Especially deep sulci may be called **fissures**, for example, the longitudinal fissure or the lateral fissure. Two prominent sulci on the lateral hemispheral surface, the **lateral sulcus** (also called the **Sylvian fissure**) and the **central sulcus** (also called the **fissure of Rolando**), are important landmarks in delineating the lobes from one another (Figure 2-16). The base, or stem, of the lateral sulcus begins as a deep cleft, the **Sylvian fossa**; the sulcus then extends posteriorly and somewhat superiorly on the lateral hemispheral surface. The central sulcus is a deep, usually continuous furrow beginning as a notch at the junction of the lateral and medial hemispheral surfaces. It runs downward and somewhat anteriorly toward the lateral sulcus but does not actually reach the latter. On the medial surface of a hemisected brain, three prominent sulci help distinguish lobes from one another: the **parieto-occipital sulcus**, the **calcarine sulcus**, and the **cingulate sulcus**. The first two form a Y lying on its side with the calcarine sulcus making up the stem and inferior wing. The superior wing is formed by the parieto-occipital sulcus that usually notches

Thought Question

Name the major fissures that are visible on the surface of the cerebrum, and indicate which lobes each divides. Some lobes do not have distinct divisions between them. Which are they, and how are these lobes demarcated?

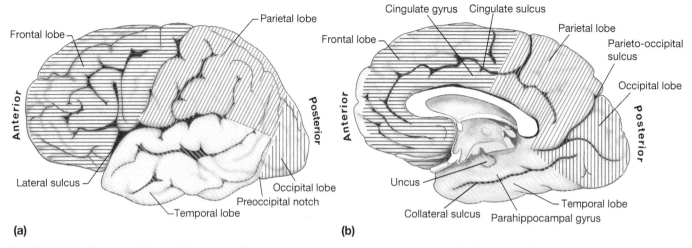

(a)   **(b)**

FIGURE 2-17 The major lobes of the cerebral hemisphere and major components of the limbic system. Note that the cingulate gyrus is present only on the medial hemispheral surface.

the dorsolateral surface of the hemisphere. Lastly, the **pre-occipital notch** on the inferolateral hemisphere surface is an important landmark in delineating lobes from one another.

The frontal lobe comprises about one-third of the lateral hemispheral surface. Extending from the frontal pole (anterior tip of the brain), it is bounded posteriorly by the central sulcus and inferiorly by the lateral sulcus (Figure 2-17 ■). Its inferior surface is termed the orbital surface.

Two imaginary lines on the lateral hemispheral surface distinguish parts of the parietal, occipital, and temporal lobes from one another. One line extends from the parieto-occipital sulcus to the preoccipital notch, while the second is a posteriorly directed line from the lateral sulcus to the point where it intersects the first line. The parietal lobe is bounded anteriorly by the central sulcus, posteriorly by the imaginary line uniting parieto-occipital sulcus with preoccipital notch, and inferiorly by the lateral sulcus and its imaginary posterior extension. The occipital lobe is posterior to the parietal lobe and extends to the posterior tip of the brain (occipital pole). Finally, the temporal lobe is anterior to the occipital lobe and inferior to the lateral sulcus and line forming the inferior boundary of the parietal lobe.

On the medial surface of a hemisphere, the frontal lobe extends posteriorly from the frontal pole to an imaginary line extending from the top of the central sulcus to the cingulate sulcus. The parietal lobe is bounded anteriorly by the frontal lobe, posteriorly by the parieto-occipital sulcus, and inferiorly by the cingulate and calcarine sulci. The posterior boundary of the temporal lobe on the medial surface is an imaginary line extending from the preoccipital notch toward the back of the corpus callosum, while its superior boundary consists mostly of the **collateral sulcus**. The occipital lobe is bounded anteriorly by the parietal and temporal lobes.

The limbic system is predominantly on the medial hemispheral surface (see Figure 2-17). Its largest component is the curved **cingulate gyrus**, immediately superior to the corpus callosum and inferior to the frontal and parietal lobes. The cingulate gyrus curves around the posterior end

of the corpus callosum, then merges with the **parahippo-campal gyrus** of the dorsal temporal lobe. At its anterior end, the parahippocampal gyrus curves back on itself to form a medial bulge, the **uncus**.

The **hippocampus**, which is contained within the parahippocampal gyrus, is part of the medial wall of the temporal lobe (Figure 2-18 ■) and is an important part of the limbic system. The limbic system plays a vital role in memory and emotion, as discussed in Chapter 22. The hippocampus and parahippocampal gyrus, in particular, are involved with memory.

An additional surface area of the cerebral cortex is the **insula**. The insula lies buried in the depths of the lateral fissure, hidden from view by and is comprised of portions of the frontal, parietal, and temporal lobes. It can be seen only by separating the frontal and temporal lobes or, better yet, by a dissection that removes portions of each of the three lobes

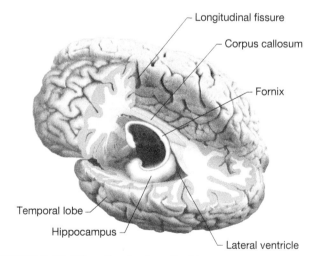

FIGURE 2-18 Dissection to show the hippocampus, a "submerged" cortical gyrus located in the medial wall of the temporal lobe. The diencephalon and brainstem have been removed. The fornix, a stout bundle of mainly efferent fibers originating from cells of the hippocampus, also is shown.

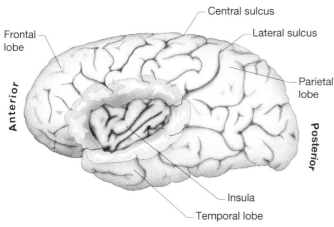

FIGURE 2-19 A dissection to show the insula buried in the depths of the lateral fissure. The portions of the frontal, parietal, and temporal lobes that cover the insula and hide it from view have been removed.

Thought Question

Which structures comprise the diencephalon?

(Figure 2-19 ■). The insula is a triangular cortical area whose apex is directed downward and forward to open into the Sylvian fossa. The insula is an important anatomical landmark when viewing the brain in frontal and horizontal sections.

Diencephalon

Very little of the diencephalon can be seen on the surface of an intact whole brain. What can be seen are several structures forming the floor of the hypothalamus. In order to view the components of the diencephalon it is necessary to look at a midsagittal section of the brain. In such a section, one can see that most of the diencephalon consists of the thalamus and hypothalamus (hypo-, Gr., under) (Figure 2-20 ■). These are paired structures lying on either side of a narrow, midline, slit-like cavity, the third ventricle (Figure 2-21 ■). (However, the hypothalami are in continuity with one another at the bottom of this ventricle.) Consequently, what we can see of the diencephalon in a hemisected brain is its medial surface. The thalamus is the largest diencephalic subdivision and consists of two egg-shaped structures on either side of the midline third ventricle. The thalamus lies superior to the **hypothalamic sulcus**, a shallow groove on the lateral wall of the third ventricle.

The hypothalamus is situated ventral to the hypothalamic sulcus. It forms the floor (inferior portion) and lateral walls of the third ventricle such that, in frontal sections, the hypothalamus has the configuration of a horseshoe. A number of ventral hypothalamic structures can be seen on the ventral surface of a whole brain. These include the **mammillary bodies**, the **infundibulum**, and **tuber cinereum**. The infundibulum (L., funnel) is a small funnel-shaped structure to which the **pituitary gland (hypophysis)** is attached (see

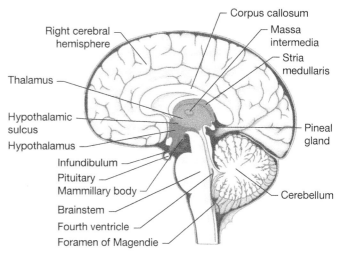

FIGURE 2-20 The medial surface of the diencephalon is revealed by a midsagittal section of the brain. The major components of the diencephalon are the dorsally located thalamus and ventrally located hypothalamus, separated by the shallow hypothalamic sulcus. The red line with arrow in the fourth ventricle illustrates the route of CSF into the subarachnoid space.

Figure 2-20). The infundibulum arises from the tuber cinereum, an elevated region forming the floor of the third ventricle (i.e., the floor of the hypothalamus) (see Figure 2-11).

Internal Organization

Ventricular System

The ventricular system is a series of four interconnected cavities within the CNS filled with **cerebrospinal fluid (CSF)**. Each brain subdivision contains its own component of the ventricular system. The four ventricles are a pair of lateral ventricles, one within each cerebral hemisphere; a midline third ventricle that is the cavity of the diencephalon; and a fourth ventricle that is positioned dorsal to the pons and medulla. Ventricular CSF can flow into the subarachnoid space surrounding the CNS via several foramina leading from the ventricular system into the subarachnoid space (see Chapter 25).

Each lateral ventricle is a long, C-shaped structure of variable width. Its C shape conforms to the shape of the cerebral hemisphere (see Figure 2-21). Each lateral ventricle is divided into four parts: an **anterior horn**, a **body**, a **posterior horn**, and an **inferior horn**. An opening, the **interventricular foramen**, connects each lateral ventricle to the third ventricle. Thus, CSF produced in the lateral ventricles can flow through these interventricular foramina (plural) into the third ventricle.

The anterior horns (of the two lateral ventricles) are situated anterior to the interventricular foramina and are within the frontal lobe. These anterior horns are parallel to one another and are separated by a thin plate of neural tissue, called the **septum pellucidum**. The body of each lateral ventricle extends posteriorly from the interventricular foramen to the

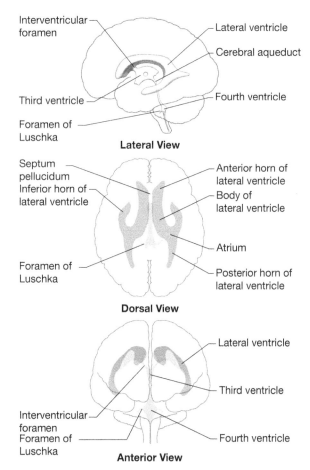

Lateral View

Dorsal View

Anterior View

FIGURE 2-21 Configuration and components of the ventricular system. Each lateral ventricle is connected to the third ventricle by an interventricular foramen, and the third ventricle is connected to the fourth ventricle by a cerebral aqueduct located in the midbrain. The fourth ventricle of the brainstem is continuous with the central canal of the spinal cord.

caudal, rounded end of the corpus callosum, the **splenium**. The body of the lateral ventricle is situated within the parietal lobe. As each body of the lateral ventricle extends posteriorly from the interventricular foramen, it is also diverging laterally, and this divergence continues through the rest of the ventricle. Thus, in progressing posteriorly, the lateral ventricles of the two sides separate. To understand this divergence, see Figure 2-21, which shows both a superior and an anterior perspective of the configurations of the lateral ventricles.

The **atrium**, or collateral trigone, is an expanded portion of the lateral ventricle that is located posterior to the thalamus. From the atrium, the inferior horn sweeps ventrally and rostrolaterally into the temporal lobe. The posterior horn, quite variable in size in different brains, extends posteriorly from the atrium into the occipital lobe.

The narrow midline cavity of the diencephalon, the third ventricle, communicates with each lateral ventricle through the interventricular foramina. In most brains, the third ventricle is partially occluded in its center by the massa intermedia, a bridge of tissue uniting the thalami of the two sides

(see Figure 2-20). Note that this bridge does not allow for neuronal projection between the two. The boundaries of the third ventricle can be seen on a hemisected brain. The roof of the ventricle attaches along a line demarcated by the **stria medullaris**, a horizontally running ridge on the dorsomedial surface of the thalamus. Posteriorly, the third ventricle tapers rapidly to communicate with the tube-like canal of the midbrain, the cerebral aqueduct. The cerebral aqueduct extends from the posterior, inferior aspect of the third ventricle to the fourth ventricle (located at the level of the cerebellum).

The fourth ventricle is a broad, diamond-shaped cavity overlying the pons and rostral portion of the medulla (this rostral portion is called the "open" portion of the medulla, or "open medulla"). The fourth ventricle is continuous rostrally with the cerebral aqueduct and caudally with a very small canal in the caudal medulla (the so-called closed medulla). The small canal in the caudal medulla is continuous with the central canal of the spinal cord. The recess at the apex of the fourth ventricle is formed by white matter of the cerebellum. From this apex, two thin laminae split at an acute angle to form the roof of the ventricle. Being diamond shaped, the fourth ventricle has a tapered lateral extension on either side; each is called the **lateral recess** (see Figure 2-21). If you inserted a probe into the lateral recess, it would emerge through an opening into what was the subarachnoid space at the **cerebellopontine angle**. This portion of the subarachnoid space is called the **cisterna magna**, and the foramen that opens into it is the **foramen of Luschka** (plural, foramina). The fourth ventricle also contains an unpaired, midline opening into the cisterna magna of the subarachnoid space, the **foramen of Magendie**. It is located in the midline of the caudal roof of the fourth ventricle (see Figure 2-20). These three foramina permit CSF from the ventricular system to drain into the subarachnoid space (see Chapter 25 for the circulation of CSF through the ventricles and subarachnoid space).

White Matter and the Basal Ganglia

Each cerebral hemisphere is composed of an inner core of white matter surrounded by a thin outer layer of gray matter, the cerebral cortex (see Figure 1-12). Axons of this inner core of white matter serve one of two functions: (1) they conduct information from neurons in the cerebral cortex to another set of distantly located cell bodies or (2) they conduct information to neurons of the cerebral cortex from a distantly located set of neurons. Many of these distantly located cell bodies are positioned inferior to the cerebral cortex; that is, they are located subcortically. The subcortical cell bodies of each cerebral hemisphere are found in structures such as the basal ganglia and the thalamus. The components of the basal ganglia will be discussed later, but their neurons are reciprocally interconnected with those of the cerebral cortex, as just discussed.

A second important aggregation of neurons reciprocally interconnected with neurons of the cerebral cortex are those in the diencephalon, a component of the cerebrum but not the cerebral hemisphere. Thus, the overall configuration of the cerebrum is an outer mantle of gray matter, the cerebral cortex, and an inner core of white matter within which are embedded the gray matter structures comprising the basal ganglia and diencephalon.

WHITE MATTER OF THE CEREBRAL HEMISPHERE If the upper parts of the hemisphere are sliced off superior to the corpus callosum, the central white substance of the hemisphere appears as an oval area, the **centrum semiovale**, surrounded by a narrow convoluted margin of gray matter. This common mass of fibers is composed of the three fiber types that characterize cerebral white matter: (1) **projection fibers** that bidirectionally connect the cerebral cortex with subcortical nuclei as well as with gray matter of the brainstem and spinal cord, (2) **association fibers** that connect different parts of the same hemisphere with one another, and (3) **commissural fibers** that reciprocally link the two hemispheres to each other. It is important to understand, in particular with reference to association and commissural fibers, that the connections between the different lobes of the same hemisphere as well as those between hemispheres represent the neuroanatomical basis of an important principle of cerebral functional organization. This is the principle that cerebral functions are organized in terms of distributed systems with different aspects of a given behavior being mediated in different areas and/or lobes. For example, portions of all four major lobes are involved in mediating language, with each region contributing a specialized function to the behavior. Similarly, higher-order processing of visual information is dependent upon parietal, frontal, and temporal lobes, not just the occipital lobes as was once believed. The concept of distributed systems contrasts with the old idea that cerebral functions are organized in terms of lobes.

Projection fibers are relatively few in relation to the enormous number of neurons confined entirely to the cerebral cortex. Fibers conveying nerve impulses to and from the entire cerebral cortex converge on the diencephalon from all directions. Within the core of each hemisphere, these fibers form a radiating mass known as the **corona radiata** (Figure 2-22 ■).

At the level of the diencephalon, fibers of the corona radiata converge further to form the **internal capsule**, a prominent fiber band making up the lateral boundary of the thalamus. The configuration of the internal capsule is best visualized in horizontal sections such as Figure 2-23 ■ . It consists of an **anterior limb** and a **posterior limb**, joined at an obtuse angle with the apex directed medially. The posterior limb is longer and larger than the anterior limb. The region where the two limbs join is called the **genu**. The genu of the internal capsule points medially.

Fibers of the internal capsule that project to the cerebral cortex arise primarily in the thalamus and project to virtually the whole of the cerebral cortex; such fibers comprise the **thalamocortical radiations**. Fibers in the internal capsule that project from the cerebral cortex are categorized according to the specific nuclear mass in which they terminate. Among others, these would include corticothalamic, corticopontine, corticoreticular, corticobulbar

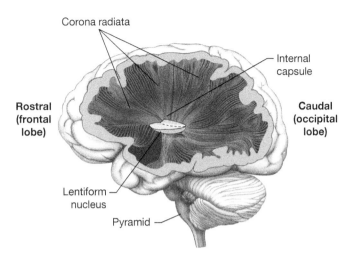

FIGURE 2-22 Projection fibers reciprocally connect neurons of the cerebral cortex with subcortical nuclei of the cerebrum and diencephalon as well as with nuclei of the brainstem and gray matter of the spinal cord. Specific origins and terminations are not shown. Note that the same projection fibers may be given different names depending on their location in the CNS. The lentiform nucleus (consisting of a medial globus pallidus and a lateral putamen) forms the lateral boundary of the internal capsule.

(projecting to cranial nerve motor nuclei), and corticospinal fibers. Projection fibers are topographically organized within the internal capsule in that fibers coming from or going to specific cortical areas are located in particular parts of the capsule. It is important to emphasize that due to the

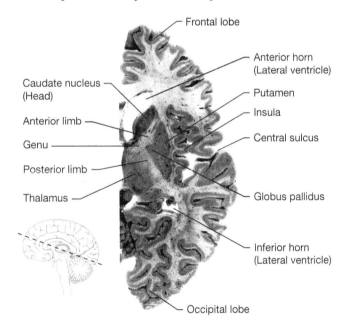

FIGURE 2-23 A horizontal section through the right cerebrum at the level indicated in the inset. The section reveals the V-shaped configuration and three major components of the internal capsule. The internal capsule is a major landmark in the interior of the cerebrum because its limbs separate well-defined components of the basal ganglia and thalamus from one another. The anterior and posterior limbs of the internal capsule carry fibers with different origins and terminations and, therefore, subserve different functions.

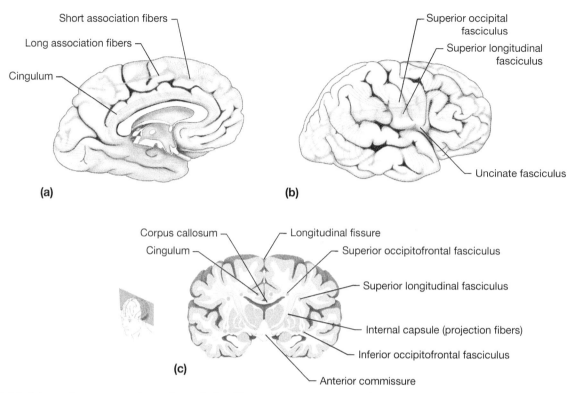

FIGURE 2-24 Schematic representations of association fibers as seen from medial (a) and lateral (b) perspectives. Commissural, projection, and association fibers as seen in a (c) frontal section.

proximity of fibers from functionally and anatomically diverse cortical areas, capsular lesions, even relatively small ones, may result in neurologic deficits involving widespread areas of the body and diverse functions.

Association fibers are the axons of cortical cells projecting from cells in one cortical area to cells in another area in the same hemisphere. These intrahemispheric fibers are divisible into short and long association fibers (Figure 2-24 ■). **Short association fibers** may be intracortical or subcortical. **Subcortical association fibers** form bundles of fibers that pass from a cortical region in one gyrus to an area of an adjacent gyrus. These fibers pass in an arc (hence the term **arcuate fibers** sometimes applied to them) within the white matter deep to the sulcus between gyri. They run transversely, not lengthwise along the long axis of the gyrus.

Long association fibers interconnect cortical areas in different lobes within the same hemisphere. These fibers organize themselves into several named bundles that can be revealed by careful gross dissection. However, none of the bundles represent point-to-point pathways linking just one cortical area with another specific area, because fibers enter and leave these bundles throughout their lengths. These long association fiber bundles are the **superior longitudinal fasciculus**, the **superior** and **inferior occipitofrontal fasciculi**, and the **cingulum**. The superior longitudinal fasciculus (also called the **arcuate fasciculus**) is the largest long association bundle and, among other things,

links language areas of the frontal and parietal lobes in the dominant (usually left) hemisphere with one another (see Figure 2-24). The superior and inferior occipitofrontal fasciculi, as their name implies, run between the frontal and occipital lobes. The fibers of the inferior occipitofrontal fasciculus that hook around the margin of the lateral sulcus and interconnect the orbital frontal cortex with the anterior temporal cortex usually are considered separately as the **uncinate fasciculus**. The cingulum is a long, curved bundle on the medial hemispheral surface lying within the cingulate gyrus. It follows the curve of the gyrus and enters the parahippocampal gyrus and adjacent temporal lobe cortex. Fibers enter and leave the cingulum all along its course. The cingulum is an important component of the **limbic system** (see Chapter 22).

Commissural fibers, reciprocally interconnecting the two cerebral hemispheres, are represented by the large corpus callosum and small anterior commissure. The **anterior commissure** is a small fiber bundle crossing the midline in front of the columns of the fornix. Most of its fibers interconnect portions of the middle and inferior temporal gyri of the two hemispheres. It is important in transmitting the emotional content of information from one hemisphere to the other. The massive corpus callosum contains more than 300 million axons and connects most of the neocortex of one hemisphere with that of the other hemisphere. Most callosal fibers connect homotopic (mirror-image) regions, but some have heterotopic connections. The

Table 2-4 **Myelinated Nerve Fibers in the Cerebral Hemisphere**

TYPE OF FIBER	NAME	FUNCTION
Commissural (transverse)	Corpus callosum Anterior commissure	Connect homologous areas of the two cerebral hemispheres
Projection	Afferent fibers	Connect the thalamus to the cerebral cortex
	Efferent fibers	Connect the cerebral cortex to the thalamus, basal ganglia, brainstem, and spinal cord

Association	Short association (U) fibers
	Long association fibers:
	    Superior longitudinal fasciculus
	    Superior occipitofrontal fasciculus
	    Inferior occipitofrontal fasciculus
	    Uncinate fasciculus
	    Cingulum
		Connect gyri, lobes, or widely separated areas within each hemisphere

corpus callosum forms boundaries for much of the lateral ventricle; for example, the genu forms the roof and rostral wall of the anterior horn.

Table 2-4 ■ summarizes the types of myelinated fibers making up the interior of each cerebral hemisphere.

BASAL GANGLIA The subcortical nuclei embedded within the white matter core of each cerebral hemisphere, the basal ganglia, have been conceptualized to include different nuclei over the years. Historically, the following nuclei were considered to make up the basal ganglia: the **caudate nucleus**, the **putamen**, the **globus pallidus**, and the **amygdala** (Figure 2-25 ■). Today, most authors consider the term *basal ganglia* to include additional nuclei, and these will be presented in Chapter 7.

Each caudate nucleus consists of three parts: head, body, and tail. These are arranged in the shape of an inverted C and closely follow the configuration of the lateral ventricle whose boundaries the nucleus helps form. The putamen is oval, and each is positioned lateral to the head and body of each caudate nucleus. The globus pallidus (again, a paired structure) is positioned medial to each putamen (see Figure 2-23). Together, the globus pallidus and the putamen are called the **lentiform nucleus**.

The amygdalae are positioned at the anterior tips of the tails of the caudate nuclei. Because of the close proximity of the caudate nuclei with the lateral ventricles, the paired amygdalae are also positioned at the anterior tips of the inferior horns of the lateral ventricles.

Over most of its length, the caudate nucleus is separated from the putamen by the thick internal capsule.

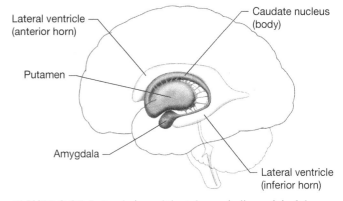

FIGURE 2-25 Lateral view of the telencephalic nuclei of the basal ganglia (the subthalamic nucleus of the diencephalon and substantia nigra of midbrain are also commonly considered to be part of the basal ganglia). Note that the C-shaped caudate nucleus helps form the boundary of the lateral ventricle. The globus pallidus (not shown in the figure) is medial to the putamen.

The caudate is medial to the internal capsule while the putamen is lateral and anterior to the internal capsule (see Figure 2-23); the head to the caudate nucleus fuses with the putamen.

Thought Question

The basal ganglia are comprised of different nuclei. Where is this structure located? Is it a single or a paired structure? Is this structure medial or lateral to the thalamus? And is the thalamus a single or paired structure?

Centrals and Cs

The topographic anatomy of the brain interior can be considered as a set of central structures and a set of C-shaped structures. Understanding their individual locations and mutual relations will help you to build a three-dimensional perspective of brain anatomy as well as help you to identify these structures when you see them in sections of the brain.

As the term implies, the *central structures* comprise a core within the cerebrum. In a medial-to-lateral sequence, this core consists of the third ventricle, the diencephalon, the internal capsule, the globus pallidus, and finally the putamen (Figure 2-26 ■; see also Figure 2-23).

These core structures, in turn, are surrounded by a set of extended C-shaped structures (Figure 2-26). Each lateral ventricle is positioned within the cerebral hemisphere as an inverted C that begins in the frontal lobe, and, after sweeping around the thalamus, ends far rostrally in the temporal lobe. The caudate nucleus is similarly positioned and, in fact, helps to form the lateral boundary of the lateral ventricle. Yet another readily identified structure, the **fornix**, has a C shape. The fornix is a robust contingent of axons composed primarily of efferent fibers from the hippocampus. As a consequence of their C shape, the lateral ventricle, caudate nucleus,

and fornix will be encountered twice in many horizontal and/or frontal (coronal) sections of the brain. See Figure 2-27 ■ for an overview of the general anatomical organization of the CNS.

CLINICAL CONNECTIONS

Association Neurons of the Cortex and Language Deficits

In Chapter 23, language is discussed in detail, and two areas related to language are identified: the area where language is formulated for speech and the area where language is interpreted. These two areas must be connected in order for a person to formulate speech in response to something that is heard. The superior longitudinal fasciculus connects these two areas. A lesion involving the superior longitudinal fasciculus disconnects the two language areas, producing a distinct aphasic syndrome known as **conduction aphasia**. People with conduction aphasia are not able to repeat words, phrases, or sentences spoken by the examiner even if they can understand the words and can use the words spontaneously (as in conversation).

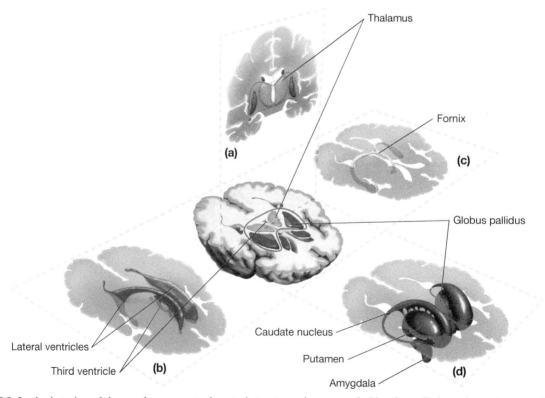

FIGURE 2-26 In the interior of the cerebrum, a set of central structures is surrounded by three C-shaped structures as depicted in both frontal (a) and horizontal (b, c, d) sections. The central structures comprise the thalamus (green), internal capsule, and globus pallidus and putamen (lenticular nucleus) of the basal ganglia (red) and are enclosed by a line. The C-shaped structures consist of the lateral ventricle (purple, b), the fornix (yellow, c), and the caudate nucleus of the basal ganglia (red, d). As a consequence of their C shape, appropriate frontal and horizontal whole brain sections will pass through each such structure twice.

(Adapted from Evans, B. *The Human Brain: Illustrations*. MS Thesis, Department of Anatomy and Neurobiology, Colorado State University, 1991.)

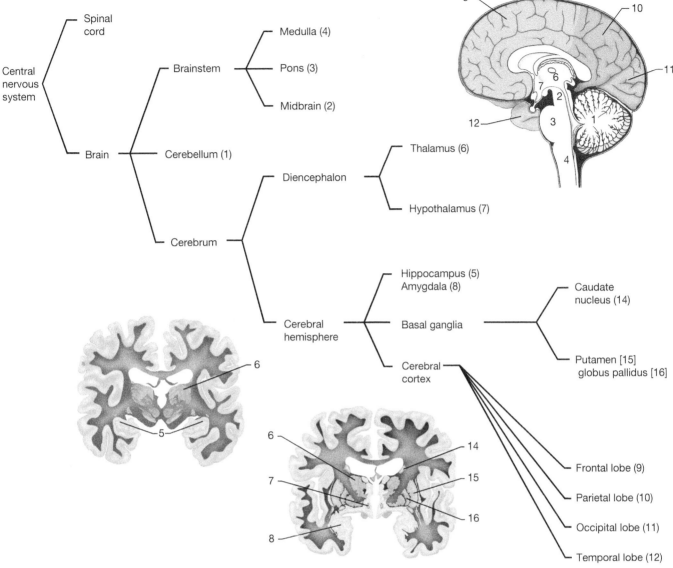

FIGURE 2-27 Summary of the subdivisions of the CNS.

(Adapted from Nolte, J. *The Human Brain*, 6th ed. Mosby Elsevier, Philadelphia, 2009.)

Clinical Preview ·················

Consider the four different patients that you "met" at the beginning of the section on the cerebrum. One had a stroke that affected the frontal cortex; the second had a stroke involving the parietal cortex; the third had involvement of his temporal cortex; and the fourth had damage to the occipital cortex. In reading through this chapter, begin to consider how knowledge of the blood supply to the cortex will assist you in determining which regions of the cortex are affected by strokes in different blood vessels.

BLOOD SUPPLY OF THE CNS

The brain makes up only about 2 percent of total body weight (three pounds or so), yet it consumes from 15 to 20 percent of the total output of blood from the heart. Why does this relatively small organ require such a large blood supply? The answer is that the energy demands of neurons are very high (including during sleep!), yet they have no mechanism by which to store significant amounts of the essential nutrients that fuel their high metabolism. The essential nutrients—oxygen and glucose—are delivered to neurons by blood; thus, the brain must receive a large and uninterrupted supply from the heart. In other words, neurons operate almost exclusively via aerobic metabolism with little energy stored as glycogen for anaerobic metabolism.

This dependence of neuron survival on a continuous and abundant blood supply is reflected in a number of facts. First, any given neuron is only a minute distance away from a blood capillary, no more than 20 to 50 micrometers. Consequently, once glucose and oxygen have crossed the wall of a capillary, they have to diffuse only minute distances to reach a neuron. Second, depriving the brain of its blood supply quickly results in disastrous consequences. When blood is totally prevented from reaching the brain, loss of consciousness will occur in about 10 seconds. If the brain is completely deprived of blood, neurons will begin to die within three to five minutes, causing irreversible brain damage. This is because the limited glucose and oxygen stores within neurons are exhausted in a matter of minutes, and the supply of molecules the neuron uses to power its metabolic activity fall to zero shortly thereafter.

Two major arterial systems deliver blood to the brain and much of the spinal cord. These are the **internal carotid arteries** and the **vertebral arteries** (Figure 2-28 ■). The internal carotid arteries arise in the neck from the common carotid arteries, ascend vertically to the base of the skull, and enter the cranial cavity through the carotid canals located in the temporal bones. The terminal branches of the internal carotid arteries supply most of the cerebral hemisphere and much of the diencephalon. The lobes supplied by these terminal branches include all of the frontal and parietal lobes as well as the lateral surfaces of the occipital and temporal lobes. The internal carotid arteries and their branches are often referred to clinically as the *anterior circulation of the brain.*

The vertebral arteries arise from the subclavian arteries and then ascend through foramina in the transverse processes of the first six cervical vertebrae. They perforate the dura and arachnoid and pass through the foramen magnum of the skull. The two arteries unite at the caudal border of the pons to form the unpaired basilar artery. The vertebrobasilar arterial system and its terminal branches are referred to clinically as the *posterior circulation of the brain.* The vertebrobasilar system supplies all of the brainstem and cerebellum as well as parts of the diencephalon and occipital and temporal lobes. In addition, the vertebral arteries supply much of the spinal cord.

The total blood flow to the brain is about 750 to 1,000 milliliters per minute (ml/min). Of this amount, about 350 ml/min flows through each of the two carotid arteries and about 100 to 200 ml/min flows through the vertebrobasilar system. These normal flow differences should not be confused with the issue of importance. Both systems are vital to a normal life; they simply supply different parts of the brain. The flow differences are due to the fact that the internal carotid system supplies a larger volume of brain tissue than does the vertebrobasilar system.

After giving off a number of branches, each system reaches the base of the brain to contribute to a set of arteries called the **circle of Willis (Figure 2-29 ■)**. From the circle of Willis, each system gives off an elaborate network of arterial branches, each of which is named and the area of brain supplied known (see Chapter 7). The circle of Willis is a ring of arteries at the base of the brain where the internal carotid and vertebrobasilar systems form anastomotic links (Figure 2-29). The internal carotid artery gives rise to two major arteries: the **middle cerebral artery (MCA)**, the largest of the three cerebral arteries and considered the direct continuation of the internal carotid, and the smaller **anterior cerebral artery (ACA)**. The internal carotids and ACAs participate in the formation of the circle of Willis. At the level of the midbrain, the basilar artery bifurcates into two **posterior cerebral arteries (PCAs)** that together form the posterior portion of the circle of Willis. The circle is completed by two communicating arteries: the **anterior communicating artery**, which links the ACAs of the two sides, and **the posterior communicating artery**, which links the posterior cerebral artery on each side with each internal carotid artery. Because the arterial pressures are about equal in the internal carotid and posterior cerebral arteries, little blood normally flows around this circle. However, in only 50 percent of people is the circle fully intact with all of its pieces of significant size. In some individuals, the structure may be such as to enable the circle of Willis to provide effective collateral circulation when there is occlusion of one internal carotid artery in the neck.

The blood supply to much of the spinal cord is derived from branches of the vertebral arteries (see Figure 5-13).

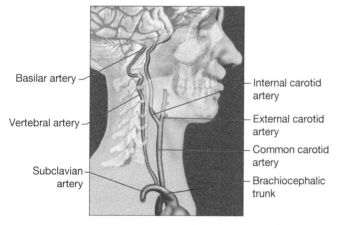

FIGURE 2-28 The two major arterial systems that deliver blood to the brain are the internal carotid and vertebrobasilar systems.

(Adapted from Bowman, J. P., and Giddings, F. D. *Strokes: An Illustrated Guide to Brain Structure, Blood Supply, and Clinical Signs.* Prentice Hall, New Jersey, 2003.)

Thought Question

What vessels are connected through the circle of Willis? Thinking ahead, why might this connection of blood vessels be of importance?

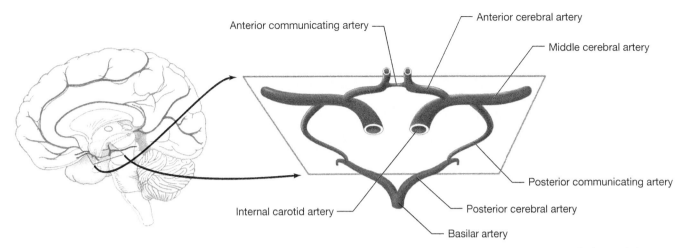

FIGURE 2-29 The vertebrobasilar and internal carotid systems, after giving off a number of branches, each reach the base of the brain where they contribute to the formation of the circle of Willis. The circle of Willis is a ring of arteries where the two systems form anastomotic links. The vertebrobasilar system gives rise to the posterior cerebral arteries, while the internal carotid system gives rise to the middle and anterior cerebral arteries. The vertebrobasilar system also supplies the brainstem and much of the spinal cord.

Upon entering the foramen magnum, each vertebral artery gives rise to a **posterior spinal artery**, each of which descends on the dorsolateral surface of the spinal cord. More rostrally, each vertebral artery gives rise to a branch that runs medially to unite with its fellow from the opposite side to form a midline, unpaired artery, the **anterior spinal artery**. The anterior spinal artery descends along the anterior median fissure of the spinal cord.

Summary

In this chapter, we have added detail to the basic design of the central nervous system that was presented in Chapter 1. We have learned that the five basic subdivisions of the CNS vary markedly from one another. Furthermore, within the structures there also is variability. The structure of the spinal cord varies systematically over its length such that the amount of white matter is greatest at cervical levels of the cord and least over sacral levels. In addition, the structure of the spinal cord varies regionally in that it exhibits focal enlargements over specific cervical and lumbosacral segmental levels. Both of these structural variations have important clinical correlates following localized spinal cord injury.

The structure of the brainstem differs dramatically from that of the spinal cord. For example, the continuous columns of sensory cells in the dorsal horn and motor neurons in the ventral horn seen in the spinal cord are replaced by discrete aggregations of sensory or motor neurons in the cranial nerve nuclei of the brainstem. The white matter of the brainstem segregates itself into discrete axonal collections of tracts as opposed to a homogeneous appearing mantle of white matter surrounding a central core of gray matter that characterizes the spinal cord. Each subdivision of the brainstem contains its own unique set of cranial nerves that lack the uniform organization of dorsal and ventral roots seen in spinal nerves. The particular set of cranial nerves residing in a given brainstem subdivision is important in determining whether the medulla, pons, or midbrain has been the site of a brain injury.

The cerebrum is the largest and most complexly organized subdivision of the brain. Its superficial gyri are parceled into four lobes, some of whose boundaries are demarcated by distinct sulci, others by imaginary lines. From a functional perspective, all lobular boundaries are arbitrary, but the lobular concept is necessary because it provides a common language for describing location in the cerebral hemispheres. In contrast to the white matter of the spinal cord and brainstem, many of whose axons run longitudinally (ascending or descending through the structure), axons of the white matter of the cerebrum course in all three dimensions, sorting themselves into association, commissural, and projection fibers. In addition, many of the structures belonging to the cerebrum, including the cerebral hemispheres, lateral ventricles, basal ganglia, and hippocampus and the fornix together, are configured in the shape of inverted Cs as a result of their developmental history.

In this chapter, we have begun to appreciate why the human brain is considered to be the most complex organ currently known. In Part II, further detail will be added to this regional anatomy. The remainder of the book addresses the systems and subsystems that reside and function within this structural framework.

Applications

1. Use the dermatome chart and the table relating muscle innervations to nerve roots from this chapter to practice sensory testing and muscle testing.

2. Describe the location of the insula with respect to the frontal, temporal, and parietal lobes and the limbic system.

3. Identify and diagram the arteries that form the circle of Willis. Explain how the circle of Willis may prevent neurological damage.

References

Alpers, B. J., Berry, R. G., and Paddison, R. M. Anatomical studies of the circle of Willis in normal brain. *Arch Neurol Psychiat* 81:409, 1959.

DeArmond, S. J., Fusco, M. M., and Dewey, M. M. *Structure of the Human Brain: A Photographic Atlas*, 3rd ed. Oxford University Press, New York, 1989.

Duvernoy, H. M. *The Human Brain: Surface, Three-Dimensional Sectional Anatomy with MRI, and Blood Supply*, 2nd ed. Springer-Verlag, Vienna, 1999.

Gluhbegovic, N., and Williams, T. H. *The Human Brain: A Photographic Guide.* Harper & Row, New York, 1980.

Ludwig, E., and Klingler, J. *Atlas Cerebri Humani.* Little Brown & Co., Boston, 1956.

Nieuwenhuys, R., Voogd, J., and van Hurjzen, C. *The Human Central Nervous System: A Synopsis and Atlas*, 3rd ed., Springer-Verlag, New York, 1988.

Nolte, J. *The Human Brain: An Introduction to Its Functional Anatomy.* Mosby Elsevier, Philadelphia, 2009.

Nolte, J., and Angevine, J. B., Jr. *The Human Brain in Photographs and Diagrams*, 2nd ed. Mosby, New York, 2000.

Parent, A. *Carpenter's Human Neuroanatomy*, 9th ed. Williams & Wilkins, Baltimore, 1996.

Roberts, M., and Hanaway, J. *Atlas of the Human Brain in Section.* Lea & Febiger, Philadelphia, 1970.

PEARSON
myhealthprofessionskit

Use this address to access the Companion Website created for this textbook. Simply select "Physical Therapy" from the choice of disciplines. Find this book and log in using your username and password to access self-assessment questions, a glossary, answers to the applications questions, and more.

Cells of the Nervous System

LEARNING OUTCOMES

This chapter prepares the reader to:

1 Recall the meaning of the following terms: synapse, axonal transport (anterograde and retrograde), and necrosis.

2 Discuss the neuron doctrine and fundamental properties of neurons.

3 Appreciate the properties associated with neurons that make them functionally unique to the NS.

4 Identify the purpose of different proteins that allow for transport of molecules into and out of neurons, including channel proteins, pump proteins, carrier proteins, transducer proteins, and neurotransmitter transporter proteins.

5 Identify and classify neurons based on shape or function.

6 Discuss the specific function of each part of a neuron.

7 Differentiate the role of the presynaptic component from the postsynaptic component of the synapse.

8 Describe the following major structures found within the neuronal cytoplasm, and identify the functional importance of each: ribosomes, Golgi complex, mitochondria, lysosomes.

9 Describe the following types of neuroglia and their roles: astrocytes, oligodendrocytes, microglia, ependyma, Schwann cells, and satellite cells.

10 Predict the prognosis for and rate of nerve regeneration, based on the site of a lesion to a peripheral nerve.

11 Use tetanus toxin to explain the process and function of retrograde transport.

12 Relate disorders of the nervous system to the specific neuroglial cells involved.

ACRONYMS

AD Alzheimer's disease

AIDS Acquired immunodeficiency syndrome

ATP Adenosine triphosphate

CNS Central nervous system

CSF Cerebrospinal fluid

DNA Deoxyribonucleic acid

ER Endoplasmic reticulum

HIV Human immunodeficiency virus

HSV Herpes simplex virus

MS Multiple sclerosis

RER Rough endoplasmic reticulum

RNA Ribonucleic acid

Introduction

The task of this chapter is to describe the types of cells that make up the adult nervous system. It has been said that the many and diverse behaviors mediated by the nervous system are, in the final analysis, to be attributed to the arrangement, function, and interaction of the individual cells of which it is composed. Equally common has been the corollary observation that behavioral dysfunctions resulting from brain disease are the expressions of the abnormal function of these individual cellular units. While both observations are true, a seemingly unbridgeable conceptual gulf exists between such statements and a rational, holistic account about how a particular neuronal organization is capable of generating behaviors that are uniquely human. Nonetheless, an understanding of cellular form and function is vital because it provides important insights into such things as the way in which specific chemicals (including medicinal and recreational). Indeed, even concentrations of specific ions affect the function of neurons as do specific and commonplace diseases. Such disruptions of normal cellular function can often result in dramatic behavioral abnormalities.

As noted in Chapter 1, two primary classes of cells comprise nervous tissue: neurons and neuroglial, or glial cells. Within both categories, one finds cells of widely varying form and size, characteristics reflective of a specialization of the cell to fulfill a particular functional role. The first section of this chapter considers neurons. According to the **neuron doctrine**, the individual neuron is the genetic, anatomic, functional, and trophic unit of the nervous system. All of the features associated with brain function, sensation, movement, speech, language, thought, emotion, and the like are mediated through the activity of neurons. The second section is devoted to a discussion of neuroglial cells. Long considered to perform functions ancillary to those of neurons, neuroglial cells are vital to the very survival of neurons. Far more numerous than neurons, glial cells occupy essentially all of the space not taken up by neurons. Additionally, they play important roles in the reactions nervous tissue displays to injury and disease.

The various cellular constituents of the nervous system along with their processes and the numerous blood capillaries combine to form what is called **parenchyma** that represents the tissue substrate of the CNS. Pathologic processes affecting the brain involve all of the constituents of CNS parenchyma either at once or sequentially.

NEURONS

Clinical Preview

You are working with Martin Herskovitz who sustained an injury that crushed his radial nerve. As you read through this section of the text, consider the information that you are learning in context of this individual. What will be the short- and long-term consequences of this injury? Will it make a difference whether only the nerve is severed or the cell body also is damaged? How will this information assist you in determining Mr. Herskovitz's prognosis for physical recovery?

The week after you begin to treat Mr. Herskoivitz, Martha Smith comes into your clinic. Mrs. Smith sustained an injury within the spinal cord that supplies the peripheral nerve root for the radial nerve. Consider the differences in prognosis, given that Mrs. Smith's injury is within the spinal cord while Mr. Herskovitz's injury is strictly to the peripheral nerve.

Properties Associated with Neurons

Some of the properties associated with neurons impart unique attributes to the nervous system—attributes not shared by any other organ system. Among these properties are the following:

1. *The number of neurons, their specialization as a class, and the specialization of individual members of the class.* The human brain has been estimated to consist of 10^{12} neurons (a million million), each independently living its own biological life but precisely interrelated with vast numbers of its fellows. As a class, neurons are highly specialized: they possess a distinctive shape; an outer membrane specialized to receive information and to support a variety of electrical signals; and a unique structure, the synapse, for communicating with other neurons or effector cells.

Furthermore, the extraordinary specialization of each neuron effectively subdivides each cell into a number of interdependent biologic compartments that will be discussed in detail later. Each functional compartment, in turn, contains its own unique constellation and proportion of organelles as well as its own particular proteins—adaptations that equip the compartment to fulfill its special functional role in the life and activity of the cell. One consequence of this specialization is to make each compartment dependent upon the others in order to successfully perform its specialized function. This, in turn, demands a vehicle by which communication between compartments can occur. Thus, a further specialization of the neuron is a phenomenon called *axoplasmic transport* (discussed later) by which the various compartments of the neuron communicate with one another.

Despite their vast numbers, it probably is true that few neurons are identical in form. Diversity in neuronal size, shape, and spatial array of processes is greater than for any other cell type in the body. Such variability is, of course, the hallmark of functional specialization in that neurons of differing form contribute differentially to overall brain function. But the specialization of the individual members of the class is so great that it may well be that no such entity as a typical neuron exists, at least insofar as there being a single cell that is uniformly descriptive of those found in the different subdivisions of the CNS. Nonetheless, it is true that with few exceptions, all neurons have common functional demands placed upon them. Thus, neurons share the common attributes of being responsive to the many stimuli impinging on their membranous surfaces; of conducting the resultant information to other parts of itself in the form of graded and nongraded electrical signals; and of precisely influencing other nerve, muscle, or glandular cells. It should not be surprising, then, to find that neurons as a class have elaborated common biologic compartments to meet these demands.

2. *A lack of capacity to divide?* Although retaining their full complement of DNA, the conventional view had been that neurons lose mitotic competency at the time of their differentiation into immature cells. In other words, conventional wisdom had it that we are born with our full complement of neurons and these must suffice for the duration. The lack of mitotic competency meant that the death of neurons through disease or injury resulted in a loss of whatever function those neurons subserved. This does not mean that recovery of function following brain damage cannot occur, only that when it does, the function is mediated by surviving neurons. It was almost as though neurons had paid a price for their ultraspecialization. The view that new neurons are not added after birth was recently shown not to be true at least in one area of the adult human brain, the hippocampus, a structure known to be important in learning and memory. Although the absolute number of new neurons is low relative to the total number in the brain, the fact that adult neurogenesis occurs to some extent in the human brain raises many tantalizing prospects for rehabilitative medicine.

3. *The complexity of connections between neurons (connectivity) and the extent to which function is dependent upon precise connectivity patterns.* The connections established between neurons (i.e., at synapses) are remarkable for the precision of their organization. This can be observed at the cellular level, at the level of sets of neurons that are linked together to form a system with a special function, and at the level of behavior.

A typical neuron may receive input from thousands of other neurons, each such input source forming synapses with a postsynaptic neuron that is unique in location and sometimes structure. For example, in motor neurons of the spinal cord, the location of a synapse on the neuronal surface establishes the effectiveness of that input in contributing to the neuron's final response to the total barrage of information it receives over all input channels at any one time. Each input is differentially weighted according to its position on the membrane of the receptive surface of the cell.

Shifting attention to systems of neurons, the specificity of connection between sets of neurons at different way stations along, for example, the visual pathway allows the final processor, the cerebral cortex, to extract meaningful patterns from incoming sensory signals. And finally, at an elementary behavioral level, it is the connectivity pattern that allows us to locate the position of a touch stimulus on our body surface, and it is the connectivity pattern that determines the form of a reflex response in which specific agonist muscles contract while their antagonists simultaneously relax.

An area of intense current research interest is determining the nature of the chemical and other signals recognized by a developing neuron that enable its processes to lengthen, seek out, locate, and finally establish precise synaptic linkages with predetermined targets, often situated centimeters away.

4. *The unique function of neurons.* As N. Wiener, the father of cybernetics, observed in 1948, "Information is information, not matter or energy." In contrast to the cells of other organ systems, neurons are only incidentally concerned with the manipulation of energy and molecular substances although clearly using both in transacting their business. The business of neurons is information: specifically they are cells uniquely concerned with the generation, processing, storage, and transfer of information. Thus, the orderly assemblage of neurons comprising the nervous system may be viewed as a highly sophisticated communication device.

The Plasma Membrane

One of the simplest but most far-reaching findings of electron microscopy has been that all neurons (including their processes) are bounded by a continuous plasma membrane. Neurons, like other cells, are separated from one another by their own membranes as well as by a narrow, fluid-filled extracellular space. This flexible plasma membrane is highly organized and dynamic. Neuronal membrane is formed by a **phospholipid bilayer**, so named because the phospholipid molecules form two distinct layers—a variety of proteins, lipids (cholesterol and glycolipids), and carbohydrates. Carbohydrate chains are found on the external side of the membrane. Those associated with membrane proteins are called **glycoproteins**. Glycoproteins are important in guiding the pathways of cell migration during development and in the outgrowth of axons towards their innervated targets, a factor of significance both during development and in adult nervous tissue following its damage.

The phospholipid bilayer is arranged such that the hydrophilic (water-attracting) polar (charged) heads of the phospholipid molecules face the aqueous solutions inside and outside the neuron while the hydrophobic (water-fearing) lipid tails face each other in the center of the membrane (Figure 3-1 ■). The consequence of this arrangement is that water-soluble substances (e.g., ions) are prevented from diffusing across the membrane by its hydrophobic center. Nonetheless, there is a continuous crossing of small molecules from one side of the membrane to the other.

Many processes carried out by neurons are initiated as a result of molecular reactions occurring within the plasma membrane. Such processes, including the trafficking of small molecules across the membrane, are mediated by the wide variety of proteins embedded in the lipid bilayer called **integral, or intrinsic, proteins**. Some face the aqueous environment on one side only, while others span the entire width of the membrane to protrude on both sides (see Figure 3-1). Because they are embedded in a solution of membrane lipids, integral proteins can move laterally within the plane of the membrane and even rotate within the bilipid layer. Such movement has been compared to icebergs floating in the ocean. This fluidity of the plasma membrane is important functionally. Significantly, membrane fluidity becomes compromised in aging and thereby changes the way neurons function in the aged brain (see Chapter 23). **Peripheral proteins**

are not embedded within the lipid bilayer. Rather, they attach to integral proteins on either the extracellular or intracellular surface of the membrane.

Membrane proteins have been classified according to the functions they fulfill. The ultraspecialization of neurons resulting in each cell being divided into compartments with unique functions (discussed later) is a consequence of a differential distribution of these functionally specific types of protein in different parts of the neuron's plasma membrane.

> **Thought Question**
>
> The plasma membrane consists of a phospholipid bilayer designed to allow only certain substances in and out of the cell. The mechanisms by which this occurs are described in Chapter 4. In preparation for understanding that material, name and identify two different mechanisms for transporting molecules across the membrane.

Channel proteins (ionophores) form membrane-spanning central pores that selectively allow specific ions to diffuse down their concentration gradients. Ions may pass across the membrane in either direction. Some channel proteins are always open, but others are open only temporarily. The latter are called **gated channels** because when the gate opens, ions pass through the channel whereas they do not when the gate is closed. **Pump proteins** maintain

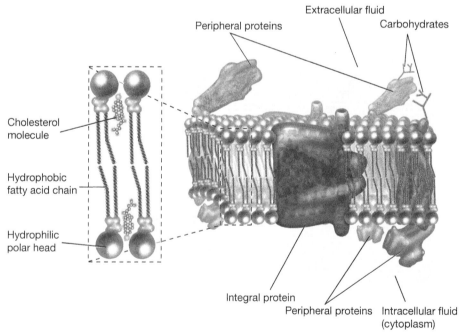

FIGURE 3-1 Modified fluid-mosaic model of the plasma membrane. The plasma membrane is a lipid bilayer composed primarily of phospholipid molecules, cholesterol, and protein molecules. The double-layered phospholipid molecules are oriented such that their hydrophobic (water-hating) fatty acid chains face each other to form the inner portion of the membrane, while their hydrophilic (water-loving) polar heads form the intracellular and extracellular surfaces of the membrane. Cholesterol molecules are incorporated within the gaps between the phospholipids on both sides of the membrane. Peripheral and integral membrane proteins are shown. Carbohydrate chains attach to both types of protein, thereby forming glycoproteins. Protein and glycoprotein molecules float in the liquid membrane. The "fluid" part of the model is the phospholipid bilayer, while the "mosaic" part consists of the protein and glycoprotein molecules. Protein molecules constitute about half the total membrane mass.

appropriate concentrations of ions on either side of the membrane by moving them against their concentration gradients. Specific ions are moved from intracellular fluid to the extracellular, while others are moved in the reverse direction. In so doing, pumps expend considerable metabolic energy. **Carrier proteins** facilitate the movement of lipid-insoluble nutrients such as glucose into neuronal cytoplasm. **Receptor proteins** provide high affinity binding sites for specific molecules present in the extracellular fluid. Such molecules are called **ligands**. Receptor proteins thus are present on the outer surface of the plasma membrane. Some enzymes are peripheral membrane proteins attached to certain types of receptor proteins called *metabotropic* receptors. This name reflects the fact that when activated, these receptors alter the neuron's metabolism via enzymatic engagement of second messenger molecule. The second messenger in turn mediates the postsynaptic response, often by opening or closing ion channels that are not physically associated with the receptor. Following the interaction of a receptor protein with a ligand, **transducer proteins** may be present to couple the receptor to enzymes within the neuron. Enzymes are peripheral proteins attached to receptor proteins. They initiate the action of intracellular second-messenger systems that actually mediate the neuron's response to an extracellular ligand. **Neurotransmitter transporter proteins** are plasma membrane glycoproteins that transport certain neurotransmitters from the synaptic cleft back into the presynaptic axon terminal (a process called *re-uptake*). These various classes are not mutually exclusive in that a given protein may, for example, function simultaneously as a receptor and channel; these types of receptors are called ionotropic, with the receptor physically part of the ion channel complex and without a second messenger system.

The plasma membrane is a highly dynamic structure. Membrane components are degraded through normal use and are constantly renewed by freshly synthesized substances. Indeed, much of the functional activity of a neuron is devoted to maintaining the protein composition of the plasma membrane.

Classification of Neurons

Neurons may be classified in a variety of ways using either structural or functional criteria. One such structural scheme classifies neurons in terms of the number of processes emerging from the cell body as being unipolar, bipolar, or multipolar (Figure 3-2 ■). **Unipolar neurons** have a single process extending from the soma. While such neurons are found in invertebrates, in humans, the single process of unipolar neurons extends only a short distance from the soma then bifurcates into two long processes. In humans, the term **pseudounipolar neuron** is often applied to these cells. Pseudounipolar neurons represent the predominant input, or sensory, neurons of the somatosensory and visceral nervous system, with one of the long processes ending in the periphery and the other in the CNS. The cell bodies of these neurons are located in the

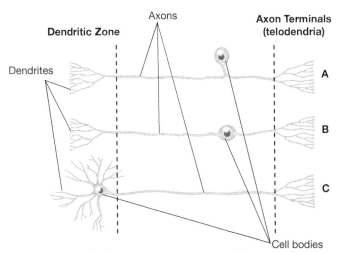

FIGURE 3-2 Classification of neurons according to the number of processes extending from the cell body. Many neurons of the CNS are multipolar (C), but multipolar neurons also occur in the peripheral autonomic nervous system. As a generalization, pseudounipolar (A) and bipolar (B) neurons are found only in the PNS where they function as sensory neurons.

spinal (dorsal root) ganglia of spinal nerves. Pseudounipolar neurons also are found in the sensory ganglia of some cranial nerves. **Bipolar neurons** have two processes extending from the cell body. Bipolar neurons are found in the retina of the eye and in several of the cranial nerves (the vestibulocochlear and olfactory). Finally, **multipolar neurons** have three or more processes extending from the cell body. By far, the vast majority of neurons in the CNS are multipolar. Multipolar neurons have numerous, short dendrites and a single, long axon. Many multipolar cells function as output, or motor, neurons of the CNS with their axons terminating in effector organs such as muscle and gland.

> **Thought Question**
>
> Most neurons are multipolar. What makes a neuron multipolar? Thinking ahead, what is the functional implication of having a multipolar neuron in terms of communication?

A common functional classification distinguishes neurons according to the direction in which they transmit (conduct) information (nerve impulses). In addition to sensory (afferent) and motor (efferent) neurons defined earlier, **ascending neurons** conduct information from structures positioned lower in the CNS to structures that are located at higher levels. **Descending neurons** conduct information in the reverse direction. Some ascending neurons are sensory and some descending neurons are motor, but certainly not all are. Thus, the terms cannot be used synonymously without reference to a specific system. Commissural neurons conduct information from one side of the CNS to the opposite side. **Internuncial neurons**, or interneurons, link other neurons—for example, sensory neurons with motor neurons. Note that these categories are not mutually exclusive.

A distinction also can be made between interneurons, which are local circuit neurons whose axon and dendrites remain within their home nucleus/cortical territory, and projection neurons, whose axons leave their home nucleus/cortical territory. In contrast to the previous categories, these categories are mutually exclusive.

> **Thought Question**
>
> Neurons have a number of major components. What is the function of each of these components: soma, axon, dendrites, nerve terminals?

Parts of the Neuron Defined According to Function

Soma (Cell Body)

The soma, or cell body, is that part of the neuron containing the nucleus and surrounding cytoplasm. The location of the cell body is not a fundamental feature of neurons as a cell class because the position of the cell body varies in different types of neurons as is shown in Figure 3-2. In multipolar neurons, the soma is interposed between dendrites and axon; in bipolar neurons, it appears as an ovoid swelling with two distinct processes emerging from the cell body; in pseudounipolar neurons, it appears as an appendage offset from the axon. Cell bodies have diameters ranging from 4 to 35 micrometers, size being roughly correlated with the length of the axonal process. Within the cytoplasm are located the nucleus and various organelles associated with the extremely high metabolic rate of neurons. Organelles will be considered later.

Characteristically positioned in the center of the cell body, the nucleus is approximately spherical and appears unusually large for the size of the soma (Figure 3-3 ■). It contains chromatin in a widely dispersed, fine granular state. Chromatin is composed of DNA, and its ubiquitous distribution is indicative of active transcriptional activity. Transfer ribonucleic acid (RNA) also comes from the nucleus. The nucleus contains a darkly staining, conspicuous **nucleolus** composed largely of RNA. Ribosomal RNA is synthesized as a consequence of nucleolar activity. A small deoxyribonucleic acid (DNA)-containing body, called the Barr body or sex chromatin, is located adjacent to the nucleolus in the neurons of females.

A **nuclear membrane**, or *nuclear envelope*, surrounds the nucleus separating its contents from that of the cytoplasm. Pores in the nuclear envelope allow the nucleus to communicate with the cytoplasm and endoplasmic reticulum (refer to Figure 3-3); they are of sufficient size to permit the easy passage of macromolecules such as messenger RNA that is synthesized in the nucleus and exported to the cytoplasm.

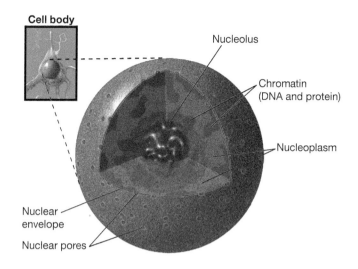

FIGURE 3-3 The nucleus of a neuron is delineated from the cytoplasm by the double-layered unit membrane called the nuclear envelope. The nuclear envelope contains numerous circular openings, called *nuclear pores*, that provide avenues for a bidirectional exchange of materials between the nucleoplasm and cytoplasm.

The cell body is the **trophic** (Gr., nursing) center of the neuron. It contains a full complement of cellular organelles. Within it are synthesized enzymes and other molecules essential to the function and life of the entire cell. Destruction of the cell body through disease or trauma results in death of the neuron, including degeneration of all its processes—a phenomenon known as **necrosis**. When injury severs an axon but leaves the cell body undisturbed, only the portion of the axon distal to the transection and isolated from the soma degenerates. This does not necessarily mean that the neuron will survive on a long-term basis (there are reasons it might not), but the occurrence of axonal degeneration demonstrates that the axon is dependent upon the cell body for its own survival. Lacking certain organelles, the axon simply does not contain the biochemical machinery, or, for that matter, the raw materials, necessary for its own maintenance. As we noted earlier, such interdependence is a consequence of the neuron's high specialization. So long as the soma remains intact, the potential for axonal regeneration and functional recovery exists (Figure 3-4 ■). However, regeneration is of practical significance only in the PNS. In addition to maintaining the structural and functional integrity of its own parts, the cell body also exerts a trophic influence on postsynaptic cells.

> **Thought Question**
>
> As a rehabilitation professional, you need to be able to predict which injuries will cause permanent damage and permanent loss of function and which will not. If a cell body is destroyed, but the axon is intact, will the axon survive? Why or why not? Conversely, what happens to the cell body if an axon is destroyed? What are the implications of these two scenarios for recovery of physical function?

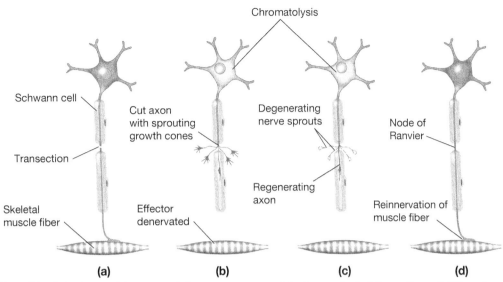

FIGURE 3-4 The cell body is the trophic center of the neuron responsible for survival of the entire cell. When, for example, an axon is cut, the portion severed from the cell body degenerates (a, b). The cell body then shifts its metabolic activity into a repair mode, as manifested by a reaction in the cell body called chromatolysis (b, c), in which the nucleus occupies an eccentric position in the cell body and endoplasmic reticulum becomes disorganized. The severed axon sprouts new growth cones as it attempts to reestablish synaptic contacts, in this case with striated muscle cells (d).

Axon

The axon comprises a distinct metabolic compartment of the neuron. Axonal membrane (axolemma) is continuous with the membrane of the cell body (plasma membrane); axonal cytoplasm (axoplasm) is likewise continuous with cytoplasm of the soma. Both axolemma and axoplasm, however, have distinguishing compositions befitting their specialized functional roles. In a typical multipolar neuron (internuncial and motor neurons), the axon arises from a cone-shaped extension of the cell body, termed the **axon hillock** (Figure 3-5 ■). The initial portion of the axon always is devoid of a myelin sheath and is called the **initial segment**. The initial segment represents the site at which nerve impulses (action potentials) are initiated (see Chapter 4). Immediately distal to the initial segment, the axon assumes the diameter that, in general, it subsequently maintains for most of the remainder of its length. Many axons become ensheathed at this point in a discontinuous layer termed the **myelin sheath**. The myelin sheath is interrupted at regular intervals by the **nodes of Ranvier**. Along

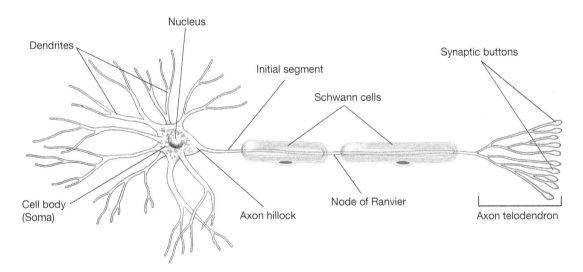

FIGURE 3-5 Structural components of an axon. The axon arises from an extension of the cell body called the axon hillock. The unmyelinated initial segment of the axon is the site at which action potentials are generated. If the axon is myelinated, the myelin sheath begins after the initial segment. Over the length of an axon, the myelin sheath is formed by many neuroglial cells (Schwann cells in the PNS and oligodendroglial cells in the CNS). Interruptions occur in the myelin sheath, resulting in gaps referred to as nodes of Ranvier. The axon branches near its termination to form the axon telodendron (G. *telos*, end + *dendron*, tree). At the end of each branch is a terminal expansion called the synaptic knob or button (bouton).

their course, axons branch only infrequently, but when they do, the branches emerge from the nodes of Ranvier and at approximately right angles to the parent fiber. Such branches often are referred to as **axon collaterals**. Near its distal end, each axon branches repeatedly (see Figures 3-2 and 3-5) to form an irregularly arranged terminal arborization (L., *arbor*, tree). Axonal diameters in this terminal arborization may be smaller than in the parent axon. The terminal *arborization* is sometimes referred to as the **axon telodendron** (Gr., *telos*, end, + *dendron*, tree). Each branch, in turn, ends in a small expansion known as the **synaptic knob or synaptic button**.

In sensory (receptor) neurons, the axon begins at the point where the dendritic processes, if multiple, assemble into a single strand (see Figure 3-2). The cell body of most sensory neurons appears in one of two general locations: as an enlargement of axonal membrane, as in the bipolar neurons of the vestibulocochlear (VIII) nerve, or as an appendage to the axon as in the pseudounipolar neurons of spinal and certain cranial nerves. Axons of sensory neurons may be myelinated or unmyelinated.

Axonal membrane is specialized to support the nerve impulse. Nerve impulses (action potentials) are electrical signals representing a state of neuronal excitation. They travel (conduct) from their site of initiation (the axon initial segment) to the terminal ends of the axon (axon telodendron). Action potentials represent the means by which information is conducted to and from the CNS and between different sites within the CNS. Thus, the axon is considered functionally to be that portion of the neuron specialized for the conduction of excitation over distance. Accordingly, it often is referred to as the **conducting portion** of the neuron. Each nerve impulse, after originating in the initial segment, is conducted the entire length of the axon without any alteration of its shape or amplitude. Axoplasm is also specialized, in this case to support and sustain a busy bidirectional molecular traffic by which a wide variety of substances are transported to and from the cell body. This will be discussed later in the section on axoplasmic transport.

Axons of different neurons vary greatly in diameter and length, depending on the functional system to which they belong. Axons also are called nerve fibers. They group themselves into more or less discrete bundles in the CNS, forming tracts and pathways (see Chapter 1). In the PNS, axons form spinal and cranial nerves. The length of some axons is remarkable. Within the CNS, giant pyramidal cells of the cerebral cortex have axons that extend from the cortex (top of the head) to lumbar segments of the spinal cord. Some sensory neurons have axons that extend from a peripheral receptor in the big toe, pass all the way up in the spinal cord, and end in the brainstem. Such axons, located partly within the PNS and partly within the CNS, would span a distance from the big toe to the nape of the neck.

Thought Question

In this chapter, the concept of the action potential is introduced in preparation for a more detailed discussion in Chapter 4. To get started, consider the following: What is an action potential, and why is the action potential the key to nervous system function? What portion of the neuron is the "conducting portion"? What is the length of this portion in comparison to other parts of the neuron?

Dendrites

Dendrites may be considered the true extensions of the cell body because they possess membrane and cytoplasmic compositions similar to the soma, although there is a progressive decrease in organelles with increasing distance from the cell body. Structurally, dendrites are relatively short, tapering, of irregular diameter, and contain many branches, contrasting in these and other aspects with the typical axon. The unmyelinated dendrites are specialized to serve as the **receptive portion** of the neuron.

Much of the variability in the form of different neurons is due to the varying lengths, complexity of branching, and spatial disposition of its dendrites. Virtually every conceivable structural array exists. Several examples follow (Figure 3-6 ■): (1) motor neurons contain large tapering dendrites that branch in all three planes; (2) giant **pyramidal cells** of the cerebral cortex contain a single robust dendrite (called the apical dendrite) extending from the apex of the pyramid-shaped cell body from which numerous smaller dendritic branches extend; and (3) **Purkinje cells** of the cerebellar cortex have a profuse, brush-like spread of dendrites, all oriented in a single plane. While neurons of given configuration tend to occur in selective regions of the nervous system, a given region typically contains many anatomical variants.

Many dendrites contain small excrescences of various sizes and shapes called **dendritic spines**, *thorns*, or *gemmules*. These do not occur on cell bodies or on the bases of large dendritic trunks. Spines participate in the formation of a synapse, usually representing the postsynaptic component. When present, spines comprise a major receptive apparatus of the neuron, receiving input from other neurons (presynaptic neurons). A typical large pyramidal cell contains some 20,000 spine synapses and a cerebellar Purkinje cell contains 200,000. However, not all synapses are associated with postsynaptic spines. In such situations, other postsynaptic (dendritic) membrane specializations exist in the area of the synapse. Spines and dendrites are generally the structural means by which the neuron gains a large membrane surface area on which to receive information from other neurons. Dendrites and spines increase in number during maturation and undergo continual remodeling as learning progresses. Increased or altered synaptic input requires expansion and/or remodeling of the receptive surface. Regrettably, late in life, once robust dendritic

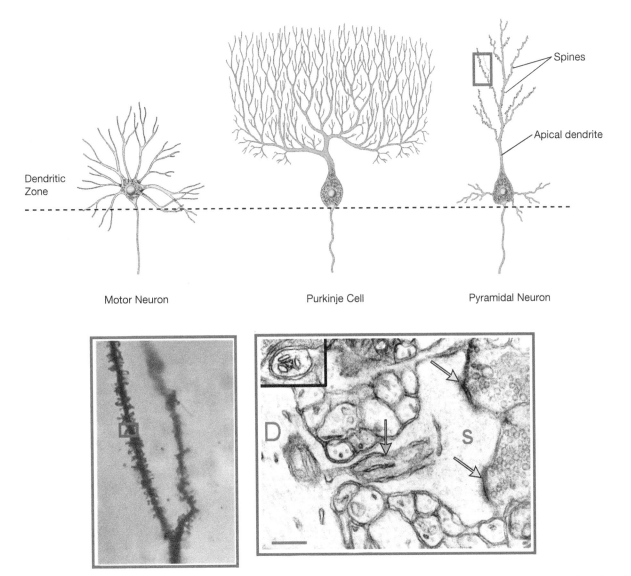

Motor Neuron Purkinje Cell Pyramidal Neuron

FIGURE 3-6 Most of the structural variability in different neurons of the CNS resides in the number and three-dimensional profile of dendrites extending from the cell body. Each dendrite may be studded with small excrescences called dendritic spines. Electron micrographs reveal that the dendritic spines are specialized for synaptic contacts, two of which are shown on the mushroom-shaped spine. Abbreviations: D, main (stem) dendrite; S, dendritic spine. Arrow points to the spine apparatus in the neck of the spine, and the inset shows the appearance of the spine apparatus in transverse section. Bar = 300 nm.

Bottom left: Photo courtesy of Bob Jacobs, Ph.D., Colorado College; bottom right: © J Spacek/Atlas of Ultrastructural Neurocytology, http://synapses.clm.utexas.edu/atlas/.

profiles begin to recede, dendrites decrease in number and shrink. The phenomenon is referred to as *pruning*. It is a manifestation of normal of aging, a fate we all share. In certain pathological conditions—Alzheimer's disease being the most notable—dendritic pruning may occur in selected neuronal populations to a rate and extent far more accelerated than that characterizing normal aging.

Other more general terms sometimes applied to dendrites are **dendritic zone** and **receptive zone**, the latter term reflective of the role of dendrites as the neuron's major receptive membrane. It must be understood, however, that synapses are not confined to dendrites: they are distributed as well on the membrane of the cell bodies and, in some instances, on axons. But their numbers at these

locations are less than on the dendrites so that, for example, of the 10,000 or so synapses studding the surface of a typical motor neuron, 8,000 will be on dendritic and 2,000 on somal membranes. Somatic membrane makes up part of the receptive zone of CNS neurons.

Sensory neurons lack true dendrites; that is, they lack structures we would recognize as dendrites under the microscope. However, they do possess receptive (dendritic) zones. The receptive zone of a sensory neuron is the peripheral receptor itself that receives and responds to some form of environmental energy (see Chapter 4). The receptor terminal transduces such external energy into the language of the nervous system, that is, into an electrical signal called a **receptor (generator) potential**.

Thus, to summarize, the term *dendritic zone* is used to designate the receptive membrane of the neuron, which may be extensions of the cell body (dendrites), the cell body itself, or a specialized receptor.

A common functional demand placed on the receptive zone of all neurons is to integrate multiple inputs. In most cases, these inputs impinge on the cell as a consequence of synaptic activity, but in sensory neurons, they arrive in the form of environmental energy that possesses multiple time-varying parameters (such as intensity, duration, and motion). The receptive zone meets this demand by generating a unique electrical signal, one that is **graded** and **nonpropagated** (see Chapter 4). This signal does *not* travel (conduct) down the axon (it is nonpropagated), and its amplitude varies in accordance with variation in the input (it is graded). In the case of sensory neurons, the signal is called a *receptor potential*; in all other neurons, it is called a **postsynaptic potential**. Its function is the same in either case: first, to encode or integrate information impinging on the cell's receptive surface, and second, to set up a pattern of nerve impulses in the axon reflective of this integration.

Nerve Terminals

Distally each axon branches into a simple or extensive terminal arborization called the axon telodendron. The distal endings of the terminal arborization are called **nerve terminals**. Nerve terminals are situated at the pole of the neuron opposite the receptive zone (see Figure 3-5). The expanded nerve terminals may be synaptic endings (knobs, boutons) on other neurons in which case they form the presynaptic component of a synapse. Other nerve terminals may be effector endings in muscle and glands. In either case, these terminals are specialized to act as the **transmitting portion** of the neuron. They accomplish this function by releasing a chemical onto the membrane of the cell on which they terminate (see Chapter 4).

Organelles

Neuronal cytoplasm contains a host of organelles that are the basis of translation as well as the numerous other biochemical processes associated with the neuron's intense metabolic rate. The exceedingly high metabolism of neurons is required for the following essential functions: (1) operation of the ionic pumps across the surface membrane that maintain the correct intracellular ionic composition; (2) the manufacture, assembly, and recycling of surface and intracellular membrane components; (3) the manufacture of chemical signaling substances such as neurotransmitters and neuromodulators; and (4) the transport of a wide variety of chemical substances along the axon to and from the cell body.

The cell body contains large amounts of **rough endoplasmic reticulum (rER)**, also known as **Nissl bodies** or *Nissl substance* (Figure 3-7 ■). Considerable variation occurs in the size, shape, and distribution of Nissl bodies in different neurons. Rough ER is the principal protein-synthesizing machinery of the neuron, and the impressive concentration of Nissl substance in the soma is reflective of the prodigious rate of protein synthesis occurring in neurons. Nissl bodies extend into dendrites, but not into the axon.

An individual Nissl body may consist of a large or small stack of flattened cisterns with a parallel arrangement. Studding the outer surface of these cisterns (and occurring

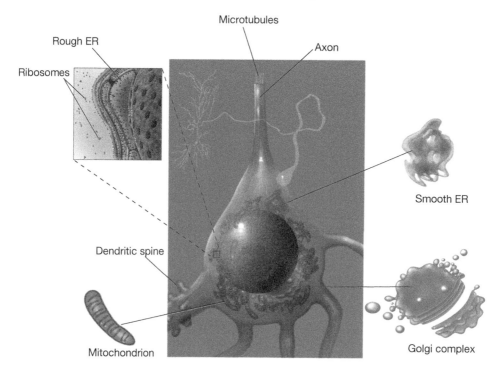

FIGURE 3-7 Organelles present in a typical neuron.

in clusters or rosettes between them) are armies of minute granules called **ribosomes** (or polyribosomes) composed of proteins and one variety of RNA (ribosomal RNA). Those mounted on the surface of the endoplasmic reticulum (ER) impart a rough appearance to the membrane, hence the name rough ER (or rER). Ribosomes function to assemble amino acids into proteins (the process of translation) in accordance with the coded instructions carried by strands of messenger RNA arriving from the nucleus of the cell.

Nissl bodies provide a sensitive index of the physiologic state of the neuron because a host of conditions alter their form and position. Nissl substance stains well in physiologically inactive neurons but poorly in neurons subjected to excessive stimulation. Damage to a neuron, most commonly to its axon, may result in **chromatolysis**, a reaction in which Nissl bodies disappear or form poorly outlined aggregations near the surface of one side of the cell (see Figure 3-4).

Thought Question

Is the distribution of different organelles within a neuron uniform? Why or why not?

A second, widely dispersed cytoplasmic organelle, again absent from the axon, is the **Golgi apparatus** or **Golgi complex** (see Figure 3-7). Its most characteristic structural component is a stack of smooth-surfaced cisternae having flattened plate-like centers and dilated rims. The Golgi apparatus is especially dense around the nucleus and is present within the proximal portions of dendrites. The Golgi complex has been described as a hub of extensive intracellular traffic (a traffic policeman, if you will) with a wide variety of substances moving into and through the complex while being processed en route.

The Golgi apparatus modifies, concentrates, and packages constituents received from the ER (from both the smooth and rough ER, which are continuous with one another). Proteins—for example, those synthesized in the rough ER—are carried to the Golgi complex in transport vesicles that bud off from rough ER membrane and fuse with the outer face of the Golgi membrane. Following appropriate modification within the Golgi compartments, the different proteins are tagged for delivery to specific sites and then packaged in vesicles targeted exclusively for that site. The ultimate destination of the protein may be an intracellular organelle such as the lysosome, insertion into the plasma membrane as, for example, an integral protein, or export from the cell as a secretory product.

Numerous **mitochondria** are distributed throughout the cell body and all of the processes of the neuron, attaining even the far reaches of the axon—the synaptic button—where, in fact, a high concentration is present (see Figure 3-7). Mitochondria are unusual organelles in that they contain their own unique bacteria-like DNA and RNA, different from that of the remainder of the cell, and their own

unique translation mechanism. (Such features have generated the interesting speculation that in the course of evolution, the cell was at one point invaded by a bacterium that then established a symbiotic relationship with the cell.) Each mitochondrion is bounded by a smooth-contoured outer membrane and by an inner membrane possessing multiple infoldings projecting into an inner cavity.

Mitochondria are the power plants of the neuron. The inner membrane is a sheet of multi-enzyme systems containing the respiratory and energy-transferring enzymes involved with energy extraction. Energy is stored in the form of high-energy phosphate bonds, especially **adenosine triphosphate (ATP)**. Mitochondria occur in the vicinity of the nodes of Ranvier and are abundant in the terminals of axons where intense activity occurs during the metabolism of neurotransmitters.

Lysosomes are spherical membrane-bound organelles that function as the primary component of the intracellular digestive system. Each contains a rich complement of digestive enzymes derived from the rough ER that are collectively capable of hydrolyzing almost all classes of macromolecules. Unlike other organelles, lysosomes are quite variable in size. Also, its contents vary, depending upon its most recent "meal" and the amount of time elapsed since ingestion. Although lysosomes may accumulate and sequester indigestible residues, sometimes for the life of the cell, they are more than garbage dumps. They are more like recycling plants because most breakdown products are available for metabolic reuse.

Two basic types of fibrillar structures, uniquely characteristic of neurons, have a widespread distribution in the cytoplasm of the cell body, axon, and dendrites. These are **neurofilaments** and the larger-diameter **microtubules** (see Figure 3-7). Both are longitudinal, unbranched organelles oriented approximately lengthwise along the axon and dendrites. These organelles form the cytoskeleton of the neuron. The cytoskeleton of a neuron forms the internal scaffolding of the cell over which the neuronal membrane is draped like a tent. In a sense, cytoskeletal elements are like the "bones" of the neuron in that they determine neuronal shape. But they are far more dynamic than the bones making up the skeleton of an adult body because they continuously assemble and disassemble, growing longer or shorter according to the needs of the neuron.

The most prominent function attributed to neurofilaments, which are separated and interconnected with one another by numerous cross bridges, is their role as a structural scaffolding for the neuron maintaining the form of the cell's long, slender processes. Microtubules are formed of a spontaneously self-assembling globular protein called **tubulin** as well as a variety of so-called microtubule-associated proteins. These dynamic and changing organelles play a variety of intracellular roles, including one in the vital phenomenon of axoplasmic transport, the process by which a variety of materials are moved between the cell body and the axon.

Axoplasmic Transport and Axoplasmic Flow

The high degree of regional specialization, or compartmentalization, existing in neurons means that the region involved in synthesizing a particular substance may be located at a distance (often considerable) from the site where the substance is actually used. Consequently, neurons possess specialized mechanisms by which to distribute molecules and materials from one part of the neuron to another. Two such distributive processes are recognized: (1) **axonal transport**, a bidirectional movement of substances between the cell body and axon terminal that occurs at the fast rate of some 400 mm/day; and (2) **axoplasmic flow**, a unidirectional movement of substances from the cell body towards the axon terminal that occurs at a slow rate of 0.5 to 6.0 mm/day. Substances moved by the two processes are different. **Anterograde** refers to movement from the cell body towards the terminal, **retrograde** to movement in the reverse direction (Figure 3-8 ■).

Because the axon and its numerous terminal appendages possess only limited biosynthetic capacities (consistent with their lack of rough ER and a Golgi apparatus), nearly all macromolecules are synthesized and packaged in the cell body. This means that virtually all membranous organelles and macromolecules present in axons and axon telodendria must originate in the soma either fully assembled or in suitable precursor form so that assembly can occur at the target destination. Such precursors may be likened to prefabricated fragments of cell membrane consisting for the most part of protein–lipid assemblages. These then are exported from the soma and loaded onto intracellular transport systems. Because normal use continually degrades axonal membrane, some of the material is deposited along the course of the axon to maintain, for example, chemical coding of the axolemma; other components reach the synaptic knobs (see Figure 3-8).

Substances are moved by fast anterograde transport at about a rate of 100 to 400 mm/day. The substances moved in this way are primarily membranous organelles, one of the most important being the synaptic vesicle. Receptor proteins, proteins involved in uptake mechanisms, and other membrane-associated proteins also are conveyed by rapid anterograde transport. Slow axoplasmic flow, on the other hand, moves such materials as the biosynthetic enzymes involved in the synthesis and storage of neurotransmitters as well as the protein constituents of microtubules and neurofilaments. This occurs at a rate of 0.5 to 6.0 mm/day. Although synthesis of low molecular weight neurotransmitters occurs in the terminal itself, the process of synaptic transmission remains dependent upon both fast and slow transport mechanisms.

Fast transport in the retrograde direction occurs at about half the rate of anterograde fast transport. This fast retrograde transport fulfills several important functions. First, axoplasmic and membrane constituents worn out through normal use are picked up by lysosomes and returned to the soma for degradation or recycling. A second major function of retrograde transport is as a feedback route helping to shape activity of the cell body, the neuron's major governing entity. Information conveyed by retrograde transport pertains to the extracellular as well as intracellular environment. Retrograde transport keeps the soma abreast of the state of biochemical affairs in its terminals. Should, for example, a long-term heavy demand be placed on transmitter use, the cell body would be signaled to accelerate its synthesis of biosynthetic enzymes. In the case of axonal injury, retrograde transport inaugurates the chromalytic reaction (referred to previously) in the cell body and elicits an accelerated synthesis of materials required for repair and longitudinal regrowth of the axon.

Fast retrograde transport also keeps the cell body informed of the status of the extracellular environment at nerve terminals. Receptor-mediated endocytosis takes up large molecules from the synaptic cleft that are then transported back to the cell body and elicit a compensatory shift in protein syntheses by affecting the nucleus. Trophic factors, such as nerve-growth factor, comprise one important category of endocytosed molecule. Some are emitted from the innervated target and are essential for the survival of the neuron, because without functional innervation of an

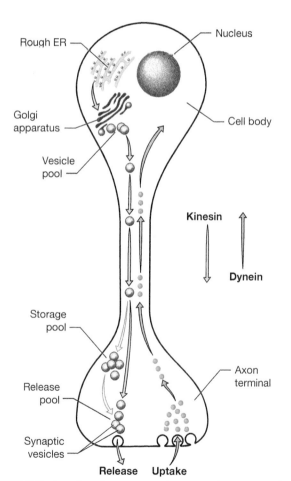

FIGURE 3-8 Axoplasmic transport. Anterograde transport is from the cell body to the axon terminal, whereas retrograde transport is from the terminal to the cell body. Microtubules serve as tracks along which materials are transported by protein "motors," a distinct one for each direction.

appropriate postsynaptic target, the neuron fails to survive. Other factors guide the growth of the axonal process and the laying down of proper synaptic contacts during development. However, retrograde transport also has a negative side (see Clinical Connections).

Fast axoplasmic transport is a microtubule-dependent process. Microtubules are polarized structures because the tubulin forming them polymerizes faster at one end [the plus (+) end than the other [the minus (−) end]. The plus end is located at the terminal of the neuron, while the minus end is located in the cell body, near the nucleus. The polarized microtubules act as tracks for microtubule-based motor proteins that distribute vesicles throughout the neuron. There are two such motor proteins, *kinesin* and *dynein*, each of which has a motor domain at one end and a "cargo" domain at the other. Kinesin is a plus-end-directed motor protein and therefore functions in anterograde axoplasmic transport. Dynein is a minus-end-directed motor protein and therefore functions in retrograde axoplasmic transport.

CLINICAL CONNECTIONS
Peripheral Nerve Regeneration

As mentioned earlier, there is potential for axonal regeneration and recovery of neuronal function within the PNS so long as the soma is intact. The axons making up peripheral nerve fibers may be myelinated by Schwann cells, which serve both to increase speed of action potential conduction and to protect the axon structurally. Further, peripheral nerves are surrounded and protected by three layers of connective tissue (see Chapter 25).

The potential for recovery is dependent upon the extent of damage to the peripheral nerve (also see Chapter 10). If damage is localized to the myelin sheath alone, prognosis for full recovery is likely. Typically, such damage is due to compression causing local ischemia. Recovery is also likely, but slower, if the damage affects the myelin and the axon but the investing connective tissues are intact. This can be caused by prolonged compression. It is estimated

that regeneration occurs at a rate of 1 mm/day, sometimes requiring months for full recovery depending on the location of the nerve injury relative to the target structures the nerve innervates. Finally, functional recovery is unlikely if the peripheral nerve damage includes the myelin, axon, and connective tissues. Such damage can occur from a penetrating injury, such as a stab or gunshot wound, or an avulsion injury. Surgical repair is often required, and not always successful.

Thought Question

Typically peripheral nerve regeneration occurs at a rate of about 1 inch/month. What is the rate-limiting factor in this process?

Retrograde Axonal Transport and Nervous System Pathology

Certain toxins, such as the tetanus toxin from the *Clostridium tetani* bacterium, are retrogradely transported from the environment to the cell bodies of CNS motor neurons, potentially causing tetanic contraction of muscles with possible death. Neurotropic viruses such as rabies, herpes simplex, and poliomyelitis also gain access to the CNS via retrograde transport.

Clinical Preview

In your clinical practice, you work with both children and adults. Over the past few months, you have worked with clients who have pathological conditions related to the following: an astrocytoma, Multiple sclerosis (MS), acquired immunodeficiency syndrome (AIDS), and Alzheimer's disease (AD). As you read through the next section, consider the similarities and differences in the pathophysiology of these four conditions and the implications for such individuals' prognoses.

Neuropathology Box 3-1: Herpes Simplex

Infection of the brain by the herpes simplex virus (HSV) results in the most common and severe from of acute encephalitis in the United States. Between 30 and 70 percent of cases are fatal, and of those who survive, the majority are left with major neurologic deficits. The virus is thought to invade the peripheral nervous system via the trigeminal nerve and be transported to the sensory ganglion of the nerve via the retrograde axoplasmic transport system. The HSV then resides latent in the sensory ganglion of the trigeminal nerve (the gasserian or

semilunar ganglion). In fact, the virus can be isolated from the ganglion in as many as 50 percent of routine autopsies. Upon reactivation, the virus spreads along trigeminal axons into the brain. Trigeminal axons innervate the pia mater and arachnoid mater of the meninges in the anterior and middle fossae of the cranium (see Chapter 13). This innervation explains the characteristic distribution pattern of hemorrhagic necrotic lesions in the inferior and medial temporal lobes and orbitomedial parts of the frontal lobes.

NEUROGLIA

Unlike the peripheral nervous system where a variety of connective tissue investments support and anchor peripheral nerve fibers in their often tortuous and long course toward innervated targets, the parenchyma of the CNS lacks an intrinsic supportive and stabilizing connective tissue network. Although three connective tissue membranes—the meninges—invest (surround) the CNS, the supportive framework for CNS neurons is provided by a subset of neuroglial cells. The term *neuroglia* is appropriate because it means "neural glue." Vastly outnumbering neurons, neuroglia occupy the spaces between neurons and thus comprise the "interstitial tissue" of the CNS. They do indeed provide structural support, separating individual neurons from one another and maintaining the form of neuronal cell groups. But we know now that they do much more, particularly in the way of providing neurons with metabolic support and controlling the environment of neurons. Additionally, they retain their mitotic competency, which makes them the primary source of intrinsic tumors of the CNS. Furthermore, evidence is evolving for signaling between neurons and glial cells.

Neuroglia are classified on the basis of their size as well as structural geometry (Figure 3-9 ■). Within the CNS, four types generally are identified: astrocytes (*astroglia*), oligodendrocytes (*oligodendroglia*), microglia, and ependyma. Sometimes astrocytes and oligodendrocytes are referred to as the **macroglia** because they are the largest of the neuroglial cells. No system of structural classification has proven entirely satisfactory. It seems that a given cell may exist in different forms because intermediate and transitional cells that defy unequivocal structural classification can be recognized in a section of brain tissue. Microglia sometimes are excluded from neuroglial membership owing to their apparent non-neural origin from cells that enter the developing CNS along with ingrowing blood vessels.

Neurons and neuroglia are separated by a narrow space filled with extracellular (interstitial) fluid. The width of this space has been variously estimated, depending on the technique used to measure it. Whatever the case, the volume of the extracellular compartment and the ionic composition of its fluid are of vital importance to the normal functioning of neurons. Even small fluctuations in extracellular volume can render neurons helpless; large fluctuations can be fatal. Neuroglia play an essential role in maintaining an appropriate extracellular ionic environment. Significantly, the size of the extracellular compartment may vary to some extent, depending on functional state, but, more importantly, it clearly varies, sometimes with disastrous consequences, following head trauma or other pathologic states.

Astrocytes

Astrocytes are the largest and most structurally elaborate of all glial cells. They are the most numerous as well. Astrocytes, as the name tells us, are star-shaped cells with numerous processes radiating in all directions from the soma. Some of the

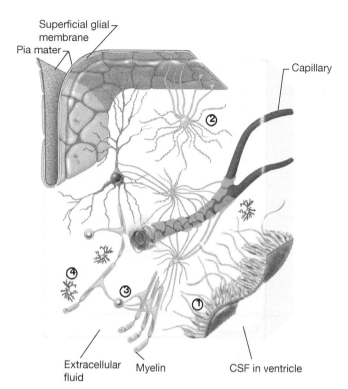

FIGURE 3-9 Neuroglia in the CNS. Note that different classes of neuroglial cells participate in forming the inner and outer boundaries of brain tissue. Ependymal cells (1) line the ventricular system in the case of the inner boundary, while the interlocking processes of astrocytes (2) form the superficial glial membrane that fuses with the pia mater in the case of the outer boundary. (3) An oligodendrocyte myelinating a portion of many axons in the CNS. (4) A microglial cell. A pyramidal neuron is shown in blue. Note that the cerebrospinal fluid (CSF) within a brain ventricle and the extracellular fluid bathing neurons and neuroglia are shown in the same color. This is to emphasize that CSF and extracellular fluid are in ionic equilibrium as the ependymal cells lining the brain ventricles do not impede that exchange of ions between the two fluids.

processes extend to a blood capillary, where their terminal expansions, known as *end feet* or *sucker feet*, end on the capillary surface (see Chapter 25). Other processes of the same cell may terminate on the nonsynaptic surface of nearby neurons, thereby interposing themselves between capillary and neuron. The processes of other astrocytes, specifically those positioned near the surface of the CNS, extend to the surface of the brain and spinal cord, where their end feet interlock to form an uninterrupted membranous outer wall of the CNS. This continuous wall is the *superficial glial membrane*, but because it fuses with the innermost meningeal layer, the pia mater, it is probably more common to refer to the covering as the pia–glial membrane (see Figure 3-9).

Two types of astrocytes are recognized that possess distinctive morphological features. The **fibrous astrocyte** is most numerous in white matter and is characterized by its thin poorly branched processes that radiate from the cell body in all directions. The **protoplasmic astrocyte** is most numerous in gray matter. Protoplasmic astrocytes have numerous, profusely branching processes and perivascular end feet. The processes are shorter than those of fibrous astrocytes. Both types contain typical cytoplasmic organelles: mitochondria, smooth and rough ER, and a nucleus.

A number of functions have been attributed to astrocytes in addition to that of providing the structural matrix for neurons. One of the major functions is to regulate and maintain the stability of the extracellular microenvironment, a role facilitated by their close contacts with neurons. Given the existence of gap junctions between astrocytes, they form a functional syncytium so that changes in the concentration of ions (such as potassium) and small solutes can be rapidly equilibrated by distributing them to other brain areas, where the concentration of the ion is lower. Astrocytes also control the extracellular concentrations of a number of neurotransmitters.

Several roles have been attributed to astrocytes in certain pathologic conditions. In one of the several mechanisms of brain edema, cells imbibe water and swell. While neurons, capillary endothelial cells, and glia are all involved, astrocytes are especially so. Astrocytes play a major role in the repair of CNS lesions characterized by necrosis. Astrocytes react to brain injury by undergoing hypertrophy and producing numerous intermediate filaments as well as by increasing in number (**fibrillary gliosis**). They may also alter their gene expression after traumatic brain injury. They play essential roles in preserving neural tissue (limiting degeneration) and restricting inflammation after moderate (but apparently not severe) brain injury. In severe injury—for example, a cerebral infarct, where neurons, blood vessels, and glial cells all die—astrocytic processes proliferate to form a meshwork wall around the lesion. Eventual phagocytosis of the dead cells leaves a cavity within the CNS. Finally, astrocytes also play an important role in the development of tumors; indeed most primary brain tumors derive from astrocytes.

Oligodendrocytes

Oligodendrocytes can be distinguished from astrocytes by several criteria. Among other things, their cell bodies are smaller and give rise to fewer, thin processes that radiate only a short distance from the soma. A number of functions have been attributed to oligodendrocytes, but many are unsubstantiated. The best-documented function of these glial cells is their role in the formation and maintenance of the myelin sheaths investing CNS axons (Figure 3-10 ■).

As would be expected from their function, oligodendrocytes are more abundant in white matter than in gray matter. A single oligodendrocyte may myelinate segments from as few as 7 up to as many as 70 CNS axons. Numerous tongue-like processes extend from the cell body to nearby axons, where each then spreads out as a flat, thin sheath of doubled cell membrane and spirals around the axon. In this spiraling process, the cytoplasm is squeezed out,

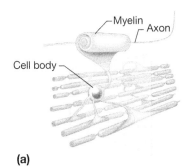

(a)

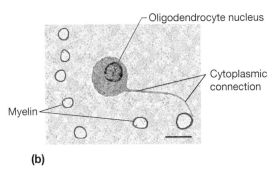

(b)

FIGURE 3-10 (a) A single oligodendrocyte is shown myelinating a portion of many axons in the CNS. Myelin is a spiral of oligodendrocyte plasma membrane surrounding an axon. During this ensheathing process, most of the cytoplasm of the oligodendrocyte is squeezed out, leaving a series of tightly wrapped, lipid-rich membranes. This compactness endows myelin with a high electrical resistance and low capacitance so that it functions as an insulator around the axon. (b) The electron micrograph shows that the cell body of the oligodendrocyte is connected to its myelin sheaths by thin processes. Calibration bar = 2μm.

leaving compacted layers of plasma membranes abutting one another. This is the myelin sheath. As in the peripheral nervous system, the sheath is discontinuous, being interrupted at the nodes of Ranvier.

Microglia

Microglial cells are estimated to comprise about 10 to 20 percent of all glial cells (see Figure 3-9). These cells resemble tissue specific macrophages and, indeed, have been thought to derive from monocytes (macrophage precursor cells) that infiltrate the nervous system during development. However, their origin is not altogether certain. Microglial cells are distributed throughout the CNS, but are most abundant in the gray matter. These small cells give off long, branched processes with sharp bends (antler-like). They are positioned between neurons in the gray matter and are parallel to axons in the white matter, but they do not contact one another. Microglia provide the nervous system with its first line of defense against damage or infection. Microglia within the brain parenchyma have resting and activated forms. Those in the resting state have been depicted as being "immunoalert," their highly branched processes presenting as much surface membrane as possible to monitor the extracellular fluid. Microglia respond within hours to a challenge of the integrity of the nervous system. They draw in their branches, divide, become ameboid, and migrate to the site of injury or surround involved neurons. Activation is local and graded and depends on the severity of the nervous system insult. Microglia are regarded as the scavenger cells of the CNS, but it is only when neuronal degeneration has occurred that they become cytotoxic phagocytes. Microglia are involved in a phenomenon called *synaptic stripping*, wherein they separate axonal terminals from postsynaptic sites on damaged neurons. By thus preventing synaptic influences on the postsynaptic neuron, the damaged neuron may be able to more readily shift to a repair mode.

Ependymal Cells

Ependymal cells line the central canal of the spinal cord and all parts of the ventricular system (see Figure 3-9). In general, adjacent ependymal cells are not joined together by tight junctions so that CSF and the brain's extracellular fluid are in free communication with one another (i.e., they are in ionic equilibrium). Highly modified ependymal cells occur at specific sites where they participate in formation of **choroid plexus** (see Chapter 25). These ependymal cells are called **choroid epithelial** cells, and they are joined together by tight junctions.

Schwann Cells and Satellite Cells

Within the *peripheral nervous system* (PNS), two types of neuroglial cells are recognized: **Schwann cells** (the most abundant) and **satellite cells**. Schwann cells in the PNS are the homologues of oligodendrocytes in the CNS. The Schwann cells form the myelin sheaths that invest axons of peripheral nerves (see Chapters 4 and 9). Satellite cells surround the cell bodies of neurons located in ganglia of the PNS. They are thought to play a role in the metabolism of ganglion cells.

Thought Question

A number of different glial cells were described. What disorders are associated with different neuroglia? Does each disorder affect cells in the PNS or CNS?

CLINICAL CONNECTIONS

Multiple sclerosis (MS) is an autoimmune disorder in which proteins expressed by oligodendrocytes are erroneously recognized by the immune system as foreign entities. The signs and symptoms of MS result in part from a loss of myelin in the brain and spinal cord. Over the years, different opinions have been expressed as to whether the loss of myelin is due to the lethal effect of the disease on oligodendrocytes or whether the loss of myelin is due to a direct attack on the myelin sheath itself. While the major target of the disease process is the myelin sheath, oligodendrocytes are vulnerable to the disease process, especially in the early phases of the demyelinazation.

Microglia and macrophages are thought to play a role in the infective process elicited by the human immunodeficiency virus (HIV) that causes the acquired immunodeficiency syndrome (AIDS). Both cells bear on their external surfaces a receptor to which the HIV binds. Unlike the situation with the helper T lymphocytes that the virus ultimately devastates, the HIV does not readily kill microglia or macrophages. Thus, these cells not only may hide the virus from the immune system, they may also be acting as a viral reservoir for the body and brain. Microglia also have been implicated in several processes in Alzheimer's disease.

Finally, glial cells maintain their mitotic capacity. The uncontrolled division of these cells results in neoplasms known as gliomas. Astrocytes are the most numerous of all the glial cells and are the most frequently occurring glioma. In children, astrocytomas appear most frequently in the cerebellum, and in adults they are more common in the lobes of the cerebrum. Even with surgical excision and radiation treatments, long-term prognosis is poor.

Summary

This chapter provides details about the two types of cells that constitute neural tissue. The structural parts of a typical neuron, broadly defined in Chapter 1, are examined further in terms of the organelles they posses and their functions. The concept that the different parts of a neuron comprise separate compartments with distinct constellations of organelles was developed to show that the different compartments depend on one another for their function, and, indeed, very survival. For example, the elaborate structure of the dendritic tree adapts to receive vast amounts of incoming information. The absence of protein-synthesizing (rough ER and free ribosomes) and protein-packaging (Golgi apparatus) machinery in the axon and its terminals means that proteins must be supplied to the axon by the cell body. This necessities the existence of a transport system from the cell body to the axon and its terminals, whereby proteins can be shipped from the cell body to other compartments of the neuron. The specific proteins that are inserted into the plasma membrane give rise to the unique properties of different compartments of the neuron to receive, process, store, conduct, and transfer information.

Like neurons, neuroglial cells come in a dazzling array of structural forms that adapt to support the activities of neurons in unique ways. Oligodendrocytes in the CNS and Schwann cells in the PNS myelinate axons, enabling them to conduct action potentials faster than in nonmyelinated axons. Astrocytes, the most numerous of the neuroglia, play of variety of roles in the normal CNS as well as in pathological states such as edema and brain repair. Microglia, the smallest of the neuroglia, are regarded as providing a first line of defense against brain injury or infection and are important to the repair of damaged brain tissue. Ependymal cells line the ventricles of the brain and are specialized in the choroid plexuses, where they secrete cerebrospinal fluid into the ventricular system.

Applications

1. Compare and contrast oligodendrocytes and Schwann cells. Include a discussion of their structure and function. Describe the consequences of demyelination. Provide an example of demyelination of the central nervous system and of the peripheral nervous system.

2. Why is it essential to brain function that neuroglia retain their mitotic competency? Does the ability of neuroglia to divide pose any potential problems to the nervous system?

3. The herpes simplex virus is the most common cause of acute encephalitis in the United States. How does this virus gain access to the peripheral nervous system, and what nerve is involved? How does the virus then seed the central nervous system?

References

Beal, M. F. Mitochondria take center stage in aging and neurodegeneration. *Ann Neurol* 58: 495–505, 2005.

Bodian, D. The generalized vertebrate neuron. *Science* 137: 323–326, 1962.

Bullock, T. H., Bennett, M. V. L., Johnston, D., et al. The neuron doctrine, redux. *Science* 310: 791–793, 2005.

Buss, A., Brook, G.A., Kakulas, B., et al. Gradual loss of myelin and formation of an astrocytic scar during Wallerian degeneration in the human spinal cord. *Brain* 127: 34–44, 2003.

Conde, J. R. and Streit, W. J. Microglia in the aging brain. *J Neuropathol Exp Neurol* 65: 199–203, 2006.

Eriksson, P. S., et al. Neurogenesis in the adult human hippocampus. *Nature Medicine.* 4: 1313–1317, 1998.

Goodman, C. C., Fuller, K. S., and Boissonnault, W. G. *Pathology: Implications for the Physical Therapist.* Saunders Elsevier, Philadelphia, 2003.

Jones, E. G., and Cowan, M. W. Ch. 8. The nervous tissue. In: *The Structural Basis of Neurobiology*, Jones, E. G. (ed.). Elsevier, New York, 1983.

Kempermann, G., Gage, F. H. New nerve cells for the adult brain. *Scientific American*, May 1999.

Lee, S. K., and Wolfe, S. W. Peripheral nerve injury and repair. *J Am Acad Orthop Surg* 8: 243–252, 2000.

Myer, D. J., Gurkoff, G. G., Lee, S. M., et al. Essential protective roles of reactive astrocytes in traumatic brain injury. *Brain* 129: 2761–2772, 2006.

Nolte, J. *The Human Brain: An Introduction to Its Functional Anatomy.* Mosby Elsevier, Philadelphia, 2009.

Pcters, A., Palay, S. L., and Webster, H. De F. *The Fine Structure of the Nervous System: Neurons and Their Supporting Cells*, 3rd ed., Oxford University Press, New York, 1991.

PEARSON myhealthprofessionskit™

Use this address to access the Companion Website created for this textbook. Simply select "Physical Therapy" from the choice of disciplines. Find this book and log in using your username and password to access self-assessment questions, a glossary, answers to the applications questions, and more.

Cellular Neurobiology

LEARNING OUTCOMES

This chapter prepares the reader to:

1 Recall the meaning of the following terms: receptor (generator) potential, equilibrium potential, action potential, modality gated ion channels, postsynaptic potentials, and gap junctions.

2 Discuss the forces that drive ions across a membrane.

3 Explain how the sensory system transduces energy into an electrical signal, including the receptor machinery of the system.

4 Describe hyperpolarization and depolarization of cells and relate these processes to the equilibrium potential of the cell.

5 Explain the factors that together determine the equilibrium potential of the cell, including the role of the sodium–potassium pump.

6 Describe the characteristic components and properties of the action potential, including the following: threshold, specific phases of the action potential, and refractory periods.

7 Contrast action and generator potentials.

8 Recall the cells that comprise the myelin sheath and explain the importance of this sheath in terms of conduction of the action potential.

9 Define postsynaptic potentials (PSPs) and differentiate excitatory from inhibitory PSPs.

10 Identify the three classes of neurotransmitters and provide examples of each.

11 Discuss the purpose of the G-protein with respect to opening and closing channels.

12 Identify five steps that occur during chemical synaptic transmission and describe the processes that occur at each step.

13 Define long-term potentiation and long-term depression and discuss these phenomena in terms of the means used to study them, the receptors of importance in generating these phenomena, and the resulting structural modifications that make them permanent.

14 Relate the occurrence of demyelination to nerve conduction velocity in the disorder of multiple sclerosis.

15 Describe the role of neurotransmitters as related to the etiology and treatment of biologic depression.

ACRONYMS

5-HT Serotonin
ACh Acetylcholine
AMPA α-amino-3-hydroxy-5-methyl-4-isoxazole propionate
AP Action potential
ATP Adenosine triphosphate
cAMP Cyclic AMP
CMT Charcot-Marie-Tooth disease
DA Dopamine
EPSP Excitatory postsynaptic potential
ER Endoplasmic reticulum
GABA Gamma-amino butyric acid
GDP Guanosine diphosphate
GP Generator potential
GTP Guanosine triphosphate
IPSP Inhibitory postsynaptic potential
LTD Long-term depression
LTP Long-term potentiation
MAO Monoamine oxidase
MS Multiple sclerosis
NE Norepinephrine
NMDA N-methyl-D-aspartate
PD Parkinson's disease
PKA Protein kinase A
PKU Phenylketoneuria
PSD Postsynaptic density
PSP Postsynaptic potential
SSRI Selective serotonin re-uptake inhibitor

Introduction

This chapter focuses on the processes that occur within and between neurons that enable them to communicate with the environment and with one another. The language of nervous system communication is one of electrical signals, and these signals contain information. The words of the language consist of two fundamentally different types of electrical signals: graded and nongraded. Despite this seeming limitation, the vocabulary is rich. This is because a graded electrical signal varies in size and shape over time according to the input the neuron receives. This enables a graded electrical change to encode the information contained in the input. Such input has virtually unlimited variability so that graded electrical signals are seemingly unlimited in terms of their temporal configuration. Graded potentials include the generator potential and postsynaptic potentials.

In contrast, the second, or nongraded, signal is designed to transmit this encoded information over distance. Thus, it is a propagated signal. It is like the activity in a fiber-optic cable or telephone line that transmits information over long or short distances from the sender to receiver but cannot itself add information to what the sender is forwarding. Nongraded potentials are action potentials. The grammar and syntax of this language derive from the rules that govern how systems of neurons are linked together at the synapses that form them. These rules vary from system to system. These, too, are almost infinitely variable. While many systems obey predictable rules, some, most notably those responsible for pain perception, do not. All electrical activity in neurons is generated by a flux of ions crossing through the plasma membrane.

The first section of this chapter discusses the membrane-spanning channels that permit ions to enter or leave the interior (cytosol) of the neuron. The next two sections analyze the specific types of electrical signals that occur in neurons beginning with the resting membrane potential.

We then discuss the communication links between neurons, that is, synapses. While synapses come in two different forms, electrical and chemical, the *vast majority* of synapses in the human nervous system are chemical. Thus, at synapses, the arrival of an electrical signal in the terminal of a presynaptic neuron initiates the release of a chemical neurotransmitter. Combined with the previous sections, this means that communication between neurons in the nervous system is by an electrochemical process. The neurotransmitter's action then sets up another electrical signal in the postsynaptic neuron. It may take time for this postsynaptic electrical signal to develop, depending on the type of postsynaptic process that creates the electrical signal. There are five distinct steps in the process by which a chemical comes to be able to mediate an exchange of information between a pre- and postsynaptic neuron. Most important is the fact that each of these steps can be influenced by an exogenous drug or toxin. Thus, not only can some steps be the target of a disease, but all can be manipulated medically in the treatment of disease.

That the brain possesses a remarkable capacity to be shaped by experience is apparent by observing an infant develop into a reasoning and communicative child or observing a person with traumatic brain injury recover under the guidance of a skilled therapist. That is, the brain is a very plastic organ, the topic of the final section of the chapter. Specific types of synaptic interactions between neurons seem a far cry from global human functions such as learning and memory. They are. Nonetheless, our reductionist Western science looks at such cellular interactions as perhaps forming a basis for learning and information storage. These intercellular phenomena are long-term potentiation and long-term depression. They reflect, respectively, either an increase or a decrease in the efficiency of synaptic transmission between pre- and postsynaptic neurons. Both are examples of neural plasticity at the cellular (synaptic) level.

ION CHANNELS AND ELECTRCIAL ACTIVITY IN NEURONS

In Chapter 3, we noted that the plasma membrane of a neuron contains channel proteins possessing membrane-spanning central pores that, when open, allow ions to move across the membrane. Such ion fluxes may occur in either direction: either into or out of the interior of the neuron. Neurons exist in two fundamentally different states: (1) processing synaptic and intrinsic membrane potentials that are making the neuron more or less likely to generate an action potential or (2) generating an action potential. The former mode involves steady-state electrical activity, whereas the latter mode is characterized by electrical activity that varies over time. Thus, in the act of processing information, neurons generate time-varying electrical signals that represent coded information. Interestingly, both states depend on the flux of ions across the membrane and, therefore, depend on open channel proteins.

The channel proteins residing in the neuron's plasma membrane are composed of different polypeptides organized into a variable number of subunits. In general, channel proteins have four to six subunits, and all such proteins have a membrane-spanning domain that can form a pore across the membrane (Figure 4-1 ■). Some channel proteins have pores that are always open, whereas others open

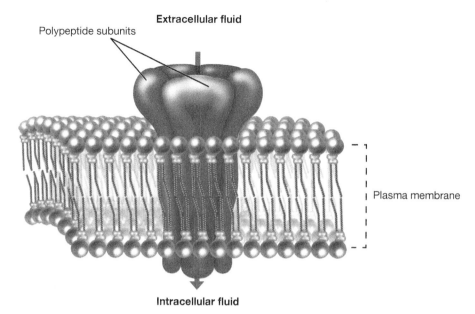

FIGURE 4-1 A membrane ion channel is an integral membrane protein that spans the neuronal plasma membrane. It consists of four to six polypeptide subunits that can form a pore across the membrane. The pore of one type of channel called leak channels is always open, whereas in other channels, the pore is gated and open only under specific conditions.

only in response to certain circumstances. The former are referred to as **nongated channels**, or **leak channels**, whereas the latter are referred to as **gated channels**.

Nongated channels (i.e., leak channels) are always open no matter the state of the neuron. These leak channels generate electrical signals by virtue of allowing ions to cross the membrane. They play a critical role in establishing the "resting" membrane potential, which is an energy-requiring steady state, not an energy-free resting condition. Leak channels also are critical components of the passive membrane properties that are part of information processing by neurons.

Gated channels open or close in response to their appropriate stimulus, be it ligand binding, membrane voltage, etc. For example, voltage-gated channels respond to changes in the transmembrane potential and are influenced by the intracellular and extracellular environments. Gated channels generate the electrical signals of neurons, whereas nongated channels participate in the generation of the neurons' steady-state, resting condition.

What is essential to understand is that conditions established during the resting state of neurons enable them to generate electrical signals and process information. All of the electrical signals generated by neurons take advantage of the fact that in the resting state, ion concentration differences are established across the neuronal cell membrane. Such ion concentration differences represent stored energy, and the electrical signals of neurons are generated by releasing this stored energy. The mechanism by which the neuron releases this stored energy is to change the ionic permeability pattern of the membrane *away* from that characterizing the resting state by opening or closing ion channels in the membrane. The nature of the altered permeability pattern allows given ion species to move down their electrochemical gradients across the

membrane (transmembrane current). This alters the membrane potential and thereby generates an electrical signal within the neuron.

> **Thought Question**
>
> Two types of channels allow for molecules to traverse the membrane of neurons: leak and gated channels. Compare and contrast the two.

THE RESTING MEMBRANE POTENTIAL

Factors That Determine Flow of Current across the Membrane

What forces act to drive ions through open channels in the membrane of a neuron? There are two: diffusion and electrical. Ions dissolved in water are in constant random motion such that, over time, they tend to distribute themselves evenly throughout the water. In achieving this even distribution, ions move, in a process called **diffusion**, from regions where they are in high concentration to regions where they are in low concentration (Figure 4-2 ■). The difference in concentration between these two regions is called a **concentration gradient** so that ions diffuse *down* their concentration gradient. In order for diffusion to propel a specific ion across a neuron's membrane down its concentration gradient, the membrane must contain channels permeable to that ion because the lipid bilayer itself is impermeable to ions.

Because ions are electrically charged particles, the second force acting to produce a net movement of ions dissolved in a solution is electrical. Given that opposite charges attract and like charges repel, when wires from

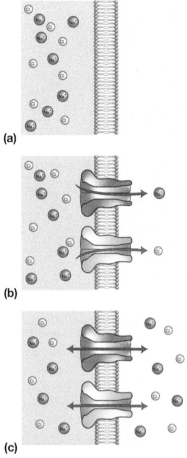

FIGURE 4-2 Diffusion drives ions through open membrane channels. (a) It contains two water-filled compartments separated by an impermeable membrane. NaCl has been dissolved in the left compartment, where the number of Na^+ and Cl^- ions indicates the relative concentrations of the ion. (b) Open channels are inserted into the membrane that allow the passage of Na^+ and Cl^-. There is a net movement of Na^+ and Cl^- from the region of high concentration to the region of low concentration because of the concentration gradient. (c) Net movement of Na^+ and Cl^- stops when the ions are equally distributed on both sides of the permeable membrane and the concentration gradient has disappeared.

the two terminals of a battery are placed in a solution of dissolved sodium chloride (NaCl), there will be a net movement of Na^+ toward the negative terminal and a net movement of Cl^- to the positive terminal. The rate at which electrical charge moves is called **electrical current**.

Two factors determine the magnitude of current flow. The force driving ion movement depends, first, on the size of the charge difference between the anode and cathode of the battery, called the **electrical potential** or voltage of the battery. The larger the difference in electrical potential, the greater the current flow. The second factor that determines the magnitude of current flow is the ease with which charged ions move from one place to another. This is called **conductance**. In the case of the neuronal cell membrane, only the channels in the lipid bilayer have any conductance because it is only via channels that ions can cross the membrane. Conductance

and permeability are generally used interchangeably in that a membrane permeable to a given ion easily conducts current carried by that particular ion. In other words, ion channels function as electrical resistors. Resistance is the inverse of conductance in that an ion channel with high conductance has little resistance to current flow and vice versa.

> **Thought Question**
>
> How do ions move across a membrane when they have to move against the concentration gradient?

Membrane Potential

The membrane potential of a neuron at rest can be measured by inserting a microelectrode into the interior of the cell (Figure 4-3 ■). The microelectrode is connected to a voltmeter that measures the electrical potential difference between the tip of the microelectrode and a ground wire outside the cell. The inside of the neuron is electrically negative with respect to the outside, which by convention is considered to be at 0 mV [1 mV = 0.001 volt (V)]. The value of the resting membrane potential is about –65 mV, meaning that the inside of the neuron has a negative voltage compared to the surrounding extracellular environment. Because of this potential difference, the resting neuron is said to be *polarized*. If the interior of the neuron becomes less negative, the neuron is said to be **depolarized**. If the interior becomes more negative than its resting membrane potential, the cell is said to be **hyperpolarized**. In order to understand the genesis of the resting membrane potential, we need to understand which ion species are available to produce it and how they are distributed on the inside and outside of the neuron.

The ion concentration differences existing across the resting neuronal cell membrane are due to two types of integral proteins in the plasma membrane. The first type consists of nongated, passive, and always open ion channels (leak channels). Leak channels are selectively permeable to specific ions, allowing them to move down their concentration gradients. The second type of protein is an energy-expending ion pump that actively moves ions in or out of the neuron against their concentration gradients. The ion channels and pump work against one another but, in so doing, generate a steady transmembrane neuronal electricity in the resting state.

The major ion species involved in the resting state are sodium (Na^+), potassium (K^+), chloride (Cl^-), and organic anions (An^-). The resting neuron has a high concentration of K^+ and organic anion and a little Na^+ on the inside and a high concentration of Na^+ and Cl^- with a little K^+ on the outside.

Consider, first, the behavior of a hypothetical cell that is permeable only to K^+ but not to any of the other ions. Under this condition, the difference in K^+ concentration on either side of the membrane establishes a chemical gradient driving K^+ out of the cell interior. But the cell does not continue to lose K^+ until the concentration gradient disappears and the K^+ concentration is equal on both sides of the

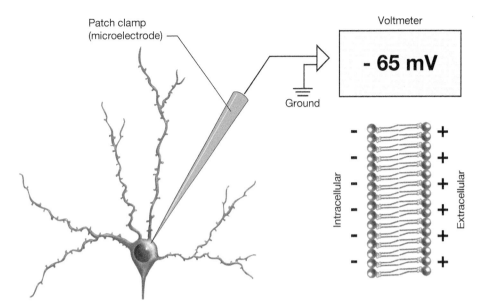

FIGURE 4-3 Measuring the resting membrane potential. The electrical potential existing across the membrane of a resting neuron is determined by measuring the difference in electrical potential between the tip of a microelectrode inside the neuron and a ground wire in the extracellular fluid. The difference, measured by a voltmeter, is about –65 mV with the interior being negative. It is due to the unequal distribution of electrical charges on the two sides of the membrane.

membrane. This is because as soon as a few K^+ ions have diffused outward, organic anions will remain inside the cell, whose negative charge will not be neutralized by nearby positive charges. While the organic anions will migrate toward the membrane along with the K^+, they cannot pass through it. As they accumulate on the inner surface of the membrane, they will tend to pull the positive ions back in. But because the membrane is permeable only to K^+, the only cation to be pulled back in is K^+. The system then quickly comes into an equilibrium in which the chemical gradient driving K^+ to diffuse outward is balanced by the electrical gradient pulling K^+ back into the cell. The potential difference required to balance a given concentration gradient is called the **equilibrium potential** (Figure 4-4 ■). In the case of K^+, the equilibrium potential is about –90mV.

This balancing process can be thought of as analogous to a weight hanging from a spring. The weight produces tension in the spring, while the tension in the spring keeps the weight from dropping further. The weight represents the concentration gradient for the ion (in this case, K^+) and the spring the electrical gradient. It should be clear that the larger the concentration gradient, the larger will be the electrical gradient required to keep the ion in equilibrium (i.e., a larger weight produces more tension in the spring).

Next let us consider the same hypothetical cell with the same ionic concentration gradients as just described but with a different permeability pattern. Suppose now the cell is permeable only to Na^+ ions. Because Na^+ is more concentrated on the outside than inside, it will diffuse inward. But because the membrane is impermeable to Cl^- the movement of Na^+ ions creates a potential difference across the membrane (Figure 4-5 ■). Sodium ion

movement to the cell interior leaves an excess of negative charge on the outside that pulls Na^+ back out. Thus, the factors limiting the inward movement of Na^+ are the same as those limiting the outward flow of K^+. The equilibrium potential for Na^+ is about +55 mV.

The equilibrium potential is simply the concentration gradient expressed in units of electricity. We have seen that the transmembrane potential of a cell with the ionic concentrations given earlier (for a squid axon) can vary from –90 mV to +55 mV, depending on whether the cell is permeable to K^+ or Na^+. The actual quantitative relation between potential and concentration gradient was worked out by physical chemists in the 19th century and is called the **Nernst equation**.

Thought Question

A membrane's potential can be negative (e.g., –75 mV) or positive (e.g., +55 mV). What does this mean in terms of the charge on the inside and outside of the cell? What produces this gradient? And how do leak and gated channels relate to this phenomenon?

In order to generate these electrical potentials, only small numbers of ions actually move across the membrane—and those that do move are lined up immediately adjacent to the membrane. The number of ions that must move across the membrane to establish large charge differences between the two sides of the membrane are exceedingly small relative to the number of each ion species on either side of the membrane. Therefore, the fluxes cause

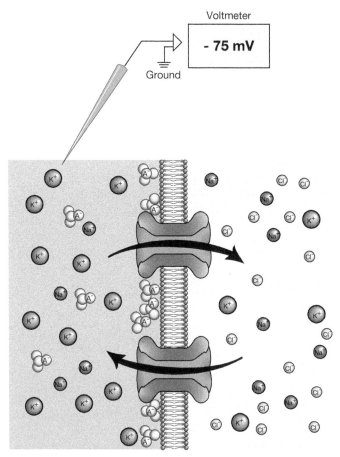

FIGURE 4-4 Establishment of the K⁺ equilibrium potential. (a) K⁺ and A⁻ are in high concentration inside this hypothetical cell whose membrane is permeable only to K⁺ and no other ions. There is a net movement of K⁺ ions down their concentration gradient from the inside to the outside of the cell. This results in a net accumulation of positive charge on the outside of the cell and negative charge on the inside. (b) This charge difference retards the movement of K⁺ until it reaches a magnitude where there is no net movement of K⁺ to the outside. The efflux of K⁺ sets up an electrical gradient (negative inside, positive outside) that creates an electromotive force that hinders K⁺ leaving the cell, and that equilibrium occurs when this electromotive force is equal and opposite to the chemical diffusion force. This is the equilibrium potential for K⁺ and establishes a specific charge difference between the two sides of the membrane — in this case, of –75 mV. Note that "A⁻" is not an ion, but rather a symbol representation of impermeable charged entities, such as proteins, and chemical compounds, such as phosphate groups.

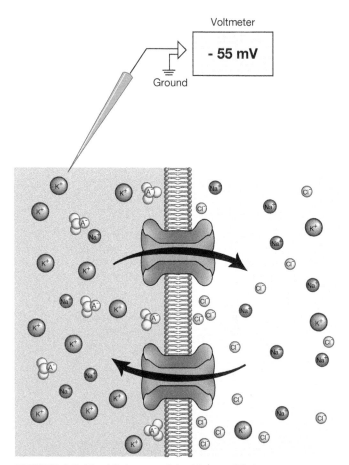

FIGURE 4-5 Establishment of the Na⁺ equilibrium potential. (a) In this case, Na⁺ has high concentrations outside this hypothetical cell whose membrane is permeable only to Na⁺ and no other ions. There is a net movement of Na⁺ ions down their concentration gradient from the outside to the inside of the cell. This results in a net accumulation of positive charge on the inside of the cell and negative charge on the outside. (b) This charge difference retards the movement of Na⁺ until it reaches a magnitude where there is no net movement of Na⁺ to the inside. This is the equilibrium potential for Na⁺ and establishes a specific membrane potential at which Na+ ions are in equilibrium across the membrane (i.e., not net movement of Na+ across membrane), which in this case occurs at a membrane potential of +55 mV.

very minor changes in ionic concentrations inside and outside the cell. The opposite charges inside and outside the cell line up immediately adjacent to the membrane because the phospholipid membrane is so thin it does not represent a barrier to the electrostatic attraction of the opposite charges. Most of the cell's cytoplasm and most of the extracellular fluid is electrically neutral.

If the resting membrane potential is not at the equilibrium potential for either Na⁺ or K⁺, this must mean that both of these ions are moving across the resting neuronal cell membrane. And they are, through the always-open

passive leak channels. But there are many more leak channels for K⁺ than there are for Na⁺. In fact, the permeability to K⁺ is about 25 times greater than that to Na⁺ at rest. This means that the resting membrane potential should be closer to the K⁺ equilibrium potential than to the Na⁺ equilibrium potential — which it is. Thus, while there is only a small net force (the concentration gradient) acting to drive K⁺ out of the cell, there are many open K⁺ channels. In contrast, there is a large net force acting to drive Na⁺ into the cell, consisting of both a concentration gradient and an electrical force. But there are relatively few Na⁺ leak channels.

It seems that with the presence of these always-open leak channels, there could be a net movement of both ion species. However, there is no net loss of K⁺ from the inside of the resting neuron or net gain of Na^+ such that the resting concentration gradients are maintained in a steady state despite the lack of ionic equilibrium. This is accomplished by the **sodium–potassium pump**, a large integral protein that spans the membrane (Figure 4-6 ■). Because it is moving ions against their concentration gradients, energy is required to drive this pump. The energy comes from the hydrolysis of **adenosine triphosphate (ATP)**. The pump has binding sites for Na^+ and ATP on its intracellular surface, while the binding sites for K^+ are on its extracellular surface. This continuously operating membrane pump transports 3 Na^+ ions out of the cell for every 2 K^+ ions transported back into the cell, resulting in a net positive flow and hyperpolarization of the membrane. Its operation exactly counterbalances the continuous passive influx of Na^+ and efflux of K^+ through the always-open leak channels.

The permeability pattern of the resting neuron, although generating the resting membrane potential of –65 mV via leak channels and the Na^+–K^+ pump, prevents the neuron from exploiting the large ion concentration differences existing between the interior of the cell and extracellular fluid. In other words, a large reservoir of stored energy is not utilized. Communication between neurons depends on releasing this stored energy. This is accomplished by changing the permeability pattern of the neuron *away* from that characterizing the resting state, as noted earlier. The fundamental mechanism for accomplishing this change is by opening gated ion channels. Each of the electrical signals discussed in the sections that follow is created by opening and closing of specific and unique types of gated ion channels.

> **Thought Question**
>
> What is the sodium–potassium pump, and why does it require ATP, which is an energy source?

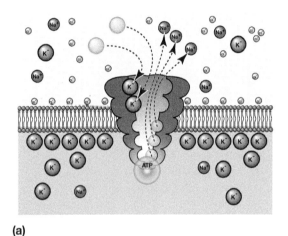

(a)

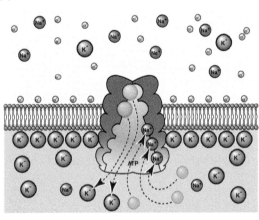

(b)

FIGURE 4-6 The sodium–potassium pump. This integral membrane-spanning protein is a pump that moves ions against their concentration gradients and, therefore, requires energy to function. The always-open leak channels in the resting membrane allow some Na^+ to leak into the cell interior and some K^+ to leak into the extracellular fluid. The bidirectional sodium–potassium pump transports three Na^+ ions out of the cell for every two K^+ transported back into the cell and maintains the resting membrane potential at about –65 mV by maintaining the unequal distribution of these ions across the membrane.

ELECTRICAL SIGNALS OF NEURONS

Clinical Preview ·················

Marney Morrison is a 45-year-old woman who was diagnosed with multiple sclerosis (MS) eight years ago. You began treating her in an outpatient rehabilitation clinic shortly after she was diagnosed with the disorder. At this point in time, she has begun to experience difficulties with gait and balance and has considerable somatosensory loss, especially of the lower extremities. All of her symptoms are exacerbated when she visits her daughter in July or August. Her daughter lives in Arizona, where the temperature frequently is over 100°F during these months. As you read through information presented in this section, consider the following:

- Why do Marney's symptoms worsen when she visits her daughter?

- Why does she now have somatosensory loss of the lower extremities?

- What is the underlying cause of deficits in neurotransmission associated with MS?

Receptor (Generator) Potential

The first task faced by all sensory systems is to transduce some form of environmental energy into an electrical change that encodes the relevant information about the environmental stimulus. This task is accomplished by sensory receptors that represent the specialized terminals of peripheral nerve fibers (see Chapter 9). This electrical change is the receptor, or generator, potential and is produced by **modality-gated ion channels** that shift the membrane potential away from its resting level. Modality-gated ion channels contain, in addition to a membrane-spanning domain, an extracellular domain that responds to an appropriate environmental stimulus—mechanical, thermal, chemical, or electromagnetic (light). Sensory receptors contain a specialized portion of membrane that contains the molecular machinery for the transduction. It is noteworthy that different sensory modalities fulfill the transduction process with distinct molecular mechanisms.

Mechanoreceptors that sense stretch of the muscle or pressure on the skin respond to the impact of the stimulus with a deformation of the receptive membrane. In these cases, ion channels in the membrane are linked to the cytoskeleton of the membrane and thus open when the membrane is deformed by a mechanical stimulus (Figure 4-7 ■). An influx of Na^+ and Ca^{2+}

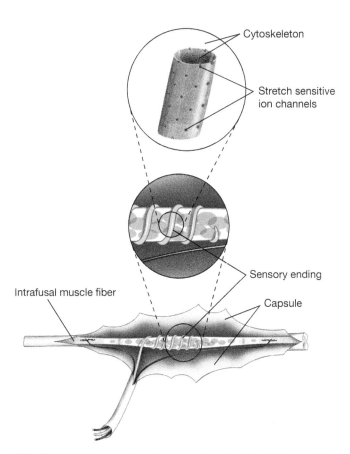

FIGURE 4-7 The receptor (generator) potential of the muscle spindle is generated by the opening of ion channels that are mechanically linked to the cytoskeleton of the membrane. Thus, when the receptor's membrane is stretched, the ion channels open and allow an influx of Na^+ and possibly other cations, which results in depolarization of receptor.

depolarizes the nerve ending, producing the receptor potential. A stronger stimulus causes the amplitude of the receptor potential to increase by opening more ion channels. When the stimulus ends, the receptive membrane is no longer deformed and the ion channels close. **Chemoreceptors** bind ambient chemicals, and this opens ion channels. However, olfactory and taste receptors employ a unique molecular mechanism, called a second-messenger system, to open the channels. **Photoreceptors** in the retina also employ a second-messenger system to create the receptor potential.

The generator potential (GP) has a number of properties. First, it is nonpropagated; that is, the GP remains in the immediate vicinity of the receptor terminal and does not self-propagate (travel) down the axon of the primary afferent neuron. Second, it *decays* (declines in amplitude) as a function of distance from the nerve terminal; that is, it spreads only passively along the membrane. This is shown in Figure 4-8 ■ , where the generator potential can still be recorded from the initial segment of the axon but cannot be recorded further down the axon. Third, the GP is a graded electrical change; that is, its amplitude varies in response to the parameters of the stimulus such as intensity. Fourth, successive or simultaneously occurring generator potentials in a given receptor can *summate* (see Postsynaptic Potentials, later). In order for successive GPs to summate, following GPs must occur before the preceding GP has decayed. Summating (adding together) results in a single GP larger in amplitude than the individual contributory potentials.

The GP fulfills two broad functions. First, it *encodes* information about the parameters of the adequate stimulus. Information that has not been encoded by the GP cannot be "added" at a later stage in the transduction process. Second, once threshold has been reached, the GP sets up a pattern of action potentials (discussed later) in the nerve fiber that contains the same information as encoded in the GP. The number and spacing of the action potentials depends on the absolute magnitude and the variation in amplitude with time of the GP.

As shown in Figure 4-9 ■ , the components of a generic, depolarizing GP that contain information about the stimulus are (1) the absolute magnitude of the depolarization, (2) the rate at which the depolarization occurs, (3) the rate of adaptation, (4) the magnitude of adaptation, and (5) the duration of the preceding threshold depolarization.

Action Potential

The action potential is the second category of electrical signal used by neurons. The action potential, commonly referred to as a *spike*, is the nerve impulse. It is designed to conduct information over distance—that is, down an axon from the receiving to the transmitting end of a neuron. The different types of ion channels that open and close to generate an action potential in the membrane of an axon do so in a specific and fixed temporal sequence. The permeability pattern characterizing the resting state is changed in such a way that allow first Na^+ and then K^+ to move down their concentration gradients.

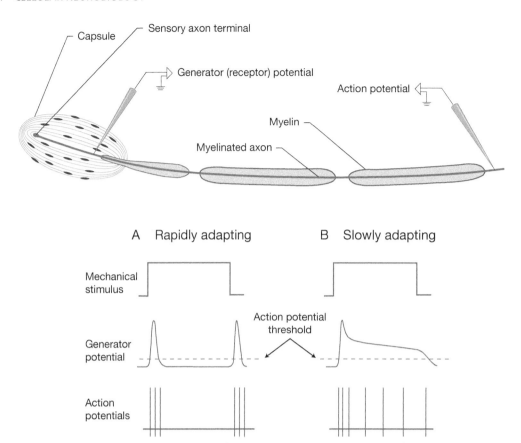

FIGURE 4-8 Properties of the receptor potential. The receptor potential is a graded response in that the number of channels that open is proportional to the magnitude of the stimulus. The receptor potential is nonpropagated. It does travel down the axon, but only passively; therefore, it decays in a short distance. It cannot be recorded beyond the trigger zone (initial segment) of the primary afferent axon unless threshold is reached in the vicinity of the receptor potential. Thus, further down the axon, only action potentials can be recorded. At the cell's trigger zone at the first node of Ranvier, recording reveals a sum of the receptor potential and the action potentials it generates.

Thought Question

Action potentials differ from generator potentials in fundamental ways. Contrast the properties of these two types of potentials.

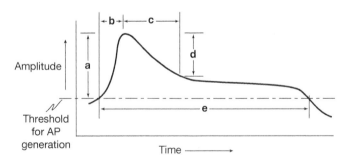

FIGURE 4-9 A representation of the information-bearing components of a depolarizing receptor potential that leads to an action potential. Information is encoded to the CNS about the stimulus parameters only so long as the depolarization exceeds the threshold required to generate action potentials in the neuron, thereby resulting in action potentials being propagated into the CNS. (a) The absolute magnitude of depolarization; (b) the rate of depolarization; (c) the rate of adaptation; (d) the magnitude of adaptation; (e) the duration of the above threshold depolarization.

This is accomplished by depolarizing the membrane of the initial segment of the axon. Distributed in the membrane of the initial segment of the axon (and throughout its remaining length) are voltage-gated ion channels. Voltage-gated channels have specialized domains that detect the electrical potential across the neuronal cell membrane. This enables the ion channel to open or close in response the level of the membrane potential (voltage). Voltage-gated channels specifically permeable to sodium (Na^+), potassium (K^+), calcium (Ca^{2+}), and chloride (Cl^-) have been identified, and subtypes of channels exist for each ion.

The necessary *depolarizing* trigger to open voltage-gated Na^+ channels can be one of several events: a receptor potential generated by specialized sensory nerve terminals, a synaptic input to the neuron causing an excitatory postsynaptic potential, or a local current that mediates the spread of the action potential down the axon. The latter two events are described in detail later. For now, it is necessary to appreciate that a preceding electrical event triggers the one that follows in a specific sequence.

In order to open sufficiently large numbers of voltage-gated Na^+ channels and initiate an action potential, a specific level of depolarization must occur at the initial segment. This critical level is called **threshold**. Action potentials never occur without a depolarizing stimulus that

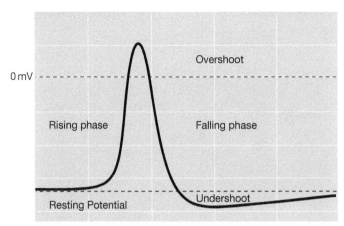

FIGURE 4-10 An action potential has a characteristic waveform and phases. During the rising phase, the axon membrane is rapidly depolarizing, and the membrane potential actually reverses polarity (becomes positive). After reaching a peak, the action potential enters a falling phase during which the magnitude of depolarization decreases and the membrane is repolarizing. There is a period of time in both the rising and falling phases during which the interior of the neuron is positive; this is called overshoot. After again reaching the resting-membrane potential, the action potential becomes hyperpolarizing for a short time before returning the resting potential; this is called undershoot.

brings the membrane to threshold. As the depolarization begins, voltage-gated Na^+ channels start to open, and a small inward Na^+ current develops. As long as the depolarization is small, this influx of Na^+ is countered by the normally greater efflux of K^+ that characterizes the resting membrane. But at some level of depolarization, enough Na^+ channels have opened such that the inward Na^+ current exceeds the driving force for the compensating outward K^+ current and the membrane has reached threshold.

The action potential has a characteristic waveform with several different phases (Figure 4-10 ■). During the *rising phase*, the axon membrane is rapidly depolarizing. The membrane potential actually reverses, with the inside of the cell positive and the outside negative, and this is called the *overshoot phase*. During the *falling phase*, the membrane is rapidly repolarizing, causing the membrane potential to become negative. During the *undershoot phase*, the membrane actually hyperpolarizes.

Once threshold is reached, massive numbers of Na^+ channels pop open. Once set into motion, an explosive sequence of events occurs that is entirely independent of the stimulus source. A number of functional properties characterize the voltage-gated Na^+ channel, and these help define the properties of the action potential (Figure 4-11 ■). They open with little delay, which accounts for the rapid rising phase of the action potential. They remain open only for about 1 msec then spontaneously close (inactivate), which helps explain why the action potential is so brief. The channels cannot open again until the membrane repolarizes toward the negative value of the resting potential (see discussion of absolute refractory period, later). Within less than 1,000th of a second, the explosive movement of sodium ions has caused the membrane to

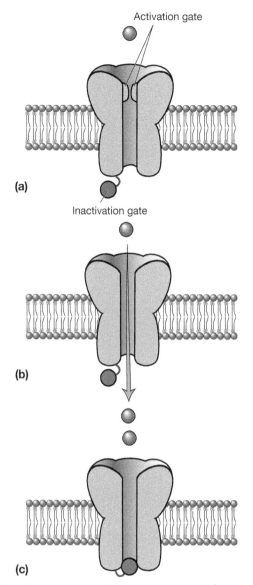

FIGURE 4-11 Properties of the voltage-gated Na^+ channels that determine the form of an action potential. The channel has two gates that respond in opposite ways to depolarization. (a) In the resting state, the activation gate is closed and the inactivation gate is open. (b) With depolarization, the activation gate opens, allowing Na^+ to enter the axon through the channel. (c) After about 1 msec, the inactivation gate closes and the channel is inactivated, or closed. With the resulting repolarization of the membrane, the activation gate closes, after which the inactivation gate opens and the channel returns to its resting state (a) in that the channel can now open in response to membrane depolarization.

rapidly depolarize and the inside of the cell to become positive and the outside negative. The membrane potential has completely reversed (Figure 4-12 ■).

Once threshold is reached, the voltage-gated K^+ channels do not open immediately: there is about a 1-msec delay before they open (see Figure 4-12). They pop open just as the Na^+ channels inactivate. Furthermore, the K^+ channels do not inactivate but remain open for a few milliseconds. K^+ ions rush out of the cell through the open channels

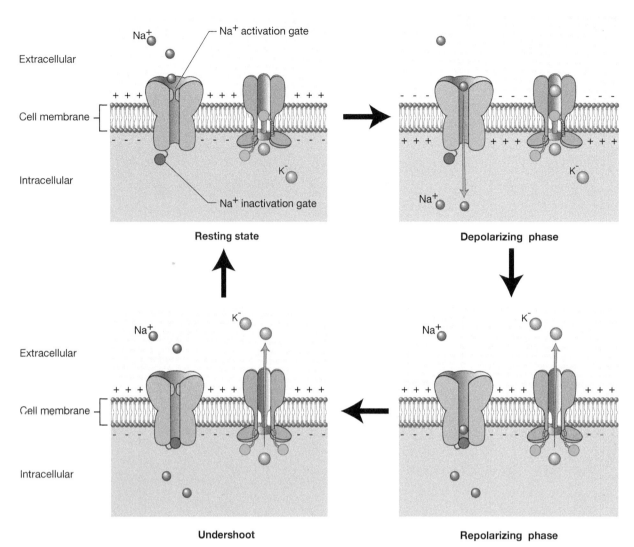

FIGURE 4-12 Phases of an action potential and the function of voltage-gated ion channels in those phases. An action potential can be divided into three phases during which the membrane's permeability to Na$^+$ and K$^+$ is changing. During the rising phase of the action potential, Na$^+$ channels are open and K$^+$ channels closed. At the peak of the action potential, Na$^+$ channels close and K$^+$ channels open. Throughout the falling phase of the action potential, K$^+$ channels remain open. During the undershoot phase, K$^+$ channels are still open because their gate opens and closes relatively slowly (compared to the Na$^+$ channel activation gate) and have not had sufficient time to close in response to repolarization of the membrane. Thus, the membrane becomes hyperpolarized beyond the resting-membrane potential due to the sustained increase in K$^+$ permeability. Within several milliseconds, the K$^+$ channel gate closes, and resting membrane potential is restored.

repolarizing the membrane, causing it to become negative again. In fact, there is a brief **after-hyperpolarization** during which the membrane potential moves even closer to the potassium equilibrium potential. The repolarization occurs rapidly because the membrane potential has reversed so that potassium ions not only move down their concentration gradient, but are also attracted to the exterior by the negative charge on the outside of the membrane.

The repolarization process has important consequences for the generation of another action potential. First, for a brief time after the peak of the action potential, so many Na$^+$ channels are in the inactivated state that another action potential cannot be generated no matter how much the membrane is depolarized. The channels cannot be opened again until the membrane potential goes sufficiently negative to

return the *channels* to their resting state. This is the **absolute refractory period**. This grades into a **relative refractory period** during which the membrane potential stays hyperpolarized until the voltage-gated K$^+$ channels close. During this period, it requires a greater depolarization to bring the membrane potential to firing threshold and initiate another action potential. The refractory period has several consequences. One is that it limits the number of action potentials that a given neuron can generate per unit time (see Chapter 9).

The concentration of ion species existing on the two sides of the resting membrane does not change in a substantive way for a given neuron. Moreover, the ion channels open in a fixed sequence and remain open for only fixed periods of time. Because of these factors, the size, shape, and duration of the action potential are fixed

Thought Question

An important feature of the nervous system is that transmitter-gated ion channels can result in either *hyperpolarization* or *depolarization* of the postsynaptic membrane. Describe what this means with respect to action potentials, and explain how these opposite responses could occur in the same neuron.

or invariant for a given neuron. Furthermore, an action potential either occurs or it does not occur. One initiated, the entire sequence of events unfolds. The action potential is, therefore, referred to as an **all-or-none electrical event**.

Propagation of the Action Potential

Action potentials must carry information from the receiving to the transmitting end of the neuron. In some neurons this means that information in the form of action potentials must be conducted over a distance of a meter or more. In order to faithfully conduct information down an axon, action potentials must not decay electrically as they move

along the axon from the site where they were generated to the transmitting end of the neuron. The property of the axon that enables it to fulfill this demand is that the mechanism for the production of an action potential is distributed over the *entire* length of the axon. Each patch of axon membrane contains all of the necessary machinery to generate an action potential of fixed size, shape, and duration. Given this, in order for action potentials to travel down the length of an axon, it is only necessary to get the trigger for an action potential to spread down the membrane. At each succeeding point on the membrane, the trigger would then evoke an action potential with fixed characteristics.

The trigger is an electrical current created at the leading edge of the action potential by the action potential itself (Figure 4-13 ■). Some of the local current generated by the action potential flows passively down the axon. This current depolarizes the downstream patch of axonal membrane. So the membrane immediately ahead of the action potential then generates its own new action potential as the preceding action potential in back of it disappears through repolarization. This sequence is then repeated down the

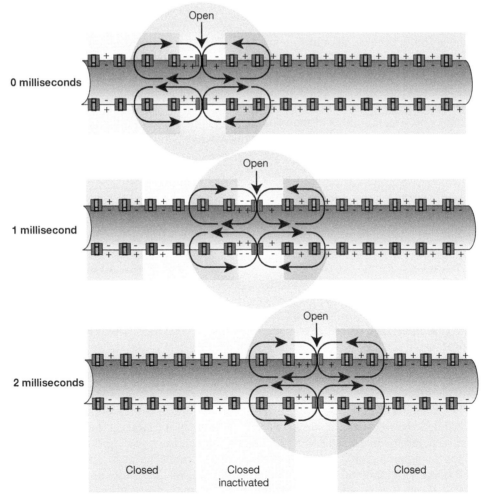

FIGURE 4-13 Conduction of the action potential. The entry of positive charge during the action potential causes electric currents (in the form of Na$^+$ ions) to flow across the membrane and longitudinally inside and outside the axon as a result of the differences in potential. These Na$^+$ currents depolarize the membrane at the site of the open Na$^+$ channels, ahead of the impulse. This leads to opening of voltage-gated Na$^+$ channels and the resulting transient change in Na$^+$ permeability that drives this patch of membrane to the action potential threshold.

length of the axon: one patch of membrane stimulating the next. The action potential, therefore, is referred to as a **self-propagating electrical event**. The refractoriness of the membrane in the wake of an action potential accounts for the fact that action potentials do not propagate back along the axon toward their point of initiation.

Years ago, the conduction of the action potential along the axon was depicted as occurring in a wave-like fashion, analogous to the ripple or wave seen to travel along a length of rope when one end of the rope is quickly flipped up and down. But this is hardly an accurate comparison. The reason is that action potential propagation is not a single wave traveling down the axon, but an entirely new bioelectrical event that is generated sequentially at each point along the length of the axon's membrane. That is why the amplitude of an action potential does not decrement as it travels down the membrane.

Myelin and Conduction in Myelinated Axons

The speed of conduction of an action potential is important behaviorally because faster conduction permits quicker reaction times. One mechanism by which speed can be increased is by increasing the diameter of the axon. This would lower its resistance to current flow. However, this mechanism has obvious limits because axonal size must be balanced by the requirement of having large numbers of axons in a small space. For example, the precise control of the small muscles of the fingers and the exquisite sensitivity of their sensory surfaces to touch depend on the innervation of the fingers by large numbers of motor and sensory nerve fibers. Thus, rapid, precise responses that are delicately tuned to prevailing environmental conditions depend on fast conduction in large numbers of axons.

The combination of fast conduction and small axon size is achieved by surrounding the axon membrane with a highly effective insulating cover, the myelin sheath. This sheath is formed by different types of neuroglial cells in the PNS and CNS: by Schwann cells in the PNS and by oligodendrocytes in the CNS. Each Schwann cell participates in myelinating a portion of only one axon, but each oligodendrocyte participates in myelinating portions of many axons. A single axon is myelinated by many neuroglial cells, many hundreds in the case of certain axons of the PNS. A small gap, the node of Ranvier, separates each myelinating cell so that there are regularly spaced gaps in the insulating myelin sheath. At each node, the axonal membrane is in direct communication with the extracellular fluid.

Voltage-gated Na^+ channels are concentrated at the nodes of Ranvier, which are the only sites along the axon where action potential–generating ion exchanges can occur (Figure 4-14a ■). Action potentials therefore skip from node to node in myelinated fibers. This mode of action potential (AP) propagation is called **saltatory conduction** (from the Latin word *saltare* meaning "to leap"). A myelinated nerve fiber conducts impulses faster than an unmyelinated fiber of the same diameter (except for very small diameter axons, which is the functional reason why the smallest diameter

axons are unmyelinated). The main reason for this marked increase in conduction speed is that the process of action potential generation consumes time: in a myelinated axon, AP generation occurs only at separated points along the axon rather than continuously as in an unmyelinated axon.

The extent to which myelination increases conduction speed depends on a number of factors: the thickness of the sheath, the diameter of the axon, and the distance between nodes. All of these factors vary in different axons. As far as size is concerned, the following comparison is instructive. A peripheral nerve containing 1,000 myelinated fibers, 10 to 20 micrometers in diameter, is about 0.04 of an inch thick (1 millimeter). To accommodate the same number of nerve fibers having the same conduction speeds, a peripheral nerve composed of unmyelinated axons would have to be 1.5 inches (38 mm) in diameter.

Conduction in myelinated axons is highly reliable and this reliability has been expressed as a *safety factor*. The safety factor is the ratio between the amount of current *available* to stimulate a node of Ranvier and the amount of current actually *required* to stimulate the node. In normal myelinated axons, the safety factor is between 5 and 6. The safety factor decreases markedly in diseases that result in the demyelination of axons. In demyelinated fibers, the myelin sheath is damaged or lost. The insulating myelin sheath normally functions to promote current flow from one node of Ranvier to the next, as illustrated in Figure 4-14b. But when an action potential approaches a demyelinated region, loss of the insulating myelin sheath allows current to leak out through the internodal axon membrane and damaged myelin sheath. This loss of current results in a decrease in the amount of current available to stimulate (depolarize) the next node of Ranvier. The safety factor has been reduced so that the reliability of propagation of the action potential is decreased. As long as the safety factor has a value above 1, the threshold for generating an action potential will still be reached. It will just take longer to reach it. Therefore, conduction of the action potential down the axon will be slowed. In more severely demyelinated axons, the safety factor falls below 1, at which point threshold will not be reached at distal nodes of Ranvier, and the action potential will fail to conduct down the axon past the site of demyelination. This is referred to as a **conduction block**.

Postsynaptic Potentials

The arrival of action potentials at the terminal of an axon sets into motion a sequence of molecular events that results in the release of a chemical, the neurotransmitter, from the axon terminal. The neurotransmitter diffuses from the presynaptic axon terminal to the receptive membrane of the postsynaptic neuron and thus causes an electrical change in the postsynaptic neuron—hence, the name *postsynaptic potential*.

Postsynaptic potentials (PSPs) are changes in the neuron's membrane potential caused by ligand-gated ion channels (receptors) interacting with a neurotransmitter. Extracellular ligand-gated channels open when an

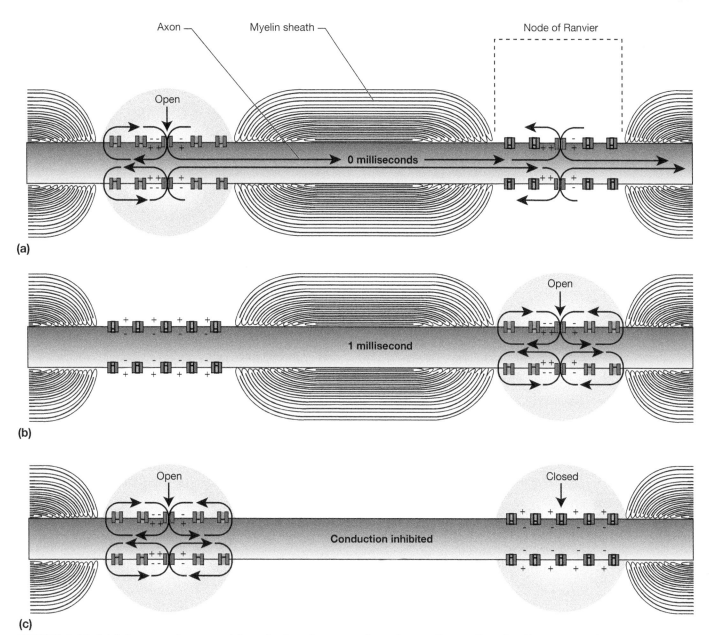

FIGURE 4-14 (a) Saltatory action potential conduction along a myelinated axon. Current flows locally. However, the presence of myelin prevents this local current from leaking across the internodal membrane. As a result, the current flows further down the axon than it would in the absence of myelin. Because voltage-gated sodium channels are concentrated at the nodes of Ranvier, active, voltage-gated currents occur only at these unmyelinated regions. (b) The action potential "jumps" from node to node, and conduction velocity is greatly enhanced. (c) The effect of demyelination on saltatory conduction. Because of its high resistance and low capacitance, myelin functions as an effective insulator that shunts current from one node of Ranvier to the next. When axons demyelinate, current leaks across exposed axon membrane to a greater extent than normal. Because there is less current making it to the next node, it takes longer to reach threshold, and conduction velocity is slowed. With severe demyelination, there may not be sufficient current to even reach threshold at the next node, and action potential propagation fails altogether at the site of demyelination.

extracellular ligand such as a neurotransmitter binds to the channel (receptor). Such channels may allow more than one ion species to flow down its concentration gradient.

Neurotransmitters released into the synaptic cleft by the presynaptic neuron affect the postsynaptic neuron by binding to thousands of receptor proteins (ligand-gated ion channels) concentrated in the patch of postsynaptic membrane that participates in the formation of the synapse. These potential changes thus occur on the dendritic

zone of interneurons and motor neurons that receive synaptic input from other neurons.

Transmitter-gated ion channels are proteins that have two functional domains: an extracellular domain that functions as the receptor for a neurotransmitter (and is the site at which a neurotransmitter binds) and a membrane-spanning domain that forms an ion channel. The membrane-spanning domain is made up of four or five subunits that come together to form a pore (Figure 4-15 ■). The pore

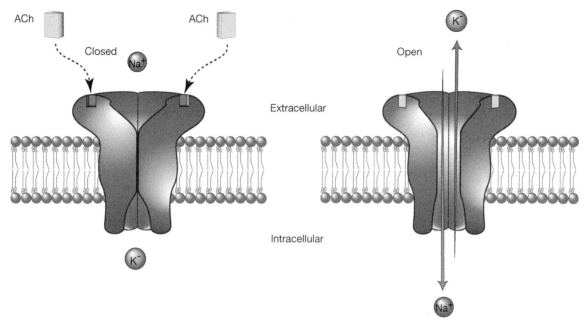

FIGURE 4-15 Model of a transmitter-gated ion channel. This channel responds to the transmitter ACh. When two molecules of ACh bind to the surface recognition unit on the channel, the inner domain changes its conformation to open a pore in the ion channel that allows cations to flow down their concentration gradients.

is closed until a neurotransmitter binds to the extracellular site. When binding occurs, it causes the membrane-spanning subunits to twist, thereby opening the pore. Depending on which ions can pass through the pore, the membrane potential of the postsynaptic neuron can be hyperpolarized, reducing the probability that an action potential will be generated, or depolarized, and increasing the probability that an action potential will be generated.

When the open channels admit Na^+ to the cell interior, the postsynaptic neuron will be depolarized, bringing the membrane potential closer to the threshold for generating an action potential (Figure 4-16 ■). The transient postsynaptic potential change is then called an **excitatory postsynaptic potential (EPSP)**.

On the other hand, when the open channels admit chloride ions (Cl^-), the membrane of the postsynaptic neuron will be hyperpolarized, driving the potential away from the threshold for generating an action potential (Figure 4-17 ■). This transient postsynaptic potential change thus is called an **inhibitory postsynaptic potential (IPSP)**. This is a basic description of the effect of chloride ions. It is important to understand that moving toward the threshold potential does not necessarily result in an action potential and moving away from the threshold potential does not necessarily inhibit an action potential. It simply means that the postsynaptic neuron is more or less likely to discharge (fire). Consider a synapse that involves gating of chloride channels. Most neurons have a chloride pump with a chloride Nernst equilibrium potential of about –65 mV. If the membrane potential is –60 mV when this synapse is active and the chloride channel opens, the PSP will be hyperpolarizing and will head in the direction of –65 mV. If the membrane potential is –70 mV when the synapse is active, the PSP will be depolarizing as it heads toward –65 mV. In both cases, the PSP is an IPSP

because its potential is negative to threshold—that is, the active synapse tends to "clamp" the membrane potential negative to threshold, which makes the neuron less likely to fire an action potential.

Finally, it should be noted that synapses that open K^+ channels are always hyperpolarizing. For this reason, these synapses also generate IPSPs.

The properties associated with postsynaptic potentials are markedly different than those associated with the action potential. For one thing, they are graded potentials, which has two consequences for the function of the postsynaptic neuron. First, the size of a PSP varies depending on the amount of neurotransmitter released into the synaptic cleft and the number of channels that open. Releasing more transmitter produces a larger PSP. Second, graded potentials can summate, that is, add together algebraically. Two types of summation are possible and may occur simultaneously. **Spatial summation** is the adding together of PSPs generated simultaneously at many different synapses on the dendritic zone (Figure 4-18 ■). **Temporal summation** is the adding together of PSPs occurring at the same synapse when they are generated within 5 to 15 msec of one another. Because neurons typically contain thousands of synapses on their dendritic zone membrane, temporal and spatial summation allow the postsynaptic neuron to integrate the electrical information provided by all excitatory and inhibitory synapses active at any given moment. Whether or not the postsynaptic neuron generates an action potential depends on the net balance between excitation and inhibition.

Another property of PSPs is that they are local membrane potential changes; that is, they are not self-propagated away from their site of generation like the action potential. Rather, PSPs decay passively as a function of distance from their site of generation. However, to be effective in controlling

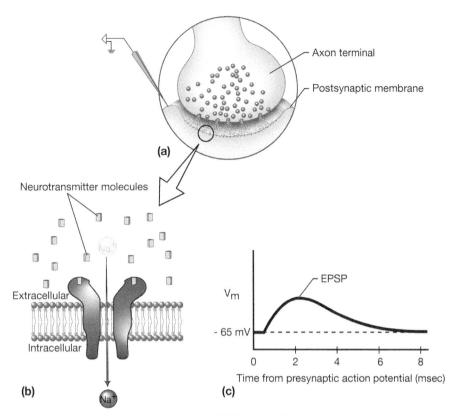

FIGURE 4-16 Generation of an excitatory postsynaptic potential. The arrival of an action potential at the presynaptic terminal causes the release of the neurotransmitter (a). Released neurotransmitter molecules bind to a postsynaptic transmitter-gated receptor that, in this case, is located on the ion channel complex. The chemical energy from this binding leads to activation of the receptor, and the channel's gate opens. If the channel is permeable to Na^+ ions, Na^+ will enter the postsynaptic neuron and depolarize this patch of membrane (b). This generates an EPSP that is recorded by an indwelling microelectrode (c).

the behavior of the postsynaptic neuron, PSPs only have to spread passively to the initial segment. And this they do, with varying degrees of effectiveness depending on the distance of the synapse from the axon initial segment and the membrane properties of the neuron. The different types of electrical signals that occur in a neuron are summarized in Figure 4-19 ■.

CLINICAL CONNECTIONS

Multiple Sclerosis

Demyelinating disorders can have a profound impact on a person's ability to function. These disorders are characterized by the following: (1) destruction of the myelin sheaths surrounding axons, (2) relative preservation of the axons themselves, (3) the presence in the lesion area of inflammatory and immune cells that mount the attack against myelin, and (4) the location of the lesions in white matter. The demyelinating diseases are a varied group, the most common member of which is multiple sclerosis (MS). MS is the yardstick by which all other diseases of myelin are measured. No other human disease condition can match the specificity of destruction of the demyelinating diseases in which a single isolated membrane becomes the primary target of a complex, largely immunologic attack. However, axonal damage and neuronal cell death also have been

identified in MS, but these features of the disorder are beyond the scope of the current discussion.

The first modern clinical description of MS occurred in 1868 when a French neurologist described multiple "brown patches" in the brain and spinal cord of autopsied patients and correlated these brown patches with the neurological symptoms of the disease. MS is an important disease because it is the leading cause of serious neurological problems in young and middle-aged adults in the United States.

The demyelination of MS is confined to the CNS. The specific signs and symptoms depend on which structures can no longer communicate with one another, which is to say, they depend on where the lesions are located. As a result, the symptoms can be quite variable from person to person. In spite of this potential variability, the lesions tend to favor certain sites in the CNS so that there are groups of symptoms and signs that are characteristic of MS. The most common symptoms are fatigue, gait and balance disturbance, bowel and bladder dysfunction, and visual problems.

The slowing down of conduction velocity from demyelination may not result in clinical problems for the individual. For example, in MS the conduction time from a light stimulus on the retina in the eye to the response in the occipital cortex where the light flash is seen can be prolonged by as much as 50 msec. But a person with such a delayed visual evoked response may experience no apparent problem with vision. This makes sense from a functional standpoint. The temperature of the body rises and falls over a 24-hour period with the overall change being about 2°C. Temperature changes affect the speed with which ion channels in the axon membrane open and close so that conduction speed changes about 2.5 percent per degree of temperature change. In spite of these normal changes in conduction speed, vision remains normal over the day. Thus, a slowing of conduction speed may not always produce noticeable clinical problems for vision.

In contrast, a conduction block occurring in a significant number of fibers in the optic nerve of a person with MS will produce clinical abnormalities. Thus, a person may complain of blurred vision or double vision.

In addition to failures of conduction, demyelination can result in naked axons that may respond abnormally to, for example, the normal mechanical stresses and strains to which the nervous system is subjected during daily behavior. People with MS who have demyelinating lesions in the cervical region of the spinal cord may experience an electric shock-like sensation extending down the back into the legs and/or into the arms when they are performing movements accompanied by forward flexion of the head. They may occur when bending over to pick up an object or to lace the shoes or when energetically nodding yes. This is called **Lhermitte's sign**, after the physician who first described it. The sensation is apparently caused by the slight stretching of the cervical spinal cord and mechanical stimulation of its denuded axons.

Heat is one of the most common factors that aggravates symptoms of MS. Elevated temperature is an aggravating factor in people with MS because the reliability of conduction in the demyelinated fibers already is reduced. As temperature is raised, the ion channels in the axon membrane open and close faster. This means that the action potential occurs faster so that less current is generated in any given region of the axon. The reduction in available current reduces the safety factor. When this temperature-dependent reduction is added to the already present disease-related reduction, the conduction of action potentials may fail altogether. Thus, the person's neurological symptoms worsen as temperature rises. People with MS should be warned about the possible worsening of symptoms when taking hot baths or showers. Increased weakness or muscular incoordination can lead to injury-causing falls that are preventable.

A "hot bath test" was once used as a diagnostic aid in MS. This test was based on the observation that filling a bath with water at a temperature of 102°F caused the patient to complain of blurred vision. When the temperature of the water was raised to 104°F, the patient complained of numbness of one hand, difficulty in moving the other hand and leg, and other problems. Visual acuity has been shown to fall when body temperature is raised by excessive exercise, while cooling has the reverse effect. The lowering of body temperature by cold baths or cold air has been shown to provide temporary relief of symptoms for people with MS.

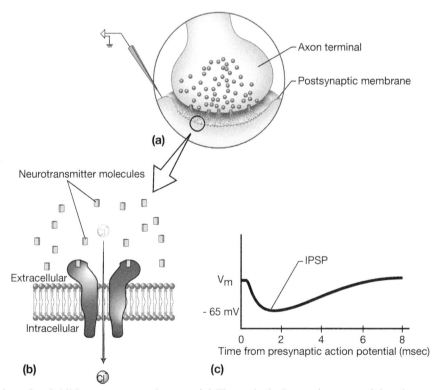

FIGURE 4-17 Generation of an inhibitory postsynaptic potential. The arrival of an action potential at the presynaptic terminal causes the release of the neurotransmitter (a). Released neurotransmitter molecules bind to postsynaptic transmitter-gated ion channels, which then open. If Cl⁻ enters the postsynaptic neuron, the membrane is hyperpolarized (b). This generates an IPSP that is recorded by an indwelling microelectrode (c).

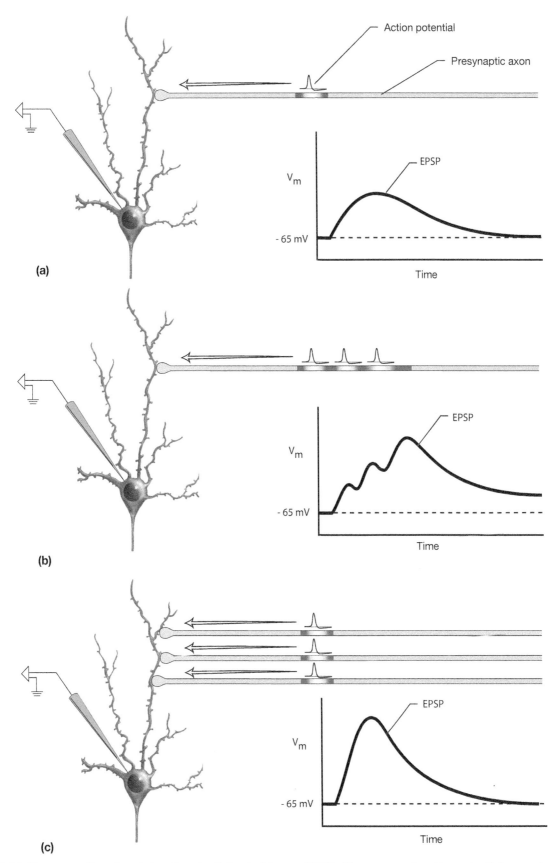

FIGURE 4-18 The summation of postsynaptic potentials—in this case, EPSPs. The presynaptic action potential generates a small EPSP (a). When the same presynaptic axon fires action potentials in quick succession before the preceding EPSP has fully decayed, the individual EPSPs sum (b). This is called temporal summation. When two or more different and contiguous presynaptic inputs are active at the same time, their individual EPSPs sum. (c) This is called spatial summation.

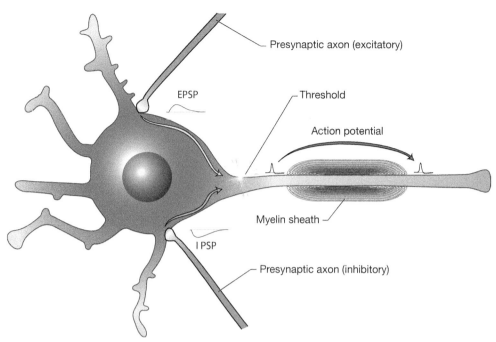

FIGURE 4-19 Summary of the signaling between neurons. Synaptic inputs generate active currents in the postsynaptic membrane. These currents spread passively (electrotonic conduction) through the membrane and extracellular fluid. When such currents spread to the trigger zone of the axon and when they are depolarizing and sufficiently large, they can trigger the generation of an action potential. The action potential generates local currents that spread passively down the axon ahead of the action potential. This leads to depolarization of the downstream membrane, which propagates the action potential, and the process repeats itself all the way down to the axon terminals.

SYNAPSES AND SYNAPTIC TRANSMISSION

Clinical Preview

You are treating two different people who have deficits related to neurotransmitters. The first, Roger Schwartz, has Parkinson's disease. The second, Marilyn Holston, has had lifelong difficulties with depression. As you read through this section, consider the following:

- What neurotransmitters are associated with each condition?

- How is knowledge about neurotransmitters and their impact on function used in developing pharmacological interventions?

- Where might dysfunction occur in the process from synthesis, storage, and release of the various neurotransmitters to their interaction with the receptor cells, and how might this influence the nature and remediation of functional problems?

In order to generate behavior, information coded by patterns of action potentials must be communicated from one neuron to another (or from a neuron to an effector cell). As noted earlier, the synapse is the specialized structure that communicates information between

neurons. Given the vast number of neurons in the human brain, the total number of synapses almost defies imagination. Synapses represent sites at which the information transfer from presynaptic to postsynaptic neuron can remain unaltered, can be stopped altogether, or can be modified in a significant way. Understanding the process of synaptic transmission is essential to understanding how the brain carries out its manifold functions, the actions of psychoactive drugs (therapeutic and recreational), and the causes and treatment of mental disorders and many other diseases affecting the nervous system.

The Synapse

Although there are a few instances in which neurons communicate with one another via a direct link (see discussion of electrical synapses later), the overwhelming majority of neuronal communication occurs at chemical synapses wherein a chemical, the neurotransmitter, is released from a presynaptic neuron onto the receptive membrane of a postsynaptic neuron. As previously noted, a single chemical synapse is structurally defined in terms of two neurons, one presynaptic and the other postsynaptic, separated by a gap, the *synaptic cleft*, that is filled with extracellular fluid. Although this two-neuron link is used to define a single synapse, it does not define the total relationship between the two neurons. Single neurons receive input from many other neurons and, in turn, establish synapses with many other

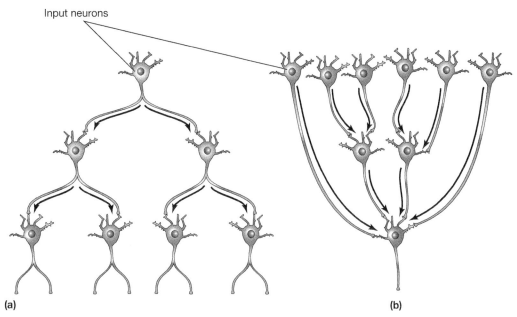

FIGURE 4-20 The synaptic relationship between any two neurons is not one-to-one because of (a) divergence and (b) convergence. Divergence is defined according to a presynaptic neuron, whereas convergence is defined according to a postsynaptic neuron, respectively.

neurons. This is called either **convergence** or **divergence**, depending on the cell of reference. The terminal arborization of a single axon branches, or diverges, to establish synapses with many postsynaptic neurons (Figure 4-20 ■). When the point of reference is the receptive zone of the postsynaptic neuron, its membrane is studded with synapses that have converged on it from many different presynaptic neurons. An average neuron may form some 1,000 synaptic connections and, in turn, receive some 10,000 synaptic inputs. Thus, while it is true that neurons communicate at synapses, neurons of the brain never speak to one another exclusively on a one-to-one basis.

Synapses are often classified anatomically according to which parts of the pre- and postsynaptic membrane are involved in forming the synapse. The primary types of synapses identified using this scheme are axodendritic, axosomatic, and axoaxonic (Figure 4-21 ■), meaning the presynaptic axon synapsing with a dendrite, with the soma (body), and with another axon, respectively.

The Presynaptic Neuron

Both the presynaptic and postsynaptic components of the synapse contain structural specializations equipping them to transfer information between neurons. In the presynaptic

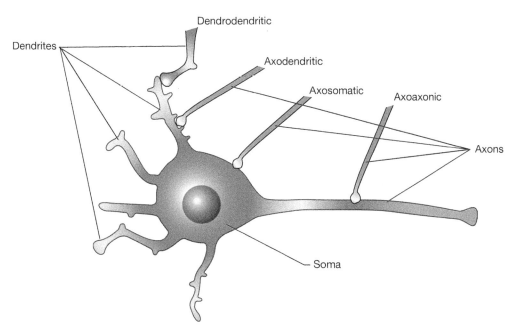

FIGURE 4-21 Classification of types of chemical synapses according to the parts of the pre- and postsynaptic membranes involved.

Thought Question

Neurons release a variety of neurotransmitters into the synaptic cleft. What three classes of these molecules exist, and how do they vary in size? How are these molecules manufactured, stored, and transported?

neuron, the axon telodendron (synaptic knob) contains thousands of small membrane-bound spherical organelles, the **synaptic vesicles**. Typically the vesicles are about 50 nm in diameter. These organelles are synthesized in the cell body of the neuron and transported to the axon terminal by the fast axoplasmic transport system. Synaptic vesicles play important roles in the synthesis, storage, and release of the molecules of neurotransmitter they contain. The synaptic knob also contains larger vesicles, some 100 nm in diameter, that contain different neurotransmitters and are referred to as **dense-core vesicles** or **secretory granules**. The synaptic vesicles cluster at regions of the intracellular presynaptic membrane specialized for releasing the neurotransmitter and are called **active zones**. In contrast, the dense core vesicles do not cluster at active zones but remain in the interior of the terminal. Because both synaptic and dense core vesicles occur in the same nerve terminal, neurons can release more than one transmitter—which they do, but under different conditions.

The neurotransmitters that are stored in the synaptic and dense core vesicles fall into one of three chemical classes: *amino acids*, *amines*, and *peptides* (Table 4-1 ■). The amino acids and amines represent small-molecule transmitters, while the peptides are large-molecule transmitters. The small-molecule transmitters are synthesized and packaged in synaptic vesicles in the terminal of the presynaptic neuron (i.e., synaptic knob). The peptides, in contrast, are synthesized and packaged in dense-core vesicles in the cell body and transported to the presynaptic terminal by fast axoplasmic transport. It is noteworthy that a mature (i.e., postmitotic) neuron releases only one type of neurotransmitter [e.g., acetylcholine (ACh), norepinephrine (NE)] and releases the same transmitter at all of its axon terminals. This is referred to as Dale's law. More recently, it has become apparent that many axon terminals also co-release neuropeptides when the firing rate is high.

It is important to understand that to classify a transmitter chemically does not classify its function (i.e., what effect it will have on the postsynaptic neuron). Transmitters are often classified as excitatory or inhibitory, but it is, in fact, the postsynaptic receptor, not the transmitter itself, that determines the nature of the response. Thus, in some cases, the same transmitter can excite or inhibit the activity of the postsynaptic neuron, depending on the type of receptor with which it binds.

The amino acid transmitters include **glycine**, **glutamate**, **aspartate**, and **gamma-amino butyric acid (GABA)**. Glycine and GABA are classified as inhibitory neurotransmitters, while aspartate and glutamate are classified as excitatory transmitters. The amine transmitters include **acetylcholine**, **dopamine (DA)**, **norepinephrine (NE)**, **epinephrine**, **serotonin [5-hydroxytriptamine (5-HT)]**, and **histamine**. Of these, dopamine, norepinephrine, and serotonin are classified as **monoamine (biogenic amine) transmitters**. The peptide transmitters include **dynorphin**, **enkephalins**, **substance P**, and a number of others. Amine and peptide neurotransmitters may be excitatory or inhibitory, depending on the receptor type with which it binds.

Some of these transmitters reside in the neurons of known sets of neurons within the brain and are released onto the neurons of identified structures. They, therefore,

Table 4-1 Major Neurotransmitters

CLASSIFICATION	MAJOR TRANSMITTERS	TYPICAL EFFECT
Amino acid (small molecule)	Aspartate	Fast excitatory
	Glutamate	Fast excitatory
	Glycine	Fast inhibitory
	Gamma-amino butyric acid (GABA)	Fast inhibitory
Amines (small molecule)	Acetylcholine (ACh)	Second-messenger effect may be excitatory or inhibitory, depending on the receptor type with which the transmitter binds
	Catecholamines	
	Dopamine (DA)	
	Norepinephrine (NE)	
	Serotonin (5-hydroxytriptamine, 5-HT)	
	Histamine	
Peptides (large molecule)	Dynorphin	Second-messenger effect may be excitatory or inhibitory, depending on the receptor type with which the transmitter binds
	Beta-endorphin	
	Enkephalin	
	Substance P	

represent functional systems of neurons. Nearly all such systems are more or less selectively targeted by specific disease processes. Moreover, appropriately designed drugs can selectively target such functional systems in the treatment of specific brain disorders. Other transmitters (the amino acid transmitters) are used ubiquitously in the brain and spinal cord and belong to many different functional systems.

Neurotransmitters may act over different time courses and in different ways. The postsynaptic response may be excitatory or inhibitory and may last tens of milliseconds. The response may be to alter the metabolism (i.e., the biochemical activity) of the postsynaptic cell and may last for minutes. Or the gene expression in the postsynaptic neuron may be changed leading to long-term or even permanent changes.

The Postsynaptic Neuron

The major specialization of the membrane on the postsynaptic side of the synapse is the **postsynaptic density (PSD)** that contains the receptors for the neurotransmitter released by the presynaptic neuron (Figure 4-22 ■). Membrane receptors are chemoreceptive protein molecules in the cell membrane that specifically interact with a neurotransmitter and cause a response in the postsynaptic neuron either directly or indirectly. Receptors may potentially contain up to four specialized functional molecular domains. All receptors contain an extracellular **recognition**, or **specificity**, **domain** that binds with a specific transmitter (ligand). Some receptors contain, in addition, a membrane-spanning **channel domain** that opens a pore (channel) in the membrane in response to the ligand. Some receptors contain a **regulatory domain** that controls the effectiveness of the binding

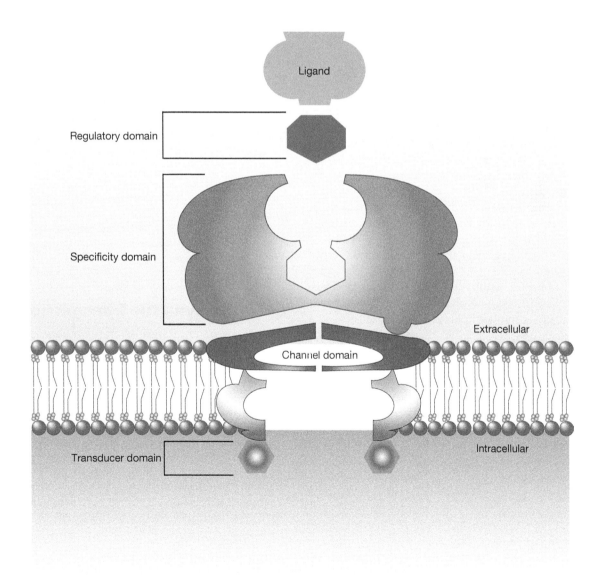

FIGURE 4-22 The postsynaptic density contains receptor proteins that contain recognition units that bind with specific neurotransmitters.

between the transmitter and receptor. For example, the antianxiety agents Librium and Valium increase the effectiveness of GABA binding with its receptor and so facilitate inhibition in specific structures of the brain. Finally, a large number of receptors contain a **coupling**, or **transducer, domain** that couples the transmitter–receptor interaction with the intracellular biochemical machinery that actually mediates the response of the postsynaptic neuron. The functioning of each of these domains is discussed in more detail next.

Thought Question

All postsynaptic membranes contain a recognition or specificity subunit. What is the purpose of this feature of the postsynaptic membrane? In addition, some postsynaptic neurons contain additional subunits. What are their names, and what role does each play?

Depending on their combination of specialized domains, receptors can be classified as either **ionotropic receptors** or **metabotropic receptors**. Ionotropic receptors are those that gate ion channels directly. That is, the receptor protein contains both recognition and channel domains. Metabotropic receptors, on the other hand, gate ion channels indirectly after first activating a membrane protein that, in turn, activates an intracellular protein called a G-protein. These are called **G-protein-coupled receptors**. Intracellular G-proteins may then open or close a separate channel.

Alternatively, the G-protein can act on enzymes that synthesize molecules called second messengers. **Second messengers**, in turn, can activate additional enzymes in the cytoplasm that open or close ion channels or alter the metabolism of the postsynaptic neuron (discussed later). As noted earlier, the transduction process that occurs in certain types of sensory receptors and generates the receptor potential may involve G-protein coupled second messengers. Thus, transduction in olfactory and photoreceptors and in some taste and visceral receptors employ second messengers.

Given receptors are specific for particular types of neurotransmitters. While this is true, a given neurotransmitter may have more than one type of receptor with which it interacts. Thus, for example, an amine transmitter like acetylcholine interacts with both ionotropic and metabotropic receptors.

What is the purpose of having different types of receptors for the same neurotransmitter? The answer is that it is the receptor that determines the kind of response the neurotransmitter will generate in the postsynaptic neuron. Imagine the following situation: in response to a particular event, the brain needs to produce different responses in its different parts. One way the brain achieves this goal is to have different receptors located on different sets of neurons. That way, the event can cause the release of a single transmitter that can then produce different kinds of responses in different parts of the brain.

The distribution of receptors across the neuron's receptive membrane is patchy because they are predominantly confined to synapses and only sparsely in nonsynaptic membrane. New receptor molecules are continually being assembled by neurons to replace those degraded by use. However, they are inserted predominantly into synaptic regions of the postsynaptic membrane. Thus, there is some sort of signal from the presynaptic neuron that guides receptor insertion in the postsynaptic neuron. This is clear from a phenomenon observed when a postsynaptic neuron is deprived of its synapses either through injury or disease. The neuron is then said to be **denervated**. Under this circumstance, the neuron often becomes hypersensitive (or supersensitive) to normal amounts of released transmitter, and the phenomenon is called **denervation hypersensitivity**. It is explained by the spread of receptors into nonsynaptic and formerly unresponsive regions of the postsynaptic membrane stemming from the loss of the presynaptic guidance signal.

Additionally, receptor numbers can either be **up-regulated** or **down-regulated** as the postsynaptic neuron attempts to maintain normal synaptic transmission in the face of changes in the amount of transmitter released. Disease or exogenous drugs (including recreational) can cause a change in the amount of transmitter release. If the amount of transmitter released declines and remains depressed over time, the postsynaptic neuron often increases its number of receptors (up-regulated). Conversely, if release is enhanced over time, the number of postsynaptic receptors often decreases (down-regulated).

Thought Question

Not all channels can be opened directly by a ligand. For those that cannot be opened directly, a specific molecule called the G-protein is important. What is the role of the G-protein?

Chemical Synaptic Transmission

Chemical synaptic transmission is broken down into five distinct steps:

1. The neurotransmitter must be synthesized or manufactured.
2. The neurotransmitter must then be packaged for storage.
3. The neurotransmitter is then released into the synaptic cleft and diffuses toward the membrane of the postsynaptic neuron.
4. Upon reaching the postsynaptic membrane, the transmitter interacts with a receptor molecule on the membrane, which is called transmitter–receptor interaction.
5. The neurotransmitter is inactivated so that its duration of action is controlled.

Of fundamental clinical significance is the fact that *each* of these steps can be manipulated by exogenously administered drugs or toxins. Some steps are specifically manipulated in given neurological disorders, and these will be pointed out as we progress through each step.

Synthesis

The synthesis of a neurotransmitter requires the presence of two ingredients: precursor molecules and enzymes. Precursor molecules are the raw ingredients for the neurotransmitter. They are readily available in our diets. In some cases, the dietary precursor undergoes a chemical change in the liver before being released into general circulation to be carried to the brain. For example, in the case of the synthesis of the transmitter serotonin (5-hydroxytryptamine), the dietary essential protein precursor molecule phenylalanine is first broken down in the liver to tyrosine (by the liver enzyme phenylalanine hydroxylase) before entering general circulation. Once in the brain, the precursor crosses the blood-brain barrier and enters the extracellular fluid surrounding neurons. The precursor is then actively transported into the interior of the neuron. Located within the neuron are enzymes that transform the precursor into the neurotransmitter. There may be only a single type of enzyme that converts the precursor to the transmitter, or there may be a number in which case the transmitter is synthesized in a series of

chemical reactions. This depends on the particular transmitter being manufactured.

Small molecule transmitters are synthesized locally within the presynaptic terminal. The enzymes required for synthesis are manufactured in the cell body and transported to the presynaptic terminal by slow axonal transport. The precursor molecules acted upon by these enzymes are actively transported into the terminal. The enzymes produce a free pool of neurotransmitter molecules in the terminal's cytoplasm.

In contrast, the enzymes and molecular machinery involved in the synthesis of peptides are found only in the cell body. Peptides are synthesized when amino acids are linked in the **rough endoplasmic reticulum (rER)** of the cell body. The peptides are cleaved to form the active neurotransmitter in the Golgi complex. Dense core vesicles containing the transmitter bud off from the Golgi complex. They are carried from the cell body to the axon terminal by the fast axoplasmic transport system. Figure 4-23 ■ illustrates the synthesis and storage of small- and large-molecule transmitters.

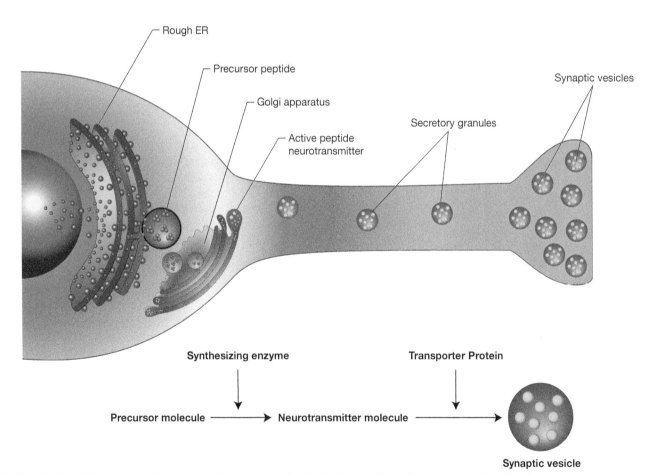

FIGURE 4-23 Different types of neurotransmitters are synthesized and stored by unique processes. Peptides (large molecule neurotransmitters) are synthesized only in the cell body. The precursor peptide is synthesized in the rough ER and cleaved in the Golgi complex to form the active neurotransmitter. Transmitter-containing secretory vesicles (granules) bud off from the Golgi complex and are conveyed down the axon via anterograde transport to the terminal where they are stored. The amines and amino acid neurotransmitters (small-molecule neurotransmitters) are synthesized and stored in the axon terminal. Precursor molecules are pumped into the terminal from the extracellular fluid, where axoplasmic enzymes convert the precursor into the neurotransmitter. The transmitter is then pumped into synaptic vesicles (by membrane transporter proteins), where the transmitter is stored until released into the synaptic cleft.

Thought Question

As you read this section, be prepared to summarize the steps that occur during chemical synaptic transmission. List the five steps and identify major processes that occur during each step.

Storage

Once synthesized, the transmitter is stored in synaptic or dense core vesicles. For the amino acid and amine transmitters, after synthesis in the cytoplasm of the terminal, the transmitter is pumped into the interior of the vesicle by a carrier-mediated transport system. There may be thousands of vesicles in a nerve terminal, each loaded with thousands of molecules of transmitter. In the case of the peptides, they are loaded into dense core vesicles in the cell body and the vesicles transported to the axon terminal.

Importantly, once a transmitter is within a membrane-bound vesicle, it is protected from enzymatic breakdown into a chemical that would no longer be able to function as a transmitter. This seems puzzling at first glance. Why should there be some enzymes inside the neuron that synthesize a neurotransmitter only to have others present that destroy it? Part of the answer is that the neuron regulates the amount of neurotransmitter it stores. It does this by enzymatically degrading the transmitter before it ever gets inside the vesicle. One such enzyme present in the presynaptic terminal of monoaminergic axons is **monoamine oxidase (MAO)**. Located on the outer membrane of mitochondria in the axon terminal, MAO breaks down the amine neurotransmitters, DA, norepinephrine (NE), and serotonin (5-HT).

Release

The mechanism responsible for the release of the neurotransmitter is activated by the action potentials that invade the presynaptic axon terminal after propagating down the axon. In essence, bioelectrical activity originating in the cell body of the presynaptic neuron is transmitted via an action potential to the axon terminal to induce transmitter release. This will alter the excitability of postsynaptic neurons as follows: The action potentials depolarize the nerve terminal. The membrane of the axon terminal contains voltage-gated ion channels, just as does the membrane of the axon. However, the channels in the nerve terminal are permeable to calcium ions (Ca^{2+}). When the nerve terminal's membrane is depolarized, it opens and allows Ca^{2+} ions to enter the nerve terminal (Figure 4-24 ■). The internal concentration of Ca^{2+} is quite low so that Ca^{2+} enters the terminal rapidly. Ca^{2+} enters through channels located at the active zones where the synaptic vesicles already are "docked" waiting to release their transmitter. The mechanism by which this occurs is complex and beyond the scope of this text. However, the fundamental process involves activation of motor proteins by Ca^{2+}. The motor proteins that lead to glycoproteins on the surface of vesicles bind to "docking" proteins, leading

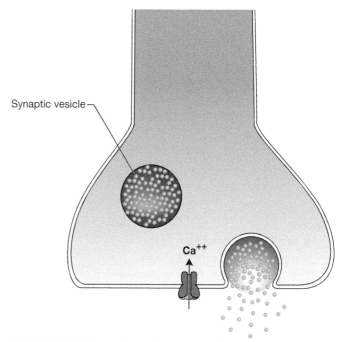

Synaptic vesicle

Ca^{++}

FIGURE 4-24 Transmitter release occurs by exocytosis. Invasion of the presynaptic terminal by an action potential opens voltage-gated Ca^{2+} channels in the terminal membrane. The influx of Ca^{2+} activates a complex of motor proteins in the active zone, resulting in the transmitter-loaded vesicle docked at an active zone to fuse with the presynaptic membrane, "rupture," and release its contents into the synaptic cleft. Vesicles that are not docked at active zones are induced to migrate toward the active zone and dock by the Ca^{2+} influx.

to fusion with the presynaptic membrane at active zone and then to exocytosis of neurotransmitters.

The vesicles release their transmitter by **exocytosis**. The membrane of the synaptic vesicle and presynaptic nerve terminal membrane at the active zone fuse and form a pore. The pore allows the neurotransmitter to escape into the synaptic cleft. The pore continues to expand until the vesicle membrane is fully incorporated into the presynaptic membrane.

The synaptic vesicles are recycled after fusing with the presynaptic membrane. They pinch off from the membrane and reenter the interior of the nerve terminal. In the case of the small-molecule neurotransmitters, the vesicles are refilled rapidly because the transmitters are synthesized in the nerve terminal. Thus, release can be rapid and sustained.

Exocytosis triggered by Ca^{2+} influx is also the mechanism by which dense-core vesicles release peptide neurotransmitters. However, exocytosis does not occur at the active zones but at a distance from the sites of Ca^{2+} entry. This means that the Ca^{2+} concentration in the nerve terminal away from the active zones must be allowed to build up to a sufficient level before release is triggered. This requires a high-frequency train of action potentials invading the axon terminal, which thus increases the time required before release is triggered. As a result, release of the peptides is a more time-consuming process and is dependent on the rate of action potentials. Unlike synaptic vesicles, dense-core vesicles are used only once.

Transmitter-Receptor Interaction

Once in the synaptic cleft, the molecules of neurotransmitter diffuse toward the membrane of the postsynaptic neuron. Once there, the transmitter binds to a receptor molecule in the postsynaptic density. Binding is chemically specific, has high affinity, and is reversible. As noted earlier, membrane receptors are either transmitter-gated ion channels or G-protein coupled receptors. In G-protein-coupled receptors, the postsynaptic neuron's response is generated by chemical events that occur inside the cell, not on the extracellular side of the membrane as in the case of transmitter-gated ion channels.

TRANSMITTER-GATED ION CHANNELS Most of the fast synaptic transmission in the brain and spinal cord is mediated by ionotropic amino acid-gated ion channels generating EPSPs and IPSPs. With the possible exception of the receptor for the transmitter glycine, the other amino acid-gated channels each have several subtypes of receptor.

Glutamate-Gated Channels There are three subtypes of receptor for the transmitter glutamate. Each subtype bears the name of the chemical compound that activates the receptor (called the **receptor agonist**). The subtype for the agonist kainate is not fully understood and will not be considered further. The two other subtypes are the AMPA receptor and the NMDA receptor. (AMPA stands for α-amino-3-hydroxy-5-methyl-4-isoxazole propionate, and NMDA stands for N-methyl-D-aspartate.) The AMPA- and NMDA-gated channels mediate most fast excitatory transmission in the brain. The EPSPs generated by the activation of AMPA receptors are faster than those generated

by the activation of NMDA receptors. Because most synapses in the brain contain both AMPA and NMDA receptors, glutamate-generated EPSPs have components resulting from both types of channel. While AMPA receptors are permeable to both Na^+ and K^+, at the negative resting membrane potential, they preferentially admit Na^+ into the cell interior due to the larger driving force on Na^+. The Na^+ influx results in a rapid and large depolarization of the membrane and an EPSP (Figure 4-25 ■).

NMDA-gated channels differ from AMPA receptors in two significant ways. First, in addition to being permeable to both Na^+ and K^+, NMDA receptor ion channels allow the entry of Ca^{2+}. As a result, EPSPs produced by NMDA receptors increase the concentration of Ca^{2+} within the postsynaptic neuron. Postsynaptically, Ca^{2+} can activate enzymes, regulate the opening of different channels, and even affect gene expression. Second, the inward ionic current through NMDA-gated channels is voltage dependent. When glutamate binds to the NMDA receptor, the gate opens but the channel is blocked by extracellular Mg^{2+} ions at the negative resting membrane potential. Mg^{2+} is extruded from the channel via electrical repulsion only when the membrane is depolarized relative to the resting membrane potential, which results from the simultaneous activation of AMPA channels at the same or neighboring synapses or the co-release of another depolarizing transmitter.

A large percentage of the brain's neurons release glutamate, and glutamate is stored in large quantities even in the cytoplasm of neurons that do not utilize the transmitter. This fact has potentially dire consequences for the survival of

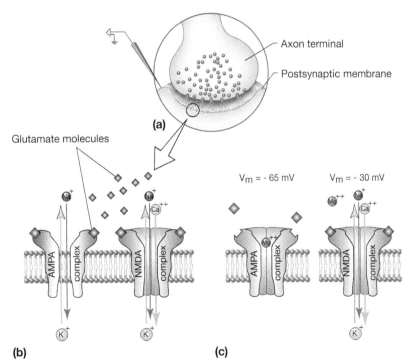

FIGURE 4-25 Glutamate-gated channels. (a) An action potential invading the presynaptic terminal triggers the release of glutamate. (b) Glutamate binds to both AMPA and NMDA receptors in the postsynaptic membrane. Na^+ enters the postsynaptic neuron through AMPA channels, and both Na^+ and Ca^{2+} enter through NMDA channels, generating a fast EPSP. (c) The inward ionic current through the NMDA-gated channel is dependent on the Mg^{2+} "block" being removed by a depolarization of the postsynaptic membrane.

neurons following brain or spinal cord damage (see Chapters 5 and 25). Specifically, ischemia leads to a cascade of damaging biochemical reactions involving excessive glutamate release and entry of Ca^{2+} into the cell, referred to as excitotoxicity.

GABA-Gated and Glycine-Gated Channels Inhibition in the brain and spinal cord is mediated primarily by GABA. Two subtypes of GABA receptor exist: the $GABA_A$ and the $GABA_B$ receptors. The $GABA_A$ receptor is an ionotropic receptor that gates Cl^- channels, generating IPSPs. It is the $GABA_A$ receptor that contains the regulatory subunit on one of its extracellular domains, referred to earlier. The $GABA_B$ receptor is a metabotropic receptor that activates a second-messenger cascade, which often activates a K^+ channel.

G-PROTEIN-COUPLED RECEPTORS AND EFFECTOR SYSTEMS Members of all three classes of neurotransmitter bind to G-coupled protein receptors. Three general steps are involved in transmission mediated by these receptors: (1) binding of the transmitter to the receptor protein, (2) activation of the G-protein, and (3) activation of an effector system. G-protein-coupled receptors contain a transmitter binding site on the extracellular side and a G-protein binding site on the intracellular side of the postsynaptic membrane. Structural variations in these two sites determine which neurotransmitter binds to the receptor, as well as which G-protein binds and is activated. The particular G-protein that is activated, in turn, determines which effector system is activated in response to the binding of the transmitter.

G-proteins, of which there are about 20 types, consist of three protein subunits, designated alpha, beta, and gamma. G-proteins exist in two conformations, wherein the alpha subunit is bound to either guanosine diphosphate (GDP) or guanosine triphosphate (GTP). When the alpha subunit is bound to GDP, the alpha subunit binds to the beta and gamma subunits and the G-protein is inactive. However, when the alpha subunit is bound to GTP, the alpha subunit dissociates from the beta and gamma subunits and the G-protein is activated. This exchange of GDP for GTP, which the alpha subunit picks up from the cytoplasm, is triggered by the binding of a neurotransmitter to the receptor (Figure 4-26 ■). The alpha subunit with its GTP

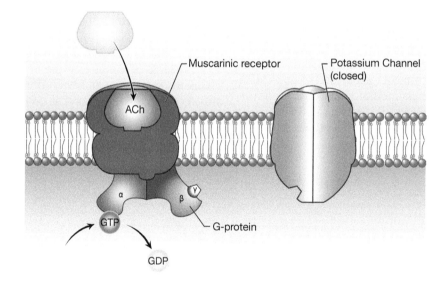

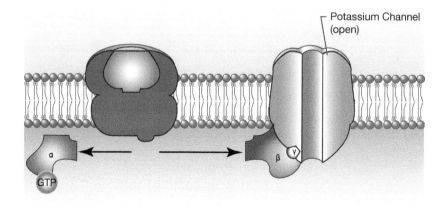

FIGURE 4-26 Direct modulation of ion channels by G-proteins is the fastest mechanism by which G-proteins act. In heart muscle, G-proteins are activated by ACh binding to muscarinic receptors. The dissociated beta-gamma subunit binds directly to the potassium channel gate.

then activates different effector proteins. However, the alpha subunit is itself an enzyme that breaks down GTP into GDP so that the alpha subunit terminates its own activity. All three subunits reassociate, and the G-protein returns to its resting state, ready for the cycle to begin again.

Direct Modulation of Ion Channels by G-Proteins The most rapid means by which activated G-proteins can affect ion movements across the postsynaptic membrane is when the beta-gamma subunit of the G-protein binds directly to an ion channel. Because multiple proteins must bind to one another in sequence to generate such a postsynaptic response, the response is considerably slower than the PSPs generated by ligand-gated ion channels, requiring tens of milliseconds as opposed to about one millisecond. Muscarinic acetylcholine (ACh) receptors on heart muscle cells are the most frequently cited example of this direct modulation. Activation of these metabotropic receptors by ACh allows the beta-gamma subunit to bind directly to K^+ channels, opening them and inhibiting the firing rate of heart muscle cells, thereby slowing the heart rate.

Second-Messenger Cascades Activated G-proteins can also interact with effector enzymes in the postsynaptic neuron. These effector enzymes, in turn, generate **second messengers** that can directly bind to ion channels and open or close them or, more typically, activate other enzymes. One of the best-understood effector enzymes is **adenylyl cyclase**, although others have been identified.

Different G-proteins can either stimulate or inhibit the effector enzyme adenylyl cyclase (Figure 4-27 ■). The transmitter NE acting via the beta receptor stimulates adenylyl cyclase to convert ATP to cyclic AMP (cAMP). Cyclic AMP then activates the downstream enzyme **protein kinase A (PKA)**. PKAs transfer phosphate from ATP present in the cytoplasm to target proteins such as ion channels. Phosphorylation of an ion channel changes its conformation and can regulate the opening or closing of the channel. However, when NE binds to a different type of NE receptor, the alpha-2 receptor, a different G-protein is activated that inhibits the activity of adenylyl cyclase.

One significant advantage offered by the coupling of metabotropic receptors to ion channels via effector enzymes is that the binding of the receptor to its membrane receptor is amplified in each subsequent step of the transduction process. When bound to its receptor, a single transmitter molecule can result in the dissociation of many G proteins. Each G protein, in turn, can activate many molecules of adenylyl cyclase, each of which results in the generation of many molecules of cAMP, and so on down the cascade. As a result, many ion channels can be influenced. Because of the additional time required for enzymes to generate their products, postsynaptic responses generated by metabotropic receptors occur on a time scale of tens of milliseconds to minutes or even hours.

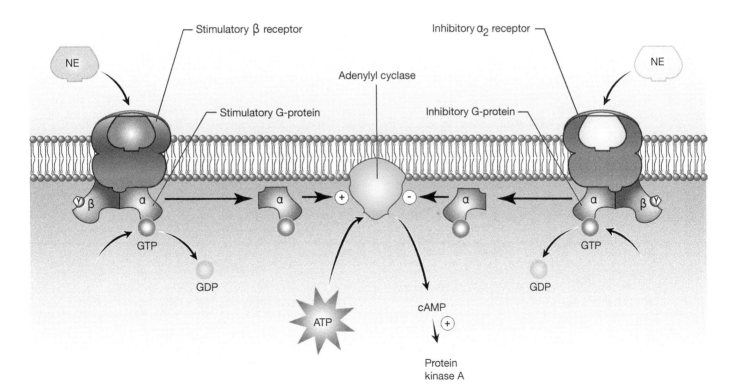

FIGURE 4-27 Different G-proteins can either stimulate or inhibit the effector enzyme adenylyl cyclase. (a) The transmitter NE acting via the beta receptor stimulates adenylyl cyclase to convert ATP to cyclic AMP (cAMP). Cyclic AMP then activates the enzyme protein kinase A. (b) When NE binds to an alpha-2 receptor, an inhibitory G-protein is activated that inhibits adenylyl cyclase.

Postsynaptic Responses Involving Gene Expression Second messengers also are capable of altering the expression of genes in the postsynaptic neuron. Specific proteins regulate gene transcription, and their phosphorylation by protein kinase A (PKA) can lead to translational changes that determine the proteins the postsynaptic neuron synthesizes. The affected genes may code for proteins involved in the synthesis of neurotransmitters, such as tyrosine hydroxylase, proteins that can modulate the state of ion channels, or even the assembly of ion channels themselves. Such responses occur on a time scale even longer than those of responses mediated by second-messenger cascades. The responses are generated in minutes to hours and may persist for weeks, months, or perhaps even permanently.

Inactivation

Once the released neurotransmitter has interacted with postsynaptic receptors, it must be removed from the synaptic cleft in a timely manner to enable new signals to get through in another cycle of synaptic transmission. It also is important to remove the transmitter from the cleft because its continued presence there at a high concentration can lead to the **desensitization** of certain receptors. When desensitization occurs, receptors no longer respond to the transmitter. The situation has been compared to two people talking. If words persisted as an echo in the space between the talker and listener, effective communication would be impossible. However, after activating the listener's auditory system, words disappear as the sound waves forming them dissipate into the surrounding air. After activating the postsynaptic receptor, a transmitter detaches from the receptor and reenters the synaptic cleft, where it will again "roam" about in search of another unoccupied receptor.

Three different mechanisms exist by which transmitter is cleared from the synaptic cleft. The first is by simple **diffusion** out of the cleft. Diffusion dilutes the concentration of transmitter in the extracellular fluid of the synapse and takes it out of the range of available receptors. To some extent, all neurotransmitters are inactivated by this

Neuropathology Box 4-1: The Addicted Brain

Two common recreational drugs, cocaine and the amphetamines, affect the inactivation of the transmitter dopamine (DA) by blocking the transporter mechanism involved in its reuptake. Amphetamines, in addition, increase the release of DA. Both of these drugs are highly addictive, and both cause changes in brain structure and function. The fundamental changes that occur at the molecular, cellular, structural, and functional levels persist long after use of the drug has stopped. For example, it has been shown that glucose metabolism remains impaired in the brains of cocaine addicts up to 100 days after withdrawal from cocaine.

Individual drugs may have certain effects specific to that drug and are not shared by other drugs of abuse, but all drugs of abuse have in common an effect on the mesolimbocortical dopaminergic system. This system is comprised of connections between the basal ganglia (of the midbrain) and limbic and prefrontal cortical areas. Cocaine sustains synaptic concentrations of DA at a high level by blocking the transporter molecule that would otherwise carry DA back into the neurons that release it. Normally, DA-producing neurons inactivate DA by transporting it back into them (re-uptake). The effect of cocaine is to keep the neurons that respond to DA responding at an abnormally high level for a longer than normal period of time. Amphetamines penetrate DA-producing cells and stimulate them to release more DA than they normally would. Amphetamines also secondarily block re-uptake.

The mesolimbocortical dopaminergic system participates in self-survival; hence, it directly or indirectly affects three types of control systems in the brain: (1) It is an essential component of the motivational control system. This system prompts the individual to take drug-seeking and drug-taking actions. (2) It affects physical control systems that result in the autonomic and somatic actions of the drug. These lead to physical dependence with continued drug ingestion and to physical withdrawal when drug-taking is stopped. (3) It affects associative memory systems that result in the occurrence of cue-dependent drug-craving. Thus, people, situations, and objects associated with previous drug-taking episodes elicit the desire to take drugs.

The pattern of drug-seeking and drug-taking behaviors that characterize addiction develop because chronic drug exposure hijacks the mesolimbocortical dopaminergic system. Chronic drug exposure causes DA-receiving neurons to adapt to the continued presence of the drug. This chronic exposure alters the functioning of individual DA-responding neurons. Because these individual neurons are members of functional systems of neurons (neuron circuits), the functioning of the circuits to which the neurons belong is altered. Bombarded by abnormally high levels of DA, DA-receiving neurons respond "defensively" by reducing the number of receptors with which DA can bind. These changes in brain function continue for months or years after the last use of the drug. This accounts for the occurrence of relapse into drug-taking after a period of abstinence. When brain levels of the drug drop in a user who had maintained prolonged, heavy use of the substance (thereby causing a decrease in brain DA), DA-receiving neurons experience a DA deficit. This may result in the appearance of unpleasant withdrawal symptoms that have a "negative-reinforcing" action. Thus, while addicts initially take a drug to feel high, they continue drug ingestion to avoid feeling low. However, not all addictive drugs produce physical dependence as manifested by a withdrawal syndrome. Significantly, withdrawal may not be readily apparent with the use of stimulants such as amphetamine and cocaine.

mechanism. It is probably most important for the large-molecule, peptide neurotransmitters. As noted in Chapter 3, astrocytes surrounding the synapse assist in removal of transmitter that has diffused from the synaptic cleft.

The second mechanism is **enzymatic degradation** of the neurotransmitter. The best-known example of this type of inactivation is for the transmitter acetylcholine. The enzyme **acetylcholinesterase** is located in the synaptic cleft. It breaks acetylcholine down into choline and acetate, making it unable to interact with ACh receptors.

The third mechanism is by a process called **re-uptake**. The term is appropriate because the nerve terminal that releases the neurotransmitter takes it back into itself after it has interacted with a receptor. The membrane of the nerve terminal contains transporters that attract the transmitter and pump it back into the terminal. Once within the terminal, the neurotransmitter can be destroyed, recycled, or pumped back into a synaptic vesicle for reuse. Re-uptake seems to be the most common mechanism for inactivating transmitters. The biogenic amines (serotonin, dopamine, and norepinephrine) and the amino acid transmitters (GABA, glycine, and glutamate) are all inactivated by re-uptake mechanisms.

Table 4-2 ■ summarizes some of the drugs and toxins that affect different steps in the process of synaptic transmission.

Table 4-2 Drugs and Toxins Affecting Different Steps in Synaptic Transmission

DRUGS THAT ENHANCE STEPS IN CHEMICAL SYNAPTIC TRANSMISSION*	DRUGS OR TOXINS THAT BLOCK STEPS IN CHEMICAL SYNAPTIC TRANSMISSION*
Synthesis The drug L-DOPA is metabolized into the transmitter dopamine thus compensating for reduced dopamine levels in Parkinson's disease.	
Storage Monoamine oxidase inhibitors (e.g., Nardil) are antidepressant drugs that increase the storage of monoamine transmitters.	
Release Amphetamines (psychomotor stimulants) stimulate dopamine-producing neurons to release more dopamine than they normally would.	Release Tetanus toxin blocks the release of GABA. Botulinus toxin, causing botulism or food-poisoning, blocks the release of acetylcholine at the neuromuscular junction.
Transmitter-receptor interaction The tranquilizers Librium and Valium (antianxiety agents called benzodiazepines) increase the frequency of opening of GABA-gated Cl⁻ channels. Barbiturate tranquilizers (sedatives) increase the duration of opening of GABA-gated Cl⁻ channels. Narcotic analgesics (opium and its derivatives—morphine and heroin—and synthetic opiates like Demerol and Darvon) bind with G-coupled opiate receptors to increase the level of cyclic-AMP generated intracellular messengers.	Transmitter-receptor interaction Curare (arrow-head poison) blocks nicotinic acetylcholine receptors at the neuromuscular junction. Strychnine blocks glycine-gated Cl⁻ channels. Phencyclidine (PCP, "angel dust") blocks NMDA-type glutamate receptors. Antipsychotic drugs like Haloperidol used to treat schizophrenia block specific G-protein-coupled dopamine receptors.
	Inactivation Antidepressant drugs such as Prozac (fluoxetine) and Zoloft (sertraline) selectively block the re-uptake of serotonin. Cocaine blocks the re-uptake of monoamine transmitters. Amphetamines secondarily block the re-uptake of monoamines. Anticholinesterases inhibitors block the degradation of the transmitter acetylcholine. Mestinon (pyridostigmine) is used to treat myasthenia gravis. Tacrine is used to treat early stage Alzheimer's disease.

*These drugs may result in increased or decreased overall activity in the nervous system. The effect depends on the nature of the specific transmitter–receptor interaction as discussed earlier for norepinephrine.

Gap Junctions and Electrical Synapses

The morphological substrate for electrical synapses between neurons is the **gap junction** (Figure 4-28 ▪). At gap junctions, the normal separation between cells is reduced from about 20 nm to only 3 nm. Gap-junction channels (called *connexons* that are formed from six cylindrically arranged transmembrane proteins called *connexins*) are present in the membranes of both the presynaptic and postsynaptic cell. The channels line up with and contact one another to form a continuous bridge between the cytoplasm of the two cells. Because the central pore in gap-junction channels is larger than in ion channels, not only can ions move easily from one cell to the next, but small molecules also can pass between cells. In electrical

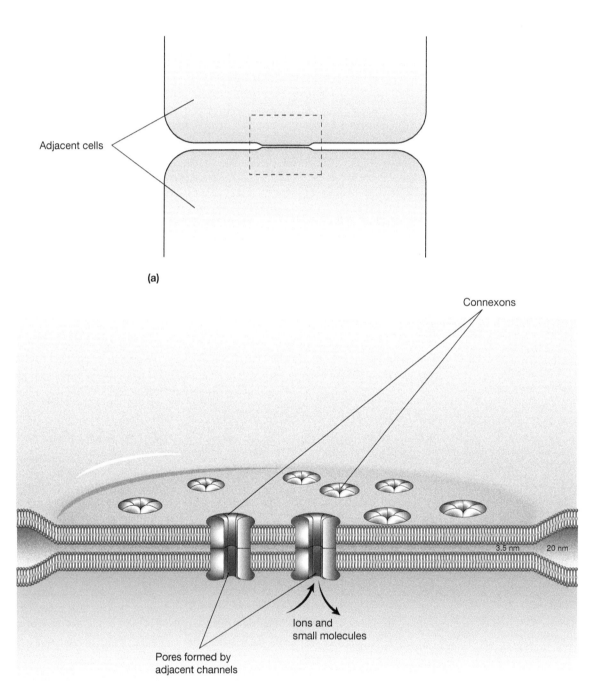

FIGURE 4-28 (a) Structure of a gap junction connecting the neurites of two cells. Each channel in the membrane is called a connexon (b) and is formed by six cylindrically arranged transmembrane proteins called connexins. Connexons are present in both membranes of a gap junction, and they line up and contact one another to form a continuous bridge between the cytoplasm of the two cells. Ions and small molecules can pass bidirectionally through the connexons.

synapses, an action potential in one neuron creates a flow of current (ions) that passes through the gap junction; if the current is large enough to depolarize the postsynaptic cell, voltage-gated channels in that cell will open to trigger another action potential. Electrical synapses produce very rapid responses and can connect large groups of neurons to create coordinated responses to stimuli. It is significant that the conductance of some gap junctions can be modulated by second-messenger effects, thereby permitting regulation of the coupling between neurons (see Chapter 18).

However, gap junctions between neurons are relatively rare in the adult human brain, perhaps because such a mode of neuronal communication eliminates the capacity of individual neurons to process information independently of one another. The latter is the hallmark of neuronal communication via chemical synaptic transmission. Also, gap junctions allow for a bidirectional communication between neurons in contrast to chemical synaptic transmission, which is unidirectional.

CLINICAL CONNECTIONS

Several disorders illustrate the use of pharmacologic approaches to managing symptoms associated with dysfunctions of neural transmission. Two of these disorders illustrate the importance of providing additional neurotransmitter in management of symptoms associated with nervous system dysfunction. Others illustrate the importance of preventing the inactivation mechanism in certain circumstances. Finally, Charcot-Marie-Tooth disease illustrates the consequences of gap junction pathology.

Parkinson's Disease

The substantia nigra, a nucleus of the midbrain, produces one of the amine transmitters, dopamine (DA), which is of particular importance in the production of movement. The substantia nigra degenerates in Parkinson's disease (PD), resulting in a dramatic reduction in the quantity of available DA and contributing to many of the signs and symptoms of PD (see Chapter 19). The synthesis of dopamine (DA) is specifically manipulated in the treatment of Parkinson's disease. The most common treatment strategy in Parkinson's disease is called replacement therapy because it seeks to replace the deficient DA. The easiest way to accomplish this would simply be to give the patient oral DA. Unfortunately, DA does not cross the blood–brain barrier. However, its precursor, L-DOPA, does. The excess L-DOPA occurring with oral administration of L-DOPA is taken into the *still-surviving* DA neurons, stimulating them to increase their synthesis of DA above their normal levels. As a result, more DA is stored and released when these surviving neurons are active.

Biologic Depression

One hypothesis concerning the etiology of **biologic depression** is that it is due to a deficiency in the brain of the amine transmitters—NE and/or 5-HT. One way

of increasing the availability of these transmitters is to store more in synaptic vesicles so that when active, NE and 5-HT neurons release more of their transmitters. One of the earliest strategies for accomplishing this (circa 1950) was to administer a drug to depressed patients that inhibits the degradative enzyme monoamine oxidase (MAO), thereby increasing the transmitter's storage pool. As a result, increased amounts of NE and 5-HT are released when the neurons discharge. Although **MAO inhibitors** still are used, they are drugs of second or third choice in the treatment of psychiatric disorders because of the possibility of unwanted side effects due to their toxicity and complex interactions with many other drugs. It should be noted that these drug treatments can require three to four weeks for efficacy, possibly as a result of the time required for changes in gene expression of reuptake blockers.

Charcot-Marie-Tooth Disorder

Although gap junction pathology (channelopathy) is not known to be involved in any disease of the human brain, such pathology does occur in the most common form of inherited peripheral neuropathy, **Charcot-Marie-Tooth disease (CMT)**. The genetic mutation in CMT affects the connexins that join adjacent layers of myelin in Schwann cells, resulting in demyelination and loss of peripheral axons. The consequence of this peripheral nerve degeneration is weakness, sensory loss, and atrophy of the distal muscles. Together, these impairments lead to difficulty walking.

Phenylketoneuria

Phenylketoneuria (PKU) is a rare, inherited, metabolic disease that prevents the essential dietary amino acid phenylalanine from being properly metabolized into tyrosine. It is due to a deficiency of the hepatic enzyme phenylalanine hydroxylase and results in the accumulation of high levels of phenylalanine in the blood and brain. The latter stunts development in the rapidly growing postnatal brain, and severe mental retardation results, along with other disorders in some people. High levels of phenylpyruvic acid also occur in the blood, CSF, and urine, the latter circumstance being the basis of a screening test required for all newborns in the United States. Infants with PKU are placed on a special diet with a severe restriction (but not a total elimination) of phenylalanine, which may be continued through adolescence or after. If instituted in infancy, intellectual development improves, but once the neurological deficit unfolds, diet has little effect on intellectual status. In countries with widespread screening for PKU and the initiation of dietary therapy in early postnatal life, neurological damage associated with PKU is less common.

Aspartame is a low-calorie artificial sweetener found in more than 6,000 food products, including carbonated soft drinks and tabletop sweeteners. Aspartame is hydrolyzed by the intestine into phenylalanine (and other products), which is then absorbed into the blood. Although it is not harmful to healthy individuals, people with PKU must consider aspartame as an additional source of phenylalanine. Aspartame-containing foods produced in the United States must state "Phenylketoneurics: Contains Phenylalanine."

Therapeutic Drugs Affecting Transmitter Inactivation

A variety of neurologic disorders characterized by a neurotransmitter deficiency are treated *symptomatically* by manipulating the inactivation mechanism. **Alzheimer's disease**, for example, is characterized by a degeneration of neurons synthesizing ACh. **Anticholinesterase** medications prolong the action of *available* ACh by blocking the action of the inactivating enzyme acetylcholinesterase. Likewise, **myasthenia gravis**, a disorder of skeletal neuromuscular transmission, is treated with anticholinesterase medication. Similarly, one of the latest generation of antidepressant medications, the **selective serotonin reuptake inhibitors (SSRIs)**, block the re-uptake of the transmitter serotonin that is deficient in some cases of biologic depression. SSRIs are preferred over the MAO inhibitors discussed earlier.

SYNAPTIC PLASTICITY

Clinical Preview ....

One of the most intriguing frontiers in rehabilitation is the possibility of neuroplasticity as a mechanism for recovery from injury. You are working with John Curry, a 14-year-old boy who sustained an incomplete spinal cord injury at the T4 level. Based on recent evidence suggesting that there may be plasticity of the nervous system, one of your colleagues has suggested using high-intensity treadmill training to assist in his recovery of walking. As you read through this section, begin to consider the mechanisms that could explain the possibility of plasticity in individuals who have incomplete spinal cord injury.

Plasticity refers to the brain's capacity to be shaped by experience. Thus, plasticity is activity dependent. Many different manifestations of plasticity have been investigated. On the level of gross anatomy, changes in the activity of different regions of the CNS in response to disease, recovery from brain injury, and therapeutic training have been analyzed using contemporary imaging technology. This is called **map plasticity** because it reflects how a normal map of brain function changes with experience. Map plasticity is discussed in Chapter 26.

At a cellular level, plasticity has been analyzed by examining the functional relationship between presynaptic and postsynaptic neurons as a result of the pattern of activity in the presynaptic neuron. At the cellular level, this means that plasticity must operate by regulating the expression and function of virtually the entire roster of molecules that mediate neuronal and synaptic function. This, in turn, results in modifications in structure and function in both pre- and postsynaptic neurons. The search for long-term experienced-induced alterations in the strengths of synaptic relationships among neurons participating in given functions has focused on two experimental phenomena, known as **long-term potentiation (LTP)** and **long-term depression (LTD)**. Both phenomena assess the strength of synaptic connection between pre- and postsynaptic neurons. The intense experimental interest in LTP and LTD has been fueled by the hypothesis that these forms of synaptic plasticity may participate in learning and information storage. Yet this goal remains elusive (but perhaps still promising) in that neither phenomena has been *unequivocally* linked to either learning or memory. Certainly, very few neuroscientists would be willing to make the claim that LTP, for example, is sufficient for either of these functions. Moreover, the cellular and molecular mechanisms underlying LTP and LTD have been studied overwhelmingly in animal models (especially in rodents) and in two brain regions (the hippocampus and cerebellum), whose neuronal organization is much more transparent than in the remainder of the CNS. In contrast, research into LTP in humans is very limited. The only direct evidence of synaptic plasticity in humans has been provided by studying brain tissue excised from patients undergoing surgery for intractable epilepsy, a condition in which the tissue studied may be abnormal to begin with.

Long-Term Potentiation and Long-Term Depression

LTP and LTD are defined as the persistent increase or decrease, respectively, in synaptic strength induced in a postsynaptic neuron by conditioning electrical stimuli delivered to its presynaptic afferents. Such conditioning stimulation is commonly referred to as a **tetany**, but the word usage is not entirely correct. LTP, at least, can last for weeks or months.

LTP and LTD are studied using the following protocol. First, a baseline is established in which the magnitude of postsynaptic EPSPs elicited by a series of test stimuli delivered every minute or so to presynaptic neurons is measured. Either LTP or LTD is then induced by electrically stimulating the same presynaptic axons with conditioning stimuli. The strength of the postsynaptic response resulting from such stimulation is then assessed by measuring the amplitude of EPSPs elicited by subsequent test stimuli applied to the presynaptic axons. The larger the amplitude of postconditioning EPSPs to a test stimulus relative to baseline (i.e., without the previous conditioning stimulation), the stronger the postsynaptic effect, and vise versa.

In order to induce LTP, the same axons to which the test stimuli are applied are given a brief burst of high-frequency stimulation (e.g., 50 to 100 stimuli at a frequency of 100/sec, a "tetany"). This causes a long-lasting increase in the amplitude of EPSPs evoked by subsequent test stimuli. Test stimuli delivered to other presynaptic inputs onto the same cell that did not receive the brief tetanic stimulation do not generate EPSPs of increased amplitude, showing that LTP is *input specific.*

In order to induce LTD, the presynaptic axons to which the test stimuli are delivered are subjected to low-frequency stimulation (about 1/sec) for long periods (10 to 15 minutes). This pattern of presynaptic activity depresses the baseline EPSPs evoked by subsequent test stimuli for several hours. Like LTP, LTD is input specific in that there is no change in the size of EPSPs evoked in the postsynaptic neuron by stimulation of an input that was not subjected to the low-frequency stimulation.

Thought Question

What are some of the cellular changes associated with LTP and LTD?

Both LTP and LTD depend on an interaction between the two types of glutamate receptors noted earlier—that is, on NMDA and AMPA receptors. And both LTP and LTD *begin* with the *same* signal—namely, the entrance of Ca^{2+} through the NMDA receptor. However, the key difference here is the effect frequency of the tetany has on the magnitude of the postsynaptic depolarization and thus on the postsynaptic NMDA receptor. NMDA receptors are activated by binding with glutamate, as noted earlier, but their channels are "clogged" by Mg^{2+} ions. Thus, even when bound with glutamate, NMDA receptors do not admit much Ca^{2+} *until* the Mg^{2+} block is fully removed. Such removal occurs only with a strong depolarization of the postsynaptic neuron. In contrast, weak depolarization of the postsynaptic neuron does not remove the Mg^{2+} block so that little Ca^{2+} enters the postsynaptic neuron. High-frequency tetanic stimulation of presynaptic neurons results in strong depolarization of the postsynaptic neuron, removal of the Mg^{2+} block, and the entry of high levels of Ca^{2+} into the postsynaptic neuron. Low-frequency tetanic stimulation of presynaptic neurons, on the other hand, does not strongly depolarize the postsynaptic neuron so that the Mg^{2+} block is not removed and little Ca^{2+} enters the postsynaptic neuron.

How much Ca^{2+} enters the postsynaptic neuron through NMDA receptors determines what happens to the number of AMPA receptors in the postsynaptic plasma membrane. AMPA receptors are subject to rapid exo- and endocytosis in the plasma membrane because there is a mobile pool of receptors residing in the postsynaptic density of dendritic spines. Recall that the postsynaptic density

(PSD) represents the plasma membrane across from the presynaptic active zone. LTP and LTD are dependent on the rapid redistribution of AMPA receptors into and out of the postsynaptic plasma membrane, respectively.

Strong depolarization of NMDA receptors and high Ca^{2+} entry leads to the delivery of AMPA receptors into dendritic spines at synapses (exocytosis). This results from the activation of intracellular protein kinases. Protein kinases also increase the effectiveness of existing AMPA receptors by phosphorylating them. This increases the effectiveness of bound glutamate leading to LTP.

Weak depolarization of NMDA receptors leads to little Ca^{2+} entry, and the activation of protein phosphatases that have the opposite effect on AMPA receptors leads to their removal from the postsynaptic plasma membrane (endocytosis). The result is a decrease in the strength of the synapse to bound glutamate.

There is, then, an activity-dependent redistribution of AMPA receptors into and out of the postsynaptic membrane. Which of these competing processes is dominant will determine synaptic strength. This, in turn, will be a function of the pattern of activity experienced by the neuron. The long-term maintenance of LTP involves alterations in gene expression and shifts in protein synthesis in the postsynaptic neuron.

Structural modifications occurring in the synapse are thought to underlie the expression LTP. One such model focuses on structural modifications occurring in the postsynaptic plasma membrane that lead to the production of new dendritic spines and new synapses. The activation of Ca^{2+}-dependent signal-transduction pathways leads to the translocation of AMPA receptors into the dendritic spine and receptor insertion into the plasma membrane via a mechanism analogous to exocytosis. The latter increases the size of the PSD, eventually resulting in its perforation. These perforated spines then split so that a second spine is generated—and still in contact with the same presynaptic terminal as its neighbor. Retrograde signaling from this multi-spine synapse to the presynaptic neuron then elicits the formation of a second presynaptic terminal. Thus, eventually, LTP results in an increase in the total number of synapses.

LTD, on the other hand, involves a cascade of events the opposite of those occurring in LTP. Thus, the activation of a Ca^{2+}-dependent signal-transduction pathway leads to the endocytosis and loss of AMPA receptors from the PSD, which decreases its size. Eventually, the dendritic spine itself disappears.

LTP research has revealed that six different cellular mechanisms may be involved in enhancing the strength of synaptic transmission, with some being located in the presynaptic neuron and others in the postsynaptic neuron:

1. The fraction of available presynaptic vesicles that actually *are* released could be increased, for example, from one out of four vesicles in a normal synapse (25 percent release probability) to two out of four

available vesicles (50 percent release probability). Note there is no structural change here, only a functional change.

2. The number of synaptic vesicles available for release could be increased.

3. The number of release sites in the presynaptic membrane could be increased. Mechanisms 2 and 3 both involve structural changes that would require the growth of new presynaptic machinery for transmitter release. Such growth, in turn, is dependent on the synthesis of new RNA and protein in the cell body and axoplasmic transport to the presynaptic axon terminal.

4. The sensitivity of available receptors on the postsynaptic membrane could be increased.

5. The number of available postsynaptic receptors could be increased by inserting new ones into the postsynaptic membrane.

6. New synaptic contacts (synaptogenesis) between the same pair of neurons could be generated by the growth of new dendritic spines in the postsynaptic neuron. Mechanisms 5 and 6 obviously are structural changes that require the synthesis of new protein and RNA, this time in the postsynaptic neuron.

The concept of "silent synapses" has received considerable attention recently. The concept relates to activity dependent development of glutaminergic synapses. These synapses become active by increasing the number of postsynaptic AMPA receptors. Early animal studies identified these synapses in the spinal cord, brainstem, and hippocampus. Subsequently these have been identified throughout the brain. Silent synapses are gradually turned on during the developmental process. In the adult, synapses that had been active can revert to silence and then may be turned on again in response to activity by insertion of the post synaptic AMPA receptors. While much remains to be learned about these synapses, it has been suggested that silent synapses provide a simple and effective mechanism for modifying neural circuits in response to synaptic activity.

Importantly, the silent synapses illustrate that the synapse itself can serve as an operational processing unit. By turning this processing unit on and off, it is possible to alter the functions of the brain itself. The complex physiology is predominantly mediated by glutamate receptors. If a given synapse has only NMDA receptors, it will be largely silent. The dynamic insertion of glutamate AMPA receptors or their removal is what turns the synapse on or off. The visual system provides an example of activation of synapses during development (Chapter 18). Finally, the turning on of silent synapses has profound implications for plasticity (and hence for learning and rehabilitation) which are discussed in Chapter 26.

Summary

Whether resting or active, all differences in electrical potential across the plasma membrane of a neuron are generated by the movement of ions across the membrane. Such ion fluxes are possible only when the membrane is permeable to one or more ion species and only when there is an electrochemical gradient that promotes ion flow. At rest, the neuron is not in a signaling mode. Nonetheless, ion fluxes are occurring across its membrane. This is because passive, always open leak channels permeable to Na^+ and K^+ are present in the membrane and because electrochemical gradients for the two ions have been established by the Na^+–K^+ pump, wherein Na^+ is in high concentration outside the neuron and K^+ is in high concentration inside the neuron. However, the number of K^+ leak channels is much greater than the number of Na^+ leak channels. Thus, the Na^+–K^+ pump, as well other pumps and other factors, maintain the unequal distribution of ions across the membrane, leaving the inside of the neuron negatively charged—that is, at a membrane potential of about –65 mV.

When a neuron shifts into an active signaling mode, all of the electrical signals it generates depend on the resting membrane potential because they involve a change in the membrane's permeability pattern away from that characterizing the resting state. Not all neurons generate the same array of electrical signals, but all generate two types: graded and nongraded. Graded potentials include receptor potentials that occur on the receptive zone of sensory neurons and postsynaptic potentials that occur on the receptive zones of postsynaptic neurons. In both cases, graded potentials function to encode and integrate the information they receive either from the environment or from other neurons. The nongraded potential is the all-or-none action potential whose function is to conduct information from the receiving to the transmitting end of the neuron and, once at the terminal, to trigger the release of neurotransmitter. An action potential is generated when there is a very brief rise in Na^+ influx across the membrane that has become dominantly permeable to Na^+. This brief rise is followed by a secondary brief rise in K^+ permeability, wherein the K^+ efflux repolarizes the membrane. When these "explosive" active permeability changes subside, the membrane potential returns to its resting level because of the high resting membrane permeability to K^+. The speed of conduction of the AP along the length of an axon is increased if the axon is myelinated.

Neurotransmitters are the essential links between neurons (and between neurons and effector cells). The structural specializations on the pre- and postsynaptic sides of the synapse that subserve synaptic transmission were addressed. Five distinct steps are involved in synaptic transmission: synthesis, storage, release, transmitter–receptor interaction, and inactivation. Importantly, each of these steps can be influenced by exogenous drugs and/or toxins, and some are the target of specific neurologic disease. The postsynaptic signaling actions of neurotransmitters are mediated by two very different families of neurotransmitter receptors. Ligand-gated ion channels (ionotropic) combine a receptor subunit with a channel subunit into a single molecular entity. As a consequence, they give rise to rapid postsynaptic electrical responses (EPSPs and IPSPs). Metabotropic receptors, on the other hand, regulate postsynaptic responses indirectly, via G-proteins, and therefore cause slower and longer-lasting electrical responses. The most rapid responses meditated by metabotropic receptors occur when the G-proteins themselves open ion channels. Slower metabotropic responses result from the activation of intracellular effector enzymes whose activity modulates the phosphorylation of intracellular proteins and/or gene transcription.

In addition to facilitating understanding of information processing and signaling in the nervous system, as well as the effects of drugs, understanding chemical synaptic transmission provides insight into a potential cellular basis of learning and memory. The phenomenon of neural plasticity has been investigated at a cellular level by studying long-term potentiation (LTP) and long-term depression (LTD). Both LTP and LTD involve NMDA and AMPA glutamate receptors.

Applications

1. Clostridium botulinum releases a potent neurotoxin. Investigate the historical use of this bacterium. Identify the mechanism of action of the neurotoxin. Identify the current medical and nonmedical uses of clostridium botulinum.

2. Diagram the synapse and outline the steps in synaptic transmission. Consider the following agents: chlordiazepoxide, phenelzine sulfate, and setraline hydrochloride. For each agent, identify the drug's impact on synaptic transmission.

3. Leslie Sorenson is a 35-year-old woman who has multiple sclerosis. One morning, while taking a leisurely hot shower, her vision seemed to dim like a fog coming over her eyes.
   a. What neuroanatomical structure is affected by multiple sclerosis, and what is the consequence?
   b. By what mechanism does temperature affect the safety factor for individuals with multiple sclerosis, and how does this relate to the change in Leslie Sorenson's vision?

References

Electrical Signals of Neurons

Koester, J., and Siegelbaum, S. A. Ch. 7. Membrane potential. In: *Principles of Neural Science*, 4th ed. Kandel E. R., Schwartz, J. H., and Jessell, T. M. (eds). McGraw-Hill, New York, 2000.

Koester, J., and Siegelbaum, S. A. Ch. 8. Local signaling: Passive electrical properties of the neuron. In: *Principles of Neural Science*, 4th ed. Kandel E. R., Schwartz, J. H., and Jessell, T. M. (eds). McGraw-Hill, New York, 2000.

Koester, J., and Siegelbaum, S. A. Ch. 9. Propagated signaling: The action potential. In: *Principles of Neural Science*, 4th ed. Kandel E. R., Schwartz, J. H., and Jessell, T. M. (eds). McGraw-Hill, New York, 2000.

Waxman, S. G., Kocsis, J. D., and Stys, P. K. (eds). *The Axon: Structure, Function, and Pathophysiology*. Oxford University Press, New York, 1995.

Synapses and Synaptic Transmission

Bullock, T., et al. The neuron doctrine, redux. *Science* 310:791–793, 2005.

Clapham, D. E. Direct G protein activation of ion channels. *Ann Rev Neurosci* 17:441, 1994.

Hahn, A. F., et al. Pathological findings in the X-linked form of Charcot-Marie-Tooth disease: A morphometric and ultrastructural analysis. *Acta Neuropath* 101:129, 2001.

Matthews, G. Neurotransmitter release. *Ann Rev Neurosci* 19:219, 1996.

Ropper, A. H., and Brown, R. H. Ch. 43. Disorders of the nervous system due to drugs, toxins, and other chemical agents. In: *Adams and Victor's Principles of Neurology*, 8th ed. McGraw-Hill, New York, 2005.

Stuart, G., Spruston, N., and Hausser, M., eds. *Dendrites*. Oxford University Press, New York, 1999.

Sudhof, T. C. The synaptic vesicle cycle. *Annu Rev Neurosci* 27:509–547, 2004.

Multiple Sclerosis

Aktas, O., Ullrich, O., Infante-Durate, C., et al. Neuronal damage in brain inflammation. *Arch Neurol* 64:185–189, 2007.

Antel, J., and Owens, T. Multiple sclerosis and immune regulatory cells. *Brain* 127:1915–1916, 2004.

Compston, A. Making progress on the natural history of multiple sclerosis. *Brain* 129:561–563, 2006.

DeLuca, G. C., Ebers, G. C., and Esiri, M. M. Axonal loss in multiple sclerosis: A pathological survey of the corticospinal and sensory tracts. *Brain* 127:1009–1018, 2004.

Kutzelnigg, A. Lucchinetti, C. F., Stadelmann, C., et al. Cortical demyelination and diffuse white matter injury in multiple sclerosis. *Brain* 128:2705–2712, 2005.

Stys, P. K. Axonal degeneration in multiple sclerosis: Is it time for neuroprotective strategies? *Ann Neurol* 55:601–603, 2004.

Synaptic Plasticity

Beck, H., Goussakov, I. V., Lie, A., et al. Synaptic plasticity in the human dentate gyrus. *J Neurosci* 20:7080–7086, 2000.

Buccino, G., Solodkin, A., and Small, S. L. Functions of the mirror neuron system: Implications for neurorehabilitation. *Cog Behav Neurol* 19:55–63, 2006.

Cooke, S. F., and Bliss, T. V. P. Plasticity in the human central nervous system. *Brain* 129:1659–1673, 2006.

Ji, R.-R., Kohno, T., Moore, K. A., and Woolf, C. J. Central sensitization and LTP: Do pain and memory share similar mechanisms? *TRENDS Neurosci* 26:696–705, 2003.

Keller, A., Iriki, A., and Asanuma, H. Identification of neurons producing long-term potentiation in the cat motor cortex: intracellular recordings and labeling. *J Comp Neurol* 300:47–60, 1990.

Kandel, E. R. Ch. 63. Cellular mechanisms of learning and the biological basis of individuality. In: Kandel, E R., Schwartz, J. H., and Jessel, T. M. (eds) *Principles of Neural Science*, 4th ed. McGraw-Hill, New York, 2000.

Luscher, C., Nicoll, R. A., Malenka, R. C., and Muller, D. Synaptic plasticity and dynamic modulation of the postsynaptic membrane. *Nature Neurosci* 3:545–550, 2000.

Nolte, J. *The Human Brain: An Introduction to Its Functional Anatomy*. Mosby Elsevier, Philadelphia, 2009.

PEARSON

myhealthprofessionskit™

Use this address to access the Companion Website created for this textbook. Simply select "Physical Therapy" from the choice of disciplines. Find this book and log in using your username and password to access self-assessment questions, a glossary, answers to the applications questions, and more.

PART II

Anatomy of the Major Regions of the Central Nervous System and Their Blood Supply

The study of neuroscience provides the basis from which we appreciate the generation and control of functional movement. In addition, neuroscience provides the basis from which we predict the signs and symptoms of disorders of the nervous system and interpret the consequences of specific injuries. Take, for example, a 17-year-old male who was diving in a shallow pool, hit the bottom, and sustained a complete cervical spinal cord injury. A second 17-year-old was riding his bicycle in the rain, skidded into an oncoming car, and sustained an incomplete injury to the thoracic spinal cord. Through an appreciation of the neurophysiology of tissue damage in the spinal cord, anatomy of the spinal cord, and the pathways connecting the spinal cord with the cortex, it is possible to anticipate the very different consequences of these two injuries. Now consider a young woman who had an accident while riding her bike, sustained some thoracic spinal cord damage, and also damaged brainstem structures. This woman's situation will be quite different from the young man who injured the thoracic spinal cord without brainstem damage. And finally consider what would have happened to the bicyclist if she also sustained damage to structures of the cerebrum!

With your understanding of clinical neuroscience, you will be prepared to compare and contrast the anticipated consequences of these four injuries, linking neurological damage with resulting signs and symptoms and inferring the implications for physical intervention. Indeed, eventually you will be able to "tell a whole story" of what happened to these different individuals from a neurophysiological and neuroanatomical perspective. You will be able to discuss the consequences of the injuries in terms of control of movement and cognitive function, to infer the likelihood of recovery, and to apply foundational information to your decisions about how to best assist each of these individuals with their physical recovery. This may sound like a tall order, but if you absorb the information in steps, the task is very manageable.

Just as children learn to read by first learning simple words and simple sentence structure, so too will you begin with the basic building blocks of the nervous system and the overall structures. Chapters 1 through 4 began the basic introduction to that language and to the way that cells interact. But there is much more to learn. You can think of the next three chapters of this text as providing more of the basic language of the nervous system and the simple sentence structure necessary to fully appreciate the situation of each of the individuals described earlier.

Chapter 5 provides the names of many of the important structures in the spinal cord and brainstem. This chapter also introduces the concept of pathways, or tracts, that link information from one part of the nervous system to another and introduces a few of the important tracts that traverse the spinal cord. Proceeding rostrally, Chapter 6 delves into the basic structures of the diencephalon (including the thalamus and hypothalamus) as well as the cerebellum. Chapter 7 introduces the basic structure and connections of the cerebral cortex and basal ganglia. Included in these three chapters are basic structures, some basic connections, and the blood supply of many of these areas. Once you have learned the basic information in Chapters 5, 6, and 7, you will be prepared to learn more detailed language and connections that are presented in the next two parts of the text. Together, this foundational knowledge will allow you to read this most fascinating story of the nervous system. You will also be prepared to compare and contrast the injuries of the three individuals described, as well as a host of other disorders and injuries.

While the task of learning the language and function of the nervous system takes patience and diligence, it will pay off in the end. You will be well positioned to understand and appreciate how diverse sensory, motor, and cognitive information is synthesized by the nervous system in order to allow us to function in this multifaceted environment in which we live.

Spinal Cord and Brainstem

LEARNING OUTCOMES

This chapter prepares the reader to:

1. Identify the following structures: lumbar cistern, conus medullaris, substantia gelatinosa, Rexed's laminae.

2. Name the membranous coverings of the spinal cord and briefly describe the characteristics of each.

3. Name major nuclei of the spinal cord and identify them in cross sections.

4. Define lower motor neurons, recall their location and identify them in cross sections of the spinal cord.

5. Characterize five tracts that traverse the spinal cord in terms of their origin and destination, location within the spinal cord, and major function.

6. Differentiate the blood vessels from which the anterior and posterior arteries of the spinal cord originate and name the segmental vessels derived from each.

7. Identify major components of vertebrae and the location of the spinal cord with respect to the vertebral column.

8. Discuss the causes and consequences associated with the syndrome of the anterior spinal artery.

9. Relate the anatomy of the vertebral column and spinal cord to lesions such as disc herniation and spondylosis that produce pain and loss of function.

10. Recognize levels of the brainstem from cross sections by correlating the shape with surface features of the brainstem.

11. Differentiate effector from interneuronal zones of the reticular formation in terms of their location and the cells that comprise them.

12. Name the major afferent, efferent, and projection systems of the reticular formation.

13. Compare seven states of consciousness that relate to reticular formation function.

ACRONYMS

AL Anterolateral system
ARAS Ascending reticular activating system
CSF Cerebrospinal fluid
LMN Lower motor neuron
STT Spinothalamic tract

Introduction

This chapter further explores the organization of the spinal cord and brainstem, concentrating primarily on the internal structures comprising each. The first major section presents the meningeal investments of the spinal cord as well as its structural features and blood supply. This section focuses on the internal structure of the spinal cord, its nuclei, and fiber tracts. Not all of the fiber tracts residing in the white matter of the spinal cord are presented although they all are enumerated in Table 5-2. The spinal cord is the route through which somatosensory information from the body enters the CNS and motor signals for controlling movement of the body exit the CNS. For example, when a person sits curled up with a blanket and pillow in front of a fire, information about the person's environment enters the central nervous system. The information travels rostrally, by way of the spinal cord, to the brain for processing, interpretation, and generation of actions. If the pillow and blanket are soft and comforting, the person might fall asleep. Sensory information travels in specific pathways, many of which have been characterized. The spinal cord also is the thoroughfare by which the CNS signals to specific muscle groups so that postures and movements can be initiated and controlled. Thus, if the fire is too hot, the person might be stimulated to move away from the fire. As with sensory information, this motor information travels in specific pathways.

The spinal cord is of particular clinical importance because of its susceptibility to injury, the final topic of this chapter's first section. Susceptibility to injury is due in part to its sheer longitudinal extent, 42 to 45 cm. Beyond this, however, is the fact that, unlike the brain, it is encased in 24 individual bony units—the vertebrae that articulate with one another. This collective articulation yields a structure—the vertebral column—possessing significant flexibility, indeed even a remarkable flexibility in certain athletes who begin to train early in life (think of the young female gymnast working the balance beam). Although the collective articulations between adjacent vertebrae at the intervertebral discs are designed to provide this flexibility, they paradoxically subject the spinal cord to injury. For one thing, intervertebral discs themselves are subject to normal wear and tear and deteriorate with aging, predisposing them to injury. For another thing, the very flexibility of the vertebral column means that it can *hyperextend* or *hyperflex*. When this occurs, the vertebral column exposes the spinal cord to injury. Unfortunately, several common activities of modern-day life, most notably contact sports and automobile accidents, result in such hyperextensions and hyperflexions, often causing fractures of vertebrae, rupture of intervertebral discs, or both, and sometimes severely damaging the spinal cord. When injury does occur, knowledge of the organizational structure of the spinal cord allows the clinician to localize the place of injury and to interpret the extent to which recovery from injury is likely to occur.

The second major section of this chapter presents the general internal structure of the brainstem. The purpose of presenting the internal structure of both the spinal cord and brainstem together in a single chapter is to emphasize that they represent linked conduits in a two-way flow of information. That is, somatosensory information from the body that travels rostrally in fiber tracts of the spinal cord must also traverse the brainstem in order to gain access to the cerebral cortex and cerebellum. Reciprocally, motor information generated in the cerebral cortex must traverse the length of the brainstem and spinal cord in order to gain access to the muscles of the body and generate behavior. This is the function of long tracts that traverse the spinal cord and brainstem. These long tracts shift position as they ascend or descend through the three brainstem subdivisions. Thus, it is important to be able to recognize the level at which a transverse section through the brainstem has been taken because this will tell us where to look for a particular tract or pathway. By correlating the surface features of the brainstem delineated in Chapter 2 with their appearance in transverse sections, the first topic of the second section, it is possible to determine the level of a brainstem section. This will lay the necessary background for understanding the sensory and motor systems of the CNS. The major focus of this second section is on the brainstem reticular formation, the largest structural component of the brainstem tegmentum. The brainstem reticular formation receives sensory information from a wide variety of sources and sends information to structures residing in all parts of the CNS: from the spinal cord to the cerebral cortex. Its neurons are involved in regulating a broad array of functions, ranging from vital ones like the control of heart rate, blood pressure, and respiration to the regulation of level of consciousness. Consideration of the brainstem's blood supply is deferred until Chapter 15 for reasons that will be explained later.

SPINAL CORD

The surface features of the spinal cord and its general internal organization were presented in Chapter 2. In this chapter, we consider the structures with which the spinal cord is associated, the meninges and vertebrae, and provide a more detailed look at the internal organization of the cord.

The gray matter is organized into nuclei and a series of laminae called Rexed's laminae. The white matter is organized into tracts that either ascend to connect the spinal cord with the brainstem or cerebellum or descend to connect the cerebral cortex or brainstem with the spinal cord. Finally, the blood supply of the spinal cord is considered.

Clinical Preview ·················

In your outpatient orthopedic practice, about 70 percent of the people you treat have low back pain. Frequently, you need to develop hypotheses regarding the underlying cause of your patients' discomfort. This is of critical importance because it assists you to determine whether it is safe to provide physical interventions for the individual as well as to estimate the likely prognosis. As you read through this section, consider how an understanding of the anatomy of the spinal column and spinal cord will assist you to:

• Develop appropriate hypotheses about the person's underlying condition.

• Help people to understand their symptoms such as weakness, numbness, stiffness, and pain.

Meninges of the Spinal Cord

Thought Question

The spinal cord has three membranous coverings. How do these coverings compare to the coverings of the cerebral hemispheres that you learned about in Chapter 1?

Three membranous coverings, the meninges, invest the spinal cord and brain, providing important supportive and protective functions to the semisolid neural tissue. From outer to inner these connective tissue sheets are the dura mater, the arachnoid, and the pia mater (Figure 5-1 ■). Because the latter two are similar histologically and are interconnected, they often are referred to as the pia-arachnoid. Two spaces are associated with the three meninges: an **epidural space** external to the dura (not present in the cranium) and a **subarachnoid space** between the arachnoid and pia. The subarachnoid space is filled with cerebrospinal fluid, as noted in earlier chapters.

Dura Mater

The most external of the meninges, the dura is thick, tough, and poorly extensible (*dura mater* from the Latin words meaning *hard mother*). Because the vertebral canal is lined by its own periosteum, the dura of the spinal cord consists of only a single layer, corresponding to the meningeal layer of cranial dura (see Chapter 25) with which it is continuous through the foramen magnum. This gives rise to an epidural space, absent in the cranium, between the dura and vertebral periosteum (Figure 5-2 ■). The epidural space contains fatty tissue, loose connective tissue, and an extensive epidural venous plexus. The spinal dura forms a cul-de-sac approximately at the level of the second sacral vertebra. It is attached rostrally to the margins

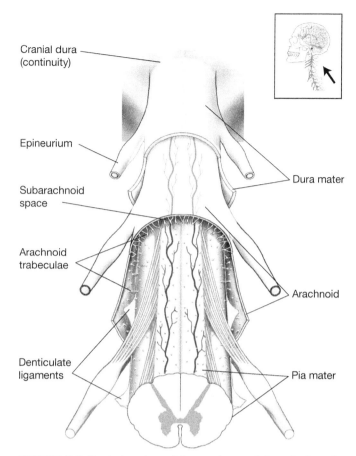

FIGURE 5-1 Posterior view of the meninges of the spinal cord. Note that the dura of the spinal cord is continuous with that of the cerebrum through the foramen magnum and that it is also continuous with the most external connective tissue investment of spinal nerves, the epineurium.

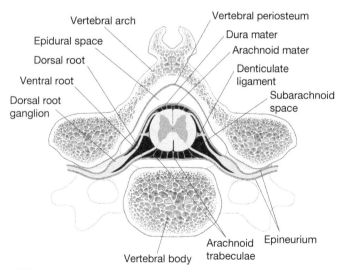

FIGURE 5-2 Cross section of a vertebra, the spinal cord, and meninges showing their mutual relations. Note the prominent epidural space between the dura mater and periosteum of the vertebra.

of the foramen magnum and caudally, via the **coccygeal ligament** (composed of pia, arachnoid, and dura mater) to the periosteum of the coccyx (see Figure 2-5). Dura invests each spinal nerve as a tubular sleeve extending approximately to the level of the intervertebral foramen. It then becomes continuous with the external connective tissue investment of the peripheral nerve, the **epineurium**.

Pia Mater

The pia is a delicate connective tissue layer representing the innermost of the meninges (see Figure 5-1) (*pia mater* from the Latin words meaning *tender mother*). It is firmly adherent to the surface of the spinal cord being anchored to neural tissue by the end feet of astrocytes. The pia consists of two layers: a superficial **epipial layer** and a deeper layer, the **intima pia**. The epipial layer is well developed around the spinal cord, and the blood vessels supplying the cord are embedded within this layer. At sites where blood vessels penetrate neural tissue, the intima pia is invaginated to form the outer wall of the *perivascular space* that persists until the vessel becomes a capillary.

The spinal cord is anchored to the arachnoid and dura by a series of flattened, triangular-shaped flanges of epipial tissue, each of which forms a **denticulate ligament** (see Figures 5-1 and 5-2). There are 18 to 24 pairs of denticulate ligaments attaching in a continuous line to the lateral aspect of the spinal cord midway between the dorsal and ventral roots. Each ligament extends laterally; its apex passes through the arachnoid and attaches to the inner surface of the dura.

Pia mater extends inferiorly from the cone-shaped termination of the spinal cord (the conus medullaris) forming part of the **filum terminale**. The latter penetrates the dural cul-de-sac, receives a dural investment, and continues caudally as with the previously described coccygeal ligament (see Figure 2-5).

Arachnoid Mater

The thin avascular arachnoid is the middle meningeal layer between dura and pia. It is closely applied to the inner surface of the dura, and thus the subdural space *in life* is really only a potential space filled with a thin film of fluid (not CSF). The CSF containing subarachnoid space intervenes between the arachnoid and pia. The space is traversed by numerous **arachnoid trabeculae**, delicate fibrous threads given off from the inner surface of the arachnoid and attaching to the pia (see Figure 5-1). This gives the arachnoid the appearance of a cobweb, hence its name (Gr, *arachne*, web).

Cells of the arachnoid are joined together by **tight junctions** that serve to isolate the general extracellular fluid of the body from the extracellular fluid of the CNS. The latter includes the cerebrospinal fluid occupying the subarachnoid space. These arachnoidal tight junctions form part of a system of barriers that collectively are referred to as the blood–brain barrier.

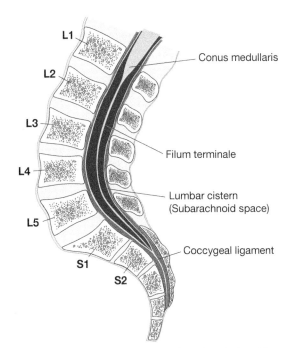

FIGURE 5-3 Midsagittal section showing the relationships between the termination of the spinal cord at the junction of the L1 and L2 vertebrae and the termination of the dura mater in a cul-de-sac at the level of the S2 vertebra. The space between the conus medullaris and dural cul-de-sac forms the lumbar cistern filled with cerebrospinal fluid. The lumbar cistern is traversed by the cauda equina (not shown), the collection of descending spinal nerve roots on their way to the intervertebral foramina through which they exit the vertebral canal. The coccygeal ligament anchors the dura to periosteum of the coccyx.

The **lumbar (spinal) cistern** is a focal enlargement of the subarachnoid space located at lower lumbar and upper sacral levels of the vertebral column (Figure 5-3 ▧). It is formed because the spinal cord and pia end at the junction of the L1–L2 vertebrae, while the arachnoid and dura continue as a membranous sac to the level of the S2 vertebra. The lumbar cistern is filled with a large amount of cerebrospinal fluid and contains only the filum terminale and nerve roots of the cauda equina. The lumbar cistern is of clinical importance because it is the site at which a **lumbar tap** is performed to measure intracranial pressure and to withdraw a sample of cerebrospinal fluid for laboratory analysis (see Chapter 25).

Nuclei of the Spinal Gray Matter and Rexed's Lamina

Despite the regularity so evident in its gross structure, the spinal cord possesses a far-reaching anatomical and functional differentiation when we begin analyzing the arrangement and connections of its cells. That we are dealing with an elaborately organized part of the CNS is apparent when the complex functions it carries out are considered. Among its functions, the spinal cord must sort, analyze, and integrate all of the diverse information arriving from the body periphery as well as that descending from suprasegmental structures of the brain. It routes this information to local and distant sites within the CNS. In addition, the spinal cord mediates the complex behavioral responses whose final expression is sensation, movement of body parts, or glandular secretion.

Two schemes have been used to describe the organization of neuronal cell bodies comprising the spinal cord gray matter: one is to describe their grouping into clusters or nuclei, while the second is to describe their cytoarchitectural organization into 10 layers or laminae, called Rexed's laminae after the developer of the scheme. Both schemes are important because they are used to describe the locations of neurons giving rise to the tracts that originate in the spinal

cord and the terminations of fibers that end (synapse) in the spinal gray. Both schemes apply to the entirety of the spinal gray: the dorsal horns having a sensory function, the ventral horns having a motor function, and the intermediate gray having an integrative and autonomic function.

Nuclei

When viewed in cross section, the cell bodies of neurons in the spinal gray are grouped into clusters called nuclei. Each dorsal horn is capped by a distinctive horseshoe-shaped region of gray matter called the **substantia gelatinosa** (Figure 5-4 ■). Compared to the rest of the spinal gray, the substantia gelatinosa appears paler in myelin-stained

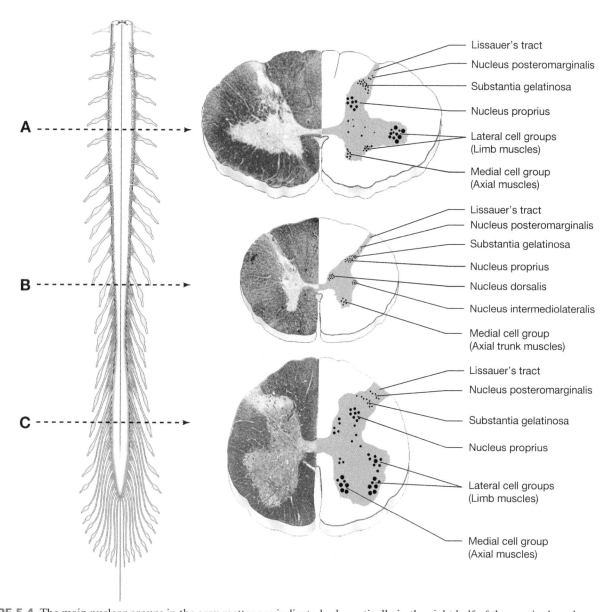

FIGURE 5-4 The main nuclear groups in the gray matter are indicated schematically in the right half of these spinal cord cross sections taken through the cervical enlargement (a), thoracic spinal cord (b), and lumbosacral enlargement (c). Note that the nucleus posteromarginalis, substantia gelatinosa, and nucleus proprius of the dorsal horn and the medial cell group of the ventral horn are represented throughout the length of the spinal cord. However, the nucleus dorsalis of the dorsal horn is seen only over spinal cord segments C8 through L2; the nucleus intermediolateralis of the intermediate gray is seen only over spinal cord segments T1 through L3, and the lateral nuclear groups of the ventral horn are seen only in the cervical and lumbosacral enlargements.

sections because its neurons receive lightly myelinated and unmyelinated sensory fibers. The substantia gelatinosa is a nucleus that extends the entire length of the spinal cord. The **nucleus proprius**, ventral to the substantia gelatinosa, comprises most of the dorsal horn. It also extends the entire length of the cord. The **nucleus dorsalis (Clarke's nucleus or column)** forms a bulge on the medial side of the base of the dorsal horn. This nucleus is present only within spinal cord segments C8 through L2.

The intermediate gray zone exhibits a pointed lateral extension over spinal cord segments T1 through L2 or L3. This is known as the **intermediolateral cell column**, or **nucleus intermediolateralis**, and contains neurons belonging to the sympathetic division of the autonomic nervous system.

Cross sections through the spinal cord reveal several distinct groups of large motor neurons in the ventral horn whose axons innervate striated muscle. The nuclear groups are particularly prominent in the cervical and lumbar enlargements. Conspicuous lateral and medial nuclear groups can be identified in the enlargements (see Figure 5-4). The medial nuclear groups form a continuous cell column extending the entire length of the spinal cord, from cervical through sacral levels. The medial nuclear groups innervate the neck, axial trunk, and girdle muscles. The lateral motor nuclei form an interrupted cell column, present only in the cervical and lumbar enlargements. They innervate the limb muscles. Ventral horn motor neurons thus are organized **somatotopically**.

> ### Thought Question
>
> Many nuclei of the CNS are organized somatotopically. The first example of this organizational feature is seen in the motor neurons of the spinal cord ventral horn. Be on the look out for this organizational feature throughout the anatomical arrangement of the nervous system from spinal cord to cortex. What might be the reason for this feature?

Individual skelctal muscles are innervated by a set of neurons called lower motor neurons (LMNs). By definition, these LMNs have their cell bodies within the CNS, and their axons travel in the PNS to directly innervate skeletal muscle. Such LMNs are distributed over several segments of the spinal cord. The entire set innervating a given muscle is called the **lower motor neuron pool** for that muscle. For example, the lower motor neuron pool for the opponens pollicis muscle is distributed over spinal cord segments C6 and C7 (Figure 5-5 ■). This muscle is responsible for the most important movement made by the thumb, namely, bringing the thumb into contact with another finger (opposition). We use this movement when buttoning a shirt or picking up an object such as lifting a teacup by the handle. The number of LMNs in a pool is related to the function of the muscle. Muscles that require precise voluntary control have large pools relative to the number of muscle fibers that they innervate (see

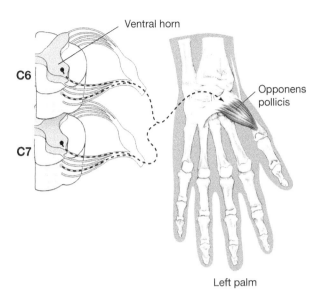

FIGURE 5-5 The opponens pollicis muscle is innervated by motor neurons distributed over spinal cord segments C6 and C7. This set of motor neurons represents the lower motor neuron pool for the muscle.

Chapter 10). The LMN pool innervating a given muscle appears to have a number of different preprogrammed (prewired) arrangements with local interneurons and peripheral receptors, depending on the role of the muscle in a particular task. The presence of this preprogrammed circuitry at the spinal level allows suprasegmental motor control centers to use more simplified commands to elicit complex movement patterns.

Neurons of the spinal gray also may be classified in terms of the destination of their axons (Figure 5-6 ■). **Intrasegmental neurons** are those with axons terminating in the same spinal segment in which the cell body is located. **Intersegmental neurons** are those with axons that

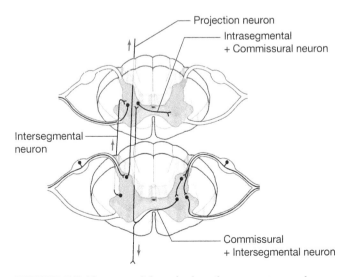

FIGURE 5-6 Neurons of the spinal cord gray matter can be classified according to the destinations of their axons. These classifications are not mutually exclusive. For example, some transmission neurons cross to the opposite side of the spinal cord before they ascend to the brainstem.

ascend or descend in the white matter to terminate in segments superior or inferior to the segment containing the cell body. The axons of **commissural neurons** cross from one side of the cord to the side opposite the location of the cell body. Finally, **projection neurons** are those with axons that ascend in the white matter from their cell of origin in the spinal cord to terminate in the brainstem, cerebellum, or diencephalon.

Rexed's Laminae

In 1952, B. Rexed developed a system for subdividing the gray matter of the cat's spinal cord into a series of 10 layers or laminae, now referred to as **Rexed's laminae**, based on cytoarchitectonic features. Rexed's system also applies to the human spinal cord and is the most precise and widely used method for describing the organization of cell populations within the spinal gray matter. The laminae are designated by Roman numerals.

The first six laminae subdivide the dorsal horn into horizontal zones that vary somewhat in configuration over the length of the spinal cord as shown in Figure 5-7 ■. Lamina I is the posteromarginal nucleus (or marginal zone) that forms a thin layer overlying the substantia gelatinosa, laminae II. Laminae III through VI make up the body of the dorsal horn and include the nucleus proprius. Lamina VII corresponds to the intermediate gray matter and includes the nucleus dorsalis medially as well as the intermediomedial and intermediolateral cell columns. Lamina VII also extends into the ventral horn. Lamina VIII makes up an interneuronal zone in the ventral horn, while the motor neuron cell groups in the ventral horn form lamina IX. Lamina X comprises a

Table 5-1 Nuclei and Laminae of Spinal Cord Gray Matter

ZONE	NAMED NUCLEI	REXED'S LAMINAE
Dorsal horn	Posteromarginal nucleus	I
Dorsal horn	Substantia gelatinosa	II
Dorsal horn	Nucleus proprius	III, IV
Dorsal horn	Neck of dorsal horn	V
Dorsal horn	Base of dorsal horn	VI
Intermediate zone	Clarke's nucleus (nucleus dorsalis), intermediolateral nucleus	VII
Ventral horn	Commissural nucleus	VIII
Ventral horn	Medial and lateral motor nuclei	IX
Gray matter surrounding the central canal		X

zone of gray matter surrounding the central canal. The correlations between named nuclei and Rexed's laminae are summarized in Table 5-1 ■.

Fiber Tracts of the Spinal Cord

We are concerned with two types of fiber tracts: (1) long ascending and descending tracts and (2) local (intrinsic) tracts. Both play important roles in the control of movement. Although a number of unique ascending and descending tracts occupy the three funiculi of the spinal cord, spinal white matter presents itself as a homogeneous mass with little evidence of segregation of nerve fibers into distinct tracts. Indeed, tracts of the spinal cord do not have sharply circumscribed boundaries: the fibers of adjacent tracts typically intermingle and sometimes overlap quite extensively. Naturally occurring spinal cord lesions, such as traumatic injury as opposed to surgical lesions such as a tractotomy, nearly always damage more than one tract because of this overlap and because of the anatomical size of such lesions, producing a complex of neurologic signs. A large number of tracts have been identified, only five of which will be considered briefly in this chapter (Figure 5-8 ■). More detailed coverage of these five tracts, as well as others, occurs in subsequent chapters. However, before

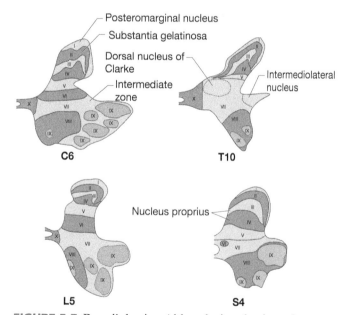

FIGURE 5-7 Rexed's lamina. Although given laminae always reside in the dorsal or ventral horns or intermediate gray, their configurations vary over different levels of the spinal cord.

(Adapted from Parent, A. *Carpenter's Human Neuroanatomy*, 9th ed. Williams & Wilkins, Baltimore, 1996.)

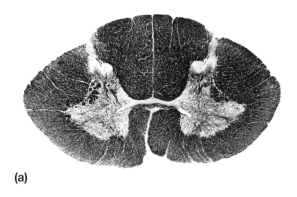

(a)

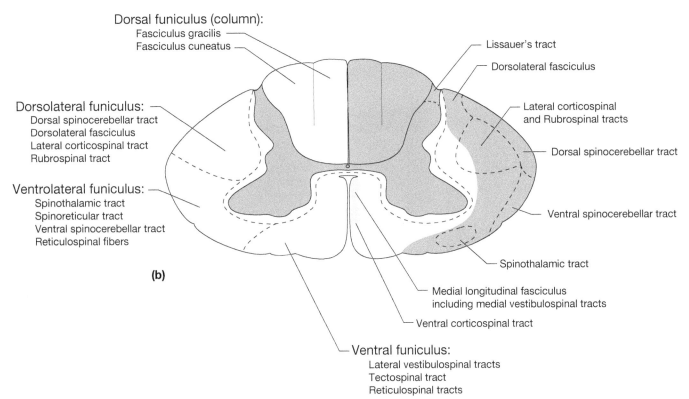

Dorsal funiculus (column):
Fasciculus gracilis
Fasciculus cuneatus

Lissauer's tract

Dorsolateral fasciculus

Lateral corticospinal
and Rubrospinal tracts

Dorsal spinocerebellar tract

Dorsolateral funiculus:
Dorsal spinocerebellar tract
Dorsolateral fasciculus
Lateral corticospinal tract
Rubrospinal tract

Ventrolateral funiculus:
Spinothalamic tract
Spinoreticular tract
Ventral spinocerebellar tract
Reticulospinal fibers

Ventral spinocerebellar tract

Spinothalamic tract

(b)

Medial longitudinal fasciculus
including medial vestibulospinal tracts

Ventral corticospinal tract

Ventral funiculus:
Lateral vestibulospinal tracts
Tectospinal tract
Reticulospinal tracts

FIGURE 5-8 (a) The myelin-stained cross section through C8 illustrates that the white matter of the spinal cord presents itself as a homogeneous mass of axons. Only the dorsal columns provide any evidence of the segregation of axons into distinctly identifiable bundles, a medial fasciculus gracilis and a lateral fasciculus cuneatus. (b) Schematic showing the positions of the major ascending and descending tracts, indicating that some overlap extensively.

we consider these long ascending and descending tracts of the spinal cord, it is important to understand that a set of fibers are local (intrinsic) to the spinal cord in that they both originate and terminate in the cord. These fibers will be considered first. This local tract of the spinal cord is called the spinospinal system.

Spinospinal (Propriospinal) System

The axons that make up the **spinospinal system** are from interneuronal cell bodies located at the border of the spinal cord gray matter (Figure 5-9 ■). Such neurons send their axons into the white matter bordering the spinal cord gray, where they bifurcate into ascending and descending branches that extend for variable numbers of segments before reentering the spinal gray to synapse. Bundles of spinospinal axons surround the spinal gray everywhere. They link segments as far distant as cervical and lumbar levels. In addition to connecting adjacent segments on the same side, axons of cells on one side may cross the midline, thus permitting an integration of activity between the right and left halves of the spinal cord. The spinospinal system represents an essential substrate for the fact that the spinal cord functions as an integrated unit, not as a series of isolated segments. (Think of stepping on a tack and your resulting arm movements that occur in conjunction with leg movements.)

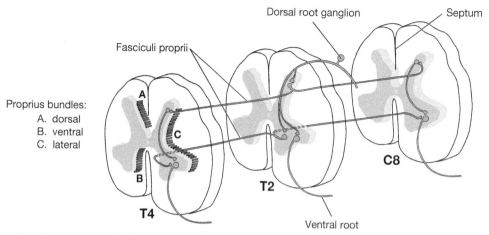

FIGURE 5-9 The spinospinal, or propriospinal, system consists of intersegmental axons that both originate and terminate in the spinal cord. The system occupies a rim of white matter that is immediately adjacent to the gray matter and is distributed in all three funiculi. Some axons of the spinospinal system extend only a few segments, but others extend virtually the length of the spinal cord.

> **Thought Question**
>
> To summarize, which part of the neuron comprises gray matter of the spinal cord, and which comprises the white matter?

Dorsal Columns

The posterior funiculi also are referred to as the **dorsal columns** (Figure 5-10 ∎; see also Figure 5-8). Most fibers running longitudinally in the **dorsal columns** terminate in the gray matter of the medulla, forming part of the pathway by which information is transmitted to the cerebral cortex, where it is consciously perceived. Many of these fibers that form the ascending dorsal columns are heavily myelinated, rapidly conducting *primary afferents* whose cell bodies are located in dorsal root ganglia. The information carried by these primary afferents comes from peripheral receptors situated in skin, muscle, tendons, and joints. The sensory modalities conveyed to the cerebral cortex by dorsal column fibers relate to certain cutaneous discriminations: the ability to identify object shape by manipulation (without the use of vision), the capacity to specify the position of an extremity and the direction in which it is moved, and to identify a stimulus as vibration.

Spinothalamic Tract

The **spinothalamic tract (STT)** is a second major pathway by which somatosensory impulses from the body are consciously perceived (see Figures 5-8 and 5-10).

> **Thought Question**
>
> Primary afferent neurons have their cell bodies in a dorsal root ganglion. What is the meaning of the word *ganglion*? Is this ganglion located in the peripheral or central nervous system?

The STT travels to the brain via the thalamus and is one of the components of the **anterolateral system (AL)**. Lightly myelinated and unmyelinated dorsal root afferents carrying **pain, temperature**, and **light (crude) touch** information synapse on neurons of the spinal cord dorsal horn such as those in the substantia gelatinosa. After this synapse, transmission neurons of the spinothalamic tract cross the midline within the spinal cord via the ventral white commissure. A clinically important fact is that the crossing is not completed until the spinal cord segment above the segmental level of entry of the dorsal root fiber. Spinothalamic tract axons form a diffuse band distributed in the anterolateral funiculus.

Spinothalamic tract function has been defined largely with respect to the tract's relevance to clinical neurology (Figure 5-11 ∎). A number of nondiscriminative sensory tests are used to reveal deficits attributable to spinothalamic tract lesions. These include fast (cutaneous, superficial) pain, as tested with a pinprick; light (crude) touch, as tested by stroking the surface of the skin with a wisp of cotton; and temperature, as tested with flasks of hot and cold water. It should be emphasized that superficial pain is the variety of pain sensibility in which the noxious stimulus is rapidly perceived, can be localized by the subject, and is without a strong affective component. Injury of the anterolateral funiculus of the spinal cord produces sensory alterations on the side of the body contralateral to the lesion beginning in associated

> **Thought Question**
>
> In this chapter, conventions are introduced related to the naming and locations of tracts. This information is necessary in preparation for learning more about the functional importance of tracts. For now, note the names of tracts and contrast them in terms of their origins, location within the cross section, and destinations. Notice that the name of the tract often tells you where the tract will end.

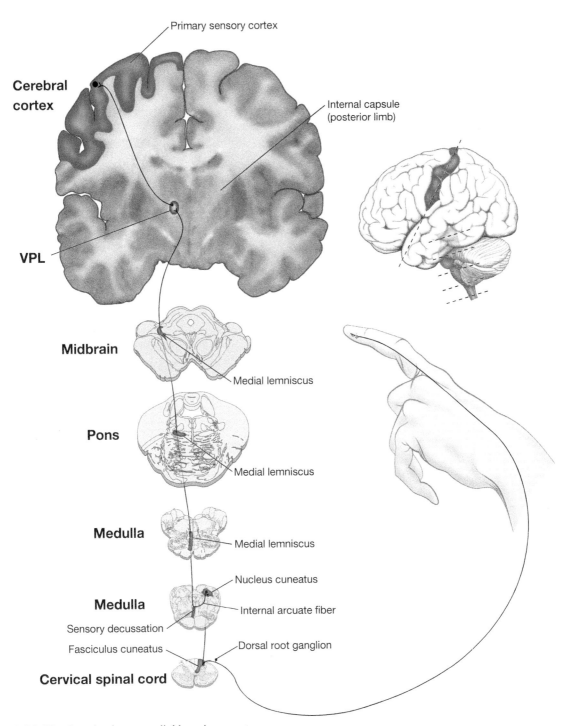

FIGURE 5-10 The dorsal column-medial lemniscus system.

dermatomes one or two segments caudal to the lesion (due to the crossing of fibers within the spinal cord, see Chapter 11).

Spinocerebellar Tracts

The **spinocerebellar tracts** connect the spinal cord with the cerebellum and convey touch, pressure, and proprioceptive information from peripheral receptors to the cerebellum. The cerebellum receives abundant sensory information, although it is considered a motor and not a sensory structure. We are not consciously aware of

cerebellar activity, but the cerebellum, which plays an important role in correcting motor errors, must necessarily have available to it information about the ongoing activity of muscles and the relative positions of body parts if it is to ensure that their movements are smooth and coordinated. The two most prominent of the spinocerebellar tracts will be considered in this chapter, but others exist and will be considered in Chapter 19.

Branches of dorsal column fibers carrying touch, pressure, and proprioceptive information (mostly the latter) mainly from the lower extremity synapse on cells

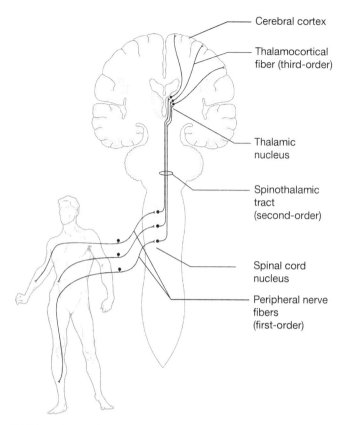

FIGURE 5-11 The anterolateral system.

Labels for Figure 5-11:
- Cerebral cortex
- Thalamocortical fiber (third-order)
- Thalamic nucleus
- Spinothalamic tract (second-order)
- Spinal cord nucleus
- Peripheral nerve fibers (first-order)

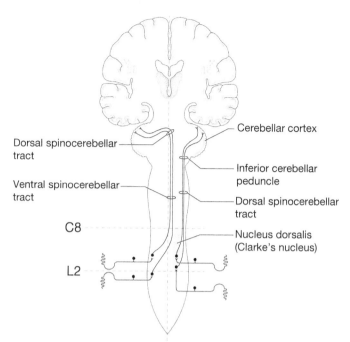

FIGURE 5-12 The spinocerebellar tracts.

Labels for Figure 5-12:
- Dorsal spinocerebellar tract
- Ventral spinocerebellar tract
- C8
- L2
- Cerebellar cortex
- Inferior cerebellar peduncle
- Dorsal spinocerebellar tract
- Nucleus dorsalis (Clarke's nucleus)

of the nucleus dorsalis (Clarke's column or nucleus) (Figure 5-12 ■; see also Figure 5-4). The **dorsal spino-cerebellar tract** arises from the cells of the nucleus dorsalis, located at the base of the dorsal horn from spinal cord segments C8 to L2. Axons of the tract run laterally into the ipsilateral lateral funiculus, coming to occupy a position at the periphery of the funiculus, where they turn rostrally to ascend to the cerebellum.

The **ventral spinocerebellar tract** is also related to proprioceptive information derived from the lower extremity, but it carries, in addition, exteroceptive information. The tract arises from cells in the dorsal horn and intermediate gray. Axons of these cells then cross to the contralateral side and take up a position at the periphery of the lateral funiculus, immediately ventral to the dorsal spinocerebellar tract. The ventral spino-cerebellar tract conveys information from a variety of sources concerning the lower extremities. Included are

all of the motor descending pathways and collaterals of spinal cord reflex circuits. Information conveyed is related more to intended movement than to unconscious proprioception.

Lateral Corticospinal (Pyramidal) Tract

The **corticospinal tract** is a substantial descending fiber system, with each tract consisting of more than 1,000,000 axons in humans. Its fibers originate in the cerebral cortex and pass uninterrupted through the brainstem. At a caudal brainstem level (caudalmost medulla), the majority of fibers of each side cross in the pyramidal decussation. These crossed fibers enter the spinal cord as the **lateral corticospinal tract** situated in the dorsal part of the lateral funiculus (see Figure 5-8). The tract gives off fibers at all spinal cord levels and thus decreases in size as it descends.

The lateral corticospinal tract is concerned with the control of voluntary movement, but most especially with skilled, independent finger movements. Damage to the tract produces weakness and an impaired capacity for voluntary movement. This is referred to as **paresis**, a partial or incomplete paralysis. When the damage is located

Neuropathology Box 5-1

Together, the spinocerebellar tracts transmit proprioceptive and cutaneous information to the specific parts of the cerebellum, enabling the latter to contribute to the control of posture and movement. While they may be damaged in demyelinating diseases such as multiple sclerosis and **Friedreich's ataxia**, they are not selectively damaged. Selective damage to a spinocerebellar tract is virtually unknown.

Table 5-2 Tracts of the Spinal Cord

NAME	ORIGIN	TERMINATION	LOCATION	FUNCTION
Dorsal column	Peripheral somatic receptors	Dorsal column nuclei of medulla	Dorsal funiculus	Conscious awareness of discriminative somatic sensation
Spinothalamic	Dorsal horn of spinal gray (Rexed's laminae I, II–V)	Thalamus and brainstem reticular formation	Anterior and lateral funiculi	Conscious awareness of pain, temperature, and touch
Spinocerebellar	Clarke's column of dorsal horn and intermediate spinal gray (Rexed's lamina VII)	Cerebellum	Lateral funiculus	Afferent somatic information for motor control and intended movement information
Corticospinal	Cerebral motor cortex	Spinal cord	Lateral (predominantly) and anterior funiculi	Voluntary control of skeletal muscle
Rubrospinal	Red nucleus of midbrain	Spinal cord	Lateral funiculus	Voluntary control of arms; may not be important in humans
Reticulospinal	Reticular formation of medulla and pons	Spinal cord	Anterior funiculus	Control of postural muscles and reflexes
Vestibulospinal	Vestibular nuclei of the brainstem	Spinal cord	Anterior funiculus	Control of postural muscles and reflexes for maintaining balance and upright stance
Tectospinal	Superior colliculus of midbrain	Spinal cord	Anterior funiculus	Control of movement of the head and upper extremity
Spinospinal (propriospinal)	Spinal cord	Spinal cord	All funiculi	Integrates activity across multiple spinal cord segments

in the spinal cord, the paresis is ipsilateral to the lesion, because this descending projection descussates in caudal medulla.

Table 5-2 ■ summaries the tracts of the spinal cord and their functions. The table contains tracts that will be considered in later chapters. Further, all of the tracts considered in this chapter will be addressed again in subsequent chapters.

Blood Supply of the Spinal Cord

Blood supply to the spinal cord is derived from two major sources: (1) from branches of the two vertebral arteries and (2) from branches of multiple segmental vessels called **radicular arteries**. Segmental vessels are branches from the vertebral arteries in the neck, from intercostal arteries in the thorax, from lumbar arteries in the abdomen, and from iliolumbar and lateral sacral arteries in the pelvis.

Posterior Spinal Arteries

Each of the paired **posterior spinal arteries** arises from a vertebral artery and/or posterior inferior cerebellar artery at the level of the medulla (Figure 5-13 ■). Passing

Thought Question

The lateral corticospinal tracts cross (decussate) in caudal medulla. Recall how this looks on the surface of the brainstem. As a rehabilitation professional, you will find that the location of the decussation is of central importance to predicting and interpreting an individual's functional deficits following spinal cord injuries and disorders. What is the functional role of this tract? If this tract is damaged, what symptoms would likely occur? If the damage is above the decussation, would the symptoms be ipsilateral (same side) as the lesion or contralateral (opposite side)? What if the damage is below the decussation?

posteriorly from its origin, each descends on the dorsal surface of the spinal cord along the dorsolateral sulcus just medial to the dorsal roots. The blood supply of each vessel is reinforced by radicular arteries derived from the segmental arteries. Each segmental artery divides into an anterior and posterior ramus. Each posterior ramus gives rise to a spinal branch that enters the vertebral canal

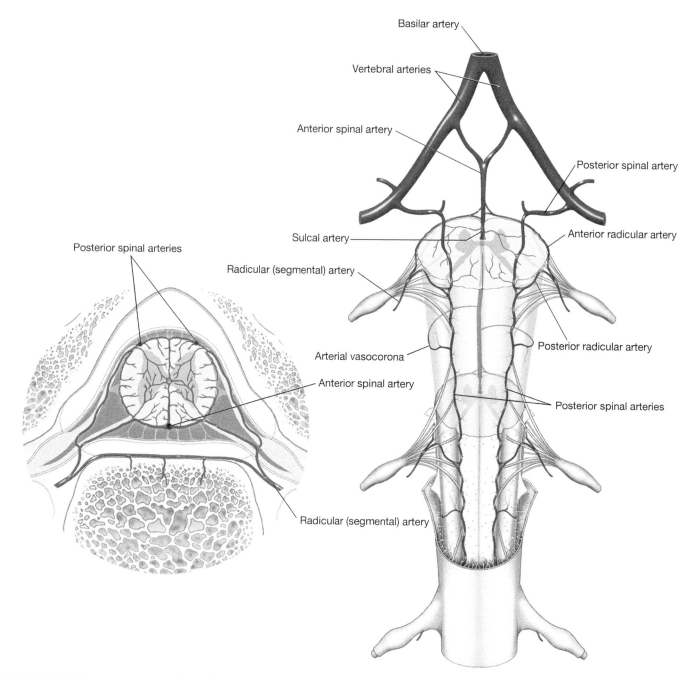

FIGURE 5-13 The spinal cord receives its blood supply from three small longitudinally running arteries that extend the length of the cord: the single anterior and paired posterior spinal arteries. These arteries originate from the vertebral arteries, and their blood supply is supplemented along their length by segmental spinal arteries that gain access to the spinal cord via the intervertebral foramina and bifurcate into anterior and posterior radicular arteries. The posterior spinal arteries supply the approximate dorsal one-third of the spinal cord, while the anterior spinal arteries supply the approximate ventral two-thirds of the spinal cord.

through an intervertebral foramen, pierces the dura mater, and supplies a dorsal root ganglion and spinal nerve roots via its anterior and posterior radicular branches. The **posterior radicular arteries** branch on the posterolateral surface of the spinal cord and join each posterior spinal artery. Thusly reinforced, the posterior spinal arteries continue to the conus medullaris and cauda

equina. Branches of each posterior spinal artery form anastomoses around the dorsal roots of the spinal nerve and communicate, via tortuous transverse branches, with vessels of the same and opposite sides. The posterior spinal arteries supply the approximate dorsal one-third of the spinal cord, comprising the dorsal funiculi and dorsal portions of the dorsal horn.

Anterior Spinal Artery

The anterior spinal artery arises from the midline union of two vessels that originate near the termination of the vertebral arteries. These two vessels descend on the anterior surface of the medulla and unite to form a single midline vessel, the **anterior spinal artery**, at the level of the foramen magnum. The anterior spinal artery descends in the pia mater along the anterior median fissure and gives off sulcal branches that enter the fissure; in general, they pass alternately to supply the right or left sides of the spinal cord. The anterior spinal artery extends the entire length of the cord and gives off branches that nourish the cauda equina. The anterior and posterior spinal arteries form anastomotic channels that run the full length of the cord and receive branches from the radicular arteries.

The blood supply within the anterior spinal artery is reinforced by a succession of **anterior radicular arteries**, derived from segmental vessels. Different levels of the spinal cord receive different numbers of anterior radicular branches. The cervical spinal cord receives the most—up to six anterior radicular branches derived from the vertebral artery. In fact, these branches provide the principal blood supply of the cervical spinal cord. The thoracic cord receives only two to four branches, derived from intercostal branches of the thoracic aorta. The lumbar spinal cord receives one or two anterior radicular branches, derived from the lumbar branches of the abdominal aorta. The largest of these is the *artery of Adamkiewicz* or the artery of the lumbar enlargement. Branches of the anterior spinal artery supply the approximate ventral two-thirds of the spinal cord.

Spinal Veins

The spinal cord is drained by six longitudinally running plexiform vessels. Veins emerging from the anterior median fissure drain into an anterior central (median) vein, whereas those emerging from the posterior median sulcus drain into the posterior central (median) vein. There are two lateral longitudinal veins on either side of the spinal cord—one along the line of attachment of the dorsal roots and one along the line of attachment of the ventral roots. All of these veins drain into radicular veins that, in turn, drain into an extensive epidural venous plexus located between the dura mater and vertebral periosteum.

Spinal Cord–Vertebrae Relations

The way in which a disease process affects a particular organ depends importantly on the relationship of that organ to surrounding structures. This is especially true with regard to the CNS because here we are presented with a soft structure encased within a rigid, nonexpansible, bony vault. While the position of the spinal cord within the bony vertebral canal clearly fulfills a protective function, minimizing the potential for CNS damage following external trauma, it paradoxically represents the mechanical basis for damage to the CNS in a variety of pathological conditions that have the effect of occupying space.

Vertebral Canal and Intervertebral Foramina

A typical **vertebra** consists of a body, a vertebral arch, and several processes for muscular and articular connections. The body of the vertebra is the portion that gives strength and supports weight. The body of each vertebra is separated from the bodies of the vertebrae superior and inferior to it by the fibrocartilaginous intervertebral discs.

Posterior to the body is the vertebral arch that, with the posterior surface of the body, forms the walls of the vertebral (spinal) foramen. These walls enclose and protect the spinal cord. Collectively, the vertebral foramina form the **vertebral canal** within which the spinal cord is situated. The vertebral arch is composed of right and left pedicles and right and left laminae. Depressions are present on the superior and inferior aspects of each pedicle or root, the superior and inferior vertebral notches. When vertebrae articulate to form the intact vertebral column, the vertebral notches of adjacent vertebrae form the **intervertebral foramina**. The spinal nerves, together with the arteries and veins supplying the spinal cord, pass through intervertebral foramina of each side. (Figure 5-14 ■).

Position of the Spinal Cord within the Vertebral Column

Invested by its meningeal coverings, the spinal cord lies loosely in the vertebral canal, situated posterior to the vertebral body (see Figure 5-2). The bony vertebral canal must accommodate fatty tissue and venous plexuses of the epidural space, the meninges, cerebrospinal fluid (CSF), roots of the spinal nerves, the spinal cord, and the arteries and veins supplying the cord. The total volume of the adult vertebral canal does not change. Although the foregoing structures do not completely fill the vertebral canal, there is little "extra" volume available to accommodate additional substances that occupy space. A tumor, swelling from trauma to the spinal cord, or hemorrhage all occupy space and represent **space-occupying lesions**. Because the total volume of the vertebral canal will not change, the additional space taken up by the lesion occurs at the expense of neural tissue. It also compresses blood vessels nourishing the spinal cord, potentially leading to ischemia. Regional variations in the size of the spinal cord render certain segments more vulnerable to space-occupying lesions than others.

The Vertebral Column and Intervertebral Discs

Consideration of individual vertebrae enables us to see how each participates in such functions as articulation with its neighbors, weight-bearing, and protection of the spinal cord. The vertebral column (spinal column) is the most obvious component of the axial skeleton. The axial skeleton is so named because it forms the longitudinal axis of the body. It

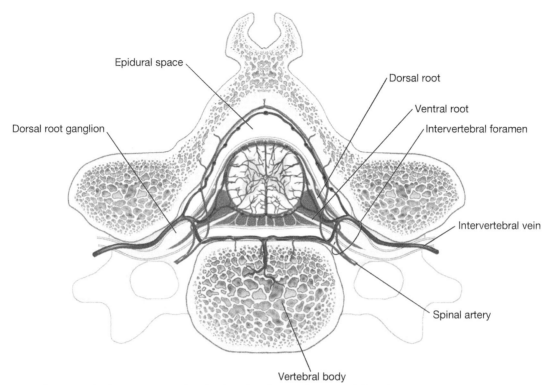

FIGURE 5-14 Each intervertebral foramen contains the dorsal and ventral roots and dorsal root ganglion of a spinal nerve plus arteries and veins supplying and draining a region of the spinal cord.

provides an extensive surface for the attachment of muscles that adjust the position of the head, neck, and trunk as well as stabilize or position structures of the appendicular skeleton (the upper and lower extremities, which include the pectoral and pelvic girdles that attach the upper and lower limbs to the axial skeleton). The vertebral column plays a key role in the static and dynamic bases of postural control and locomotion. The osseous forms of the vertebrae are important if we are to understand their coordinated action and mutual mobility. Significant roles are played also by the soft tissue parts between adjacent vertebrae. **Intervertebral discs** are situated between adjacent surfaces of the vertebral bodies. They fulfill important articular and shock-absorbing functions. Finally, the articulation between adjacent vertebrae produces a segmental column that protects the spinal cord, thereby assuring sensory and motor integrity.

Each fibrocartilaginous disc is composed of an outer, laminated fibrous ring known as the **annulus fibrosus** that is firmly attached to the rims of the vertebral bodies. The annulus surrounds a central homogenous mass of gelatinous substance known as the **nucleus pulposus**. The normal interplay between these two disc components is such that the nucleus pulposus exerts pressure on all sides of the annulus fibrosus, thereby maintaining a distance between adjacent vertebral bodies.

The nucleus pulposus is the central point in the disc for weight-absorption and distribution. During rest (i.e., unloading), it tends to assume a rounded form as it

imbibes water. The application of a sudden force in, for example, a superior-to-inferior direction causes a flattening and distension of the nucleus that, in turn, stretches the surrounding annulus. Pressure is thus equalized across the whole intervertebral surface and the shock absorbed. The strong attachment of the annulus fibrosus to the rims of adjacent vertebrae and the dynamic interplay between it and the nucleus pulposus fulfill two functions: they exert a restraining influence on the mobility of the vertebral column, while, at the same time, equalizing the forces placed on the column during rest, static stress, and motion. The articulations between adjacent vertebrae allow only slight individual vertebral movement. Nonetheless, when this slight movement between pairs takes place in all the joints of the vertebral column, the total range of movement is considerable.

Spinal Cord Segments and Their Relation to Adjacent Vertebrae

In the adult, a rather specific anatomical relationship exists between given spinal cord segments and vertebrae of the same number. This relationship is a product of developmental changes in the length of the vertebral column relative to the spinal cord. In the embryo, development of the vertebral column and spinal cord are closely related events so that the spinal nerves attaching to the spinal cord are on virtually the same level as the intervertebral foramina through which they course. The first seven cervical spinal nerves emerge from the vertebral canal above each respective cervical vertebrae. Because there are only seven cervical vertebrae, the eighth cervical nerve emerges from the intervertebral foramen between the seventh cervical and first thoracic vertebrae. All more caudal spinal nerves emerge from the intervertebral foramina below the vertebrae of its type and number. However, during fetal development, the vertebral column elongates more rapidly than does the spinal cord. The net result of this disproportionate growth is as though the spinal cord were "pulled" superiorly in the vertebral canal owing to the cord's attachment to the brainstem (Figure 5-15 ■). Consequently, the segments of the spinal cord in the adult do not correspond levelwise to their respective vertebrae. The disparity between cord segment and vertebra of the same number increases progressively in a superior-to-inferior direction. Thus, for example, all sacral segments of the spinal cord lie in the

vertebral canal of the L1 vertebra. This cord segment–adjacent vertebrae relation is of diagnostic importance, for example, in the case of performing a lumbar spinal puncture (see Chapter 25).

CLINICAL CONNECTIONS
Vascular Disorders of the Spinal Cord

Vascular disorders produce their effects by depriving the spinal cord of its arterial blood supply (**ischemia**). The vascular anatomy of the spinal cord accounts for the most common clinical features observed with spinal cord infarction (necrosis of nerve tissue resulting from a lack of arterial blood). First, major differences exist in the anterior and posterior spinal arteries. The paired posterior spinal arteries supply only a small area of the spinal cord (one-third), and they are longitudinally continuous and anastomotic vessels. In contrast, the unpaired anterior spinal artery supplies most of the spinal cord (two-thirds), but the continuity of its blood supply depends on its reinforcement from the anterior radicular arteries. Second, certain areas of the spinal cord are more vulnerable to interruption of their blood supply than others. Thoracic segments are vulnerable for several reasons. One is the result of the long distance between adjacent anterior radicular artery branches (only two to four branches to nourish 12 segments) such that thoracic circulation can be effectively compromised by occlusion of a single branch. Another reason is that the sulcal branches of the anterior spinal artery are small in the upper four thoracic segments, making these segments dependent for their nourishment upon the anterior radicular branches derived from the intercostal segmental arteries of the thoracic aorta. L1 is another vulnerable spinal cord segment.

Because vascular disorders affect the area supplied by the vessel involved, it is essential to know the territory perfused by each of the major vessels associated with the spinal cord. Vascular disease involving the spinal cord characteristically is limited to the territory supplied by the anterior spinal artery involving thoracic or upper lumbar segments, the resultant deficits being called the **syndrome of the anterior spinal artery**. Symptoms associated with infarction of the anterior spinal artery are summarized here in order to illustrate the relationship between location of the vessels and the resulting consequences of injury.

The neurologic signs are usually acute in onset. Typically, they include a flaccid paraplegia (both legs) characteristic of spinal shock due to interruption of the corticospinal and other descending motor tracts; a bilateral deficit in pain and temperature sensation below the level of the lesion due to interruption of the spinothalamic tracts; a preservation of proprioception, the capacity to discriminate the direction of a moving tactile

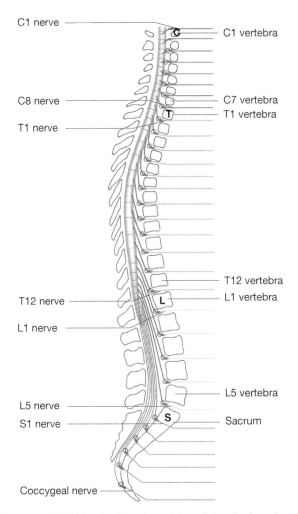

FIGURE 5-15 Midsagittal section of the adult spinal cord and vertebral column showing the relationship between spinal cord segments and vertebrae of the same number. The lateral position of the intervertebral foramina by which spinal nerves exit the vertebral canal are indicated by circles. Abbreviations: C, cervical; L, lumbar; S, sacral; T, thoracic.

stimulus, and vibration because the dorsal columns are spared; and a loss of bowel and bladder control due to interruption of descending autonomic tracts. These symptoms will be discussed in detail in later chapters (see Chapters 9 through 12).

After recovery from spinal shock, a spastic paraplegia may develop, provided the lower motor neurons in the anterior horn have not been damaged, along with associated hyperactive tendon reflexes, clonus, and Babinski signs. When the anterior horns have been infarcted, flaccid paralysis continues, and the prognosis for any recovery of function usually is poor.

Extrinsic–Intrinsic Spinal Cord Lesions

The spinal cord is the target of a large number of disease processes that may be of extrinsic or intrinsic origin. With the exception of vascular disorders and direct lacerations resulting from knife or penetrating missile wounds, *extrinsic lesions* involve structures associated with the spinal cord and produce their effects by compression of the cord and its nutrient arteries. Extrinsic lesions include the following: direct cord compression due to fracture dislocations of vertebra, prolapsed intervertebral discs, cervical spondylosis, neoplasms invading the vertebrae and epidural space, and meningiomas (Figure 5-16 ■). Extrinsic compressive disorders produce a variety of clinical effects, depending on the rapidity and severity of cord compression. When fully developed, extrinsic lesions tend to involve the spinal cord at a particular level in a relatively complete bilateral or hemisectional manner. A variety of extrinsic lesions are presented next.

Intrinsic lesions, on the other hand, arise from or within neural tissue itself. These tend to involve functional systems or parts of the spinal cord in a more or less selective manner. Syringomyelia (see Chapter 10), for example, can produce a dissociated sensory disturbance in which pain and temperature sensations are lost but vibration and position sense are preserved. Poliomyelitis and amyotrophic lateral sclerosis (see Chapters 10 and 11) both involve anterior horn motoneurons but leave sensory systems intact. Intrinsic lesions include the following: a variety of inflammatory processes collectively referred to as myelitis; various degenerative diseases, some of known (subacute combined degeneration), others of unknown (multiple sclerosis) etiology; and intrinsic tumors (gliomas) arising from neuroglial cells (primarily astrocytes and ependymal cells).

Herniation of the Vertebral Disc

The displacement of disc tissue from its normal position between vertebral bodies is often called a slipped or **herniated disc.** The formal name for a slipped disc is **herniated nucleus pulposus.** Because the herniated disc tissue occupies space, it may compress the spinal cord against the bony vertebral canal, or the spinal nerve roots against the walls of the intervertebral foramen,

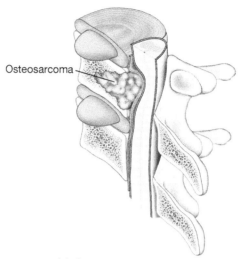

(a) Osteosarcoma

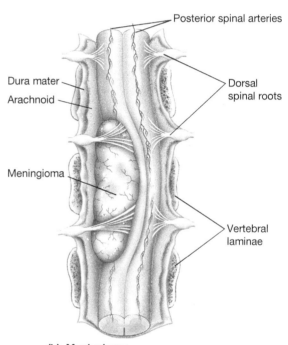

(b) Meningioma

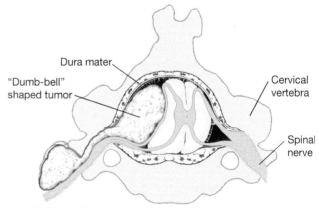

(c) Neurofibroma

FIGURE 5-16 Neoplastic external lesions of the spinal cord. (a) and (b) Neoplasms that invade the vertebral canal. (c) A meningioma that arises from cells of the arachnoid within the vertebral canal. All compress the spinal cord and/or spinal nerve roots.

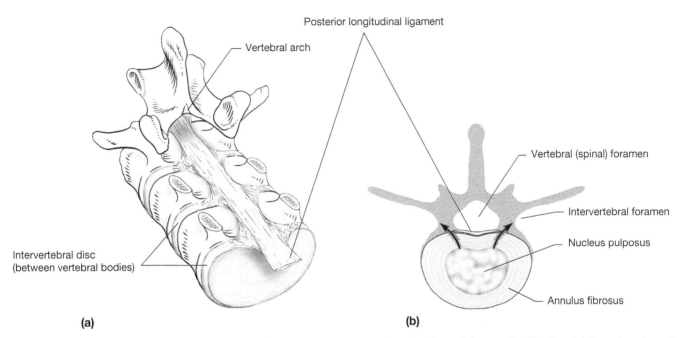

FIGURE 5-17 The posterior longitudinal ligament is positioned along the dorsal surface of the vertebral bodies. (a) Posterior view of the ligament with the vertebral arches removed. (b) Transverse section showing how the ligament routes herniated nucleus pulposus tissue laterally into the intervertebral foramina containing the spinal nerve roots.

and thus lead to neurologic symptoms. Herniations potentially may occur in any direction although certain directions are favored owing to the position of the **posterior longitudinal ligament** within the vertebral canal (Figure 5-17 ■). Thus, most herniations involve the posterolateral or posterior displacement of the nucleus pulposus toward the spinal nerve roots within the intervertebral foramen or spinal cord. With its associated soft tissues, the intervertebral foramen is small so that the blood vessels and nerve roots contained within it are readily susceptible to compression. Herniations may also involve varying amounts of disc tissue.

Only rarely is a single, acute trauma sufficient to cause a normal, healthy disc to rupture in the absence of predisposing factors. Generally, when a disc prolapse does occur as a result of sudden stress, degenerative changes in the annulus and/or nucleus already have occurred either as a result of previous trauma, advancing age, normal wear and tear, or certain diseases. Given the position of the intervertebral disc ventral to the spinal cord, involvement of the cord or spinal nerve roots may follow a posterior or posterolateral herniation in which disc tissue extrudes into the vertebral canal.

The mildest from of herniation is referred to as a **nuclear protrusion** in which the nuclear material does not breach the outer annulus but creates a bulge on the posterior annulus and/or posterior longitudinal ligament that presses on the spinal cord (Figure 5-18 ■). Next in severity is the **disc prolapse**. Here, the herniated nucleus pulposus reaches the outer edge of the annulus, but again does not physically breach it. But the bulge in the posterior annulus is more pronounced, exerting greater pressure on the

spinal cord or spinal nerve roots. More severe herniations, extrusions and sequestrations, involve a physical breaching of the annulus, allowing the herniated nucleus pulposus to escape into the epidural space and exert direct pressure on

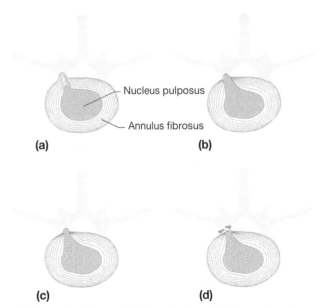

FIGURE 5-18 Types of disc herniations. (a) Protrusion where the annulus fibrosus bulges but is not breached by the herniated nucleus pulposus. (b) Herniation where the extruded nucleus pulposus has incompletely breached the annulus fibrosus resulting in a more pronounced bulge. (c) Herniation in which the annulus has been completely breached and pulposus tissue has been extruded into the vertebral canal. (d) Sequestration in which herniated pulposus tissue is free within the vertebral canal and becomes lodged within the epidural space.

neural tissue, a process aided by the fact that the annulus normally maintains the nucleus under pressure.

Considerable variability occurs in the size, position, and appearance of a herniated nucleus pulposus. This variability accounts for the lack of a common and constant neurologic picture. If the cleft in the annulus remains open, the herniated nucleus pulposus may extrude into the vertebral canal with certain movements but move back into the intervertebral space with other movements. This is known as a recurrent herniation and is characterized by a waxing and waning of neurologic symptoms. If the tear in the annulus closes, prolapsed tissue may become trapped in the vertebral canal (an incarcerated herniation) and either remain in a fixed position (a fixed herniation) or migrate superiorly or inferiorly from its site of origin (a free herniation). With so much potential variability in the size and position of a posterior herniation, one could hardly anticipate that all patients would present with a common list of complaints or a given patient necessarily with the same set of neurologic signs over time.

Movements of the vertebral column are freest in the cervical and lumbar regions. While symptom-producing intervertebral disc herniations are most common in the lumbar region, they are almost as common in the cervical region. The most common cause of acute mid and low back pain radiating down the posterolateral aspect of the thigh and leg is posterolateral herniation of a lumbar intervertebral disc at the L5/S1 level that compresses and compromises the L5 or S1 nerve root. In the cervical region, the discs that most commonly herniate are those between the C5/C6 and C6/C7, compressing spinal nerve roots C6 and C7, respectively. This results in pain in the neck, shoulder, arm, and hand.

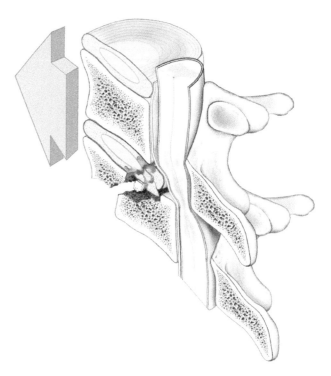

FIGURE 5-19 When causing spinal cord damage, the fracture dislocation of a vertebral body is an extrinsic lesion. The figure shows an anterior displacement of the entire intact vertebra rostral to the fracture (indicated by the arrow), resulting in its vertebral arch compressing the spinal cord.

variable degree of hemorrhage, further damaging the cord. Damage is maximal at the level of injury and for one or two segments on either side. The cord is seldom cut in two.

Thought Question

The spinal cord only extends as far as the L2 (lower border of L1) vertebrae, although the vertebral column extends all the way to the sacral vertebra. Explain why the spinal cord stops short of the spinal column. What might be the ramifications of this anatomical arrangement with regard to traumatic damage to the vertebral column below the level of L2?

Thought Question

Trauma to neural tissue often results in a cascade of events, beginning with damage to the tissue itself and extending into other tissues because of release of molecules that are destructive to neurons. We will see these physiological responses when we learn about strokes and traumatic brain injuries. Several neurotransmitters and other molecules are associated with secondary damage to the spinal cord. Give three examples. In addition, edema can lead to further damage. What causes the edema?

Vertebral Fractures and Their Consequences for the Spinal Cord

In dislocations or fracture dislocations, an anterior displacement of the vertebral column rostral to the site of vertebral damage occurs. In the absence of vertebral body fracture, there must be a break in the posterior longitudinal ligament and intervertebral disc in order for such displacement to happen. In either case, the sharp angulation of the axis of body support markedly narrows the vertebral canal, compressing the spinal cord between the laminae of the vertebra above and the body of the vertebra below the site of dislocation (Figure 5-19 ■). Such crush injury destroys gray and white matter and is accompanied by a

Not all of the tissue damage resulting from spinal cord trauma is sustained immediately. Some results from delayed events or so-called secondary injury that acts to expand the extent of the initial traumatic injury. Trauma-induced neurochemical changes represent one of the proposed mechanisms to account for such delayed and irreversible tissue damage. The endogenous acidic amino acid neurotransmitters glutamate and aspartate, which function as excitatory transmitters in many parts of the CNS (including the spinal cord), become **neurotoxic** following trauma due to their excessive release. In **excitotoxic** neuronal cell death, extracellular amino acid concentrations increase markedly following spinal cord trauma. Most of the amino acid probably originates from the cells of the spinal cord itself, but some may derive from a trauma-induced disruption of the blood–brain barrier, allowing free amino acids in the plasma to enter the extracellular space of the spinal cord. Several hypotheses have been advanced to explain how these excitatory amino acids produce their neurotoxic actions, and both involve receptor-mediated changes in intracellular ion concentrations of spinal cord neurons. The initial event entails an influx of sodium and chlorine ions and results in cellular **edema** (**cytotoxic edema**). This is followed by an increase in the intracellular concentration of calcium ions that leads to cell death, perhaps by damaging cell membranes, activating proteolysis, or causing protein cross-linking. The combination of trauma and secondary injury may result in the syndrome of spinal shock. Spinal shock is discussed in Chapter 11.

Cervical Spondylosis

Chronic compression of the cervical spinal cord and its associated spinal nerve roots can result from degeneration of the intervertebral disc accompanied by osteophytic (bony) outgrowths and changes in surrounding ligaments. This is a slow, intermittently progressive disorder with long periods of unchanging symptomatology. When this occurs in the cervical cord, it is referred to as **cervical spondylosis**.

The basic lesion in cervical spondylosis is degeneration and tearing of the annulus fibrosis with extrusion of the nucleus pulposus into the spinal canal. The disc becomes covered with fibrous tissue, partly calcifies, or covered with bone. Alternatively, the annulus may bulge without the extrusion of nuclear material and this may be associated with bony overgrowth of adjacent vertebrae (osteophytes) and the formation of transverse bony ridges (Figure 5-20 ■). Whatever the specific combination of pathological changes, the cervical spinal cord and/or nerve roots are compromised by compression. The posterior longitudinal ligament anteriorly and the **ligamentum flavum** posteriorly both undergo hypertrophy and contribute to the compression.

The particular vulnerability of the lower cervical spine to these degenerative changes is related to its high degree of mobility. Lower cervical vertebrae are positioned between the atlanto-occipital joint that allows nodding (flexion and extension) with slight lateral movements, and the C7–T1 interspace that is relatively immobilized by the thoracic cage. Degenerative changes are maximal at the C5–C6, C6–C7, and C4–C5 interspaces, respectively. Additionally, the volume of the cervical spinal cord is expanded over these vertebrae owing to the cervical enlargement, and the vertebral canal is relatively narrow ranging from 15 to 20 mm in anteroposterior diameter. People with a diameter of less than 13 mm may develop cord compression with quite mild degrees of spondylosis.

The mechanism of spinal cord injury is primarily one of compression and compromise of blood supply (ischemia). However, the high mobility of the neck in natural motions

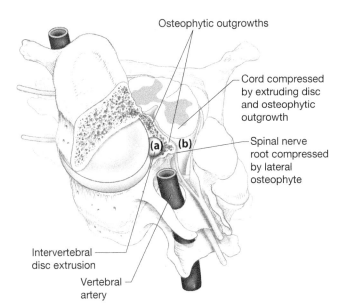

FIGURE 5-20 When compressing the spinal cord or spinal nerve roots, cervical spondylosis represents an extrinsic lesion. Here, the extruded nucleus pulposus (a) elicits a vertebral body reaction in which the vertebral body develops a ridge (bar) of bone over time that compresses spinal nerve roots and/or (b) the spinal cord.

of flexion and extension place a considerable demand on the cervical spinal cord and contribute to the cord and root damage. The spinal cord is not entirely free to ride these natural motions because it is held forward by the anteriorly directed nerve roots and is restrained from moving backward by the denticulate (dentate) ligaments at each side that tether the spinal cord to the dura mater. In forward flexion, the length of the spinal canal may increase by as much as 2 cm, and the cord stretches and tends to pull forward and is dragged over protruding osteophytes. When the neck is extended, the spinal cord, which is displaced posteriorly by the osteophytes, will be compressed by the infolding ligamentum flavum. The nerve roots are pulled in and out of the intervertebral foramina during neck flexion and extension and would be dragged over protruding osteophytes. Such intermittent trauma progressively injures the spinal cord or nerve roots. Additionally, neck extension or flexion may induce pain resembling a sudden electrical shock throughout the body called **Lhermitte's sign** (actually a symptom rather than a sign).

The most characteristic symptoms associated with cervical spondylosis are (1) painful, stiff neck; (2) arm pain (**brachialgia**) and numb hands; (3) spastic leg weakness and unsteadiness of gait with **Babinski signs**; and (4) **paresthesias** of the distal limbs and trunk. Paresthesias are abnormal sensations often described by the patient as burning, pricking, tingling, or tickling.

With respect to neck pain, it is important to note that approximately 40 percent of middle-aged persons (beyond 50 years of age) have some clinical abnormality of the neck, most commonly pain or **crepitus** with restricted mobility of movement. Furthermore, approximately 75 percent of people over age 50 with no neurological complaints have been found to have a narrowed cervical spinal canal due to osteophytosis. These bony changes can then place the individual at risk for injury to the cervical spinal cord from such events as falls or motor vehicle accidents.

BRAINSTEM

Clinical Preview

Some of the most tragic of situations that you see in your rehabilitation practice involve those individuals who sustained traumatic brainstem injuries as a result of an automobile or sports accident. In some cases, you are called upon to treat these people in the intensive care unit (ICU) and sometimes while they are still in a coma. As you read through this section, consider the brainstem mechanisms that are critical to awakeness and alertness of such individuals.

The brainstem represents the conduit whose fiber tracts link the spinal cord with the cerebellum and cerebrum. These tracts either originate in the spinal cord and ascend or originate in the cerebral cortex or the brainstem itself and descend. Additionally, the brainstem contains fibers that link structures confined to the brainstem in analogy with the propriospinal system of the spinal cord. Although not organized into a named tract, these fibers link structures that regulate functions such as respiration, cardiovascular activity, micturition, and movement. The surface features of the three divisions of the brainstem (medulla, pons, and midbrain) were presented in Chapter 2. Chapter 2 also discussed the general internal organization of the brainstem and how this organization differs from that of the spinal cord.

This chapter has two objectives related to the brainstem. The first is to correlate the surface features with the internal structures that produce them. The second is to introduce the organization and function of the brainstem reticular formation; the major component of the tegmentum; and the homologue of the spinal cord intermediate gray matter, but with a neuronal organization far more elaborate and a functional diversity far greater than the spinal intermediate gray.

The blood supply to the brainstem is not considered in this chapter but is deferred to Chapter 15 because the numerous vessels that nourish the brainstem have fairly distinct regional distributions. When a given artery is occluded, it results in ischemia in a particular region of the brainstem. An understanding of the clinical signs such an occlusion would produce depends on knowing the set of structures that reside in the vascular territory of the particular artery. Chapters 13 and 14 detail these structures. Consideration of the brainstem's blood supply and the clinical signs that follow occlusion of particular vessels provides an excellent way to review the regional anatomy of the brainstem and is a major topic of Chapter 15.

Cross-Section Correlations: Recognizing Level

The ability to easily recognize the brainstem level through which a particular transverse section was taken is of particular importance because this will reinforce learning the location of clinically relevant nuclei and tracts within the brainstem. The ability to quickly recognize brainstem level is accomplished by correlating specific surface features of the brainstem with the underlying structures that produce them. Subsequent chapters in this text will describe numerous clinically important structures of the CNS. Many of these are in the brainstem. Some reside only at specific levels of the brainstem (e.g., specific cranial nerve sensory and motor nuclei), whereas others can be found throughout the brainstem, although their positions change significantly as the structure traverses the medulla, pons, and midbrain (e.g., the medial lemniscus).

Thought Question

The brainstem has a highly complex organizational structure. Rehabilitation professionals who specialize in both neurological and orthopedic rehabilitation are likely to treat patients with brainstem related deficits. This structure is discussed in detail in later Chapters 13, 14, and 15. In preparation for assimilating this complex structure and its functional importance, it is useful to develop an understanding of overall brainstem structure. As a first step, identify levels of the brainstem by relating surface features and major internal features to the shape of the cross section. What structures can you use to differentiate cross sections through the medulla, pons, and midbrain? Can you differentiate sections through the caudal (low) versus rostral (high) medulla? What about the caudal versus rostral midbrain?

Caudalmost medulla is characterized by its essentially cylindrical shape, mimicking that of rostral cervical segments of the spinal cord, by the pyramidal decussation, and by the formation of the medullary pyramids (Figure 5-21a ■). The pyramids, initially separated by the deep anterior median fissure, are a constant feature of the ventral surface of the medulla throughout its extent (Figure 5-21b, c). Three major changes occur in moving rostrally through the medulla. First, the central canal of caudal medulla moves dorsally and expands into the

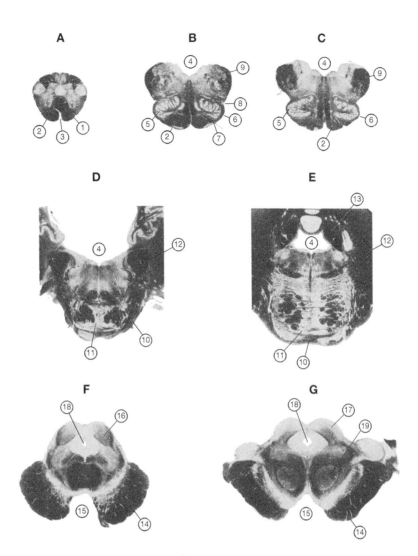

FIGURE 5-21 Histologic sections, stained for myelin, through caudal and rostral levels of the three brainstem subdivisions. Numbers indicate the structures key to determining whether the section is in the medulla, pons, or midbrain and then identifying whether the section is caudally or rostrally located in that subdivision.

(a) Spinomedullary junction; (b) caudal medulla; (c) rostral medulla; (d) caudal pons; (e) rostral pons; (f) caudal midbrain; (g) rostral midbrain.

1. Pyramidal decussation
2. Pyramid
3. Anterior median fissure
4. Fourth ventricle
5. Inferior olivary nucleus
6. Olivary eminence (olive)
7. Preolivary sulcus
8. Postolivary sulcus
9. Inferior cerebellar peduncle
10. Transverse fibers of the pons
11. Pontine nuclei
12. Middle cerebellar peduncle
13. Superior cerebellar peduncle
14. Cerebral peduncle
15. Interpeduncular fossa
16. Inferior colliculus
17. Superior colliculus
18. Cerebral aqueduct

(Sections from *Fundamental Neuroanatomy* by Walle J. H. Nauta and Michael Feirtag. © 1986 by W. H. Freeman and Company. Used with permission.)

fourth ventricle (Figure 5-21b). Caudally, the fourth ventricle is a narrow, deep trough but rostrally it expands and the trough appears flatter (Figure 5-21c). Second, the inferior olivary nucleus (the crumpled-bag-looking band of cells) appears (Figure 5-21b), expands tremendously (Figure 5-21c), and then rather abruptly decreases in size.

The nucleus produces the bulging olivary eminence. Note that you can see the pre- and postolivary sulci (recall which cranial nerves attach to each). Third, the inferior cerebellar peduncle appears (Figure 5-21b) and increases progressively in size. The lateral surface of rostral medulla thus comes to feature two large bulges (Figure 5-21c): a dorsal one formed by the inferior cerebellar peduncle and a ventral one formed by the inferior olivary nucleus.

Entry into caudal pons is signaled by a covering over of the pyramids by the transverse fibers of the pons (Figure 5-21d), and this feature characterizes the ventral surface of the pons throughout its extent (Figure 5-21e). Note that in the ventral third or so of caudal pons there are wide expanses of lightly stained, clear areas. These contain the cell bodies of the diffuse **pontine nuclei** whose axons form the transverse pontine fibers and then the middle cerebellar peduncles (same axons, just given different names). The axons run laterally and come together as the large middle cerebellar peduncles, appearing as the massive dark area on the lateral aspect of the pons. The ventral region of the pons, consisting mainly of the pontine nuclei and transverse pontine fibers, is the basilar portion of the pons. Note that in moving rostrally, the basilar portion increases markedly in size but it decreases in size again in rostralmost pons. Progressing rostrally through the pons, several other changes are valuable keys to recognizing level. First, the fourth ventricle narrows progressively, actually becoming the cerebral aqueduct before entering the midbrain. Second, it can be seen that the lateral walls of the ventricle are formed by the superior cerebellar peduncles (Figure 5-21e).

Throughout its caudal to rostral extent, the ventral surface of the midbrain is characterized by two massive bundles of fibers—the cerebral peduncles—separated by a midline interpeduncular fossa (Figure 5-21f, g). The presence of the inferior and superior colliculi provide a landmark that can be used to differentiate the caudal and rostral midbrain because the long axes of the inferior and superior colliculi have different orientations. The long axis of each inferior colliculus is tilted at an acute angle (Figure 5-21f), whereas that of the superior colliculus is more horizontal (Figure 5-21g).

Reticular Formation

The reticular formation forms the core of the entire brainstem, where it makes up the bulk of the tegmentum. The term *reticular formation* refers to the fact that its cells come in a wide variety of sizes; are not aggregated into well-defined groups as are, for example, the cranial nerve sensory and motor nuclei; and are enmeshed in a complicated network of fibers traveling in all directions, as opposed to the defined longitudinal ascending and descending tracts that traverse the brainstem. Despite this net-like appearance, the brainstem reticular formation possesses a far-reaching structural and functional differentiation. Different parts of the reticular formation contain cells that have distinctive cytoarchitectural features, and the different cell groups have specific connections.

Anatomicofunctional Zones

In general, the reticular formation is subdivided into two anatomicofunctional zones. The approximate medial two-thirds comprises the **effector zone**. This zone contains numerous large neurons (the zone is also called

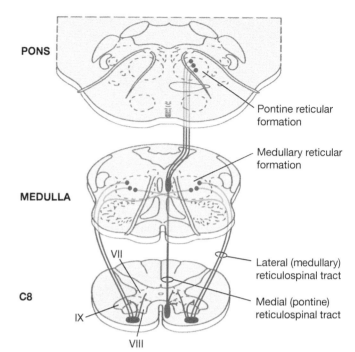

FIGURE 5-22 Section through rostralmost medulla showing the subdivisions of the reticular formation. Magnocellular neurons in the medial subdivision give rise to the long descending (reticulospinal) tracts. In contrast, parvocellular neurons in the lateral reticular formation function as interneurons involved, for example, in integrating reflexes mediated by local cranial nerves. Abbreviations: MLF, medial longitudinal fasciculus; ML, medial lemniscus; PYR, pyramids; MCP, middle cerebellar peduncle.

the **magnocellular zone**) that are the cells of origin of the long ascending and descending projections of the reticular formation (Figure 5-22 ■). The approximate lateral one-third comprises the **interneuronal zone**. These lateral portions contain primarily small neurons (hence, this zone is also called the **parvocellular zone**) whose axons have intrareticular projections that serve to integrate and pattern intrareticular formation activity.

Connections of the Reticular Formation

Not all connections of the reticular formation will be delineated in this section. For example, efferent projections from the reticular formation project to the cerebellum, and the reticular formation receives afferents from the cerebellum. These connections are important in mediating the motor functions of the cerebellum and are discussed in Chapter 19. Likewise, the vestibular nuclei are reciprocally connected to reticular formation neurons, and efferent projections from the reticular formation are important to the vestibular control of posture and equilibrium and will be discussed in Chapter 17.

AFFERENT PROJECTIONS Neurons of the reticular formation receive projections from the cerebral cortex—in particular from the somatosensory and motor cortices—but all areas of the cortex, including those on the basal and medial surfaces, contribute to these projections. These projections subserve two functions. First, they influence the transmission of activity that ascends from the reticular formation back to the cerebral cortex. Second, corticoreticular projections influence the activity of the descending reticulospinal systems that modulate both sensory and motor function.

Afferents from the spinal cord reach reticular formation neurons via two routes. First, reticular neurons receive collaterals from most sensory tracts ascending through the brainstem including those that originate from cranial nerve sensory nuclei. (The one exception is the medial lemniscus which does not send collaterals to reticular neurons.) Second, there are direct **spinoreticular projections** that ascend in the ventrolateral funiculus of the spinal cord medial to the spinothalamic tract.

Reticular neurons receive input from all sensory cranial nerves, but the most important functionally are the auditory, vestibular, and trigeminal nerves. This input is from collaterals of secondary sensory neurons associated with these cranial nerves. Finally, a considerable amount of visceral information reaches neurons of the reticular formation.

EFFERENT PROJECTIONS Efferent projections from the reticular formation include axons that descend into the spinal cord as well as axons that ascend to the diencephalon. Two named and long-recognized tracts descend into the spinal cord from the effector zone of the reticular formation. The **medial (pontine) reticulospinal tract** originates from neurons in the pons and descends ipsilaterally close to the midline to enter the ventral funiculus of the spinal cord (Figure 5-23 ■). The **lateral (medullary) reticulospinal tract** originates from neurons in the effector zone of rostral medulla. Its neurons descend bilaterally to enter the ventral part of the lateral funiculus of the spinal cord. These tracts play a vital role in the regulation of motor function. Two other tracts that, among other things, descend into the spinal cord are identified by the neurotransmitter they release. These descending projections relate importantly (but not exclusively) to the modulation of pain and are discussed in Chapter 16. Finally, **reticulobulbar connections** project to all of the cranial nerve sensory and motor nuclei.

A major ascending projection of the reticular formation terminates in the thalamus. The recipients of this input are a collection of thalamic nuclei (the midline, intralaminar, and reticular nuclei) referred to as the **generalized thalamocortical system** because these nuclei influence widespread areas of the cerebral cortex. Projections, in particular from the reticular formation of the midbrain, also terminate in the hypothalamus.

Functions of the Reticular Formation

The reticular formation participates in regulating a broad array of functions. These include motor function (discussed in Chapters 15, 17, and 19), autonomic activity (discussed in Chapter 12), and the modulation of pain (discussed in Chapter 16). Additionally, a major function of the reticular formation is as a participant in regulating the level of consciousness.

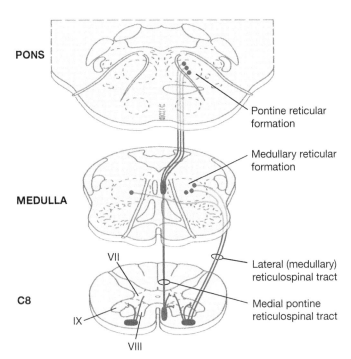

FIGURE 5-23 The origin, course, and terminations of the medial and lateral reticulospinal tracts. Fibers of the medial (pontine) reticulospinal tract (red) terminate in Rexed's lamina VIII and adjacent parts of lamina VII. Fibers of the lateral (medullary) reticulospinal tract (blue) terminate primarily in lamina VII, with some ending in lamina IX. Note: Although pontine reticulospinal tract is ipsilateral, it has bilateral influences via spinal cord interneurons that cross the midline; this is not represented in the diagram. The medullary reticulospinal tract is bilateral, with some fibers decussating in the medulla; as represented in the diagram.

The brainstem reticular formation plays an essential role in the regulation of two different aspects of consciousness. First, the reticular formation is a part of a neuronal system by which the brain regulates its own excitability or level of consciousness. Second, the reticular formation is an essential part of the mechanism by which the brain programs its own cyclic oscillations between sleep and wakefulness.

Thought Question

When comas occur, they usually indicate that damage has occurred within the brainstem. What portion of the brainstem is likely involved if a person is in a coma?

CLINICAL CONNECTIONS
Control of the Level of Consciousness

Different levels of consciousness are recognized clinically, some of which are not sharply demarcated from one another. Beginning with the most excitable state, these levels are attention, alertness, relaxed mood, drowsiness, sleep, stupor, and coma. **Attention** is the state of directing or concentrating one's consciousness on only one object or an internal or external stimulus. **Alertness** is the state of being aware and mentally functional. **Drowsiness** is the state of almost falling asleep. **Stupor** is a state of impaired consciousness in which the patient shows a marked diminution in reactivity to environmental stimuli. **Coma** is a state of profound unconsciousness from which the patient cannot be roused.

Clinical evidence confirms that the brainstem reticular formation plays an essential role in regulating consciousness, sleep, and wakefulness, although it is not the only brain area so involved. Neurosurgeries to treat intractable epilepsy or neoplasms indicate that large areas can be removed from any one hemisphere, or indeed, one entire hemisphere can be removed without loss of consciousness or disruption of normal sleep–wakefulness patterns. Brainstem lesions, on the other hand, have quite different sequelae. They often produce alterations not only in the level of consciousness but also disrupt the sleep–wakefulness cycle. For example, bilateral damage to the midbrain reticular formation and the projections traversing it results in a comatose state. The portion of the reticular formation producing this general arousing effect is called the **ascending reticular activating system (ARAS)** and occupies the pontomesencephalic reticular formation. It is an important component of a more widely distributed system of neurons having the same effect and termed the **ascending arousal system**. The ascending arousal system has additional components in the basal forebrain and hypothalamus.

The influence of the cerebral cortex on the activity of the reticular formation is dramatic. Widespread areas of multimodal association cortex, including the basomedial limbic cortex, project to the pontomesencephalic reticular formation. Our general alertness is influenced by words we hear, events we see, and sensations we experience. Daydreaming and mental imagery and their associated emotions are phenomena generated in specific areas of the cerebral cortex involved in memory. Both can have a general alerting effect on the entire cerebral cortex that is as marked as that which occurs in response to the actual sensory experience upon which the memory is based. Thus, mental imagery replicates the effect of environmental afferent input to the reticular formation and is able to maintain an attentive state. These corticoreticular projections are also involved in facilitating and inhibiting sensory inputs that impinge on reticular neurons. Auditory input has a particularly pronounced effect on the reticular formation. This facilitatory and inhibitory input enables us to concentrate on particular sensory experience and neglect others, such as, for example, attending to a single speaker's voice against a background of noise or other speakers at a party. It also is responsible for differentiated behavioral arousals, such as when a sleeping mother responds to the cry of her infant while not responding to other louder sounds generated by a passing train or honking car horn.

Summary

This chapter expanded on organizational features of the spinal cord and brainstem addressed initially in Chapter 2. Beyond its organization into dorsal and ventral horns and intermediate gray, neurons of the spinal cord gray matter are organized into nuclei and layers, or Rexed's laminae. Nuclei contain neurons whose axons either give origin to ascending sensory tracts (transmission neurons) or innervate specific groups of striated muscle. Some nuclei, such as the substantia gelatinosa and nucleus proprius of the dorsal horn and medial nucleus of the ventral horn, extend the entire length of the spinal cord, whereas others are located only in specific segments such as the nucleus dorsalis (T1–L2) in the intermediate gray and lateral nuclei in the ventral horn of the cervical and lumbosacral enlargements. The 10 laminae of Rexed represent the most detailed analysis of the cytoarchitecture of the spinal gray. Neurons residing in particular laminae have specific sensory inputs or motor outputs. Chapter 16, for example, discusses how different types of input from pain receptors terminate on neurons in different Rexed laminae whose neurons, in turn, give origin to different ascending pain tracts. The

homogeneous-appearing white matter of the three funiculi contains a variety of ascending and descending tracts that subserve different functions. Axons of some of these different tracts overlap. Only five of the tracts were outlined structurally and functionally. These are considered in more detail in later chapters along with the introduction of other tracts.

The surface features of the brainstem detailed in Chapter 2 were considered again in the context of the internal structures that produce them. The correlation between internal structure and surface anatomy is key to recognizing different levels of transverse sections through the brainstem that are used to describe the trajectories of ascending and descending tracts that link the spinal cord with the cerebellum and cerebrum. The major focus of this section was a description of the brainstem reticular formation that comprises the central core of the brainstem and occupies most of the tegmentum. Four major functions of the reticular formation were introduced. Most will be discussed in later chapters, with the exception of the role of the reticular formation in regulating the level of consciousness.

Applications

1. A 38-year-old construction worker suffered acute onset of back pain while lifting a wheelbarrow filled with concrete. The pain radiated down the posterior aspect of his left thigh and into the ventral surface of his foot. Coughing or sneezing made the pain worse. He experienced numbness and "pins and needles" over the same area of his leg and foot. He had difficulty walking and was unable to stand on his toes with his left foot, which he attributed to the pain. The neurological examination revealed weakness in the left gastrocnemius and hamstrings muscles and loss of the Achilles tendon reflex on the left. Sensory examination showed a marked diminished responsiveness to light touch and pinprick in the left lateral calf, lateral foot, including the outer toes and sole of the foot. He was found to have a herniated intervertrebral disc.
   a. What nerve root appears to have been damaged?
   b. Identify the most likely vertebral level of the disc herniation.

2. Maria, a 59-year-old woman, underwent an abdominal angiogram to evaluate an aortic aneurysm. Following the procedure, she had severe pain around her waist. She developed paralysis of both legs and was incontinent of bowel and bladder. Her knee and ankle reflexes were absent. She had a diminished response to pain and temperature over her legs below the 12th thoracic dermatome on the right and below the 1st lumbar dermatome on the left. She had normal and accurate response to discriminative touch and position sense.
   a. What does paralysis indicate?
   b. What sensory tracts are damaged?
   c. Identify where the lesion occurred. Which blood vessel(s) could be obstructed, and which were spared to give this pattern of motor and sensory losses?

References

Spinal Cord

Beres-Jones, J. A., and Harkema, S. J. The human spinal cord interprets velocity-dependent afferent input during stepping. *Brain* 127: 2232–2246, 2004.

Cheshire, W. P., Santos, C. C., Massey, E. W., and Howard, J. F. Spinal cord infarction: Etiology and outcome. *Neurology* 47: 321, 1996.

Crock, H. V., and Yoshizawa, H. *The Blood Supply of the Vertebral Column and Spinal Cord in Man*. Springer-Verlag, Berlin, 1977.

Herrick, M., and Mills, P. E., Jr. Infarction of the spinal cord. *Arch Neurol* 24: 228, 1971.

Schoenen, J., and Faull, R. L. M. Ch. 2. Spinal cord: Cytoarchitectural, dendroarchitectural, and myeloarchitectural organization. In: Paxinos, G., ed. *The Human Nervous System*. Academic Press, New York, 1990.

Waxman, S. G., and Kocsis, J. D. Spinal cord repair: Progress towards a daunting goal. *Neuroscientist* 3: 263–269, 1997.

Brainstem

Brodal, A. *The Reticular Formation of the Brainstem. Anatomical Aspects and Functional Correlations.* Charles C. Thomas, Springfield, IL, 1957.

Nolte, J, *The Human Brain: An Introduction to Its Functional Anatomy*. Mosby Elsevier, Philadelphia, 2009.

Plum, F., and Posner, J. B. *The Diagnosis of Stupor and Coma*, 3rd ed. Davis, Philadelphia, 1980.

Diencephalon and Cerebellum

LEARNING OUTCOMES

This chapter prepares the reader to:

1. Name the four major subdivisions of the diencephalon.

2. Locate the pineal gland and identify its postulated functional roles.

3. Identify the thalamus in cross section.

4. Name the major nuclei of the thalamus and the prominent lamina that separate major groups of nuclei.

5. Differentiate specific inputs from regulatory inputs to the thalamus.

6. Contrast the role of three types of nuclei associated with the thalamus: relay, association, and regulatory.

7. Discuss the major functions of the hypothalamus.

8. Identify the major inputs to and outputs from the hypothalamus.

9. Describe the blood supply of the thalamus, hypothalamus, and subthalamus.

10. Discuss clinical syndromes related to damage to the thalamic and hypothalamic structures.

11. Describe the role of the cerebellum with regard to movement.

12. Identify the input and output fibers of the cerebellum.

13. Name the nuclei of the cerebellum.

14. Discuss the subdivisions of the cerebellum phylogenetically and functionally.

15. Describe the blood supply of the cerebellum.

16. Discuss some of the causes and characteristic features of cerebellar dysfunction.

ACRONYMS

AICA Anterior inferior cerebellar artery

ADH Antidiuretic hormone

GABA Gamma-amino butyric acid

MFB Medial forebrain bundle

PCA Posterior cerebral artery

PICA Posterior inferior cerebellar artery

SCA Superior cerebellar artery

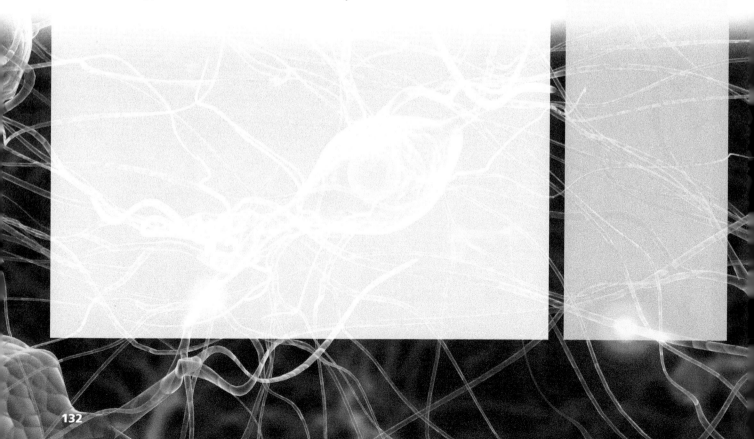

Introduction

This chapter builds on previous information, providing additional background details on the structural organization and functions of two important subcortical divisions of the CNS: the diencephalon and cerebellum. Both structures maintain extensive and critical relationships with the entire neuraxis, and these will be explored further in subsequent chapters. We focus here on general organizational and functional concepts.

The first section of this chapter discusses the diencephalon. This component of the cerebrum consists of four major subdivisions, each having a specialized function or set of functions. These are the epithalamus, thalamus, hypothalamus, and subthalamus. The thalamus is by far the largest subdivision, making up about 80 percent of the diencephalon. The thalamus and hypothalamus, and their separation on the medial wall of the third ventricle by the hypothalamic sulcus, were introduced in Chapter 2 (see Figure 2-20). The thalamus is divisible into more than two dozen distinct nuclei. It represents the gateway to the cerebral cortex. All sensory systems, with the exception of olfaction, synapse in the thalamus before gaining access to the cerebral cortex for conscious analysis. It also is the gateway by which the cerebellum and basal ganglia access the cerebral cortex. The hypothalamus, despite its small size, is organized into a number of rather indistinct nuclei and is intimately involved in the regulation of activity of the autonomic nervous system and the control of emotion and its behavioral manifestations. It also functions as the chief gland of the endocrine system, regulating the activity of all endocrine glands through its control of the pituitary gland.

The second section considers the cerebellum, a structure whose gross anatomical organization is simplistic compared to the much larger cerebrum. The general anatomy of the cerebellum is addressed first. The subject of intensive research over the years, the cerebellum is considered to be concerned foremost with the regulation of movement. Four different anatomical schemes are discussed by which the anatomy of the cerebellum is subdivided into different regions that subserve different aspects of movement. None of these has been entirely successful in correlating structure with motor function. This chapter's discussion of the cerebellum lays the groundwork for a more detailed consideration of its motor functions in Chapter 19. Recently, the cerebellum has been discovered to have certain cognitive functions and these are considered in Chapter 21.

DIENCEPHALON

Clinical Preview • • • • • • • • • • • • • • • •

Mr. Coulter, Mrs. Yang, and Mrs. Yancey are three people who live in the skilled nursing facility where you work. All three of them complain of the following: they have difficulty sleeping and are never able to "get warm." In addition, Mrs. Yancey sustained a small stroke. Her only additional deficit following this stroke is intractable pain in her right shoulder. As you read through this section, consider the anatomical areas that contribute to these distressing symptoms experienced by these three individuals.

Thought Question

A number of functions of the epithalamus have been inferred from disorders of the pineal gland. What are they?

The pineal gland has no known output via neuroanatomical pathways. Rather, the pineal is an endocrine gland whose secretory product is the hormone **melatonin**. Melatonin is secreted cyclically under the influence of the hypothalamus and so displays a circadian rhythm in which secretion is highest in darkness. The gland thus may play some role in the regulation of circadian rhythms, including the sleep–wakefulness cycle. Melatonin is synthesized from the neurotransmitter serotonin. Significantly, serum melatonin concentration is sometimes decreased in cases of biologic depression, indicating that one possible cause of depression is decreased serotonin content in the brain.

An unusual feature of the pineal gland, and one of potential clinical importance, is its tendency to accumulate calcareous deposits in individuals after they reach about 16 years of age. Such deposits render the gland visible in brain imaging. Because the gland normally lies in the midline, shifts in its position can be useful in the diagnosis of space-occupying intracranial masses of different types.

The anatomy of the habenular nuclei and its afferent connections via the stria medullaris and its efferent

Epithalamus

The **epithalamus** consists of the pineal gland, habenular nuclei, stria medullaris, and epithelial roof of the third ventricle. The **pineal gland** (see Figure 2-20), its most prominent member, is an unpaired, midline structure positioned just rostral to and in between the superior colliculi. The precise function of the pineal gland in humans is not well defined. Tumors involving cells of the pineal gland increase normal secretions of the gland and tend to result in hypogonadism and delayed pubescence. In contrast, lesions that destroy the gland tend to be associated with precocious puberty. Thus, one function of the pineal is that it likely plays some role in sexual development.

projections via other pathways are known in some detail. Although the functions of these nuclei in humans have not been well studied, it appears from studies of other mammals that their role includes diverse functions related to circadian rhythm and cognitive/emotional behaviors.

Thalamus

The thalamus is a bilaterally symmetrical egg-shaped structure situated on either side of the midline third ventricle (see Figure 2-26). It is subdivided into a large number of variably distinct nuclei with different functions that are discussed in the next section. Such subdivision reflects the fact that the thalamus is part of a large number of neural pathways, each of which incorporates a distinct nucleus (or several nuclei) in its pathway. The thalamus is the gateway to the cerebral cortex and has been described as a relay station. It is important to recognize that the thalamus serves both to relay and to process information. For example, all sensory systems (with the exception of olfaction) relay in the thalamus before gaining access to the cerebral cortex. Such **sensory relay nuclei** function as processing stations in the main sensory pathways and are located in the caudal half of the thalamus. They are discussed in relation to the ascending sensory pathways in Chapters 9, 12, 16, 17, and 18. Other nuclei are parts of circuits used by the cerebellum and basal ganglia and represent **motor relay nuclei**, whereby cerebellar and basal ganglia information is forwarded to the cerebral cortex. The motor relay nuclei are located in the rostral half of the thalamus and are discussed in Chapter 19. Still other thalamic nuclei have their own unique functions, and these will be introduced later in this chapter.

Topographical Organization

Situated between the posterior limb of the internal capsule laterally and the third ventricle medially, this largest subdivision of the diencephalon is subdivided into groups of nuclei by fibers of the **internal medullary lamina**, a complexly arranged thin sheet of myelinated axons (Figures 6-1, 6-2 ■). Anteriorly, the internal medullary lamina splits and encloses an **anterior group (a)** of nuclei that is separate from the other groups. The anterior nuclei form a visible rostromedial bulge on the thalamus called the *anterior tubercle*. More posteriorly, the lamina separates medial and lateral groups of nuclei from one another. However, inferiorly, the lamina splits again to enclose a set of nuclei called the **intralaminar nuclei**. The name of each nucleus (as discussed next) designates its position in the thalamus.

Table 6-1 ■ summarizes the topographic organization of the major thalamic nuclei. The medial nuclear group contains a single large nucleus, the **dorsomedial (DM)** (or **mediodorsal (MD)** nucleus) (see Figure 6-1). The lateral nuclear group is further divided into dorsal and ventral tiers of nuclei. The most rostral nucleus of the

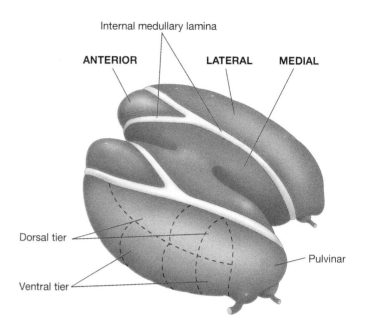

FIGURE 6-1 View of the thalamus from a dorsal perspective. On the right side, the division of the thalamus into anterior, lateral, and medial nuclear groups by the internal medullary lamina is indicated. The left side shows that the lateral nuclear group is further subdivided into a dorsal tier of nuclei and a ventral tier of nuclei. There are few obvious macroscopic landmarks to indicate this subdivision. The pulvinar is the largest nucleus of the dorsal tier. The medial and lateral geniculate bodies belong to the ventral tier of nuclei.

dorsal tier is the **lateral dorsal nucleus (LD)**, followed by the **lateral posterior nucleus (LP)** in an intermediate position, and finally by the **pulvinar (P)**, the greatly expanded caudalmost nucleus. The ventral tier consists in rostrocaudal sequence of a **ventral anterior nucleus (VA)**, a **ventral lateral nucleus (VL)**, a **ventral posterior nucleus (VP)**, and the **medial** and **lateral geniculate bodies (MGB and LGB)**. The VP nucleus is subdivided into a **ventral posterolateral nucleus (VPL)** and **ventral posteromedial nucleus (VPM)**. The largest of the intralaminar nuclei is the **centromedian nucleus (CM)**, wedged between the DM and VPM nuclei.

A narrow band of cells located immediately adjacent to the internal capsule lines the anterior and lateral surface of the thalamus like a shield. This is the **reticular nucleus** of the thalamus. It is uncertain whether its embryological derivation is the same as that of the other thalamic nuclei. Functionally, as well as with respect to its connections, the reticular nucleus differs markedly from other thalamic nuclei. The nucleus exerts a profound control over the function of other thalamic nuclei, which makes it appropriate to consider the reticular nucleus as part of the thalamus. The reticular nucleus, despite its name, is not related to the brainstem reticular formation. The ventricular surface of the thalamus is covered by a layer of cells called the **midline nuclei** that represent a rostral continuation of the midbrain periaqueductal gray matter. In 80 percent of

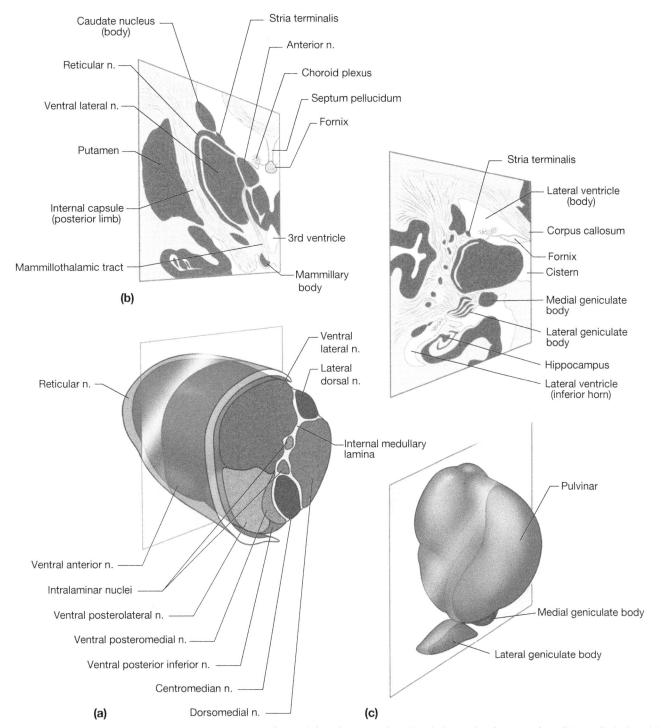

FIGURE 6-2 (a) The left thalamus viewed from a posterior and dorsal perspective. The thalamus has been sectioned frontally in its middle to reveal the internal medullary lamina and its associated nuclei as well as the fact that the lamina defines the anterior, medial, and lateral divisions of the thalamus. (b) An anterior section through the diencephalon that includes the mammillary bodies of the hypothalamus and mammillothalamic tract projecting to the anterior nucleus. Note the orientation of the posterior limb of the internal capsule. (c) A posterior section through the thalamus that passes through the medial and lateral geniculate bodies as well as the pulvinar.

brains, the midline nuclei fuse in the midline to form the massa intermedia (interthalamic adhesion), a cell bridge between the thalami; however, in spite of this cell bridge, there are no axonal projections between the left and right thalamus.

General Functional Organization

There is a general organizational pattern common to all thalamic nuclei (with the exception of the reticular nucleus) although the details of this pattern vary in different nuclei (Figure 6-3 ■). Each nucleus contains **projection neurons**.

Table 6-1 Topographic Organization of Major Thalamic Nuclei

NUCLEAR GROUP	MAJOR NUCLEUS OR NUCLEI	ABBREVIATION
Anterior	Anterior	A
Medial	Dorsomedial (mediodorsal)	DM (MD)
Lateral	Dorsal tier	
	Lateral dorsal	LD
	Lateral posterior	LP
	Pulvinar	P
	Ventral tier	
	Ventral anterior	VA
	Ventral lateral	VL
	Ventral posterior	VP
	Ventral posterolateral	VPL
	Ventral posteromedial	VPM
	Medial geniculate body	MGB
	Lateral geniculate body	LGB
Intralaminar	Centromedian	CM
	Parafascicular	PF
Reticular	Reticular nucleus	R

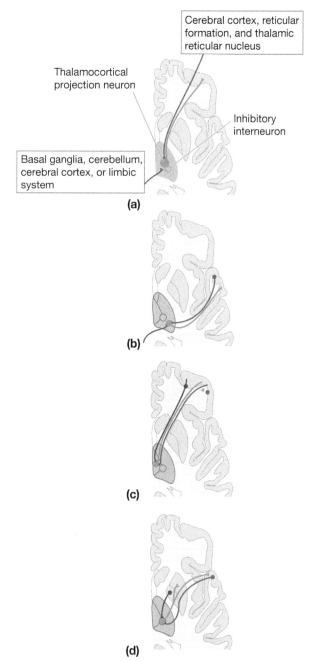

(a)

(b)

(c)

(d)

FIGURE 6-3 Horizontal sections through the right cerebral hemisphere and thalamus. (a) Overview of the organization of the connections of thalamic nuclei except for the reticular nucleus. All thalamic nuclei contain inhibitory interneurons (orange) and projection neurons (green) that project the cerebral cortex and synapse on a variety of cells. All nuclei receive specific subcortical inputs (blue), most of which usually originate from one major source. Each thalamic nucleus also receives a set of regulatory inputs (red), most of which originate in the cortical area to which that thalamic nucleus projects. (b) Thalamic relay nuclei receive specific inputs from subcortical structures (such as the cerebellum) or pathways (such as the medial lemniscus) and project to a well-defined area of the cerebral cortex. (c) Association thalamic nuclei receive specific inputs from association areas of the cortex and project back to association cortex. (d) Midline and intralaminar nuclei receive specific inputs from structures such as the basal ganglia or limbic system and project to the cerebral cortex as well as to the basal ganglia and limbic system.

Projection neurons comprise at least 75 percent of the neurons in a nucleus and convey output from the nucleus primarily to the cerebral cortex, although some nuclei project to other sites as well. An exception is the reticular nucleus of the thalamus, which has no projections to the cerebral cortex but receives topographically organized input from other thalamic nuclei and the cerebral cortex and has inhibitory projections back to the thalamus (e.g., inhibitory feedback and feedforward circuitry, respectively). All influences received by the cerebral cortex originate in thalamic nuclei, with the exception of olfactory information and the diffuse cholinergic and monoaminergic projections from the forebrain and brainstem. Thus, the thalamus is considered to be the primary gateway to the cerebral cortex. In addition, thalamocortical projections involve precise reciprocal corticothalamic projections. For example, the VPL nucleus receives somatosensory input from medial lemniscus, spinothalamic, and trigeminal tracts and projects to somatosensory cortex; somatosensory cortex projects back onto the VPL nucleus. Hence, the thalamus is not just a "relay" to cerebral cortex; rather, thalamus and cerebral cortex are best considered as a functional unit with many different subunits/channels involving separate thalamic nuclei and their reciprocal projections to distinct cortical areas.

With respect to projections to the thalamus, all thalamic nuclei receive afferent input from at least one extrathalamic source. Some of the inputs are categorized as **specific inputs** in that they carry information typically from one primary source that the thalamic nucleus forwards on to a specific area of the cerebral cortex for additional processing. For example, auditory input synapses on neurons in the medial geniculate body located in the posterior thalamus, whereas visual input synapses on neurons of the lateral geniculate body, also located in the posterior thalamus but, as the name suggests, a bit more laterally. Other inputs are categorized as **regulatory inputs**, and they far outnumber the specific inputs. Regulatory inputs determine, first, whether information received by a thalamic nucleus will be forwarded on to the cerebral cortex and, if so, in what form. Most regulatory input comes from the cerebral cortex, from the same area that received the projection from the nucleus,

but some comes from the reticular nucleus of the thalamus, and some from the diffuse noradrenergic, serotonergic, and cholinergic projections originating in the brainstem reticular formation. In Chapter 5, these neurotransmitter-specific systems were introduced in the context of their direct projections to the cerebral cortex. Some of these axons, however, give off collateral branches to the diencephalon.

The pattern of inputs and outputs from a given thalamic nucleus allows most of the nuclei to be placed into one of three categories. These patterns are summarized in Table 6-2 ■. The **specific relay nuclei** receive specific inputs from well-defined tracts and project to (and receive fibers from) well-defined cortical areas related to specific sensory, motor, or limbic system functions. The particular cortical projection field subserves the same general function relay nucleus; that is, it is unimodal. The specific relay nuclei have few, if any, interconnections with one another. **Association nuclei** do not receive a dominant input from a single specific source, but receive multimodal inputs and project to areas of the cerebral cortex classified as

Table 6-2 Inputs to and Cortical Outputs from Selected Thalamic Nuclei

TYPE AND NUCLEI	PRINCIPAL INPUT	CORTICAL OUTPUT
Relay Sensory		
VPL	Medial lemniscus, spinothalamic tract	Somatosensory cortex
VPM	Trigeminothalamic tracts	Somatosensory cortex
MGB	Auditory via inferior colliculus	Auditory cortex
LGB	Visual via optic tract	Visual cortex
Relay Motor		
VA	Basal ganglia	Motor cortex
VL	Cerebellum	Motor cortex
Relay Limbic		
A	Mammillothalamic tract, hippocampus	Cingulate gyrus
LD	Hippocampus	Cingulate gyrus
Association Limbic		
DM	Prefrontal cortex, olfactory and limbic system structures (e.g., amygdala)	Prefrontal cortex
Association Sensory		
P	Parietal, temporal, and occipital lobes; visual system	Parietal, temporal, and occipital lobes
LP	Parietal lobe	Parietal lobe
Diffuse Cortically Projecting		
Intralaminar	Cortex of the frontal and parietal lobes, basal ganglia, cerebellum, spinal cord, reticular formation	Widespread areas of the cerebral cortex, basal ganglia, especially striatum
CM		
Pf		
Regulatory		
R	Collaterals of thalamocortical and corticothalamic axons	None

association cortex. Association areas of the cerebral cortex concurrently process several different types of information; that is, they are multimodal. The two largest nuclei of the human thalamus, the dorsomedial nucleus and the pulvinar, are association nuclei and are discussed in more detail in Chapter 21. The final set of nuclei distinguish themselves by projecting to widespread areas of the cerebral cortex as well as by their subcortical reciprocal relations with parts of the basal ganglia and limbic system. These are (primarily) the **intralaminar nuclei**, and they are extensively interconnected. They are considered to be rostral extensions of the brainstem reticular formation into the diencephalon.

Functions of the Thalamus

The thalamus subserves a variety of functions. A major function is sensory integration. The thalamus receives, processes, and then forwards sensory information to the cerebral cortex, including both the primary sensory and association cortices. Important exceptions are olfaction and the monoaminergic

> ### Thought Question
>
> The thalamus is considered the major way station for sensory information except for olfactory information. Explain what this implies. In addition, the thalamus plays other critical roles. What are they and why are they important?

and cholinergic projections originating in the brainstem reticular formation whose afferents attain the cerebral cortex directly without first synapsing at a thalamic level. (These projections also give off collateral branches to the diencephalon.) Recognition of the affective quality of sensation is believed to occur at the thalamic level. This attribute of sensory experience has to do with pain sensibility as well as with the agreeableness or disagreeableness of sensations. Such aspects of sensory experience are thought to contribute importantly to the perception of general bodily well-being or malaise. Although profoundly modulated by cortical activity, clinical evidence indicates that the affective dimension of sensation enters consciousness at a thalamic level.

A second major function of thalamic nuclei is motor integration. The major outputs from the subcortically positioned basal ganglia and cerebellum are processed in the thalamus prior to their projection to the motor executive areas of the cerebral cortex (see Chapter 19). Finally, along with a host of other structures distributed within various subdivisions of the brainstem, the thalamus participates in governing the level of consciousness, alertness, and attention by virtue of influencing neural activity within the cerebral cortex via thalamocortical projections (also see Chapter 5).

Blood Supply

The primary blood supply to the thalamus is derived from branches of the posterior cerebral (PCA) and posterior communicating arteries (Figure 6-4 ■). These are called

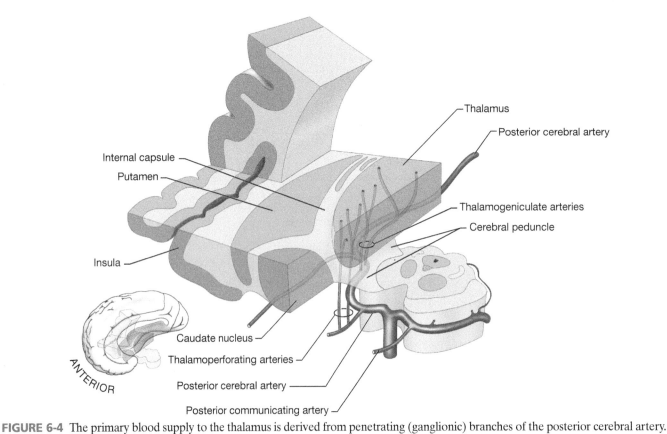

FIGURE 6-4 The primary blood supply to the thalamus is derived from penetrating (ganglionic) branches of the posterior cerebral artery.

(Bowman, J. P., and Giddings, D. F. *Strokes: An Illustrated Guide to Brain Structure, Blood Supply, and Clinical Signs.* Prentice Hall, New Jersey, 2003.)

ganglionic or **penetrating branches** because they branch at right angles from their parent artery to penetrate deeply into the substance of the brain. The anterior and medial portions of the thalamus are nourished by a posteromedial group of penetrating branches that arise from the most proximal portions of the PCAs and from the whole extent of the posterior communicating arteries. They enter the tuber cinereum, mammillary bodies, and interpeduncular fossa and course dorsally and medially. These are called the **thalamoperforating arteries**. The caudal half of the thalamus—including the lateral geniculate body, pulvinar, lateral nuclear group, and most of the ventral tier of thalamic nuclei—is nourished by penetrating branches called the **thalamogeniculate arteries**. These branches are given off from the PCAs further distally, as they wind around the cerebral peduncles. Occlusion of the thalamogeniculate arteries results in the thalamic syndrome (see Clinical Connections).

Hypothalamus

The hypothalamus is small, weighing only 4 grams and making up less than 1 percent of total brain weight. Despite its small size, the hypothalamus mediates a number of complex functions (Figure 6-5 ■). It influences the activity of the viscera via projections to the preganglionic motor neurons of the sympathetic and parasympathetic nervous systems; regulates the activity of endocrine glands; and, as the chief effector of the limbic system, elicits the behavioral manifestations associated with emotions. As noted in Chapter 2, the hypothalamus lies on either side of the ventral portion of the third ventricle and is continuous across its floor.

Subdivisions and Nuclei of the Hypothalamus

The hypothalamus extends from the lamina terminalis anteriorly to the mammillary bodies posteriorly. The elevated inferior surface of the hypothalamus, bounded anteriorly

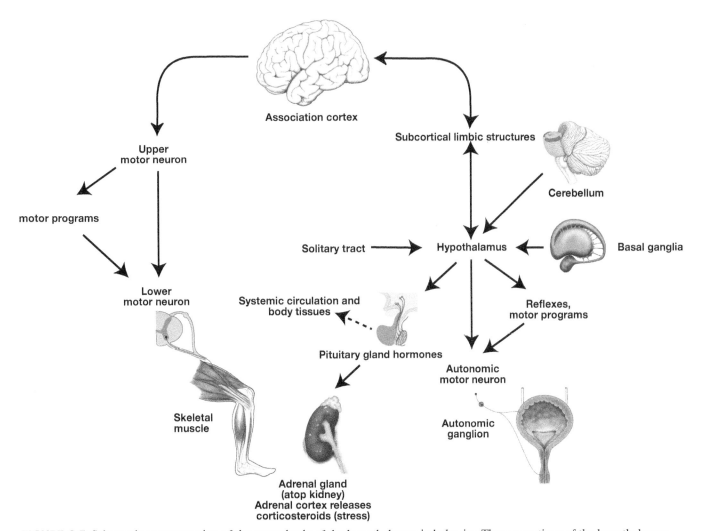

FIGURE 6-5 Schematic representation of the central role of the hypothalamus in behavior. The connections of the hypothalamus enable it to influence autonomic as well as somatic activities. Autonomic motor neurons in the spinal cord and brainstem are influenced directly as well as indirectly. Autonomic responses also are mediated by hypothalamic control of the pituitary gland. The hypothalamus is also able to generate somatic responses via its connection with limbic structures that, in turn, are reciprocally connected with the neocortex. The neocortex controls motor neurons that innervate skeletal muscle. And, via its return projection to limbic structures, the neocortex is able to modulate hypothalamic function.

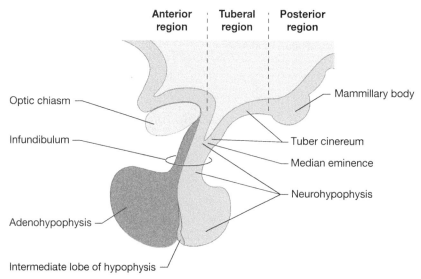

FIGURE 6-6 Schematic midsagittal section, illustrating the three anteroposterior regions of the hypothalamus and divisions of the pituitary gland.

by the optic chiasm, laterally by the optic tracts, and posteriorly by the mammillary bodies is called the **tuber cinereum** (Figure 6-6 ■). The **median eminence** is a swelling on the surface of the tuber cinereum from which emerges the pituitary stalk to connect the hypothalamus to the pituitary. The hypothalamus has been subdivided in both longitudinal and medial-lateral dimensions. In the longitudinal dimension, the hypothalamus is subdivided into an **anterior**, or **supraoptic**, **region**, above the optic chiasm; a **middle**, or **tuberal**, **region**, above and including the tuber cinereum; and a **posterior**, or **mammillary**, **region**, above and including the mammillary bodies.

The hypothalamus also is divided into three sagittal zones on either side of the midline. It is subdivided into **medial** and **lateral zones** by a parasagittal plane passing through the fornix, a prominent fiber bundle that traverses the hypothalamus on its way to the mammillary body.

The region of the hypothalamus immediately adjacent to the ependyma of the third ventricle makes up the third sagittal zone, the **periventricular zone**. Named nuclei lie within each of these nine zones, but the boundaries of many are not well defined. The lateral zone consists primarily of scattered cells interspersed by the longitudinally running fibers of the **medial forebrain bundle (MFB)**, a diffuse system of axons reciprocally interconnecting the septal region, hypothalamus, and brainstem.

The medial and periventricular zones contain a number of identified nuclei. These are summarized in Table 6-3 ■. Their functions will be discussed in connection with lesions of the hypothalamus (see Clinical Connections).

Input to the Hypothalamus

Neural input to the hypothalamus (Figure 6-7 ■) originates primarily from structures of the limbic system, a set of interconnected cortical (limbic lobe) and subcortical

Table 6-3 Hypothalamic Nuclei

REGION	MEDIAL AND PERIVENTRICULAR ZONES
Anterior (supraoptic)	Preoptic nucleus
	Supraoptic nucleus
	Paraventricular nucleus
	Anterior nucleus
	Suprachiasmatic nucleus
Middle (tuberal)	Dorsomedial nucleus
	Ventromedial nucleus
	Arcuate nucleus
Posterior (mammillary)	Mammillary body
	Posterior nucleus

structures concerned with emotions, learning, and memory and discussed in Chapter 22. Afferent projections from the hippocampus travel via the **fornix** and terminate largely in the mammillary body. The mammillary bodies make up the most posterior part of the hypothalamus. Fibers from the amygdala (see Chapter 7) reach the hypothalamus via two projections. One is via the **stria terminalis**, a long curved fiber bundle that travels with the caudate nucleus. The other is the **ventral amygdalofugal pathway** that passes beneath the globus pallidus. Projections from the orbitofrontal cortex, septal nuclei (located adjacent to the septum pellucidum), and ventral striatum reach the lateral hypothalamus in the medial forebrain bundle. Various sensory inputs from the spinal cord and brainstem terminate in the hypothalamus. There is a direct projection from the solitary nucleus of the medulla

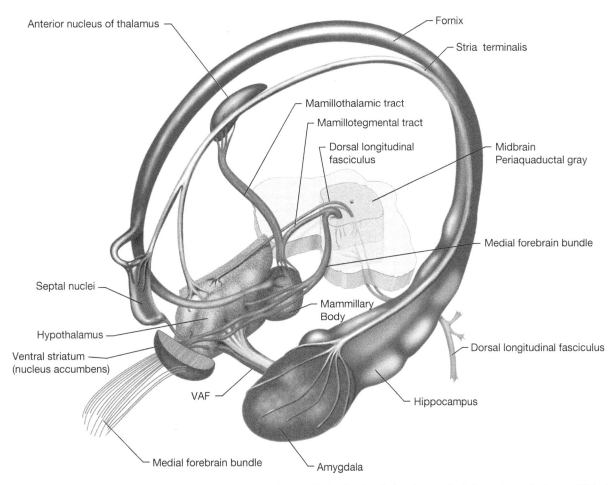

FIGURE 6-7 Principal inputs to and outputs from the hypothalamus. Only circuitry belonging to the left cerebrum is shown. With the exception of the mammillothalamic and mammillotegmental tracts that are composed of hypothalamic efferents, input to and output from the hypothalamus are via the same fiber bundles. Not shown are the retinohypothalamic projection, input to the hypothalamus from the solitary nucleus, and connections of the hypothalamus with the pituitary gland. Abbreviation: VAF, ventral amygdalofugal pathway.

that reaches the hypothalamus in the medial forebrain bundle. The medial forebrain bundle also contains axons of the ascending neurons containing serotonin and norepinephrine that arise from the raphe nuclei and locus coeruleus that project to the cerebral cortex. Collaterals of these axons are given off to cells of the hypothalamus (and thalamus) as the medial forebrain bundle traverses this structure. Collaterals of spinothalamic tract axons project to the hypothalamus. There also is a direct projection to the suprachiasmatic nucleus from the retina (the **retinohypothalamic projection**).

Other important input reaches the hypothalamus via a vascular route. Physically and chemically sensitive hypothalamic neurons respond to blood glucose levels, blood-borne hormones, blood osmolality, and blood temperature. In addition, there are isolated sets of neurons surrounding the ventricular system that lack a blood–brain barrier. These individual groups of neurons are called the **circumventricular organs** and are located primarily around the borders of the third ventricle. In lacking a blood–brain barrier, neurons of the circumventricular organs are able to detect chemical changes in the cerebrospinal fluid and blood. Their neurons then convey this information to the adjacent hypothalamus.

Output from the Hypothalamus

Much of the neural output from the hypothalamus is via the same pathways and to the same structures as provide input to the hypothalamus (see Figure 6-7). This is the case for efferent projections to the septal nuclei, widespread areas of the cerebral cortex, hippocampus, amygdala, and the brainstem and spinal cord autonomic projections. The neural projection to the pituitary gland is discussed later. The *mammillothalamic tract*, projecting to the anterior nucleus of the thalamus, and the *mammillotegmental tract*, projecting to the midbrain reticular formation, are primarily efferent.

Structural Links to the Pituitary Gland

The pituitary gland consists of two structurally and functionally distinct components: an anterior lobe and a posterior lobe. Both lobes are involved in the release of hormones, but the means by which they do this are vastly different. The posterior lobe does not manufacture the hormones it releases. Rather, it receives these hormones from neurons of the hypothalamus. In contrast, cells of the anterior lobe actually manufacture the hormones they release. This difference is a product of the distinct embryological origins of the two lobes. This differential origin also results in very different ways by which the hypothalamus communicates with the two lobes of the pituitary gland.

The **posterior lobe (neurohypophysis)** develops from the infundibulum, a downward evagination in the floor of the diencephalon. In contrast, the **anterior lobe (adenohypophysis)** is not part of the brain at all. It develops from an outpocketing of ectodermal tissue (Rathke's pouch) from the roof of the embryonic oral cavity. Accordingly, the links between the hypothalamus and the two lobes are different. The anterior lobe is endocrine, while the posterior lobe is neural (CNS).

The link between the hypothalamus and posterior lobe is entirely neural (Figure 6-8a ■). The posterior lobe of the pituitary gland does not manufacture hormones, and the two released by the posterior lobe are supplied to it by axons of hypothalamic nuclei. The link begins in the magnocellular neurosecretory cells of the **supraoptic** and **paraventricular nuclei** whose axons descend through the infundibular stalk to terminate in a dense plexus of capillaries in the posterior lobe.

The link between the hypothalamus and anterior lobe of the pituitary is indirect (refer to Figure 6-8b ■). It is established by a network of blood vessels. Hypophyseal arteries (branches of the internal carotid) enter the median eminence of the hypothalamus and form a set of looping capillaries that then form veins that drain into the anterior lobe of the pituitary where they divide into a second set of capillaries. This system of vessels is called the **hypothalamopituitary portal system**. Hypothalamic neurons in the tuberal region close to the wall of the third ventricle send axons into the median eminence where they terminate on the highly fenestrated capillaries therein. They release

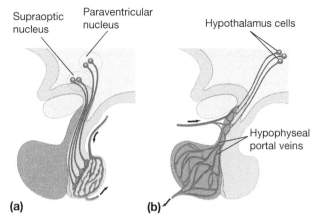

FIGURE 6-8 (a) The posterior lobe of the pituitary gland (the neurohypophysis) manufactures no hormones but releases two that are supplied to it by axons from the hypothalamus. Neurons in the supraoptic and paraventricular nuclei manufacture vasopressin and oxytocin. Their axons project to the posterior lobe and release their hormone into the capillary bed of portal blood vessels. (b) Cells of the anterior lobe of the pituitary (the adenohypophysis) manufacture a number of hormone releasing and inhibiting factors that either promote or inhibit hormone release by glandular cells in the anterior pituitary. Releasing factors are secreted by axons from neurons of the hypothalamus. Releasing factors enter the hypothalamopituitary portal system. The system comprises, first, a capillary bed in the median eminence, then a venous drainage channel in the infundibulum, and, finally, a second capillary bed in the anterior lobe.

chemical products, called releasing and inhibiting factors, or hormones, into the hypothalamopituitary portal system that then transports them into the capillary bed of the anterior lobe. The endocrine cells of the anterior lobe of the pituitary synthesize and store a number of hormones. They release them under the influence of the releasing factors secreted by hypothalamic neurons. The pituitary hormones and target organs upon which they act are summarized in Figure 6-9 ■.

Clinical Application Box 6-1: Vasopressin and Oxytocin

The peptide hormones, vasopressin and oxytocin, are stored in the bulbous axon terminals of cells of the supraoptic and paraventricular nuclei. The arrival of action potentials in cells of the nuclei releases the hormones into the highly fenestrated capillaries of the posterior lobe. This allows the hormones to enter into the systemic circulation. Vasopressin (antidiuretic hormone, ADH) controls water balance by increasing the reabsorption of water in the kidney, thereby decreasing the production of urine. Oxytocin causes contraction of the smooth muscle in the uterus and myoepithelial cells in the mammary glands and so is involved in parturition and milk ejection. While nearly all of the cells of the supraoptic nucleus project axons into the posterior lobe, only some 30 percent of paraventricular neurons send their axons into the lobe. Many paraventricular neurons have axons that enter a pathway that descends directly from the hypothalamus to the spinal cord and terminate on preganglionic sympathetic motor neurons of the intermediolateral cell column.

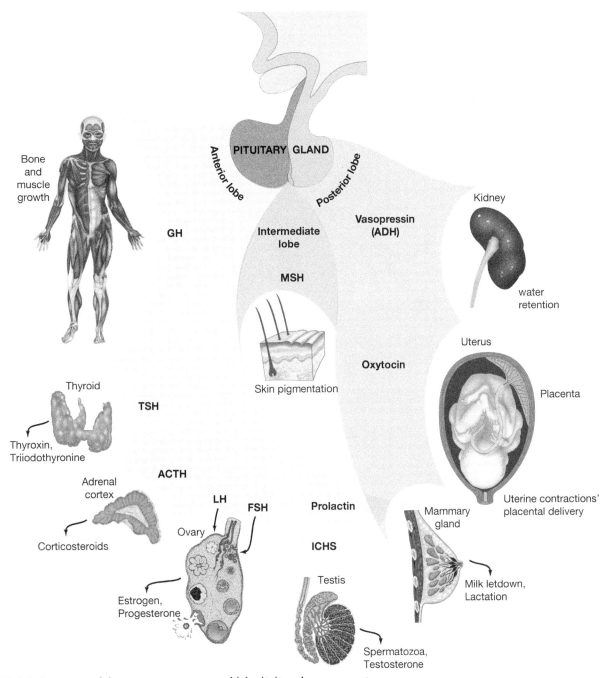

FIGURE 6-9 Summary of the target organs upon which pituitary hormones act.
Abbreviations: ACTH, adrenocorticotropic hormone; ADH, anti-diuretic hormone; FSH, follicle-stimulating hormone; GH, growth hormone; ICSH, interstitial cell-stimulating hormone; LH, luteinizing hormone; MSH, melanocyte stimulating hormone; TSH, thyroid-stimulating hormone.

Blood Supply

Two groups of penetrating branches supply most of the hypothalamus (Figure 6-10 ■). The **anteromedial group** arises from the anterior cerebral arteries and anterior communicating artery. They enter the medial part of the anterior perforated substance and nourish the anterior hypothalamus, including the preoptic and supraoptic regions. The **posteromedial group** arising from the posterior cerebral arteries and posterior communicating arteries, some whose branches supply parts of the thalamus as already mentioned, have shorter branches that nourish the caudal parts of the hypothalamus, including the mammillary region as well as the subthalamic region.

Functions of the Hypothalamus

The hypothalamus subserves a number of functional roles including endocrine function, body temperature regulation, sleep–wakefulness cycles, and emotional and behavioral

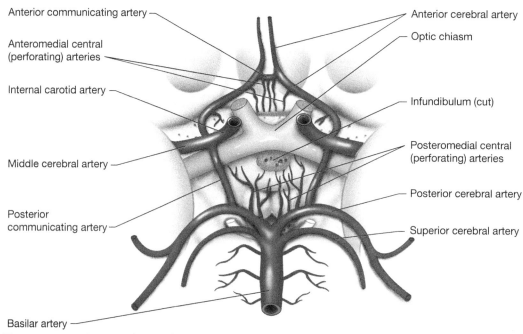

FIGURE 6-10 The two groups of penetrating arteries that nourish the hypothalamus. The anteromedial group of penetrating arteries arises from the anterior cerebral artery, while a posteromedial group arises from the posterior cerebral and posterior communicating arteries.

Thought Question

What are the consequences of damage to the hypothalamus? How do they differ from the consequences of damage to the subthalamus?

---

functions. These functions are listed in Table 6-4 ■, and the nuclei associated with each functional role are identified.

These functions are considered again in conjunction with hypothalamic lesions.

Subthalamus

The subthalamus is a wedge-shaped subdivision of the diencephalon, representing a zone of transition between the thalamus (dorsal thalamus) and the midbrain tegmentum. It is located medial to the cerebral peduncle

Table 6-4 Functions and Nuclei of the Hypothalamus

ANTERIOR		MIDDLE		POSTERIOR	
Function	**Nucleus**	**Function**	**Nucleus**	**Function**	**Nucleus**
Heat loss	Preoptic	Endocrine activity	Tuberal and arcuate	Heat conservation	Posterolateral
Drinking	Preoptic	Satiety	Ventromedial (?)		
Sleep	Preoptic (?)	Feeding	Lateral (?)	Waking cortical activation	Posterior
Water balance	Supraoptic and paraventricular	Emotions	Dorsomedial (?) Lateral (?)	Recent memory	Mammillary body
Milk ejection and uterine contraction	Supraoptic and paraventricular				
Circadian rhythms	Suprachiasmatic				
Parasympathomimetic				Sympathomimetic	

Note that the question marks (?) indicate uncertainty in the scientific literature.

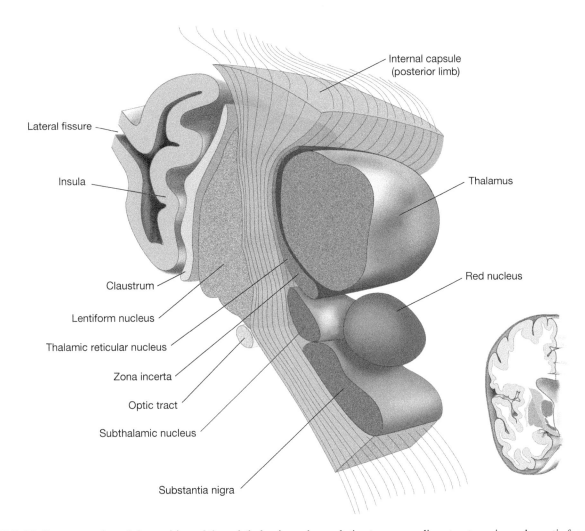

FIGURE 6-11 Representation of the position of the subthalamic nucleus relative to surrounding structures in a schematic frontal section. Note that the nucleus is positioned between the midbrain and thalamus rostrocaudally and medial to the internal capsule.

and internal capsule and contains the rostral extensions of the substantia nigra and red nucleus. It is traversed by prominent pathways projecting from the cerebellum and basal ganglia. Its most prominent constituent is the **subthalamic nucleus**, a biconvex, lens-shaped nucleus lying immediately dorsal to the projection fibers at the transition from the internal capsule to the cerebral peduncle (Figure 6-11 ■). The nucleus is an integral component of the circuitry of the basal ganglia, and its function is discussed in Chapter 19.

Blood Supply

The thalamoperforating (thalamoperforate) branches of the PCA were noted in conjunction with the blood supply of the thalamus. In addition to nourishing the anterior and medial parts of the thalamus, a thalamoperforant branch supplies the subthalamic nucleus (see Figure 6-10). Occlusion of this branch results in **hemiballismus**, an involuntary movement disorder discussed in Chapter 19. Hemiballismus is characterized by unilateral, uncontrolled, wild, flinging movements of the extremities. The symptoms present on the side of the body contralateral to the lesion.

CLINICAL CONNECTIONS
Thalamic Syndrome

In Chapters 8 and 9, we will learn the detailed pathways by which sensory information travels from the periphery to the cortex by way of the thalamus. For now, it is important to recognize that lesions of the somatosensory cortex—even the complete destruction of the sensory cortical areas of both hemispheres—leave intact the appreciation of pain, crude touch, and some thermal sense. Individuals with such lesions can still recognize that they have been touched or have received a painful stimulus, but they can neither localize the stimulus nor discriminate its intensity.

Extensive lesions of the posterior thalamus, usually from a stroke involving the thalamogeniculate branches of the posterior cerebral artery, produce the **thalamic syndrome** whose symptoms manifest themselves on the side contralateral to the lesion. The syndrome consists of three components that occur in variable proportion in different people: *hemianesthesia*, *sensory ataxia*, and *thalamic pain*. Hemianesthesia is a profound, sometimes total, loss of somatic sensation over the contralateral head and body. Pain, temperature, and crude touch sensibility usually return after a variable period of time. In sensory ataxia, the person displays a motor incoordination due to a loss of the proprioceptive information derived from muscles, joints, and tendons. Deprived of information about the prevailing status of the motor periphery (such as muscle length, velocity of limb movement, etc.), central motor structures have no effective way of successfully planning, coordinating, and executing movement. Thalamic pain is excruciating and may be triggered by normally innocuous somatic stimuli. Significantly, it is unresponsive to narcotic analgesics, whose site of action is within the brainstem and spinal cord. Neurogenic pain of this nature may be due to deficient pain modulation rather than to excessive activation of pain afferent systems. A **dysesthesia** may be manifest in which somatic stimuli are perceived abnormally. The affective quality of sensation also may be altered.

Hypothalamic Syndromes

Many pathologic processes can damage the hypothalamus and pituitary gland. Tumors are the most common. Primary tumors of the pituitary gland most often expand in a dorsal direction because it is the pathway of least resistance. Thus, the earliest signs of a pituitary tumor often are due to involvement of the hypothalamus. Lesions must be bilateral to affect most hypothalamic functions. The functions of the hypothalamus are listed in Table 6-4 and will be considered in conjunction with hypothalamic lesions. Hypothalamic lesions can produce a global hypothalamic syndrome in which all or many hypothalamic functions are disordered. Alternatively, a hypothalamic lesion can result in a partial hypothalamic syndrome in which a selective loss of a particular hypothalamic function is observed due to a discrete lesion and a deficiency or overproduction of a single hormone. The global hypothalamic syndrome is characterized by diabetes insipidus, deficits in endocrine function, disordered body temperature regulation, disordered sleep–wakefulness cycles, and emotional and behavioral changes.

Diabetes insipidus is caused by lesions that involve the supraoptic and paraventricular nuclei or their projections. This reduces the production of vasopressin so that ADH is not released into bloodstream of the posterior lobe. ADH increases the permeability of the distal convoluted tubules and collecting ducts of the kidney so that, in its absence, water is not reabsorbed by the kidney. Thus, there is excessive urine production and urination (**polyuria**) that, in turn, causes excessive thirst and drinking (**polydipsia**).

Damage to the hypothalamus or to the hypophyseal portal system can result in a decreased secretion of all anterior lobe hormones (except prolactin) due to the loss of releasing factors. This causes deficits in endocrine gland function that are manifest clinically by signs such as those associated with hypothyroidism and menstrual cycle irregularities.

Disturbances in temperature regulation can result from damage in either the anterior or posterior hypothalamus. Temperature-sensitive neurons in the anterior hypothalamus respond to small increases in the temperature of blood circulating in the capillary bed near these neurons. They initiate responses that lower blood temperature—namely, cutaneous vasodilation and sweating—and therefore, these neurons comprise a heat loss center. Damage to these neurons in the anterior heat loss center results in **hyperthermia**. If pronounced, hyperthermia may lead to the death of the patient within hours or days. Postoperative hyperthermia is sometimes seen in patients operated on for the removal of pituitary tumors. Conversely, neurons in the posterior hypothalamus are sensitive to decreases in blood temperature. These neurons comprise a heat gain center because they initiate cutaneous vasoconstriction and shivering, responses designed to increase body temperature. Damage to these neurons results in **hypothermia**. However, bilateral lesions in the posterior hypothalamus are more likely to result in poikilothermia, a condition in which body temperature varies with that of the surrounding environment. Poikilothermia occurs because not only are the neurons of the heat gain center damaged, but the posterior lesion also damages fibers from the anterior heat loss center en route to the brainstem reticular formation.

Both sleep and the sleep–wakefulness cycle are influenced by the hypothalamus. The circadian rhythm of sleep is controlled by the **suprachiasmatic nucleus** of the anterior hypothalamus. Damage to the posterior hypothalamus causes hypersomnia such as occurred during the post–World War I influenza pandemic (encephalitis lethargica, Von Economo disease, sleeping sickness). In contrast, damage to the anterior hypothalamus results in insomnia. Bilateral damage in or near the ventromedial nuclei of the hypothalamus may result in a patient exhibiting spells of spontaneous and extreme anger, sometimes accompanied by aggressive and violent behavior toward anyone in the patient's presence (doctors, relatives, etc.).

Dystrophia adiposogenitalis results from damage to the ventromedial hypothalamic nuclei and resulting in hyperphagia and, eventually, obesity. The ventromedial nucleus, therefore, was called a *satiety center*. The adiposity (excessive fat deposition) may be associated with underdevelopment of the genitalia, and the condition is then called **Froehlich syndrome**. These signs may be combined with antisocial behavior, unprovoked rage, or aggression.

CEREBELLUM

The term *cerebellum* is the diminutive form of cerebrum and means "little brain." The cerebellum is indeed a little brain in that while it accounts for only a fraction of the total volume of the brain, it contains more than half of all its neurons. Traditionally, the human cerebellum has been considered to function exclusively in the motor domain. It unquestionably does have indispensable functions for normal motor behavior, but within the past decade or so, the

Clinical Preview ················

Gordon Black was referred to your orthopedic clinic because of right foot pain that interfered with his ability to run marathons. When you first saw him, you noticed that he had difficulty controlling his movements. Indeed, at first you thought he might be intoxicated. However, during the history and interview, it became evident that these problems had been developing gradually over the previous two years and that they were not related to alcohol abuse. As you read through this section, you will begin to understand the anatomical basis for his deficits. (Note that you will learn much more about the anatomy underlying this gentleman's problems in Chapter 19.)

Anatomy of the Cerebellum

The general anatomical organization of the cerebellum is similar to that of the cerebral hemisphere covered in Chapter 7. The cerebellum consists of an outer mantle of cortex whose cells are arranged into distinctive layers. The cortex surrounds an inner core of white matter whose axons carry information to and from cells of the cortex. Like the cerebral hemisphere, embedded within this central core of cerebellar white matter is a set of cerebellar nuclei.

Given this organizational similarity, our overall approach to the anatomy of the cerebellum will be the same as that to the anatomy of the cerebral hemisphere in the next chapter. We first consider the surface appearance of the cerebellum and its division into lobes. Next neurons of the cerebellar cortex are considered and their arrangement into distinct layers discussed. Then the deep cerebellar nuclei are presented.

Folia, Fissures, Lobes, and Lobules

The hallmark of cerebellar gross anatomy is its surface. The surface area of the cerebellum has been tremendously expanded relative to its volume by an extensive infolding into numerous narrow leaf-like folds separated by sulci. Each such fold is termed a **folium** (L., leaf; pl. folia). Folia are like the gyri of the cerebral hemisphere, but are of a much finer grain. The folial pattern typically is characterized as being oriented in the transverse or coronal plane. While this is true, in particular, for the pattern on the superior surface of the cerebellum, it is not true for all folia on the posterior and inferior cerebellar surfaces where many folia are oriented in a near sagittal and variety of other orientations (see Figure 2-14). The orientation of cerebellar folia is the macroscopic expression of the orientation of a set of underlying cortical fibers called parallel fibers (see Chapter 19). Extending from the anterior to the posterior limit of the cerebellum, the folia are organized into a continuous succession of quasi-parallel ridges.

The fissures and lobes of the cerebellum can best be visualized by unfolding the cerebellum and laying it flat as depicted in Figure 6-12 ■. Two transversely oriented fissures divide the cerebellum into three major lobes. The first fissure to appear in the developing embryo is the **posterolateral fissure**. The posterolateral fissure separates the small **flocculonodular lobe** from the much larger body of the cerebellum (called the **corpus cerebelli**). The **primary fissure** appears next in development. Seen best from a midline perspective, it divides the body of the cerebellum into an **anterior lobe**, located rostral to the primary fissure, and a much larger **posterior lobe**, situated between the primary and posterolateral fissures. As noted in Chapter 2, each lobe consists of an unpaired midline vermis and lateral hemispheral portions on either side of the vermis. Although not evident except on the superior surface, the vermal and hemispheral components are structurally continuous with one another.

A series of additional transverse fissures subdivide the cerebellum into 10 primary lobules, designated by Roman numerals as well as by name. These numerals and names are of limited clinical utility but are widely used in research literature.

view that the cerebellum also performs significant nonmotor functions has been evolving. Recently, an anatomical substrate for involvement of the cerebellum (and basal ganglia) in higher cognitive function has been defined experimentally (see Chapter 21).

The cerebellum is involved in a number of aspects of motor behavior, in a modulatory and regulatory capacity. In contrast to other components of the motor system, cerebellar damage does not result in paralysis or paresis (muscle strength is not impaired), although hypotonia is common. Even its total removal does not abolish movement. Movement still can be performed by persons with cerebellar damage, but they may lose their smoothness, accuracy, and coordination. People with cerebellar damage may exhibit postural instability because the normal cerebellum helps maintain muscle tone and the body's position and balance in space during the execution of movement. Motor incoordination may be apparent in limb, orofacial, and eye movements following cerebellar damage.

Located in the posterior cranial fossa, dorsal to the medulla and pons, the cerebellum is positioned to monitor descending motor signals from the cerebral cortex, and ascending sensory information from the spinal cord and vestibular system. This is commonly referred to as the "comparator" function of the cerebellum. Specifically, the cerebellum compares the intended movement with the actual movement, which permits detection of motor errors when these two signals do not match. When motor errors are detected, the cerebellum plays a role in correcting them in ongoing and subsequent movements. Hence, the cerebellum also has an important role in motor learning (see Chapter 18). Despite receiving a massive input derived from peripheral somatosensory receptors, patients with isolated cerebellar damage do not complain of alterations in somatosensation. They may stagger, reel, and fall, but they do not report dizziness. Their movements may deviate to one side of the desired target, but their sense of position in space is not defective. For this reason, the sensory function of the cerebellum is referred to as unconscious proprioception.

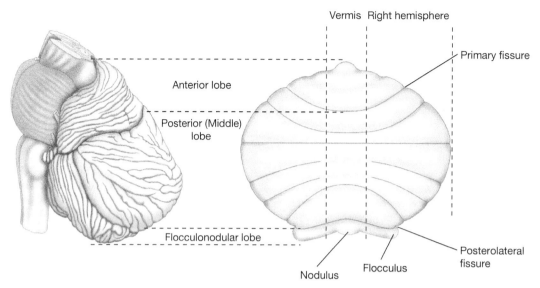

FIGURE 6-12 The cerebellum unfolded and flattened (right) to reveal the major landmarks and terminology.

Cerebellar Cortex

Each folium of the cerebellum is made up of a mantle of cortex surrounding a slender ray of white matter containing the fibers going to or coming from cells of the cortex. The arrangement of cells and fibers within the folia is structurally the same throughout the cerebellum so that any folium is representative of all others. However, as we shall discuss in Chapter 19, not all folia receive the same kind of afferent information, nor do they send their information to the same more deeply placed structures.

The cerebellar cortex is made up of three distinct layers (Figure 6-13 ■). The outermost layer is the **molecular layer**. It is made up of the dendrites of cerebellar neurons named *Purkinje cells* along with certain types of interneurons. The **Purkinje cell layer** is deep to the molecular layer. It consists of a single layer of regularly arranged Purkinje cells. The extensive dendrites of each Purkinje cell ascend through the molecular layer forming therein a flattened, leaf-like arborization oriented perpendicular to the long axis of the folium. The thinner dendritic branches of the Purkinje cells are densely beset with spines, thus providing an enormous surface area for synaptic contacts. Each Purkinje cell is estimated to contain some 200,000 spiny synapses. The innermost cortical layer is the **granular layer**, so named because of the densely packed, small granule cells composing it. The granular layer is densely packed with small-sized neurons, and has been estimated to contain 10 to 50 percent of all the neurons in the human CNS. Like the molecular layer, the granular layer contains characteristic interneurons.

Cerebellar Input and Output Fibers

Fibers afferent to cells of the cerebellar cortex are of two types, both of which are excitatory: **climbing fibers**, which originate from the contralateral inferior olivary nucleus

> ### Thought Question
>
> What are climbing fibers and mossy fibers? Compare and contrast the origins and destinations of each.

and end directly on Purkinje cells, and **mossy fibers**, which originate from cell bodies in the spinal cord and brainstem (e.g., the pontine nuclei) and influence Purkinje cells indirectly, via a granule cell relay (Figure 6-14 ■). Both types of afferents also end on cells of the deep cerebellar

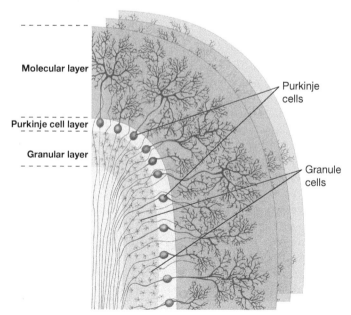

FIGURE 6-13 The three layers of the cerebellar cortex. The outermost molecular layer contains dendrites of Purkinje cells, the cell bodies of which reside in the Purkinje layer. The innermost granular layer is densely packed with small granular cells.

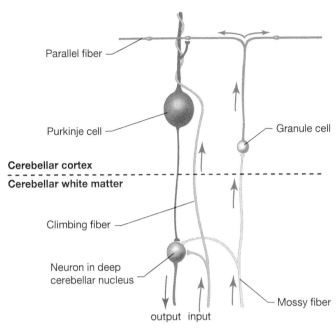

FIGURE 6-14 Cerebellar input (climbing and mossy fibers) and output (Purkinje cell) fibers. Climbing fibers wind around and synapse upon the Purkinje cells; mossy fibers synapse upon granule cells. The Purkinje cell is the only efferent route from the cerebellar cortex, shown here to a deep cerebellar nucleus.

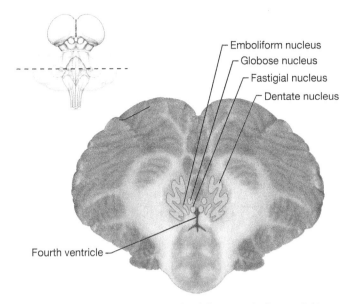

FIGURE 6-15 There are four paired deep cerebellar nuclei buried in each cerebellar hemisphere. The fastigial nucleus is most medial, the dentate nucleus most lateral. Between these two nuclei are two additional nuclei, a more medial globose nucleus, and a more lateral emboliform nucleus.

nuclei, providing them with a background excitatory drive (see Chapter 18).

Purkinje cell axons represent the *sole output* from the *cerebellar cortex*. The vast majority of these axons terminate on neurons of the deep cerebellar nuclei, forming the *corticonuclear projection system* (as discussed later). However, a small contingent of Purkinje cell axons leave the cerebellum to end on neurons of the vestibular nuclei. Purkinje cells are inhibitory to their target neurons so that the net result of Purkinje cell activity is inhibition of the spontaneous background activity occurring in cells of the deep cerebellar nuclei and vestibular nuclei.

Cerebellar Nuclei

Four distinct paired nuclei are buried in the white matter of each half of the cerebellum (Figure 6-15 ■). The **fastigial nucleus (FN)** is most medial and the **dentate nucleus (DN)** most lateral. Between these two nuclei are two smaller cellular masses, a more medial **globose nucleus** and a more lateral **emboliform nucleus**. The DN is by far the largest nucleus; its ventrolateral portion has undergone a tremendous expansion in the human. Although there are, in fact, four nuclei in the cerebella of subhuman primates, two of these nuclei—the globose and emboliform nuclei—are commonly referred to as the **nucleus interpositus** (interposed nucleus), the term we will use. The output fibers from the cerebellum originate from neurons of the cerebellar nuclei, with one notable exception mentioned earlier—the contingent of Purkinje cell axons that project directly from the cerebellar cortex to the vestibular nuclei of the brainstem.

There is a somatotopic representation of the body within each of the cerebellar nuclei. In each representation, the caudorostral dimension of the body is mapped onto the sagittal dimension of the nucleus: the legs are represented anteriorly and the head posteriorly, with the distal limbs medial and the proximal limbs lateral. Each of the deep cerebellar nuclei subserves a different function. This results from the fact that each nucleus receives its input from Purkinje cells located in different regions of the cerebellar cortex and projects its output to unique targets in the CNS. This is elaborated in more detail in Chapter 19.

Cerebellar Peduncles

Three cerebellar peduncles contain the afferent and efferent fibers that join the cerebellum to the rest of the nervous system (Figure 6-16 ■). Many different types of receptors send afferent information to the cerebellum. Conversely, the cerebellum influences, via its efferent fiber system, levels of the nervous system extending from the cerebral cortex to the spinal cord. Afferent fibers outnumber efferent fibers in a ratio of about 40:1. Additionally, the functional diversity and number of cerebellar inputs indicates the extent to which the coordination of motor patterns is dependent on multiple factors.

Thought Question

The cerebellar peduncles were identified previously in Chapter 2, and in more depth in this chapter. What are the pathways associated with each peduncle?

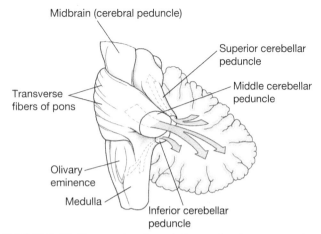

FIGURE 6-16 Three pairs of cerebellar peduncles connect the cerebellum to the brainstem.

The inferior cerebellar peduncle (restiform body) connects the spinal cord and medulla with the cerebellum. The majority of its fibers are afferent, and most of these originate in the inferior olivary nucleus of the contralateral medulla. The middle cerebellar peduncle (brachium pontis) is the most massive of the cerebellar peduncles. It connects the pons with the cerebellum. This peduncle contains some 20 million fibers, all of which are afferent to the cerebellum. Most of these afferents are derived from the pontine nuclei, which are collections of cells distributed throughout the basilar portion of the pons. The superior cerebellar peduncle (brachium conjunctivum) is the major efferent pathway from the cerebellum and distributes its fibers to nuclei of the brainstem and thalamus. These latter structures then convey cerebellar influences to other parts of the CNS.

Subdivisions of the Cerebellum in Relation to Function

The functions of the cerebellum, like those of so many other brain structures, were originally defined in terms of the behavioral deficits resulting from its damage as a result of naturally occurring pathology. The most obvious signs and symptoms occurred during movement, and the cerebellum was considered to function in three aspects of motor control: the regulation of equilibrium; the control of posture and muscle tone; and the coordination of voluntary movement. Because the cerebellum represents one of the more intensively studied structures of the CNS, it should not be surprising that numerous attempts have been made to understand the motor functions of the cerebellum in terms of its anatomic organization. Such attempts have produced four major schemes for subdividing the cerebellum into different regions that mediate unique aspects of motor behavior. Unfortunately, each scheme generated its own terminology, and all remain in more or less common usage. Hence, it is necessary to know the terminology for each scheme and to be able to contrast the different terminologies. None of these schemes is particularly successful in correlating structure and function with clinical applicability.

The first scheme developed from initial efforts to understand cerebellar function in terms of its gross anatomy—specifically, the subdivision of the cerebellum into the three lobes noted earlier. The flocculonodular lobe was considered to be concerned with equilibrium, the anterior lobe with posture, and the posterior lobe with voluntary movement. The evidence supporting this anatomic lobular organization as the fundamental pattern of cerebellar functional organization is weak indeed. It is immediately apparent, for example, that posture is fundamental to all movement, from the maintenance of equilibrium to voluntary movement that only can be executed from a suitably adjusted postural base. It is illogical to parcel posture to one cerebellar subdivision and voluntary movement to another. Furthermore, lesion studies in experimental animals do not support such a scheme.

A second concept of cerebellar organization, based on the phylogenetic order of appearance of various subdivisions, grew out of comparative anatomic work. The phylogenetically oldest part of the cerebellum present in all vertebrates, the flocculonodular lobe, is termed the **archicerebellum**. The **paleocerebellum**, next in order of appearance, is represented by the vermal part of the anterior lobe and several small regions of the posterior lobe (Figure 6-17 ■). It comprises the largest subdivision in lower forms but only a small portion of the human cerebellum. The phylogenetically youngest parts of the cerebellum are designated as the **neocerebellum**. The latter is represented primarily by the lateral regions corresponding approximately to the hemispheres. These areas increase in size commensurate with the development of apical motor organs capable of skilled movement and, in man,

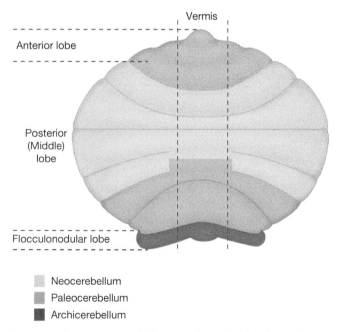

FIGURE 6-17 The cerebellum can be subdivided into three lobes noted earlier: the flocculonodular lobe, the anterior lobe, and the posterior lobe. The cerebellum can also be subdivided based on the phylogenetic order of appearance: the archicerebellum, paleocerebellum and neocerebellum.

completely overshadow other cerebellar parts. While the greatest expansion occurs in the lateral parts of the posterior lobe, lateral parts of the anterior lobe also increase in size so that, like the paleocerebellum, the neocerebellum cuts across lobular boundaries.

A third approach subdivides the cerebellum in terms of the distribution of afferent fibers within the cerebellar cortex (Figure 6-18 ■). Three major categories of afferent projection were defined for this purpose: pathways from the vestibulocochlear nerve and vestibular nuclei (vestibulocerebellar), pathways from the spinal cord (spinocerebellar), and pathways primarily from the cerebral cortex that reach the cerebellum after synapsing the pons (pontocerebellar). This approach led to the delineation of a **vestibulocerebellum**, a **spinocerebellum**, and a **pontocerebellum**. Because at least some correspondence exists between this subdivision and that derived from phylogenetic data, the vestibulocerebellum is sometimes considered analogous to the archicerebellum, because the latter receives the terminals of vestibular afferents. Similarly, the spinocerebellum equates with the paleocerebellum and the pontocerebellum with the neocerebellum. This correspondence, however, is inexact. While pontocerebellar fibers project primarily to the neocerebellum, they also have abundant connections with the spinocerebellum. Likewise, spinocerebellar afferents connect with the vestibulocerebellum and vestibular afferents invade the spinocerebellum. Indeed, the vestibular system even influences the neocerebellum. Other afferent systems, such as that originating in the inferior olivary complex, project to all parts of the cerebellar cortex.

A fourth approach to cerebellar functional organization, which excludes the flocculonodular lobe, is to subdivide the cerebellum into longitudinal zones that cut across anterior and posterior lobes (Figure 6-19 ■). This

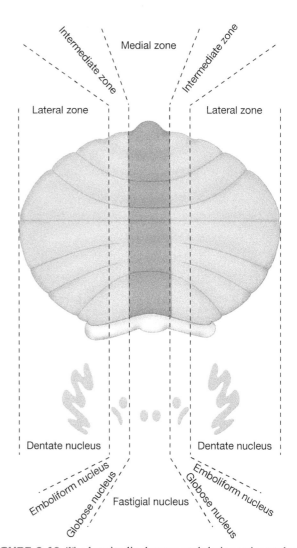

FIGURE 6-19 The longitudinal zones and their corticonuclear projections to related deep cerebellar nuclei.

approach is based on the pattern of projections from the cerebellar cortex to the deep cerebellar nuclei, the **corticonuclear projection** pattern. The phylogeny of the nuclei parallels that of the cerebellar cortex so that in man the dentate nucelus is by far the largest. Corticonuclear projections are made up of the axons of Purkinje cells that terminate on neurons of the underlying deep nuclei. By mapping degeneration patterns in the nuclei resulting from discrete cortical lesions, the cerebellum can be subdivided into three zones, each consisting of a longitudinally oriented strip of cortex and a corresponding deep nucleus to which the overlying cortex sent its fibers. The medial zone consists of the vermal cortex and fastigial nuclei, the intermediate zone is composed of paravermal cortex and the interposed nuclei, the lateral zone consists of hemispheral cortex and the dentate nucleus. Within each zone, the projections have a rostrocaudal organization so that the anterior part of the zone projects to the rostral part of the corresponding nucleus and the posterior to the caudal.

Early stimulation and ablation experiments in animals have elaborated the zonal concept in terms of its

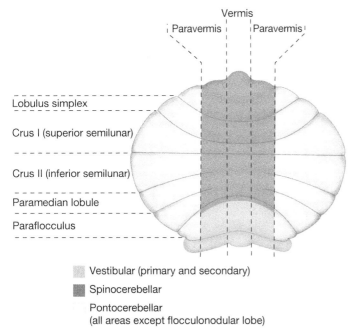

FIGURE 6-18 There are three major categories of afferent projections: vestibulocerebellar, spinocerebellar, and pontocerebellar.

Neuropathology Box 6-1: Ethanol Intoxication

The locomotor behaviors associated with ethanol intoxication implicitly implicate the cerebellum as a site of ethanol's action. The roadside sobriety test is used to detect staggering, reeling, uncoordinated gait of the drunk. This pattern of gait, combined with slurred uncoordinated speech and nystagmus (rhythmic conjugate deviations of the eyes) are similar to motor deficits resulting from cerebellar damage (see Chapter 19). Altered cerebellar function appears to be caused in large part by increased activity of the inferior olivary complex. (See Chapter 17 for details about the nystagmus.) In experimental animals, ethanol increases climbing fiber bursts to Purkinje cells and alters their basal pattern of firing. This would substantively change cerebellar cortical output. Ethanol's action appears to be through activation of $GABA_A$ receptors within the cerebellum. GABA (gamma-amino butyric acid) is used as a neurotransmitter by Purkinje cells and many cerebellar interneurons.

functional correlates. The three bilaterally symmetrical zones reflect a medial to lateral gradient from the control of gross postural movements toward the regulation of spatially organized skilled movement of the extremities. Each medial zone regulates the tone, posture, locomotion, and equilibrium of the entire body. Each intermediate zone governs spatially organized and skilled movements of the ipsilateral extremities, as well as the posture and tone associated with these movements. Each lateral zone controls similarly spatially organized and skilled movements of the ipsilateral limbs but without apparent involvement of their posture and tone.

Ensuing studies with more sophisticated techniques have shown that the zonal concept is less rigid than originally assumed. Thus, a given cortical zone projects to more than one nucleus, and the lateral zone has important functions in the regulation of posture and tone in addition to its role in controlling skilled movement. Nonetheless, the zonal concept has been more successful in correlating anatomy with function than any other scheme of cerebellar subdivision. It emphasizes a general theme of intracerebellar organization that is preserved in the extracerebellar efferent projections arising from the three zones (see Chapter 19).

Inferior Olivary Nucleus

The inferior olivary nucleus, located in the medulla, is one of the best-understood nuclei of the CNS in terms of its anatomical connections and cellular physiology. Yet the behaviors this large nuclear complex modulates have remained elusive to researchers.

The inferior olivary complex is a convoluted band of cells in the medulla appearing as a folded bag with its opening (or *hilus*) directed medially. Fibers exiting the nucleus pass through the hilus, traverse the medial lemnisci, and course through and around the opposite inferior olivary complex. After traversing the reticular formation and spinal trigeminal complex, olivary axons enter the contralateral inferior cerebellar peduncle and make up the bulk of its axons.

In contrast to other cerebellar afferent systems that terminate as mossy fibers within particular parts of the cerebellum, olivary afferents terminate as climbing fibers in *all* areas of the cerebellar cortex. Because each functionally specialized region (equilibrium, posture, voluntary movement, vision, audition, etc.) of the cerebellum is subject to olivary regulation, this means that the inferior olive must modulate all behaviors in which the cerebellum participates.

The inferior olivary complex receives afferents from a wide variety of sources. Among these are the following: the cerebral cortex, the spinal cord, the trigeminal nuclei, the red nucleus, the reticular formation, the superior colliculus, and the cerebellum itself.

A number of functions have been proposed for the inferior olive. Lesions of the nucleus have been shown to produce motor deficits similar to those following cerebellar ablations, including ataxia, tremor, and disorganization of voluntary movement. Through its interactions with the flocculonodular lobe, the inferior olive is thought to regulate eye movements required to compensate for the slip of visual images on the retina. It also has been proposed that the inferior olive is involved in motor learning (see Chapter 19).

Blood Supply

Blood supply to the cerebellum is provided by three branches of the vertebrobasilar system (Figure 6-20 ■). From caudal to rostral, the first branch, the **posterior inferior cerebellar artery (PICA)**, is given off from the vertebral artery; the second branch, the **anterior inferior cerebellar artery (AICA)**, is given off as the first branch of the basilar artery; while the rostralmost branch, the **superior cerebellar artery (SCA)**, is given off from the top of the basilar artery, just before the latter's bifurcation into the posterior cerebral arteries. These three cerebellar arteries, via penetrating branches, take part in the vascularization of the brainstem as they wind around it from their origins on the ventral brainstem surface toward the dorsally positioned cerebellum.

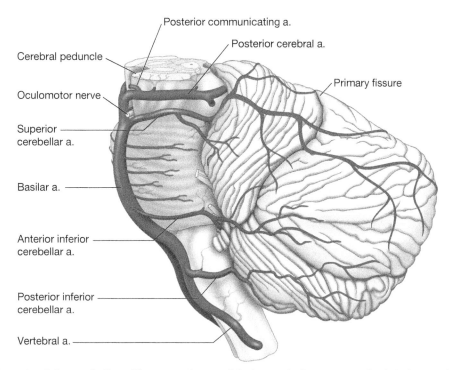

Posterior communicating a.

Posterior cerebral a.

Cerebral peduncle

Primary fissure

Oculomotor nerve

Superior cerebellar a.

Basilar a.

Anterior inferior cerebellar a.

Posterior inferior cerebellar a.

Vertebral a.

FIGURE 6-20 Blood supply of the cerebellum. Three arteries nourish the cerebellum: a posterior inferior cerebellar artery, a branch of the vertebral artery; an anterior inferior cerebellar artery, a branch of the inferior portion of the basilar artery; and a superior cerebellar artery, a branch of the rostral portion of the basilar artery.

(Bowman, J. P., and Giddings, D. F. *Strokes: An Illustrated Guide to Brain Structure, Blood Supply, and Clinical Signs*. Prentice Hall, New Jersey, 2003.)

The PICA gives rise to two branches that nourish the inferior vermis and inferior and posterior surfaces of the cerebellar hemispheres. The AICA supplies a strip of inferior and posterior vermal and hemisphere cortex anterior to those supplied by the PICA. The SCA divides into medial and lateral branches that nourish the superior half of the vermis and cerebellar hemispheres. These hemispheric arteries give rise to numerous branches that penetrate deeply into the cerebellum. These vessels nourish the middle and superior cerebellar peduncles as well as the deep cerebellar nuclei.

CLINICAL CONNECTIONS
Cerebellar Dysfunction

In Chapters 19 and 20, the contributions of the cerebellum to voluntary movement are discussed in detail, as are the clinical manifestations of disorders of the cerebellum. For now, it is important to recognize that cerebellar dysfunction can stem from a variety of causes such as acute and/or chronic alcohol intoxication, developmental disorders, brainstem strokes that extend into the cerebellum (as well as strokes specifically within the cerebellum), and trauma (e.g., gunshot wounds to the back of the head, specifically affecting the cerebellum or traumatic brain injury involving cerebellar structures).

Characteristic symptoms of cerebellar dysfunction typically include hypotonicity (abnormally low tone), incoordination (e.g., evident with problems such as "past pointing" when attempting to point to a target), tremors with intentional movement (referred to as "intention tremors"), and ataxia. Additional symptoms can occur related to the cerebellar/vestibular connections that result in difficulties with eye movements (e.g., nystagmus) and poor oculomotor control. Lastly, cerebellar dysfunction can also result in changes in cognition that will be discussed in Chapter 21.

Summary

In this chapter, further anatomical features of the diencephalon and cerebellum beyond those presented in Chapter 2 are discussed, along with general functional aspects of both structures. The diencephalon consists of four major components: the epithalamus, thalamus, hypothalamus, and subthalamus. The epithalamus is the smallest subdivision and lies dorsal to the thalamus. Its most conspicuous component is the unpaired pineal gland that apparently functions in sexual development and plays some role in regulating the sleep–wakefulness cycle. The topographic organization of the largest component of the diencephalon, the thalamus, was presented, and a functional grouping of its nuclei into relay, association, and intralaminar nuclei was developed. Specific functions of these nuclei are elaborated in later chapters. Despite its small size, the hypothalamus plays a vital role in regulating the functions of the endocrine and autonomic nervous systems. These functions are explored in more detail in Chapters 12 and 22. The subthalamic nucleus is the most prominent structure of the subthalamus and plays an essential role in the regulation of movement, a topic discussed in Chapter 19.

The cerebellum, like the cerebral hemispheres, consists of an outer mantle of cortex surrounding a central core of white matter within which deep nuclei are embedded. The three-layered cerebellar cortex is organized as a large number of transverse folds, the folia, all of which possess an identical structure. Input to the cerebellum is via climbing and mossy fibers, and output originates predominantly from the four deep cerebellar nuclei. The gross anatomy of the cerebellum is organized in both anterior-to-posterior and medial-to-lateral dimensions. The former divides the cerebellum into anterior, posterior, and flocculonodular lobes, while the latter organizes the cerebellum into midline, intermediate, and lateral zones. These anatomical subdivisions have functional counterparts wherein the cerebellum controls equilibrium, posture, and voluntary movement.

Applications

1. Mrs. Jeffries is a 53-year-old woman whose medical history included migraine headaches and hypertension. She reported right-sided pain that began a year ago; she became progressively worse over the last several months. She described her pain as continuous, burning, and stabbing. She rated her pain as 9/10, with 0 indicating no pain and 10 indicating the worst pain imaginable. A neurological examination revealed patchy areas of tactile hyperesthesia and loss of thermal sensation along the right arm, leg, and trunk. Her reflexes and motor examination were normal throughout. She demonstrated mildly ataxic gait and transfers.

   a. Damage to what neuroanatomical structure could cause her loss of thermal sensation and hyperesthesia?
   b. What type of lesion might this be?
   c. On which side of the brain is the lesion located that produced these right-sided symptoms?

2. Jacquelyn is a 6-year-old girl who became lethargic and difficult to arouse. Her parents took her to the emergency room. They reported that over the previous few days she had become irritable, had a decreased appetite, and sudden onset of emesis. Upon neurological examination, she walked with a wide base of support staggering pattern and was unable to carry objects while walking. She had difficulty focusing visually and had gaze nystagmus. Neuroimaging revealed a posterior fossa hemorrhage due to an astrocytoma in the right cerebellar hemisphere.

   a. What is an astrocytoma?
   b. Investigate the incidence and prognosis of astrocytomas in children.
   c. For Jacquelyn, which symptoms are attributable to damage of the vestibulocerebellum? Which are attributable to damage of the spinocerebellum? And which symptoms are attributable to damage of the cerebrocerebellum?

References

Diencephalon

Allen, L. S. et al. Two sexually dimorphic cell groups in the human brain. *J. Neurosci* 9:497, 1989.

Bergland, R. M., and Page R. B. Pituitary-brain vascular relations: a new paradigm. *Sci* 204:18, 1979.

Braak, H., and Braak, E. The hypothalamus of the human adult: Chiasmatic region. *Anat Embryol* 175:315, 1987.

Carrera, E., and Bogousslavsky, J. The thalamus and behavior: Effects of anatomically distinct strokes. *Neurol* 66:1817–1823, 2006.

Cotton, P. L., and Smith, A. T. Contralateral visual hemifield representations in the human pulvinar nucleus. *J Neurophysiol* 98:1600–1609, 2007.

Hofman, M. A. Zhou, J.-N., and Swaab, D. F. Suprachiasmatic nucleus of the human brain: Immunocytochemical and morphometric analysis. *Anat Rec* 244:552, 1996.

Koutcherov, Y. et al. Organization of the human paraventricular hypothalamic nucleus. *J Comp Neurol* 423:299, 2000.

Nolte, J. *The Human Brain*, 5th ed. Mosby, St. Louis, 2002.

Paradiso, G., Cunic, D., Saint-Cyr, J. A., et al. Involvement of human thalamus in the preparation of self-paced movement. *Brain* 127:2717–2731, 2004.

Pinault, D. The thalamic reticular nucleus: Structure, function, and concept. *Brain Res Rev* 46:1–31, 2004.

Ropper, A. H., and Brown, R. H. Ch. 27. The hypothalamus and neuroendocrine disorders. In: *Adams and Victor's Principles of Neurology*, 8th ed. McGraw-Hill, New York, 2005.

Swaab, D. F. et al. Functional neuroanatomy and neuropathology of the human hypothalamus. *Anat Embryol* 187:317, 1993.

van Esseveldt, L. E., Lehman, M. N., and Boer, G. J. The suprachiasmatic nucleus and the circadian timekeeping system revisited. *Brain Res Rev* 33:34, 2000.

Young, J. K. and Stanton, G. B. A three-dimensional reconstruction of the human hypothalamus. *Brain Res Bull* 35:323, 1994.

Cerebellum

Jansen, J., and Brodal, A. *Aspects of Cerebellar Anatomy*. Johan Grundt Tanum Vorlagm, Oslo, 1954.

Larsell, O. Morphogenesis and evolution of the cerebellum. *Arch Neurol Psychiat* 31:580–607, 1934.

Larsell, O., and Jansen. J. *The Comparative Anatomy and Histology of the Cerebellum: The Human Cerebellum, Cerebellar Connections, and Cerebellar Cortex*. The University of Minnesota Press, Minneapolis, 1972.

Nolte, J. *The Human Brain: An Introduction to Its Functional Anatomy*. Mosby Elsevier, Philadelphia, 2009.

Tatu, L., Moulin, T., Bogousslavsky, J., and Duvernoy, H. Arterial territories of human brain: Brainstem and cerebellum. *Neurol* 47:1125–1135, 1996.

Thach, W. T., Goodkin, H. P., and Keating, J. G. The cerebellum and the adaptive coordination of movement. *Annu. Rev. Neurosci.* 15:403–442, 1992.

Cerebral Hemispheres and Vascular Supply

LEARNING OUTCOMES

This chapter prepares the reader to:

1. Identify the major lobes, gyri, and sulci of the cerebral hemispheres.

2. Discuss the cell types of the cerebral neocortex.

3. Identify three phylogenetically distinct regions of the neocortex and the structures that comprise them.

4. Compare and contrast cortical organization according to phylogeny, horizontal layers, and vertical columnar structures.

5. Discuss the relevance of Brodmann's areas and relate selected areas to their functional roles.

6. Describe the location and function of the primary motor area and five primary sensory areas.

7. Name the five nuclei of the basal ganglia; compare and contrast the different nomenclature for characterizing these structures.

8. Identify major origins and destinations of basal ganglia circuitry and name the major fiber bundles.

9. Describe the different types of disordered movement (tremor, dyskinesia, athetosis, chorea and ballismus) associated with basal ganglia dysfunction.

10. Locate the four portions of the internal capsule in cross sections and identify the destination of the fibers related to each portion.

11. Explain major contributions to the blood supply of the cerebral hemisphere.

12. Differentiate between penetrating and cortical arterial branches and central and peripheral territories of vascularization.

13. Contrast the major clinical consequences of occlusion of each of the following vessels: MCA, ACA, IC, and PCA.

14. Discuss the clinical consequences of occlusion of the major blood vessels in the context of Brodmann's areas.

ACRONYMS

ACA Anterior cerebral artery

BA Brodmann's area

DM Dorsomedial thalamic nuclei (or mediodorsal)

GPi Internal segment of the globus pallidus

IC Internal carotid

MCA Middle cerebral artery

PCA Posterior cerebral artery

SNpr Pars reticulata of the substantia nigra

VA Ventral anterior thalamic nucleus

VL Ventral lateral thalamic nucleus

VPL Ventral posterolateral thalamic nucleus

VPM Ventral posteromedial thalamic nucleus

Introduction

This chapter builds on the basic information presented in earlier chapters, providing a more in-depth presentation of the cerebral hemispheres. Enveloping the surface of the cerebrum, the cerebral cortex is a multilayer sheet of some 25 billion neurons. Its thickness varies from 1.5 to 4.5 mm because different regions of the cortex are made of different numbers of neurons whose size and shape vary. This highly convoluted sheet of gray matter has a total area of about 2.5 ft^2, but only about one-third to one-half of this total occupies the surface gyri of the cerebrum, the remainder being hidden in the depths of sulci and fissures. Each of the four lobes of a cerebral hemisphere identified in Chapter 2 is characterized by a reasonably consistent pattern of gyri and sulci.

The first major section of this chapter deals with the cerebral cortex. This section begins with major features, including sulci and gyri. Next, the histology of the cerebral cortex is considered. The organization of cortical cells can be conceptualized along two spatial dimensions—first, in horizontal layers and, second, in vertical columns oriented perpendicular to the surface of the hemisphere. In addition to this dimensional organization, the cells making up the cortex of different areas of each hemisphere vary in terms of their size, shape, and packing density as just noted. This variation affects the width, appearance, and even presence of the different horizontal layers making up the cortex. This variation was studied exhaustively in 1909 by an anatomist named Korbinian Brodmann. He produced a detailed map of the cerebral cortex containing some 50 different areas. Each different Brodmann's area was given a distinct number. Many of these areas are of functional importance and clinical relevance, and these will be discussed. The last section on the cerebral cortex considers its organization in terms of the modality of information different parts of each hemisphere process. This functional organization shows that cerebral cortex can be classified as being association cortex, motor cortex, or sensory cortex. As might be expected, this method of classifying cortex correlates with Brodmann's map. For example, the different types of sensory cortex (somatosensory, auditory, visual, and vestibular) consist of different Brodmann areas (BAs) have different Brodmann numbers with distinctive histological attributes.

The second and third major sections of this chapter consider structures that reside in the interior of each hemisphere. The basal ganglia are the topic of the second major section of this chapter and are discussed in more detail than in Chapter 2 where they were first introduced. Also noted in Chapter 2 was that the internal capsule consists, in large measure, of axons that enter and exit the cerebral cortex and is a major anatomical landmark in understanding the organization of the interior of the hemisphere. This structure is explored in more detail in the third major section of this chapter, and some of the clinically important projection fibers running in the internal capsule are pointed out.

The final section of this chapter presents the blood supply of the cerebral hemispheres. Because of its vast anatomical extent, the blood supply of the cortex is the most frequent target of cerebrovascular disease in the entire brain. The cortical localization of function is covered in detail in Chapter 24.

Clinical Preview

You are working with three individuals, each of whom sustained a stroke. These strokes are in different areas of the brain, yet each of these patients has a resulting problem with balance. Amit Mohammed had a stroke affecting his parietal cortex. Sharon Warren had a stroke primarily affecting her medial frontal lobe. And Barbara Nishimura had a small stroke in the internal capsule. As you read through this section of the text, consider the following:

- What are the basic functional roles of the regions of the brain involved for each individual?
- Compare the probable losses that each person will have as a result of his or her stroke.

Later in this chapter, you will learn much more about the relationships among blood supplies, regions supplied, and expected clinical consequences. In later chapters, you will learn about the complex contributions to balance dysfunction, which will assist you to understand why these three people have a similar problem with balance control.

CEREBRAL CORTEX

Gyri and Sulci of the Cerebral Cortex

Lateral Hemispheral Surface

The most prominent sulci on the lateral hemispheral surface are the lateral and central sulci. These were presented in Chapter 2 along with other landmarks used to delineate the lobes of each hemisphere.

In the frontal lobe, four main gyri make up its lateral surface. One gyrus is oriented approximately vertically, while the other three are oriented horizontally. (Figure 7-1 ■). The vertically oriented convolution is the **precentral gyrus**, located immediately anterior to and paralleling the central sulcus. It is a continuous band of cortex (but generally contains several depressions) whose anterior boundary is formed by the **precentral sulcus**. The latter may be broken up into superior and inferior segments.

The three horizontally oriented convolutions are the **superior**, **middle**, and **inferior frontal gyri**. These are somewhat difficult to differentiate from one another for several reasons. First, they do not seem to consist of superficially continuous gyri. Second, each seems to be composed of more than one convolution. And, third, the sulci

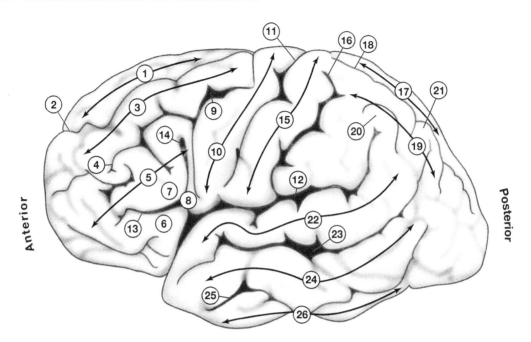

FIGURE 7-1 Gyri and sulci of the lateral hemispheral surface. Arrows indicate the rostrocaudal or dorsoventral extent of a gyrus. (Note that the numbers on the figure correspond to the numbers in this legend and are not Brodmann's areas.) (1) Superior frontal gyrus. (2) Superior frontal sulcus. (3) Middle frontal gyrus. (4) Inferior frontal sulcus. (5) Inferior frontal gyrus. (6) Pars orbitalis of inferior frontal gyrus. (7) Pars triangularis of inferior frontal gyrus. (8) Pars opercularis of inferior frontal gyrus. (9) Precentral sulcus. (10) Precentral gyrus. (11) Central sulcus. (12) Lateral sulcus. (13) Anterior horizontal branch of lateral sulcus. (14) Anterior ascending branch of lateral sulcus. (15) Postcentral gyrus. (16) Postcentral sulcus. (17) Superior parietal lobule. (18) Intraparietal sulcus. (19) Inferior parietal lobule. (20) Supramarginal gyrus. (21) Angular gyrus. (22) Superior temporal gyrus. (23) Superior temporal sulcus. (24) Middle temporal gyrus. (25) Inferior temporal sulcus. (26) Inferior temporal gyrus.

separating them—the **superior** and **inferior frontal sulci**—are tortuous. The inferior frontal gyrus is subdivided into three regions by the short **anterior horizontal** and **anterior ascending branches** of the lateral sulcus. The most anterior subdivision is the **pars orbitalis** and is followed by the **pars triangularis** and **pars opercularis**.

The boundaries of the parietal lobe on the lateral convexity of the hemisphere are imprecise, except for the anterior border formed by the central sulcus. Sulci of the parietal lobe vary from brain to brain, but two main sulci usually can be distinguished: the **postcentral** and **intraparietal sulci**. These subdivide the parietal lobe into three parts.

The postcentral sulcus runs parallel to the central sulcus and forms the caudal boundary of the vertically oriented **postcentral gyrus**. Both the sulcus and gyrus may be discontinuous. The more or less horizontally oriented intraparietal sulcus, usually continuous with the postcentral sulcus, arches backward toward the occipital

lobe. It divides the portion of the parietal lobe posterior to the postcentral gyrus into a **superior** and **inferior parietal lobule**. The inferior parietal lobule consists of two, often horseshoe-shaped, gyri, the **supramarginal** and **angular gyri**. The supramarginal gyrus caps the posterior, ascending branch of the lateral sulcus, while the angular gyrus, caudal to the supramarginal gyrus, surrounds the ascending terminal part of the superior temporal sulcus (discussed later).

The convexity of the temporal lobe is composed of three major, horizontally oriented convolutions: the **superior**, **middle**, and **inferior temporal gyri**. The superior temporal gyrus is bounded above by the lateral sulcus and below by the **superior temporal sulcus** (it runs upward and backward into the parietal lobe). The superior temporal gyrus has a broad superior surface that is hidden from view deep within the lateral sulcus. The boundaries of the middle and inferior temporal gyri are poorly defined in most brains and are separated by the **middle temporal sulcus**. Much of the inferior temporal gyrus lies on the inferior surface of the temporal lobe.

The **insula** lies buried in the depths of the lateral sulcus. It is triangular shaped with the apex of the triangle directed forward and downward and opening into the Sylvian fossa (see Figure 2-20). The insular surface consists of a number of short gyri anteriorly and one or more long posterior gyri.

Thought Question

Which of the major gyri and sulci can be viewed on the lateral, medial, and inferior surfaces, respectively?

Medial Hemispheral Surface

Lobular boundaries on the medial surface are essentially arbitrary (with the exception of part of the occipital lobe) as many gyri continue uninterrupted from one lobe to another. The corpus callosum is separated from the overlying **cingulate gyrus** by the **callosal sulcus** that follows the superior surface of the corpus callosum (Figure 7-2 ■). The outer, mostly superior, border of the cingulate gyrus is formed by the **cingulate sulcus** that runs parallel to the callosal sulcus. The cingulate sulcus has one constant branch, the **marginal branch**, that turns upward and attains the superior border of the hemisphere a short distance posterior to the central sulcus. At the level of the splenium of the corpus callosum, the cingulate gyrus turns inferiorly as the narrow *isthmus* of the cingulate gyrus and continues anteriorly into the temporal lobe as the **parahippocampal gyrus**. As noted earlier (Chapter 2), the cingulate and parahippocampal gyri that appear to ring the thalamus are major components of the limbic system (L., *limbus*, border). The limbic system is a functionally defined area comprised of parts of the frontal, parietal, and temporal lobes. The limbic system is involved in mediating emotion and memory (see Chapter 22).

The cingulate sulcus divides the medial hemispheral surface into two major tiers: an inner tier consisting of the cingulate gyrus and an outer tier represented by the extensions of the frontal and parietal lobes onto the medial hemispheral surface. The portion of the outer tier belonging to the frontal lobe is made up primarily by the medial extension of the superior frontal gyrus, whose inferior boundary is the cingulate sulcus but includes also the medial extension of the precentral gyrus.

The boundary between the frontal and parietal lobes is formed by a vertical imaginary line extending from the central sulcus to the cingulate sulcus. The posterior boundary of the parietal lobe is the deep parieto-occipital sulcus, while the inferior boundary is the corpus callosum. The medial surface of the parietal lobe contains the extensions of the postcentral gyrus and superior parietal lobule.

The medial hemispheral portions of the pre- and postcentral gyri together make up the **paracentral lobule**, whose posterior boundary is the marginal branch of the cingulate sulcus. The portion of the parietal lobe between the marginal branch of the cingulate sulcus and the parieto-occipital sulcus is the **precuneus** (sometimes called the quadrate lobule).

The deep **calcarine sulcus**, confined to the occipital lobe, extends anteriorly from the occipital pole toward the temporal lobe. At the point where it is joined by the distinct parieto-occipital sulcus, the calcarine sulcus bends inferiorly, thereby forming the stem of a Y-shaped formation. The wedge-shaped area bounded in front by the parieto-occipital sulcus and

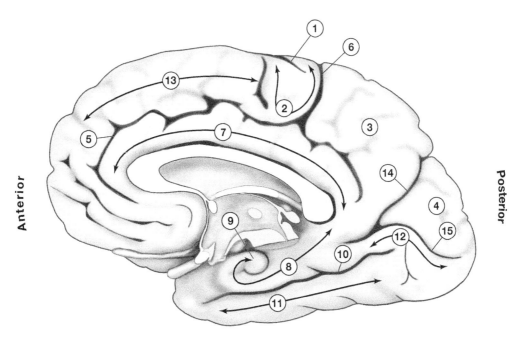

FIGURE 7-2 Gyri and sulci of the medial hemispheral surface. Arrows indicate the rostrocaudal or dorsoventral extent of a gyrus. (Note that the numbers on the figure correspond to the numbers in this legend and are not Brodmann's areas.) (1) Central sulcus. (2) Paracentral lobule. (3) Precuneus of parietal lobe. (4) Cuneus of occipital lobe. (5) Cingulate sulcus. (6) Marginal branch of cingulate sulcus. (7) Cingulate gyrus. (8) Parahippocampal gyrus. (9) Uncus. (10) Collateral sulcus. (11) Occipitotemporal gyrus. (12) Lingual gyrus. (13) Superior frontal gyrus. (14) Parietooccipital sulcus. (15) Calcarine sulcus.

below by the calcarine sulcus is the **cuneus**. The **lingual gyrus** of the occipital lobe is located ventral to the calcarine sulcus.

Inferior Hemispheral Surface

The inferior hemispheral surface is composed of two parts, the point of division being the Sylvian fossa. The anterior part is the smaller of the two and consists of the orbital surface of the frontal lobe. The larger posterior part is composed of the inferior surfaces of the temporal and occipital lobes in which gyri run interrupted between the two lobes. Among the constant landmarks is the **collateral sulcus** that begins near the occipital pole and extends anteriorly, roughly paralleling the calcarine sulcus (see Figure 7-2). The collateral sulcus continues into the temporal lobe and separates the **occipital-temporal gyrus** laterally from the parahippocampal gyrus medially. Anteriorly, the parahippocampal gyrus is continuous with the hook-like **uncus**.

Further Organization of the Cortex

Layers of the Cerebral Cortex

One hallmark of cortical organization is that its cells are arranged in layers. The number of layers varies markedly in different parts of each hemisphere because of the phylogenetic development of major parts of the hemisphere.

The cerebral cortex can be visualized as consisting of three regions that develop in a phylogenetic sequence. The innermost region, consisting of the hippocampus (see Figure 2-18), is the most primitive and has only three layers. The cortex in this region is referred to as **archicortex** (also called **allocortex**). The next region of cortex, consisting of the parahippocampal gyrus, is considered transitional between cortex of the hippocampus and that of the outer region. The parahippocampal gyrus is made up of three to five horizontal layers. This cortex is referred to as **mesocortex** (or **juxtallocortex**). The outermost region is phylogenetically the newest and is referred to as **neocortex** (or **isocortex**). The neocortex occupies about 90 percent of cerebral cortex volume in humans. It has six horizontal layers and represents the vast majority of the cortical surface, consisting of the frontal, parietal, occipital, and temporal (with the exception of the parahippocampal gyrus) lobes. These features are summarized in Table 7-1 ■.

CELLS AND LAYERS OF THE NEOCORTEX A variety of different cell types have been identified in the neocortex, but two types predominate. Most distinctive are the pyramidal neurons, often referred to as **pyramidal cells**. This name reflects the conical shape of their cell bodies. A long apical dendrite extends from the top of the cell and ascends vertically toward the surface of the cortex, while a series of basal

> **Thought Question**
>
> Compare and contrast the shapes and functions of pyramidal and nonpyramidal cells.

Table 7-1 Types of Cerebral Cortex

TYPE OF CORTEX	MAJOR STRUCTURES	PHYLOGENETIC AGE
Archicortex (three layers)	Hippocampus Dentate gyrus	Oldest
Mesocortex (three to five layers)	Parahippocampal gyrus	
Neocortex (six layers)	Primary motor cortex Primary sensory cortices Association cortex	Newest

dendrites extend from the base of the cell body and spread horizontally (Figure 7-3 ■). Pyramidal cells have long axons that leave the cerebral cortex to reach other cortical areas in the same or opposite hemisphere or to terminate in various subcortical structures. They vary widely in size and are the principal output neurons of the neocortex.

Nonpyramidal neurons in the cerebral cortex also come in a variety of sizes and shapes. Most numerous are the **stellate**, or **granule**, neurons (Figure 7-4 ■). These small, star-shaped cells have numerous short dendrites that extend in all directions and a short axon that arborizes on nearby cortical neurons. Granule neurons are the primary interneurons of the neocortex.

> **Thought Question**
>
> The association cortex is a phylogenetically newer portion of the cerebral cortex. What does this imply regarding its function.

Neurons of the neocortex form primary sensory, primary motor, and association areas, among others. The primary somatosensory cortex receives afferent information that originated from the opposite side of the body and is conveyed to the cortex via specific sensory relay nuclei of the thalamus. The primary motor cortex gives rise to the corticospinal tracts that control movement of the opposite side of the body. In contrast to these cortices, the association cortices provide for integration of afferent and efferent inputs from a variety of sources and are responsible for higher-level information processing. These association areas are involved in the analysis and elaboration of sensory information, in integrating the different sensory modalities into a coherent perception, and in the planning of motor action. The pathways for primary somatosensory and primary motor areas are

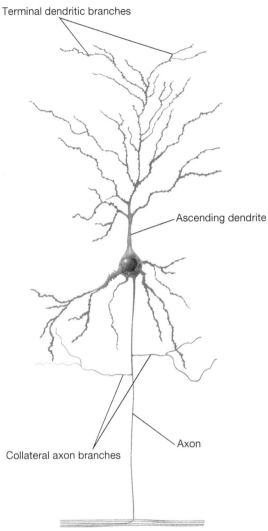

Terminal dendritic branches

Ascending dendrite

Collateral axon branches

Axon

FIGURE 7-3 Pyramidal neuron of the cerebral cortex. Note that the dendrites are studded with synaptic spines. The axon gives off numerous collateral branches shortly after emerging from the cell body. It then extends into the white matter of the cerebrum.

discussed in detail in Chapters 9, 10, and 11. The primary sensory areas for special senses (e.g., vision, hearing) are discussed in Chapters 17 and 18.

Neurons of the neocortex are arranged in horizontal layers oriented parallel to the cortical surface. The disposition of cells in these layers varies in different parts of the neocortex, but in most areas it is possible to distinguish six layers. The most superficial layer is the fiber-rich but cell-poor **molecular layer** (I), and the deepest layer is the **multiform layer** (VI). In between these layers are granular and pyramidal layers, so named because either granule or pyramidal cells dominate the layer. Granule and pyramidal layers alternate with one another. Each of these layers is subdivided into an external and internal layer. Thus, the alternating sequence is the **external granular layer** (II) followed by the **external pyramidal layer** (III), then the **internal granular layer** (IV) followed by the **internal pyramidal layer** (V) (see Figure 7-4).

The six cell layers are not equally apparent in all cortical areas. Two extremes are identified, called agranular and granular cortex. Areas of the neocortex that give rise to numerous long axons (output cortex)—such as neurons of the motor cortex that give rise to axons that descend all the way to the spinal cord—have many large pyramidal cells (including the largest of the neocortex). As a result, layers II through V are dominated by the presence of pyramidal cells, whereas granule cells are comparatively few. As a consequence, layers II through V are difficult to distinguish from one another. The end result is that a six-layered organization is no longer readily apparent. This output cortex is, therefore, called **agranular** because of the reduction of granule cells (see Figure 7-4). Agranular motor cortex is thick, up to 4.5 mm in width.

At the opposite extreme are cortical areas whose axonal projections are mostly adjacent to areas of the neocortex. As a result, they do not give rise to many long output axons. Such connections characterize the primary sensory cortices. Consequently, large pyramidal neurons are markedly reduced in number, whereas granule cells are increased in number for the reception of sensory input. In primary sensory cortices, layers II through V are dominated by granule cells in layers II and IV that appear almost as one continuous layer. Primary sensory areas are therefore called **granular** cortex. Granular cortex is thinner than agranular cortex. It may be as narrow as 1.5 mm. In between these two extremes of the thick agranular motor cortex and the thin granular sensory cortex is a continuum of structural types in which six layers can be discerned.

The different layers of the neocortex have different patterns of connections. Input to the neocortex originates either from other cortical areas in the same or opposite hemispheres or from subcortical structures. Subcortical structures include the thalamus, basal ganglia, cholinergic basal forebrain nuclei, and the brainstem aminergic nuclei. Each has a distinctive laminar pattern of termination in the neocortex. For example, afferents from the specific sensory relay nuclei in the thalamus terminate on granular neurons in the internal granular layer (IV). Similarly, cortical efferents have distinctive patterns of laminar origin, depending on the destination of their axons. For example, layer III is the major source of corticocortical fibers (commissural fibers); layer V of corticostriate projections (from the cortex to the caudate nucleus and putamen of the basal ganglia), corticobulbar, and corticospinal fibers; and layer VI of corticothalamic fibers.

Cortical Columns

In addition to its laminar (horizontal) organization, the neocortex is organized in a vertical (perpendicular to the surface) dimension called **cortical (functional) columns**. Cortical columns extend from the pial surface of the cortex to the white matter, and the neurons forming a column have extensive interneuronal connections. The discovery of this columnar organization was greeted with great enthusiasm because of the possibility that it represented a basic

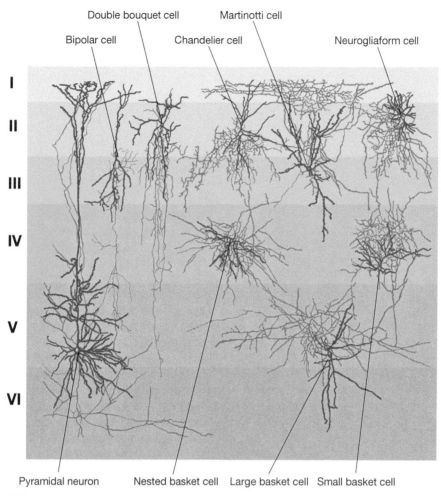

FIGURE 7-4 Neurons within the six layers of the neocortex.

structural–physiological principle underlying all cortical activity. However, definitive cortical columns with specified functions have been identified only in the primary sensory cortices. In both the primary somatosensory (postcentral gyrus) and primary visual cortices, functional columns are defined by the focused input of mode- and place-specific thalamocortical projections from the ventral posterolateral thalamic (VPL) and ventral posteromedial thalamic (VPM) nuclei and lateral geniculate bodies, respectively. Thus, when a microelectrode is advanced along a trajectory perpendicular to the cortical surface from layer II through layer VI in the primary somatosensory cortex, all of the cells recorded from respond to the same type of peripheral stimulus—for example, they are activated by a single type of sensory receptor (mode-specific) such as touch or the position of a joint, have the same receptive field on the body surface (place-specific), and respond with about the same latency. Likewise, the primary visual cortex is organized in columns, each of which is specific to a particular orientation of a light stimulus and responds selectively to stimulation of one or the other of the eyes (see Chapter 18). Whether such a columnar organization defines function in other areas of the neocortex has been difficult to assess. This is because a column is defined as being composed

of mode- and place-specific neurons and the vast majority of neocortical neurons do not receive modality-specific thalamocortical input; therefore, it is impossible to define what the best peripheral stimulus is for a particular neuron.

> **Thought Question**
>
> Contrast the purpose of differentiating cortical structures according to horizontal layers and vertical columns. What are the commonalities between these two organizations?

Brodmann's Map

The neocortex is structurally heterogeneous and can be subdivided into different areas based on variations in the size, shape, arrangement, and densities of cells in its different layers. The most widely adopted such cytoarchitectural map is that of Korbinian Brodmann, published in 1909, in which he identified more than 50 different cortical areas (Figure 7-5 ■ and Table 7-2 ■). It is important to note that Brodmann numbered different areas simply in the order in which they were studied. Thus, there is no systematic relationship between Brodmann's numbers

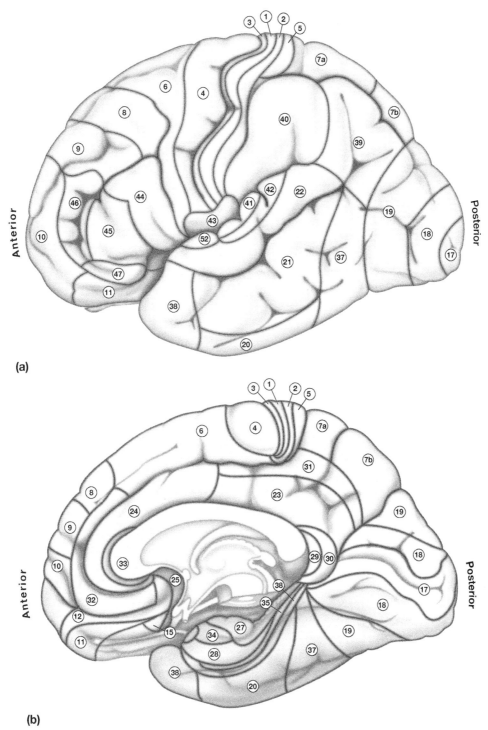

(a)

(b)

FIGURE 7-5 Brodmann's cytoarchitectonically defined areas of the cerebral cortex. (a) Lateral view of the left cerebral hemisphere. (b) Medial view of the right cerebral hemisphere.

(Adapted from Duvernoy, H. M. *The Human Brain: Surface, Blood Supply, and Three-Dimensional Anatomy*, 2nd ed. SpringerWein, New York, 1999.)

and their location in the cerebral cortex: for example, areas 1, 2, 3, 5, and 7 are in the parietal lobe, but areas 4, 6, and 8 are in the frontal lobe. Many of the areas defined by Brodmann have been found to correspond nicely to functions of the cortex as defined by other measures—such as subjective accounts and objective responses of patients who have areas of the cortex damaged or irritated by lesions or surgical ablations, or in whom cortical sites have been stimulated electrically. Indeed, many of the numbers proposed by Brodmann are commonly used by clinicians and researchers for reference purposes, as will be discussed here and in other chapters.

Several caveats should be borne in mind as we consider Brodmann's map of the cerebral cortex. First, there is structural variability among human brains. Thus, the relationships between Brodmann's numbers and specific gyri and sulci shown in his map of the cerebral cortex does not apply precisely to all brains. Second, the boundaries between different cytoarchitectonic areas are not as distinct as implied in the map. Third, as is discussed in detail in Chapter 26, the brain is a plastic organ such that training and use can slightly change the physical size of specific areas. Size can be influenced by the degree of training and functional use of the area. Thus, the physical size of a given **Brodmann's area** can vary across the brains of different people, depending on their life experiences.

> **Thought Question**
>
> Brodmann's maps are of great importance when communicating about cortical pathology and functional consequences. Can you think of two applications of this information that will be important to you as a clinician?

Functional Areas

The division of the neocortex of each hemisphere into motor, sensory, and association areas is based in large measure on differences in cytology and on microstimulation studies dating back to the 1870s. It should be noted that

Table 7-2 Selected Brodmann's Areas

LOBE	NUMBER	LOCATION	NAMES
Frontal	4	Precentral gyrus, paracentral lobule	Primary motor cortex; M1
	6	Precentral gyrus, middle and superior frontal gyri	Premotor cortex, supplementary motor area*
	6, 8	Middle and superior frontal gyri	Frontal eye field*
	9-12	Superior, middle, and inferior frontal gyri rostral to area 6 to the frontal pole	Prefrontal cortex, dorsolateral prefrontal cortex*
	44, 45	Opercular and triangular parts of inferior frontal gyrus	Broca's area; anterior speech area (in dominant hemisphere)*
Parietal	3, 1, 2	Postcentral gyrus, paracentral lobule	Primary somatosensory cortex; S1
	5, 7	Superior parietal lobule	Somatosensory association cortex*
	39	Inferior parietal lobule	Angular gyrus; posterior speech area (part of in dominant hemisphere)*
	40	Inferior parietal lobule	Supramarginal gyrus; posterior speech area (part of in dominant hemisphere)*
Occipital	17	Banks of calcarine sulcus	Primary visual cortex; V1; striate cortex
	18, 19	Surrounding 17	Visual association cortex; V2, V3, V4, V5; extrastriate cortex*
Temporal	41	Transverse temporal gyri	Primary auditory cortex; A1
	42	Transverse temporal gyri	Auditory association cortex; A2*
	22	Superior temporal gyrus	Auditory association cortex; posterior portion is Wernicke's area; posterior speech area (part of in dominant hemisphere)*
Limbic	23, 24	Cingulate gyrus	Limbic association cortex*
	28	Parahippocampal gyrus	Limbic association cortex*

*These terms will be defined in later chapters and are included in the table for future reference.

this view of cortical function is an oversimplification. The distinction between primary areas (or projection areas in the traditional view) and association areas (or nonprojection areas in the traditional view) is not distinct in terms of projections. Association areas, like primary areas, are massively and reciprocally connected with the thalamus and other subcortical structures such as the basal ganglia. The corticospinal tract arises from neurons not just in the primary motor cortex, but from neurons in a number of other cortical regions including the primary somatosensory cortex and association cortex. Our consideration of neocortical function will be separated into the primary areas, the topic of this chapter, and the association cortices, the topic of Chapters 21 and 22. The primary motor and sensory cortical areas are summarized in Figure 7-6 ■.

The **primary motor area** is located in the frontal lobe. It consists of the precentral gyrus on the lateral hemispheral surface and the anterior portion of the paracentral lobule on the medial surface. The primary motor area corresponds to Brodmann's area 4. It is concerned in particular with the control of voluntary movement. The primary motor area contains a comprehensive representation of the body, or **somatotopic** map, that is known as the **motor homunculus** (Figure 7-7 ■). The homunculus follows the medial-lateral orientation of the precentral gyrus, with the representation of the head close to the lateral sulcus and the feet dangling down on the medial hemispheral surface. This orderly representation of different parts of the body is highly significant clinically. The reason is that these areas are differentially supplied by distinct cerebral arteries and

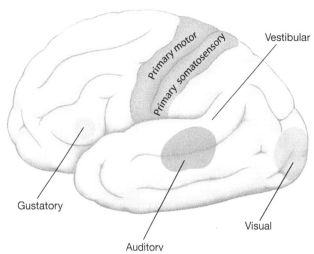

FIGURE 7-6 Primary motor and sensory areas of the cerebral hemisphere. These areas have a general bilateral symmetry structurally as well as functionally.

therefore can be selectively affected by cerebrovascular disease (as discussed later). The motor homunculus also is quite distorted because the body map is related not to actual body geometry, but to innervation density. For example, parts of the body requiring precise motor control, such as the tongue and fingers, have disproportionately large cortical representations reflecting the large numbers of pyramidal neurons dedicated to their control. In contrast, the trunk musculature is primarily postural in nature and capable only of coarse, gross movement. Therefore,

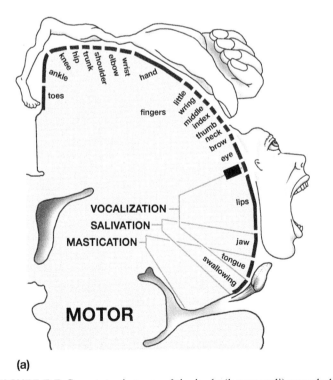

(a)

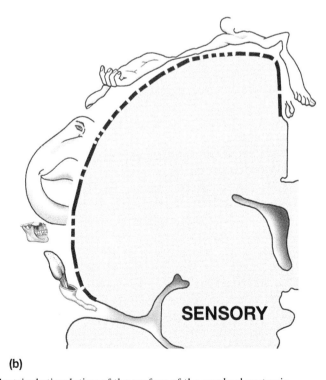

(b)

FIGURE 7-7 Somatotopic maps of the body (homunculi) revealed by electrical stimulation of the surface of the cerebral cortex in conscious human patients undergoing neurosurgery. In both the motor (a) and somatosensory (b) homunculi, the size of the cortical representation is related to the innervation density of that body part and not to its physical geometry.

the trunk musculature has a low innervation density and a small representation in the precentral gyrus.

Primary sensory areas in the neocortex receive their inputs from the specific sensory relay nuclei of the thalamus. The postcentral gyrus on the lateral hemispheral surface and the posterior part of the paracentral lobule on the medial surface constitute the **primary somatosensory area**. This area corresponds to Brodmann's areas 3, 1, and 2. Collectively, these three parallel strips of neocortex occupy nearly all of the postcentral gyrus and the posterior part of the paracentral lobule. Each strip is concerned with its own modality of somatosensory input. The primary somesthetic area receives superficial and deep mechanoreceptive information from the body periphery necessary for the appreciation of position and movement, certain forms of tactile discrimination, as well as the ability to identify an object by manipulation without the use of vision. Like primary motor cortex, primary somatosensory cortex contains a medial-laterally oriented homunculus (somatotopic map), but in this case, the homunculus is related to sensory innervation density (see Figure 7-6). Lips, tongue, and fingertips have disproportionately large somatosensory cortical representations because of their dense receptor populations per unit of tissue area. Hence, sensory discrimination is much more acute in these structures than, for example, on the back or abdomen. The motor and somatosensory homunculi are arranged in direct correspondence with one another across the central sulcus and are reciprocally interconnected via short association fibers.

> **Thought Question**
>
> The motor and somatosensory homunculi are "distorted." What are the anatomical reason and the functional implications?

Primary auditory cortex is located in the temporal lobe. The superior surface of the superior temporal gyrus is within the lateral sulcus and can be seen by pulling down on the temporal lobe and pulling up the frontal lobe to increase the separation of lateral fissure, thereby exposing the insula. The portion of the superior temporal gyrus that is within the lateral fissure then can be visualized (see Figure 7-6). Such a dissection reveals the **transverse (temporal) gyri of Heschl**. These contain the **primary auditory cortex**, which corresponds to Brodmann's areas 41 and 42. Just as there is an orderly arrangement of the body surface in the primary somatosensory cortex (somatotopic organization), so an orderly arrangement of the spectrum of audible frequencies is mapped onto the primary auditory cortex (**tonotopic** organization).

Primary visual cortex is located in the occipital lobe. The primary visual area occupies the cortex superior and inferior to and deep within the calcarine sulcus, as well as the walls of the sulcus, on the medial hemispheral surface. It corresponds to Brodmann's area 17, which consists of long strips of cortex positioned within and on either side of the calcarine sulcus and extending onto the pole of the

occipital lobe. Just as in the primary somatosensory and auditory cortices, there is an orderly map of the retina in the primary visual cortex (a **retinotopic** map).

Several areas of the neocortex receive vestibular input, but it is uncertain whether a **primary vestibular area** can be defined. Electrical stimulation of the parietal lobe in the region of the intraparietal sulcus in conscious patients undergoing neurosurgery elicits vestibular sensations of being rolled with motion of the visual surroundings. Also, focal infarctions involving the posterior insula and operculum of the parietal lobe result in a tilt of the patient's internal representation of gravity. This area is referred to as the **parieto-insular vestibular cortex**.

Gustatory sense (taste) also has a cortical representation. It is located in the anterior insula and adjacent operculum of the frontal lobe. Table 7-2 presents selected Brodmann's areas that have been successfully correlated with function.

BASAL GANGLIA

Clinical Preview

Robert O'Reilly had a small stroke affecting his basal ganglia. As a rehabilitation professional, it will be important to know what signs and symptoms he is likely to have and to relate these symptoms to specific areas of the basal ganglia. As you proceed through this text, it will become evident that this information will assist you in determining functional consequences of different types of strokes and will guide your thinking about intervention. For now, it is important to understand the basic anatomy and major functional consequences of damage to the basal ganglia. As you read through this section, consider the following:

1. Where are the basal ganglia located?
2. What are the names of the associated nuclei?
3. What blood vessels supply the basal ganglia?
4. What are some of the major clinical findings associated with damage to these structures?

The term *basal ganglia* has been used differently over the years. Historically, the basal ganglia were considered to consist of the caudate nucleus, putamen, and globus pallidus, as noted in Chapter 2. However, many authors consider the term *basal ganglia* to include additional nontelencephalic nuclei, specifically, the **subthalamic nucleus**; part of the diencephalon, located at the junction of the thalamus and midbrain; and the **substantia nigra** of the midbrain (Figure 7-8 ■). We shall include all of these structures as components of the basal ganglia.

The caudate nucleus and putamen are the largest nuclei of the basal ganglia and together are referred to as the **striatum**. Over most of its length, the caudate nucleus is separated from the putamen by the thick **internal capsule**. The caudate

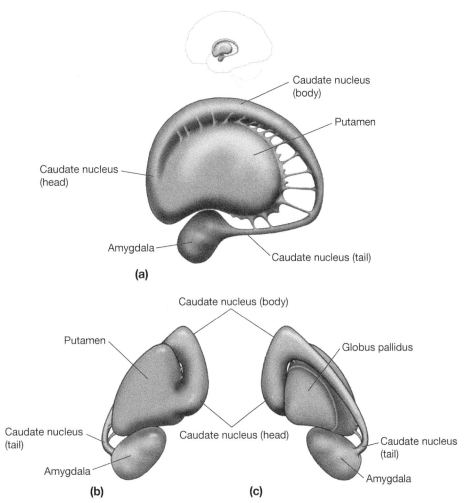

FIGURE 7-8 Telencephalic components of the basal ganglia and terminology applied to them. (a) Lateral view. (b) Anterolateral view. (c) Posteromedial view.

is medial and the putamen lateral to the internal capsule (see Figures 2-22 and 2-23). However, anterior to the internal capsule, the head to the caudate nucleus fuses with the putamen. The histology and connections of the caudate and putamen are similar and lend credence to considering these two nuclei as being one nucleus—the striatum—that is penetrated and divided by fibers of the internal capsule. Also lateral to the internal capsule is the globus pallidus. These three structures—the caudate, putamen, and globus pallidus—make up the **corpus striatum**. The globus pallidus also is called the **pallidum**.

Prefixes and suffixes derived from these names are used to designate inputs to and outputs from these nuclei. Thus, *strio–* and *–striate* are applied to the striatum so that, for example, *striopallidal* refers to projections from the striatum (caudate nucleus and/or putamen) to the globus pallidus, and *corticostriate* refers to projections from the cerebral cortex to the striatum. *Pallidothalamic* refers to projections from the globus pallidus to the thalamus. *Nigrothalamic* applies to projections from the substantia nigra to the thalamus.

Historically, the primary function of the basal ganglia was considered to be motor. This is because initial concepts of basal ganglia function were derived from clinical neurology, and, specifically, from the correlation of documented behavioral deficits during life with pathologic findings at autopsy. At the time of these early observations, clinical testing lacked its present-day sophistication, and concepts of brain function were rudimentary. As a result, only the most obvious symptoms were catalogued and described, and these were motor in nature. Over the years, the idea that the basal ganglia functioned first and foremost in the regulation of somatic motor activity became firmly entrenched in the clinical as well as experimental literature.

While it definitely is the case that the basal ganglia subserve important motor functions, this is true only for certain components. The advent and growth of neuropsychology, together with the capacity to study brain physiology in behaving subjects using contemporary imaging technologies (e.g., functional magnetic resonance imaging), have resulted in a dramatic revision of concepts of basal ganglia function. This revision focuses on the caudate nucleus, now regarded as the predominantly nonmotor component of the basal ganglia. Within the past several years, a whole host of cognitive functions have been attributed to the caudate nucleus. The cognitive functions of the basal ganglia are discussed in Chapter 21.

Among the key concepts that are important to understanding basal ganglia function is the idea of *parallel processing*. Each of the diverse functions of the basal ganglia is mediated by a more or less dedicated circuit through the basal ganglia that is segregated functionally and structurally from the circuits mediating other behaviors. Overall, then, the basal ganglia are organized into an array of simultaneously operating parallel circuits such that multiple behaviors are capable of being regulated at one time. Another key concept is that the basal ganglia have massive and specific connections, both afferent and (via the thalamus) efferent, with the cerebral cortex such that the functions of the basal ganglia cannot be considered independent of those of the cortical areas to which they are connected. The connections between a specific part of the basal ganglia and a specific part of the cerebral cortex, in fact, form a functional system. Thus, for example, the functional specialization in different parts of the caudate nucleus reflects the functional specialization of the cortical region to which that part of the caudate is connected. These concepts are developed in detail in Chapter 19.

Gross Anatomy

This section builds on the anatomy of the basal ganglia presented in Chapter 2. The putamen and globus pallidus (together sometimes referred to as the **lentiform nucleus** due to being shaped like a lens in coronal sections) appears in horizontal sections as a wedge-shaped structure with the apex (pallidus) directed medially into the internal capsule (see Figure 2-22). A thin, somewhat curved vertical layer of white matter divides the lentiform nucleus into the more laterally located **putamen** and the more medially located **globus pallidus**. Positioned deep to the insula, the putamen is the largest of the basal ganglia with a volume of about 15 cc, the same as that estimated for the thalamus. Abutting the lateral surface of the internal capsule (largely its posterior limb), the globus pallidus is itself composed of two segments—an **internal** and an **external segment** separated from one another by another thin lamina of myelinated axons. In fresh specimens, the globus pallidus appears paler than the adjacent putamen owing to its being traversed by numerous myelinated fibers. The term *globus pallidus* means pale ball.

Thought Question

Different terms are used with respect to naming the basal ganglia. Two terms commonly used are *lentiform nucleus* and *corpus striatum*. Compare and contrast nuclei that comprise the lentiform nuclei (Chapter 2) with the nuclei that comprise the corpus striatum.

The **caudate nucleus** is derived embryologically from the same cells that give rise to the putamen, and the two have a similar appearance in sectioned fresh or fixed gross specimens as well as in myelin-stained histologic

Thought Question

It is important to identify cortical and subcortical structures in different cross-sectional views of the cerebral hemispheres. You will use this information as clinicians when you identify structures on CT and MRI scans. Can you identify all the parts of the basal ganglia in cross section and relate these components to the internal capsule and the thalamus? Can you explain why they show up as disconnected segments in cross section? Recall the "central Cs" described in Chapter 2. What part of the basal ganglia has this C-shape and why? What other structures in the brain have this shape? Can you identify these structures in cross section? Finally, can you explain why the appearance of these structures changes, depending on the orientation of the cross section?

sections. In the adult, the caudate attains a volume of some 12 cc which, added to the 15 cc volume of the putamen, makes the striatum the largest single subcortical mass of the brain. The elongated, C-shaped caudate nucleus is related throughout its extent to the walls of the lateral ventricle. The *head of the caudate* nucleus is the enlarged rostral portion that forms the bulging wall of the anterior horn of the lateral ventricle (Figure 7-9 ■). Tapering rapidly in size posteriorly, the head extends approximately to the level of the interventricular foramen. The *body of the caudate* is positioned dorsolateral to the thalamus and forms the lateral wall of the body of the lateral ventricle. Still lying within the ventricle, the thin *tail of the caudate* arches around the posterior surface of the thalamus, then extends anteriorly into the temporal lobe within the inferior horn of the lateral ventricle. Hence, wherever you see a lateral ventricle, the striatum will be visible nearby.

Continuous with the head of the caudate nucleus, and present at the level of the anterior limb of the internal capsule, is a structure called the **nucleus accumbens**. The nucleus accumbens along with adjacent ventral parts of the caudate nucleus and putamen form the **ventral striatum**, a functionally unique subdivision of the striatum. A second important nucleus, the **amygdala**, is continuous with the tip of the tail of the caudate nucleus. Note that the amygdala is a component of the limbic system and is anatomically and functionally distinct from the basal ganglia, even though the tail of the caudate blends into the caudal aspect of the amygdala.

Despite its location in the midbrain, functionally the substantia nigra is considered to be a component of the basal ganglia. The **substantia nigra** is the largest nucleus of the midbrain, extending its entire rostrocaudal length as a band of cells between the cerebral peduncle ventrally and midbrain tegmentum dorsally. In primates, the substantia nigra has a dark appearance in fresh tissue due to the dense accumulation of a neuromelanin pigment in the cell body of dopaminergic neurons (from which the nucleus derived its name of *black substance*). The substantia nigra

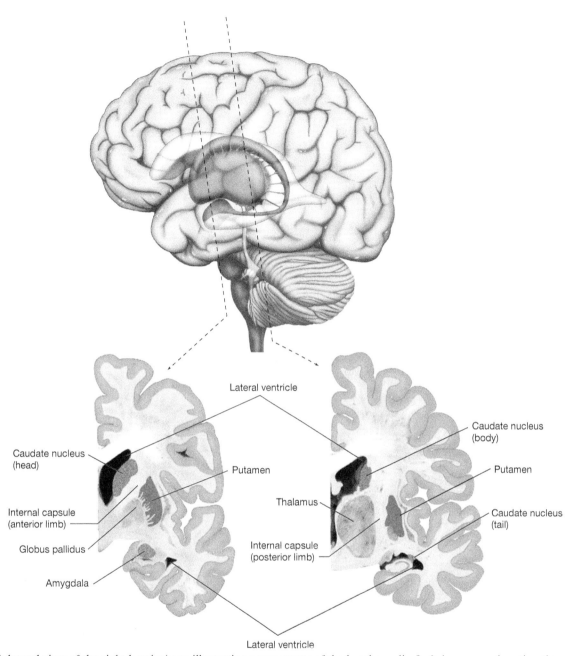

FIGURE 7-9 A lateral view of the right hemisphere, illustrating components of the basal ganglia. Left, in a coronal section through the frontal and temporal lobes, the head of the caudate nucleus can be visualized. Right, in a more posterior section, the body and tail of the caudate can be seen.

is subdivided into two distinct regions: the **pars compacta**, a cell-rich region, and the **pars reticulata**, a cell-sparse region with a well-organized neuropil. The pars reticulata comprises the bulk of the nucleus and lies ventral to the pars compacta. Neurons of the pars compacta are the ones containing the neuromelanin pigment and release the neurotransmitter dopamine onto striatal neurons. Both components of the substantia nigra, but in particular the pars reticulata, transmit basal ganglia influences to other parts of the CNS. The substantia nigra, then, along with the globus pallidus, is an important component of the basal ganglia efferent system. In fact, the pars reticulata of the substantia nigra represents a part of the internal segment

of the globus pallidus that has been artifactually displaced by fibers of the internal capsule.

The **subthalamic nucleus** (body of Luys) was presented in Chapter 6. Despite its location at the junction of the thalamus and midbrain, it is considered to be a member of the basal ganglia. The nucleus definitely is an integral component of basal ganglia circuitry. The subthalamic nucleus is involved in mediating the clinical signs of several important diseases (Parkinson's disease and Huntington's disease) that will be discussed in Chapter 19. The nucleus possesses a rich blood supply. When this blood supply is compromised, hemiballismus (a motor disorder) may result (see Chapter 6).

General Anatomy of Circuits through the Basal Ganglia

The general organization of a circuit through the basal ganglia is a loop that originates in the cerebral cortex, projects to the basal ganglia, and is then routed via the thalamus back to the area of the cerebral cortex from which it originated (Figure 7-10 ■). This circuit provides for critical modulation of efferent output as will be discussed in Chapter 19.

The cerebral cortex provides the single most massive input to the striatum. From the striatum, this information is processed and transmitted to the output nuclei of the basal ganglia via the internal segment of the globus pallidus (GPi) and the pars reticulata of the substantia nigra (SNr). Other projections within (intrinsic to) the basal ganglia will be discussed in Chapter 19. Between three and five separate but parallel loops through the basal ganglia

have been described. Each basal ganglia loop starts in a distinct region of the cerebral cortex; projects to a distinctive region of the striatum; then to a distinctive region of the GPi/SNr; and finally, via different thalamic nuclei, projects back to its place of origin in the cerebral cortex. In general, the different loops selectively involve the caudate nucleus, the putamen, and the ventral striatum. These loops are discussed in Chapters 19 and 21.

> ### Thought Question
>
> The basal ganglia have motor and cognitive functions that you will learn about in Chapter 19. In preparation for understanding the complex circuitry, it is important to begin to recognize some of the circuitry. What structures connect with the basal ganglia, and what are the names of some of the fiber bundles?

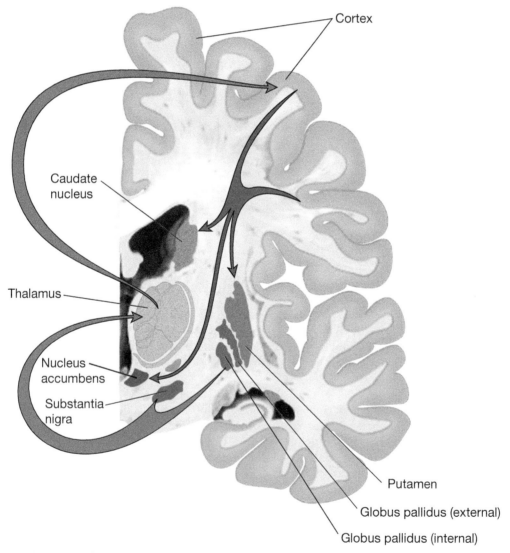

FIGURE 7-10 Major connections of the basal ganglia. The principal input originates in the cerebral cortex and projects to the caudate nucleus, putamen, and ventral striatum (nucleus accumbens). Output derives from the internal segment of the globus pallidus and pars reticulata of the substantia nigra, whose efferents terminate in the thalamus. The thalamus, in turn, projects back to the cerebral cortex.

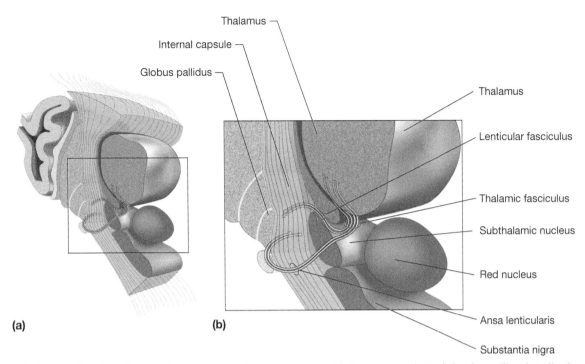

Thalamus
Internal capsule
Globus pallidus

Thalamus
Lenticular fasciculus
Thalamic fasciculus
Subthalamic nucleus
Red nucleus
Ansa lenticularis
Substantia nigra

(a)   **(b)**

FIGURE 7-11 (a) The fiber bundles positioned near the internal capsule. (b) The ansa lenticularis is a large fiber bundle situated on the ventral surface of the globus pallidus. Some fibers originating from cells in the internal segment of the globus pallidus penetrate the internal capsule forming the lenticular fasciculus. The ansa and lenticular bundles join to form a common bundle, the thalamic fasciculus.

Fibers comprising the output from the basal ganglia are common to each loop. Those originating in the internal segment of the globus pallidus organize themselves into grossly visible fiber bundles (Figure 7-11 ■). These convey information primarily to the thalamus, specifically to the ventral anterior thalamic (VA) and ventral lateral thalamic (VL) nuclei, for the control of movement (see Chapter 19) and to the dorsomedial thalamic (DM) nuclei for cognitive functions (see Chapter 21).

The **ansa lenticularis** is a large fiber bundle situated on the ventral surface of the globus pallidus. Fibers are added progressively to the ansa in moving anteriorly through the globus pallidus. Initially positioned lateral to the internal capsule, upon reaching the latter's anterior limit, the ansa loops around the internal capsule's posterior limb to assume a position medial to the capsule. (The Latin word *ansa* means loop.) Ansal fibers then project posteriorly toward their target thalamic nuclei.

Some fibers originating from cells in the internal segment of the globus pallidus penetrate directly through the internal capsule. These form the **lenticular fasciculus**. Initially it is positioned dorsal to the ansa, and, further posteriorly, dorsal to the subthalamic nucleus.

Axons of the lenticular fasciculus and ansa lenticularis join to help form a common fiber bundle, the **thalamic fasciculus**, situated dorsal to the zona incerta. In addition to fibers from the globus pallidus, the thalamic fasciculus contains projections to the thalamus from the cerebellum.

CLINICAL CONNECTIONS

Involuntary Movements Attributed to Basal Ganglia Dysfunction

A number of the pathological processes and disease entities affecting the basal ganglia produce significant and often debilitating motor deficits. The most common diseases affecting the basal ganglia are discussed in Chapter 19. For now, it is helpful to recognize some of the typical motor symptoms that occur with disorders affecting the basal ganglia.

Patients with lesions of the corpus striatum and related nuclei typically have alterations of **muscle tone** that may present as hypertonia, hypotonia, or variable combinations of the two. In addition, these individuals may have various abnormal, involuntary movements including dyskinesias, athetosis, chorea, and ballismus. Collectively, these abnormalities are referred to as movement disorders.

Four types of dyskinesia are distinguished clinically, although they may represent nothing more than different points on a spectrum of dyskinetic movement. Dyskinesias may occur in variable combination and some are rather difficult to differentiate from one another.

Tremor, derived from the Latin word meaning *a shaking*, may be defined as a more or less regular, rhythmic, alternating movement of a body part around a fixed point that is of variable frequency and amplitude. The tremor of basal ganglia disease is observed most clearly in Parkinson's disease (see Chapter 19).

Athetosis, derived from the Greek word meaning *changeable* or *unfixed*, is characterized by slow, sinuous, writhing movements that have a tendency to blend with one another to give the appearance of a continuous, mobile spasm. In general, these purposeless movements are most pronounced in the fingers and hands, face, tongue, and throat, but all muscles may be involved. Athetosis is commonly associated with variable degrees of paresis, spasticity, and chorea. Among the causes of athetosis are anoxia, perinatal insults, and kernicterus (a neurological condition of infants associated with jaundice).

Chorea, derived from the Greek word meaning *dance*, is characterized by brisk, graceful, sometimes complex involuntary movements affecting primarily the distal extremities and face. The movements are well coordinated and may resemble fragments of purposeful voluntary movements, but they never are combined into a coordinated act. The person may, on occasion, incorporate them into a voluntary movement, perhaps to make them less conspicuous. Athetoid movements are slower than those in chorea. However, in some cases, it is impossible to distinguish between the two—hence, the term **choreoathetosis**.

Ballismus, derived from the Greek word meaning *a jumping about*, is the most violent of the dyskinesias and stands at the opposite end of the severity spectrum from tremor. It consists of forceful, flinging movements occurring predominantly in the proximal musculature and muscles of the shoulder and pelvic girdles. In given individuals, ballismus may be difficult to distinguish from choreoathetosis.

INTERNAL CAPSULE

Our earlier discussion of the striatum and globus pallidus mentioned their relationship to the projection fibers of the internal capsule. Indeed, the internal capsule is a key structure in understanding the topographic organization of the interior of the cerebrum (Figure 7-12 ■). In addition to the basal ganglia, the interior of the cerebrum includes the diencephalon. The V-shaped configuration in the horizontal plane of the internal capsule with its apex directed medially toward the third ventricle was presented initially in Chapter 2 along with its three parts: an *anterior limb*, a *posterior limb*, joined at the *genu* (knee or apex).

An oblique section through the superior level of the internal capsule reveals that its anterior limb separates the medially located head of the caudate nucleus from the laterally positioned putamen, while its posterior limb separates the medially located thalamus from the laterally positioned putamen (Figure 7-13 ■). The globus pallidus lies lateral to the internal capsule in the wedge between anterior and posterior limbs. Thus, the internal capsule separates the globus pallidus from both the head of the caudate nucleus and diencephalon. A more inferior section would reveal that the anterior limb of the internal capsule disappears with only the posterior limb remaining. This is because the anterior limb of the internal capsule is made up mostly of thalamocortical (and corticothalamic) fibers, and at caudal levels of the internal capsule, the thalamus no longer is present. In contrast, the posterior limb of the internal capsule contains not only thalamocortical (and corticothalamic) projections, but also projection fibers that descend from the cortex to the brainstem and spinal cord. In fact, fibers of the posterior limb of the internal capsule become the crus cerebri of the midbrain (some of which become the longitudinal fibers of the pons, which become fibers of the pyramids of the medulla, which become fibers of the corticospinal tracts).

> ### Thought Question
>
> What part of the cell comprises the internal capsule? What does this tell you about the function of that structure?

A number of clinically important sets of fibers run in the internal capsule. These include thalamocortical fibers subserving sensation and corticospinal fibers subserving movement, as well as other sets of fibers. Given sets of fibers have specific distributions in the anterior and posterior limbs of the internal capsule, and these are discussed in later chapters.

BLOOD SUPPLY OF THE CEREBRAL HEMISPHERE

> ### Clinical Preview • • • • • • • • • • • • • •
>
> Recall from earlier in this chapter that you met three individuals, each of whom sustained a stroke. These strokes were in different areas of the brain, yet each of these patients had a resulting problem with balance. Amit Mohammed had a stroke affecting his parietal cortex. Sharon Warren had a stroke primarily affecting her medial frontal lobe. And Barbara Nishimura had a stroke in the internal capsule. As you read through this section of the text, for each person:
>
> - Recall the basic functional roles of the affected region of the brain.
> - Consider how knowledge of the vascular supply of the cortex allows you to interpret the relationship between the vessel involved and the functional consequence of a stroke affecting that vessel.
> - Finally, consider whether the damage will likely be constrained to a small area or will be extensive.

As noted in Chapter 2, each side of the circle of Willis gives off three major branches that vascularize each hemisphere: the internal carotid artery divides into a larger middle cerebral artery (MCA) and a smaller anterior cerebral artery (ACA), while the basilar artery bifurcates into the two posterior cerebral arteries (PCAs).

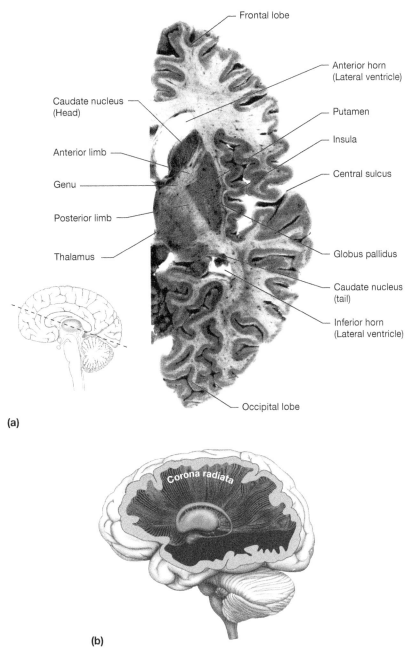

Frontal lobe

Anterior horn
(Lateral ventricle)

Caudate nucleus
(Head)

Putamen

Anterior limb

Insula

Genu

Central sulcus

Posterior limb

Globus pallidus

Thalamus

Caudate nucleus
(tail)

Inferior horn
(Lateral ventricle)

Occipital lobe

(a)

Corona radiata

(b)

FIGURE 7-12 (a) An oblique horizontal section (see inset). In this view, the anterior and posterior limbs of the internal capsule appear in V-shaped configuration. (b) A lateral view exposing the internal capsule and cortical projections.

Two types of arterial branches arise from the circle of Willis and the three major cerebral arteries. The first type is called a **penetrating branch**, and there are many. Penetrating branches (also called **central** or **ganglionic**) arise from all parts of the circle of Willis and from the proximal parts of the three cerebral arteries. There are many penetrating branches, for example, the **lenticulostriate (lateral striate) arteries** and the **thalamogeniculate arteries** (see Figure 6-4). They dip perpendicularly into the substance of the brain and supply structures located deeply in the brain interior such as the basal ganglia, internal capsule, and thalamus. The second type of arterial branch is called a **cortical branch**. Again, there are many—for example, the **Rolandic artery** and **calcarine artery**.

Cortical branches are larger than penetrating branches. Cortical branches divide repeatedly, finally giving off terminal branches of variable length that enter the brain. The shorter terminal branches supply the cerebral cortex. The longer branches supply the immediately adjacent subcortical white matter. The territory of any artery, penetrating or cortical, may be involved as a result of cerebrovascular disease.

Each of the major cortical arteries is responsible for nourishing a specific region of the cerebral cortex. The region of cerebral cortex supplied by each artery is broken down into a central territory and a peripheral territory (see Figure 7-13). The *central territory* is the region of cortex for which the particular artery is the sole source of supply. No

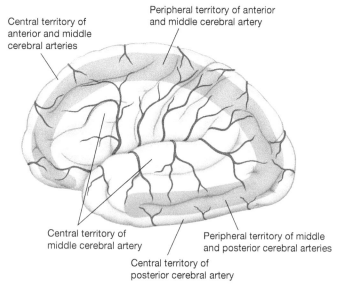

Central territory of anterior and middle cerebral arteries

Peripheral territory of anterior and middle cerebral artery

Central territory of middle cerebral artery

Peripheral territory of middle and posterior cerebral arteries

Central territory of posterior cerebral artery

FIGURE 7-13 The central and peripheral (shaded) territories of supply of the major cerebral arteries depicted on the cortex of the left cerebral hemisphere.

(Adapted from Bowman, J. P., and Giddings, D. F. *Strokes: An Illustrated Guide to Brain Structure, Blood Supply, and Clinical Signs*. Prentice Hall, New Jersey, 2003.)

other artery contributes to the nourishment of neurons lying in the central territory of a major cortical artery. As a result, the central territory invariably undergoes extensive infarction when the vessel is severely occluded. In contrast, the *peripheral territory* of any of the major cerebral arteries also receives a blood supply from another major artery. That is, the peripheral territory of an artery is the region of cortex that also is in the peripheral territory of one or more of the other major cerebral arteries. When a vessel is severely occluded, the peripheral territory is not usually as severely infarcted because it also receives a blood supply from another, unoccluded vessel. Because the infarction in the peripheral territory is less extensive and fewer brain cells die, the resulting neurologic deficits would be correspondingly less severe. This is discussed in detail in Chapter 24.

The reason this distinction between central and peripheral territories is so important is that the central and peripheral territories of certain arteries supply areas of the cortex that receive information from, or control the movements of, distinct and different parts of the body. By noting the distribution and severity of neurologic deficits in different body parts, a clinician can often determine the specific vessel that has been occluded.

Thought Question

Thinking ahead, why would occlusion of a vessel near its origin cause a much greater deficit than occlusion of a vessel near the end of its territory? Note that deficits associated with occlusion of these vessels will be discussed in much greater detail in Chapter 24.

Another feature of the cerebral blood supply that is clinically important is that natural communications, called **anastomoses**, occur between cerebral blood vessels (Figure 7-14a ■). These anastomoses unite branches of the three major cerebral arteries end-to-end. They occur within the sulci of each hemisphere and are not visible on the surface of the adult brain. They are referred to as meningeal anastomoses and they occur in the border zones of the territories of each artery (Figure 7-14b). There are many individual variations in the number and size of these anastomotic channels. In some individuals, when there is occlusion of one of the major arteries, these interarterial anastomoses may be sufficiently robust to carry enough blood into the compromised territory to lessen the degree of ischemic infarction. But only rarely are the end-to-end anastomotic channels that are large enough to support instant retrograde blood flow from one territory to another sufficient to prevent some ischemic damage. In other individuals, the anastomoses may be insufficient to prevent ischemia from occurring over the entire vascular territory of the occluded vessel.

Middle Cerebral Artery

Cortical Branches

The main stem of the MCA passes laterally and reaches the surface of the insula, where it divides into a number of cortical branches. The main stem of the MCA on the surface of the insula divides into two main cortical divisions (Figure 7-15 ■): a **superior division** and an **inferior division**. Each division, in turn, is composed of a number of branches that individually supply different areas of the cortex. Figure 7-16 ■ shows the branches of the MCA. Figure 7-17 ■ illustrates the functional areas of the cerebral cortex and their Brodmann's areas/numbers (BAs) supplied by the various branches of the MCA.

There are three clinically important branches of the superior division. A **pre-Rolandic branch** supplies the premotor cortex, BA 6, including a region of the cortex responsible for turning the head and deviating the eyes laterally to the contralateral side (BA 8), and, in the dominant hemisphere only, the motor **language area of Broca** (BAs 44 and 45). A **Rolandic branch** supplies the primary motor area (BA 4) of the precentral gyrus and some of the primary somatosensory area of the postcentral gyrus. An **anterior parietal (post-Rolandic) branch** supplies most of the primary somatosensory cortex of the postcentral gyrus (BAs 3, 2, 1).

Branches of the inferior division of the MCA are named after the cortical area supplied. These include **anterior**, **middle**, and **posterior temporal branches**; a **posterior parietal branch**; and an **angular branch**. In the dominant hemisphere (usually the left), a number of these branches contribute to the supply of the **sensory language area of Wernicke** (BAs 22, 40, 39). In the nondominant hemisphere (usually the right), these same branches contribute to the supply of an area of cortex that is responsible for visuospatial functions. Such visuospatial

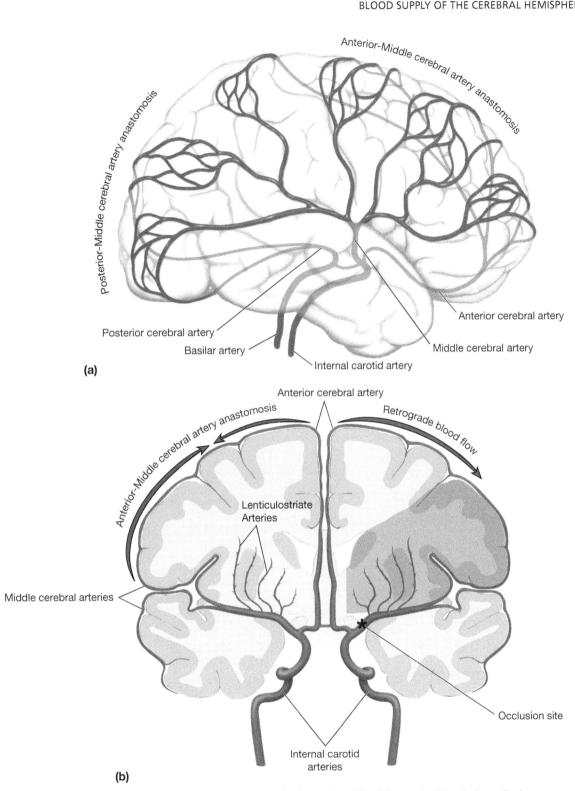

FIGURE 7-14 (a) End-to-end anastomoses between the major cerebral arteries of the right cerebral hemisphere. Such anastomoses lie within the sulci of the hemisphere and are not visible on the surface of the adult brain. The extent and size of these anastomoses influence the potential severity of an infarct resulting from blockage of just one of the arteries participating in the anastomosis. (b) Coronal section. Arrows in the left half indicate one of the sites where, at each systole of the heartbeat, blood flows meet at a "dead point" in potential collateral channels formed by end-to-end arterial anastomoses between the middle and anterior cerebral arteries. An occlusion is shown near the origin of the MCA in the right half. The territory supplied by the penetrating branches of the MCA will be infarcted (dark shading). However, the extent of the infarct in the peripheral territory of the MCA's cortical branches depends on the capacity of the meningeal anastomoses with the unoccluded ACA for retrograde (collateral) flow as shown by the arrow and light shading.

(Adapted from Bowman, J. P., and Giddings, D. F. *Strokes: An Illustrated Guide to Brain Structure, Blood Supply, and Clinical Signs.* Prentice Hall, New Jersey, 2003.)

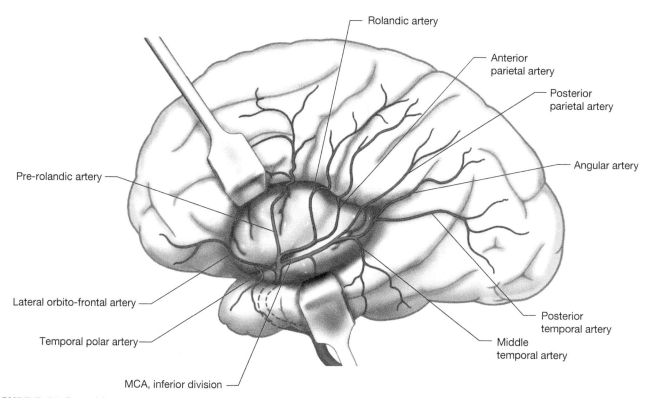

FIGURE 7-15 Branching of the middle cerebral artery on the insula of the left cerebral hemisphere. Portions of the frontal, parietal, and temporal lobes have been retracted to show how the branches of the MCA are distributed over the surface of the insula to form the Sylvian triangle. After dividing, the branches reach the lateral surface of the hemisphere via the lateral sulcus (Sylvian fissure).

(Adapted from Bowman, J. P., and Giddings, D. F. *Strokes: An Illustrated Guide to Brain Structure, Blood Supply, and Clinical Signs*. Prentice Hall, New Jersey, 2003.)

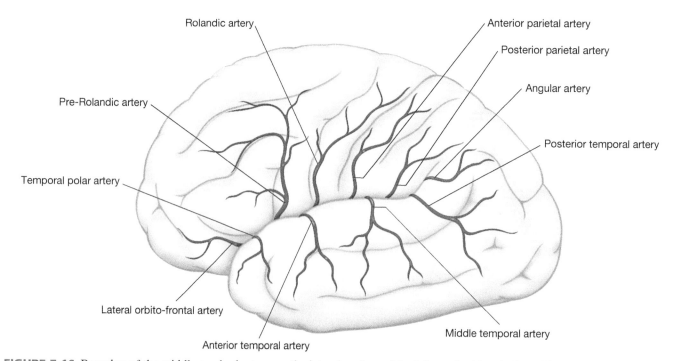

FIGURE 7-16 Branches of the middle cerebral artery on the lateral surface of the left cerebral hemisphere. These branches arise from either the superior or inferior division of the MCA.

(Adapted from Bowman, J. P., and Giddings, D. F. *Strokes: An Illustrated Guide to Brain Structure, Blood Supply, and Clinical Signs*. Prentice Hall, New Jersey, 2003.)

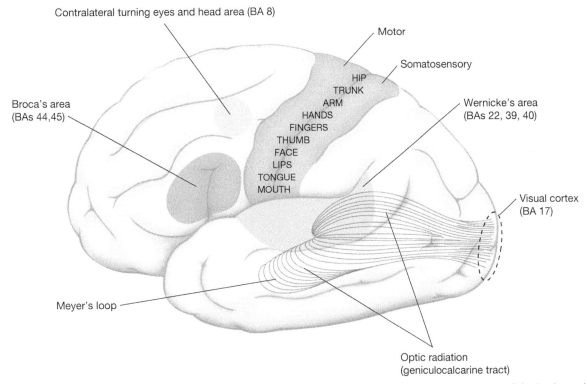

FIGURE 7-17 Location of areas in the left cerebral hemisphere that, when damaged, produce focal neurological deficits. In the majority of people, the speech-language areas of Broca and Wernicke are located only in the left (dominant) hemisphere. Corresponding areas in the nondominant (usually right) hemisphere have different functions. The Brodmann's numbers associated with these cortical areas are indicated. Parts of the body (homunculi) represented in the precentral (motor) and postcentral (somatosensory) gyri are indicated.

(Adapted from Bowman, J. P., and Giddings, F. D. *Strokes: An Illustrated Guide to Brain Structure, Blood Supply, and Clinical Signs.* Prentice Hall, New Jersey, 2003.)

functions include the ability to understand and use visual representations and spatial relationships in learning and in performing a task, such as dressing or drawing a three-dimensional object.

Penetrating Branches

From its origin at the base of the brain, the middle cerebral artery (MCA) travels in a lateral direction toward the surface of the brain. As it does so, this main stem of the MCA gives off a number of penetrating branches (see Figure 7-14b). The penetrating branches are called the **lenticulostriate arteries**. The lenticulostriate arteries ascend perpendicularly to supply a number of structures, including the clinically important basal ganglia and posterior limb of the internal capsule (discussed later).

Thought Question

As a simplification, occlusion of the MCA often produces motor and somatosensory deficits of the upper extremity, while occlusion of the ACA often produces motor and somatosensory deficits of the lower extremity, whereas occlusion of the PCA does not affect either motor or somatosensory function. Can you explain these findings drawing on your understanding of Brodmann's areas?

Anterior Cerebral Artery

Cortical Branches

The cortical branches of the ACA supply the anterior three-quarters of the medial surface of the cerebral hemisphere as well as the anterior four-fifths of the corpus callosum. Named cortical branches supply the medial and orbital surfaces of the frontal lobe, the frontal pole, the medial surface of the parietal lobe, and a strip of the lateral surface of the cerebral hemisphere along the superior border (Figure 7-18a ■). Figure 7-18b shows important Brodmann's areas supplied by the ACA.

Penetrating Branches

The **medial striate artery (recurrent artery of Heubner)** most often arises from the ACA just distal to the anterior communicating artery. The artery courses laterally, then doubles back on its parent artery. It branches repeatedly and penetrates the anterior perforated substance as multiple vessels. The medial striate artery supplies the anteromedial and inferior part of the head of the caudate nucleus (including the nucleus accumbens), adjacent parts of the anterior limb of the internal capsule and putamen, and portions of the septal nuclei. It also gives rise to branches that supply deep white matter of the inferior frontal lobe.

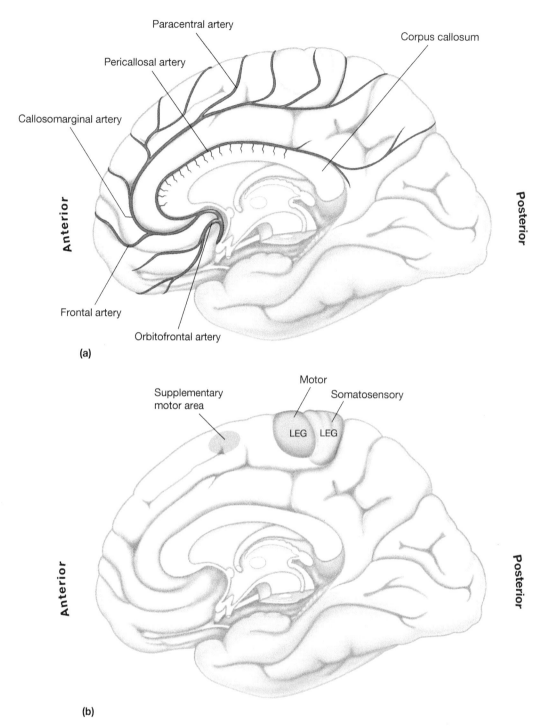

FIGURE 7-18 The medial surface of the right cerebral hemisphere is shown. (a) The named cortical branches of the anterior cerebral artery ACA supply the anterior three-fourths of the medial cortical surface and the anterior portions of the corpus callosum. (b) Several of the functional areas in the central territory of the ACA. In particular, note that the lower extremity is represented in the paracentral lobule. Abbreviation: BA, Brodmann's area.

(Adapted from Bowman, J. P., and Giddings, D. F. *Strokes: An Illustrated Guide to Brain Structure, Blood Supply, and Clinical Signs.* Prentice Hall, New Jersey, 2003.)

Internal Carotid Artery

Recall from Chapter 2 that the internal carotid artery gives rise to both the middle and anterior cerebral arteries that form the anterior circulation of the brain. The MCA is considered to be the direct continuation of the internal carotid artery.

Thought Question

Review the vessels that comprise the circle of Willis (Chapter 2). How do the penetrating and cortical branches of major vessels relate to the circle of Willis?

Posterior Cerebral Artery

The posterior cerebral arteries (PCAs) are a part of the vertebrobasilar system, the second of the two major systems that supply blood to the brain. In about 70 percent of autopsied brains, the PCAs originate as the direct continuations of the basilar artery upon its bifurcation (see Figures 6-10 and 6-20). As a result, occlusive disease of the basilar (or vertebral) artery may result in the development of symptoms in the territories of both PCAs.

Cortical Branches

The various cortical branches of the PCA supply the inferior and medial parts of the temporal lobe and the medial surface of the occipital lobe. Figure 7-19 ▧ shows the

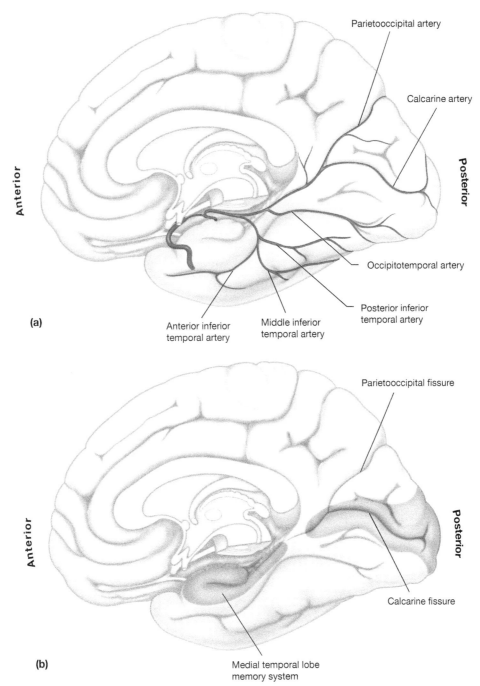

(a)

Parietooccipital artery

Calcarine artery

Posterior

Anterior

Occipitotemporal artery

Posterior inferior temporal artery

Anterior inferior temporal artery

Middle inferior temporal artery

(b)

Parietooccipital fissure

Posterior

Anterior

Calcarine fissure

Medial temporal lobe memory system

FIGURE 7-19 Medial surface of the right cerebral hemisphere is shown. (a) Cortical branches of the posterior cerebral artery supply the inferior and medial parts of the temporal lobe and the medial surface of the occipital lobe via the named branches indicated. (b) Functional areas in the central territory of the PCA. The medial portion of the temporal lobe is concerned with recent memory. The medial portion of the occipital lobe is concerned with vision. The cortex bordering the calcarine fissure on either side represents the primary visual cortex.

(Adapted from Bowman, J. P., and Giddings, D. F. *Strokes: An Illustrated Guide to Brain Structure, Blood Supply, and Clinical Signs.* Prentice Hall, New Jersey, 2003.)

cortical branches of the PCA. The medial portion of the temporal lobe, including BA 28, is concerned with the learning of new information (recent memory). The medial portion of the occipital lobe, supplied by the **calcarine artery**, is concerned with vision. Marked differences in symptoms occur when the occlusion involves just one side (unilateral) as opposed to occlusions that involve both sides (bilateral).

Penetrating Branches

The penetrating branches of the PCA supply the rostral portion of the midbrain and thalamus. Occlusion of the penetrating thalamogeniculate branches supplying the thalamus was presented in Chapter 6. The penetrating branches that nourish the midbrain are discussed in Chapter 15, as are the syndromes that follow their occlusion.

Blood Supply of the Internal Capsule and Basal Ganglia

Given that fibers of the **internal capsule** intervene developmentally between the **caudate** and **lentiform nuclei** (hence the name *corpus striatum*), it should not be surprising that these three structures share common blood supplies. For learning purposes, we present the arterial supplies of these structures individually.

Thus far, we have not considered the **anterior choroidal artery**, but it provides an important blood supply to the posterior limb of the internal capsule and basal ganglia (as well as to other structures such as the hippocampal formation). The artery usually arises from the internal carotid artery distal to the origin of the posterior communicating artery. However, it may also arise from the middle cerebral artery. The anterior choroidal artery pursues a long course in the subarachnoid space and is of relatively small diameter. For these reasons, it is susceptible to thrombosis. Interestingly, surgical occlusion of the proximal portion of the anterior choroidal artery was used at one time as a treatment for the tremor and rigidity of Parkinsonism.

Internal Capsule

The primary blood supply to both the anterior and posterior limbs of the internal capsule is from the lenticulostriate (lateral) penetrating branches of the middle cerebral artery (see Figure 7-14). However, specific portions of the internal capsule are supplied by other arteries. Fibers of the rostral and ventral part are nourished by a penetrating branch of the anterior cerebral artery, also called the medial striate (Heubner) artery. The genu is supplied by direct branches of the internal carotid artery, while fibers of the ventral part of the posterior limb and the entire retrolenticular part of the internal capsule are nourished by the anterior choroidal artery.

Basal Ganglia

Both the caudate nucleus and putamen are nourished primarily by the lenticulostriate branches of the middle cerebral artery, while most of the globus pallidus is supplied

mainly by the anterior choroidal artery. Again, there are regional exceptions in all of these structures. The ventral portion of the head of the caudate nucleus (including the nucleus accumbens) and the adjacent ventral and rostral portion of the putamen that fuses with the head (ventral to the anterior limb of the internal capsule) is supplied by the anterior cerebral artery (medial striate artery). The tail of the caudate is nourished by the anterior choroidal artery, as is the amygdala.

CLINICAL CONNECTIONS

The clinical consequences of occlusion or hemorrhage of arteries to the cerebrum are distinct and relatively complex. They are a major topic of Chapter 24, which discusses strokes. However, it is possible to begin to appreciate the clinical symptoms associated with occlusion of these arteries, based on the information that has already been presented and drawing on knowledge of Brodmann's areas in particular. Appreciation of these symptoms provides an important basis for mastering the content of Chapter 24.

Middle Cerebral Artery

The superior and inferior divisions of the MCA can be occluded separately. When this occurs, two distinct clinical syndromes result. Occlusion of the superior division is illustrated in Figure 7-20a ■. Such an occlusion would affect Brodmann's area 4 on the precentral gyrus and areas 3, 1, and 2 on the postcentral gyrus. Relating this damage to the layout of the motor and sensory homunculi (see Figure 7-10), it can be seen that the cortical motor and sensory deficits would relate to the upper extremity and face. The lower extremity would not be involved because it is represented on the medial surface of BA areas 4 and 3, 1, 2 in the paracentral lobule. In addition, a superior division occlusion would affect BA 8, resulting in deficits in voluntary eye movement, and BAs 44 and 45 resulting in a motor aphasia if the left hemisphere was involved (see Chapter 22).

Occlusion of the inferior division of the MCA is shown in Figure 7-20b. Such an occlusion would affect BAs 22, 39, and 40. If the occlusion involved the inferior division in the dominant left hemisphere, a sensory aphasia would result (see Chapter 22). On the other hand, if the occlusion were located in the inferior division in the nondominant right hemisphere, deficits in visuospatial function would occur (see Chapter 21).

It was noted earlier that the posterior limb of the internal capsule contains upper motor neuron projection fibers. These upper motor neuron fibers control voluntary movements of the body and face. Thus, the classic clinical syndrome associated with occlusion of the lenticulostriate arteries on one side is a pure motor syndrome that involves the face, arm, trunk, and leg in a **spastic (capsular) hemiplegia**. Occlusion of the main stem of the MCA before it gives off any branches blocks the flow of blood into

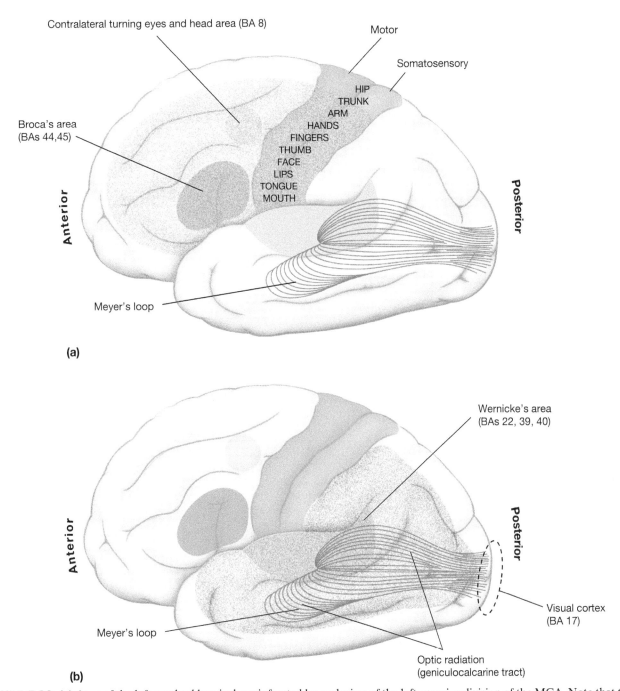

FIGURE 7-20 (a) Area of the left cerebral hemisphere infarcted by occlusion of the left superior division of the MCA. Note that the damage is confined to the frontal lobe and postcentral gyrus of the parietal lobe. (b) Area of the left hemisphere infarcted by occlusion of the inferior division of the MCA. Note that the damage is confined to the posterior portion of the parietal lobe and the temporal lobe.

Abbreviation: BA, Brodmann's area.

(Adapted from Bowman, J. P., and Giddings, D. F. *Strokes: An Illustrated Guide to Brain Structure, Blood Supply, and Clinical Signs.* Prentice Hall, New Jersey, 2003.)

the penetrating lenticulostriate arteries, as well as into the superficial cortical branches belonging to both the superior and inferior divisions. The resultant syndrome would be a summation of the lenticulostriate and cortical branch syndromes. The cortical deficits resulting from occlusion of the main stem of the MCA would be a combination of those discussed for involvement of the superior and inferior divisions of the MCA.

Anterior Cerebral Artery

Occlusion of one ACA is illustrated in Figure 7-21 ■. Occlusion of the ACA is much less common than occlusion of the larger middle cerebral and internal carotid (IC) (see Chapter 24). The cortical area involved includes medial aspects of BAs 4 and 3, 1, 2. Note that the paracentral lobule involvement on the medial hemispheral surface is in the central

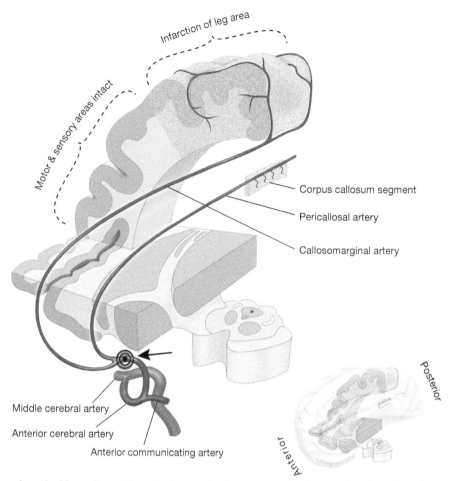

FIGURE 7-21 The named cortical branches of the anterior cerebral artery supply the anterior three-fourths of the medial cortical surface and the anterior portions of the corpus callosum. In particular, note that the lower extremity is represented in the paracentral lobule. With infarction of the main branch of the ACA, the cortical area representing the leg will be affected.

(Adapted from Bowman, J. P., and Giddings, D. F. *Strokes: An Illustrated Guide to Brain Structure, Blood Supply, and Clinical Signs.* Prentice Hall, New Jersey, 2003.)

territory of the ACA, as is a strip of cortex along the superior border of the lateral hemispheral surface. Because the sole source of blood supply to these regions is the ACA, these regions will be the most severely affected by an occlusion of one ACA distal to the anterior communicating artery. The part of the body represented in the paracentral lobule is the lower extremity. Consequently, such an occlusion results in cortical somatosensory and motor deficits that are most severe in the leg. Recall that in contrast, the upper extremity representation lies in the peripheral territory of the MCA. Moreover, the extent of upper extremity involvement would be variable from patient to patient, depending on the robustness of the leptomeningeal anastomoses between the ACA and MCA. There would be no involvement of the face because its representation is in the central territory of the MCA.

Internal Carotid Artery

One of the more common patterns of carotid artery insufficiency occurs with occlusion of one carotid artery and is called the **watershed area**. The internal carotid artery must

be occluded by at least 70 percent in order to produce the carotid border syndrome. With this degree of occlusion, blood flow in the artery distal to the occlusion is decreased significantly but is not eliminated. In this situation, the peripheral territories of both the middle and anterior cerebral arteries represent the zone of maximal ischemia (Figure 7-22 ■).

Maximal ischemia occurs in the watershed area because it requires the greatest pressure for blood to reach the terminal ends of the two arteries where the vessels have the smallest diameter. The area of maximal ischemia is also referred to as the **border zone** between the middle and anterior cerebral arteries, hence the clinical name of **carotid border syndrome**. The portion of the body represented in the pre- and postcentral gyri belonging to this border zone includes the shoulder and hip. The border zone is also the most vulnerable cortical area in cases of transient ischemia attacks with stenosis of the internal carotid artery. The symptoms in the carotid border syndrome include contralateral numbness and weakness.

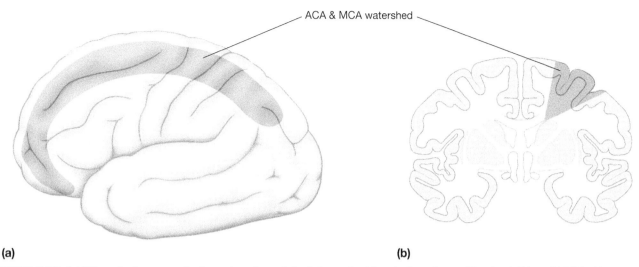

FIGURE 7-22 (a) Watershed area on the lateral surface of the left cerebral hemisphere formed by the ACA and MCA. The watershed area is in the peripheral territories of each artery and represents the zone of maximal ischemia with stenosis of the internal carotid artery on that side. (b) Coronal section of the brain showing the watershed area for the ACA and MCA. Note that in addition to the cortex, the subjacent white matter is in the watershed area.

(Adapted from Bowman, J. P., and Giddings, D. F. *Strokes: An Illustrated Guide to Brain Structure, Blood Supply, and Clinical Signs.* Prentice Hall, New Jersey, 2003.)

Posterior Cerebral Artery

Unilateral involvement of the calcarine branch of the PCA affects the primary visual cortex, BA 17 (see Figure 7-19). This results in a loss of vision in one-half of the visual field in each eye (see Chapter 18). Because a small collateral from the MCA perfuses the area of the cortex that receives afferents from the fovea, there may be sparing of foveal vision, referred to as macular sparing (see Chapter 18).

Summary

This chapter began with a survey of the gross organization of the cerebral cortex into gyri and sulci. Although there are slight variations from brain to brain, a general pattern of organization is discernable. From the perspective of cytoarchitecture, the cerebral cortex is organized in both horizontal and vertical dimensions. Organization in the horizontal dimension is into layers. In the neocortex, six horizontal layers can be discerned that vary in terms of their thickness and cellular density in different areas of the cortex. Motor cortex, for example, is characterized as being agranular because of the thinness of its two granular layers, while primary sensory cortex is characterized as granular because of the thinness of its two pyramidal layers. Brodmann developed his map of the cerebral cortex by examining the detailed regional variation in neocortical cytoarchitecture. Brodmann's map contains some 50 different cortical areas. Importantly, many of these have rather clearly defined functional and clinical correlates.

The anatomical components of the basal ganglia and their regional variations and subdivisions were analyzed in more detail than in Chapter 2. A generalized circuit through the basal ganglia was defined in terms of its origin in the cerebral cortex, then via a sequence of relays first in the caudate nucleus and putamen, then in the globus pallidus and substantia nigra pars reticulata, and finally in the thalamus whose axons return to the cortical origin of the circuit. The internal capsule is an important structure in terms of an anatomical landmark, as well as clinically. The latter was discussed in terms of the contingent of upper motor neuron projection fibers it contains in its posterior limb.

Finally, the blood supply of each cerebral hemisphere was detailed in terms of the three major vessels that supply the cerebral cortex as well as the penetrating branches arising from these arteries and the circle of Willis that nourish structures residing in the interior of each hemisphere. The correlation between the functions of different Brodmann's areas and their blood supply—including the concepts of central and peripheral territories of supply—enable a clinician in many cases of cerebrovascular disease to localize the site of a lesion and the blood vessel involved. All this, even in the absence of a brain scan!

Applications

1. Mr. Brown, a 76-year-old gentleman, suddenly developed right arm and leg weakness and was unable to speak. He was brought to the emergency department by ambulance. On admission, he could not utter words and did not understand simple commands. The right side of his face was "droopy." He was unable to move his right arm or leg volitionally. Although difficult to test, he seemed to have somatosensory losses of the right arm, leg, and face. The left arm, leg, and face seemed unaffected. He had a medical history of hypertension, diabetes, and hypercholesterolemia.
   a. What is the diagnostic term to describe Mr. Brown's language deficits?
   b. Where is the lesion, and which Brodmann's areas were damaged?

2. Andrea Andrews, a 56-year-old attorney, had several episodes of right arm tingling and weakness. During these episodes she had difficulty with finding the right words. This was transient, but seemed to happen at the most inopportune of times, such as while she was in court. She did not seek medical care due to her busy work schedule and because the episodes always quickly and fully resolved. One day at work, she had a severe headache, blurred vision, and right arm weakness. She asked a colleague to take her to the hospital. Upon arrival, she had great difficulty talking, but could shake her head yes/no appropriately and follow simple commands. Her colleague reports Andrea is a heavy drinker and smoker.
   a. What is the diagnostic term to describe Ms. Andrews' language deficits?
   b. Where is the lesion?

3. Consider the two cases in problems 1 and 2. Both Mr. Brown and Ms. Andrews experienced sudden vascular events. Discuss the significance of their respective medical and social histories. Note that you may need to read basic information about risk factors for stroke to answer this question.

References

Cerebral Hemisphere

Bense, S., Bartenstein, P., Lochmann, M., et al. Metabolic changes in vestibular and visual cortices in acute vestibular neuritis. *Ann Neurol* 56:624–630, 2004.

Bertrand, G., Blundell, J., and Musella, R. Electrical exploration of the internal capsule and neighboring structures during stereotaxic procedures. *J Neurosurg* 22:333–343, 1965.

Hanaway, J., and Young, R. R. Localization of the pyramidal tract in the internal capsule of man. *J Neurol Sci* 34:63–70, 1977.

Nolte, J. *The Human Brain: An Introduction to Its Functional Anatomy*. Mosby Elsevier, Philadelphia, 2009.

Parent, A. *Carpenter's Human Neuroanatomy*, 9th ed. Williams & Wilkins, Philadelphia, 1996.

Penfield, W., and Rasmussen, T. *The Cerebral Cortex of Man*. Macmillan, New York, 1950.

Blood Supply

Bowman, J. P., and Giddings, F. D. *Strokes: An Illustrated Guide to Brain Structure, Blood Supply, and Clinical Signs*. Prentice Hall, New Jersey, 2003.

Duvernoy, H. M. *The Human Brain Surface, Blood Supply, and Three-Dimensional Sectional Anatomy*, 2nd ed. SpringerWien, New York, 1999.

Schaller, B. Physiology of cerebral venous blood flow: from experimental data in animals to normal function in humans. *Brain Res Rev* 46:243–260, 2004.

PART III

Somatosensory and Motor Systems for the Extremities and Trunk

Together, the somatic sensory and motor systems allow us to interpret our environment and move within it. One function of the somatic sensory system is to provide us with descriptions of our immediate external environment. In some cases, such descriptions are of survival value—for example, a painful stimulus warning us of impending danger. In other cases, such descriptions enhance the comfort and quality of our existence—for example, informing us of warmth of an environment or the texture of softness. The somatosensory system also is essential to movement and function, providing our nervous system with knowledge of the body's position in space and providing feedback and adjustments for movement as it occurs. Somatic motor systems, in regulating the contractions of striated (voluntary) muscle, allow us to successfully negotiate within our physical environment. Together, the somatic sensory and motor systems collaborate intimately in mediating behaviors ranging from the simplest, such as reflexes, to the most complex.

The interplay between the sensory and motor systems is particularly well illustrated by the hand, with its seemingly inexhaustible repertoire of dexterity. So important is the hand to ordinary human behavior that the major function of the shoulder and arm is to place the hand in a position where it can perform its specific function of precision grasping, writing, or playing a musical instrument. Human perception and the way we classify objects are importantly determined by how we handle them. But how is it that the motor act of performance, for example, of object manipulation, is a vehicle by which we gain knowledge; how is it that movement can provide data by which objects are known? The answer is that the hands are not simply motor organs for doing, they also are sense organs for feeling and exploration.

We explore the world around us with our eyes and hands. In this exploration, vision dominates our perception to such an extent that we do not usually attend to the sensory data simultaneously being sent to the brain from the hand. However, hands offer a number of significant advantages over eyes in environmental exploration. In being attached to long, highly flexible arms, they can see around corners. They also can see in the dark, as when retrieving a quarter from the bottom of a backpack or feeling with extraordinary precision a violin's strings, spaces between them, and positions along them as the violinist plays with her eyes closed. And, having perceived the environment, a hand can immediately alter it because the equipment for feeling is anatomically the same as the equipment for doing. It thus should not be surprising to find that the central nervous system has evolved mechanisms for the control of hand function wherein a strict distinction between sensory and motor systems becomes behaviorally irrelevant.

The first chapter in Part III, Chapter 8, provides an overview of the somatic sensory and motor systems. The main components of the somatosensory system are summarized from the sensory receptors in the periphery to the cortex. The main components of the somatic motor system likewise are summarized, starting in the cortex and ending at the muscle. Chapter 9 elaborates on the components of the somatosensory system and illustrates the pathways that information travels, using two important senses: those associated with proprioception and those associated with pain and temperature. Chapters 10 and 11 elaborate on the motor systems, with emphasis on the tracts that motor information follows. Finally, Part III of the text ends with Chapter 12, an overview of the autonomic nervous system. One might question the logic of including the autonomic nervous system along with the somatic sensory and motor systems, given that the autonomic is involuntary (autonomous, self-governing), while somatic sensory and motor are voluntary. However, both systems originate in the brain. Our ongoing experiences and memories dictate not only the contractions of striated muscle, but simultaneous functional shifts in the body's internal organs. Indeed, such shifts may even occur in anticipation of voluntary movement. The functions of the autonomic nervous system are fully integrated with voluntary movement and emotion.

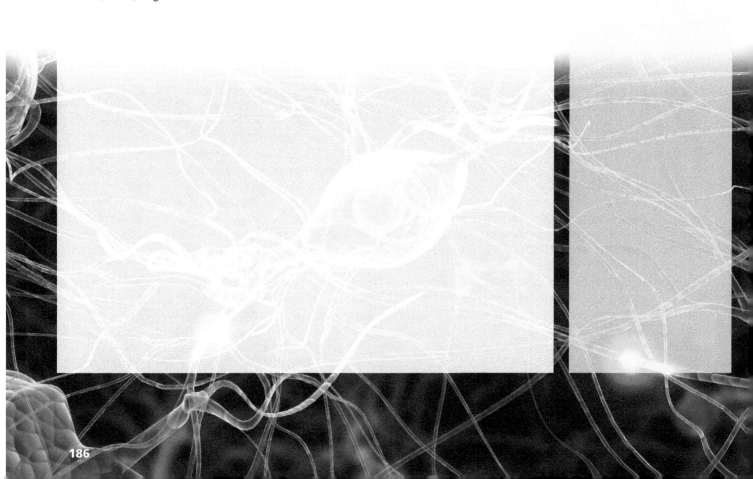

Introduction to the Somatic Sensory and Motor Systems

LEARNING OUTCOMES

This chapter prepares the reader to:

1. Identify the anatomy and functions of six structural components of the somatosensory system.

2. Explain the role of parallel processing in the somatosensory system.

3. Explain the nature and purpose of efferent modulation.

4. Identify the anatomy and function of five structural components of the somatic motor system.

5. Differentiate upper motor neurons from lower motor neurons.

6. Name the cortical region and brainstem nuclei from which upper motor neurons (UMNs) originate.

7. Discuss how UMNs are modulated by the thalamus, basal ganglia, and cerebellum.

8. Differentiate positive and negative neurological signs.

9. Differentiate feedforward and feedback control systems and their functional roles.

10. Define the concepts of reciprocal innervation, synergistic movement, and central motor patterns.

11. Define muscle tone and discuss the factors that can influence tone.

12. Discuss the four aspects of voluntary movement that differentiate it from reflexive movement.

ACRONYMS

CPG Central pattern generator
CST Corticospinal tract
DRG Dorsal root ganglion
LMN Lower motor neuron
UMN Upper motor neuron

Introduction

Purposeful movement involves many aspects of motor control and requires precise integration of both the somatosensory and motor systems. This chapter lays the groundwork for understanding how the somatosensory and motor systems work together. The first major section introduces basic components and organization for the somatosensory system. The somatosensory system includes six structural components that take sensory information from the periphery to the somatosensory cortex. Each component of the system is described. The second major section introduces five structural components of the motor system and the general functional plan by which they are integrated together. This information is followed by an overview of types of movement, contrasting reflexive from volitional movements. Next we introduce different types

of motor control that subserve daily functional activities and the role of sensation in each. Finally, a functional example is used to illustrate the interplay of different types of movement and the role of sensory information in each.

This overview provides an anchor for understanding the somatosensory and motor systems. The following three chapters (Chapters 9, 10, and 11) on the somatosensory and motor systems provide a detailed explanation of these critical systems and, in addition, provide a functional framework from which to understand other chapters in the text on special functional systems of the CNS that mediate somatosensory and motor functions. The control of voluntary movement will be revisited in Chapter 20 after all components of the system, from muscle to cerebral cortex, have been presented.

SOMATOSENSORY SYSTEMS

Clinical Preview

James McNabb has diabetes and, as a result, developed a peripheral neuropathy, affecting his peripheral sensory nerves. One of the consequences of this neuropathy is that he is no longer able to feel touch or pressure from the soles of his feet. In this chapter, you will learn about the pathways that transmit information from his feet (where the information is received) to his cortex (where information is perceived). Consider the following:

- What is the role of the receptor in this process of transfer of information?
- What is the difference among first-, second-, and third-order neurons involved in the transfer of information?
- Given that the neuropathy is peripheral, which neuron is affected?

Note that you will revisit these topics again in Chapter 9.

General Anatomical Plan

The sensory systems allow the organism to sense the body and environment—and to respond appropriately. The term *sense* means to feel, to perceive, or to be aware of. All sensory systems follow a similar general anatomical plan and exhibit similar organizational (functional) principles in carrying information from the periphery to the cerebral cortex for conscious awareness, although the details vary from system to system. Components of

the nervous system involved in mediating somatic sensation are numerous and are distributed in both the peripheral and central nervous systems. Somatosensory systems generally consist of six structural components. In the PNS, these include (1) receptors (sensory end organs) and (2) primary afferent fibers and their ganglia. In the CNS, they include (3) a prethalamic "relay nucleus," (4) a decussation or crossing, (5) a thalamic relay nucleus, and (6) a cortical projection target (Figure 8-1 ■). As we will see throughout the chapter, a variety of other terms may be applied to some of these structural components. With respect to gross anatomy, the CNS components of somatosensory systems are located in the spinal cord, brainstem, diencephalon (thalamus), and cerebral hemisphere. Each of these subdivisions contains somatosensory nuclei and ascending tracts that link them.

Receptors

A major task faced by sensory systems is to transduce some form of environmental energy into the language of the nervous system—namely, an electrical change that encodes the relevant information about the environmental stimulus (see Chapter 4). This function is fulfilled by **receptors** or **sensory end organs**. Anatomically, receptors represent the terminals of peripheral nerve fibers. Although the nerve terminal often is associated with a variety of non-neural cells that direct a stimulus in a stereotyped way toward the terminal, it is the nerve terminal itself that is the receptor. This electrical change is the **receptor**, or **generator**, **potential** and is produced by modality-gated ion channels. Sensory receptors contain a specialized portion of membrane that contains the molecular machinery for the transduction. It is noteworthy that different sensory modalities fulfill the transduction process with distinct molecular mechanisms.

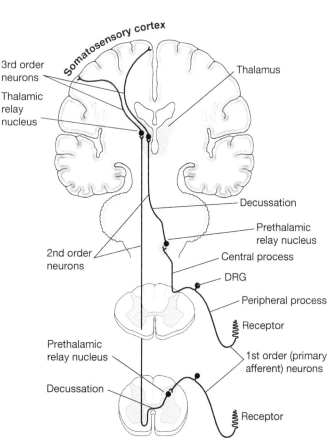

FIGURE 8-1 The general anatomical plan of a somatic sensory system for the extremities and trunk. Six structural components are illustrated. The components in the PNS are receptors and primary afferent neurons, while those in the CNS include a prethalamic relay nucleus, a decussation, a thalamic relay nucleus, and a cortical projection site. Note that first-order neurons always are components of the PNS with cell bodies in a dorsal root ganglion (DRG) of a spinal nerve. The prethalamic relay may be located either in the spinal cord or brainstem, as may the origin of second-order neurons and location of the system's decussation. Third-order neurons that project to the primary sensory cortex always have their cell bodies in the thalamus.

Primary Afferent Neurons

The environmental information encoded by receptors is conveyed to the CNS over **primary afferent fibers** (axons), also called **first-order fibers**. The terms *primary* or *first-order* derive from the fact that such neurons represent the first link in a chain of neurons that carry information from peripheral receptors to specific sites in the brain where it will be analyzed to generate perceptions and influence some behavioral function. Each primary afferent neuron related to a receptor in the body has its cell body in a **dorsal root ganglion (DRG)** of the PNS located adjacent to the spinal cord. Each ganglion neuron has a peripheral process that ends as a somatic receptor in a tissue of the body wall and a central process (see Figure 8-1). The central process of a ganglion neuron enters the CNS, where it will synapse in a prethalamic relay nucleus.

Thought Question

First-order neurons were introduced in Chapter 2. In this chapter, you learn about second-order neurons. In what fundamental ways do first- and second-order neurons differ? What term is used to describe the nucleus of the second-order neurons, and where are these neurons located in the spinal cord?

Prethalamic Relay

A **prethalamic relay nucleus** is a collection of cell bodies within the spinal cord or brainstem aggregated into an identifiable group on which first-order neurons synapse. The nucleus is prethalamic in that it occupies a position in the sensory system that is caudal to the thalamus. The prethalamic relay nucleus contains the cell bodies of **second-order neurons** that represent the second neuron in the chain linking the sensory system to its cortical projection site (see Figure 8-1). In the case of somatosensory systems, the prethalamic relay nucleus is located in the posterior horn of the spinal cord or in the brainstem, depending on the specific somatosensory system. The prethalamic relay nucleus is linked to a nucleus in the thalamus via an ascending sensory tract.

Decussations

In all sensory systems, at least some of the second-order neurons that leave the prethalamic relay nucleus in tracts cross (decussate) to the contralateral side of the CNS. In some systems, virtually all of the axons cross. Because of this decussation, damage to a sensory system on one side of the CNS may result in symptoms on the opposite side of the person's body (as discussed later). Thus, knowing the level in the CNS at which fibers of a specific sensory system cross is critical to an accurate interpretation of where in the CNS damage has occurred.

For example, the **ventral white commissure** of the spinal cord is a structure of unquestionable clinical significance because it is the site where a set of ascending somatosensory axons crosses from one side of the spinal cord to the other. This crossing, or decussation, takes place along the entire length of the spinal cord, with specific fibers decussating according to their entry to the spinal cord (see Chapter 11). The ventral white commissure must always be taken into account when determining the location of a lesion based on the somatosensory symptoms displayed by a patient. Pain, temperature, and crude touch are important somatosensory modalities tested in the neurologic workup of a patient, and axons conveying these sensations cross in the ventral white commissure of the spinal cord. For these somatosensory modalities, a lesion *caudal* to the commissure at which those fibers decussate would produce **ipsilateral signs**; that is, the patient's symptoms would occur on the side of the body that is the *same* as the side of the spinal cord

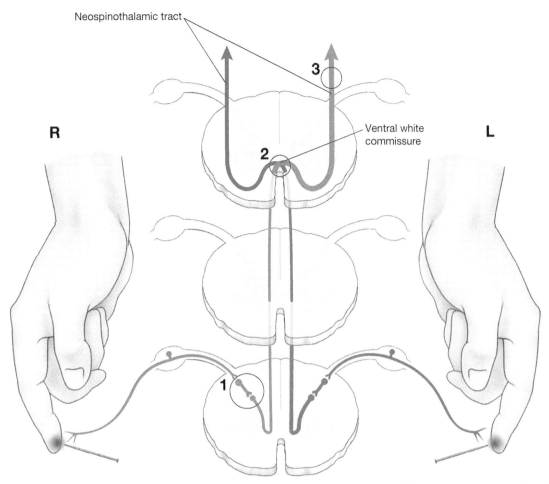

Neospinothalamic tract

R

L

Ventral white commissure

3

2

1

FIGURE 8-2 Knowing the site in the CNS where the axons of a sensory system decussate is critical to interpreting the location of a lesion based on the patient's clinical signs. For example, the integrity of the neospinothalamic component of the anterolateral system is tested by the determining a subject's ability to locate the site of a pinprick applied to the body surface. This system's axons decussate in the ventral white commissure of the spinal cord. A lesion caudal (distal) to the decussation (site 1) would result in ipsilateral signs; a lesion in the ventral white commissure (site 2) would result in bilateral signs; while a lesion rostral to the decussation (site 3) would result in contralateral signs.

lesion (Figure 8-2 ■ , site 1). A lesion *rostral to* the commissure at which those fibers decussate would produce **contralateral signs**; that is, the patient's symptoms would occur on the side of the body that is the *opposite* to the side of the spinal cord lesion (Figure 8-2, site 3). A lesion *in* the ventral white commissure would result in **bilateral signs**; that is, the patient would display a loss of pain, temperature, and light touch on both sides of the body. Such a lesion occurs in a degenerative disorder of the spinal cord called **syringomyelia** (Figure 8-2, site 2) (see Chapter 11).

Thought Question

Which components of the somatosensory system are in the PNS, and which are in the CNS? Which decussate? What does this mean in terms of the location of symptoms when lesions occur in the PNS versus the CNS?

Thalamic Relay

A number of sensory systems contribute to conscious awareness of environmental events. With the exception of olfaction, all tracts of these sensory systems synapse in the thalamus before their information reaches the cerebral cortex, where it is interpreted. As discussed in Chapter 6, each such system has its own, unique thalamic nucleus or set of nuclei within which its second-order prethalamic axons terminate. As a group, these aggregations of thalamic cells often are referred to as the **specific relay nuclei** because of their role in relaying ascending sensory information to the cortex for perception. Specific relay nuclei of the thalamus contain the cell bodies of third-order neurons (see Figure 8-1).

Cerebral Cortex

The final link between receptor and cerebral cortex is represented by **third-order neurons** in the thalamus. Third-order neurons also are called **thalamocortical projection fibers** because they link the thalamus with the cerebral cortex (see

Figure 8-1). Thalamocortical projection fibers ascend to the cerebral cortex in the **internal capsule**. Each specific relay nucleus of the thalamus projects to a specific area (or areas) of the cerebral cortex within which conscious analysis of the sensory input begins. These cortical areas are designated in several ways. One is by the lobe and specific gyri in which the fibers terminate. Another is by the system of Brodmann's numbers, which are presented in Chapter 7. Brodmann's areas are important clinically because many can be associated with specific behavioral functions. Thus, specific clinical signs result from the damage of given Brodmann's areas.

Topographic Organization

The distribution of receptors in the body periphery is replicated over and over again in maps within each sensory system. Orderly maps of the receptive surface exist within each relay nucleus, as well as in the cerebral cortex. The precision of the map varies across different systems but is always elaborated in greatest detail in the cerebral cortex. The maps are named with reference to the specific sensory system as noted in Chapter 7: **somatotopic** for the somatosensory system, **retinotopic** for the visual system, and **tonotopic** for the auditory system.

Other Connections of Sensory Pathways

So far, we have considered the parts of the sensory system that allow the individual to consciously perceive the environment. It is important to recognize that perception of sensory stimuli requires cortical processing. However, not all tracts carrying information from peripheral receptors to suprasegmental structures are used in perception. For example, the spinocerebellar tracts go to the cerebellum, which does not possess the neural machinery to perceive, but rather utilizes so-called unconscious proprioception in the control of movement. The spinocerebellar tracts are indispensable to normal movement. This sensory information is used in a comparator fashion, allowing the nervous system to compare the ongoing movement that is occurring with the movement that was intended. When discrepancies arise, the system then takes corrective action. The comparator function of the cerebellum is discussed in detail in Chapter 19.

Thought Question

Not all sensory information is destined to reach the cerebral cortex. What is another major destination for these neurons, and what is the functional significance of these connections?

General Functional Plan

Parallel Processing

In everyday behavior, single sensory systems are never activated in isolation. Rather, multiple sensory systems are activated simultaneously, or *in parallel*. This is readily apparent in the case of somatic sensation. For example,

when you grasp and manipulate an object, it is obvious that superficial receptors for touch, as well as deep receptors in muscles, are activated along with those that tell you whether the object is warm or cold, hard or soft, etc. Thus, if the receptors for temperature and those for touch are different and they send information into sensory systems that are separate, those systems must be activated in parallel.

Thought Question

Parallel processing and efferent modulation are two important features of CNS organization of the sensory system. Can you think of functional examples illustrating the importance of these two features?

Efferent Modulation

Efferent modulation refers to the fact that each relay structure in a sensory system is subject to regulation by descending fibers from higher-order structures, in particular the cerebral cortex. The term *efferent* derives from the fact that the axons that descend from the higher-order structure are efferent fibers from that structure. Efferent modulation means that the CNS regulates its incoming information. Such descending control increases alertness, filters out background noise, sharpens contrast, enhances discrimination, and improves acuity. For example, in the system responsible for pain perception, efferent modulation may act not only to augment the perception of pain, but also to suppress it. Efferent modulation also acts on the information conducted by the auditory hair cells.

SOMATIC MOTOR SYSTEMS

Clinical Preview

Earlier in this chapter, you met James McNabb, who has diabetes. In addition to the sensory loss described previously, the peripheral neuropathy also affected his motor system. As you read through this section of the chapter, consider the following:

- What is the difference between upper and lower motor neurons?

- Given that the neuropathy is peripheral, which neuron is affected?

- What might be the ramification for reflex responses?

Note that you will revisit these issues in greater detail in Chapters 10 and 11.

The term **motor system** is a generic term in that it refers to all of the structures of the central and peripheral nervous systems that contribute to motor activity. In the case of central control of skeletal muscle activity, we define **motor activity** as the occurrence of action potentials in the nerve fibers that run from the CNS directly to muscles. We tend to think of motor activity in the context of overt movement of some sort—that is, as behavior. Common observation and experience tell us that motor behaviors manifest themselves in a variety of different types of overt movement. Overt movements range from reflexes, such as the patellar tendon reflex, at one extreme to complicated skilled voluntary actions, such as playing a piano, at the other. However, motor activity is not limited to specification of overt movement. For example, motor activity also can result in sustained postures and changes of underlying tone (as discussed later). The motor system engages distinct neural mechanisms and structures by which it mediates different types of motor activity. These different types of motor activity will be enumerated after we discuss the general anatomical and functional plan of the motor system.

General Anatomical Plan and Definitions

The somatic motor system includes descending pathways from the cerebral cortex and brainstem to the spinal cord (as discussed later). The motor system includes five structural components. In the CNS, these components include (1) an origin (either in the cerebral cortex or brainstem) called the upper motor neuron; (2) a decussation, or crossing, of some pathways; and (3) a synapse on an alpha motor neuron called the lower motor neuron. In the PNS, the structural components include (4) the efferent fibers of lower motor neurons and (5) the neuromuscular junction. In addition, the motor system involves complex circuitry utilized to plan, program, coordinate, and modulate descending motor pathways.

> **Thought Question**
>
> How do the five structural components of the motor system compare to the six components of the sensory system? Which are located in the PNS and which in the CNS?

Before discussing the structural components, we need to define two terms: upper and lower motor neurons. **Lower motor neurons (LMNs)** have their cell bodies in the CNS—either in the anterior horn of the spinal cord or in the cranial nerve motor nuclei of the brainstem. Their individual axons are distributed to groups of striated skeletal muscle fibers. In the case of the spinal cord, the axon of an LMN leaves the CNS via a ventral root, becomes part of a spinal nerve, and synapses directly with skeletal muscle fibers. In the case of the brainstem, LMN axons course to striated muscles of the head and neck via cranial nerves. LMNs are also called **alpha motor neurons** because their cell bodies are the largest

cell bodies in the structures in which they reside. **Upper motor neurons (UMNs)** have their cell bodies situated in structures rostral to the spinal cord (Figure 8-3 ■). Both their cell bodies and axons reside entirely within the CNS. The motor pathways begin with upper motor neurons. UMN axons influence—either directly or, more commonly, indirectly via interneurons—the discharge patterns of alpha LMNs.

Upper Motor Neurons

The term *UMN* is generic because it designates literally everything upstream that gives rise to projections that converge on alpha LMNs. Because all of the structures that represent sources of UMNs are located superior (rostral) to the location of alpha LMNs in the spinal cord, the projections from UMN to spinal cord LMN are called descending tracts. There are numerous descending motor tracts, each originating from distinct cortical areas or brainstem nuclei, and each is unique in terms of the type of regulatory influence it exerts on alpha LMNs.

Upper motor neuron systems are organized into two groups of structures. The first group consists of the *motor areas of the cerebral cortex* (see Figure 8-3). Some axons from these motor areas descend to the spinal cord and cranial nerve motor nuclei of the brainstem, where they influence alpha LMNs. Examples are the lateral *corticospinal tract (CST)* discussed in Chapter 11 and the corticobulbar projections discussed in Chapter 14. These systems are responsible for voluntary movement.

The second group of UMNs consists of neurons in the *brainstem nuclei*. Four different sets of UMNs comprise the brainstem nuclei. These are the red nucleus, the vestibular nuclei, nuclei of the reticular formation, and the superior colliculus. Axons from cells in these nuclei descend to the spinal cord in six distinct, identified descending tracts (see Table 5-2). All descending motor tracts originate from these sets of UMNs in the brainstem, with the exception of descending tracts from the motor areas of the cerebral cortex. Some of these brainstem UMN systems also influence alpha LMNs innervating the cranial nerve motor nuclei. It is important to note that these brainstem UMNs, like those of the cerebral cortex, are influenced by other structures (see Figure 8-5). The brainstem nuclei are responsible for (1) influencing voluntary movement, particularly of the trunk and proximal extremities; (2) posture; (3) activity that sets the background tone of muscles; and (4) the regulation of reflexes.

> **Thought Question**
>
> Compare and contrast the location of the cell bodies for LMN and UMNs. How many locations can you think of for each? Thinking ahead, can you predict whether the symptoms associated with lesions of these cell bodies would be contralateral or ipsilateral to the site of the lesion?

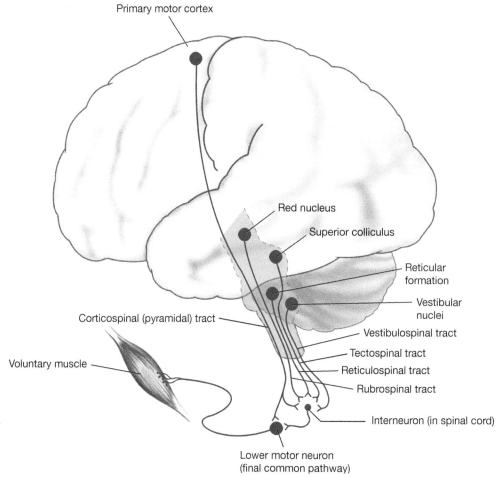

FIGURE 8-3 Schematic overview of somatic motor systems. Upper motor neurons are located in the cerebral cortex and brainstem, and their activity is modulated by association cortex, the cerebellum, and basal ganglia. Lower motor neurons are located in the brainstem and spinal cord, and their activity is modulated by UMNs both directly and indirectly by interneuronal networks. Note that UMN cell bodies and axons are confined to the CNS, whereas LMN cell bodies reside in the CNS but their axons run in the PNS.

Decussations and Laterality

Like ascending sensory tracts, many descending motor tracts may have axons that cross the midline. As discussed in Chapter 11, many descending axons of the corticospinal tract cross the midline just once, in the pyramidal decussation located in caudalmost medulla. In such a system, a lesion *rostral* to (i.e., above) the decussation produces motor signs on the *contralateral* side of the body. For example, damage located in the brainstem or cerebrum rostral to the pyramidal decussation typically results in contralateral motor signs. A lesion *caudal* to (i.e., below) the pyramidal decussation (e.g., damage in the spinal cord) typically results in motor signs *ipsilateral* to the lesion. Note that this is a general rule that applies most specifically to the lateral corticospinal tract Thus, when specific clinical signs of abnormal motor function are lateralized to only one side of the patient's body, knowing where a decussation occurs in the descending tract responsible for that sign is critical to accurately interpreting the location of damage in the CNS.

Synapse on Lower Motor Neurons

UMNs, whose axons form descending motor tracts, synapse directly on LMNs or on interneurons that in turn synapse on the LMNs whose axons enter peripheral nerves. Each alpha LMN receives input from many neurons, hence alpha LMNs are referred to as the **final common pathway** (see Figure 8-3). Any motor activity that depends on the discharge of alpha LMNs results from the summation of the inputs they receive from a wide variety of sources. Although the array of specific structures that send information to alpha LMNs varies depending on the type of motor activity that is to be generated, the input from those multiple sources converges on this common motor neuron. This converging input can be derived from regions of the cerebral cortex, from a variety of structures in the brainstem, or from primary somatosensory afferents that are conveying signals that originated in peripheral receptors. However, not only is the convergence from structurally (and therefore functionally) diverse sources, it may exert opposite influences on different LMNs. Some of this input

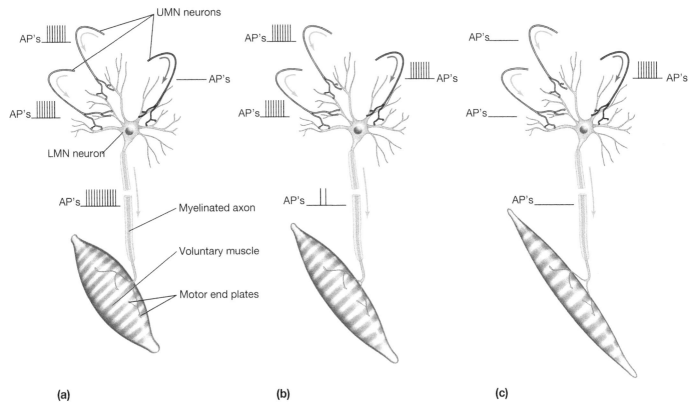

(a)   (b)   (c)

FIGURE 8-4 The net balance of active excitatory (green) and inhibitory (red) synapses impinging on the dendritic zone of a neuron, in this case a LMN, determines whether the postsynaptic neuron discharges action potentials (APs). In (a), only excitatory inputs are active, the LMN generates many APs, and the muscle contracts strongly. In (b), an inhibitory input is added to the excitatory inputs, and the summation yields a net excitation; however, the LMN generates fewer APs, and there is a less forceful contraction of the muscle. In (c), only the inhibitory input is active, the LMN does not discharge, and the muscle relaxes.

may excite particular LMNs, while another component of the input may inhibit other LMNs (see Reciprocal Innervation). But beyond this, a given LMN ultimately may be either excited or inhibited depending on the net balance of excitatory and inhibitory inputs synapsing on its receptive membrane (Figure 8-4 ■). When the summation of inputs to the final common pathway is excitatory, the LMNs increase their spike activity, and the skeletal muscle cells to which they project will likewise be excited and will contract. When the summation is inhibitory, LMNs decrease or cease spike activity, and their targeted muscle cells will relax.

Efferent Fibers

As noted earlier, efferent fibers of the somatic motor system represent axons that originate from the cell bodies of alpha LMNs in the CNS. They run directly to striated

muscle in a peripheral nerve. All of these axons are myelinated and have fast conduction velocities. As each axon enters the belly of a skeletal muscle, it divides into a variable number of terminal branches, each of which directly innervates a single muscle fiber. A single alpha LMN and its axon thus can innervate many striated muscle fibers (see Chapter 10).

Thought Question

What is the functional importance of myelination of efferent fibers? Are the myelinated fibers in the PNS or CNS? What cell type produces the myelin of these efferent fibers?

Neuromuscular Junction

Each of the terminal branches of an LMN axon ends on the membrane surface of a single skeletal muscle fiber (cell). The junction between the axon terminal and muscle fiber membrane is a highly specialized structure called the **neuromuscular junction**. It functions as a chemical synapse (see Chapter 10). Indeed, because of the neuromuscular junction's ready accessibility to experimental manipulation, it was used as the first model of a chemical synapse to understand the nervous system.

Thought Question

A muscle innervated by a single group of alpha motor neurons might contract or relax. How can this be? Explain this feature of the motor system in terms of the types of inputs to the alpha motor neuron pool.

Modulation of Upper Motor Neuron Systems

Modulation of upper motor neuron systems is complex, involving the thalamus, basal ganglia, and cerebellum. The concept of modulation is introduced here for completeness, and the topic is developed in Chapters 19 and 20. The thalamus modulates motor areas of the cerebral cortex. In turn, the thalamus is modulated by sensory systems, the cerebellum, and the basal ganglia. The cerebellum modulates motor areas of the cerebral cortex indirectly, by way of the thalamus. It also directly modulates the activity of many UMN brainstem nuclei. In turn, the cerebellum is modulated by the cerebral cortex and by sensory inputs. The cerebellum coordinates motor activity by producing synergistic patterns of muscle contraction. It functions as an error-correcting device for *goal-directed* movement. The cerebellum does this by receiving descending motor cortical control signals specifying the intended movement and comparing this information with returning somatosensory signals specifying the actual movement. When the actual movement deviates from its intended trajectory, the cerebellum takes corrective action.

The basal ganglia indirectly modulate the motor cortex via the thalamus. In turn, the basal ganglia are modulated within themselves and by the cerebral cortex. The exact contribution made by the basal ganglia to motor control is not altogether clear, but disorders such as Huntington's disease involve certain parts of the basal ganglia and severely disrupt motor activity by causing uncontrollable, involuntary movements and disturbances in posture.

> **Thought Question**
>
> UMNs can by influenced by the thalamus, basal ganglia, and cerebellum. Identify which of these structures influence UMNs directly and which influence them indirectly.

Topographic Organization

The motor system is topographically organized in that maps of the body musculature are laid out across the neurons making up UMNs and LMNs. An important way in which this reflects itself is that groups of neurons controlling the same body part are interconnected with one another. For example, neurons of the cerebral motor cortex that control arm movement project to neurons that control arm movement in the brainstem nuclei, basal ganglia, and cerebellum as well as to alpha LMNs in the spinal cord that control arm movement.

General Functional Plan

Purposeful movement is orchestrated through precise integration of a number of different types of motor control—all of which eventually have an impact on the final common pathway to the relevant muscles. Some of these controls occur reflexively or automatically, while others occur under the direction of conscious attention. Some are directed by sensory stimuli, while others are directed by prespecified motor instructions (motor programs) in the absence of sensory stimuli. Furthermore, all processes must be integrated. Chapter 20 provides an in-depth discussion of the complex processes involved in the control of purposeful movement. In preparation for that information, this chapter introduces a few of the key concepts, both in terms of mechanisms of controlling movement and in terms of the types of movement that are generated.

Parallel Operation and Locus of Control

UMNs of the cerebral cortex and each of the six brainstem descending tracts exert a unique but simultaneous influence on the final common pathway. For example, skilled voluntary movement can only be performed from an appropriate postural base. Therefore, the lateral corticospinal tract acts simultaneously with the brainstem nuclei that regulate posture. Parallel operation may, in some situations, facilitate compensation by intact systems when others are compromised by disease or injury.

The simplest motor behaviors tend to be organized at lower levels of the motor system. The very simplest is the monosynaptic deep tendon reflex (such as the patellar tendon reflex) in which a sensory stimulus leads directly to motor output. However, more complex motor behaviors also can be organized at lower levels. A good example is the stepping movements that can be generated in the spinal cord of newborn infants. As discussed later, the neural circuits that mediate reflex movements, stepping movements, and other prewired movements can be voluntarily regulated by UMN systems.

Feedback and Feedforward Control Systems

Some movements require ongoing sensory feedback, while others may be initiated by a sensory stimulus but proceed without further sensory input. For example, when we run to catch a ball, we use visual information about the ball's initial movement to estimate its future trajectory and time of interception. Our effort to catch the ball incorporates this anticipation of the ball's trajectory in determining our own movement. This anticipatory relation between motor system and environment defines a **feedforward system**. Because of this anticipatory regulation, the motor system is never allowed to deviate from its desired state. The great advantage of a feedforward system is speed because the motor system's response is generated *before* the impact of the ball on the catcher's hand. But a cost is paid in terms of the feedforward controller's complexity because an accurate response depends on the controller having precise

> **Thought Question**
>
> Based on the information presented so far, how might parallel processing be used when pitching a baseball?

knowledge of the actual state of the motor system and its functional capacities, as well as prior experience (memory) of the trajectories of thrown balls and the factors potentially influencing trajectory. Thus, a control signal defined by its intended effect may not achieve that effect because the controller's knowledge of the controlled system is inaccurate.

Figure 8-5 ■ contains an example of the operation of a feedforward system. Here, the sailor sees a wave approaching and adjusts his posture as it arrives under the boat. To prevent postural tilt, the feedforward controller must have prior experience with waves and boats under a wide variety of conditions.

By contrast, a **feedback system** is dependent on sensory information in determining the motor response that will occur. The feedback system is not anticipatory because it is activated only *after* an environmental event has disturbed

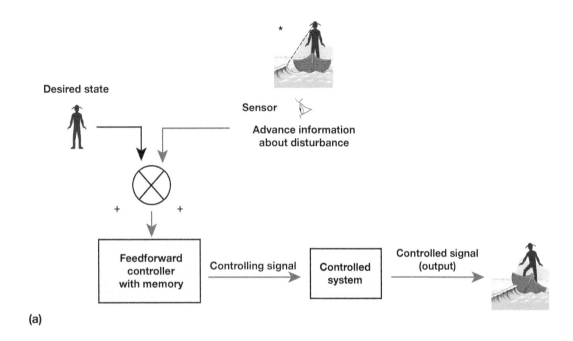

(a)

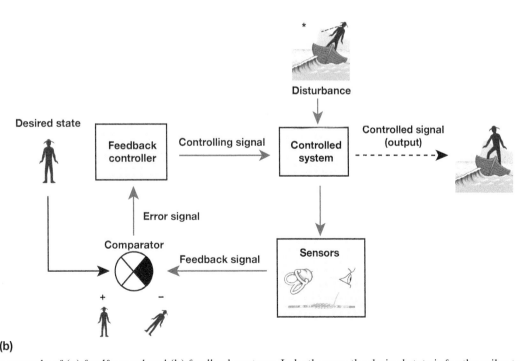

(b)

FIGURE 8-5 An example of (a) feedforward and (b) feedback systems. In both cases, the desired state is for the sailor to maintain an upright stance.

Note that the asterisks (*) represent the onset signal that initiates activity in the control system.

the controlled system. Thus, a feedback system can only correct an error that has already occurred. Feedback depends on sensors that continually monitor the status of the motor periphery, such as limb position and muscle tension (the somatosensory system), or sensors that monitor body position relative to gravity (the vestibular system) or relative to the environment (the visual system). Whether or not a compensatory control signal is generated depends on a reference signal representing a desired state of the motor periphery, such as joint angle. In a negative feedback system, the signal from peripheral sensors is compared with the reference signal (the desired state), and any difference generates an error signal that produces a compensatory change in the activity of the controller. In the case of catching a thrown ball, feedback control is activated only after the ball has reached the catcher's hand and the elbow and wrist have been displaced from a desired position. In the case of the sailor and boat depicted in Figure 8-5, the sailor did not see the wave approaching and detects its arrival only after some tilting has occurred as registered by his vestibular (tilting from the gravitational vertical), visual (sighting on a distant reference object), and somatosensory (proprioceptive detection of changes in muscle length and joint angles) systems. A corrective postural adjustment opposing the disturbance then takes place.

Feedback systems have several potential disadvantages. One is speed in that a corrective action must wait for the results of the disturbance to occur. This means that the delay time in conducting information around the control loop may itself become disadvantageous. If the delay time is long and the external environment is changing rapidly, the corrective signal may be inappropriate by the time it is executed. Second, excessive corrective action—that is, too high a gain in the feedback loop—can cause oscillations to develop by propagating a corrective signal around the loop in a nonending cycle. Third, correction may not be complete, because the compensatory signal depends on the presence of an error.

> **Thought Question**
>
> Humans use feedforward and feedback control systems to produce and modulate posture and movement. Why are both types of control necessary? Identify which system is fastest and why.

Reciprocal Innervation

During movement, muscle groups need to function in a coordinated way, often requiring one group of muscles to relax while another group contracts. For example, in contracting the quadriceps muscles to extend the knee, it may be important for the antagonistic hamstring muscles to relax. To accomplish this coordinated relaxation/excitation, alpha LMNs innervating agonist and antagonist muscles may receive influences of opposite sign—that is, excitation versus

inhibition. This is called **reciprocal innervation** and is a hardwired property of the way neurons are interconnected with one another. These opposite influences on the final common pathway come from several sources: directly from descending UMN systems and from local circuits of interneurons situated adjacent to LMNs. Local circuits are influenced both by UMN systems and by peripheral receptors. Inhibitory connections to LMNs of antagonistic muscles ensure that when an agonist contracts to produce a specific movement, the antagonist relaxes to a proportionate degree. To understand this functional system, it is important to recognize that LMNs only have excitatory influences on muscle fibers. Therefore, the CNS motor system relaxes muscle by inhibiting the LMN; as a consequence, the muscle is not excited.

Synergistic Movements

During purposeful movements, muscle groups may serve in a variety of different roles, depending on the task. Furthermore, a given muscle may function as an agonist for one task but might serve as an antagonist or stabilizer (supporter) for other tasks. The muscle group may be engaged in phasic or tonic movement or in dynamic or static motor acts. Purposeful muscular activity requires the coordinated interplay of groups of muscles. Muscles that normally act in unison in the execution of any given motor act are called **synergists**.

Synergists include the agonist (or prime mover) and associated muscles that either promote the same movement (secondary movers and helping synergists) or that reduce unnecessary movements (stabilizers) as the prime mover contracts. Examples of helping synergists are the anterior and posterior deltoid, working together in abduction of the shoulder. Regarding stabilizers, when a prime mover passes over more than one joint, its contraction causes movement of all the spanned joints unless synergists contract to stabilize a particular joint. For example, the finger flexor muscles cross both the wrist and phalangeal joints. However, you can make a fist without bending the wrist because synergist muscles contract to stabilize the wrist joint.

Complex purposeful movements, such as throwing a ball, require coordinated actions of a wide variety of movers, stabilizers, and helping synergists. Synergy is a distributive property in the organization of the motor system. At the lowest level, synergy is a product of the way in which alpha LMNs of the spinal cord (cranial nerve motor nuclei of the brainstem) are connected with peripheral receptors and local interneurons. At a higher level, synergy is a product of activity in the cerebellum.

Pattern Generator–Dependent Movements

The nervous system has a number of mechanisms to reduce the complexity of signals that are required to specify routines for purposeful movement. One such example is the central pattern generator (CPG). Central pattern generator–dependent movements are executed from central motor programs. Such programs are thought to depend on hard-wired connections among interneurons (local circuit neurons) of the spinal cord and brainstem that, in turn, influence the final common pathway. That rhythm-generating neuronal networks capable of producing complex stepping motor patterns in the absence of sensory feedback exist has been amply demonstrated in the spinal cord of animals. For example, with appropriate stimulation, an overall locomotor gait rhythm can be recorded electromyographically in cats with transection of the spinal cord. Recent evidence suggests that such stepping CPGs even exist in bipedal humans (see Chapter 20).

Central motor programs store and automatically play out patterns of muscular activity. To one degree or another, these are subject to conscious control via UMNs. In some cases, voluntary effort may regulate the rate and amplitude of the movement sequence, but not its occurrence. Respiration is one example. In other cases, the occurrence of the sequence may be initiated voluntarily, but once initiated, the sequence plays out automatically. Stepping, swallowing, and chewing are examples. Feedback from peripheral receptors sharpens the timing and performance of the movement sequence but is not essential to its execution. A peripheral stimulus may trigger the movement pattern, as in swallowing that is not voluntarily initiated.

Cats with transected spinal cords illustrate this concept very well. If supported by a harness, these cats demonstrate appropriate stepping movements on a treadmill. The movements are initiated by the sensory stimulus of the treadmill on the pad of the foot and appear to be run using hard-wired routines once the movement is initiated.

Types of Motor Activity in Functional Movement

Human function is directed by a continuous repertoire of routines required for purposeful movement. These purposeful movements are themselves organized by careful orchestration and integration of different types of motor control, utilizing all of the mechanisms described earlier. Some of the key concepts are defined here and are synthesized in the context of movements related to playing baseball at the end of this chapter.

Background Muscular Activity (Tonus)

Certain muscle groups are maintained in a more or less continuous state of mild contraction thought to be due to low levels of spontaneous spike activity by alpha LMNs innervating the muscle. This is called **tone (tonus)**. Tonicity is

assessed clinically by noting the resistance a muscle offers to passive stretching. Muscle fibers and their connective tissue investments possess an inherent elasticity. However, the resistance due to tonus is in addition to the normal recoil of muscle following its release from a stretch because of this inherent elasticity.

The neural mechanisms maintaining tone are not well understood, in part because tone cannot be measured electromyographically. It is known, however, that peripheral sensory structures, such as mechanoreceptors of the somatosensory system (particularly the neck and hair cells of the vestibular system), influence activity of UMNs, spinal cord interneurons, and/or LMNs and thereby indirectly influence muscle tone, as do inputs from visual centers.

The tone of a muscle depends on the position of the person, his or her ability to relax muscles voluntarily, and the person's state of alertness. Tone of a muscle is most pronounced in the antigravity muscles of the trunk and proximal limbs and increases as demands increase for maintaining posture and resisting gravity. Complete relaxation can occur when the skeleton is fully supported, but it requires practice and is increasingly difficult in elderly individuals.

Excessive increases or decreases in muscle tone are hallmarks of many neurological diseases and are typically assessed by resistance to passive movement of the limbs. Although the assessment of resistance in the limbs seems relatively straightforward, it requires considerable clinical experience to accurately assess normal and abnormal tone.

Types of Movement from Reflexive to Voluntary

Everyday functional movements are controlled by a combination of voluntary movement and reflexive responses. Voluntary movements can be further differentiated into those that are under conscious control and those that occur as automatic routines. The degree to which the sensory and motor systems work coordinately depends on the type of movement under consideration.

REFLEXES Reflexes are the simplest and most stereotyped overt movements executed by the motor system. By definition, reflexes are set into motion by a peripheral stimulus and do not occur without such peripheral receptor input. Reflexes are mediated by hard-wired neuronal connections among peripheral receptors, interneurons, and LMNs. Perhaps the most familiar example is the patellar tendon reflex that is often tested as part of the general physical examination. The patellar tendon is struck with a reflex hammer, resulting in knee extension when the reflex is functioning normally. Another familiar example is the quick withdrawal of the hand when a person accidentally touches a hot pot. In concept, reflexes are obligatory motor responses to a sensory stimulus. However, *all* somatomotor reflexes are subject to regulation by UMNs (see Chapter 11). Indeed, most people can modulate the patellar tendon reflex by deciding beforehand not to allow the knee to extend, and many can keep the hand on a hot surface if the need arises.

VOLUNTARY MOVEMENTS All **voluntary movement** is unique in four respects: (1) voluntary movement involves a decision to act; (2) purposeful voluntary movement is learned; (3), in being learned, voluntary movement initially is under conscious control; and (4) voluntary movement exploits hard-wired subroutines such as reflexes, reciprocal innervation, and automatic postural adjustments in its execution. Beyond this, however, the nature of a voluntary movement must be qualified. Thus, some voluntary movement remains under a high degree of conscious control throughout the movement sequence. Think, for example, of a skilled furniture maker using a hand plane to shape a wooden armrest to a specific aesthetically pleasing curve. Although the act of planning is repetitive, the specific parameters of the act are always novel as the desired curve is finally approached. Other voluntary movements have been learned through extensive practice such that they are under little or no conscious control as they evolve. Here, we may include movements such as speaking, shooting a basketball into the hoop, or playing a musical instrument. The position of the hoop does not change, nor do the positions of the keys or strings of a musical instrument. The act of walking has its own unique neurological attributes that are discussed in Chapter 20. But, clearly, the infant learns to deploy locomotion voluntarily toward the attainment of a goal. The term **goal-directed purposeful movement** in this text refers to voluntary movement with a functional purpose. The goal may be an object in the individual's immediate sensory field (as opposed to surrounding objects), or may be represented in the person's memory. This definition is significant in terms of rehabilitation. For example, in some cases, an individual may be able to reach into a cupboard to retrieve a specific item but may not be successful in lifting the arm without a functional context.

During the period when the movement is being learned, peripheral receptor feedback guides the motor learning process and remains capable of monitoring the movement even after it has been learned. This feedback is required to correct the course and velocity while the movement is being executed. Once initiated, a learned movement may be run by central programs and reflex mechanisms.

The degree to which sensory feedback is used depends on the type of voluntary movement. So-called **ballistic movements** are learned movements with a time course too short to be modified by peripheral feedback during the movement. Examples are movements involved in serving a tennis ball or swinging a bat at a hard pitch.

Associated movements are those that occur as part of the motor pattern but are ancillary to fulfillment of the motor pattern's purpose. Associated movements provide for subtle adjustments of posture in order to control the body center of mass in relation to the support surface during the goal-directed part of the movement. For example, in the seemingly simple task of reaching into a high cupboard, the goal-directed part of the movement is the reaching of the hand into the cupboard. Simultaneously, there are adjustments of weight from one extremity to the other and adjustments of the spinal segments for postural control.

Thought Question

Goal-directed movements require a combination of reflexive and voluntary movement. Furthermore, voluntary movements may be under conscious control or may be generated automatically. Explain how these different mechanisms interact for initiating and controlling functionally relevant movement. These distinctions will frequently be important in your clinical practice. Can you think of reasons for this importance?

Another example of an associated movement is the swinging of the arms during walking. When gait is sufficiently fast, the arms hang loosely at the sides, each moving gracefully and rhythmically forward with the opposite leg. In many respects, associated movements impart an individualistic style to a person's motor behavior (strutting, sashaying, bobbing the head rhythmically while walking, etc.).

It is not known whether associated movements are generated in one or several sites in the CNS. However, they disappear in certain CNS disorders such as Parkinson's disease, a disorder that affects the functioning of the basal ganglia.

CLINICAL CONNECTIONS
Negative and Positive Neurological Signs

If damage occurs in the PNS or in the anterior horn cells of the spinal cord, the final common pathway itself can be disrupted. The signs of weakness or paralysis are clearly evident in these cases. Disruption of the spinal cord can also prevent signals from reaching the anterior horn cell. Damage to other parts of the CNS results in signs and symptoms that are more complex. A stroke, for example, can result in an inability to *access* intact motor programs, an inability to *execute* intact motor programs, or sometimes a *loss* of the motor program itself.

Lesions to motor structures of the CNS produce two types of clinical signs: negative and positive. **Negative signs** are motor deficits due to the loss of function of damaged neural structures. Weakness, loss of speed of movement, loss of dexterity, fatigability, and paresis are examples of negative signs. In essence, they impair or prevent a motor act the person would like to perform but is no longer able to accomplish. The absence of movement can be due to a variety of problems.

Positive signs are at the opposite extreme. Also called **release phenomena**, positive signs involve an excess of neural activity and the expenditure of energy. Examples of positive signs are hyperreflexia, hypertonicity, and the positive Babinski sign. Positive signs are of two primary causes. The first is overactivity of an intact structure due to its excessive stimulation. Spasticity is an example (see Chapter 11). The second is overactivity in an intact structure due to its being released from inhibitory control by the damaged structure. This is called **disinhibition**, and the dyskinesias are examples (see Chapter 19). In essence, a positive sign designates a motor act the person does not want to perform or a posture the he or she does not want to assume but is unable to prevent.

It is important for the rehabilitation specialist to identify both the positive and negative signs associated with CNS damage. Because positive signs are more easily observed than are negative signs, they can be mistaken for the underlying problem, with intervention directed at reducing the positive signs. In fact, the main problem with respect to functional movement most often is that which is missing (e.g., weakness, slowness of movement). Unless intervention is directed toward the negative signs, restoration of functional movement may be limited.

Functional Movements—A Synthesis

A whole host of physiological steps are required in the production of actual functional movements, several of which occur before the movement itself is actually initiated. For example, functional movements typically begin with the conscious decision to act. This decision may be initiated by the thought of completing an action, or it may be initiated in response to something seen (e.g., a bicycle out of control, careening onto the pavement where you are standing) or something heard (e.g., a request that you do the dishes). Once the decision is made to act, the nervous system plans the movement before execution is actually initiated. Once execution begins, the movement evolves, sometimes under sensory feedback and sometimes using preprograms without further sensory feedback. In addition, postural control mechanisms come into play before and during the movement. Finally, functional movements must be terminated

effectively. The game of baseball easily illustrates the interplay of these different types of movement.

Take, for example, the act of pitching a baseball. Before even pitching the baseball, the pitcher decides to act (cognitive processing, which is discussed in detail in Chapter 20). He uses visual information to determine the goal of the pitch (see Chapter 18) and may incorporate responses to auditory information (Chapter 17) as well. Before actually pitching the ball, his nervous system takes into account sensory information from the ground such as hardness of the support surface and slope of the ground. This information plays a role in determining which automatic routines will be required for postural control so that the ball is pitched with the right speed, direction, and velocity. Some of these postural adjustments occur before the pitcher even begins the arm movements associated with the pitch. When the pitcher winds up to pitch the ball, muscles of the lower extremities, trunk, and neck all fire. The pitch itself is a ballistic action, without time or room for feedback. Once the pitch is completed, routines are used to terminate the movements, including stabilizing the body in relation to the support surface and stopping the motion of the arm.

The act of catching likewise requires cognitive processing (decision to catch), as well as visual information regarding the direction and speed of the ball. In addition, however, this action can be highly feedback dependent. The impact of the ball in the catcher's glove can result in adjustments both of the hand and of the whole body to smoothly execute the catch. As with pitching, the termination of the movement also must be specified.

Summary

This chapter presented overviews of the anatomical and functional organizations of somatosensory and motor systems. We began with sensory systems, noting that each system consists of six anatomical components differentially distributed in the PNS and CNS. Thus, in the PNS, each somatosensory system begins with a peripheral receptor that converts environmental energy into action potentials that are then forwarded to the CNS over primary afferent fibers. Within the CNS, each primary afferent synapses in a prethalamic relay nucleus that contains the cell bodies of the second-order neurons of the system. Some, or virtually all, of the second-order neurons may cross to the opposite side of the CNS in an identified sensory decussation such as

the ventral white commissure of the spinal cord. The tract originating in the prethalamic relay nucleus then projects to a specific relay nucleus of the thalamus, which contains the cell bodies of the third-order neurons of the system that ascend in the thalamocortical projection to terminate in the cerebral cortex, where conscious analysis of the sensory information begins. Naturally occurring environmental stimuli simultaneously engage more than one ascending sensory system so that these systems function in parallel, each contributing something unique to the overall sensory experience. Additionally, there is a cascade of control of ascending sensory information, with each higher station controlling those located at lower levels of the neuraxis.

Somatic motor systems were discussed next, and the terms upper and lower motor neuron were defined. UMNs have their cell bodies either in the motor areas of the cerebral cortex or in motor-related nuclei such as the brainstem, including the red nucleus, the vestibular nuclei, nuclei of the reticular formation, or the superior colliculus. Each of these descending motor systems converges on the LMN, the final common path, but exerts a unique influence on the LMN. Many of these descending systems also decussate in known locations of the CNS so that damage to a given descending motor tract results in deficits on a specific side of the body, depending on the location of the lesion in the tract. UMN systems are modulated by the thalamus, cerebellum, and basal ganglia. Thus, the cerebellum contributes importantly to the regulation of movement as do the basal ganglia (discussed at length in Chapter 19). Like somatosensory systems, somatic motor systems operate in parallel. Feedforward and feedback motor control systems were introduced and discussed. Feedforward systems are anticipatory and ensure that the motor system is governed so as to effect the smooth attainment of its intended goal. Feedback systems are error regulated such that the motor system has already erred in the attainment of its intended goal. The principle of reciprocal innervation ensures that antagonistic muscle groups do not interfere with one another in the attainment of a specific goal. The concept of pattern generator–dependent movements was introduced and includes such motor acts as respiration, swallowing, and stepping. But as we will learn in Chapter 20, the term *generator* should not be taken to imply that a specific movement is actually generated (initiated) by a system of hard-wired connections in a localized part of the CNS, only that the pattern of the movement may be determined by that wiring. Finally, different categories of movement were discussed as were positive and negative signs.

Applications

1. Descending motor tracts have axons that decussate (cross the midline). Where would motor symptoms occur if damage to the tract occurs *rostral* to the decussation, and where would symptoms occur if damage occurs *caudal* to the decussation?

2. Chris, a 38-year-old bartender, was stabbed in the back while attempting to break up a fight. Immediately after the injury, he had neurological symptoms. One year after the injury, signs of neurological damage to his spinal cord remained. Neurological examination revealed atrophy of the intrinsic muscles of his right hand. He had paresis of the right leg with exaggerated knee-jerk reflexes on that side. There was a loss of all cutaneous sensibility over a strip along the ulnar side of the right arm. There was a loss of kinesthesia and vibration sensibility in the right leg and trunk. Finally, there was a loss of pain and temperature sensibility over his entire left leg and trunk, as high as the level of his third rib.

   a. What sensory tracts have been disrupted?
   b. What segments of the spinal cord have been damaged?
   c. What side of the spinal cord sustained damage?
   d. Compare the symptoms that would accompany injury to the spinal nerves of the leg or to their cell bodies with the symptoms that Chris experienced.

References

Gurfinkel, V., Cacciatore, T. W., Cordo, P., et al. Postural muscle tone in the body axis of healthy humans. *J Neurophysiol* 96:2678–2687, 2006.

Minassian, K., Persy, I., Rattay, F., Kern, H., and Dimitrijevic, M.R. Human lumbar cord circuitries can be activated by extrinsic tonic input to generate locomotor-like activity. Human Movement Science 26, 275–295, 2007.

Nolte, J. *The Human Brain: An Introduction to Its Functional Anatomy.* Mosby Elsevier, Philadelphia, 2009.

Pearson, K., and Gordon, J. Ch. 37. Locomotion. In: Kandel, E., Schwartz, J. H., and Jessell, T. M. *Principles of Neural Science*, 4th ed. McGraw-Hill, New York, 2000.

PEARSON
myhealthprofessionskit™

Use this address to access the Companion Website created for this textbook. Simply select "Physical Therapy" from the choice of disciplines. Find this book and log in using your username and password to access self-assessment questions, a glossary, answers to the applications questions, and more.

9

The Somatosensory System for the Extremities and Trunk

LEARNING OUTCOMES

This chapter prepares the reader to:

1. Recognize the different ways that somatosensory receptors are classified and provide examples of each, including structure, source of stimulus, location of the receptor, sensitivity of the receptor to specific types of stimulus energy, and rate of adaptation to constant and varying stimuli.
2. Name four main classes of somatosensory receptors (based on adequate stimulus) and discuss their functional importance.
3. Describe five different types of receptors that respond to pain and temperature.
4. Discuss the role of mechanoreceptors and identify examples.
5. Discuss the mechanoreceptors that provide information about posture and movement (i.e., proprioception).
6. Describe the components of the muscle spindle and explain why this receptor has both a sensory (afferent) and motor (efferent) component.
7. Explain how sensitivity of the muscle spindle is modulated.
8. Describe alpha-gamma co-activation and explain why this phenomenon is of critical functional importance.
9. Contrast the anatomy and function of the Golgi tendon organ (GTO) to the anatomy and function of the muscle spindle.
10. Explain the role of myelin as it relates to nerve conduction velocity and discuss the manner in which cells myelinate axons in peripheral nerves.
11. Recall relative conduction rates of different types of nerve fibers.
12. Describe the relationship between the receptive field and function.
13. Name all components from the receptor to the cerebral cortex of two major pathways that convey somatosensory information from the periphery to the cerebral cortex (i.e., dorsal column–medial lemniscal pathway [DC-ML] and the spinothalamic tract [STT]).
14. Discuss the functional roles of the DC-ML pathway and STT.
15. Explain the meaning of efferent modulation and provide an example.
16. Correlate the following clinical conditions to the location within the somatosensory system of the damage producing the following syndromes: radiculopathy, Brown-Sequard syndrome, sensory loss associated with diabetes mellitus (DM).

ACRONYMS

AL Anterolateral system
AP Action potential
DC Dorsal column
DC-ML Dorsal column–medial lemniscal system
DCN Dorsal column nuclei
DM Diabetes mellitus
GP Generator potential
GT Golgi tendon organ
MI First motor area (in Brodmann's area 4)
ML Medial lemniscus
SI First somatosensory cortex (within Brodmann's areas 3, 1, 2)
SII Second somatosensory cortex (within Brodmann's areas 3, 1, 2)
SMA Supplementary motor area (Brodmann's areas 6)
STT Spinothalamic tract
VPL Ventral posterolateral thalamic nucleus
WDR Wide, dynamic range

Introduction

This chapter is the first to undertake a more detailed consideration of nervous system structures introduced in earlier chapters. Building on information introduced in Chapter 8, this chapter considers the sensory systems mediating somatic sensation in the extremities and trunk.

The first major section of this chapter begins with a presentation of somatic receptors. The peripheral nerve terminals detect, determine the quality (modality), scale the intensity, and inform the brain about the timing of environmental stimuli that impinge on the surfaces of the body or arise from the movement of body parts. Each of the different somatic receptors is adapted to respond to a particular type of environmental energy. As was discussed in Chapter 4, the function of a receptor is to transduce this energy into the language of the nervous system—in this case, the generator (receptor) potential. As noted there, the generator potential is the first in a series of electrochemical events enabling our brains to experience the real world. Interestingly, receptors have a punctate (dot-like) distribution over the body surface, sometimes with wide intervening areas devoid of a particular receptor type. Yet, we perceive continuity in response to stimulation.

The second major section of this chapter analyzes the structure and function of the two somatosensory systems that carry information to the cerebral cortex for conscious discrimination. These are the dorsal column–medial lemniscal system (DC-ML) and the anterolateral system (AL). Within the anterolateral system is the spinothalamic tract (STT), which is the major focus of this chapter. Although naturally occurring somatic stimuli activate both systems simultaneously, each plays a unique role in somatic sensibility as can be determined from their markedly different structural and functional organizations.

As we shall see, our experience of the real world is actually an abstraction because we are linked to the real world only indirectly, via receptors, their primary afferent fibers, and the sensory tracts and pathways that carry this information to consciousness. What that experience consists of is an awareness of the state of the neural pathways that convey to the brain information normally encoded by somatic receptors. Neurogenic pain illustrates this concept dramatically. Neurogenic pain is that which is experienced in a peripheral body part but that, in fact, is due to a pathological process occurring in a peripheral nerve or in the pain pathways in the CNS. The receptors themselves are not activated. A herniated intervertebral disc, for example, causes neurogenic pain by compressing on a spinal nerve, but the patient could experience the pain in, for example, his or her neck or arm (as illustrated by cervical spondylosis, discussed in Chapter 5).

SOMATIC RECEPTORS

General Patterns of Organization

In nearly all somatic receptors, it is the nerve terminal of the peripheral nerve fiber that is the transducer of environmental energy. In general, the type of environmental energy to which a specific receptor responds is unique. That is, each receptor is specific with regard to the type(s) of peripheral stimulus to which it will respond. Most somatic receptors respond to just one type (submodality) of peripheral stimulus, although some respond to more than one type (called polymodal receptors). But even such polymodal receptors are specific with respect to the array of submodalities to which they respond (see discussion of pain receptors later). The specific stimulus modalities to which receptors respond are determined by the particular molecular machinery residing in the membrane of the nerve terminal (Chapter 4).

The term **sensory end organ** refers to the nerve terminal plus the accessory non-neural cells, if any, with which the nerve terminal is associated. Somatosensory end organs exhibit three different patterns of organization. In some somatosensory end organs, there are no non-neural cells associated with the receptor. Thus, the bare nerve terminal itself represents the entire sensory end organ. The free nerve ending is an example. In other somatosensory end organs, the peripheral nerve terminal is associated with non-neural cells. The non-neural cells serve to direct the peripheral stimulus to the nerve terminal in a uniquely stereotyped way so that they determine how the receptor responds to its adequate stimulus but not the type (submodality) of stimulus energy to which the receptor responds. Such receptors come in a dazzling array of forms, sizes, and structural specializations. Examples of this pattern of organization abound and include Pacinian corpuscles, Golgi tendon organs, and muscle spindles. In still other receptors, a non-neural cell is the transducer, and it synapses with the terminal of the peripheral nerve fiber. In the case of somatic receptors, the Merkel cell–neurite complex is an example. All of these receptor types will be described in more detail later.

The Classification of Receptors

Somatosensory receptors have been classified in a variety of ways, all of which overlap to some extent and none of which completely integrate structure, function, and location. Each type of peripheral somatic receptor may be distinguished by its structure, by the source of the stimulus and location of the receptor, by the sensitivity of the receptor to specific types of stimulus energy, and by the rate of adaptation of the receptor to a constant and unvarying stimulus. Additionally, receptors can be distinguished by the size of the receptor's receptive field and by the nature of the primary afferent fiber projecting from the receptor into the CNS.

Classification by Structure

This anatomical system of classification recognizes two broad categories of receptors. The first category is composed of the free and diffuse nerve endings that have no accessory structures surrounding the naked axon terminal. The second category consists of the encapsulated receptors, all of which are enclosed in a capsule of supporting cells.

Classification by the Source of the Stimulus and Location of the Receptor

This anatomical system of classification recognizes three main types of receptors. **Exteroceptors** respond to changes in the immediate external environment. In the case of somatic sensation, exteroceptors include those end organs distributed in the skin. **Interoceptors** are stationed in the walls of the digestive and respiratory tracts and in the walls of the heart and blood vessels. They do not mediate somatic sensation. Rather, interoceptors give rise to poorly localized sensations, including visceral pain, thirst, hunger, excretion, and sexual feelings. They contribute importantly to visceral reflexes and the generalized feeling of well-being or malaise. **Proprioceptors** respond to stimuli originating within the body itself. With respect to somatic sensation, proprioceptors are positioned within the deeper portions of the body wall and in muscles, tendons, and joint capsules. They mediate such sensations as movement, position of the body and limbs in space, and muscle tension.

Classification by the Type of Stimulus Energy That Most Readily Excites the Receptor

Most receptors are uniquely adapted to respond best to a particular type of stimulus energy. They thus exhibit a preferential sensitivity to one form of stimulus energy and either complete or relative insensitivity to others. Preferential sensitivity to a particular kind of stimulus energy is an intrinsic property of the nerve terminal, not the accessory cells with which the terminal may be associated. The adequate stimulus is the stimulus that elicits a generator potential at the lowest threshold. On the basis of their selective responses to stimuli, four classes of somatic receptors may be distinguished.

Mechanoreceptors respond preferentially to mechanical stimuli that physically deform the receptor terminal membrane. This is an extremely heterogeneous group of

> ### Thought Question
>
> What differentiates interoception, proprioception, and exteroception? Provide examples of each, and explain the functional importance of each in relation to rehabilitation.

receptors having members with widely varying structures, having distributions in many different body regions, and subserving a wide variety of somatosensory submodalities. Proprioceptors are an example and are found in joints, tendons, muscle, and the sliding planes between layers of smooth muscle tissue.

Thermoreceptors respond to temperature gradients across the skin. Thermal sensibility has a punctate distribution over the body surface. Discrete spots (points) of skin exist, each about 1 mm in diameter, in which thermal stimulation elicits either a warm or cold sensation.

Nociceptors respond to tissue-damaging stimuli. Nociceptors are all free nerve endings and are the most numerous and widely distributed type of receptor in the body. Some nociceptors respond to intense mechanical stimuli such as crushing pressure or to thermal stimuli such as burning heat or freezing cold, others to the chemicals released by damaged body tissues such as prostaglandin, and some to all three modalities.

Chemoreceptors respond preferentially to chemical constituents in a body fluid, for example, the blood or saliva. This category also includes those nociceptors (free nerve endings) that respond to chemicals released by damaged tissue.

> ### Thought Question
>
> What is meant by "adequate stimulus"? Drawing from information in Chapter 4, what is the physical basis for this phenomenon?

Classification by the Rate of Adaptation

All somatic receptors eventually adapt to a stimulus in that the generator potential decreases in amplitude in response to a maintained and constant stimulus and a corresponding decrease in the rate and number of action potentials that were generated by receptor stimulation. Adaptation of the generator potential was discussed in Chapter 4. Speed of adaptation is important in signaling the time parameters of physical stimuli. This physiological system of classification recognizes two categories of receptors: slowing and rapidly adapting (Figure 9-1 ■). Rate of adaptation is important because it defines the receptor's capacity to signal the duration of a stimulus. Slowly adapting receptors have a generator potential of above threshold magnitude so long as a stimulus continues to be applied to the receptor. The threshold referred to is the threshold required for the axon to generate action potentials. An example of a slowly adapting receptor is the type of muscle spindle that signals static muscle length. However, the generator potential of a slowly adapting receptor may decline in amplitude during a maintained, constant stimulus. Rapidly adapting receptors respond transiently to a stimulus and only at the onset and offset of stimulation. Their generator potentials decline to a subthreshold magnitude soon after the stimulus is applied or withdrawn. An example is the Pacinian corpuscle that responds to the application and removal of

FIGURE 9-1 Classification of receptors according to their rates of adaptation. (a) The generator potential of a rapidly adapting receptor declines to zero so that the receptor can signal only the application and removal of the stimulus, but not its maintained presence. (b) The generator potential of a slowly adapting receptor remains above threshold as long as the stimulus is applied to the receptor. However, it may decline in amplitude during the maintained stimulus in which case the frequency of action potentials in the axon decrease. (c) The intact Pacinian corpuscle is a rapidly adapting receptor. However, if the connective tissue layers surrounding the nerve terminal are removed, the sensory terminal is transformed to a slowly adapting receptor to the same mechanical stimulus.

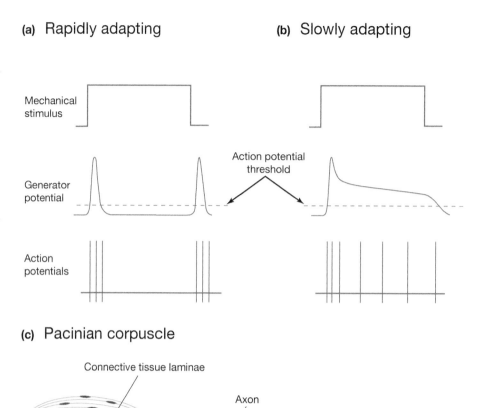

Thought Question

Some receptors are slow adapting and others are fast adapting. Think of examples where each might be of functional importance.

a mechanical stimulus, but not to its continued presence. Rapidly adapting receptors signal changes of intensity and movement of the stimulus along their receptive field.

The Receptive Field

Different receptors can be distinguished by the size of their receptive fields, but this is not a system of receptor classification. The receptive field of a somatic receptor is the area of the body within which a stimulus of appropriate quality and magnitude will cause an afferent neuron to discharge. The nature of a receptor's receptive field depends on the structure and function of the receptor as well as its tissue environment. The receptive field of a cutaneous receptor is represented by an area of skin in which a mechanical stimulus will produce a generator potential. In the case of the fingertips, cutaneous receptive fields are very small, whereas in the skin of the trunk, they are large. In the case of a receptor located in a joint capsule, the size

and location of the receptive field may relate to the angle of the joint, or its movement within a certain range.

Specific Somatosensory Receptors

We begin our survey of somatic receptors by considering those that mediate pain and temperature sensibility. We do this for several reasons. First, these sensory modalities are mediated by receptors that have the simplest structure of all receptors. And, second, these sensory modalities are readily understood, being among the most commonly encountered sensations in everyday behavior.

Receptors for pain and temperature are embedded in the skin, which makes up about 16 percent of body weight and is the largest sensory organ of the body. It provides our most direct contact with the environment. Skin consists of two main layers, a surface epithelium, or **epidermis**, and a deeper connective tissue layer, the **dermis** (Figure 9-2 ■). Skin is continuous with several mucous membranes. These mucocutaneous junctions are located at the lips, nares, eyelids, vulva, prepuce, and anus. The junction between the epidermis and dermis is uneven. The superior surface of the dermis contains nipple-like projections called **dermal papillae**. The dermal papillae indent the overlying epidermis to form epidermal ridges between

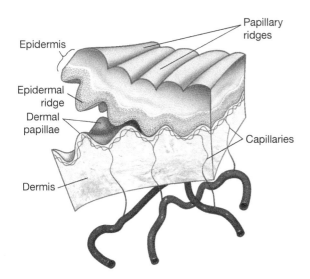

FIGURE 9-2 The basic organization of skin. The epidermis is the outermost protective layer. It is composed of epithelial cells and is avascular. The thickness of the epidermis varies in different parts of the body, being thickest on the surfaces of the palms and soles. The underlying dermis is composed of fibrous connective tissue and, unlike the epidermis, is vascularized.

adjacent dermal papillae. This tongue-and-groove arrangement helps hold the dermis and epidermis together. On the palmar surface of the hands and soles of the feet, the dermal papillae are large and arranged in ridge-like lines. Because the epidermis follows the corrugated pattern of the underlying dermis, this arrangement produces papillary ridges in the epidermis that are arranged in individually unique fingerprint patterns.

Pain and Thermal Receptors

Free nerve endings are distributed virtually everywhere in the body but are most numerous in the skin (Figure 9-3 ■). They are derived from small myelinated and unmyelinated peripheral nerve fibers. In the skin over the entire body, the free nerve endings are formed by branching terminals that end between epithelial cells of the epidermis. As a group, the free nerve endings appear similar under the light microscope, but some are mechanoreceptors, others thermoreceptors, and still others nociceptors (depending on the properties of the nerve terminal's membrane).

Both pain and temperature sensibilities are mediated by free nerve endings. Which of these modalities is signaled by a particular free nerve ending depends on the properties of the nerve terminal's membrane. As noted, free nerve endings are the most widely distributed receptors in the body. They are most numerous in the skin but are found also in mucous and serous membranes, muscles, deep fascia, joints, and the connective tissue of many visceral organs.

Free nerve endings are derived from lightly myelinated and unmyelinated primary afferent fibers. If myelinated, the terminals are invested with Schwann cells, except near their tips where they are bare. These small axons penetrate into the epithelium, divide further, and wind vertically

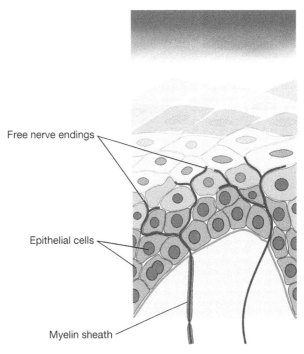

FIGURE 9-3 Free nerve endings. The fiber on the left is a lightly myelinated afferent fiber, while that on the right is unmyelinated. The terminations of these afferent fibers ramify among the epithelial cells of the lower layers of the epidermis.

through the epidermis (see Figure 9-3). They end in small knob-like thickenings on the surface of epithelial cells.

Nociceptors (L., nocere, to *injure*) are receptors that respond selectively to stimuli that damage tissue. Four types exist. Thermal nociceptors respond to burning heat (above 45°C) or to extreme cold (below 15°C) that damages tissue. Mechanical nociceptors respond to strong mechanical stimulation, especially sharp objects. Chemically sensitive nociceptors respond to chemical agents. Such agents can be derived from the blood or from the environment or be released by damaged tissue. For example, following inflammation or trauma, chemical agents are released locally from damaged tissue that can sensitize and/or activate free nerve endings. Polymodal nociceptors respond to combinations of chemical, mechanical, and thermal stimuli.

Non-nociceptive temperature sensations are highly punctate in distribution; that is, there are separate spots on the skin, about 1 mm wide, that will respond to either hot or cold stimuli, but not both. The fact that the location of hot and cold spots is different indicates that each sensation is mediated by a separate receptor. The afferent axons of non-nociceptive warm receptors begin firing at about 30°C and progressively increase their firing rate up to about 45°C. Temperatures above 45°C result in decreased firing of the warm receptors, but at these temperatures, thermal nociceptors begin to fire. This is consistent with the perceptual change from hot to painful scalding and the resultant tissue damage. Cold receptors respond over the temperature range of 33°C to about 10°C.

Mechanoreceptors in the Skin and Subcutaneous Tissues

Hairy (nonglabrous) skin covers the vast majority of the body's surface. The principal mechanoreceptor of hairy skin is the **peritrichial ending** (Figure 9-4 ■). Peritrichial endings respond to movement of the hair and evoke the sensation of touch. Several myelinated fibers approach the hair follicle just beneath its sebaceous gland, lose their myelin sheath, and divide into several branches that encircle the outer root sheath of the hair (Figure 9-5 ■). From these branches, numerous fine fibers run for short distances up and down the outer root sheath and terminate in flattened or bulbous endings. Bending of the hair causes a distortion of the follicle, which deforms the peritrichial ending and thus results in a generator potential.

Hairless (glabrous) skin contains two main types of mechanoreceptors: the **Meissner's corpuscle** and the **Merkel cell–neurite complex receptor**. Meissner's corpuscles are mechanically coupled to surrounding tissue by connective tissue strands. Each Meissner's corpuscle is encapsulated by a thin connective tissue sheath (Figure 9-6 ■). They are thus encapsulated mechanoreceptors. The interior of the capsule contains many flattened epithelial-like cells that are oriented transversely to the long axis of the capsule. One to four myelinated fibers supply each corpuscle. The myelin sheath disappears as each fiber enters the capsule and the axons wind spirally among the epithelial-like cells, giving off numerous branches that end in flattened expansions. Meissner's corpuscles are found in the dermal papillae at the junction of the dermis and epidermis. Their association

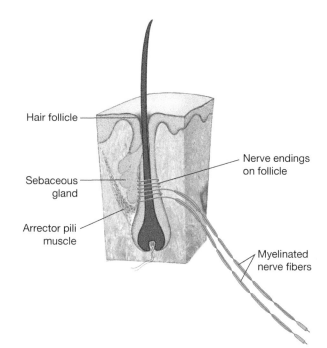

FIGURE 9-5 Peritrichial endings. Several lightly myelinated afferent fibers are shown. After losing their myelin, the axons encircle the outer root sheath of a hair follicle. Hair follicle receptors discharge in response to movements of the hair and signal a form of touch.

with the dermal papillae plays a role in their response to stimulation. One surface elevation of the epidermis, a papillary ridge, is in line with the long axis of the corpuscle, so that vertical pressure on a dermal papillae optimally

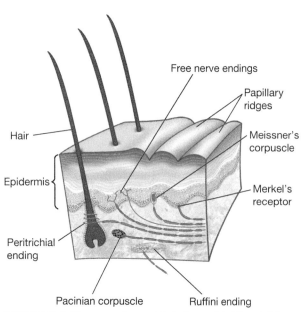

FIGURE 9-4 Receptors located in hairy and hairless (glabrous) skin. Glabrous skin contains three types of receptors: free nerve endings, Meissner's corpuscles, and Merkel's receptors. Hairy skin also contains three types of receptors: free nerve endings, peritrichial endings, and Merkel's receptors. The subcutaneous tissue of both hairy and glabrous skin contains Pacinian and Ruffini's corpuscles.

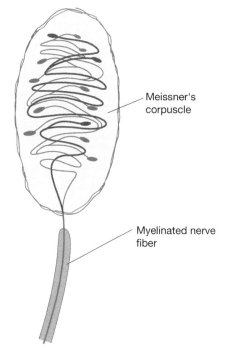

FIGURE 9-6 Meissner's corpuscles are encapsulated mechanoreceptors located in dermal papillae. Each receptor is innervated by one or more afferent fibers whose unmyelinated endings wind spirally between the stacked, transversely oriented cells within the capsule.

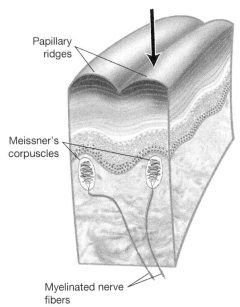

FIGURE 9-7 The long axis of a Meissner's corpuscle is in line with a papillary ridge so that vertical pressure on a ridge (arrow) optimally compresses the nerve endings between the stacked cells of the capsule. Meissner's corpuscles signal fine touch.

compresses the nerve endings between the stacked cells of the capsule (Figure 9-7 ■). Meissner's corpuscles are most dense on regions of highest tactile sensitivity. Thus, they are most numerous on the volar surfaces of fingers, hands, toes, and feet. They are numerous also in the lips and anterior tip of the tongue. Meissner's corpuscles are rapidly adapting mechanoreceptors whose rate and degree of adaptation are determined by the capsule. Meissner's corpuscles contribute to our capacity to perform fine tactile discriminations.

The deep layer of the epidermis in glabrous skin contains numerous specialized epithelial cells called **Merkel's cells** (Figure 9-8 ■). Each Merkel cell is innervated by a

single large myelinated fiber, but one fiber may innervate several Merkel's cells. Electron microscopy suggests that a synaptic junction exists between the Merkel cell and the terminal of the peripheral nerve fiber (the neurite), hence the term *Merkel cell–neurite complex*. It is hypothesized that synaptic transmission occurs. Processes extend from the upper surface of the Merkel cell and indent the epidermal cells just superficial to it. These processes may be distorted during mechanical deformation of the skin. The Merkel cell–neurite complex is a slowly adapting mechanoreceptor that responds to deformation of the surface epidermis and subserves tactile sensibility. Movement of the skin adjacent to the cell does not activate the receptor unless the stimulus is strong enough to spread to the cell.

The subcutaneous tissue beneath both hairy and glabrous skin contains two types of mechanoreceptors: the **Pacinian corpuscle** and the **corpuscle of Ruffini**. The Pacinian corpuscle is an egg-shaped, encapsulated mechanoreceptor up to several millimeters in length (Figure 9-9 ■). Each is innervated by a single, large, myelinated fiber that loses its myelin sheath soon after penetrating the corpuscle. The peripheral nerve fiber ends as a bare terminal in the center of the corpuscle. The corpuscle is composed of numerous concentric layers of connective tissue cells. The connective tissue is loosely organized around the outer portion of the corpuscle with an abundance of extracellular fluid in the spaces between cellular layers. This arrangement produces a poor mechanical coupling between the connective tissue of the corpuscle and the nerve ending such that only changes of pressure are transmitted effectively from the exterior of the corpuscle to the nerve terminal. For example, a maintained deformation results in activation of a Pacinian corpuscle both at its onset and termination, but not during the steady state deformation (see Figure 9-1). This is because a maintained force results in progressively less deformation of the nerve terminal due to transverse slippage between the layers

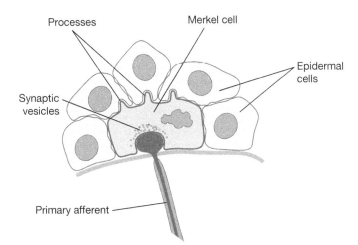

FIGURE 9-8 A Merkel cell is a modified epidermal cell located in the basal layer of the epidermis. Note the processes extending from the upper surface of the Merkel cell that indent the epidermal cells superficial to it. Each Merkel cell is innervated by a myelinated afferent fiber synapsing as a free nerve ending with the Merkel cell.

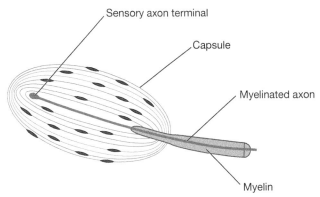

FIGURE 9-9 The afferent terminal of a Pacinian corpuscle is surrounded by up to 60 concentric layers of flattened connective tissue cells that, in turn, are enclosed by a connective tissue capsule. These rapidly adapting mechanoreceptors respond to the onset and offset of a pressure stimulus, and their stimulation is thus perceived as vibration (an "on-off" pressure stimulus).

of the capsule. Transverse slippage increases with time so that, eventually, the terminal is not deformed at all. Pacinian corpuscles are thus rapidly adapting mechanoreceptors with a generator potential only at the onset and offset of a pressure stimulus. Because Pacinian corpuscles respond only to rapid changes in pressure, their stimulation is perceived as vibration. Pacinian corpuscles are the most widely distributed of the encapsulated mechanoreceptors and are especially numerous in the subcutaneous tissues of the hand and foot. However, they also occur in other tissues (including the aponeuroses and tendon sheaths of skeletal muscle), in fascial planes, around ligaments, in the periosteum, in interosseous membranes, and in muscle tissue itself.

The encapsulated Ruffini ending consists of multiple, branched, unmyelinated terminals of a single, large, myelinated axon (Figure 9-10 ■). The nerve terminals are intimately associated with tightly packed collagen fibers in the capsule that merge with the dermal collagen. The Ruffini ending is exquisitely sensitive to stretch of the skin directly over the receptor as well as to stretch of adjacent skin.

The receptive field of each of the preceding mechanoreceptors is the area of skin that, when adequately stimulated, activates the receptor. The receptive field thus includes not only the area of skin innervated by the terminals of the receptor but also any region of surrounding tissue through which stimulus energy is transmitted to the receptor's terminals. The size of the receptive fields of a population of receptors is significant because size determines the capacity of the population to resolve spatial detail. The superficially located Meissner's corpuscle and the Merkel cell–neurite complex receptor both have small receptive fields (only a few millimeters wide), and thus these receptors are capable of resolving fine spatial differences (Figure 9-11 ■). Meissner's corpuscles are rapidly adapting receptors that respond to the onset of a stimulus but not throughout its duration, while Merkel

cell–neurite complex receptors are slowly adapting receptors that respond continuously throughout the duration of the stimulus. Merkel cell receptors and Meissner's corpuscles are of significance to individuals who are blind in reading Braille because of their capacities to resolve fine spatial differences. Particular regions of the skin are exquisitely sensitive to mechanical stimulation from objects measuring only 0.006 mm high and 0.04 mm wide, which can be felt on the fingertip. A Braille dot is about 167 times larger. The subcutaneously located Pacinian corpuscles and Ruffini endings have large receptive fields that can cover an entire finger or nearly half of the palm of the hand. The Pacinian corpuscle is a rapidly adapting receptor, whereas the Ruffini ending is slowly adapting. The Pacinian corpuscle is involved with the sense of vibration, felt as a diffuse humming sensation in deep tissues. Vibratory sense is poorly localized owing to the large receptive fields of Pacinian corpuscles. The slowly adapting Ruffini endings are associated with the sense of touch-pressure (stretching of the skin).

> **Thought Question**
>
> Based on the ability to resolve mechanical information by use of the fingers versus on the torso, how would you expect the receptive fields for their mechanoreceptors to compare?

Mechanoreceptors in Deep Tissues: Proprioceptors

Unlike superficial mechanoreceptors that provide us with sensory descriptions of the external environment, proprioceptors (L., *proprius, one's own*) provide us with information about the position of our limbs in space, whether they are moving or stationary, and, if moving, about the direction and rate of movement. Thus, the proprioceptive sensory modality consists of two submodalities: the sense of the static position of a limb in space and the sense of limb movement. The latter is called **kinesthesia**.

Proprioceptive information that signals the position of our limbs in space and their dynamic movement through that space contribute importantly to what is known as the **body schema**. The body schema is a dynamic three-dimensional mental construct of the body generated by integrative activity occurring in the parietal lobe. Such integrative activity allows us to form a coordinated image of the relationship of the parts of the body to one another and to perceive the portion of space occupied by our bodies. Proprioceptors in the deep tissues of the body wall, however, are not the only sensory modalities that contribute to the body schema. Both visual and vestibular receptors are also vital contributors to the body schema (Chapters 17 and 18).

Proprioception functions in two clinically relevant capacities. First, such information is essential in order for the brain to accurately control and guide movement. Thus, the elimination of proprioceptive information from the limbs caused by a peripheral or central nervous system lesion

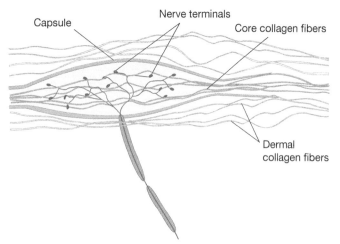

FIGURE 9-10 The multiple branched terminals of the Ruffini ending (corpuscle) wind among collagen fibers enclosed in a connective tissue capsule. Note that the collagen fibers of the Ruffini ending are continuous with dermal collagen. These slowly adapting mechanoreceptors signal touch-pressure.

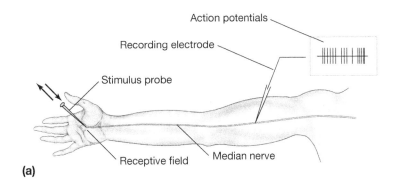

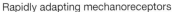

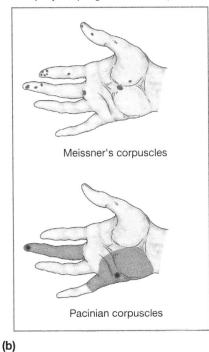

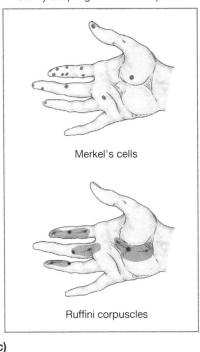

FIGURE 9-11 (a) Placing a microelectrode into the median nerve of the arm makes it possible to record the action potentials from a single afferent axon and determine its receptive field on the hand using a fine stimulus probe. (b) Receptive fields of rapidly adapting mechanoreceptors. (c) Receptive fields of slowly adapting mechanoreceptors.

results in uncoordinated limb movement. The movement incoordination is referred to as **ataxia**. Because it is due to the loss of proprioceptive sensibility, the disorder is specifically referred to as **sensory ataxia**. Second, the position and angles of our joints are used by the brain in identifying objects by manipulation, as, for example, when an object in the hand is manipulated in order to identify it. As we know, one of the main purposes of movement is to generate new or additional sensory information. Object identification by manipulation (without the use of vision) is called **stereognosis**.

Skeletal muscle and associated tendons contain two important mechanosensitive proprioceptors, the muscle spindle (neuromuscular spindle) and Golgi tendon organ (GTO). Both receptors are encapsulated and both are slowly adapting, although the muscle spindle, in addition, also has a rapidly adapting response component.

> **Thought Question**
>
> To what extent might people who are blind from birth likely be able to accurately perform movements that require specific and skilled positioning of their limbs in space? What receptor(s) might be of importance in this ability?

Muscle spindles are scattered throughout all striated (skeletal, voluntary) muscles, being distributed both superficially and deep. The number present in any given muscle is not related solely to muscle size. Muscles involved in fine, skilled voluntary movements, such as those of the thumb and fingers, contain proportionately more spindles than do those involved in producing only gross movements, such as the girdle muscles of the limbs. The muscle spindle is the most complex of all the encapsulated somatic receptors. The adequate stimulus for a muscle spindle is stretch or lengthening of the receptor. Muscle spindles signal to conscious awareness the ongoing status of muscle activity.

Each muscle spindle consists of a group of from 2 to 10 specialized muscle fibers surrounded by a connective tissue capsule (Figure 9-12 ■). The center (equatorial) portion of the capsule is expanded into a fluid-filled chamber imparting to the whole end organ a fusiform, or spindle, shape. The small, specialized muscle fibers within the capsule are called intrafusal (*intra*, meaning within, *fusus*, meaning spindle) fibers to distinguish them from extrafusal fibers. Extrafusal fibers are the striated, large skeletal muscle fibers responsible for contraction of voluntary muscle and movement. Intrafusal fibers also are capable of contracting, but their contraction does not produce movement of a body part. The intrafusal fibers are distributed among the extrafusal fibers in a parallel arrangement. In some cases, the nuclei are collected in an expanded region in the center of the extrafusal fiber, whereas in other cases, the nuclei of two to six intrafusal fibers are lined up in single file. The former are referred to as nuclear bag fibers, and the latter are referred to as nuclear chain fibers.

Of utmost importance to understanding the functions of the muscle spindle is the fact that each spindle is attached at both of its ends to the connective tissue investment (epimysium) of the extrafusal fibers. This *in parallel* structural relation between the spindle (and its intrafusal fibers) and the extrafusal muscle fibers means that when the extrafusal fibers lengthen, the muscle spindle lengthens (stretches), and when extrafusal fibers shorten, the muscle spindle becomes slack (Figure 9-13 ■). Lengthening of extrafusal fibers and stretching of muscle spindles occurs either by passively stretching the muscle, as when the arm is passively extended thus stretching the biceps muscle, or by the contraction of muscles that are antagonistic to the muscle in which the spindles are situated, as when the biceps muscle is lengthened when the triceps muscle contracts. Shortening of the whole muscle is caused by contraction of its extrafusal fibers. Potentially, this could cause the muscle spindles to go slack or unload. The reason muscle spindles do not actually unload is because the intrafusal fibers themselves are capable of contracting and thus shortening along with the shortening of the extrafusal fibers. This simultaneous shortening of the extra- and intrafusal fibers is known as alpha-gamma co-activation and is discussed later.

Two different types of afferent fiber (sensory) terminals occur on the intrafusal fibers: primary (annulospiral) endings and secondary (flower spray) endings (Figure 9-14 ■). A primary ending coils around the central, equatorial region of all intrafusal fibers. While these fibers coil around both nuclear bag and nuclear chain fibers, they do so more on the nuclear bag fibers. Secondary endings occur on either side of the primary ending, predominantly on nuclear chain fibers. Efferent nerve terminals (motor endings) also occur on the intrafusal fibers. These are called gamma (fusimotor) endings. The muscle spindle is thus among a unique group of receptors in the body whose activity can be controlled by the CNS. These motor endings are distributed on the polar regions of the intrafusal fibers. The polar regions, in contrast to the equatorial region, of an intrafusal fiber are striated and capable of contracting. Contraction of an intrafusal fiber shortens the polar regions of the fiber, which stretches (lengthens) the equatorial region, which is noncontractile (Figure 9-15 ■). The motor neurons associated with the intrafusal fibers are referred to as **gamma motor neurons**. The motor endings on an intrafusal fiber are small in diameter and are called **gamma, or fusimotor, fibers**. The cell bodies of the gamma fibers are located in the ventral horn of the spinal cord (and in cranial nerve motor nuclei of the brainstem) (Figure 9-16 ■).

Lengthening of a whole muscle causes the primary and secondary endings to be mechanically stretched, resulting in generator potentials in the endings. As a consequence of their positions on the intrafusal fiber, the primary and secondary endings respond differently to lengthening of the muscle. The primary ending is exquisitely sensitive to the dynamic phase of muscle lengthening. The dynamic phase is the time during which muscle length is actually increasing. The secondary

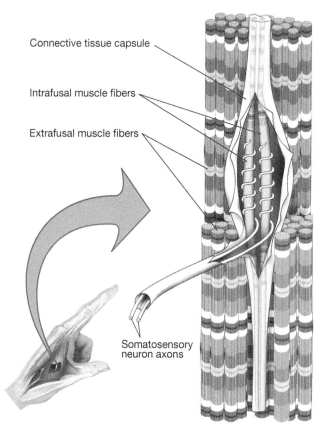

Connective tissue capsule

Intrafusal muscle fibers

Extrafusal muscle fibers

Somatosensory neuron axons

FIGURE 9-12 Each muscle spindle consists of a group of from 2 to 10 slender, specialized striated muscle fibers (intrafusal fibers) surrounded by a thin connective tissue capsule that is attached at both ends to the epimysium or to ordinary striated muscle fibers.

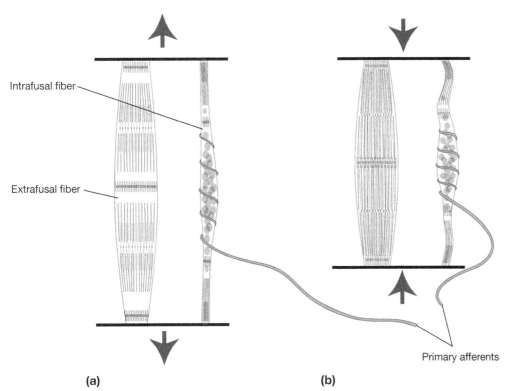

(a)   **(b)**

FIGURE 9-13 Each muscle spindle is arranged in parallel with extrafusal muscle fibers. Thus, when extrafusal muscle lengthens (a), the muscle spindle and its intrafusal fibers also are lengthened. In contrast, when extrafusal muscle shortens as, for example, during muscle contraction (b), the muscle spindle becomes slack, or "unloads."

Primary afferents

ending is relatively insensitive to the dynamic phase of muscle lengthening. Rather, secondary endings are most sensitive to the static, or steady-state, length of muscle. Primary endings are also sensitive to static muscle length but less so than the secondary endings. The sensory information sent to the brain by the muscle spindle sensory endings is about instantaneous muscle length and the velocity of muscle lengthening, as well as sustained changes in muscle length via group II (secondary) fibers. When the brain processes this information from all of the muscles acting across a given joint, it can determine the angle of the joint as well as whether the joint is moving and in what direction. Thus, muscle spindles are the most important (but not the only) receptors giving rise to the perception of limb position and kinesthesia.

Thought Question

Consider the role of the muscle spindle in proprioception and kinesthetic awareness. How do the primary and secondary endings relate to these two different functions of the muscle spindle?

Recall that when gamma motor neurons are active, they cause contraction of the polar ends of the intrafusal fibers, which stretches the equatorial region thus mechanically distorting the primary and secondary endings. This action of the gamma system produces an effect on the

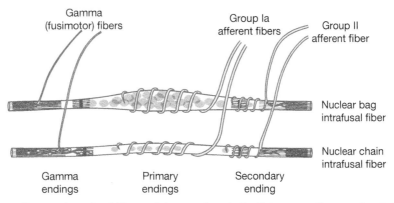

Gamma (fusimotor) fibers

Group Ia afferent fibers

Group II afferent fiber

Nuclear bag intrafusal fiber

Nuclear chain intrafusal fiber

Gamma endings   Primary endings   Secondary ending

FIGURE 9-14 Sensory and motor endings on intrafusal fibers of the muscle spindle. Primary endings are located on the equatorial region of all intrafusal fibers. Secondary endings are located on either side of the primary ending (juxtaequatorial). These endings predominantly occur on nuclear chain intrafusal fibers but also occur on nuclear bag fibers. Motor endings (gamma or fusimotor endings) occur on the striated, polar regions of all intrafusal fibers.

FIGURE 9-15 (a) Resting length of an intrafusal fiber before its contraction. (b) Contraction of an intrafusal fiber resulting from activation of the gamma system shortens both polar (contractile) regions, which stretches the noncontractile equatorial region of the intrafusal fiber, thereby causing generator potentials in the spindle's sensory endings.

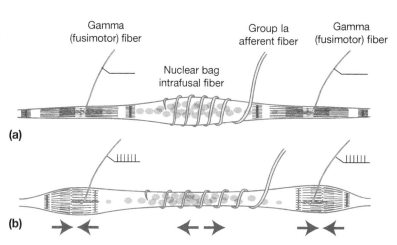

muscle spindle similar to that resulting from lengthening of the whole muscle. However, the effect is produced by the brain itself and not by any actual change in muscle length. The gamma system subserves two functions. First, it sets the sensitivity of the muscle spindle to lengthening of the whole muscle. By varying its rate of discharge, the gamma system determines the tautness of the intrafusal fibers. Increasing the tautness increases the sensitivity

of the spindle to stretch, whereas decreasing the rate of gamma system discharge decreases the sensitivity of the spindle to stretch.

The second function of the gamma system depends on its activation in conjunction with the alpha motor system, discharge of the latter producing contraction, and shortening of extrafusal muscle. The simultaneous discharge of alpha and gamma motor neurons is called **alpha-gamma**

FIGURE 9-16 (a) The cell bodies of gamma motor neurons are located in the ventral horn of the spinal cord along with the larger alpha motor neurons. (b) The axons of gamma motor neurons innervate the intrafusal muscle fibers in the muscle spindle, while the axons of alpha motor neuron innervate extrafusal muscle fibers. (c) Gamma motor endings on the polar regions of an intrafusal fiber are located on either side of a primary ending.

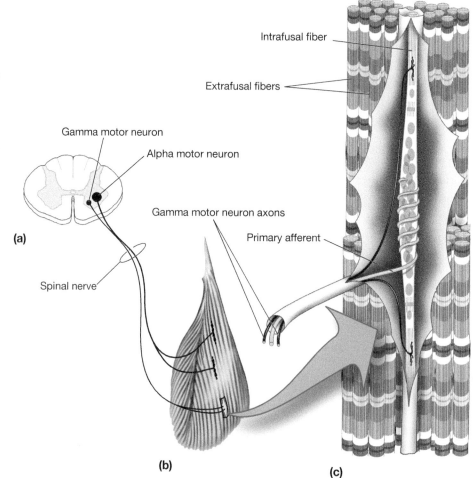

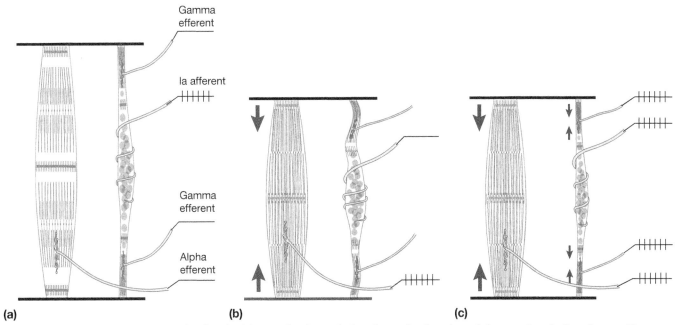

FIGURE 9-17 Alpha-gamma co-activation. In (a), extrafusal muscle is at its resting length, and the muscle spindle primary afferent (Ia afferent) is signaling this resting muscle length. The alpha motor efferent is stimulated in (b), causing the extrafusal muscle to shorten, which unloads the muscle spindle, causing the Ia afferent to stop signaling muscle length to the brain. However, when gamma motor efferents are activated at the same time as the alpha efferents as in (c), the muscle spindle is not unloaded and is thus able to signal to the brain this new, shortened muscle length.

Thought Question

The muscle spindle has both a sensory component and a motor component. Describe these two components. Why would a sensory receptor require a motor component?

co-activation. By causing the intrafusal fibers to shorten at the same time the whole muscle is contracting and shortening, the gamma system prevents unloading of the muscle spindle (Figure 9-17 ■). By preventing spindle unloading, gamma system activity ensures that the flow of sensory information from the muscle into the CNS is maintained despite contraction and shortening of extrafusal muscle. It is essential that the brain receive a continuous flow of information about what the muscle is doing if it is to effectively control movement on a continuing basis. Clearly, movement control would be compromised if every time a muscle contracted and shortened, the brain lost information about what the muscle was doing. Thus, it is essential that the brain continually receive information about muscle length, not only when the muscle lengthens, but also when it contracts and shortens.

A second major muscle mechanosensitive proprioceptor is the **Golgi tendon organ (GTO)**, situated, as the name implies, at the junction of striated muscle with its tendons. These slowly adapting encapsulated mechanoreceptors have been identified in virtually all voluntary muscle. The adequate stimulus for the GTO is muscle tension. In contrast to muscle spindles, GTOs are arranged in series with extrafusal skeletal muscle fibers. As a consequence, the tension on the GTO is increased either by stretching the whole muscle or by contracting the muscle, which increases tension on its tendons (Figure 9-18 ■). The structure of the GTO confirms that this is, indeed, a stretch receptor sensitive to increasing muscle tension.

The cells forming the capsule of the GTO resemble those of the perineural sheath surrounding peripheral nerve fibers so that the capsule is regarded as a continuation of the perineural sheath (Figure 9-19 ■). The interior of the capsule contains longitudinally oriented collagen fibers that arise from muscle and attach to the tendon. The collagen bundles spiral about one another like the strands of a braided rope. A single, large, myelinated afferent fiber innervates each GTO. After the fiber enters the lumen of the capsule, it loses its myelin sheath and divides into numerous unmyelinated fibers that thread their way through the collagen bundles. Stretch of the GTO, caused indirectly by muscle contraction or muscle stretch, tightens the braided strands of collagen, thereby pinching the axonal branches trapped between them. This mechanical deformation sets up generator potentials in the terminal, resulting in action potentials in the afferent axon. The GTO is exquisitely sensitive to tension in a muscle, the contraction of a single motor unit being sufficient to increase the discharge rate of a GTO afferent axon. Muscle contraction causes GTOs to discharge in proportion to the tension developed. Contractions that shorten the muscle without developing significant tension on the tendon cause only a modest discharge of the

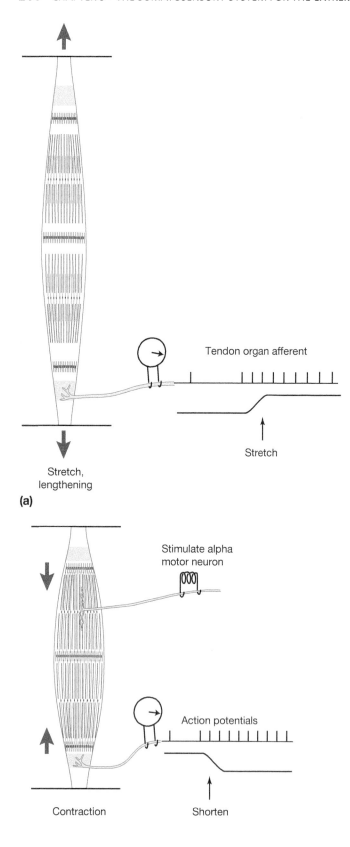

(a)

(b)

FIGURE 9-18 The Golgi tendon organ (GTO) is arranged in series with extrafusal muscle. Therefore, stretching the muscle increases tension on the GTO (a), as does contracting the muscle (b), both resulting in increased discharge of the tendon organ afferent.

GTO. Contractions that develop significant tension on the tendon cause a vigorous discharge of the GTO.

Mechanoreceptors in Joints

The final group of mechanoreceptors to be considered includes those distributed within the joint capsules and ligaments. Such receptors have had a checkered history in terms of the way in which they have been presented in different textbooks. For years, they were not considered as a separate group of receptors largely because structurally they resemble those distributed in other deep somatic structures. The joint capsules themselves contain Ruffini-like and Pacinian-like corpuscles, and a Golgi tendon organ–like receptor is distributed within the ligaments. The term *like* is used because structurally they are less complex than those distributed in subcutaneous tissues and tendons presented previously.

At one time, it was believed that joint receptors were responsible for mediating limb position sensibility and kinesthesia. Joint proprioceptors were then often presented as a separate receptor group. At that time, the prevailing, but incorrect, view was that information from muscle spindles did not reach consciousness and, therefore, could not be responsible for kinesthesia.

The view that joint receptors were responsible for limb position–movement sensibility never could be reconciled with the clinical observation that people who have undergone joint-replacement surgery retain position sense at that joint despite the absence of receptors, or the observation that injection of a local anesthetic into the knee joint of a human subject does not overtly affect kinesthesia of the knee. It also is notable that kinesthetic sensibility is acutely developed in the tongue, a structure that contains muscle spindles but obviously no joint receptors. It is now known that kinesthesia is subserved most importantly by the primary endings of muscle spindles. This has been confirmed by the fact that illusory movements are elicited in a human subject by mechanically vibrating the tendons of muscles, a procedure that selectively activates muscle spindle primary endings. Thus, while the slowly adapting Ruffini-like and the rapidly adapting Pacinian-like endings of the joint capsule may contribute to kinesthesia, their role is more limited than that of the muscle spindle.

Function

Peripheral Receptor Information: Uses and Actions in the CNS

Information generated by peripheral receptors is used by the CNS for four different broadly defined functions. These functions can be carried out simultaneously because they are mediated by parallel pathways projecting to different structures of the brain and spinal cord.

1. Peripheral receptor information may have a general arousing and alerting effect (or conversely a soporific effect) on consciousness by acting on neurons of the reticular formation comprising the ascending

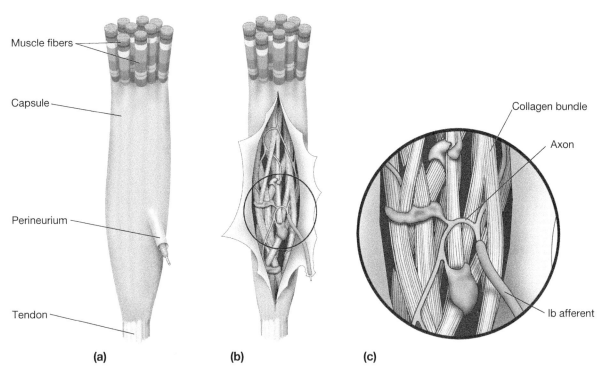

(a)   (b)   (c)

FIGURE 9-19 The GTO is located at the junction of muscle with its tendons. Note that the capsule of the GTO is a continuation of the perineural sheath surrounding the peripheral nerve innervating the receptor (a). Collagen fibers in the tendon organ attach to muscle fibers. After entering the capsule, the single Ib afferent branches into many unmyelinated endings that wrap around and between the collagen bundles (b). The bundles of collagen do not run a straight parallel course through the tendon organ but twist like the strands of a braided rope (c). When the tendon organ is stretched by contraction of the muscle, the collagen bundles straighten and twist, which compresses the endings, causing the Ib afferent to increase its firing rate.

activating system. Some peripheral receptor information is more effective than others, pain and auditory information being notable examples (Chapter 5).

2. Peripheral receptor information represents the basis for the conscious discrimination of environmental events by acting on neurons of the cerebral cortex via ascending sensory systems. The ascending systems subserving somatic sensation for the body are discussed later, while those for the head are discussed in Chapter 14. The auditory and vestibular systems are discussed in Chapter 17 and the visual system in Chapter 18.

3. Peripheral receptor information may elicit reflexes involving muscles of the body or head by acting directly or indirectly on motor neurons of the spinal cord or brainstem. Reflexes involving striated muscles innervated by spinal cord motor neurons are discussed in Chapter 11, those of the autonomic nervous system in Chapter 12, those of the striated muscle of the head innervated by brainstem motor neurons in Chapter 14, those of the auditory and vestibular systems in Chapter 17, and those of the visual system in Chapter 18.

4. Peripheral receptor information enables the brain to perform coordinated movement by acting on neurons belonging to the motor control system, such as those of the cerebellum and basal ganglia (Chapter 19) and cerebral cortex (Chapter 20).

Thought Question

Summarize a number of distinct functional roles of peripheral receptors.

Information Coding in the Receptor and Its Axon

The first step in all sensory perception relates to the overall process by which energy of a stimulus is converted into an electrical signal in a sensory neuron. This step relies on conversion of the **generator potential (GP)** to the **action potential (AP)**. As discussed in Chapter 4, a receptor's GP has two functions. First, it encodes information about the receptor's adequate stimulus. The information-bearing components of a GP were illustrated in Figures 4-8 and 4-9. Only information that is encoded by the GP can be used in the transduction process. Second, once the threshold is reached, the GP sets up patterns of APs that contain the same information as the GP. This occurs only if the membrane depolarization created by the GP is great enough to exceed the threshold for AP generation. Therefore, an intimate relationship exists between GPs and APs, as would be expected if they are to encode the same information. The neural encoding of primary afferent somatosensory information involves not only the frequency of firing, but also onset/offset, duration, and pattern of the action potentials. A number of different factors influence the strength of the stimulus. First is the rate of action potential discharge. Secondly, it is important to recognize that some receptors fire rapidly when first stimulated, but then fall silent as the stimulus continues, whereas other receptors generate a sustained discharge. An example is the dynamic versus static phase of muscle lengthening detected by primary and secondary endings of the muscle spindle. As discussed previously, this difference in adaptation is critical to providing information about both dynamic and static qualities of the stimulus. In general, rapidly adapting or phasic receptors respond briefly but maximally to a stimulus; the response then decreases if the stimulus is sustained. In contrast, when the stimulus is sustained, slowly adapting, or tonic, receptors fire as long as the stimulus is present.

The capacity to discriminate stimulus intensity thus depends on a frequency code in the axon of tonic receptors. However, this relationship between stimulus intensity and frequency applies only over a certain range of stimulus intensities. At some stimulus intensity, the receptor becomes saturated such that its GP cannot increase further in amplitude with continued increases in stimulus intensity. When this occurs, another coding mechanism comes into play. This is best illustrated by a mechanical stimulus such as touch-pressure. A more intense stimulus causes a greater area of the body surface to be deformed and, thus, more receptors to be activated. When more than one receptor and its primary afferent axon are active simultaneously, the information code is a population or ensemble code.

Cutaneous Receptive Fields

A **cutaneous receptive field** is defined as the area of the skin that, when stimulated by an adequate stimulus, will activate a single primary afferent neuron (Figure 9-20 ■). The dimensions of a receptive field are generally larger than the area of skin directly innervated by the primary afferent because of the transmission of stimulus energy by body tissues. The size of cutaneous receptive fields exhibits an orderly variation over the body surface. Receptive fields are smallest in areas of highest innervation density. They are smallest on the fingertips and tongue tip and up to 100 times larger on the trunk.

Receptive fields possess a sensitivity gradient so that the discharge pattern of the afferent fiber carries information about the location of the stimulus within the receptive field. The center of the field is maximally sensitive, with progressively less sensitivity moving toward the periphery. The center of the field has the lowest threshold, and, when stimulated, gives rise to the shortest latency, highest frequency, and most prolonged discharge in the primary afferent. In areas of the body with the highest innervation density, receptive fields overlap so that stimulation of a single point on the body may activate multiple somatosensory afferents.

The idea that the distribution of receptors in the body periphery is preserved in sensory systems of the CNS was

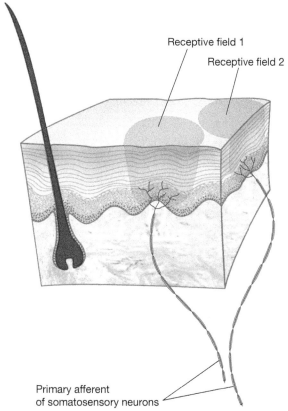

Receptive field 1

Receptive field 2

Primary afferent
of somatosensory neurons

FIGURE 9-20 Receptive fields for two cutaneous receptors. Each is the area of skin that, when stimulated, will activate a single primary afferent axon. The area of skin making up the receptive field is larger than the area of skin within which the terminal itself is located due to the transmission of stimulus energy through body tissues.

introduced in the previous chapter under topographic organization. Actually, it is the peripheral organization of receptive fields that is preserved within the CNS in the form of somatotopic maps of the body.

Point Localization and Two-Point Discrimination

The fact that certain types of incoming somatosensory messages act on a map of the body that is laid out in neural space is what enables us to discriminate the location of a stimulus on the body surface. Locus discrimination is best developed in areas of highest innervation density.

Two-point discrimination is a simple example of spatial discrimination. This is the ability to distinguish two points from one and can be tested using a compass whose tips are at various degrees of separation. The distance at which two stimuli can be discriminated varies tremendously over the body surface due to variation in innervation density. The following figures are subject to individual variability:

1 mm on the tip of the tongue

2–3 mm on the lips

3–5 mm on the fingertips

8–15 mm on the palm

20–30 mm on the dorsal surfaces of the hand and foot

40–70 mm on the trunk

Two-point discrimination depends on what is called an **ensemble code**; that is, on the distribution of the intensity–frequency relationship across a population of receptors. Two points can be discriminated as long as the points of the stimulating compass fall in separate receptive fields and the frequency profile of nerve impulses from the active primary afferents contains two peaks (Figure 9-21 ■). As the distance between the tips of the stimulating compass is progressively narrowed, a distance will eventually be reached where two points would be perceived as only one point.

Primary Afferents and Their Receptors

Primary afferent axons (first-order fibers) that carry information from the receptor into the CNS may be classified in a variety of ways: for example, they may be classified according to the peripheral tissues they innervate, the stimuli to which their terminal endings are selectively sensitive, their axon diameters (hence, conduction velocities), and their biochemical composition. A peripheral nerve contains many different types of primary afferent neurons. The most basic distinction between fiber types is whether or not they are myelinated (Chapter 4). Unmyelinated axons, however, also have a relationship with Schwann cells. In contrast to a myelinated fiber that is ensheathed by its private set of Schwann cells, unmyelinated fibers (up to 20) share

Thought Question

It is possible to discriminate two stimuli (such as a light touch) that occur in closer proximity on the hands than on the torso. What distinguishes the difference in localizing ability of these two body segments, and what is the functional importance of this difference?

single Schwann cells (Figure 9-22 ■). Each unmyelinated axon is embedded in its own trough of a Schwann cell's plasma membrane so that individual axons are separated from one another. In contrast to unmyelinated axons whose range of diameters is restricted to small diameters, myelinated axons vary greatly in diameter, from 1 to 22 micrometers (μm) in diameter. The thickness of the myelin sheath also varies.

One of the major systems of classifying peripheral nerve fibers is based on the conduction velocity of the constituent axons in a particular nerve. Conduction velocity is related to axon diameter and the presence and thickness of the myelin sheath. Large myelinated axons conduct action potentials faster because the internal resistance to current flow along the axon is low and the nodes of Ranvier are more widely spaced along its length. The factor for converting axon diameter to conduction velocity in large, myelinated axons is about six times the axon diameter. In thin, myelinated axons, the factor is five times the axon diameter. However, in unmyelinated axons, the factor is only 1.5 to 2.5.

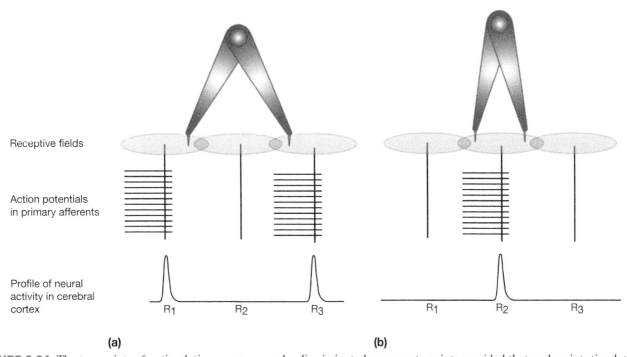

(a)   (b)

FIGURE 9-21 The two points of a stimulating compass can be discriminated as separate points provided that each point stimulates a separate receptive field (a). When both points of the compass activate the same receptive field, the brain can no longer discriminate the points as separate (b) because the profile of neural activity in the cerebral cortex from the three receptors (R) contains only a single peak.

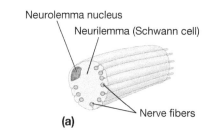

(a)

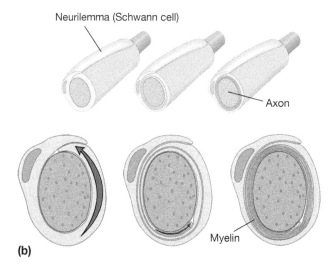

(b)

FIGURE 9-22 (a) In the PNS, single or multiple unmyelinated axons are located within troughs on the surface of Schwann cells. Although associated with a Schwann cell, these axons are not insulated by a myelin sheath. (b) Myelinated PNS fibers are surrounded by a myelin sheath that is formed by a spiral wrapping of the axon by a Schwann cell. Note that the direction of growth (arrow) occurs at the inner part of the sheath.

When a peripheral nerve is activated using a stimulus of sufficient intensity to activate all of the fibers in the nerve, a distant recording electrode will detect a compound action potential. **A compound action potential** represents the summated action potentials of all of the fibers in the nerve. The first deflection in a compound action potential is produced by the fastest conducting fibers in the nerve, the last by the slowest conducting axons. Each nerve has a characteristic pattern of conduction velocities that corresponds to the pattern of fiber diameters contained in the nerve. Therefore, different nerves generate compound action potentials with different numbers of deflections. Based on conduction velocity, nerve fibers are grouped into three main classes, designated A, B, and C (with A fibers being the fastest conducting and C fibers the slowest). The A deflection is itself complex and may contain alpha, beta, gamma, and delta peaks.

Studies on different types of nerves (muscular, cutaneous, and autonomic) allow the three groups to be correlated with function (Table 9-1 ■). Insofar as primary afferents are concerned, the largest and most rapidly conducting myelinated fibers, the A-alphas, are from stretch receptors in muscles and tendons (primary muscle spindle afferents and GTO afferents). A-beta fibers are from a variety of mechanoreceptors that mediate discriminative touch, pressure, joint rotation, and secondary muscle spindle afferents. The slowest conducting myelinated fibers, the A-deltas, transmit impulses from certain pain receptors (sharp, fast pain), thermal receptors, and tactile receptors. C fibers are unmyelinated and consist of primary afferents related mostly to certain nociceptors (diffuse, slow pain) and temperature receptors. These are the slowest conducting afferents due to their small diameter.

Thought Question

What determines whether a nerve fiber will be fast or slow conducting?

It is noteworthy that the height of the wave does not correspond to the number of fibers in the nerve. For example, the C wave is small-voltage amplitude compared to the A wave, but there are usually many more C fibers in a peripheral nerve. The C wave is small because the magnitude of extracellular currents generated by small-diameter axons is much lower than that from the larger-diameter A fibers.

That the primary afferents innervating the skin of humans are selectively sensitive to different stimulus modalities

Table 9-1 Peripheral Nerve Fiber Classification

FIBER TYPE		FUNCTION	SIZE (µm)	CONDUCTION VELOCITY (m/sec)
By Conduction Velocity	By Fiber Diameter	Proprioception, stretch	12–22	70–120
Aα	Ia	Primary muscle spindle afferents Motor efferents to extrafusal muscle		
Aα	Ib	Golgi tendon organ afferents: contractile tension (force)	12–22	70–120
Aβ	II	Mechanoreception: discriminative touch, pressure, joint rotation Secondary muscle spindle afferents (static muscle length)	5–12	30–70
Aγ	II	Motor efferents to muscle spindle intrafusal fibers	2–8	15–30
Aδ	III	Mechanoreception: touch Nociception: discriminative pain	1–5	5–30
B		Autonomic preganglionic axons	<3	3–15
C	IV	Nociception: in inflammatory or visceral pain, thermal sense Autonomic postganglionic axons	0.1–1.3	0.6–2.0

is shown by the electrical stimulation of isolated fibers in peripheral nerves in waking humans (Table 9-2). The A-beta fibers as a group innervate rapidly adapting Meissner's and Pacinian corpuscles as well as slowly adapting Merkel cell–neurite complexes and Ruffini corpuscles. Isolated stimulation of identified rapidly adapting Meissner afferents evokes sensations of moving stimuli and low-frequency vibration (flutter). These afferents signal the slip of objects held between the fingers and elicit adjustments in manual grip force in order to maintain a steady hold. Stimulation of identified, rapidly adapting Pacinian afferents evokes sensations of contact, movement, and high-frequency vibration. Stimulation of slowly adapting Merkel cell–neurite complex afferents evokes sensations of contact, pressure, texture, and two-dimensional form. These slow-adapting, type I (SA-I) afferents are especially sensitive to the corners, edges, and curvatures of objects palpated by the hand and thus contribute to the sensing of a three-dimensional form of grasped objects (stereognosis). But SA-I afferents contribute to form perception by working together with muscle spindle primary afferents. Note that stimulation of Ruffini afferents, which are slow-adapting Type II afferents (SA-II), evokes no distinct and consistent sensations.

These SA-II afferents, given their high sensitivity to stretch of the skin, are important to the control of the position and movement of joints throughout the body. Lightly myelinated A-delta fibers and unmyelinated C fibers innervate thermal receptors and nociceptors. Isolated stimulation of these fibers in humans evokes sensations of coolness, warmth, cold pain, heat pain, slow burning pain, and mechanical pain. Most A-delta fibers evoke a sensation of short latency pricking pain, and most C fibers a sensation of slow, burning pain.

There is a remarkable modality specificity of primary afferents innervating the skin of the hand. However, it is important to realize that in everyday life, where the hand is involved in the reception of passively applied stimuli or in the active acquisition of stimuli as in the manipulation of an object or exploration of an environmental surface, individual receptor classes are not usually activated in isolation. Rather, there is a population response in primary afferents wherein a variety of large-diameter, low-threshold afferents work in concert with higher-threshold, small-diameter afferents to inform the brain about all of the attributes of a stimulus acquired by the hand: size, shape, texture, hardness, slipperiness, stickiness, and temperature. Thus, concurrent sensory influx is the rule in normal behavior. It may well be that the reason isolated stimulation of, for example, muscle spindle primary afferents or Ruffini afferents does not elicit a sensation of kinesthesia is because these receptors must act together to generate such a sensory experience.

Table 9-2 Classification and Properties of Afferents Innervating the Skin

CLASS	AXON CONDUCTION VELOCITY	STATE OF MYELINATION	ADEQUATE STIMULUS	ADAPTATION RATE	SENSORY EXPERIENCE EVOKED
Mechanoreceptors					
Meissner corpuscle (RA-I)*	A-beta, 25–75 m/sec	Myelinated	Moving, displacement, velocity	Rapid	Velocity, horizontal movement, contact, flutter (best at 20–30 Hz)
Pacinian corpuscle (RA-II)*	A-beta, 25–75 m/sec	Myelinated	Contact, vibration, lateral movement	Rapid	Contact, movement, vibration (best at 250 Hz)
Merkel–neurite complex (SA-I)*	A-beta, 25–75 m/sec	Myelinated	Contact, pressure, lateral movement	Slow	Contact, pressure, texture, two-dimensional form
Ruffini corpuscle (SA-II)*	A-beta, 35–75 m/sec	Myelinated	Contact, displacement, skin stretch	Slow	None
Peritrichial ending	A-beta, 35–75m/sec	Myelinated	Contact, movement	Rapid	Contact, movement
Thermoreceptors					
Cooling, unencapsulated	A-delta, 5–30 m/sec	Thinly myelinated	Mild thermal cooling, range 15–45°C	Slow	Sense of cooling
Warming, unencapsulated	C fibers, 0.5–2 m/sec	Unmyelinated	Mild thermal warming, range 20–40°C	Slow	Sense of warming
Nociceptors					
Polymodal, unencapsulated	C fibers, 0.5–2 m/sec	Unmyelinated	Noxious heat, 45°C, chemical	Intermediate	Slow, burning pain, heat pain
High-threshold, unencapsulated	A-delta, 5–40 m/sec	Thinly myelinated	Destructive mechanical, heat >52°C	Slow	Mechanical, intense heat pain, hyperalgesia
Cold nociceptors, unencapsulated	C fibers, 0.5–2 m/sec	Unmyelinated	Extreme cooling	Slow	Cold pain
Heat nociceptors	C-fibers, 0.5–2 m/sec	Unmyelinated	Extreme heating	Slow	Heat pain

*RA-I, rapidly adapting Type I afferents; RA-II, rapidly adapting Type II afferents; SA-I, slowly adapting Type I afferents; SA-II, slowly adapting Type II afferents

CLINICAL CONNECTIONS

Peripheral Neuropathies

In general, in neuropathies involving somatosensory axons in nerves, there is impaired autonomic function in the same areas as the somatosensory impairment. Autonomic dysfunction such as anhydrosis (localized loss of sweating) and orthostatic hypotension occur most frequently and are major features of certain polyneuropathies such as diabetic polyneuropathies. Bowel and bladder incontinence and sexual impotence are other examples of manifestations of autonomic dysfunction in peripheral neuropathies (see Chapter 12).

In polyneuropathies affecting the somatosensory neurons, sensory ataxia may occur. The term *ataxia* refers to abnormally uncoordinated and inaccurate movements. This ataxic movement results not because of a specific motor system involvement, but because of somatosensory loss and its consequences. Specifically, degeneration of proprioceptive afferents occurs with a relative sparing of motor fibers so that at least a reasonable degree of motor function is retained. Because of the proprioceptive loss, the individual has impaired awareness of the position and movement of his legs and slaps his feet on the ground in an attempt to generate more proprioceptive input. Additionally, the cerebellum is deprived of the proprioceptive input it needs to properly coordinate movement.

Herpes Zoster (Shingles)

Certain diseases attack the dorsal root ganglia of the spinal cord. One such example is **herpes zoster (shingles)**, a common viral infection of the somatosensory ganglia of spinal and cranial nerves. In the majority of patients the rash is limited to the area of one dermatome (see Figure 2-6). In two-thirds of patients, thoracic dermatomes are involved, especially T5 to T10. In approximately 20 percent of cases, the somatosensory ganglia of the trigeminal and facial nerves are involved, and the disease symptoms are more severe (Chapter 13). The initial symptom may be a **dysesthesia** (i.e., a usually disagreeable paresthesia) or severe localized pain in the involved dermatome(s). Within three to four days, the involved dermatome(s) become red, and a vesicular eruption appears that resembles the generalized eruption of chickenpox. In most patients, the pain and dysesthesia last for one to four weeks, but in as many as one-third of patients, the pain may persist for months or even years after the skin lesions have disappeared.

Thought Question

What is meant by sensory ataxia? Is the motor system involved? Thinking ahead to clinical practice, why might this be important later?

SYSTEMS MEDIATING SOMATIC SENSATION FROM THE BODY

Clinical Preview

You are treating two teenage boys in your orthopedic clinic who have sports injuries that affected both their musculoskeletal and neuromuscular systems. John Carey sustained a fall on his outstretched right arm while sliding to first base. He sought your assistance because of pain throughout his entire right arm and shoulder. Martin Chung is a football player who sustained an injury affecting the left side of his lumbar spinal cord. He complains of loss of sensory awareness in both lower limbs.

As you read through the content in this section, consider the following:

- Which neuroanatomical structure, from the receptor to the third-order neuron, was involved in each situation?

- Is this structure located in the peripheral or central nervous system?

- Why would sensory loss be restricted to the side of injury for John, but would be bilateral for Martin?

Two major systems are involved in carrying information from somatic receptors to the cerebral cortex for conscious recognition and discrimination of the attributes of environmental stimuli. These are the **dorsal column–medial lemniscal (DC-ML) system** and the **anterolateral system (AL)**. The AL system includes a number of pathways, one of which is the **spinothalamic tract (STT)**. In this chapter, when discussing pain, we focus only on the STT, which is important in the localization of painful or thermal stimuli. In Chapter 16, we address pain more broadly, including other important tracts of the anterolateral system.

The name of the AL system reflects the fact that the axons of second-order neurons are located in the anterolateral funiculus of the spinal cord. The name of the STT reflects the fact that the tract begins in the spinal cord and ends in the thalamus. The name of the DC-ML system reflects the fact that the first-order neurons are located in the dorsal columns (DCs) of the spinal cord, while the second-order neurons are located in the medial lemniscus (ML) of the brainstem. Pathways that make up the DC-ML system and the STT include all six of the structural components of the general anatomical plan identified Figure 8-1.

The DC-ML system and STT mediate our conscious somatic interactions with the external environment. When this interaction involves objects, it is immediately apparent that an object possesses a texture (smoothness, roughness), a hardness (softness), a temperature, a slipperiness (or stickiness), and, if manipulated by the hand or enveloped by the whole body in a hug, a shape and size in addition to the other sensibilities. What this means in practical terms is that it is artificial to imply that the activity in these two systems takes place independently. Nevertheless, the information from the systems is largely conveyed separately, from the spinal cord up to the initial point of cortical processing. For example, vibration sense is processed solely in the DC, whereas clinical evidence suggests that joint sense and light touch are conveyed predominantly by the DC but also to a minor extent by the AL system. Furthermore, the distinction of processing at the cortical level is evident by response properties of neurons in the thalamus and cerebral cortex to somatosensory stimuli. In this chapter, we address the DC-ML pathway and the STT. We begin with the DC-ML pathway. One reason we do so is because parts of this system have the most direct, and thus easily understood, access to perceptual centers of the cerebral cortex.

Dorsal Column–Medial Lemniscal System

General Information

The dorsal column–medial lemniscal system (DC-ML) comprises a set of neurons ascending in the dorsal columns of the spinal cord and in the medial lemniscus of the brainstem that carry somatosensory information from the body periphery to the cerebral cortex for conscious discrimination and interpretation (see Chapter 5). The term *lemniscus* means a fillet, or band. Thus the medial lemniscus is a band of nerve fibers that ascends through the brainstem.

The DC-ML system mediates specific types of discriminative tactile sensations, kinesthesia, and stereognosis all essential to sensory exploration of the environment and movement control. A subset of DC-ML fibers (1) exhibits a high degree of somatotopic organization, (2) responds selectively to one modality of sensory stimulus, (3) possesses the capacity to respond precisely to stimuli whose parameters vary rapidly in time (e.g., movement of a tactile stimulus across the skin surface, lengthening of muscle), and (4) possesses an exquisite capacity for spatial discrimination (because the neurons have small peripheral cutaneous receptive fields).

The dorsal columns carry all types of proprioceptive information from the upper extremity but only certain types from the lower extremity. Consequently, with discrete DC lesions, the arm and hand are impaired more than the leg and foot. A subset of dorsal column fibers is capable of signaling noxious stimuli.

The overall anatomy of the component of the DC-ML system that carries information from the fingers is depicted in Figure 9-23 ■ .

Sensory End Organs

Both slowly and rapidly adapting mechanoreceptors distributed in skin, subcutaneous tissues, muscle, tendon, and joints send information into the DC-ML system. These include muscle spindles, Golgi tendon organs, Pacinian corpuscles, Meissner's corpuscles, Merkel cell–neurite complexes, Ruffini endings, peritrichial (hair follicle) endings, free nerve endings, and articular receptors (few). The numerical majority are rapidly adapting cutaneous mechanoreceptors, such as hair follicle receptors activated by hair displacement and receptors activated by touch-pressure stimulation of the skin. The sensations elicited by stimulation of the primary afferent fibers of cutaneous receptors were summarized in Table 9-2.

Primary Afferents (First-Order Neurons)

Primary afferents are segregated into different portions of the dorsal column according to the segmental level at which they enter the spinal cord. Ascending primary afferents entering the dorsal columns at successively more rostral segmental levels are added laterally to those already ascending from more caudal cord segments. This orderly lamination of fibers gives the DC a somatotopic organization in which fibers from contiguous body parts are located in adjacent lamella of the DC (Figure 9-24 ■). Axons from sacral, lumbar, and lower thoracic segments are located sequentially in a medially positioned fiber bundle called the **fasciculus gracilis**. The fasciculus gracilis carries afferents from all spinal cord segments below T6. Axons from upper thoracic and cervical segments are located sequentially in a laterally positioned (and larger) fiber bundle called the **fasciculus cuneatus**. The fasciculus cuneatus carries afferents from spinal cord segments above T6. Based on the number of primary afferents received from each body region, which depends on the density of receptors in that body part, the fasciculus gracilis carries information primarily from the

foot, while the fasciculus cuneatus carries information primarily from the hand (especially the fingertips).

A significant subset of primary DC afferents leaves the DCs within 2 to 12 segments from their level of entry to synapse in the dorsal horn of the spinal gray. After synapsing in the dorsal horn, some of these axons reenter the DC. This subset of DC fibers, therefore, is not primary but second-order afferents.

Projections

SECOND-ORDER NEURONS Long, ascending primary afferents traveling in the DC terminate uncrossed in the ipsilateral **dorsal column nuclei (DCN)**. The DCN represent the cell bodies of second-order neurons of the DC-ML system. The two major DCN (on each side of the brainstem) are positioned in the dorsal and medial region of caudal medulla. The medially situated nucleus gracilis receives afferents mainly from the fasciculus gracilis. The adjacent, laterally positioned main cuneate nucleus receives afferents mostly from the fasciculus cuneatus.

> **Thought Question**
>
> Somatotopic organization becomes even more obvious in the manner by which the DC-ML system is constructed. Contrast the relative location of the fibers that originate in the lower extremity with those that originate in the fingertips. Then contrast the location of the cell bodies that form the second order neurons from these two parts of the body.

The contingent of second-order (postsynaptic) afferents in the DCs also synapse in the DCN. These postsynaptic afferents arise from dorsal horn cells of the cervical and lumbar enlargements. Second-order DC afferents, unlike primary afferents, are activated by more than one type of peripheral cutaneous stimulus and also respond to noxious stimulation (pinching of the skin or intense mechanical stimulation of deep structures). Lesions of the dorsal roots do not cause degeneration of all DC fibers because some have their cell bodies in the spinal cord and not in the dorsal roots (see Clinical Connections, Tabes Dorsalis, later).

The DCN do not function as simple relays transmitting unaltered information from DC afferents to second-order neurons of the medial lemniscus. Only a minority of the synapses in the DCN is made by long ascending fibers of the DC. Information processing occurs in cells of the DCN as a consequence of the excitatory and inhibitory actions of DCN interneurons.

Most second-order axons from cells of the major DCN enter the medial lemniscus on the contralateral side of the brainstem. These axons first sweep ventromedially as the internal arcuate fibers, then cross the midline as the decussation of the

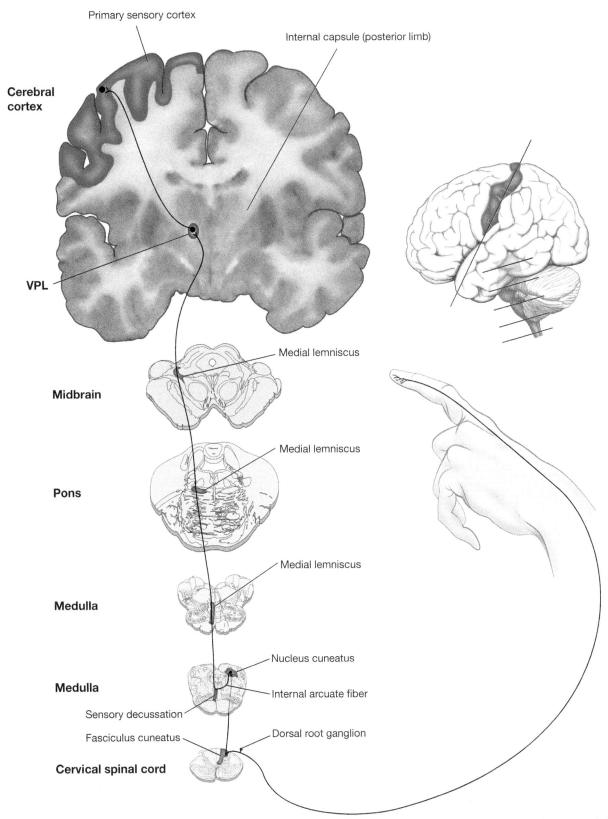

FIGURE 9-23 The overall trajectory of the dorsal column–medial lemniscal system through the spinal cord, brainstem, and thalamus (VPL) en route to its termination in the primary somatosensory cortex of the postcentral gyrus. Only one component of the system, that related to the upper extremity, is illustrated.

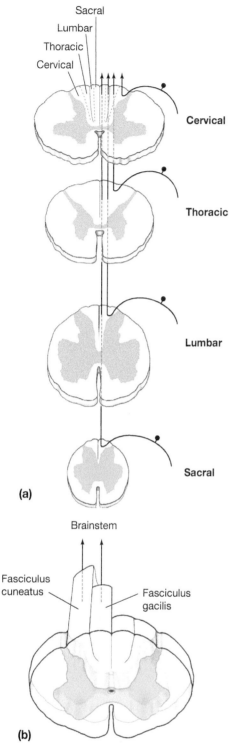

FIGURE 9-24 (a) Laminar organization of the dorsal columns. Longer ascending fibers from more caudal spinal cord segments are progressively displaced medially by shorter ascending primary afferents entering the dorsal columns at successively more rostral segments. Only the afferents above T6 are shown entering the fasciculus cuneatus; afferents arising below T6 would enter the fasciculus gracilis. (b) Posterior view of the dorsal columns showing the medially located fasciculus gracilis, related to spinal cord segments caudal to T6, and laterally located fasciculus cuneatus, related to spinal cord segments rostral to T6.

medial lemniscus to form the contralateral ML. Axons from the **nucleus gracilis** cross first (at a lower brainstem level), followed by axons from the main cuneate nucleus, giving the ML a somatotopic organization (Figure 9-25 ▪). Thus, fibers from sacral levels that synapse within the nucleus gracilis are the first to enter the forming ML. These are followed successively by fibers from each progressively more rostral spinal cord segment, with fibers from uppermost cervical levels being the last to enter the ML.

Located in the caudalmost medulla, the decussation of the ML occupies a short rostrocaudal expanse. Lesions situated caudal to the decussation produce sensory alterations on the side ipsilateral to the lesion (same side). These would be lesions of the spinal cord, DCN, or internal arcuate fibers. A lesion involving the decussation would yield bilateral symptoms. Lesions situated rostral to the decussation produce somatosensory alterations on the side opposite (contralateral) to the lesion. These include lesions to the ML anywhere in the brainstem, in the thalamic nucleus (ventral posterior lateral, VPL) to which the ML projects, and in the region of the internal capsule in which these fibers traverse as a component of the thalamocortical radiations, to primary somatosensory cortex.

Five anatomical constituents of the DC-ML system can be identified in the medulla, but not all are present throughout this brainstem subdivision: the gracile nuclei, the cuneate nuclei, the internal arcuate fibers, the decussation of the ML, and the ML. The ML is positioned between the inferior olivary nuclei. Its somatotopic organization at the level of the medulla is such that sacral fibers are most ventral, cervical most dorsal.

The major change in the DC-ML system in the pons is that the ML shifts its orientation to become a mediolaterally distributed band of fibers in the ventral part of the pontine tegmentum. Fibers from sacral segments of the spinal cord are now most lateral, those from cervical segments are most medial (see Figure 9-25).

In its ascent through the midbrain, the ML shifts progressively dorsally and somewhat laterally to assume the shape of an arc in rostralmost midbrain. Fibers from sacral segments of the spinal cord are dorsolateral, while those from cervical segments are ventromedial.

THIRD-ORDER NEURONS   Most fibers of the ML end on cells of the ventral posterior lateral (VPL) nucleus of the thalamus (see Figure 9-23). The VPL nucleus is situated posteriorly and laterally in the ventral tier of thalamic nuclei, as the name indicates. The cell bodies of the third-order neurons of the system are located in the VPL nucleus of each side. The nucleus is somatotopically organized, with neurons receiving information from sacral segments being positioned laterally and neurons receiving information from cervical segments being medially (see Figure 9-25).

The axons of VPL neurons ascend in the ipsilateral internal capsule to terminate on neurons in the somatosensory (and motor) cortices of the hemisphere contralateral to the side of primary afferent fiber origin (see Figure 9-23).

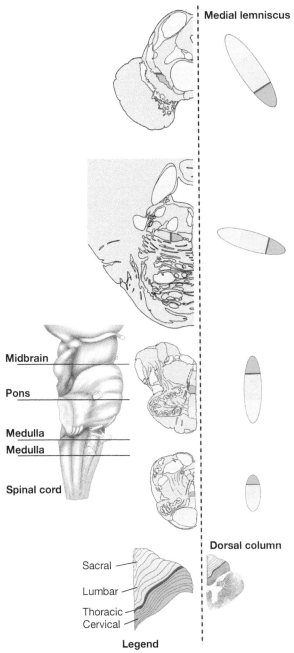

FIGURE 9-25 Somatotopic organization of the dorsal column–medial lemniscal system within the brainstem. Note that in the medulla the medial lemniscus is oriented vertically, but in the pons it is oriented horizontally.

Axons from the VPL nucleus project to the cerebral cortex via the posterior limb of the internal capsule. These axons form part of a more extensive thalamocortical radiation.

VPL axons terminate in many areas of the cerebral cortex. Most end on specific cells of the **primary somatosensory cortex (SI)** located in the postcentral gyrus (Brodmann's areas 3, 1, 2). Some end in the **second somatosensory cortex (SII)** located at the base of the postcentral gyrus on the superior bank of the Sylvian fissure. Some end in the **primary motor cortex (MI)** located in the precentral gyrus (Brodmann's area 4). Cortical motor neurons of area

4 respond with short latencies to joint movement, skin contact, and changes in muscle length or tension in the contralateral limb. Some end in the **supplementary motor area (SMA)** located on the medial hemispheral surface (part of Brodmann's area 6). Some terminate in the **superior parietal lobule** (Brodmann's areas 5 and 7).

Cells of the postcentral gyrus possess a detailed somatotopic organization referred to as the somatosensory homunculus (see Figure 7-7). In the classical somatosensory homunculus, the representation of the body is inverted medial-laterally with respect to the somatotopic organization of the VPL, due to a medial-lateral inversion of the thalamocortical projection. Somatosensory cortex neurons receiving information that originated from receptors of the hand are located most laterally (and ventrally) in the gyrus. Those receiving information from the trunk are located most dorsally in the gyrus. Those receiving information from the legs are located on the portion of the gyrus situated on the medial surface of the hemisphere.

Multiple representations of each body part actually exist in the postcentral gyrus so that the somatotopic map is quite complicated. Each representation of a given body part receives information from different receptors. However, the different representations in Brodmann's areas 3, 1, and 2 are in register with each other (e.g., the hand regions are adjacent to each other in these Brodmann areas and occupy the same medial-lateral position, resulting in parallel homunculi). Each representation plays a unique role in sensation. Thus, for example, information about limb position from muscle and joint receptors terminates in Brodmann's areas 2 and 3a, whereas tactile sensation, conveyed by mechanoreceptors, terminates in Brodmann's areas 1 and 3b. All somatotopic maps on the postcentral gyrus are anatomically distorted because they are based on innervation density and not body geometry. Those parts of the body with disproportionately large cortical volumes and cortical processing have the largest representation. This explains the distorted homuncular view of the hands/fingers, lips/tongue, and genitals as compared with the trunk.

Efferent Modulation

The thalamic nuclei play important modulatory roles in relation to processing both somatosensory and motor information. The activity of neurons of the DCN is regulated by projections descending from the cerebral cortex. These projections arise from neurons in the primary somatosensory cortex, the secondary somatosensory cortex (fewer), the primary motor cortex, and the supplementary motor cortex. Descending control also derives from the reticular formation, the cerebellum, and the caudate nucleus. Descending control may set the activity of DCN interneurons so that they influence relay neurons in a way enabling the relay neurons to extract that information most relevant to a particular sensory discrimination. For example, descending control may sharpen the spatial resolution of somatosensory signals. Descending control may inhibit the transmission of cutaneous information before and during a voluntary limb movement so as to enhance continued transmission of the proprioceptive information that is most relevant to the brain's capacity to control movement.

VPL neurons, like DCN neurons, are subject to descending modulatory inputs originating from the cortical regions to which they project. They also are subject to modulation originating in other thalamic nuclei as well as from the brainstem reticular formation. Thus, neither VPL nor DCN neurons are simple relays transmitting unaltered information from peripheral receptors.

Thought Question

What is efferent modulation, and where do the projections come from that are used for modulation of sensory stimuli?

Function

The function of the DC-ML system is best appreciated by discussing its role in everyday behavior and in functional collaboration with the motor system. The inactive hand is a poor communicator of information about an object placed in it. But once it begins to manipulate the object, once the hand is transformed into a structure that is active and exploratory in controlling the amount and kind of sensory information its receptors generate, the object is readily identified. A succession of exploratory finger movements is used in which the fingers curve around the surface of the object, fit into its cavities, explore its contours and texture by gentle rubbing, etc. The size, shape, and texture of the object are rapidly and accurately conveyed by the DC-ML system from the hand's somatic receptors to the brain's centers for perception. It is a sequential integration of this spatial and temporal information by the brain that makes form perception possible. Thus, somatosensory input, in the absence of movement, is of limited use in many aspects related to sensory perception. The parallel involvement of sensation and movement is illustrated by the size of those hand representations in the areas of the cerebral cortex that control hand movement (the primary motor cortex) and those that analyze the sensory input received from its somatic receptors (the primary somatosensory cortex). The latter includes not only sensory information that is passively received but, more importantly, that which is generated as a consequence of the hand's own movements. Neurons in the somatosensory and motor cortices are massively interconnected by short association fibers.

With respect to everyday, normal behavior, then, the DC-ML and motor systems are considered as a single neural complex, a functional entity in which the activity of one system is inseparable from that of the other. The function of this complex is to increase the precision of somatosensory guidance of motor activity and to increase the precision of motor guidance of somatosensory-generated activity. Thus, to define the function of the DC-ML system solely in terms of its role in discriminative somatic sensation does not adequately define its overall behavioral significance.

The intimate relationship between the DC-ML system and movement is, in fact, reflected in certain of the sensory discriminations uniquely mediated by the system. Such discriminations demand a sequential analysis of stimulus features and a simultaneous transformation over time and space of somatosensory information for successful discrimination. Typically, this is achieved by self-initiated contactual movement (scanning) and/or active palpation of a stimulus object. There is then a dynamic interplay of movement with superficial (i.e., cutaneous) and deep (e.g., muscle) somatic mechanoreceptors. Thus, for example, monkeys with isolated DC-ML lesions can no longer discriminate between discs that have complex shapes cut into their surfaces. Successful discrimination requires active exploratory movements of the fingers in which the skin surface is sequentially moved along the edges of the engraved pattern. Stereognosis likewise is impaired in patients with DC-ML lesions.

As discussed later, some tests used in the neurologic examination of sensation to assess DC-ML function do not depend on self-initiated contactual movement. Rather, they involve a sequential analysis of stimulus features and a simultaneous spatiotemporal analysis of mechanoreceptive information. One such test is the ability to discriminate the direction in which a tactile stimulus is moved across the skin; another is the capacity to identify a geometric figure, letter, or number drawn on the skin (graphesthesia).

Spinothalamic Tract

General Information

The STT, a component of the AL system, the second of the two major pathways projecting information from the body periphery to the cerebral cortex for conscious awareness, consists of two components that subserve different functions. These are a **neospinothalamic** component, the topic of this section, and a **paleospinothalamic** component, discussed in Chapter 16. As the name implies, the neospinothalamic component appears later in phylogeny. It attains its greatest elaboration in humans. The paleospinothalamic component is present in all mammals, including humans, and appears earlier in phylogeny. Both components have access to consciousness and thus involve neurons of the cerebral cortex.

The neospinothalamic component of the STT mediates touch, temperature, and a type of pain that is rapidly perceived, can be accurately scaled in its intensity, can be accurately localized on the body surface, and is of short duration. This type of pain is called *fast pain* and is conveyed by A-delta fibers. It is the type of pain tested in the neurologic examination with the prick of a pin to the skin surface. But we all know there is another type of pain, one that is enduring, aching, intense, and associated with a strong emotional component (stop!). This type of pain is called *slow pain*, and it is conveyed by C fibers. Slow pain is the exclusive province of the paleospinothalamic tract. We see now that the pain experience is dual in nature and that its separate components are mediated by separate sensory systems.

Because of their anatomical positions, these two pain systems have been called a lateral (neospinothalamic) pain system (which projects to the VPL) and a medial (paleospinothalamic) pain system (which projects to the medial thalamus). Unfortunately, nature does not allow us to distinguish between these two systems at the spinal cord level because the ascending fibers of the two systems intermingle with one another in the anterolateral funiculus of the spinal cord and because naturally occurring lesions to the spinal cord never are discrete enough to selectively damage just one system. However, the two pain systems can be distinguished anatomically in the brainstem (Chapter 16). Unless otherwise specified, in this section when the term STT is used, it applies to the neospinothalamic component.

Thought Question

What fiber type conveys fast pain? What is a typical conduction velocity for fast pain? What is the difference in the fibers and conduction velocity compared with those that convey slow pain?

This component of the STT comprises a set of neurons ascending in the anterolateral funiculus of the spinal cord that carry somatosensory information from the body periphery to the cerebral cortex for conscious discrimination. The neospinothalamic tract mediates the sensations of fast pain, temperature, and light touch as well as certain types of discriminative cutaneous sensibility. In contrast to the DC-ML system, the STT:

1. Is composed entirely of ascending fibers that are postsynaptic to the primary afferent neurons in the peripheral nerves.
2. Consists mostly of axons that cross in the spinal cord, but contains a clinically significant contingent of uncrossed ascending fibers.
3. Contains more neurons, and, therefore, more synaptic junctions, in the projection from the receptor to the cerebral cortex.
4. Is composed of smaller-diameter, more lightly myelinated, and, therefore, more slowly conducting fibers.
5. Does not exhibit a high degree of somatotopic organization.
6. Is composed primarily of neurons that respond to more than one modality of peripheral stimulation.
7. Processes information more in terms of the pattern of neural activity within the system rather than in terms of the somatotopic organization of the system.
8. Sends collateral branches into the brainstem reticular formation.

Neospinothalamic tract function, unlike that of the DC-ML system, has been defined largely with respect to the tract's relevance to clinical neurology.

Sensory End Organs

As noted earlier, some of the receptors that send information into the DC-ML system also send information into the neospinothalamic component of the STT. These would include free nerve endings, Pacinian corpuscles, Meissner's corpuscles, and articular receptors. However, not all receptors that feed information into the neospinothalamic system have been identified. Thus, it is more common to indicate the peripheral stimuli to which STT fibers respond than it is to specify the types of receptors sending information into the system. While not all such peripheral stimuli to which STT neurons respond have been identified, they include pressure, heat, joint rotation, distortion of muscle–fascia relations, hair displacement, and light mechanical distortion of the skin.

Primary Afferents (First-Order Neurons)

Primary afferents of the STT consist predominantly of smaller-diameter, lightly myelinated, A-delta nerve fibers. They enter the spinal cord over the lateral division of the dorsal root. Most of these dorsal root fibers then enter the dorsolateral fasciculus of the spinal cord, where they ascend or descend for variable numbers of segments (usually one to three). The dorsolateral fasciculus is present at all spinal cord levels. These fibers and their collateral branches terminate on neurons in various laminae of the dorsal horn (discussed later). Within the dorsal horn are low-threshold neurons, high-threshold neurons, and wide, dynamic-range (WDR) neurons (Chapter 16). The low-threshold neurons respond to innocuous stimuli, the high threshold neurons respond to noxious stimuli, and the WDR neurons respond to both noxious and innocuous stimuli.

Some of the primary afferents that synapse on neurons whose axons enter the AL system are collateral branches of fibers in the DCs. These fibers are of larger diameter and are more heavily myelinated than those of the dorsolateral fasciculus. They convey information from touch, pressure articular, and other types of mechanoreceptors.

Primary afferents synapse in several locations in the dorsal horn (Figure 9-26 ■). Some terminate on cells of the marginal layer (Rexed's lamina I) that form a thin band capping the substantia gelatinosa (Rexed's lamina II). Others end on cells of the substantia gelatinosa. Some afferents of the AL system, and especially the A-delta and A-beta afferents, terminate in the deep layers of the dorsal horn (and in particular in lamina V, where the WDR neurons are located).

Projections

SECOND-ORDER NEURONS The cell bodies of the second-order neurons of the STT are located in the Rexed's laminae I (marginal layer of the dorsal horn) and II (substantia gelatinosa) and wide, dynamic-range neurons in lamina V. Axons from cells in the marginal layer cross in the anterior (ventral) white commissure and enter the contralateral anterior funiculus, where they turn rostral and ascend to the thalamus as the anterolateral tract. Axons from cells in the substantia gelatinosa project deeper into the dorsal horn,

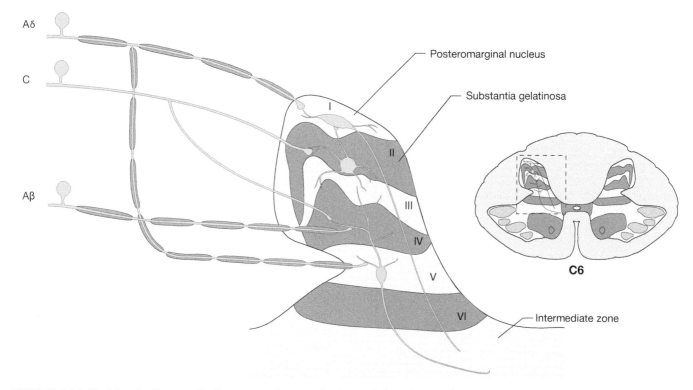

FIGURE 9-26 Peripheral afferent pain fibers enter the posterior horn of the spinal cord and synapse in laminae I–V. The axons that enter the spinothalamic tract (STT) are derived from neurons located in different lamina of the spinal gray.

where they synapse on third-order neurons located in the nucleus proprius (Rexed's laminae III and IV) and/or in the intermediate zone of the spinal gray (Rexed's lamina VII) (see Figure 9-26). Additional synapses with other interneurons may occur in the spinal gray. Axons from cells of the nucleus proprius or intermediate zone enter either the contralateral (most) or ipsilateral anterolateral fasciculus, in which they ascend to the thalamus. The synapses that occur in the spinal cord gray matter make it impossible to say whether specific neurons in the anterolateral system are second-, third-, or higher-order neurons. Some are true second-order neurons, but not all.

Most axons originating from neurons of the dorsal horn and intermediate gray matter cross in the anterior white commissure to enter the contralateral anterolateral fasciculus; most of these axons decussate after ascending no more than two spinal levels from their origin. New, crossing fibers from each more rostral cord level are added to the forming anterolateral tract at its medial edge. This gives the neospinothalamic tract a somatotopic organization such that in the cervical levels, the longest fibers—those from the leg (e.g., sacral and lumbar levels)—are located most superficially (dorsolaterally), while those from the arm (cervical levels) are positioned most ventromedially. The somatotopy is not as precise as that characterizing the DC-ML system but, nevertheless, is clinically important. A small subset of axons enters the anterolateral fasciculus on the ipsilateral side, also a fact of clinical importance (see Clinical Connections). Neospinothalamic fibers, both ipsilateral and contralateral, ascending in the

anterolateral funiculus intermingle with those of other ascending and descending systems.

Throughout the medulla, neospinothalamic fibers are positioned near the lateral edge of the brainstem between the inferior olivary complex ventrally and the spinal trigeminal complex dorsally. They are considerably lateral to the medial lemniscus at the level of the medulla. Neospinothalamic afferents retain the same relative brainstem position in the pons as they occupied in the medulla. In caudal pons, the STT is still well lateral to the medial lemniscus, which has not yet flattened out into a horizontally oriented ribbon. It is separated from the ML by a clear area occupied by the superior olivary nucleus. However, at a midpontine level and in more rostral pons where the ML has assumed a definitive mediolateral orientation, the ML and STT are adjacent to one another with the STT system positioned immediately lateral to the ML. Neospinothalamic afferents continue to be located at the lateral edge of the ML throughout the midbrain. As a result, they shift somewhat dorsally in their midbrain ascent. Thus, the brainstem trajectory, beginning in the pons of the neospinothalamic tract, follows that of the ML. In its ascent through the brainstem, the neospinothalamic tract, unlike the ML, gives off collateral branches to the reticular formation (Figure 9-27 ■).

Thought Question

Contrast the origin of the second-order neurons for the DC-ML pathway with those of the STT.

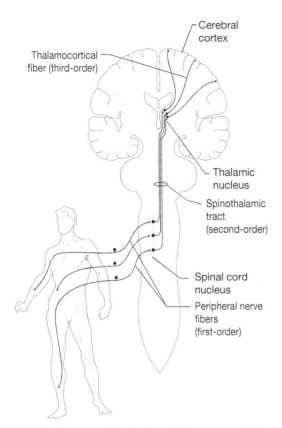

Cerebral cortex

Thalamocortical fiber (third-order)

Thalamic nucleus

Spinothalamic tract (second-order)

Spinal cord nucleus

Peripheral nerve fibers (first-order)

FIGURE 9-27 The overall trajectory of the neospinothalamic component of the anterolateral system through the spinal cord, brainstem, and thalamus en route to its termination in the primary somatosensory cortex of the postcentral gyrus. In contrast to the DC-ML system, most axons of the STT tract decussate in the spinal cord.

THIRD-ORDER NEURONS The cell bodies of the third-order (and higher-order) neurons are located in the VPL nucleus of the thalamus. Prior to entering the VPL nucleus, neospinothalamic and ML afferents merge into a common topographic pattern. Most neurons in VPL nucleus that respond to noxious peripheral stimuli also respond to innocuous mechanical stimulation, befitting the role of the STT in both touch and pain. (This is the wide, dynamic-range neuron channel of the AL system.) However, there are some neurons in VPL that only respond to noxious peripheral stimuli. (This is the nociceptive-specific neuron channel of the AL system.) Moreover, these VPL neurons have a somatotopic organization that parallels that of the cells that receive DC-ML input.

Third-order axons from the VPL nucleus ascend in association with those of the DC-ML system in the posterior limb of the internal capsule to terminate in the primary somatosensory cortex (i.e., the postcentral gyrus). Recall that this information originated predominantly from the the contralateral side of the body.

Efferent Modulation

Descending control of afferent transmission in the neospinothalamic tract is more pronounced, specific, and complex than in the DC-ML system. The control is

Thought Question

Now is a good time to synthesize the structure and functional implications of the DC-ML pathway and STT. Draw these two pathways. Where does each system decussate, and what is the functional implication with respect to nervous system lesions? Where are the cell bodies for the third-order neurons? What is the functional implication of the final destination in the cortex?

exerted on interneurons and cells of origin of the STT located in the dorsal horn and intermediate gray. The effects may be excitatory or inhibitory and may be exerted either presynaptically or postsynaptically. Structures that influence transmission in the neospinothalamic tract include the sensorimotor cortex, the cerebellum, the brainstem reticular formation, and the dorsal column nuclei. Descending control from the sensorimotor cortex, for example, inhibits the transmission of tactile stimuli without affecting the transmission of noxious stimulation.

Function

The neospinothalamic tract and the DC-ML system are interdependent and operate in parallel. Their parallel operation derives from the following features:

1. Naturally occurring stimuli activate receptors whose primary afferents engage both systems.
2. A subset of primary dorsal column afferents that synapse in the DCN give off collateral branches that synapse as well on cells of origin of the STT.
3. Some dorsal horn neurons that send information into the STT also send information into the DC-ML system (postsynaptic afferents in the DCs).
4. Neurons of the dorsal horn and DCN are linked reciprocally by interneurons.

Tactile sensibility thus survives lesions confined to one of the two systems, even though careful testing will reveal specific deficits. The occurrence of specific types of deficits following a lesion to one tract means that the two systems do not provide cortical analyzing centers with redundant information. Each system's relay nuclei perform unique operations on sometimes similar peripheral input.

Neospinothalamic system function, unlike that of the DC-ML system, has been defined largely with respect to the system's relevance to clinical neurology. The neospinothalamic tract mediates (1) fast (cutaneous, superficial) pain as defined earlier, (2) temperature sensibility, and (3) a number of aspects of tactile sensibility. The latter includes not only the detection and recognition of having been touched on the body surface but also certain aspects of discriminative tactile sensation such as the ability to localize where on the body surface contact has occurred (point localization), the capacity to discriminate the texture (roughness) of an object or surface, and the capacity to discriminate whether the skin has been contacted by one or two points (two-point discrimination).

Table 9-3 ▦ summarizes the differences between the DC-ML pathway and neospinothalamic component of the STT.

CLINICAL CONNECTIONS
Disorders of Peripheral Nerves

The term **neuropathy** is a general one meaning a disease of peripheral nerves. The location of neuropathy can be focal, involving a single peripheral nerve (**mononeuropathy**), or general, involving many peripheral nerves (**polyneuropathy**). A neuropathy affecting spinal nerve roots is called a **radiculopathy**. In general, neuropathies affect both sensory and motor fibers in the nerve, although one or the other may be preferentially involved. Any neuropathy involving sensory nerves usually causes a loss of autonomic function in the same zones as the somatosensory loss (Chapter 12).

Diabetes mellitus (DM) is the most common cause of polyneuropathy. And the most common polyneuropathy in diabetes mellitus is the distal, symmetrical, primarily sensory type. The patient complains of persistent and often distressing pain, numbness, and tingling affecting the feet and lower legs symmetrically. Deep Achilles tendon reflexes are absent as are, occasionally, knee jerk reflexes (Chapter 11). Somatosensory loss (**analgesia**) is most effectively tested with pin prick. The sensory loss can lead to injury because the individual may not be aware of damaging situations. A classic example is the frequent breakdown of tissue of the foot in people with diabetes because they are not aware of blisters and sores resulting from poorly fitting shoewear. In some people, a loss of deep sensation predominates, resulting in sensory ataxia, an uncoordinated gait due to the loss of proprioception from the lower extremities, and autonomic signs (e.g., loss of bladder muscle tone). The symptoms in the latter individuals resemble those seen in tabes dorsalis (see Clincial Connections).

Diabetes can also result in a radiculopathy. However, by far the most common cause of radiculopathy is intervertebral disc herniation (Chapter 5). Neuropathies affecting the motor system are discussed in Chapter 10.

Table 9-3 Differences between the DC-ML Pathway and the Spinothalamic Tract

FEATURE	DC-ML PATHWAY	STT*
Position in the spinal cord	Dorsal funiculi	Anterior and lateral funiculi
Ascending spinal cord fibers	Primary afferents	Second- or higher-order afferents
Modality specificity	Each sensory modality is carried by a separate set of afferents	Polymodal neurons that respond to more than one modality of sensation
Somatotopic organization	High	Low
Diameter of nerve fibers	Larger diameter and more heavily myelinated	Smaller diameter and more lightly myelinated
Number of synapses	At most, three neurons in the cerebral cortex	At least three neurons in the cerebral cortex
Speed of transmission	Fast	Slower
Collateral branches to the reticular formation	Few	Many
Sensations mediated (as tested in the neurologic exam)	Kinesthesia, stereognosis, graphesthesia, direction of tactile stimulus, vibration	Fast pain, temperature, light touch, some discriminative touch
Level of decussation	Brainstem	Spinal cord
Size of receptive fields	Smaller	Larger
Efferent modulation	Yes, but less extensive	Yes, and more extensive

*Neospinothalamic component

Syndromes Related to the DC-ML Pathway

Considerable variability is found in the clinical presentation of people with damage to the dorsal columns. This variability may be accounted for by several factors. First, if even a small proportion of fibers in the DC escape destruction, it appears that much discriminative sensibility survives. Conversely, lesions in humans seldom limit themselves just to the DC.

Tabes dorsalis is a tertiary form of syphilis and is often cited as a model of dorsal column disease. However, tabes dorsalis is essentially an inflammation of the dorsal roots, not a primary affliction of the DC (Figure 9-28 ■). It is this posterior radiculitis that is responsible for the degeneration of the long ascending fibers in the DC and the consequent somotosensory losses. Such peripheral degeneration is not expected to substantively affect the structure of second-order fibers in the DC or the second-order fibers of the dorsolateral fasciculus; nonetheless, these fibers would be deprived of input from peripheral receptors, and therefore, they are functionally compromised.

Spinal Cord Pathology

A number of spinal cord disorders have been described that are helpful for understanding the clinical anatomy of the spinal cord. These disorders affect ascending somatosensory tracts. However, they also invariably involve descending upper motor neuron (UMN) tracts and lower motor neurons (LMNs) in the ventral horn as well. Hence, these disorders result in both somatosensory and motor signs. In this chapter, we focus only on the somatosensory findings associated with three classic "teaching disorders." The full clinical pictures characterizing such disorders therefore are deferred to Chapter 11 where the motor system is presented along with illustrations of each disorder.

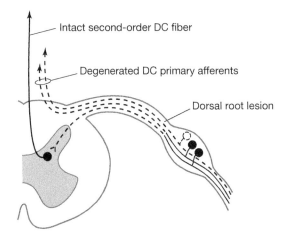

FIGURE 9-28 The degeneration of dorsal root fibers from tabes dorsalis (dotted) would result in a degeneration of primary, but not second-order afferents in the dorsal columns. This means that tabes dorsalis is not an entirely accurate model of dorsal column disease.

Traumatic injury involving one-half of the spinal cord produces the **Brown-Sequard syndrome**. Such injury affects a number of spinal cord structures mediating sensation. First, the injury would interrupt all fibers entering the spinal cord over the dorsal roots in the segments of injury. Consequently, there is an ipsilateral zone of somatosensory anesthesia (loss of all sensation) in the dermatomes innervated by the damaged segments. Second, the interruption of dorsal column fibers would cause an ipsilateral loss of proprioception (e.g., position sense, kinesthesia, and vibration sensibility) in dermatomes below the lesion. A loss of proprioception from the legs, as by a thoracic lesion, would result in a sensory gait ataxia. Third, damage to fibers of the spinothalamic tract would result in a loss of pain and temperature sensibility below the level of the lesion on the contralateral side of the body. The somatosensory loss would begin one or two segments below the level of the lesion. This is because pain and temperature afferents destined to enter the contralateral spinothalamic tract ascend one or two segments from their level of entry before completing their decussation.

Syringomyelia is a disease process resulting in a lesion that begins in the center of the spinal cord, usually over a variable number of cervical segments. Thus, the lesion first interrupts pain and temperature fibers that cross in the anterior (ventral) white commissure. Syringomyelia, therefore, is characterized by an early bilateral loss of pain and temperature sensibility typically in the hands and arms.

Subacute combined degeneration is a disorder that typically first involves fibers of the dorsal columns of the spinal cord, only later involving the motor system. Early on, the patient complains of paresthesias localized to the fingers and toes with a symmetric bilateral distribution. Typical dorsal column deficits then appear especially in the legs. The loss of proprioception results in an unsteady, ataxic gait.

Examination of the Somatosensory Systems

Testing of somatic sensation can be the most difficult part of the neurological examination, largely because it relies so much on the capacity and cooperation of patients to report what they are feeling. Several facts should be borne in mind in conducting an evaluation of somatosensory systems. For one thing, these sensory tests are only remotely related to the sensory transactions that occur in everyday life. The stimuli themselves are very artificial, and each test, with the exception of stereognosis, is preceded by verbal instruction of expected responses and "do this" demonstration.

Furthermore, it is important to understand that testing of these systems alone cannot precisely localize damage but must be interpreted in combination with other information. For example, loss of proprioception can result from damage anywhere from the peripheral receptors (as in burn injuries), to the afferent peripheral neurons, to the dorsal columns of the spinal cord, to the medial lemniscus of the brainstem, or to the primary somatosensory cortex. Hence, testing of proprioception in isolation may be of little value for purposes of localizing a lesion to a particular subdivision of the nervous system.

When disease or injury does affect the spinal cord, a number of specific tests can be used to further locate the lesion. See Table 9-4 ■ for examples.

Interventions Related to the Somatosensory Systems

Physical Interventions That Utilize the Somatosensory Systems

Rehabilitation specialists frequently utilize the somatosensory system in physical intervention. Many of the techniques utilizing the somatosensory system can either excite or inhibit muscle activity, depending on speed, degree of pressure, and direction of movement. Examples include stretch of muscles across a joint (e.g., by rotating the joint into flexion, extension), compression of joints, and touch and pressure to the belly of the muscle. Transcutaneous electrical stimulation utilizes the somatosensory systems to reduce pain (Chapter 16).

Surgical Interventions for Somatosensory Problems

So-called **spinothalamic tractotomies** are occasionally performed for the relief of intractable pain—most often in the lower trunk or leg, particularly in terminally ill patients. This produces an analgesia and thermoanesthesia on the side opposite the lesion, beginning at least one segment caudal to the lesion (this is the upper border of the somatosensory loss). Some reduction of tactile sensibility also occurs.

The procedure is more properly referred to as a **cordotomy** because a section of the entire anterior quadrant of the spinal cord is necessary to produce an effective analgesia. The procedure may be accomplished as an open operation (involving a laminectomy) or transcutaneously in which a radio-frequency lesion is produced by an electrode. Analgesia and thermoanesthesia persist for varying periods of time (perhaps a year or longer), after which some degree of pain sensibility returns and pain recurs. The recurrence of pain is attributed to the uncrossed ascending fibers that gradually take over the function previously subserved by crossed fibers.

Table 9-4 Tests to Assess Somatosensory System Integrity

MODALITY	TEST	COLUMN OR TRACT
Pain (fast pain)	Examiner randomly alternates stimulating the skin with the sharp (pin prick) or dull end of a safety pin.	Anterolateral
Temperature	Examiner places tubes with hot or cold water on the skin of the patient.	Anterolateral
Light touch	Examiner strokes the skin of the patient with a wisp of cotton.	Anterolateral
Point localization	Examiner touches points on the body and patient places index finger on point stimulated.	DC-ML
Two-point discrimination	Distances between two points stimulated on the skin are determined.	DC-ML/AL
Position sense	Patient has eyes closed and examiner moves body segments (e.g., finger, ankle, toe) into flexion or extension. The patient identifies the position of the body part.	DC-ML
Kinesthesia	Patient has eyes closed and the examiner moves one extremity through space. The patient mimics the movement with the contralateral extremity.	DC-ML
Graphesthesia	Patient has eyes closed and the examiner draws a geometric symbol, number, or letter on the skin, or draws a line in a specific direction.	DC-ML
Stereognosis	Without the use of vision, patient identifies objects (e.g., coins, a key) placed in the hand by manipulation.	DC-ML
Vibratory sense	Examiner places a vibrating tuning fork over a bony prominence.	DC-ML

Neuropathology Box 9-1: Is it really possible to test the STT and DC-ML Systems?

The dorsal column–medial lemniscal (DC-ML) system typically is thought of as the system that carries information about discriminative touch in the CNS. Indeed, testing of discriminative touch is considered a standard test of the DC-ML system in the neurological examination. However, complete transection of the dorsal columns in monkeys does not eliminate their ability to respond to certain discriminative touch sensations, indicating that the anterolateral (AL) system also carries some discriminative cutaneous sensations. Assuming that the function of the DC-ML system of humans is analogous to that of monkeys, loss of discriminative touch sensibility does not specifically identify lesions in this system. From a clinical perspective, this distinction between the

DC-ML pathway and STT in conveying discriminative touch is not of tremendous significance, because no single system typically is impaired by neurological damage. Two sensory tests, typically used in patients who have peripheral or spinal damage, to identify damage in the DC-ML system are stereognosis and graphesthesia.

From a clinical perspective, it is important to use tests of the somatosensory system because the presence, absence, or diminution of these modalities is of functional importance. Furthermore, from a learning perspective, it is helpful to relate tracts with tests, as outlined in this text. The caveat is that we may not definitively know which specific tracts are involved, based on the findings.

Summary

This chapter began with a survey of somatic receptors, that is, receptors residing in structures of the body. A variety of schemes have been developed by which to classify different receptor types, ranging from purely structural to purely functional (adaptation rate). All such schemes overlap to some extent. Regardless of receptor type, transduction in somatic receptors always occurs in the membrane of the peripheral nerve terminal of a primary afferent fiber. Non-neural cells associated with some types of mechanoreceptors may condition how the terminal transduces environmental energy, but they do not determine the type of stimulus energy to which the receptor responds, which is determined by molecular mechanisms in the nerve terminal itself. Information coding in receptors by generator potentials is analog coding, whereas information coding in axons by action potentials is digital in nature. Primary afferent fibers in peripheral nerves can be classified by axon diameter and conduction velocity, the two being related. Many different primary afferent fibers can be classified by the sensations they evoke when stimulated electrically.

Two major ascending sensory systems, the DC-ML and AL, are involved in carrying somatic information to the cerebral cortex for conscious interpretation. Within

these systems, we focused on the DC-ML pathway and STT. Their structure varies markedly, and this conditions their functional properties. Moreover, the STT has two markedly different structural components: a neospinothalamic and a paleospinothalamic, whose functions are dramatically different. This chapter concerns only the neospinothalamic component of the STT. The DC-ML system is adapted for high-speed transmission with a high degree of spatial resolution. It thus is specialized for transmitting mechanical information that varies rapidly over time, such as the direction and speed of limb movement and the capacity to discriminate the three-dimensional shape of an object by manipulating it in the hand. In contrast, the capacity for spatial resolution and high-speed transmission of mechanoreceptive information in the STT is limited by its smaller-diameter axons, more synapses, and fewer fibers. Additionally, different receptor types preferentially feed into the STT, namely, thermoreceptors and A-delta nociceptors. Thus, the neospinothalamic component of the STT is adapted to transmit low-resolution tactile information, as well as temperature and fast pain information. This chapter ends with a discussion of clinical connections related to the somatosensory systems.

Applications

1. Jason, 20 years old, noticed that he frequently burned his fingers when cooking, although he did not experience discomfort. Later, he developed ulcers on the fingers. These were slow to heal and were relatively painless. The only neurological finding following a careful examination was a bilateral loss of sensitivity to pain and temperature over his hands, forearms, elbows, and upper arm.

   a. What sensory tract carries the pain and temperature information?
   b. Describe the pathway of the tract.
   c. James has loss of pain and temperature bilaterally. What single lesion could cause James's bilateral symptoms?
   d. On a drawing of the spinal cord, shade the area of the lesion, and explain the neurological findings.

2. The two major pathways mediating somatic sensation from the body are the dorsal column–medial lemniscal (DC-ML) tract and the spinothalamic tract (STT). Damage anywhere along the major somatic sensation pathways can result in abnormalities in sensory function.

   a. Identify the sensory deficits that would be associated with damage to each of these major pathways.
   b. With injury in each of the following locations, indicate the specific losses that would occur:
      i. Right radial nerve.
      ii. Right C6 nerve root.
      iii. Right dorsal column at C5.
      iv. Right anterolateral fasciculus at C5.
      v. Anterior white commissure at C5.
      vi. Right VPL of thalamus.
      vii. Right postcentral gyrus.

References

Somatic Receptors

Berrymann, L. J., Yau, J. M., and Hsiao, S. S. Representation of object size in the somatosensory system. *J Neurophysiol* 96:27–39, 2006.

Bodegard, A., Geyer, S., Herath, P., et al. Somatosensory areas engaged during discrimination of steady pressure, spring strength, and kinesthesia. *Hum Brain Mapp* 20:103–115, 2003.

Bodegard, A., Geyer, S., Naito, E., Zilles, K., and Roland, P. E. Somatosensory areas in man activated by moving stimuli. Cytoarchitectonic mapping and PRT. *Neuro Report* 11:187–191, 2000.

Bodegard, A., Geyer, S., Grefkes, C., Zilles, K., and Roland, P. E. Hierarchial processing of tactile shape in the human brain. *Neuron* 31:317–328, 2001.

Collins, D. F., Refshauge, K. M., Todd, G., and Gandevia, S. C. Cutaneous receptors contribute to kinesthesia at the index finger, elbow, and knee. *J Neurophysiol* 94:1699–1706, 2005.

Edin, B. B., and Johansson, N. Skin strain patterns provide kinesthetic information to the human central nervous system. *J Physiol* 15:243–251, 1995.

Gilhodes, J. C., Roll, J. P., and Tardy-Gervet, M. F. Perceptual and motor effects of agonist-antagonist muscle vibration in man. *Exp Brain Res* 61:395-402, 1986.

Golaszewski, S. M., Siedentopf, C. M., Koppelstaetter, F., et al. Modulatory effects on human sensorimotor cortex by whole-hand afferent electrical stimulation. *Neurol* 62:2262–2269, 2004.

Goodwin, A. W. Paradoxes in tactile adaptation. Focus on "vibratory adaptation in cutaneous mechanoreceptive afferents" and "time-course of vibratory adaptation and recovery in cutaneous mechanoreceptive afferents." *J Neurophysiol* 94:2995–2996, 2005.

Goodwin, G. M., McCloskey, D. I., and Matthews, P. B. The contribution of muscle afferents to kinesthesia shown by vibration induced illusions of movement and by the effects of paralyzing join afferents. *Brain* 95:705–748, 1972.

Johansson, R. S., and Vallbo, A. B. Tactile sensibility in the human hand: Relative and absolute densities of four types of mechanoreceptive units in the glabrous skin area. *J Physiol* (London) 286:293–300, 1979.

Kawashima, N., et al. Alternate leg movement amplifies locomotor-like muscle activity in spinal cord injured persons. *J Neurophysiol* 93:777–785, 2005.

Macefield, V. G., Hager-Ross, C., and Johansson, R. S. Control of grip force during restraint of an object held between fingers and thumb: Responses of cutaneous afferents from the digits. *Exp Brain Res* 108:155–171, 1996.

Mahns, D. A., Perkins, N. M., Sahai, V., Robinson, L., and Rowe, M. J. Vibrotactile feequency discrimination in human hairy skin. *J Neurophysiol* 95:1442–1450, 2006.

Mountcastle, V. B. *The Sensory Hand: Neural Mechanisms of Somatic Sensation*. Harvard University Press, Cambridge, 2005.

Naito, E., Ehrsson, H. H., Geyer, S., Zilles, K., and Roland, P. E. Illusory arm movements activate cortical motor areas: A PET study. *J Neurosci* 19:6134–6144, 1999.

Reinisch, C. M., and Tschachler, E. The touch dome in human skin is supplied by different types of nerve fibers. *Ann Neurol* 58:88–95, 2005.

Roland, P. E., and Mortensen, E. Somatosensoy detection of microgeometry, macrogeometry and kinesthesia in man. *Brain Res Rev* 12:1–41, 1987.

Dorsal Column–Medial Lemniscal System

Connor, C. E., and Johnson, K. O. Neural coding of tactile texture: compairson of spatial and temporal mechanisms for roughness perception. *J Neurosci* 12:3414–3426, 1992.

Davidoff, R. A. The dorsal columns. *Neurol* 39:1377–1385, 1989.

Gibson, J. J. *The Senses Considered as Perceptual Systems*. Houghton Mifflin Company, Boston, 1966.

Golaszewski, S. M., Siedentopf, C. M., Koppelstaetter, F., et al. Modulatory effects on human sensorimotor cortex by whole-hand afferent electrical stimulation. *Neurol* 62:2262–2269, 2004.

Johnson, K. O., and Hsiao, S. S. Neural mechanisms of tactual form and texture perception. *Annu Rev Neurosci* 15:227–250, 1992.

Mountcastle, V. B. Neural mechanisms in somesthesis. In: Mountcastle, V. B. (ed.), *Medical Physiology*, Vol 1, 13th ed. C. V. Mosby, St. Louis, 1974.

Naito, E., Roland, P. E., Grefkes, C., et al. Dominance of the right hemisphere and role of area 2 in human kinesthesia. *J Neurophysiol* 93:1020–1034, 2005.

Wall, P. D. The sensory and motor role of impulses traveling in the dorsal columns toward the cerebral cortex *Brain* 93:505–524, 1970.

Wall, P. D., and Noordenbos, W. Sensory functions which remain in man after complete transection of dorsal columns. *Brain* 100:641, 1977.

Anterolateral System (Neospinothalamic)

Asbury, A. K., McKhann, G. M., McDonald, W. I., Goadsby, P. J., and McArthur, J. C., eds. *Diseases of the Nervous System: Clinical Neuroscience and Therapeutic Principles*, 3rd ed. Cambridge University Press, London, 2002.

Bradley, W. G., Daroff, R. B., Fenichel, G. M., and Jankovic, J., eds. *Neurology in Clinical Practice: Principles of Diagnosis and Management*, 4th ed. Butterworth Heinemann, 2004.

Brodal, A. *Neurological Anatomy in Relation to Clinical Medicine*, 3rd ed. Oxford University Press, New York, 1981.

Campbell, W. W. *DeJong's The Neurologic Examination*, 6th ed. Lippincott Williams & Wilkins, 2005.

Nolte, J. *The Human Brain: An Introduction to Its Functional Anatomy*. Mosby Elsevier, Philadelphia, 2009.

Heimer, L. *The Human Brain and Spinal Cord*, 2nd ed. Springer-Verlag, 1995.

10

Peripheral Components of the Motor System

LEARNING OUTCOMES

This chapter prepares the reader to:

1 Name the parts of the motor unit.

2 Explain the relationship of the motor unit to the striated muscle.

3 Explain how motor unit potentials are measured and describe the triphasic response.

4 Differentiate three muscle fiber types: red, white, and intermediate.

5 Discuss the relationship of the following: fiber type, motor unit lower motor neuron size, and synaptic current.

6 Describe the size principle in the recruitment of motor units and explain the functional significance of this principle.

7 Describe components of the neuromuscular junction and explain the functional importance.

8 Explain the role and significance of the sarcolemma end plate and junctional folds.

9 Explain generation of the end-plate potential and contrast this potential to the EPSP in the CNS.

10 Identify the consequence of damage to the lower motor neuron.

11 Differentiate the causes of paresis versus paralysis of a muscle.

12 Differentiate neurogenic from disuse atrophy.

13 Compare and contrast fibrillations and fasciculations in terms of underlying cause and expression of each.

14 Contrast neurogenic and myopathic disorders in terms of their origin and the resulting effects on the motor unit potential.

15 Identify the major categories of neuropathic disorders.

16 For the following disorders, identify the nature of the disorder (e.g., infectious, autoimmune), the part of the peripheral nervous system component affected, and the consequences of the disorder: diabetes mellitus (DM), Guillain-Barré syndrome (GBS), herpes zoster infection, and myasthenia gravis (MG).

17 Differentiate diseases of the upper motor neuron from diseases of the lower motor neuron.

18 Relate the pathology of common motor system diseases to the resulting symptoms.

ACRONYMS

ACh Acetylcholine

AChE Acetylcholinesterase (enzyme)

AIDP Acute inflammatory demyelinating polyneuropathy

ALS Amyotrophic lateral sclerosis (Lou Gehrig's disease)

DM Diabetes mellitus

EPP End-plate potential

EPSP Excitatory postsynaptic potential

GBS Guillain-Barré syndrome

LMN Lower motor neuron

MG Myasthenia gravis

UMN Upper motor neuron

Introduction

The marked structural and functional differences between the peripheral and central nervous systems have profound implications for rehabilitation of people with nervous system disorders. The basic differences between these two systems were outlined in Chapter 8, where the terms *upper* and *lower motor neuron* (UMN, LMN) were defined and the basic elements of the motor system were introduced. This chapter focuses on the motor components of the peripheral nervous system, building on the information that was presented previously.

The first section of this chapter discusses lower motor neuron innervation of muscles. We begin by defining the motor unit, which is an anatomical and functional entity by which alpha LMNs regulate the activity of striated muscle. The motor unit includes a single alpha LMN, its axon, and the group of muscle fibers it innervates. Each of these components is discussed. The different types of muscle fibers making up skeletal muscle and their unique functions are then discussed, followed by the structure and function of the neuromuscular junction.

With this information as background, disorders of the motor unit are considered in the second section of this chapter. Disorders of the motor unit are differentiated into those of muscle (myopathic) versus those of nerve (neurogenic). In this section of the chapter, we begin proximally (with disorders of the cell body) and proceed distally to the myopathies (diseases of muscle). We end this section with motor system diseases that affect both lower and upper motor neurons.

THE MOTOR UNIT: LOWER MOTOR NEURON INNERVATION OF MUSCLE

Clinical Preview · · · · · · · · · · · · · · · ·

In your wellness clinic, you work with a number of young girls from a variety of sports teams at the local high school. Carly is a long-distance runner, while Allegra is a sprinter. As you read through this section, consider the following:

- What types of motor unit does each girl rely upon most heavily for her specific sport?
- What types of muscle fibers are most utlized in each sport?
- How might the differences in motor unit requirements affect your strategy for training?

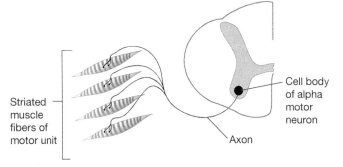

FIGURE 10-1 Each motor unit consists of a single alpha motor neuron and the group of striated muscle fibers it innervates. Alpha lower motor neurons reside in the CNS, and their axons extend to muscle in a peripheral nerve. Within the muscle, each axon divides repeatedly into a number of branches, each of which has a terminal on a single muscle fiber. The muscle fibers comprising the motor unit are distributed within the muscle.

Lower motor neuron (LMN) innervation of muscle involves a number of peripheral nervous system structures from the alpha motor neuron pool to the motor unit. We begin our description with the motor unit and progress proximally.

The Motor Unit

The **motor unit** is the fundamental structural and functional element of muscle. Each motor unit consists of a single alpha LMN, its axon, and the *group* of muscle fibers it innervates (Figure 10-1 ■). Each lower motor neuron innervates a single muscle; hence, a motor unit likewise innervates muscle cells within a single muscle. A striated muscle may be thought of as an assemblage of motor units, which collectively are referred to as the **motor pool** to that muscle. The muscle fibers innervated by a single lower motor neuron are not generally adjacent to one another in a muscle. Transmission across the neuromuscular junction is so efficient that a single action potential in the axon causes all of the muscle fibers comprising motor unit to contract.

A needle electrode inserted into muscle is able to record **motor unit potentials**. Motor unit potentials in normally innervated muscle are shown in Figure 10-2 ■ and later in Figure 10-6 under three conditions: at rest, where no potentials are recorded; during slight voluntary contraction, where a series of regularly spaced *triphasic* **muscle action potentials** are recorded; and during maximal voluntary contraction, where a complete interference pattern is recorded. In a complete **interference pattern**, previously inactive motor units have been recruited and the motor unit potentials overlap so that individual motor units can no longer be distinguished.

From a clinical perspective, it is important to understand that motor units can be made to discharge in the absence of input from UMNs. Therefore, the contraction of striated

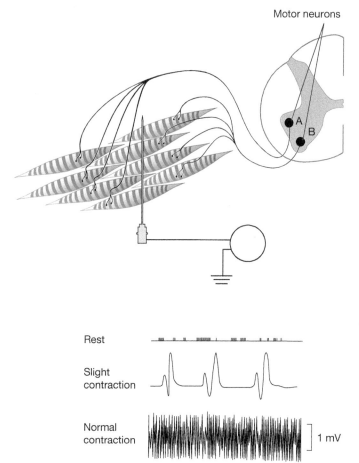

Motor neurons

Rest

Slight contraction

Normal contraction

1 mV

FIGURE 10-2 A motor unit potential is recorded by a needle inserted into healthy muscle. Trace patterns shown at rest, during slight contraction, and under a normal maximal contraction.

muscle is not dependent solely on activity in UMNs. This is because alpha LMNs (and motor units) are also innervated by input from peripheral receptors whose activity can elicit reflex contractions of skeletal muscle either by influencing LMNs directly or via local interneuronal networks, or both. This issue is discussed in detail in Chapter 11.

A given skeletal muscle may be contracted for different purposes. The gastrocnemius (the most superficial of the calf muscles), for example, must contract weakly, but for sustained periods, as we maintain an upright stance. In running, it must contract more forcefully, but its contraction cannot be maintained as long as in standing. Finally, in the most strenuous activities, such as jumping, gastrocnemius must contract still more forcefully (i.e., maximally) but even more briefly. These different purposes are fulfilled by the fact that this single muscle is made up of three

different kinds of striated muscle fibers, called red, white, and intermediate fibers. Indeed, all voluntary muscles are made up of a mixture of these three fiber types, although their proportions vary in different muscles.

Red fibers are thin because they have relatively few contractile filaments and can produce small amounts of tension for long periods without running down their energy stores. They are called *slow-twitch fibers*. This fatigue resistance is due to their reliance on oxidative catabolism wherein glucose and oxygen from the bloodstream can be used virtually indefinitely to regenerate the ATP that fuels the fiber's contractile machinery. Red fibers are surrounded by an extensive capillary network and contain large amounts of myoglobin (an oxygen-binding protein) that has a reddish color. **White fibers**, on the other hand, are larger, have fewer capillaries with red blood cells, and have relatively little myoglobin. They contract in brief, powerful twitches and rely exclusively on anaerobic catabolism to sustain force output. They are called *fast-twitch, fatigable fibers*. Their relatively large stores of glycogen are burned quickly, resulting in a rapid accumulation of lactic acid and muscle fatigue as they run out of fuel. **Intermediate fibers** have properties in between those of red and white fibers. They combine fast and relatively powerful twitch dynamics with sufficient aerobic capacity to resist fatigue for several minutes. They are called *fast-twitch, fatigue-resistant fibers*.

All of the muscle fibers within a given motor unit are of the same type so that there are three different types of motor units. Each type of motor unit is associated with an alpha LMN of unique size. Slow-twitch motor units, composed of red muscle fibers, are innervated by small alpha LMNs. The cell bodies of these alpha LMNs have small surface areas and their axons are of small diameter with relatively slow conduction velocities. Fast-twitch, fatigable motor units, composed of white muscle fibers, are innervated by the largest alpha LMNs. Their cell bodies have the largest surface area of any alpha LMNs and their axons the largest diameters with the fastest conduction velocities. Fast-twitch, fatigue-resistant motor units are composed of intermediate muscle fibers, innervated by alpha LMNs of intermediate size.

The association of the three types of motor unit with alpha LMNs of different sizes is the basis of the mechanism by which the nervous system grades the force of muscle contraction. Alpha LMNs making up a motor neuron pool innervating a given muscle have similar resting membrane potentials. Because the smallest alpha LMNs have the smallest surface area, they have the fewest number of leak channels and the greatest resistance to transmembrane

Thought Question

A motor unit can be made to discharge in the absence of input from the UMN. Explain this in terms of reflex arcs that you learned about in Chapter 8.

Thought Question

The amount of force produced by a muscle can be graded, depending on the type of fiber involved. What explains this observation?

current flow. An initially small excitatory synaptic current will produce large excitatory postsynaptic potentials (EPSPs) in small LMNs that reach threshold and generate action potentials (APs). But the same initially small excitatory drive does not generate an EPSP that reaches threshold in larger alpha LMNs. This is because the larger LMNs have larger surface areas, more leak channels, and a lower transmembrane resistance. Therefore, the small excitatory synaptic current generates smaller, subthreshold EPSPs, and the larger LMNs do not generate APs. As the synaptic drive to the motor neuron pool is increased, larger LMNs are recruited into the contraction as their EPSPs reach threshold magnitudes. They are recruited in a remarkably precise order, originally described by Elwood Henneman, according to the size of the alpha LMN. This is referred to as the **size principle** in the **recruitment** of motor units.

Figure 10-3 ■ shows how the size principle operates in building up force in a cat's gastrocnemius muscle during normal activities. During quiet standing, the small force required is generated by the exclusive discharge of slow-twitch motor units. More force is required as the cat begins to walk, then run. This is provided by the recruitment of fast-twitch, fatigue-resistant motor units. Maximal force is required when the cat jumps, and this requirement is met by the recruitment of fast-twitch, fatigable motor units into the discharge. Operation of the size principle is automatic. It is not under voluntary control and is preserved even in fast, ballistic movements.

In addition to recruitment, muscle tension is regulated by the firing rate of active motor neurons. During voluntary isometric contraction, as the force of contraction is increased, each motor unit that is recruited into the contraction progressively increases its firing rate up to a maximum of about 20 to 25 spikes per second.

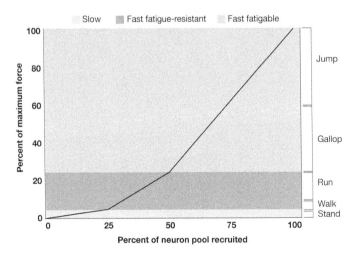

FIGURE 10-3 Recruitment of motor units in order of size in a cat's medial gastrocnemius muscle during different motor behaviors. Slow-twitch, small-motor units provide the tension for quiet standing. Fast, fatigue-resistant units are recruited next to generate the force required for running and walking. Fast, fatigable motor units are recruited last to provide force for more strenuous behavior such as galloping, and finally, to generate maximal forces for jumping.

Thought Question

Now is a good time to synthesize information. How many fiber types comprise a single motor unit? What is the relationship among fiber types, motor unit size, and alpha motor neuron size? Contrast the type of fibers that are most likely to be recruited for fine motor control (e.g., finger control when playing a piano) versus jumping activities.

The alpha LMNs of motor units also are involved in counteracting the effects of muscle fatigue. Prolonged and weak isometric contractions can result in neuromuscular fatigue. Alternating periods of activity and rest in individual motor units with *similar thresholds* (termed *rotation*) minimize neuromuscular fatigue by providing periods for the now-silent motor unit to undergo metabolic recovery of its contractile elements. The phenomenon of rotation applies to postural muscles, in which low-threshold units are expected to be active for prolonged periods of time, as well as to distal muscles of both the arm and leg in humans.

Neuromuscular Junction

The **neuromuscular junction** is a chemical synapse between the axon terminal of an alpha LMN and the sarcolemma of the striated muscle fiber. As with chemical synapses in the CNS, the neuromuscular junction exhibits both presynaptic and postsynaptic membrane specializations. Communication is mediated by a chemical released from the presynaptic neuron onto the receptive membrane of the postsynaptic neuron.

As the myelinated axon of an LMN approaches a muscle, it divides repeatedly. Once within the belly of the muscle, it branches even more extensively so that this single LMN axon is able to innervate all of the extrafusal muscle fibers comprising the particular motor unit. Each terminal branch loses its myelin sheath as it nears the sarcolemma, but the Schwann cell sheath continues to invest even the smallest terminal branches (Figure 10-4 ■). Each terminal branch forms multiple expansions, or varicosities, called *synaptic boutons*, each of which is covered by the Schwann cell sheath. The boutons contain numerous synaptic vesicles loaded with the neurotransmitter acetylcholine (ACh). The vesicles cluster around active zones, the sites of transmitter release. Voltage-gated Ca^{2+} channels are embedded in the presynaptic membrane immediately adjacent to the active zones.

Each bouton lies over a specialized region of the sarcolemma called the **end plate**, which is a trough created by an infolding of the sarcolemma. The bouton is separated

Thought Question

What is the physiological basis for the importance of a rest period to avoid muscle fatigue? How might this be applicable to clinical practice?

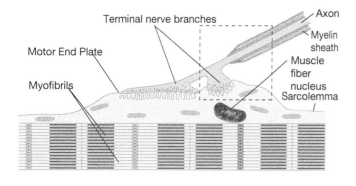

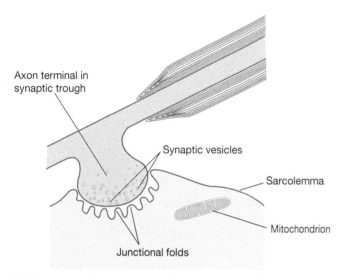

FIGURE 10-4 The neuromuscular junction is made up of multiple chemical synapses between a lower motor neuron and the sarcolemma of a skeletal muscle fiber. The presynaptic motor terminals lie over a specialized region of the sarcolemma called the end plate. The sarcolemma participating in the synapse is corrugated with junctional folds.

from the sarcolemma by the synaptic cleft. The floor of the trough is corrugated by secondary infoldings of the sarcolemma, called **junctional folds**. The presynaptic active zones are precisely aligned with the postsynaptic junctional folds. Near the crests of the junctional folds are high densities of nicotinic ACh receptors, while near the base of the folds are high densities of voltage-gated Na^+ channels. A basal lamina (basement membrane) consisting of collagen and glycoproteins occupies the synaptic cleft. The enzyme acetylcholinesterase (AChE), which inactivates ACh by hydrolyzing it into choline and acetate, is anchored to the collagen fibers of the basal lamina. These postsynaptic specializations ensure that the presynaptically released ACh molecules act on a large chemoreceptive membrane surface and that the ACh is rapidly inactivated. This means that transmission across the neuromuscular junction proceeds with a high safety factor.

Each action potential that invades the presynaptic terminal of the LMN opens the voltage-gated Ca^{2+} channels, permitting Ca^{2+} to enter the terminal and trigger

fusion of the synaptic vesicles in the active zones with the presynaptic membrane. The fusion leads to the release of ACh into the synaptic cleft. The binding of ACh to the postsynaptic nicotinic ACh receptors opens channels permeable to both Na^+ and K^+ (Figure 10-5 ■). The flow of these ions into and out of the muscle cell (there being a net influx of Na^+) depolarizes the cell, producing an excitatory postsynaptic potential called the **end-plate potential (EPP)**. The amplitude of the EPP is much larger (by about 70 times) than an EPSP in the CNS and, under nonpathological conditions, is always large enough to rapidly activate the voltage-gated Na^+ channels in the junctional folds as well as those near the end-plate region. This converts the EPP into an action potential that then actively propagates over the surface of the entire muscle fiber and into the interior of the fiber along the transverse tubules. This causes the release of Ca^{2+} from the sarcoplasmic reticulum, which stimulates all of the myofibrils in the muscle cell to contract at the same time.

The ACh is then rapidly inactivated by AChE in the synaptic cleft. Rapid inactivation is important because of the phenomenon of **desensitization** (as will be discussed

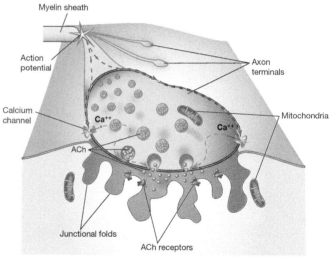

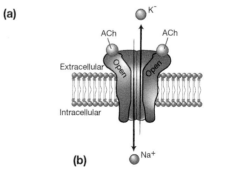

FIGURE 10-5 Synaptic transmission at the neuromuscular junction. (a) The presynaptic active zone where acetylcholine (ACh) is released into the synaptic cleft. (b) The binding of ACh to the postsynaptic nicotinic ACh receptors opens channels permeable to K^+ and Na^+ ions, resulting in a depolarization sufficient to induce an action potential in the postsynaptic muscle cell.

Neuropathology Box 10-1: Toxins and Drugs That Interfere with Neuromuscular Transmission

The bacterium *Clostridium botulinum* produces one of the most potent blockers of neuromuscular transmission known. C. botulinum bacteria grow in improperly canned foods and produce botulinum toxins that, when consumed, cause botulism. The neurotoxin blocks neuromuscular transmission at cholinergic terminals by being taken into the presynaptic terminal and destroying proteins involved in the fusion of synaptic vesicles with the presynaptic membrane. As a result, acetylcholine release is prevented, and weakness or paralysis ensues along with a variety of autonomic symptoms. Localized injections of botulinum toxin, called Botox, may be used clinically to treat conditions characterized by tonically contracted muscles as, for example, in cerebral palsy. Localized Botox injections also are widely used as a cosmetic procedure.

The venom of certain snakes contains an active compound called *α-bungarotoxin* that blocks neuromuscular transmission by binding tightly to nicotinic ACh receptors, thereby preventing ACh from opening postsynaptic ion channels. Paralysis ensues. A class of chemical compounds called *organophosphates* has been developed as a result of research to develop debilitating chemical warfare agents. Organophosphates desensitize ACh receptors by binding directly to them and also are irreversible inhibitors of AChE. By preventing the degradation of AChE, they kill their victims by causing a desensitization of ACh receptors or by binding directly to the receptor. Organophosphates like parathion also are used as insecticides. South American Indians use a mixture of plant toxins called *curare* as an arrowhead poison to immobilize their prey by blocking nicotinic ACh receptors.

in the box on myasthenia gravis). Nicotinic ACh receptors progressively inactivate in the continued presence of ACh.

A fundamental structural difference exists between the presynaptic innervation of a single striated muscle fiber compared with the innervation of a single alpha. Recall that large alpha LMNs may contain as many as 10,000 synapses on their receptive membrane. Single alpha LMNs represent a final common pathway in that these multiple synaptic inputs are derived from a wide variety of different sources: from the many UMN systems as well as from a variety of local interneurons and peripheral receptors. Contrast this with the innervation of a single striated muscle fiber. The striated muscle fiber is innervated by only one alpha LMN.

This difference is very important clinically because presynaptic neurons release not only chemical neurotransmitter molecules, but also trophic factors onto the membranes of postsynaptic cells. Trophic factors are molecules (e.g., proteins) that promote cell survival. Because of the diversity of presynaptic input to alpha LMNs, it is virtually impossible to completely denervate an alpha LMN when upper motor neurons are damaged. This means that with UMN damage, alpha LMNs continue to receive sufficient trophic factors to survive their partial denervation. But this is not true for striated muscle fibers. The destruction of one alpha LMN can lead to the death (degeneration) of all the striated muscle cells it innervates.

CLINICAL CONNECTIONS

The diagnosis of particular diseases that affect the motor unit is based on a combination of careful documentation of the clinical signs and symptoms presented by the patient together with the critical analysis of data derived from a number of laboratory techniques. Useful laboratory techniques in diagnosing disorders of the LMN include **electromyography** (see Figure 10-2) and nerve conduction velocity studies, and are discussed in the following sections.

Collectively, a constellation of definitive clinical signs define an **LMN syndrome** that results from damage either to LMNs or their axons. Certain of these signs express themselves as an alteration in the presence and/or status of reflexes. Consideration of these latter changes will be deferred until Chapter 11 after spinal cord reflexes have been presented.

Paralysis and Paresis

As discussed in Chapter 5, voluntary movement is controlled by specific UMNs, including those of the corticospinal tracts. In order to perform a voluntary movement, LMNs must be

---

Thought Question

Drawing on information that you learned in Chapter 8, describe the composition of the lower motor neuron. Now explain the relationship of the LMN to the neuromuscular junction. Then, drawing on information that you learned in Chapter 4, explain the importance of ACh and Ca^{2+} in synaptic transmission at the neuromuscular junction. Finally, compare and contrast synaptic transmission at the neuromuscular junction with synaptic transmission within the CNS.

Thought Question

Explain why damage to the LMN axon produces paralysis of the innervated muscle, whereas damage to the LMN cell body itself produces paresis.

intact so that the UMN command can be transferred to striated muscle. Thus, damage to LMNs reflects itself in a loss of voluntary movement. Such a loss may follow either damage to alpha LMN cell bodies in the CNS or to their axons in the PNS. When there is a complete loss of the capacity for voluntary movement, the term **paralysis** is used. When the loss is only partial, the term **paresis** is used. Paralysis of a single striated muscle resulting from a spinal cord lesion can occur only when the damage involves all of the spinal cord segments that supply that particular muscle. This ranges from two to six segments, depending on the particular muscle. Because the LMNs that supply a single muscle are distributed over several segments of the spinal cord, damage confined to just one spinal cord segment will cause paresis (weakness) but not complete paralysis. In contrast, PNS lesions involving LMN axons can be very discrete and still cause a paralysis of a single muscle. This is because single peripheral motor nerves contain axons from multiple spinal cord segments.

Atrophy and Denervation

Destruction of the LMN cell body or axon causes a number of clinical signs as a result of the loss of the trophic influence the LMN exerts over striated muscle. When striated muscle is no longer innervated by the LMN as a result of the latter's destruction, the denervated muscle is deprived of trophic factors normally released by the LMN. In their absence, striated muscle undergoes a severe atrophy and degeneration. Because the atrophy is of neural origin, it is referred to as **neurogenic atrophy**. The atrophy of denervated muscle proceeds slowly over several months. Its extent is proportional to the number of damaged LMNs. Neurogenic atrophy reaches a maximum in 90 to 120 days when muscle volume is reduced by 75 to 80 percent. Atrophy also results from disuse of the muscle, but such **disuse atrophy** in itself does not reduce muscle volume by more than about 25 percent. In neurogenic atrophy, degeneration and loss of muscle fibers begin in 6 to 12 months, a process that may be complete in three to four years. Hence, loss of muscle fibers occurs considerably later than the process of neurogenic atrophy.

Denervated muscle becomes overly sensitive to normal amounts of the transmitter acetylcholine (ACh) that are released by active LMNs onto the sarcolemma. This is referred to as denervation supersensitivity (hypersensitivity). New ACh receptors are continually being manufactured by striated muscle fibers to replace old receptors that have degraded with use. As long as the muscle fiber is normally innervated, the new receptors are inserted into the sarcolemma only in the region of the neuromuscular junction. However, when the fiber is denervated, these new receptors are inserted everywhere in the muscle fiber membrane. This makes the fiber overly sensitive to circulating ACh; hence, it fires spontaneously, producing fibrillations or fasciculations.

Fibrillations are the spontaneous contractions of *single muscle fibers*. They cannot be observed through the skin and produce no detectable shortening of the muscle. Fibrillations can only be detected electromyographically by recording the electrical activity of muscle with indwelling needle electrodes. The fact that muscle cells are firing in the absence of LMN stimulation is explained by the occurrence of denervation sensitivity. Fibrillation potentials begin 10 to 25 days after denervation and continue until the denervated fibers are reinnervated or until the atrophied muscle fibers degenerate and are replaced by connective tissue, a process that may take many years. **Fasciculations** are the spontaneous contractions of the muscle fibers belonging to an *entire motor unit*. Because many muscle fibers are involved, fasciculations can be observed through the skin and are sometimes referred to as twitches. The exact origin of fasciculation potentials is uncertain, but it appears that damaged LMNs may leave still intact LMN axons in a state of hyperirritability.

A variety of changes can occur in the **biochemical composition** and **histological appearance** of muscle when it is denervated. The specific changes depend on the dynamics of denervation and whether or not reinnervation of the muscle occurs by still-intact LMNs. The histochemical properties of red and white striated muscle fibers are distinct, as would be expected from their different metabolic mechanisms that fuel contraction, the former relying on oxidative catabolism and the latter on anaerobic (glycolytic) catabolism. The histochemical properties of a muscle fiber are determined by the motor neuron that innervates it. Therefore, muscle histochemistry and its appearance change following LMN damage.

DISEASES OF THE MOTOR SYSTEM

Clinical Preview ················

Meredith Balazar is a computer programmer who has begun to experience excruciating pain in her forearm and weakness in muscles of the hand. She was diagnosed with carpal tunnel syndrome, with compression on the median nerve as it crosses the wrist. She would like to avoid surgery and has decided to first attempt a course of rehabilitation. In reading through this section, consider the following:

* Why would pressure on the median nerve at the wrist cause pain?

* What would be the consequences of long-term compression?

* Relating this situation to information you learned in Chapter 4, how long might it take for symptoms to completely resolve if the pressure is removed in time?

Disorders of the motor system are helpful in understanding the neurophysiology of the peripheral motor system. Furthermore, by understanding the nature of these disorders, the rehabilitation specialist is in a good position to develop well-reasoned intervention strategies. Examples of common motor unit disorders are provided in this section.

Neurogenic and Myopathic Disorders

The motor unit provides a systematic and rational basis for the classification of a significant number of diseases that affect the motor system. Four different sites in the motor unit may be attacked by specific disease entities: the cell body of the lower motor neuron, its axon, the neuromuscular junction, or the muscle fibers it innervates. Specific diseases affecting the motor unit typically fall into one of two major categories: **neurogenic**, affecting the cell bodies or their axons in peripheral nerve, or **myopathic (myopathies)** that affect striated muscle. Neurogenic diseases are further divided into those that affect the cell bodies, called **motor neuron diseases**, and those that affect axons in peripheral nerve, called **neuropathies**. Neurogenic and myopathic diseases have different effects on the motor unit (Figure 10-6 ■).

In addition, there is a class of diseases that specifically affects the neuromuscular junction and, therefore, **synaptic transmission**. These diseases do not easily fall into either category because neither the structural changes alone on the presynaptic side of this synapse (i.e., in the motor nerve axon) nor the changes in the sarcolemma alone on the postsynaptic side (i.e., the muscle) explain the widespread and severe weakness that characterizes these disorders.

A needle electrode inserted into muscle is able to record motor unit potentials as noted earlier. Motor unit potentials in normally innervated muscle were shown in Figure 10-2. In neurogenic disorders such as disease of the cell body or its axon, the muscle fibers supplied by the degenerated neuron are denervated and undergo atrophy. Surviving lower motor neurons sprout new axon collaterals that reinnervate some of the denervated fibers. This creates larger-than-normal motor units, and when active under slight contraction, the motor unit potentials they generate are larger than normal, more prolonged, and *polyphasic* rather than triphasic. At rest, the fibrillation potentials are recorded. The interference pattern occurring during maximal contraction is reduced because there are fewer motor units in the muscle.

In myopathic disorders, the number of muscle fibers per motor unit is reduced. When such a unit is active under slight contraction, its motor unit potential is smaller in amplitude and shorter in duration than normal, and it may also be polyphasic. During maximal voluntary contraction, a full interference pattern is generated, but because fewer muscle fibers are firing, its amplitude will be smaller than

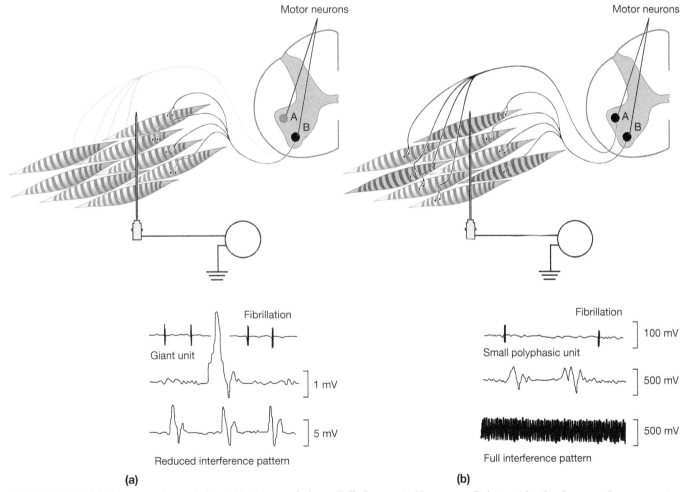

FIGURE 10-6 (a) Denervated muscle in which the muscle is partially innervated by neuron B, but not by the degenerating neuron A. This results in a reduced interference pattern. (b) Myopathy resulting in a full interference pattern.

normal. While electromyography is capable of differentiating between neurogenic and myopathic disorders, it is not capable of distinguishing among the different diseases that make up each class.

CLINICAL CONNECTIONS

Disorders of the Motor Unit

A Disease of the LMN Cell Body: Polio

The classic example of disorders of the alpha LMN is poliomyelitis. The cardinal clinical sign in poliomyelitis is weakness or paralysis of muscles, most commonly of both legs or an arm and both legs. Coarse fasciculations occur as the muscles weaken. As the weakness evolves, tendon reflexes decrease in strength and then are lost. Within about three weeks of onset of the paralysis, atrophy of muscle begins and attains its peak within three to four months. The atrophy is permanent. These clinical signs result from the destruction of LMNs in the ventral horn of the spinal cord over the segments that innervate the affected muscles.

Today in the United States, poliomyelitis is rare. This was not always the case. Prior to the development of effective vaccines in the mid-1950s, acute anterior poliomyelitis reached epidemic proportions, leaving in its wake, if they survived the lethal effects of the disease, thousands of disabled children. In one of the truly exceptional accomplishments of modern medicine, antipoliomyelitic vaccines have virtually eliminated **paralytic poliomyelitis**. However, occasional cases still occur in unvaccinated children and in unvaccinated adults exposed to a recently vaccinated infant. Moreover, 20 to 30 or more years after the acute paralytic disease, a gradual increase in weakness occurs in some cases. This is called the **postpolio syndrome** and is attributed to the additional loss of LMNs that occurs with aging as well as the metabolic stress from overuse.

Diseases of LMN Axons in the Peripheral Nerve: Neuropathies

The term *peripheral neuropathy* is most broadly defined as disease of the peripheral nervous system. Certain of the hundred or so diseases of peripheral nerves are characterized by special pathological changes in the nerve cells, but the basic pathologic processes that affect peripheral nerves are only three in number. These are segmental demyelination, axonal degeneration, (Figure 10-7 ■) and Wallerian degeneration. Myelin is the most vulnerable element of the nerve fiber; not only does it break down as part of a primary process affecting the Schwann cell itself, but it can break down secondarily due to a disease affecting the axon. In **segmental demyelination**, myelin degenerates, but the axon is spared. In such cases, recovery of function may be rapid because the intact axon only has to be remyelinated to restore function. In **axonal degeneration**, there is a distal degeneration of the axon and, secondarily, the myelin as a consequence of the disease process (see the "dying-back" phenomenon discussed later). Transection of the axon by cutting or crushing divides the axon into a proximal portion that remains connected to the cell body and a distal portion that is isolated from the cell body. Given that protein synthesis is confined largely to the cell body, the isolated distal segment undergoes degeneration. Because the myelin sheath requires contact with the

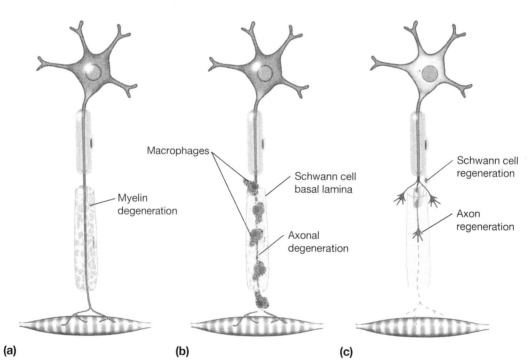

FIGURE 10-7 The basic pathological processes affecting peripheral nerves. (a) Segmental demyelination with axonal sparing. (b) Axonal degeneration with distal degeneration of the axon with secondary degeneration of myelin. (c) Schwann cell and axonal regeneration.

axon for its maintenance, it, too, undergoes degeneration. This pattern of degeneration is termed **Wallerian degeneration**. With axonal and Wallerian degeneration, recovery of function is slower and may require a year or more because the axon must first regenerate and establish synaptic contract with its target structure, then remyelinate. Axonal transection also causes chromalytic changes in the nerve cell (see Figures 3-4, 10-7). The cell body receives a signal via retrograde transport that it needs to increase its metabolic activity and to produce growth factors required for axonal regeneration. In chromatolysis, the cell body swells, the nucleus moves to an eccentric position, and the rough endoplasmic reticulum appears dispersed or dissolved.

Neuropathies are caused by a wide variety of diseases. These include infections by the herpes zoster virus (shingles); infection followed by inflammation as an expression of altered immunity, such as the Guillain-Barré syndrome; malnutrition and vitamin deficiency; toxicity to medicines, excessive vitamins, or industrial products; and metabolic complications from diabetes mellitus, liver disease, kidney failure, hypothyroidism, or hereditary disorders.

Most **polyneuropathies** result in an impairment of both motor and sensory functions, although one may be affected more than the other. The most prevalent of the polyneuropathies affecting both motor and sensory axons is associated with **diabetes mellitus (DM)**. The long-term complications of diabetic polyneuropathy may lead to limb amputations and sudden cardiac death from involvement of autonomic nerves. There still is no effective therapy for somatic and autonomic diabetic polyneuropathies associated with DM.

Another common disorder that affects both motor and somatosensory axons is the **Guillain-Barré syndrome (GBS)**. Also called **acute inflammatory demyelinating polyneuropathy (AIDP)**, GBS involves the demyelination of peripheral nerves. The clinical manifestations of GBS are the result of a cell-mediated immunologic reaction directed at the myelin of peripheral nerve. Usually, the legs are affected first and the weakness ascends to involve the trunk, arms, and finally cranial muscles. In 3 to 5 percent of patients, the weakness progresses to total motor paralysis in a matter of days, with death resulting from respiratory failure. Paresthesias and numbness are common early signs. Tendon reflexes are reduced and then lost. Nerve conduction testing reliably yields a reduction in the amplitude of muscle action potentials, slowed conduction velocity, or conduction block in motor nerves. In the Guillain-Barré syndrome, motor paralysis is more prominent than somatosensory loss.

In contrast, in many of the toxic and metabolic neuropathies, somatosensory loss is affected more than motor loss (weakness). All somatosensory modalities (kinesthesia, vibration, touch-pressure, and pain and temperature) may eventually be lost, or there may be a primary loss of pain and temperature (with sparing of kinesthesia, touch-pressure, and vibration) or a less severe loss in these latter modalities. In most types of polyneuropathy, the sensory impairment is bilaterally symmetrical, and the longest and largest fibers are affected first. Sensory loss is thus most severe in the hands and feet, referred to as a **glove-and-stocking sensory loss**. This distal pattern of sensory loss is caused by impaired axonal transport, or the dying-back phenomenon, wherein the parts of the axon most affected are those most remote from the cell bodies in the dorsal root ganglia. **Paresthesias** are an early symptom in segmental demyelination. These are spontaneously occurring (i.e., there is no proximate sensory stimulus) abnormal, sometimes unpleasant, sensations described by patients as prickling, tingling, pins-and-needles, numbness, deadness, Novocain-like, band-like, or tightness.

In most of the nutritional, metabolic, and toxic polyneuropathies, muscles of the feet and legs are affected first and more severely than those of the hands and forearms. This predominantly distal pattern of motor dysfunction is also explained by the dying-back phenomenon. Typically, tendon reflexes are either depressed or lost. Other motor signs occur, such as muscle atrophy, and will be discussed later in this chapter.

In general, in neuropathies involving sensory nerves, there is a loss of autonomic function in the same areas as the somatic sensory loss. Anhydrosis and orthostatic hypotension occur most frequently and are major features of certain polyneuropathies such as diabetic polyneuropathies. Bowel and bladder incontinence, sexual impotence, blurring of vision with an inability to focus, lack of tears and saliva, and vomiting of retained, undigested food are other manifestations of autonomic dysfunction (Chapter 12).

In polyneuropathies affecting the primary somatosensory neurons, sensory ataxia may occur. The sensory ataxic gait, for example, is characterized by brusque, flinging movements of the legs and slapping of the feet (recall Shelley's Frankenstein monster). This ataxic movement results not because of a specific motor system involvement, but because of somatosensory loss and its consequences. Specifically, degeneration of proprioceptive afferents occurs with a relative sparing of motor fibers so that at least a reasonable degree of motor function is retained. Because of the proprioceptive loss, the individual has impaired awareness of the position and movement of his legs and slaps his feet on the ground in an attempt to generate more proprioceptive input. Additionally, the cerebellum is deprived of the proprioceptive input it needs to properly coordinate movement.

A Disease of the Neuromuscular Junction: Myasthenia Gravis

Several diseases interfere with neuromuscular transmission, the most common of which is myasthenia gravis. **Myasthenia gravis (MG)** is a disorder of the neuromuscular junction, resulting in muscular weakness (not fatigue) that increases in severity with repeated or sustained activity with a partial restoration of function after rest. In more than 90 percent of cases, the eye muscles are involved first, and some 15 percent of all people with MG will manifest only ocular signs. The involvement of the levator palpebrae, which elevates the upper eyelid, and extraocular muscles, which align the visual axes of the two eyes, are responsible for an individual's initial complaints of **ptosis** (drooping of the upper eyelids) and **diplopia** (double vision). The muscles of facial expression, mastication, swallowing, and speech are the next most frequently affected. Facial expression is altered. The jaw may hang and the chewing of tough food is difficult or becomes impossible. Swallowing may become impaired during the course of a meal (**dysphagia**). As the person continues talking, the voice fades, speech becomes nasal as the soft palate fails to close off the nasal cavity, and a frank **dysarthria** develops wherein articulation becomes slurred. In advanced cases, all muscles are weakened, including the diaphragm, abdominal, and intercostal muscles. Fatalities then result as a consequence of respiratory complications.

In MG, there are no clinical signs or electromyographic abnormalities indicating denervation of muscle such as are seen with diseases of the LMN cell body or axon. Weakened muscles in myasthenia gravis do not atrophy to any significant degree. Tendon reflexes remain unaltered.

Myasthenia gravis is an **autoimmune disease** in which the circulating antibody combines with the nicotinic ACh receptor, destroying the receptor. The number of functional receptors in neuromuscular junctions is thereby reduced so that the effectiveness of ACh as a transmitter is reduced. The antibody–receptor complex provides a binding site for circulating complement protein, leading to activation of the *complement cascade*. A final product of the complement cascade is a *membrane attack complex* that punches holes in the sarcolemma at the receptor site. Only some 15 to 20 percent of the normal receptor population remains in myasthenia gravis. In addition to reducing receptor density, this focal lysis is responsible for the structural changes that are observed at the neuromuscular junction in MG (Figure 10-8 ■). In the sarcolemma, the junctional folds are simplified and reduced in number, and the synaptic cleft is wider. When the density of ACh receptors is reduced, the probability that a molecule of ACh will encounter a receptor before it is inactivated by acetylcholinesterase is reduced. When the normal infolding of the sarcolemma is reduced and the synaptic cleft widened, diffusion of ACh from the cleft is increased. These factors combine to markedly reduce the amplitude of the end plate potential to a size just above threshold.

Collectively, these changes, coupled with the concept of ACh receptor desensitization, explain the major clinical features of MG. The weakening of contraction with repeated or sustained activity is explained by the few remaining functional receptors being desensitized as they are exposed to sustained levels of ACh. The end-plate potential then falls below the threshold for generating a muscle action potential. The partial restoration of contraction with rest is explained by the recovery of ACh receptor sensitivity.

Diseases of Muscle: Myopathies

The **muscular dystrophies** are progressive, hereditary degenerative diseases of skeletal muscle. A number of clinical features common to all of the muscular dystrophies

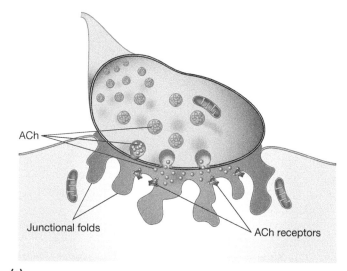

(a)

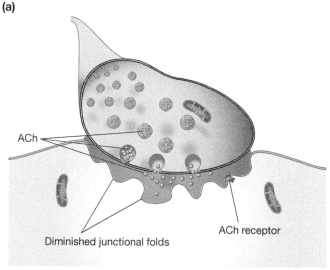

(b)

FIGURE 10-8 (a) A healthy neuromuscular junction with corrugated junctional folds and numerous ACh receptors. (b) The neuromuscular junction in myasthenia gravis with diminished junctional folds and fewer ACh receptors.

serve to set them apart as a distinct clinical entity. There is a symmetrical distribution of muscle weakness and atrophy, somatosensation is intact, and cutaneous reflexes are retained. That the disease is due to involvement of the muscle fibers themselves is demonstrated by the fact that LMN cell bodies are intact and peripheral nerves are normal as are their terminal endings, yet there is severe degeneration of muscle. Up to 11 different diseases fall into the category of muscular dystrophy, one of the most common being **Duchenne muscular dystrophy**.

Duchenne muscular dystrophy results from a defect in a gene that normally encodes for a muscle membrane–associated structural protein called **dystrophin**. Because the disease is inherited as a sex-linked recessive trait, it is transmitted from the mother only to male children. Boys with this type of muscular dystrophy either lack dystrophin or have less than 5 percent of the normal amount. The loss

Neuropathology Box 10-2: Spasticity

Spasticity is a characteristic component of the upper motor neuron syndrome that includes a velocity-dependent increase in the tonic stretch reflex (e.g., response to slow stretch of the muscle) and a hyperactive phasic stretch reflex (e.g., deep tendon reflex, DTR). Spasticity commonly occurs in clinical disorders involving damage to the upper motor neuron, such as in stroke, multiple sclerosis, and spinal cord injury. Spasticity is discussed in detail in Chapter 11.

of dystrophin renders the sarcolemma vulnerable to breaks and tears during muscle contraction. Muscle biopsy reveals a randomly distributed loss of muscle fibers with replacement by fat cells and fibrous tissue. Some of the surviving muscle fibers may be hypertrophied. Signs of muscle fibers that have attempted regeneration may also be observed, particularly in less affected parts of the muscle. Duchenne muscular dystrophy begins in infancy or, more commonly, in early childhood and progresses rapidly so that people require a wheelchair for mobility by their early teens. The weakness and atrophy begin in the muscles of the thigh, then specific muscles of the lower leg become involved, with eventual spread to muscles of the trunk, shoulder girdle, and upper limb. Finally, these individuals become bedfast, with death generally occurring during late adolescence; only a minority survive beyond the age of 25.

A Disorder of the Motor System Affecting Both the LMN and UMN

In the previous section, we considered diseases of the motor unit, beginning at the cell body and progressing to the muscle. In this section, we consider how disease affects LMNs within the spinal cord and/or brainstem and UMNs. The term *motor system disease* is a general term that applies to a progressive degenerative disease of LMNs in the spinal cord and brainstem and UMNs in the cerebral cortex. Motor system disease is manifest clinically by weakness, atrophy, and spasticity in varying combinations. Generally, these are diseases of middle to late life, but there are exceptions. Some 50 percent of cases progress to death in two to three years and 90 percent in six years. In exceptional cases, individuals live longer, one of the more notable being physicist Stephen Hawking.

Amyotrophic lateral sclerosis (ALS) (Lou Gehrig's disease) is the most frequent of the motor system diseases with an incidence rate of 0.4 to 1.76 per 100,000 population. *Amyotrophy* refers to the weakness and denervation atrophy of muscle, while *lateral sclerosis* pertains to focal areas of hardness felt by the pathologist on the lateral funiculus of the spinal cord at autopsy. Generally, the disease begins with slight weakness and wasting of the hand muscles as the individual experiences awkwardness with tasks requiring fine movements of the fingers. Cramping and fasciculations of the muscles of the forearm, upper arm, and shoulder girdle also appear. Eventually, the triad of atrophic weakness of the hands and forearms, slight spasticity of the arms and legs, and generalized hyperreflexia without accompanying somatosensory signs stamp the disorder as ALS. The disease is relentlessly progressive, with the atrophic weakness spreading to involve the muscles of the trunk and legs and the neck, tongue, and laryngeal and pharyngeal muscles so that the person exhibits dysarthria (difficulty speaking) and dysphagia (difficulty swallowing). Dysarthria is discussed in Chapter 14. There is no effective treatment for ALS. Death results when the weakness spreads to the respiratory and swallowing musculature, resulting in aspiration pneumonia and inanition. However, respiratory therapy (noninvasive positive pressure ventilation) improves an individual's quality of life as well as cognition, despite the progression of ALS, and without increasing caregiver burden or stress.

ALS no longer is considered to be a disorder confined just to the motor system. Rather, a range of behavioral and cognitive changes characterize ALS. People with ALS exhibit signs of extramotor frontal lobe deterioration, including alterations in personality, behavior, planning, organization, and language. All people with ALS demonstrate frontal, temporal, and parietal lobe atrophy on neuroimaging that is disproportionate to that seen in normal aging.

Summary

Our detailed analysis of the motor system begins in this chapter with a discussion of the components residing for the most part in the peripheral nervous system. Strictly speaking, not all of the components addressed in this chapter belong just to the PNS; the origin of the motor unit is an alpha LMN whose cell body lies in the ventral horn of the spinal cord or in a cranial nerve motor nucleus in the brainstem. The motor unit is an extremely valuable structural and functional entity for two reasons. First, because it represents the basis by which the CNS controls and grades the contraction of striated muscle. Second, because different neurologic diseases selectively attack different parts of the motor unit.

Motor units are recruited into a muscular contraction of increasing force according to a size principle, where the smallest motor units are activated first followed by larger motor units, each of which begins its discharge at a low frequency and increases its discharge rate to a maximal frequency of about 25 Hz. Each motor unit is composed of a unique set of striated muscle fibers whose contraction subserve distinct levels and speeds of contraction: red slow-twitch, fatigue-resistant fibers, white fast-twitch, fatigable fibers, or intermediate fast-twitch, fatigue-resistant fibers.

Six distinct clinical signs follow damage to LMNs or their axons in peripheral nerves and result from the loss of the capacity of the LMN to influence striated muscle in both a controlling capacity (e.g., voluntary movement) and a trophic capacity. Neurologic disease that affects the LMN cell body include poliomyelitis, diseases that affect the axon in peripheral nerve include a wide variety of neuropathies such as diabetes mellitus and Guillain-Barré syndrome, diseases that affect the neuromuscular junction include myasthenia gravis, and those that affect striated muscle itself include the muscular dystrophies. Lastly, motor system diseases such as amyotrophic lateral sclerosis affect not only LMNs of motor units, but also UMNs in the cerebral cortex.

Applications

1. At age 7, Frances contracted poliomyelitis. This is a virus that attacks a certain part of the spinal cord.

   a. What part of the spinal cord does this virus attack?
   b. Will damage to this part of the spinal cord result in an upper motor neuron lesion, a lower motor neuron lesion, or both? Why?
   c. Is poliomyelitis a neurogenic or myopathic disorder?
   d. People with poliomyelitis may have involvement of a wide variety of muscles, which may include extremities, muscles of the torso, those of the face, and those specific to respiratory function. Furthermore, some individuals may have severe motor loss while others may have mild losses. What explains this variability?
   e. What is the treatment for poliomyelitis?
   f. Some individuals who have had contracted poliomyelitis have the potential to regain strength. As Frances recovers from polio, her nerves attempt to reinnervate the muscles. Describe the role and consequences of collateral sprouting in recovery from nerve damage associated with polio.
   g. A new syndrome has been described that occurs in people previously infected with polio. Name the syndrome and describe the main features. Explore the literature to learn more about this syndrome.

2. Larry is a 48-year-old man who began to experience weakness in both of his lower extremities. He then noticed problems with coordination and balance. He was unable to participate in his favorite activities involving running, hiking, and biking. A neurological examination revealed weakness in both lower extremities, with key muscle groups testing at a manual muscle test strength score of 4-/5. Mild atrophy was present in his anterior tibialis muscles. Larry was hyperreflexic in both knees and ankles. He had fasciculations of his tongue, and he spoke with a mild dysarthria. Larry's sensation was normal throughout his face and extremities.

   a. What type of lesion is involved: UMN, LMN, or both?
   b. What disease could cause both UMN and LMN symptoms?
   c. What is the treatment for this disorder?
   d. What is the prognosis for Larry's condition?
   e. Hypothesize the role of rehabilitation professionals in caring for Larry.

3. Mark, a 37-year-old math teacher, sought physical therapy for neck pain with fatigue. He reported that his fatigue was the worst at the end of the day. Furthermore, he described difficulty with his speech that worsened over the course of the day such that his afternoon students complained that they could not fully understand him. His eyelids were droopy and his smile was affected. Examination revealed normal vital signs, sensation, coordination, and cognition. Mark was eventually diagnosed with myasthenia gravis.

   a. What type of disorder is myasthenia gravis, and what is the neuroantomical site of dysfunction?
   b. What are the current medical treatments for myasthenia gravis, and how are these treatments related to the disorder?
   c. Do you think Mark could benefit from rehabilitation? Explain your answer.

References

Al-Chalabi, A., and Leigh, P. N. Trouble on the pitch: are professional football players at increased risk of developing amyotrophic lateral sclerosis? *Brain* 128:451–453, 2005.

Beghi, E., and Morrison, K. E. ALS and military service. *Neurology* 64:6–7, 2005.

Ghez, C. and Krakauer, J. Ch. 33. The organization of movement. In: Kandel, E. R., Schwartz, J. H., and Jessell, T. M., eds. *Principles of Neural Science*, 4th ed. McGraw-Hill, New York, 2000.

Heiman-Patterson, T. D., and Miller, R. G. NIPPV: A treatment for ALS whose time has come. *Neurology* 67:736–737, 2006.

Kaminski, H. J. Restoring balance at the neuromuscular junction. *Neurology* 69:626–630, 2007.

Kaufmann, P., Pullman, S. L., Shungu, D. C., et al. Objective tests for upper motor neuron involvement in amyotrophic lateral sclerosis (ALS). *Neurology* 62:1753–1757, 2004.

Loeb, G. E., and Ghez, C. Ch. 34. The motor unit and muscle action. In Kandel, E. R., Schwartz, J. H., and Jessell, T. M., eds. *Principles of Neural Science*, 4th ed. McGraw-Hill, New York, 2000.

Mendell, L. M. The size principle: A rule describing the recruitment of motoneurons. *J Neurophysiol* 93:3024–3026, 2005.

Moritz, C. T., Barry, B. K., Pascoe, M. A., and Enoka, R. M. Discharge rate variability influences the variation in force fluctuations across the working range of a hand muscle. *J Neurophysiol* 93:2449–2459, 2005.

Murphy, J., Henry, R., and Lomen-Hoerth, C. Establishing subtypes of the continuum of frontal lobe impairment in amyotrophic lateral sclerosis. *Arch Neurol.* 64:330–334, 2007.

Nolte, J. *The Human Brain: An Introduction to Its Functional Anatomy*. Mosby Elsevier, Philadelphia, 2009.

Olney, R. K., and Lomen-Hoerth, C. Exit strategies in ALS: An influence of depression or despair? *Neurology* 65:9–10, 2005.

Ropper, A. H., and Brown, R. H. Ch. 50. The Muscular Dystrophies. In: Ropper, A. H., and Brown, R. H. *Adams and Victor's Principles of Neurology*, 8th ed. McGraw-Hill, New York, 2005.

Rowland, L. P. Diseases of the motor unit. Ch. 35. In: Kandel, E. R., Schwartz, J. H., and Jessell, T.M., eds. *Principles of Neural Science*. McGraw-Hill, New York, 2000.

Traynor, B. J., Bruijn, L., Conwit, R., et al. Neuroprotective agents for clinical trials in ALS. *Neurology* 67:20–27, 2006.

Central Components of Movement

LEARNING OUTCOMES

This chapter prepares the reader to:

1. Recall the meaning of the following terms: afferent, efferent, effector, interneuronal pool, suprasegmental control, and autogenic inhibition.

2. Discuss the anatomical arrangement of the nervous system in terms of three hierarchical structural levels.

3. Discuss distal—proximal and flexor—extensor organization of the spinal cord.

4. Compare and contrast the short and long propriospinal systems.

5. Identify one tract associated with the dorsolateral system and five tracts associated with the ventromedial system.

6. Explain the functional importance of cortical inputs to the alpha motor neuron pool.

7. Identify five components of the reflex arc and explain the role of each.

8. For each of the following reflexes, identify the name of the receptor, the interneuronal connections, the functional response, and how the reflex is elicited: stretch reflex, "inverse myotatic" reflex, and flexion reflex with crossed extensor reflex.

9. Define areflexia, hyperreflexia, and hyporeflexia and discuss how these phenomena are used in clinical evaluation of reflexes.

10. Describe the pyramidal tract in terms of cells of origin, cortical area of origin, pathways to the spinal cord, and final destination in the cord.

11. Contrast the anterior and lateral corticospinal tracts in terms of their pathways and functional roles.

12. Give examples of the role of suprasegmental control in modifying reflexes and the contribution of the tonic descending inhibitory pathway.

13. With respect to spasticity, discuss the current understanding and limitations to the definition, causes, consequences, measurement, and interventions.

14. Discuss the basis for the transition from spinal shock to spasticity and other forms of hyperreflexia following spinal cord injury.

15. Contrast shock following spinal cord and cortical injury.

16. Utilize the Brunnstrom stages to describe motor control during recovery from stroke.

17. Differentiate UMN from LMN symptoms in terms of paresis and paralysis, atrophy, and abnormal reflexive states.

18. Discuss testing of reflexes in UMN injury and relate findings to reflex pathways.

19. Explain the basis for central deficits following total knee arthroplasty and the implications for rehabilitation.

20. Discuss the combined sensory and motor consequences that occur with spinal cord injury.

ACRONYMS

ACL Anterior cruciate ligament

ACST Anterior (or ventral) corticospinal tract

AL Anterolateral system

ANS Autonomic nervous system

CVA Cerebrovascular accident

DC-ML Dorsal column-medial lemniscal system

GTO Golgi tendon organ

LCST Lateral corticospinal tract

LMN Lower motor neuron

MLR Medium latency response

NMES Neuromuscular electrical stimulation

ROM Range of motion

SLR Short latency response

TDIP Tonic descending inhibitory pathway

TKA Total knee arthroplasty

UMN Upper motor neuron

Introduction

Our exploration into production and control of movement continues with a more detailed presentation of the anatomical structures that subserve movement. This chapter builds on Chapter 8, in which two extremes of movement were defined, reflexive movement being the simplest and voluntary movement the most complex. Both extremes of movement are conditioned by the hard-wiring of the motor system in the CNS.

The first major section of this chapter explains how the neural systems that subserve movement are hard-wired at three different hierarchical levels of the motor system: the spinal cord, brainstem, and the primary motor cortex of the cerebral hemisphere. This hard-wiring is such that the components at each level of organization are constrained to mediate particular types of overt movement. The hard-wiring is exploited in the generation of both reflexes and voluntary movement.

In the second major section of the chapter, several reflexive responses are examined that are based on hard-wiring in the spinal cord. Alteration of specific reflexes results in clinical signs that can indicate whether lower motor neurons (LMNs), upper motor neurons (UMNs), or both have been affected by pathology. Furthermore, excitation of specific reflexes can be used in rehabilitation to facilitate movement in individuals with neurological dysfunction as well as individuals with weakness from other causes. Spasticity, a consequence of upper motor neuron damage, is discussed in detail, including its definition and possible causes.

In the third major section, we turn to the pyramidal tract. The pyramidal tract is the major descending UMN motor system from the cerebral cortex to the spinal cord LMNs that mediates voluntary movement and is the focus of this chapter. Normal structure and function of the pyramidal tract are presented first, followed by the consequences of damage to the pyramidal tract and related structures. These consequences include a reduction or loss

of the capacity for voluntary movement in the limbs and increased responsiveness of reflexes. Spasticity is discussed with respect to examination and implications for the rehabilitation specialist.

We end this final major section by considering clinical consequences of damage to the spinal cord, integrating information presented previously on the somatosensory system (Chapters 8 and 9) with information presented in Chapters 10 and 11 on the motor system. Specifically, we illustrate how lesions in different components of the CNS can affect both sensory and motor systems. This is most readily visualized in the case of spinal cord injury, where the axons of somotosensory and motor systems run in close proximity to one another. As we noted in Chapter 9, a number of spinal cord disorders affect the DC-ML and AL systems. Such disorders also affect descending motor tracts of the spinal cord and so are considered again in the last section of this chapter. Additionally, spinal cord lesions may involve components of the autonomic nervous system (ANS) and may cause medically significant (sometimes urgent) disability.

This chapter focuses considerable attention on the hard-wiring that forms the basic substrate on which the motor system controls purposeful movement. However, such movement is not restricted to the framework of these specific hard-wired pathways. Hence, this chapter only begins to introduce structures involved in the control of movement. Other descending tracts of importance, such as the rubrospinal and reticulospinal tracts, will be discussed in later chapters. Furthermore, other structures including the cerebellum and basal ganglia (Chapter 19) modulate the descending control systems; hence they play a key role in control of movement. Chapter 20 provides a synthesis of many components of importance in the control of purposeful movement, putting the different parts of the system together in context of purposeful movement, including those that transcend the hard wiring.

INTERNAL ORGANIZATION OF THE MOTOR SYSTEM

From an anatomical perspective, the motor system is organized in several important ways. First, there is an anatomical organization from the spinal cord to cerebral cortex; second, there is a somatotopic organization. Both of these concepts are described in the following sections.

Anatomical Organization

The anatomical organization of motor system anatomy may be depicted hierarchically in terms of three levels of the motor system. The first, and lowest on the hierarchy,

consists of built-in (hard-wired) patterns of neural connections in the spinal cord. The second, and intermediate level, consists of the descending UMN pathways originating in the brainstem that govern the activity of LMNs either directly or via the built-in neural connections. The third, and highest level, of the hierarchy consists of the cerebral cortex that modulates the activity of the UMN pathways descending from the brainstem as well as LMNs themselves. It is this level that transcends the hard wiring.

The reader should recognize from the start that this hierarchical anatomical organization does not mean that in the execution of voluntary movement we rigidly progress from the deployment of cerebrocortical UMNs, to brainstem UMNs, to spinal cord LMNs. Significant contributions also are made by the reticulospinal, vestibulospinal, and tectospinal pathways, by the cerebellum and basal ganglia, as well as by sensory systems—all of which are explored in later chapters. The cerebellum and basal ganglia, which are particularly important regulators of cerebrocortical UMN activity, are not included in the anatomical hierarchy mentioned previously. In fact, there are ongoing parallel exchanges among the cerebral cortex, basal ganglia, and cerebellum not only in the generation and initiation of voluntary movement but also in its execution. These topics will be introduced and discussed in Chapter 19. Thus, our approach to the motor system follows that of the entire book: namely, to introduce background concepts first and then build on them in subsequent chapters. This chapter focuses only on the hard-wired components of the motor system. We begin with organization at the spinal cord level, progress to the brainstem, and then to the cortex. Within the hierarchical levels of the nervous system, neurons are further organized around their functional roles, as described next.

> **Thought Question**
>
> What are the three hierarchical levels of the CNS motor systems, and what might be their role?

Somatotopic Organization

Throughout the nervous system, information is organized in a logical and systematic manner so that like information is found in common locations at different sections and travels together through the nervous system. This is referred to as *somatotopic organization*, meaning the information from different parts of the body are arranged systematically.

Spinal Cord

Within the spinal cord, neurons are organized to preferentially subserve either distal or proximal muscle groups. We should emphasize that the following organizational features are dominant trends, not absolutes. First, alpha LMNs of the ventral horn are organized according to two rules: a **distal-proximal rule** and a **flexor-extensor rule**. When segments of the cervical enlargement are telescoped into a single segment (Figure 11-1 ■), the cell bodies of LMNs in the ventral horn innervating hand muscles are most lateral, while those innervating the axial-trunk musculature are most medial. LMNs innervating flexor muscles, essential for fine movements of the fingers and hand, are more dorsal than those innervating extensor muscles, which is of particular importance to postural activity. Thus, alpha LMNs are organized into dorsolateral and ventromedial groups, subserving largely flexor-mediated discrete movements of the hand and largely extensor-mediated postural movements of

the axial musculature, respectively. Similarly, interneurons of the intermediate gray matter of the spinal cord are organized into dorsolateral and ventromedial groups. The axons of dorsolaterally positioned interneurons synapse preferentially on ipsilateral LMNs innervating the distal flexors, while ventromedially stationed interneurons have axons that synapse preferentially on LMNs innervating proximal extensors. Furthermore, the latter interneurons project not only to ipsilateral LMNs, but also to proximal extensor LMNs on the contralateral side of the spinal cord. Finally, neurons of the propriospinal system (see Figure 5-9) organize themselves into separable subsystems: a short system and a long system. Interneurons giving rise to the short propriospinal system are positioned laterally, and their axons extend only a few spinal cord segments before synapsing on dorsolaterally positioned interneurons and/or LMNs. In contrast, the long propriospinal system is derived from ventromedially positioned interneurons whose axons interconnect many spinal cord segments, some extending the entire length of the cord, to finally synapse on ventromedially located interneurons and/or LMNs.

Brainstem

The anatomical organization of neurons designated to preferentially subserve flexor and extensor muscle groups continues in the brainstem. With regard to this intermediate level of the motor hierarchy, descending UMN systems originating in the brainstem were first investigated in monkeys. These investigations demonstrated that in monkeys, the descending systems could be grouped into two functional systems: the dorsolateral system and the ventromedial system. The **dorsolateral system** consists of the rubrospinal tract. The dorsolateral system descends in the dorsal part of the lateral funiculus of the spinal cord and synapses preferentially on interneurons of the dorsolateral intermediate gray whose axons, in turn, synapse on LMNs innervating distal flexors. In contrast, the **ventromedial system** consists of five descending UMN tracts: a tectospinal tract originating from the superior colliculus, medial and lateral vestibulospinal tracts originating from the vestibular nuclei (Chapter 17), and medial and lateral reticulospinal tracts originating from the medial effector zone of the reticular formation (Chapter 5). These tracts descend in the medial part of the anterior (ventral) funiculus of the

> **Thought Question**
>
> Describe the organization of LMNs that innervate distal and proximal muscles and the organization of neurons that innervate flexors and extensors. Is this organization similar or different in the spinal cord and brainstem? Which tract(s) arises from the dorsolateral system of the brainstem and which from the ventromedial system?

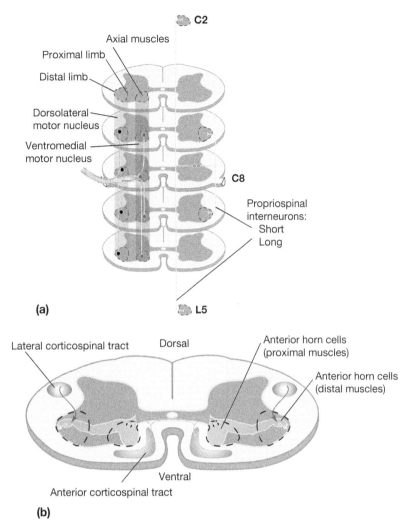

(a)

(b)

FIGURE 11-1 Lower motor neurons of the spinal cord are organized along a lateral-to-medial axis according to the location of the muscles they innervate. LMNs in the lateral nuclei form a dorsolateral group that innervates distal flexor muscles. LMNs in the medial nuclei form a ventromedial group that innervates proximal extensor muscles (axial muscles of the neck and trunk). Interneurons of the intermediate gray also are organized into dorsolateral and ventromedial groups. For example, interneurons of the propriospinal system that are located dorsolaterally and interconnect LMNs of the dorsolateral group have short axons that interconnect just a few spinal segments, whereas those propriospinal interneurons that are located ventromedially and interconnect LMNs of the ventromedial group have long axons that interconnect many spinal cord segments.

spinal cord (Figure 11-2 ■). Many of their axons terminate bilaterally in the spinal gray. Further, as individual axons descend, they send collateral projections to multiple segments of the spinal cord and they terminate on interneurons of the long propriospinal system. The organizational features of the ventromedial descending systems in humans parallel the features elucidated in the monkey. However, in humans the dorsolateral system, comprised of the rubrospinal tract, is small and of unknown significance to movement. In humans, the magnocellular part of the red nucleus giving rise to the rubrospinal tract is small; only a few fibers project to the spinal cord, and they cannot be traced caudal to upper cervical segments. In humans, the functions of the rubrospinal tract appear to have been largely taken over by the last of the descending UMN systems to be considered—namely, the corticospinal tract originating in the motor areas of the cerebral cortex.

Thought Question

Differentiate the short and long propriospinal systems in terms of their locations in the cord, the connections that they make, and the functional role of each.

Cerebral Cortex

The highest level of the motor hierarchy consists of the motor areas of the cerebral cortex. The motor system depends on motor areas of the cerebral cortex to generate complex, precisely timed and discrete movements, especially of the hands and speech muscles. Areas of the cortex that subserve different anatomical areas of the body can be identified as the homunculus. The organization of fibers related to the head, face, and neck (especially the tongue

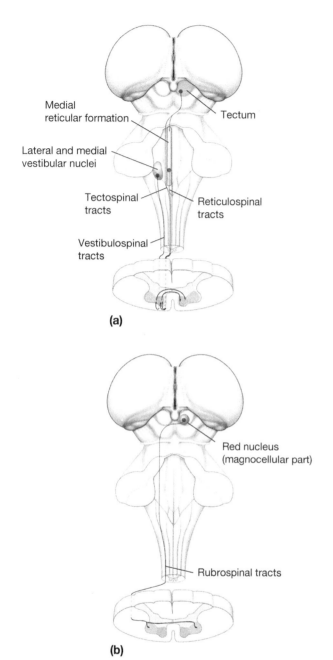

FIGURE 11-2 The dorsolateral and ventromedial descending motor systems that originate in the brainstem.

fibers to the LMNs of different distal extremity muscles originate from distinctly different groups of precentral cortical neurons. This allows the cerebral motor cortex to *selectively* activate individual distal extremity muscles by firing only those cortical motor cells that innervate that specific muscle. Therefore, the corticomotoneuronal component of the corticospinal tract represents a highly differentiated system within a more generalized motor apparatus. Note that this high degree of topographic organization contrasts markedly with the organization of the medial pathways from UMN nuclei of the brainstem. Here, small numbers of UMN cell bodies—for example, those of the magnocellular portion of the reticular formation—give rise to reticulospinal axons that influence LMNs at virtually *all* levels of the spinal cord.

The anatomical organization of the motor hierarchy is consistent at all three of its levels, and the organization's meaning is clear. The hard-wiring at each level constrains the type of motor activity its components are capable of mediating. When active, the ventromedial component can only generate bilateral, synergistic movements involving large numbers of proximal limb and trunk muscles. It represents the basic system by which the brain controls movement, being responsible for maintaining erect posture, integrating limb and body movement, integrating synergic whole limb movement, mediating orienting movements of the body and head, and directing the course of forward progression. In contrast, when active, the dorsolateral component generates fractionated voluntary movement, meaning that muscles are activated in nonstereotypical patterns to permit isolated or unique patterns of movement. In everyday behavior, of course, the two components operate in parallel.

> **Thought Question**
>
> What is the main topographic organization of the motor systems at the level of the cerebral cortex? Is the differentiation of neurons to proximal versus distal muscles and flexors versus extensors easily visualized in the cortex?

Behavioral Organization

The organization of the motor system also can be described in terms of behavior. For example, with respect to voluntary movement, the behavior begins with selecting the intended goal of the movement and generation of an overall strategy by which to attain the goal. This occurs independent of the specific effector used or the particular way the movement's goal is achieved. As an example, sign your name, with your forearm resting on the table. Then sign it on a whiteboard. The two signatures are clearly written by the same person, even though the muscles used to control the movement are substantially different. In the former case, the forearm is stabilized and muscles of the hand control the movement. In the latter case, muscles stabilize the shoulder and forearm, and the movement is from both the

area) can be differentiated from those related to the upper extremities (and especially the hands) and those related to the torso and lower extremities. In contrast to the spinal cord and brainstem, nuclei and tracts are not easily differentiated into those areas specific for flexors and extensors, or proximal versus distal muscles, at the level of cortex.

Corticospinal tract axons access LMNs of the ventral horn both directly and indirectly, via interneurons of the intermediate gray. While axons of the direct corticomotoneuronal projection synapse on LMNs innervating *both* distal extremity and proximal limb muscles, most terminate on the former group of LMNs. These projections show a high degree of topographic organization in that cortical

Thought Question

Even though the motor system can be differentiated into three hierarchical levels, purposeful movements are not hierarchically controlled. Explain the role of the anatomical hierarchy. Thinking ahead, how might the nervous system permit flexibility of movement despite the anatomical hierarchy?

hand and the shoulder. Yet, the output is so similar as to be clearly recognizable. This observation can be explained by the concept of the *motor program* to specify movement tactics. A motor program represents the spatial features of the movement, including the extent of the movement and angles through which particular joints must move. The program also dictates the selection of specific muscles, their sequence of contraction, and contraction forces that are to be used in achieving the goal. Hence, the program can operate through very different groupings of muscles. Finally, the body parts, muscles, and joints that actually execute the movement are engaged. This level of organization of the motor system will be described in greater detail in Chapter 20, but it is introduced here for completeness.

SPINAL CORD REFLEXES

Clinical Preview

In your orthopedic practice, you frequently treat individuals who have compression or other damage to spinal nerves associated with injuries to the back. As part of the examination, you test deep tendon reflexes (DTRs) and rely on the information that you obtain in order to determine your course of intervention. As you read through this section, consider the following:

- What are the structures involved in the DTR?
- When would the DTR be hyperactive, and when would it be hypoactive?
- What can you infer about the level of injury, based on reflex testing?
- What other reflexes could be affected in people who have back injuries?

As noted in Chapter 8, reflexes are the simplest and most stereotyped of all functional movement. Somatic reflexes operate through motor units and result in the contraction of striated muscle. These reflexes can be confined just to the striated muscles or to the autonomic division of the nervous system. Reflexes also may have one of their components in the somatic division and others in the autonomic division of the nervous system. Many of the autonomic reflexes are of importance to survival, as we shall see in Chapter 12.

Thought Question

Stereotypical motor responses can be initiated through reflex arcs. What five components make up the reflex arc?

A **reflex** is an involuntary, relatively short-latency, and stereotyped motor response set into motion by an environmental stimulus. Reflexes are nonvolitional motor responses that may serve protective needs of the organism. They represent preprogrammed responses mediated by neuron circuits consisting of five components collectively called the **reflex arc**. The components of a reflex arc are:

1. A *receptor* that receives and transduces the environmental stimulus.
2. An *afferent fiber* that conducts the information to the CNS.
3. A *reflex center* within the CNS consisting of a variable number of interneurons.
4. An *efferent fiber* that conducts the response from the reflex center to the effector organ in the periphery.
5. An *effector* that produces the response.

The effector may be muscle (striated, cardiac, or smooth) or a gland. The reflex center is where the afferent message from the receptor may converge with afferent impulses from other receptors, or with afferents from other sources, such as the brainstem. This integration can influence the reflex input and response in various ways (Figure 11-3 ■).

Reflexes vary tremendously in terms of their complexity, ranging from simple ones involving contraction of a single muscle to those involving the contraction of many muscles in a precisely timed sequence. Complexity is determined by the neuronal arrangements existing among the interneurons of the reflex center. Virtually all reflex actions can be modified by learning and conscious effort, although most transpire without our conscious awareness, as discussed later.

Although consisting of a specific set of synaptically connected neurons, reflex circuits are not isolated from the remainder of the nervous system. That is, specific sets of neurons dedicated just to reflexes do not exist. Rather, the neurons in reflex circuits are used for other functions as is shown by the convergence of peripheral receptor (segmental), suprasegmental, and local influences onto the neurons belonging to reflex arcs. In other words, the same circuits that are triggered from the periphery by a stimulus may also be volitionally triggered to produce patterned movement sequences. A given muscle may participate in more than one type of reflex.

The Anatomical Substrate of Reflexes

Reflex arcs utilize circuits distributed in the spinal cord, brainstem, cerebral cortex, or combinations of these structures. The afferent fiber in a spinal cord reflex arc is the axon of a spinal nerve. The *cell body* of this primary

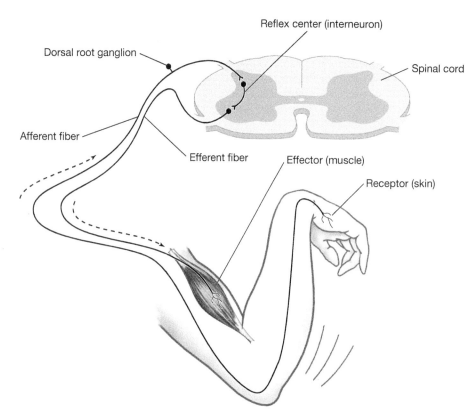

FIGURE 11-3 The five components of a typical spinal cord reflex arc. The reflex center is composed of interneurons (only one is shown) in the dorsal horn and intermediate gray.

afferent axon is located in a dorsal root ganglion. The central process of the dorsal root ganglion neuron synapses in the reflex center that is located either in the dorsal horn or intermediate gray matter, or both, of the spinal cord. The reflex center consists of one or more synaptically linked *interneurons*. As discussed later, interneurons also receive input from sources other than the dorsal root axon of the reflex arc.

Axons from these interneurons project to different parts of the spinal gray matter. When the reflex response involves striated muscle, interneurons of the reflex center project to the ventral horn of the spinal gray to synapse on alpha LMNs. The somatic axons of LMNs enter the ventral root of a spinal nerve and pass to the effector muscle in the nerve. When the reflex response involves autonomic reflexes (i.e., cardiac muscle, smooth muscle, or glandular secretion), the interneurons project to preganglionic autonomic neurons in the lateral aspect of the intermediate zone of the spinal cord (T1–L2 for sympathetic system, S2–S4 for parasympathetic system) whose axons exit the spinal cord via the ventral roots.

Immediately after they enter the spinal cord, all dorsal root fibers divide into branches that can ascend and/or descend for one or two segments before terminating, with some extending over more segments (Figure 11-4 ■). At the segment of entry and along their ascending and descending courses, these dorsal root branches give off collaterals that extend into the dorsal and/or ventral horns

to synapse. These branches and their collaterals establish an extensive network of interconnections between neighboring spinal cord segments. The spinal cord neurons that serve to distribute the reflex input over multiple spinal cord segments are those of the spinospinal, or propriospinal, system (Chapter 5).

The terms *intrasegmental* and *intersegmental reflex mechanisms* are used to describe these connections. Note that no naturally occurring reflex exists whose neurons are confined just to one segment of the spinal cord. Several anatomical arrangements function to distribute the reflex input entering the cord at one segment to affect multiple spinal cord segments.

The Interneuronal Pool

To fully understand the reflex response, it is important to further understand the **interneuronal pool**. The interneuronal pool is the set of interneurons making up the reflex center of the reflex arc. All reflex arcs contain at least one interneuron, with the exception of one component of the reflex arc belonging to the stretch (myotatic) reflex that lacks an interneuron, as discussed later. The interneuronal pool is significant for several reasons. First, the synaptic linkages of interneurons with one another and with LMNs in the case of somatic reflexes determine the pattern of the reflex response. The pattern of the reflex refers to the mechanics of the reflex behavior: which muscles contract and which relax, whether muscles on one or both sides of

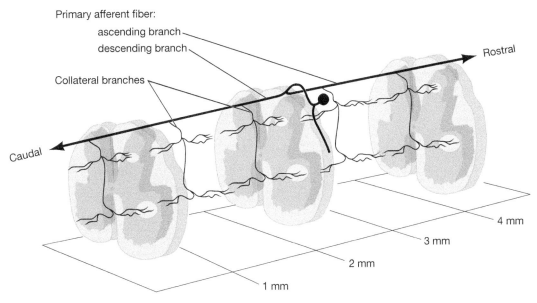

Primary afferent fiber:
ascending branch
descending branch
Collateral branches
Rostral
Caudal
1 mm
2 mm
3 mm
4 mm

FIGURE 11-4 One example of the structure of a primary afferent neuron after entering the spinal cord. Note that the collateral branches have a regular arrangement, one being given off approximately every 1 mm.

> **Thought Question**
>
> Some reflexes make synapses with interneurons, which permit them to influence muscle activity in groups of muscles—exciting some and inhibiting others. Explain how these connections operate, and give examples that illustrate the functional importance of these connections.

the body contract, which muscles are influenced and for how long, and the temporal sequence in which different muscles contract or relax. The interneuronal pool also is important because it is one of the major sites at which the brain is able to modify the characteristics of the reflex. In the case of spinal cord reflexes that are carried out by the segmental level of the nervous system, this modifying influence of the brain is referred to as **suprasegmental control** and will be discussed later in this chapter.

Examples of Common Reflexes

Comprehensive neurology textbooks can present up to 30 different reflexes involving the spinal and cranial nerves. The examples presented here illustrate the general principles governing the operation of spinal reflexes. Importantly, many of these reflexes are utilized in the context of rehabilitation.

Stretch Reflex

The simplest and best studied of the spinal reflexes is the **stretch (myotatic) reflex**, so-called because it is elicited by the stretch of the muscle. Muscle stretch is most often elicited by tapping the tendon of a muscle with a reflex hammer, which simultaneously stretches the muscle's full complement of muscle spindle stretch receptors. The response consists of a brief and brisk contraction of the stretched muscle. Virtually all muscles of the body have stretch reflexes, many of which may be tested in the neurologic examination. Table 11-1 ■ summarizes four commonly tested myotatic (stretch) reflexes.

The most commonly tested of the spinal stretch reflexes is the **quadriceps**, **patellar**, or **knee-jerk reflex** (Figure 11-5 ■). The patellar reflex is elicited by tapping the patellar tendon, which stretches the quadriceps muscle and its complement of muscle spindles. This reflex circuit causes the quadriceps muscle to briefly contract, which extends the leg at the knee. Note that only a single muscle contracts and that it is the *same one* that was stretched by the stimulus. Note also that this is a highly artificial type of stimulus—one that does not occur under normal physiological conditions—so that the normal functional significance of this reflex is not clear. Because the reflex response is so brief, this is called a **phasic stretch reflex**. It involves a fast stimulus and fast response. Despite questions about

Table 11-1 Commonly Tested Myotatic Reflexes

MUSCLE OR TENDON	NERVE	KEY SPINAL CORD SEGMENT
Biceps	Musculocutaneous	C6
Triceps	Radial	C7
Patellar	Femoral	L4
Achilles	Tibial and sciatic	S1

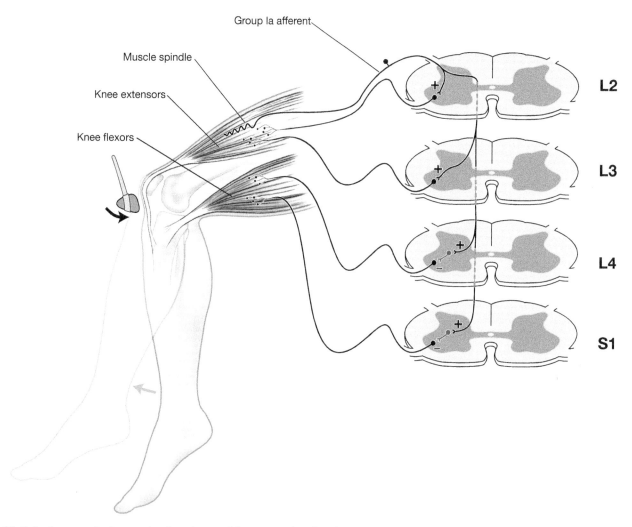

FIGURE 11-5 In the neurologic examination, the quadriceps stretch reflex (tendon jerk) is elicited by tapping the patellar tendon with a reflex hammer. This stretches the muscle spindles in the quadriceps, whose synchronous discharge directly excites LMNs innervating that muscle. This results in extension of the leg at the knee. In order for extension to occur, the antagonistic knee flexor muscles (hamstrings) must relax. This is accomplished by the muscle spindle primary afferent fibers synapsing on inhibitory interneurons that, in turn, synapse on knee flexor lower motor neurons to inhibit their activity.

the functional significance of the phasic knee-jerk reflex, the reflex is extremely useful clinically. (See Clinical Connections.)

Thought Question

The simplest reflex is the patellar stretch reflex. How is this reflex elicited, and what is its clinical importance? You can consciously modify this reflex response. Demonstrate this with a partner, and explain what this implies in terms of the circuitry controlling the reflex response.

The muscle spindles in the quadriceps respond to the tendon tap by simultaneously lengthening and sending a synchronous volley of action potentials in Group Ia afferents to the spinal cord over the appropriate dorsal roots. Once within the spinal cord, these afferents establish

highly specific synaptic connections on neurons in the ipsilateral side of the spinal gray matter. One set of branches from these primary afferents extends through the dorsal horn and intermediate gray to synapse *directly* on lower motor neurons in the ventral horn. Because only one synapse intervenes between the primary afferent and the motor neuron, the stretch reflex is called a **monosynaptic reflex**. The monosynaptic connections are made with the LMNs that innervate the quadriceps muscle, and these are distributed over several spinal cord segments (L2–L4). The synchronous volley of impulses in the muscle spindle afferents elicits an equally synchronous and brief discharge of quadriceps alpha LMNs, resulting in a sharp contraction of the quadriceps muscle and knee extension. But note that the term *monosynaptic* applies only to this particular part of the reflex arc and that another part of the arc exists in which the linkage between the primary afferent and LMN involves more than one synapse.

In order for the leg to extend at the knee, the muscles antagonistic to the quadriceps—the knee flexors (hamstrings)—must relax at the same time quadriceps contracts. This is referred to as **reciprocal innervation**. Reciprocal innervation is accomplished by inhibiting the LMNs innervating the flexor hamstring muscles (L4–S2). The group of muscle spindle primary afferent branches that mediate this inhibition synapse first on **inhibitory interneurons** in the intermediate gray that, in turn, synapse on the hamstring LMNs in the ventral horn. Thus, this part of the reflex arc is disynaptic (see Figure 11-5). The inhibitory interneuron converts the excitatory muscle spindle input into inhibition of the flexor LMNs. The excitatory innervation of the extensor (agonist) and inhibitory innervation of the flexor (antagonist) LMNs is an example of reciprocal innervations, which is a property of all somatic spinal reflex arcs. In this context, excitation of the skeletal muscle is accomplished by exciting its alpha motor neurons. In contrast, relaxation of skeletal muscles is accomplished by inhibitory interneurons such that the LMN cannot cause excitation of the muscle.

As noted, the phasic stretch reflex is elicited by a highly artificial stimulus. There are, however, **tonic stretch reflexes** that are elicited by the natural stretches imposed on muscles by gravitational forces in the act of maintaining a normal upright posture. Tonic stretch reflexes involve long-duration stimuli and long responses. In maintaining an upright stance, we actually sway slightly to and fro in opposite directions. The muscles stretched by a sway in one direction will reflexively contract to bring us back to the desired position. These tonic stretch reflexes are continuously active but, by themselves, are not strong enough to elicit a phasic reflex contraction of muscle. Quiescent motor neurons can be brought to the reflex firing level only by highly synchronized volleys in many afferent fibers, as occurs in the phasic stretch reflex. In contrast, tonic stretch reflexes work to augment the strength of muscle contraction only when the alpha LMNs themselves are *already* active, as when maintaining an upright stance.

The sensitivity of the muscle spindle, and thus the sensitivity of the stretch reflex to increases in muscle length, can be controlled by the brain. As discussed in Chapter 9, this is the function of the gamma system that provides a motor innervation to the muscle spindles themselves. During the act of sitting, for example, the sensitivity of the stretch reflex is decreased by the brain so that a reflex is not elicited, despite the fact that the length of the quadriceps muscle is increasing.

Inverse Myotatic Reflex

A second muscle receptor, which responds to muscle tension (as opposed to stretch), is the Golgi tendon organ (GTO) located in tendons near their junctions with striated muscle. Although muscle tension can increase with lengthening of a muscle, the significant aspect of increased muscle tension is that which results from *contraction of the*

muscle. GTOs are exquisitely sensitive to minute increases in tension generated by contraction of even a few of the fibers making up a whole muscle.

Like muscle spindles, GTOs have reflex connections onto alpha LMNs in the spinal cord. Stimulation of GTO Group Ib afferents results in the *relaxation of the muscle* in which the receptors reside and is due to the *inhibition* of the appropriate alpha LMNs. The effect of Group Ib stimulation is referred to as **autogenic inhibition** because the muscle stimulated is the one that is inhibited. Note that the reflex effect is the opposite of that following stimulation of Group Ia afferents.

The reflex connections established by Group Ib afferents onto alpha LMNs involve interneurons (Figure 11-6 ■). One branch of the Group Ib primary afferent synapses on inhibitory interneurons that, in turn, synapse on alpha LMNs that project back to the muscle of afferent origin. The other branch of the Group Ib afferent synapses on excitatory interneurons that, in turn, synapse on alpha LMNs that innervate the muscle antagonistic to the muscle of afferent origin. Thus, the reflex evoked by GTOs causes relaxation of the agonist and contraction of the antagonist muscle. Again, the principle of reciprocal innervation is used. However, these connections are the inverse of those made by afferents from muscle spindles. For this reason, the reflex mediated by GTOs has been called the **inverse myotatic reflex**.

> ### Thought Question
>
> Compare and contrast reflexes arising from the muscle spindle and the Golgi tendon organ in terms of the location of the receptor and influence on muscles.

The inverse myotatic reflex was originally envisioned as being protective in nature: it was thought to prevent muscle from developing potentially damaging levels of tension that could result in tearing of the muscle or tendon. However, GTOs are so sensitive to contraction tension that the reflex would be activated long before dangerous levels of tension were ever reached. So, these reflex connections must serve other functions in normal motor behavior. Possibly they function as a tension feedback system, counteracting small changes in tension by increasing or decreasing the inhibition to motor neurons (e.g., during muscle fatigue). It also has been speculated that the connections may provide a spinal mechanism for the control of exploratory movements. For example, when the hand first contacts an object, muscle force may be inhibited by the activation of GTOs in order to soften the contact.

Flexion Reflex

A suddenly applied noxious (L., *noxius*, injurious) stimulus to the skin of the arm or leg elicits a specifically patterned movement that is adapted to withdraw the limb from the

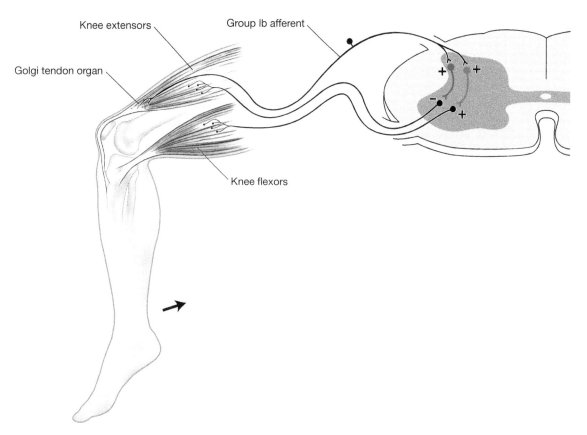

FIGURE 11-6 The inverse myotatic reflex elicited by Golgi tendon organs. These disynaptic reflex connections mediate autogenic inhibition, so-called because the muscle whose tension has increased is the one that is inhibited (−).

offending stimulus. The classic example of such a spinal defense reaction is the **flexion withdrawal reflex**, which is a much more complex reflex than the stretch reflex. The stretch reflex limits its excitatory discharge to just a few spinal cord segments. In contrast, the excitatory discharge of the nociceptive flexor reflex spreads through many segments of the spinal cord so that flexion at all joints of an extremity is elicited. Indeed, the reflex discharge may spread throughout the length of most of the spinal cord. This is true even though the reflex input enters the spinal cord over as few as two dorsal roots. Thus, the spinospinal (propriospinal) system is massively engaged in the flexor reflex.

The full response of the flexion reflex is actually a flexion reflex with extension of the contralateral extremity, and it involves both sides of the body. The reflex response is illustrated by a person stepping on a sand burr when the legs are supporting the body weight. On the stimulated side, the leg is withdrawn from the painful stimulus by flexion at all joints of the extremity (Figure 11-7 ■). Relaxation of the antagonistic extensor muscles occurs concurrently with flexor muscle contraction so that limb flexion is unimpeded by antagonistic extensor muscle contraction. At the same time, on the contralateral side, the extremity is extended, providing body weight support. These two processes are discussed next.

The excitatory influence on ipsilateral flexor and inhibitory influence on ipsilateral extensor LMNs are both

mediated by complex chains of interneurons that help determine the properties associated with multisynaptic spinal reflexes. These two properties are divergence and after-discharge. Diverging interneuronal circuits reciprocally engage lower motor neurons distributed over spinal cord segments L2–S2 so that the leg flexes at all joints. This involves not only intrasegmental interneurons but also intersegmental neurons of the spinospinal system. Additionally, these interneuronal circuits are organized in such a way that they continue to excite and inhibit motor neurons even after the painful stimulus has stopped. This prolonged output discharge that outlasts the stimulus is called after-discharge. After-discharge ensures that the extremity is held away from the painful stimulus even after it is over so that other reflexes and CNS actions can move the entire body away from the stimulus.

After-discharge occurs as a result of the patterns of synaptic linkages established by groups of interneurons in the reflex center. One pattern is characterized by the input reaching an LMN through routes containing different numbers of interneurons (Figure 11-8 ■). The signal induced by the stimulus input is delayed by about 0.5 msec at each synapse. Thus, signals that pass through successive interneurons reach the motor neuron one-by-one after varying periods of delay. After-discharge also occurs as a result of positive feedback in which the output of an interneuronal circuit feeds back to re-excite

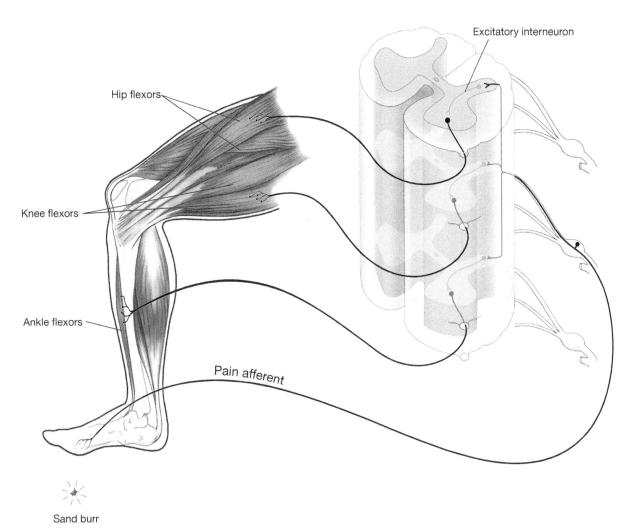

FIGURE 11-7 Ipsilateral reflex connections mediating flexion of the lower extremity at all joints following noxious stimulation of the foot.

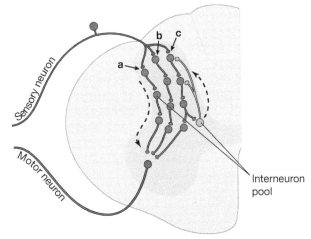

FIGURE 11-8 One possible arrangement of neurons in the interneuronal pool responsible for after-discharge. The primary afferent simultaneously activates pathways a, b, and c, but each pathway contains different numbers of interneurons before reaching the LMN. Each synapse in the pathway delays arrival of activity at the LMN by about 0.5 msec.

the same circuit. The duration of the after-discharge depends on the intensity of the painful stimulus. A weak stimulus causes almost no after-discharge, whereas the after-discharge elicited by a strong stimulus may last for several seconds. Flexion of the ipsilateral leg is accompanied by extension of the opposite leg, as described earlier. This is called the **crossed extensor reflex**. The crossed extensor reflex is properly part of the withdrawal reflex because not only does it support the body as the ipsilateral limb flexes and withdraws, but it can move the body away from the harmful stimulus. The crossed extensor component of the withdrawal reflex is mediated by interneurons that cross to the opposite side of the spinal cord. These contralaterally projecting interneurons influence flexor and extensor LMNs but in a pattern opposite to that on the ipsilateral side of the cord: extensor motor neurons are excited and flexor motor neurons inhibited (Figure 11-9 ■). Because the extension of the opposite limb begins only after the stimulated limb has started to flex, even more interneurons are involved. However,

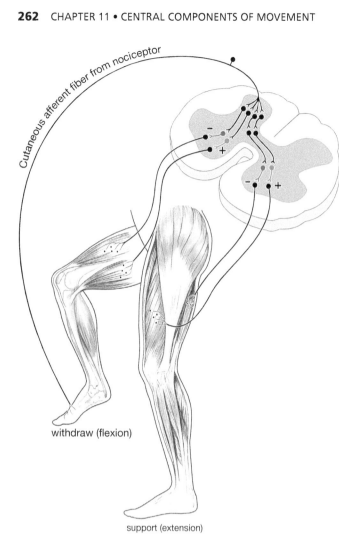

FIGURE 11-9 The flexor withdrawal–crossed extension reflex. The interneurons that cross to the opposite side of the spinal cord excite (+) extensor motor neurons and inhibit (–) flexor motor neurons, resulting in extension of the opposite leg.

their organization is such that the discharge spreads intersegmentally and creates after-discharge.

The exact pattern of a flexor withdrawal reflex in a limb varies, depending on the part of the limb that has been stimulated. This variation is called local sign. Thus, with a painful stimulus on the inside of the arm, the response will include some abduction in addition to flexion of the arm. Stimulation of the lateral surface of the arm results in some adduction along with flexion. Local sign is really a fixed spatial relationship between the locus of a stimulus and the particular set of muscles and force with which they contract. In addition to influences arising in the periphery,

Thought Question

The flexion reflex and crossed extensor reflex often go together. Explain the circuitry that allows these reflexes to operate simultaneously, and explain the functional importance of this arrangement.

such as stimulus intensity and location (local sign), the spinal flexion reflex may also be modified by suprasegmental control. Response intensity can be varied by hypnosis and attentive or apprehensive state.

ADAPTABILITY OF REFLEXES When a noxious stimulus is applied, the appropriate response is to withdraw from that stimulus. This often involves flexion and, therefore, the flexor withdrawal reflex. However, in some cases, the appropriate response is extension. Consider, for example, a noxious stimulus to the front of the thigh in which the leg would withdraw away from the stimulus and hence into extension. This illustrates that the spinally mediated flexion reflex is not the only reflex elicited by a noxious stimulus.

Other Reflexes

The stretch and flexor reflexes utilize only the somatic division of the nervous system—thus, they are **somatomotor reflexes**. Such reflexes are initiated by somatic receptors of the body wall (exteroceptors and proprioceptors) and result in the contraction of skeletal (striated, voluntary, somatic) muscles. In contrast, **visceromotor reflexes** (Figure 11-10 ■) are confined to the autonomic division of the nervous system (ANS). The receptors are situated in the viscera and the action potentials are conducted to the CNS over the general visceral afferent component of spinal nerves. These fibers synapse on autonomic motor cells of the intermediolateral cell column whose preganglionic axons then course out of the CNS in the ventral root and synapse in an autonomic ganglion. The postganglionic axon then passes to the target viscera and terminates in an effector structure. An example of a spinal visceromotor reflex is the regulation of bladder muscle tone (Chapter 12). Other visceromotor reflexes include participation of the brainstem parasympathetic component of the ANS. An example is the change of blood pressure and heart rate as a result of changes in the carotid sinus and arch of the aorta.

Autonomic activity is closely related to somatic activity. Autonomic motor neurons can be activated by visceral sensory signals arising from receptors in organs. And, somatic LMNs can be activated by receptors located in visceral organs. **Somatovisceral reflexes** are composed of somatic afferents and visceral efferents. The pilomotor reflex is an example. Cooling of the body surface is detected by thermoreceptors of the skin. The reflex response is mediated by fibers of the sympathetic division of ANS and consists of erection of the body hair to increase surface insulation. The response of blood vessels to temperature changes is another example of a somatovisceral reflex. **Viscerosomatic reflexes** utilize the autonomic division of the nervous system as the afferent limb of the reflex arc and the somatic division as the efferent limb of the reflex arc. An example of such a reflex is the muscular rigidity of the abdominal wall as a result of acute inflammation in the abdominal viscera. These reflexes are discussed further in Chapter 12.

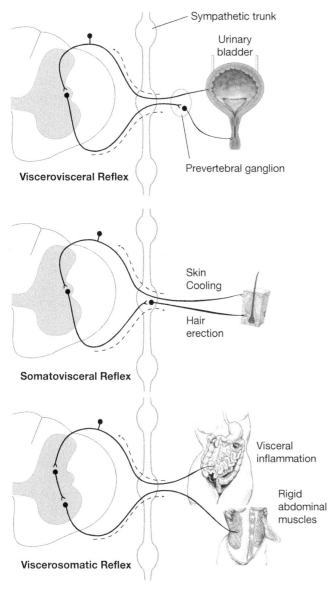

Viscerovisceral Reflex

Sympathetic trunk

Urinary bladder

Prevertebral ganglion

Somatovisceral Reflex

Skin Cooling

Hair erection

Viscerosomatic Reflex

Visceral inflammation

Rigid abdominal muscles

FIGURE 11-10 Reflexes involving the autonomic and somatic divisions of the nervous system.

CLINICAL CONNECTIONS
Clinical Evaluation of Reflexes

A variety of reflexes can be elicited in the neurological examination. Three aspects of reflex function are assessed. First, is the reflex present or absent? When the reflex cannot be elicited, then the term **areflexia** is applied. Second, if the reflex is present, has its **status** been altered? This involves the interpretation and **grading of reflexes**. The clinician must assess the strength of the minimal stimulus necessary to elicit the reflex and then must assess three interrelated components of the resulting muscle contraction: (1) the speed of contraction and relaxation, (2) the force of contraction, and (3) the

degree of shortening. When the reflex is less active than normal, the term **hyporeflexia** is applied, and when the reflex is exaggerated, the term **hyperreflexia** is applied. The third aspect of reflex function assessed is whether pathological reflexes are present. A **pathological reflex** is defined as a reflex that normally does not occur in a patient of the age being examined. Some of these reflexes have functional or diagnostic importance. Two examples that are normally expressed in infants, but not in adults, are the Babinski reflex (sign) and the stepping response discussed in the next section.

Hamstring Stretch Reflexes, Anterior Cruciate Ligament, and Knee Stability

The hamstring muscles (semitendinosus, semimembranosus, and long head of the biceps femoris) play a critical role in maintaining knee stability and directly protect the anterior cruciate ligament (ACL) from rupture under normal physiological conditions. From a mechanical standpoint, the ACL prevents the femur from sliding posteriorly on the tibia, thus preventing hyperextension of the knee. When the knee is moderately hyperextended and excessive anterior displacement of the tibia occurs, the hamstrings are stretched, thereby stretching their contingent of muscle spindles and eliciting hamstring stretch reflexes. The contracting hamstrings apply a posteriorly directed force to the proximal tibia that limits its anterior displacement, thereby relieving strain on the ACL.

Two hamstring stretch reflexes are elicited. First, a monosynaptic short latency response (SLR) occurs and is due to the primary endings of muscle spindles and Group Ia afferents. A second and later response then occurs and is called the medium latency response (MLR). This is a polysynaptic reflex and is mediated by secondary endings of the muscle spindle and Group II afferents. In addition, a third hamstring reflex has been shown to exist, and it is elicited by mechanical stretch of the ACL itself. The ACL contains a variety of mechanoreceptors, including Golgi and Pacinian corpuscles. Intraoperative (during arthroscopy) direct mechanical stimulation of the ACL elicits both short- and medium-latency hamstring reflexes. That these reflexes arise from ACL mechanoreceptors is shown by the fact that injection of a local anesthetic into the ACL results in a significant decrease in the reflex response. While this direct ACL–hamstring reflex contributes to the SLR and MLR stretch reflexes, the contribution is not large.

Thought Question

How would the reflex response of the triceps muscle change if the dorsal root carrying sensory information from that muscle was transected? What if the alpha motor neuron pool or the efferent nerve was transected?

These hamstring reflexes are differentially affected following rupture and successful surgical repair of the ACL. The SLR is not affected, but the MLR undergoes a significant increase in its latency. This latency increase has been interpreted to mean that there is a decrease in the excitability of the MLR due to a change in the polysynaptic reflex circuitry in the spinal cord.

Following ACL rupture and successful surgical repair, knee stability is decreased relative to healthy knees. Furthermore, one group of such patients complains of a subjective feeling of knee instability referred to as the "giving-way" phenomenon, whereas a second group does not. Significantly, the extent of knee instability is the same in both groups. One difference between these two groups is the length of the latency increase to the onset of the MLR following anterior–posterior tibial translation in standing patients bearing full body weight. The MLR has a significantly longer latency in patients experiencing the giving-way phenomenon than in those who do not.

The significant therapeutic question, then, is can this latency be reduced by physiotherapy? Can the excitability of the polysynaptic MLR be increased? Possibly so. Appropriate physiotherapy may increase the activity of the gamma motor system by causing changes in its suprasegmental control. By causing augmented responses of the secondary spindle endings and increased activity of Group II afferents, heightened gamma activity would result in an increased excitability of the MLR hamstring stretch reflex.

PYRAMIDAL TRACT

Clinical Preview ·················

You work in a hospital in a small rural community that provides both emergent care and rehabilitation services. You first encountered Laura Wolinsky in the intensive care unit (ICU). She had sustained a spinal cord injury during a skiing accident. Your treated her for a few days during her initial recovery from surgical stabilization of the spine. At that time, her lower extremities were flaccid. Laura then was transferred to a regional spinal cord injury rehabilitation unit for inpatient rehabilitation. She returned to your hospital for outpatient rehabilitation four months later. At that time, her lower extremities were hyperreflexive (exhibited spasticity), and her legs tended to go into flexion patterns with mild stimulation on the foot. As you read through this section, consider the following:

- What is the mechanism that caused Laura's extremities to be flaccid initially but hyperreflexive later?

- What is the time frame in which these changes occur?

- What types of interventions are available for spasticity?

By its historical definition, the **pyramidal tract** is an anatomical entity: it consists of those fibers that originate in the cerebral cortex and descend longitudinally through the pyramids of the medulla to reach the spinal cord, hence its name. (Although axons of the pyramidal tract arise from large pyramidal cells of the cerebral cortex, the tract is not named after these cells.) Recall from Chapter 2 that the white matter of each hemisphere is made up of association, commissural, and projection fibers, and from Chapter 7 that pyramidal neurons, the most numerous neurons of the neocortex named for their shape, are the principal output neurons of the cerebral cortex. Thus, fibers that leave the cerebral cortex to terminate either in another area of the cortex or in a subcortical structure are mostly the axons of pyramidal neurons.

In this text, we shall adhere to this historical definition—and add to it a function in accordance with our definition of a tract. The pyramidal tract is a UMN tract originating in the cerebral cortex and terminating in the spinal cord that regulates the activity of spinal cord LMNs in the course of controlling voluntary movement. The term **corticospinal tract** is synonymous with pyramidal tract. There is a functional equivalent of the pyramidal tract that controls LMNs of cranial nerve motor nuclei in the brainstem. This is the **corticobulbar tract**, so named because the brainstem was at one time referred to as the bulb. It is discussed in Chapter 14.

In the human, approximately 60 percent of pyramidal tract axons originate from the primary motor cortex that makes up the bulk of the precentral gyrus, Brodmann's area 4. Area 4 contains the **giant pyramidal cells of Betz**. Betz cells give rise to the largest and fastest conducting myelinated axons of the pyramidal tract (with diameters between 9 and 22 μm), but comprise only a little more than 3 percent of the total number of axons in the tract. The remaining pyramidal tract axons arise from the **premotor cortex** located on the lateral hemispheral surface in Brodmann's area 6, from the **supplementary motor cortex** located on the medial hemispheral surface of area 6, and from the postcentral gyrus of Brodmann's areas 3, 1, and 2. Although we classify areas 3, 1, and 2 as primary somatosensory cortex, they are an important UMN source of the pyramidal tract. Additionally, there are limbic-motor contributions from the cingulate gyrus.

Pyramidal tract axons leave the cortex grouped in a somatotopic order as shown in Figure 11-11 ■ . They descend through the **corona radiata** to enter the internal capsule, where they are confined to a compact region in the posterior half of the posterior limb of the capsule (Figure 11-12 ■). The somatotopic organization of the pyramidal tract as it descends through the brainstem is essentially unknown. Upon entering the midbrain, pyramidal fibers are distributed in the approximate middle third of the cerebral peduncles (crus cerebri). Each cerebral peduncle contains some 21 million axons, only 1 million of which continue on into the ipsilateral pyramid to form the corticospinal tract. The majority of the other descending axons in each cerebral peduncle terminate in

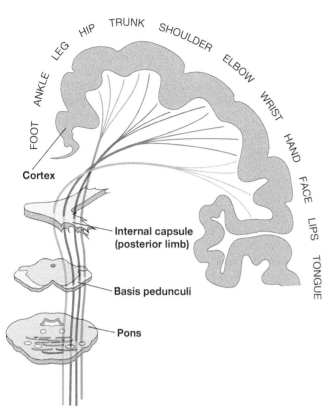

FIGURE 11-11 Somatotopic organization of the pyramidal system from its origin in the precentral gyrus to the posterior limb of the internal capsule. Note how the fibers twist in their descent toward the internal capsule.

Thought Question

Pyramidal tract fibers originate in the cerebral cortex and then follow specific pathways through brainstem to spinal cord and other destinations. By now, you should be able to describe the location of these fibers as they descend from cortex. Specifically, differentiate the pathways by which the lateral corticospinal tract (LCST) and anterior corticospinal tract (ACST) travel.

Corticospinal Tracts

At the level of caudalmost medulla, the majority (75 to 90 percent) of corticospinal tract fibers cross in the pyramidal decussation (Figure 11-13 ■). The percentage of fibers that cross not only varies across individuals, but the number of decussating axons from each side is most often asymmetrical. The fibers that cross continue their descent in the spinal cord as the **lateral corticospinal tract (LCST)**. The smaller contingent of uncrossed axons descend as the **anterior (or ventral) corticospinal tract (ACST)**. Given the typical asymmetry in the number of fibers from each side that cross, the size of these descending fibers systems on either side of the spinal cord usually varies.

The crossed LCST is located in the dorsal portion of the lateral funiculus. Its axons are spread so extensively in the cervical cord that many lesions, whether surgical or pathological, are likely to damage numerous LCST axons. The tract extends caudally in the lateral funiculus to the caudalmost sacral segment. LCST axons have a differential distribution over the longitudinal extent of the spinal cord. The majority of axons, 55 percent, terminate at cervical levels, and the bulk of these end within the cervical enlargement. Such an innervation pattern underscores the extent to which the corticospinal tract (and, of course, the motor cortex itself) focuses on the innervation of a single

the pons (pontine nuclei). Descending corticobulbar fibers are also located in the cerebral peduncle. Within the pons, pyramidal tract fibers split into a number of more or less discrete bundles of variable size known as the longitudinal fibers of the pons. These fibers then reassemble upon approaching the medulla and, within it, appear superficially positioned as the **pyramids** of the medulla.

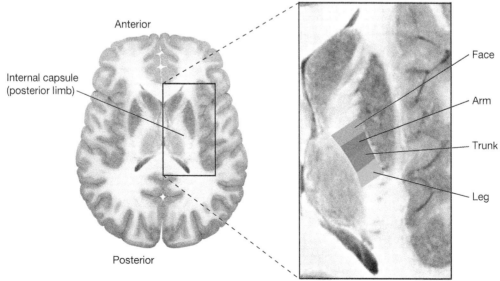

FIGURE 11-12 The trajectory of the lateral corticospinal tract through the posterior limb of the internal capsule.

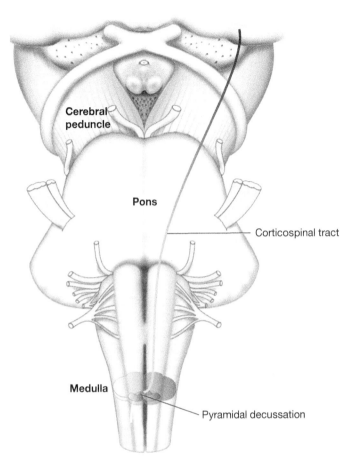

Cerebral peduncle

Pons

Corticospinal tract

Medulla

Pyramidal decussation

FIGURE 11-13 Decussation of the corticospinal (pyramidal) tract in caudal medulla.

motor structure, the hand. The next largest group of axons, 25 percent, end at lumbosacral levels innervating the lower extremity, while the fewest, 20 percent, terminate at thoracic levels innervating the trunk.

Axons of the uncrossed ACST occupy an oval area of the ventral funiculus adjacent to the anterior median fissure. Fibers of the ACST extend only to upper thoracic levels of the cord, contributing to the regulation of the neck, trunk, and proximal upper extremities. Most of these fibers cross in the anterior white commissure in cervical spinal segments to influence contralateral LMN activity.

Corticospinal tract axons influence lower motor neurons either directly, in which case cortical access to the LMN is monosynaptic, or indirectly via ventral horn interneurons, in which case cortical access is polysynaptic. The different modes of termination (direct versus indirect) are employed to achieve different functional ends. One is not more important than the other, simply different. Direct endings occur on motoneurons innervating both proximal and distal musculature but are most densely distributed to lower cervical LMNs innervating the hand muscles located in the dorsolateral ventral horn. Such direct **corticomotoneuronal** connections arise from the Betz cells of the primary motor cortex and provide for secure, precise, and rapid control over LMN activity. They are responsible for independent

movements of the fingers. In addition to ending directly on alpha LMNs, pyramidal tract axons also end on gamma motoneurons that innervate the intrafusal fibers of muscle spindles. As noted in Chapter 9, alpha and gamma motor neurons innervating the same muscle are co-activated.

The vast majority of corticospinal axons make indirect connections, synapsing first on interneurons of the intermediate gray rather than on motoneurons themselves. Routing control through an interneuronal network provides a more diffuse mode of regulation, but presumably one with greater integration. This integration would pertain to the activity of a wider array of muscle groups and contributes to the mediation of multijoint movements such as occur in walking and reaching. Also, by being routed through interneurons, corticospinal input to LMNs can be integrated with other kinds of descending and segmental influences that likewise impinge on the interneuronal pool. Many of these interneurons are intercalated in reflex pathways that, in turn, influence alpha and gamma motor neurons.

Finally, a small number of axons, fewer than in nonhuman primates, end in the dorsal horn of the spinal cord. These fibers of the pyramidal tract originate in the primary sensory cortex of the postcentral gyrus. They function to influence the transmission of sensory information through dorsal horn neurons.

To summarize, even though there is a hard-wired substrate in the spinal cord, motor responses are not restricted to that wiring. By either facilitating or inhibiting interneurons, the primary motor cortex has a wide range of influences on the final common pathway and, therefore, on the muscle contractions that occur. This system of wiring allows for complex patterns of motor behavior, despite the fact that the substrate is hard-wired.

Lesions affecting the pyramidal tract usually do so in concert with involvement of other tracts and systems, making it impossible to define the set of deficits representing true pyramidal tract signs. For example, a cerebrovascular accident involving the posterior limb of the internal capsule would interrupt not only fibers of the pyramidal tract, but also a variety of other fiber systems descending from the cerebral cortex. Such a lesion could include corticostriate, corticothalamic, corticopontine, and corticoreticular projections from which reticulospinal projections originate. The only site in the CNS where a naturally occurring lesion might selectively and completely damage the pyramidal tract is in the medulla, where the medullary pyramids occupy its ventral surface. No such lesion has been reported in the clinical literature, at least to our knowledge, with adequate histological confirmation that, in fact, all axons descending in the pyramids were interrupted bilaterally. This is not to say that lesions confined primarily, even entirely, to the medullary pyramids in humans have not been reported, only that such lesions have never been confirmed to have interrupted all pyramidal tract fibers bilaterally. If even some fibers remain intact, some capacity for voluntary control of the limbs may survive. Consequently,

Thought Question

What is the importance of having a hard-wired system for control of movement when movement itself is quite flexible?

researchers turned to placing discrete and verified surgical lesions in the pyramidal system of nonhuman primates.

In one of the more widely cited studies of this nature, the medullary pyramids were sectioned bilaterally in monkeys in a procedure called a bilateral **pyramidotomy**. One of the primary initial deficits observed was a hypotonic, or flaccid, paresis or paralysis. With time, the hypotonia gave way to a set of what were considered to be permanent deficits consisting of three elements: a reduction of movement speed, a slight muscular weakness along with an easy fatigability of muscles, and a loss of the ability to **fractionate movements** of the hand (i.e., the monkeys could no longer perform independent movements of the fingers). But considerable voluntary movement was retained, showing that an intact pyramidal tract was not necessary for voluntary movements, only for their speed, agility, and fractionation. There was no enduring paresis, and no spasticity was observed either initially or as a permanent sequela. Such findings seemed to fly directly in the face of clinical teaching, which has always considered paralysis, paresis, and spasticity as representing cardinal signs of pyramidal tract damage. Because spasticity is of such importance and complexity, this issue is discussed later in a separate section.

Following incomplete pyramidal tract lesions, recovery of voluntary movement often occurs in a characteristic pattern. Coarse movements involving the proximal muscles recover more than do fine movements mediated by distal muscles, and isolated movements of the fingers often are permanently lost. Recovery of locomotor function following chronic spinal cord injury is mediated by spared pyramidal tract fibers.

Suprasegmental Control of Reflexes

Reflexes may be modified using suprasegmental control under a variety of circumstances. For example, when you grasp a pot of boiling water, the normal rapid withdrawal response (flexion reflex) to splashing some of it on your hand may result in spilling of the hot water. This withdrawal reflex may be completely suppressed via supraspinal modulation by your knowledge of the presence of a young child standing by your side. General attentive and motivational states, as well as sleep, may determine not only the occurrence of a reflex, but its entire pattern. In some people, the intensity of even the simplest of all reflexes may be modified by conscious effort.

The prerequisite for effective **supraspinal control** (also called **suprasegmental control**) is that the brain structures controlling reflexes must receive information about the neural events transpiring in the reflex center. Thus, some of the information ascending through the long tracts of the spinal cord and brainstem comes from interneuronal components of the reflex arc and enables these suprasegmental structures to continuously monitor activity taking place in the reflex centers. Suprasegmental structures may control the amount of inhibition, the amount of excitation, or the balance of excitation and inhibition existing in the interneuronal pool. For example, a variety of peripheral stimuli are potentially capable of eliciting a flexor response in an extremity. However, only strong painful (noxious) stimuli are normally effective. This is because the spinal reflex center of the flexion reflex arc is usually held in an inhibited state by the brainstem via the **tonic descending inhibitory pathway (TDIP)** so that only noxious stimuli are strong enough to evoke the flexion reflex (Figure 11-14 ■). When the spinal cord is damaged, this descending inhibitory control may be lost so that even harmless cutaneous stimulation of the thigh may result in a massive flexion reflex (see Spinal Shock).

A variety of suprasegmental structures exert control over reflexes, including the brainstem reticular formation, cerebellum, and cerebral cortex. Importantly, each of these structures exerts a different type of control over reflex activity. Thus, by testing spinal cord reflexes in a neurologic exam, a clinician may be able to determine which of these structures has been damaged by the nature of the change in a specific reflex pattern.

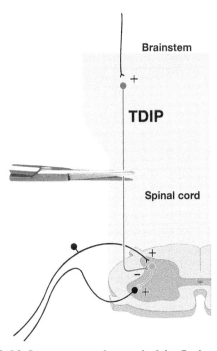

FIGURE 11-14 Suprasegmental control of the flexion reflex pathway. The tonic descending inhibitory pathway (TDIP) is continuously active and normally inhibits (−) the interneurons mediating the flexion reflex. The cells of origin of the TDIP are in the lower brainstem, and they receive a continuous excitatory (+) input. Transection of the spinal cord eliminates the influence of the TDIP and increases the excitatory activity of the flexion reflex interneurons. Thus, paraplegic patients display overly active flexion reflex responses and may develop a chronic posture of flexion.

Thought Question

Here's a question to stretch your mind! Some corticospinal fibers make direct connections, and others make indirect connections. Can you relate this organizational feature to the following concepts: fractionation of movement, regulation of multijoint muscles, supraspinal control of movements, and the ability of humans to produce novel voluntary movements?

Spasticity and Stretch Reflexes

Spasticity, which often accompanies upper motor neuron damage, is one of the most perplexing of all disorders associated with nervous system damage. Spasticity commonly develops in clinical disorders such as stroke, multiple sclerosis, and spinal cord injury. Immediately following a UMN lesion in the cerebral hemisphere, brainstem, or spinal cord, the affected limbs are usually without muscle tone (flaccid), and the stretch reflexes are reduced or absent altogether. After a variable period of time (weeks, days, or hours in some cases), muscle tone in the affected limbs gradually returns and typically exceeds that of the less affected side. The stretch reflexes are exaggerated, and there is a velocity-dependent increased resistance of the limb to passive stretching. The affected limbs are then said to demonstrate spasticity.

Despite its critical importance in clinical practice, spasticity is not consistently defined. One of the more accepted definitions of spasticity—and the one used in this textbook—is that spasticity is a "motor disorder, characterized by a velocity-dependent increase in tonic stretch reflexes (muscle tone) with exaggerated tendon jerks, resulting from hyperexcitability of the stretch reflex, and is one component of the upper motor neuron syndrome" (Lance, 1980, p. 485). However, this definition is by no means the only one used in the literature, and furthermore, many authors use the term *spasticity* without explicitly defining it. Additionally, this definition of spasticity applies only to a person in a passive state, yet the term is sometimes also used in clinical practice in the context of voluntary movement—for example, spastic gait.

The pathophysiological basis of spasticity is only partially understood. The condition was traditionally considered a pyramidal sign (implying involvement of the pyramidal or corticospinal tract). However, selective lesions of the CST or primary motor cortex more often lead to hypotonicity as opposed to spasticity. It is likely that the primary causes of spasticity are damage to cortical projections to brainstem areas that send motor projections to the spinal cord (as occurs with a cerebrovascular accident [CVA] affecting the motor cortex or internal capsule) and/or damage to the descending brainstem motor pathways to the spinal cord (as occurs with spinal cord injury). Such damage results in abnormal processing of suprasegmental influences, and especially of the reticulospinal inputs, leading to increased excitability at the spinal cord and to impairment of the interneuronal system. In spasticity of spinal cord origin, a decrease in inhibitory amino acids (in particular, GABA and glycine) has been demonstrated, resulting in presynaptic and disynaptic inhibition of interneurons, leading to spinal disinhibition.

To summarize, fundamentally, spasticity is a central phenomenon that results in hyperexcitability of the stretch reflexes and, therefore, an increased responsiveness of muscle to passive stretch. Also referred to as *spastic hypertonia*, this condition results from abnormal spinal processing of proprioceptive input and increased activity of alpha motor neurons that innervate particular muscles. This probably arises from a lowered threshold of activation for alpha motor neurons, secondary to adaptations by these neurons in response to the loss of supraspinal inputs from the brainstem/motor cortex and alterations in spinal cord interneuron activity. Thus, it is largely changes within the synaptic network of the spinal cord ventral horn in response to the loss of supraspinal inputs that gives rise to spasticity.

Thought Question

Spasticity is defined as a velocity-dependent response to stretch. What does this definition imply about the role of the sensory system in the expression of spasticity?

Spasticity is only one of a number of important signs of upper motor neuron disorders. It may be accompanied by other signs, such as a positive Babinski reflex, the clasp-knife effect, and clonus (all discussed later). In addition to abnormalities directly related to the neurophysiological system, it is increasingly evident that spasticity may be influenced by secondary changes to muscle and tendon that follow central nervous system damage. Specifically, there are changes in sarcomere number, fibrotic changes within muscles, and changes to viscoelastic properties of tendon. Additionally, shortening of muscle fibers often occurs such that complete relaxation becomes difficult. All of these changes can influence the responsiveness of the muscle to stretch. Finally, it should be noted that spasticity, a positive sign of UMN disorders (Chapter 8), often co-occurs with weakness, loss of dexterity, and inability to fractionate movement (negative signs of UMN disorders). Despite efforts to link spasticity to these negative signs and to functional deficits, no evidence has been forthcoming of a relationship.

Spasticity associated with one condition is not necessarily the same as spasticity associated with another condition, either in appearance or in response to pharmacologic agents. For example, in spinal cord injury, spasticity can occur in muscles corresponding to myotomes below the level of the lesion, potentially affecting both flexors and extensors. In stroke, not all of the muscles in the affected limbs demonstrate spasticity so that, typically, there is increased resistance to passive stretch of the muscle in *one direction only*. The spasticity associated with stroke usually selectively affects the **antigravity muscles**, for example, the flexors of the elbow, wrist, and digits, and the extensors of the hip and knee. Furthermore the response of spasticity to pharmacological agents depends on the site and nature of the CNS damage.

Finally, although spasticity is often the most obvious manifestation of CNS damage, it may not be the most significant problem faced by the person with UMN injury. This has been shown in the following way. Small axons, like those of the gamma motor neurons, are more sensitive to local anesthetics than are large axons, like those of alpha LMNs. Thus, it is possible (with an appropriately titrated dose of local anesthetic) to selectively block gamma motor neurons in a peripheral nerve. This anesthetic block desensitizes muscle spindles and depresses stretch reflexes. When this procedure is used for patients with spasticity, the spasticity is attenuated along with the hyperactive stretch reflexes, but the impaired motor performance (negative signs) resulting from the paresis does not improve and may even worsen. This suggests that the spasticity per se is not the most troublesome symptom.

Spinal Shock and the Emergence of Spasticity

With UMN damage, spasticity does not emerge immediately. Rather, the initial response to damage is described clinically as flaccidity; spasticity may develop over time. The patient may remain in a state of flaccidity, spasticity may become full blown and severe, or the patient may develop less severe spasticity. For example, in stroke, patients may remain in a state of hypotonia or flaccidity. In contrast, with spinal cord injury, spasticity typically develops.

Spinal shock following complete transection or compression of the spinal cord illustrates the transition from spinal shock to spasticity. In spinal cord injury, the initial response to spinal cord injury is hyporeflexia and hypotonia. Over time, hyperreflexia, referred to as spasticity, develops (discussed later). Three disorders characterize spinal shock: (1) all sensation, somatic as well as visceral, from dermatomes below the lesion is immediately and permanently lost; (2) all voluntary movement is abolished in parts of the body below the lesion; and (3) reflex activity in all segments of the traumatized spinal cord is completely lost. In other words, a total loss of neural function occurs in the isolated cord caudal to the lesion. The cause of this loss is thought to be the sudden interruption of facilitatory suprasegmental descending fibers that keep spinal motor neurons in a state of response readiness—that is, in a continuous state of subliminal depolarization—resulting in acute hyperpolarization of LMN and the concomitant reduced firing rate and responsiveness to excitatory afferent inputs. A number of descending tracts seem to be involved, including the corticospinal tract.

In addition to loss of skeletal muscle function, bowel and bladder function are lost, leading to fecal and urinary retention. These both demand immediate and continued medical attention to avoid infection. Finally, sexual function (genital reflexes) and vasomotor (thermoregulatory) control are lost. The skin is dry and pale; ulcerations may develop over bony prominences. The duration of spinal shock varies from one to six weeks, with an average of about three weeks.

After the period of spinal shock, intrinsic spinal cord circuits may begin to display autonomous activity, and the patient goes through a fairly orderly sequence of recovery stages as the local circuitry resumes function. The stage of minimal reflex activity is characterized initially by weak flexor responses to painful stimuli. These appear first in the distal musculature. Flexor reflexes gradually become stronger and more easily excitable and spread to include more proximal muscle groups. The Babinski sign can be elicited bilaterally, but deep tendon reflexes cannot.

As recovery continues, spasticity may emerge and evolve. Specifically, tone may become stronger in the flexor muscles, with a resulting increase in the hyperactive flexor responses to nociceptive stimuli. A mild pinprick on the foot may elicit withdrawal of the whole extremity in which there is flexion at the ankle, knee, and hip. This reflex is called the **triple flexion reflex** (Figure 11-15 ■). After several months, the withdrawal reflexes may become greatly exaggerated, and stimulation of the skin of the legs (or an interoceptive stimulus such as a full bladder) can elicit a so-called mass reflex. The **mass reflex** is characterized by bilateral powerful triple flexion reflexes, a rise in blood pressure, bradycardia, profuse sweating, piloerection, and automatic emptying of the bladder (and sometimes bowel).

Some months after spinal cord transection or compression (typically, around four months), extensor muscle tone begins to increase gradually. This marks a stage in which alternate flexor and extensor muscle spasms occur. In most cases, extensor spasms come to predominate, but this does not lead to the disappearance of flexor reflexes. Extensor overactivity, the stage of predominant extensor spasms, appears about six months after the injury, first in the proximal (hip and thigh) and then in distal muscles (leg). In some cases, such extensor activity may be sufficient to support the patient's weight, but only in a transitory manner. The patient cannot stand on his or her own without support. Whether flexor or extensor reflexes are evoked depends on the intensity and duration of the stimuli used to elicit the reflex.

The factors underlying the alterations of intrinsic neuronal activity in progressing from the stage of spinal shock through eventual overt spasticity are uncertain, but the resultant profound alteration in suprasegmental

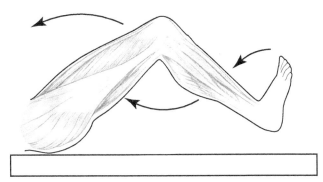

FIGURE 11-15 The triple flexion reflex involving flexion at the hip and knee and dorsiflexion at the ankle.

influences exerted on spinal cord neurons is significant. Suprasegmental control of spinal cord neurons is of two types: excitatory and inhibitory. Initially, there is a complete loss of both descending facilitatory pathways and descending inhibitory pathways. Because the loss of descending facilitatory pathways is sudden and depresses LMN excitability to such a great extent, the accompanying loss of *descending inhibition* cannot manifest itself. Emergence from spinal shock is associated with a spontaneous recovery of excitability, thereby allowing the loss of inhibition to express itself. Motor neurons are then in a state of hyperexcitability so that quantitatively normal afferent input arriving from the periphery elicits exaggerated LMN responses, expressed as hyperactive withdrawal and deep tendon reflexes. A second factor is the development of increased sensitivity of spinal interneurons and motor neurons to transmitter substances. This is the phenomenon of denervation hypersensitivity discussed earlier.

Another contributory factor underlying the late development of hyperreflexia may be the **sprouting** of collateral branches from segmental afferents entering the cord over the dorsal roots at levels caudal to the injury. The degeneration of descending suprasegmental fibers below the transection leaves synaptic vacancies on the membrane of interneurons and motor neurons. This, in turn, elicits the sprouting of collateral branches from the still-intact segmental primary afferent fibers synapsing on these ventral horn neurons. These collateral sprouts then grow to occupy the vacated synaptic sites. The abnormally augmented segmental synaptic input would necessarily yield an exaggerated reflex response to a peripheral stimulus of normal intensity. The phenomenon of collateral sprouting has been observed to occur in a number of CNS structures.

The preceding discussion focuses on the progression from spinal shock to spasticity following spinal cord injury. Sometimes, a similar process occurs when there is cortical damage, such as a stroke. One way to characterize the transition from initial injury is by the Brunnstrom stages of recovery (Table 11-2 ■). It is important to note that clinical progression of different individuals can stop at different Brunnstrom stages.

Thought Question

What physiological changes transpire following CNS injury between the period of spinal shock and development of hyperreflexia? What mechanisms have been postulated to be associated with these events?

Lower Motor Neuron versus Upper Motor Neuron Damage

To appreciate clinical consequences of damage to the pyramidal tract and motor system, it is important to recall the difference between lower and upper motor neuron damage (Chapter 8). With lower and upper motor neuron damage, one of these changes involves the stretch reflex mediated by muscle spindles. The status of the stretch reflex is altered in opposite ways, depending on whether damage has occurred in the LMN component of its reflex arc or in the UMNs that innervate the LMNs of the reflex arc, the latter remaining intact and functional after the damage. Note that this distinction applies to the chronic condition (as discussed later). We will consider LMN damage first.

In LMN damage, paralysis or paresis occurs due to damage to LMN cell bodies in the CNS or to their axons in the PNS (Chapter 10) with potential for neurogenic atrophy. In addition, certain of the clinical manifestations of LMN damage are the result of an alteration in reflex status. These clinical signs comprise additional components of the LMN syndrome that follows LMN damage. The first clinical sign of such damage is due to the interruption of the stretch reflex arc. Such interruption results in **hypoactive** or **absent tendon (stretch) reflexes**, depending on the extent of damage. The second sign manifests itself in the tone of the muscles innervated by the damaged LMNs. Tone is assessed clinically by noting the degree of resistance a muscle offers to its passive stretch (Chapter 8). An important contributor to muscle tone is the stretch reflex, especially in the postural antigravity muscles that are maintained in a stretched state by the forces of gravity. With interruption of the stretch reflex arc, muscle tone is diminished in the

Table 11-2 Brunnstrom Stages of Recovery of Movement following Stroke

STAGE	TONE	VOLUNTARY MOVEMENTS
1	Flaccidity	No voluntary movements can be initiated.
2	Spasticity begins to develop	Minimal voluntary movements are possible in basic limb synergies.
3	Spasticity severe	Voluntary control of gross movements occurs in synergistic patterns.
4	Spasticity begins to decline	Some basic movement combinations are possible that are not limb synergies.
5	Spasticity continues to decrease	More complex combinations of movement are possible.
6	Spasticity disappears	Individual joint movements become possible.

affected muscle(s), a condition described by the term **hypotonicity**. When loss is complete, the term **flaccidity** is used. Thus, coupled with the loss or impairment of voluntary movement (Chapter 10), which is referred to as paralysis or paresis (weakness), is a hypoactive or absent tendon reflex. Clinically, this combined condition is sometimes referred to as a **flaccid paralysis** or **flaccid paresis**.

With upper motor neuron damage, the situation is more complicated. A paresis may occur following UMN damage, just as it can with LMN damage. However, the nature of the paresis is different in the two cases, in part because of the different effects UMN and LMN damage have on reflexes (as discussed later). Because LMN innervation of striated muscle is intact after UMN damage, the LMN continues to liberate essential trophic factors onto the sarcolemma. Therefore, neurogenic atrophy and degeneration does not occur following UMN lesions. Although there is no neurogenic atrophy, disuse atrophy may occur, but this is slower in onset and less severe than neurogenic atrophy. Furthermore, because LMNs continue to innervate striated muscle with UMN lesions, electromyographic signs of degeneration (fibrillation and fasciculation potentials) are not present. In addition, in the acute-stage muscle retains its essential biologic and histologic integrity. Over time, atrophy may result in some structural change in muscle, and in addition, changes can occur to viscoelastic properties of muscle. Also in the acute stage, immediately following UMN damage, hypotonicity typically occurs. However, over time, spasticity often develops.

An important distinguishing feature of LMN and UMN syndromes is the pattern of involvement of muscles. In LMN damage, individual muscles or groups of muscles are affected, whereas in UMN damage, muscles that are supplied by motor nuclei below the level of the lesion are affected in synergistic groups; muscles are never affected individually. Table 11-3 ■ summarizes the differences between chronic lower and upper motor neuron damage.

Lesions confined to the PNS result only in LMN signs, as documented in Chapter 10. With damage to the spinal cord or brainstem, however, clinical signs of both LMN and UMN lesions typically co-exist, depending on the extent to which the alpha motor neuron pools are damaged and the spinal segments involved.

CLINICAL CONNECTIONS
Pathological Reflexes

With damage to the nervous system, the expression of reflexes can be abnormal. As discussed earlier in this chapter, the neuroanatomical substrate of reflex control provides a basis for routine movements that can be altered in a variety of ways through supraspinal control. In pathological situations, the reflexes may become obligatory (always occur in response to a particular sensory stimulus) and inalterable. Furthermore, certain abnormal reflexes emerge. Examples of each situation are provided throughout this section.

The Babinski Reflex

The **Babinski reflex** is the most reliable of the pathological reflexes because its meaning is considered unequivocal. This reflex can be elicited in healthy babies as a bilateral extensor plantar response during the first year of life, before the corticospinal tract has completed its development. When it is elicited beyond infancy, it is considered to be a reliable clinical sign of damage to the corticospinal (pyramidal) tract.

The Babinski reflex is elicited by stroking the sole of the foot, beginning on the lateral side of the heel and continuing forward toward the little toe. When the level of the

Table 11-3 Topography of Lower and Upper Motor Neuron Syndromes

FEATURE	UMN SYNDROME	LMN SYNDROME
Structures involved	Upper motor neurons in cerebral cortex, descending brainstem tracts, or CST of the spinal cord.	CNS: Spinal cord or brainstem alpha motor neurons (LMNs). PNS: Motor axons in all spinal nerves and cranial nerves (axons of LMNs).*
Distribution of abnormalities	Muscles that are supplied by motor nuclei below the level of the lesion are affected *in groups*: contralateral limb muscles are affected when the lesion is above the decussation; ipsilateral muscles are affected when the lesion is below the decussation. Note that individual muscles are never affected.	Effects are always segmental and limited to muscles innervated by damaged alpha motor neurons or their axons. Individual muscles or groups of muscles are affected.

*Note that all cranial nerves contain motor axons with the exception of I, II, and VIII (see Chapter 13).

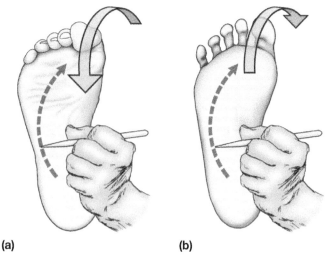

(a)　　　　　　**(b)**

FIGURE 11-16 (a) The normal response to stroking the sole of the foot. (b) The abnormal Babinski sign.

ball of the foot is reached, the stimulus is applied medially toward the base of the big toe. It may be necessary to firmly stroke the sole of the foot with a sharp object, such as a key or nail file, to elicit the reflex. In such cases, the stimulus is considered unpleasant by the patient. The sign of Babinski consists of dorsiflexion of the big toe usually accompanied by a fanning (abduction) of the other toes (Figure 11-16 ■).

Flexion Reflex

The flexion reflex can be manifested pathologically in a variety of ways. In this regard, it is important to note that the flexion reflex described earlier in this chapter (the response to stepping on a sand burr) cannot be elicited in an individual with a healthy nervous system by any of the stimuli used in clinical neurology for eliciting reflexes. Some of these stimuli such as scratching the sole of the foot in an attempt to elicit the Babinski reflex may be considered unpleasant, but none of these stimuli produce significant discomfort to the patient. This inability to elicit a flexion reflex in an adult with a healthy nervous system is because flexion reflexes are maintained in a somewhat suppressed state by the tonic descending inhibitory pathway (TDIP) descending from the brainstem as noted earlier (see Figure 11-14). However, in cases where the function of UMN systems is impaired, the interneurons mediating flexion reflexes are released from this inhibitory control so that flexion reflexes may be elicited by the stimuli normally used in the neurologic examination (e.g., scratching, stroking, pinprick). The flexion reflex is then considered pathological. Indeed, in extreme cases of UMN deficits, as when the spinal cord has been transected (see Spinal Shock), the complete flexion reflex may be exhibited spontaneously and continuously: the patient lies in bed with the hip and knee flexed and the great toe dorsiflexed. In infants, the stepping response results with weight bearing. This is a normal part of development but should not occur beyond infancy.

Clasp-Knife Phenomenon

Another clinical sign sometimes accompanying spasticity is the **clasp-knife reaction** (Figure 11-17 ■). When a spastic muscle is rapidly stretched (by extension of the arm or flexion of the leg at the knee), the limb at first moves freely for a short distance, but then a rapidly increasing muscular resistance to the stretch is encountered. Increasing the stretch still further may cause the resistance to suddenly melt away. If the upper extremity is being extended, the

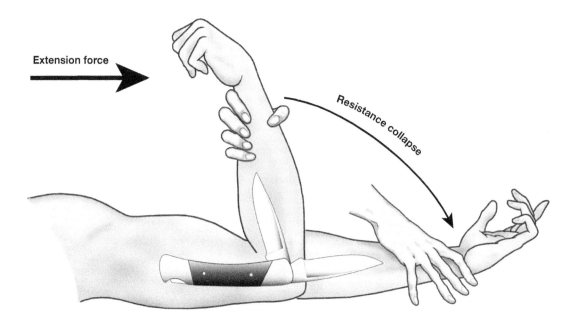

Extension force

Resistance collapse

FIGURE 11-17 The clasp-knife reflex in the upper extremity of a person with spasticity consists of a sudden collapse of the resistance to limb extension.

Neuropathology Box 11-1: Quantification of Spasticity

The Ashworth Scale was developed to grade spasticity on a four-point scale:

0   Indicates no increase in tone.
1   Indicates a slight increase.
2   Is more marked tone.

3   Indicates considerable tone.
4   Indicates that the limb is rigid in flexion or extension.

Subsequently, a modified scale was developed that attempts to quality these categories further (the modified Ashworth scale).

---

reaction would be like a clasp-knife snapping open. If the lower limb is being flexed, the leg collapses in flexion like a clasp-knife snapping shut. The clasp-knife reaction is believed to reflect the length dependence of hyperreflexia. Hyperreflexia is most intense when muscles are in a shortened position and gradually attenuates as the muscle is lengthened. As the muscle is lengthened, and when it reaches a critical length, there is a sudden giving way, reminiscent of a clasp-knife, hence the name of the response.

Clonus

The exaggerated stretch reflexes also are responsible for a second clinical sign observed in spasticity, namely, **clonus**. Clonus is routinely tested at the ankle and is elicited in the gastrocnemius and soleus muscles (Figure 11-18 ■). Ankle clonus is elicited by an abrupt and sustained dorsiflexion of the ankle, resulting in a *sustained stretch* of the gastrocnemius and soleus muscles. Ankle clonus consists of a series of rhythmic involuntary muscle contractions at a frequency of five to seven beats per second.

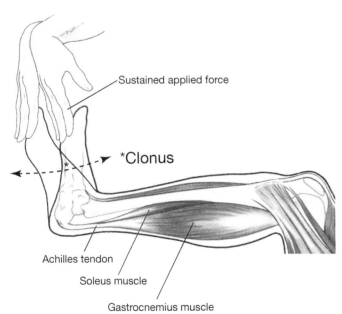

FIGURE 11-18 Ankle clonus in an individual with spasticity consists of rhythmic contraction–relaxation cycles of the ankle extensor muscles (plantar flexors of the foot) in response to their sustained stretch (i.e., stretch of the Achilles tendon).

Examination and Interventions for Spasticity

There is no consistent and agreed-upon approach to quantifying spasticity, and measurement approaches vary, depending on the author and the setting. In a clinical context, spasticity is most often assessed in terms of response to passive movement and frequently is quantified using the Ashworth scale (see accompanying box). Because spasticity is *velocity dependent*, the speed of movement is important when testing for spasticity. Rapid movements are more effective than slower movements in eliciting hyperactive stretch reflexes in patients with spasticity. In a patient with mild spasticity, slow movements may fail altogether to elicit a hyperactive stretch reflex. It is important to recognize that spasticity, by definition, is a response to an afferent stimulus to the muscle. Thus, spasticity cannot be identified by simply watching a person move, although as noted earlier, the term *spastic movement* still is used, despite being a misnomer.

Thought Question

Can spasticity be identified by observing a person's movement? What key components should be present before an individual is said to exhibit spasticity? Why is spasticity considered a positive sign associated with upper motor neuron disorders, and what is the functional implication of this terminology?

Because spasticity is accompanied by abnormalities of reflex behavior, as well as changes to the muscle itself, a number of other features should be tested when examining an individual with spasticity. In addition to quantifying spasticity (as with the Ashworth scale), it is important to palpate the muscle groups, determine available range of motion, evaluate DTRs, and perform clinical tests for accompanying signs (e.g., Babinski sign, clonus). These additional tests assess other aspects of the UNM disorder and related sequelae (e.g., loss of muscle length, altered viscoelastic properties of muscle).

In experimental studies, spasticity has been measured using both neurophysiological and biomechanical techniques. For example, some authors used the H-reflex and F-wave response of a muscle, as measured electrophysiologically in response to transcutaneous nerve stimulation.

Thought Question

Spasticity is one of the most prevalent findings following CNS damage. Yet this phenomenon is not consistently defined or measured. What is a commonly used definition? What types of approaches are used to measure spasticity, and what are their limitations?

Thought Question

A dorsal rhizotomy may be performed to reduce spasticity, especially in children who have cerebral palsy. What is a dorsal rhizotomy? To what extent would this procedure eliminate spasticity and why?

Others use instrumented approaches to quantifying stiffness, posture at rest, or range of movement.

A number of factors can aggravate spasticity. Examples include infections (e.g., urinary tract infection, pneumonia), pain (as from an ingrown toenail or a poorly fitting footwear), bladder distention, bowel impaction, fatigue, and cold weather. Hence, these should all be considered when a person has a sudden and substantial change in the presentation of his or her spasticity.

Treatments fall into three broad categories: pharmacological, surgical, and physical management. Pharmacological interventions depend on the location of lesion. For example, spasticity associated with spinal cord injury is likely to be responsive to baclofen or benzodiazepines; spasticity associated with cortical lesions, including multiple sclerosis, may respond to benzodiazepines or clonidine; and spasticity associated with traumatic brain injury and cerebral palsy may respond to clonidine or dantrolene. Injection of botulism toxin (Botox) into spastic muscles provides a prolonged (three- to six-month) but reversible relief from spasticity because it inhibits action potential mediated acetylcholine release at the neuromuscular junction. This differential response to pharmacologic agents further emphasizes the complexities associated with the term *spasticity*.

In those instances in which pharmacological interventions are not effective, surgical intervention may be considered. Selective dorsal rhizotomy may be used, in which the dorsal roots are cut for specific spinal levels (e.g., L2–S2) in order to eliminate the somatosensory stimulus for the spasticity. Unlike Botox injections, the surgical approach cannot be reversed. Also among the surgical approaches is a group of procedures directed at the orthopedic complications arising from long-term spasticity such as contracture releases, tendon transfers, osteotomies, and arthrodesis.

Of particular importance to the rehabilitation specialist are the physical interventions, designed to temporarily reduce spasticity or to counteract the secondary complications. For example, stretching tight muscles can be used to improve range of motion. Progressive casting (especially of the foot and ankle) can be used to gradually increase range of motion and alignment. This technique is particularly applicable to people who have sustained a traumatic brain injury or have cerebral palsy. The sensory stimuli of slow rhythmical rotation of a joint or application of a neutral warmth can reduce spasticity during application of the technique. These techniques may be important in preparation for treatments designed to improve range of

motion and alignment. Finally, physical interventions are necessary adjuncts to pharmacological approaches such as Botox and surgical interventions such as osteotomies in order to enhance the person's ability to maintain the range of motion and alignment achieved and to utilize the available range of motion and alignment for improved function.

Total Knee Arthroplasty and Central Activation of Muscles

Following total knee arthroplasty (TKA), patients have limitations in lower extremity muscle strength that affects their ability to perform functional tasks such as getting up from the seated position, climbing stairs, and walking. An understanding of central activation and its role in force production provides the basis for understanding possible mechanisms underlying the deficits. Reduced lower extremity muscle strength results, in part, from impaired central activation of muscle. **Central activation** refers to the neural drive from the motor cortex necessary to activate lower motor neurons, whose spike activity elicits muscle contraction; deficits in activation reflect limitations in the ability of the motor cortex to activate spinal cord LMNs in order to elicit maximal muscle forces. Measurement of central activation of the quadriceps is accomplished by first testing force produced voluntarily by the patient and then by delivering an electrical stimulus during a maximal muscle contraction. If electrical stimulation results in an overt increase in the force of muscle contraction compared to voluntary effort alone, the implication is that the muscle is not being fully activated centrally during voluntary action.

Although the neurophysiologic mechanisms underlying central activation deficits following knee surgery are not fully understood, experiments have implicated several different factors. First, spinal reflex activity from swelling or pain in the knee joint may alter afferent input from the injured joint and diminish the efferent motor drive to the quadriceps muscle required for force production. Experimentally induced pain-free, knee-joint effusions with as little as 20 to 30 ml of saline have been shown to increase quadriceps activation deficits. Experimental muscle pain has been also found to reduce force production due to central mechanisms. There is evidence that knee-joint receptors—such as Ruffini endings within the joint capsule—contribute to the regulation of muscle tone and movement through their influence on the gamma muscle loop (via muscle spindles) to regulate joint stiffness and stability. Inhibition of spinal neurons receiving nociceptive afferent inflow through descending pathways is well established in experiments on felines and may be another potential source of quadriceps activation deficits. Although investigations to date do not completely explain the underlying neurophysiologic mechanism for central activation deficits, they do suggest the involvement of a central mechanism in regulating the excitability of the motor neuron pool responsible for muscle activation deficits.

Thought Question

What can you infer from the observation that an electrical stimulus to the femoral nerve, applied during maximal contraction of the quadriceps muscle, results in a greater amount of force than contraction of the muscle alone? Why might this be particularly evident in people following surgical procedures such as a TKA?

Central activation of muscles is also being implemented in rehabilitation approaches for certain patients. Specifically, some patients with large muscle activation deficits have been reported to have negligible improvements in force, even after intensive rehabilitation focused on traditional, voluntary exercise paradigms. This may be because people with large deficits in muscle activation may have difficulty training their muscles at intensities sufficient to promote strength gains. Neuromuscular electrical stimulation (NMES) can be used as a clinical treatment to address muscle activation deficits—and often more effectively than voluntary exercise alone because it has the potential to override muscle activation deficits and re-educate muscle to contract more effectively. Thus, NMES serves to both re-educate muscle (neural improvements) and facilitate muscle hypertrophy. Changes in strength as well as functional performance (e.g., walking speed, stair climbing speed) have been demonstrated using NMES with individuals who have a number of disorders, including stroke, cerebral palsy, and spinal cord injury. Similar improvements are anticipated and are being investigated in people who have had a TKA.

Combined Sensory and Motor System Damage

To this point, we have focused on damage within the motor system from the spinal cord to the cerebral cortex. It is important to recognize that damage very often affects both the motor and sensory systems. This is apparent, for example, in spinal cord injury and in many types of strokes. Here, we consider the overall implications for damage, both in terms of the initial response to injury and the combined motor and sensory ramifications.

Brown-Sequard Syndrome or Spinal Cord Hemisection

A transverse lesion involving only one-half of the spinal cord is rarely encountered in clinical neurology. Spinal hemisection is included in most texts because of its value in helping the student learn to correlate lesion site with the side of the body on which neurologic signs are expressed: this is done by relating lesion site to the location of a tract's decussation. The **Brown-Sequard syndrome**, resulting from spinal hemisection, includes the following (Figure 11-19 ▣):

1. Ipsilateral **flaccid paralysis** (lower motor neuron syndrome) of muscle in the areas supplied by the injured segments due to the destruction of ventral horn LMNs.
2. **Spastic paralysis** (upper motor neuron syndrome) of muscles below the lesion site on the ipsilateral side due to interruption of the corticospinal and other descending motor pathways.
3. An ipsilateral zone of cutaneous anesthesia (loss of all somatic and visceral sensation) in the segments of the lesion due to damage of afferent fibers that have entered the spinal cord but not yet crossed.
4. Loss of proprioception (kinesthesia and vibration sensibility) below the lesion on the ipsilateral side due to interruption of dorsal column fibers.
5. Loss of pain and temperature sensation below the level of the lesion on the contralateral side of the body due to interruption of the spinothalamic tract fibers that have already decussated below the lesion.

The loss begins one or two segments below the lesion because afferents destined to enter the spinothalamic tract ascend one or two segments before completing their decussation to the opposite side of the spinal cord, as shown in Figure 11-19 and Figure 8-2.

Syringomyelia

Syringomyelia (G., *syrinx*, tube or pipe) is a chronic progressive degenerative disorder of the spinal cord characterized pathologically by the development of an irregular fluid-filled cavity (syrinx) in a central or paracentral location (Figure 11-20 ▣). It is a rare disease, but is important because it epitomizes the signs and symptoms associated with a lesion in the center of the spinal cord. Cavitation occurs most commonly in the lower cervical and upper thoracic levels of the cord and extends through several segments. Occasionally, the cavity extends rostrally into the brainstem (**syringobulbia**) or caudally into lower thoracic segments. Despite several theories, a pathogenesis has not been definitely established. Symptoms appear most commonly in early adulthood and then progress irregularly, sometimes remaining stationary for months or years.

The syrinx develops first in relation to the central gray matter of the cervical cord and interrupts pain and temperature fibers crossing in the ventral white commissure at several consecutive segments. The hallmark of this disease is thus early loss or impairment of pain and thermal sense, typically in the hands and arms because lower cervical levels are most commonly involved. Because tactile and proprioceptive sensations are preserved, this selective loss of pain and temperature sensibility is referred to as a dissociated sensory loss. The cavity may enlarge symmetrically

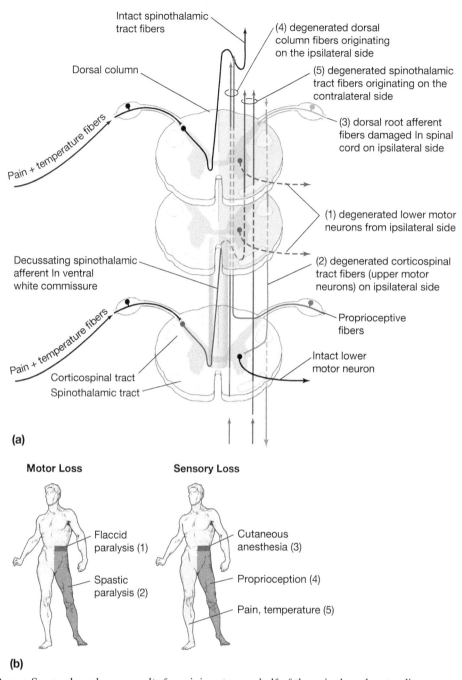

Intact spinothalamic tract fibers

Dorsal column

Pain + temperature fibers

Decussating spinothalamic afferent In ventral white commissure

Pain + temperature fibers

Corticospinal tract
Spinothalamic tract

(4) degenerated dorsal column fibers originating on the ipsilateral side

(5) degenerated spinothalamic tract fibers originating on the contralateral side

(3) dorsal root afferent fibers damaged In spinal cord on ipsilateral side

(1) degenerated lower motor neurons from ipsilateral side

(2) degenerated corticospinal tract fibers (upper motor neurons) on ipsilateral side

Proprioceptive fibers

Intact lower motor neuron

(a)

Motor Loss

Flaccid paralysis (1)

Spastic paralysis (2)

Sensory Loss

Cutaneous anesthesia (3)

Proprioception (4)

Pain, temperature (5)

(b)

FIGURE 11-19 The Brown-Sequard syndrome results from injury to one-half of the spinal cord, extending over several spinal cord segments (shaded). (a) Degeneration (broken lines) associated with spinal cord hemisection. The ventral white commissure is represented as a tube to illustrate the oblique crossing of spinothalamic tract afferents before they enter the anterolateral funiculus on the opposite side of the cord. (b) Motor and somatosensory losses associated with the Brown-Sequard syndrome.

or asymmetrically, extending into the dorsal or ventral horns and eventually into the dorsal or lateral funiculi. The exact clinical picture depends on the cross-sectional and vertical extent of the cavitation. However, it is common for the cord destruction to extend into the ventral horn, producing segmental weakness and atrophy (**amyotrophy**) of the hands and arms with a loss of deep tendon reflexes. These symptoms are due to destruction of ventral horn LMNs. Autonomic disorders result when the cavity involves the intermediolateral cell column in thoracic segments. These may include painless ulcers, dry coarse skin,

and painless neuropathic joints in the shoulder and elbow. Involvement of the lateral corticospinal tract produces a spastic paraparesis and occasionally a spastic paraplegia.

The evaluation of the benefits of any form of therapy for syringomyelia is difficult. This is because the natural course of the disease is characterized by unpredictable aggravations and long periods where the symptoms do not progress. There also is the possibility of spontaneous arrest.

As mentioned, syringomyelia is rare, though important from the perspective of understanding damage to the central cord. Another related condition that occurs more

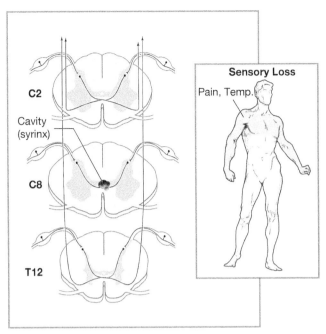

FIGURE 11-20 The cavity in syringomyelia often interrupts spinothalamic afferents crossing in the ventral white commissure.

commonly is the **central cord syndrome** in which a central cord hematoma (hematomyelia) occurs in association with spinal cord trauma.

Subacute Combined Degeneration

The majority of people with **pernicious anemia** display symptoms of nervous system disease. The peripheral nerves, optic nerves, brain, and spinal cord all may be involved, but the spinal cord is the region affected first and most commonly. Pernicious anemia results from an inability to absorb vitamin B12 from the intestine, resulting in a failure of gut mucosa to secrete sufficient intrinsic factor—an enzyme required for the transport of vitamin B12 across the intestinal mucosa. Defective DNA synthesis occurs with a consequent failure of red blood cells to mature normally, leading to pernicious anemia. The term **subacute degeneration** is applied to the spinal cord disease of pernicious anemia and is characterized by a combination of posterior and lateral column (funiculi) degeneration. The mechanism by which the vitamin B12 deficiency results in the degeneration of myelin and axons in the spinal cord is unclear, but it may involve a biochemical abnormality in myelin.

The individual first notices paresthesias such as numbness, sensation of pins and needles, and tingling, along with a general weakness. The paresthesias, which are constant and steadily progressive, are localized to the fingertips and toes with a symmetric distribution. As the disease progresses, neurologic examination discloses posterior column deficits, loss of vibration, and position sensations, especially (and most typically) in the legs. An unsteady, ataxic (sensory ataxia) gait is evident. Later, signs of lateral column involvement appear: loss of strength, spasticity, clonus, increased deep tendon

reflexes, and bilateral extensor plantar responses (bilateral Babinski signs). Motor signs are usually confined to the legs. With further progression of the disease, the pathology may spread to the spinothalamic tracts, but this is rare.

The pathologic process involves a diffuse, but uneven, degeneration of spinal cord white matter, beginning usually in the lower cervical and upper thoracic segments. The degeneration starts in the posterior columns and spreads up and down the cord as well as anterolaterally into the lateral columns (Figure 11-21 ■). Myelin is initially most affected, but eventually axons degenerate as well. Pernicious anemia often involves cerebral white matter leading to the development of mental signs.

Subacute combined degeneration is treatable, even to the point of reversing neurological signs if treatment is initiated within a few weeks after symptom onset. Early diagnosis is, therefore, of the utmost importance. A major obstacle to early diagnosis is the lack of a one-to-one relationship between the hematologic and neurologic signs. A severe degree of neurologic involvement may be present, with little evidence of anemia. Treatment consists of parenterally administered vitamin B12.

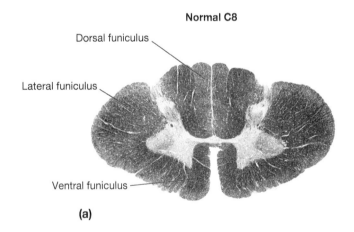
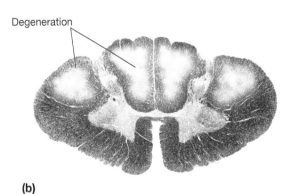

FIGURE 11-21 Myelin stained sections from the lower cervical spinal cord. (a) Normal. (b) Lesions in subacute combined degeneration involve degeneration of the white matter in the posterior and lateral funiculi of the spinal cord. The degenerated fibers lose their myelin and, hence, are unstained.

Summary

This chapter added detail to the neural substrates mediating the two extremes of movement: spinal cord reflexes and voluntary movement. The five components making up a typical reflex arc were presented. The reflex center is that component of the reflex arc that consists of a pool of interneurons within the spinal gray whose synaptic connections determine the pattern of a reflex response. The reflex center also is the site where suprasegmental control over reflexes is exerted. The hard-wiring responsible for three specific somatic spinal reflexes was detailed. The stretch reflex (mediated by muscle spindles), the inverse myotatic reflex (mediated by Golgi tendon organs), and the flexion-crossed extension reflex (mediated by nociceptors) all have significant clinical application, both to understand the neurological diseases and for rehabilitation.

Adhering to the original definition of the pyramidal tract, the terms *pyramidal tract* and *corticospinal tract* are synonymous. The pyramidal tract, originating in motor areas of the cerebral cortex (as well as somatosensory cortex, Brodmann's areas 3, 1, and 2), is the major UMN descending system mediating voluntary movement. Without compensatory structural and functional reorganization in the motor system (occurring spontaneously or through rehabilitation training), it remains an open question whether the capacity for voluntary movement in the limbs would be possible following complete and bilateral pyramidal tract lesions. This does not mean, however, that other descending UMN pathways or other structures and systems do not contribute importantly to normal voluntary movement. Significant contributions are made by the reticulospinal, vestibulospinal, and tectospinal pathways; by the cerebellum and basal ganglia; as well as by sensory systems—all of which are explored in later chapters. But voluntary movement survives damage to these components of the CNS (there is no paralysis); it's just that it is no longer normal. Besides paralysis, damage to the corticospinal tract and related motor structures results in two of the major and most reliable clinical signs occurring in the UMN syndrome. These are the Babinski sign (a pathological reflex) and spasticity (due primarily to hyperactive stretch reflexes), both signs being expressions of the loss of suprasegmental control.

The last section of this chapter discusses four distinct clinical conditions that involve both somatosensory and motor signs. Two of these are spinal shock and subacute combined degeneration. The other two are not common, the Brown-Sequard syndrome and syringomyelia. However, these two syndromes are very instructive in terms of understanding the correlation of clinical signs with lesion site.

Applications

1. Describe and diagram the typical components of a so-called monosynaptic reflex, and provide an example.

2. Describe and diagram a polysynaptic reflex, and provide an example.

3. You are walking barefoot along the beach. You step on a sharp piece of broken coral with your right foot.
   a. Describe your likely response.
   b. Draw the reflex arc(s) that control this response. Identify the receptor and fiber types involved in this response.

4. Now consider a woman who has diabetes and associated peripheral neuropathy. Peripheral neuropathy results in damage to the peripheral nerves with a loss of pain, temperature, and touch sensibility in the lower extremities. Imagine if she was walking along the beach and steps on the same sharp coral with her right foot.
   a. What sensory tracts are affected by a peripheral neuropathy in the lower extremities?
   b. Will she demonstrate a flexion withdrawal and crossed extension response? Explain your answer.
   c. What concerns might you have for an individual with peripheral neuropathy with regard to shoes, balance, and environmental surfaces?

References

Spinal Cord Reflexes

Clarke, R.W., and Harris, J. The organization of motor responses to noxious stimuli. *Brain Res Rev* 46: 163–172, 2004.

Friemert, B., et al. Intraoperative direct mechanical stimulation of the anterior cruciate ligament elicits short- and medium-latency hamstring reflexes. *J Neurophysiol* 94:3996–4001, 2005.

Gorassini, M. A., Knash, M. E., Harvey, P. J., et al. Role of motoneurons in the generation of muslce spasms after spinal cord injury. *Brain* 127: 2247–2258, 2004.

Holloway, R. The Babinski sign: Thumbs up or thumbs down? *Neurology* 65:1147–1148, 2005.

Landau, W. M. Plantar reflex amusement. *Neurology* 65:1150–1151, 2005.

Melnyk, M., et al. Changes in stretch reflex excitability are related to "giving way" symptoms in patients with anterior cruciate rupture. *J Neurophysiol* 97:474–480, 2007.

Nickolls, P., Collins, D. F., Gorman, R. B., et al. Forces consistent with plateau-like behavior of spinal neurons evoked in patients with spinal cord injuries. *Brain* 127:660–670, 2004.

Solomonow, M., and Krogsgaard, M. Sensorimotor control of knee stability. A review. *Scand J Med Sci Sports* 11:64–80, 2001.

Pyramidal System and Other Descending UMN Pathways

Bortoff, G. A., and Strick, P. L. Corticospinal terminations in two new-world primates: Further evidence that corticomotoneuronal connections provide part of the neural substrate for normal dexterity. *J Neurosci* 13:5105–5118, 1993.

Davidoff, R. A. The pyramidal tract. *Neurology* 40:332–339, 1990.

Hanaway, J., and Young, R. R. Localization of the pyramidal tract in the internal capsule of man. *J Neurologic Sci* 34:63–70, 1977.

Jagiella, W. M., and Sung, J. H. Bilateral infarction of the medullary pyramids in humans. *Neurology* 39:21–24, 1989.

Lance, J. W. Symposium synopsis. In: Feldman, R. G., Young, R. R., and Koella, W. P., eds. *Spasticity: Disordered Motor Control*. Year Book, Chicago, 1980.

Lawrence, D. G., and Kuypers, H. G. J. M. The functional organization of the motor system in the monkey. I. The effects of bilateral pyramidal lesions. *Brain* 91,1:1–14, 1968.

Malhotra S., Pandyan A. D., Day C. R., et al. Spasticity, an impairment that is poorly defined and poorly measured. *Clin Rehabil* 23:651–658, 2009.

Marx, J. J., Iannetti, G. D., Thomke, F., et al. Somatotopic organization of the corticospinal tract in the human brainstem: A MRI-based mapping analysis. *Ann Neurol* 57:824–831, 2005.

Nathan, P. W. and Smith, M. C. The rubrospinal and central tegmental tracts in man. *Brain* 105:223–269, 1982.

Nathan, P. W., Smith, M. C.. and Deacon, P. The corticospinal tracts in man. Course and location of fibres at different segmental levels. *Brain* 113:303–324, 1990.

Nolte, J. *The Human Brain: An Introduction to Its Functional Anatomy*. Mosby Elsevier, Philadelphia, 2009.

Paus, T., Zijdenbos, A., Worsley, K., et al. Structural maturation of neural pathways in children and adolescents: In vivo study. *Science* 283:1908–1911, 1999.

Thomas, S. L., and Gorassini, M. A. Increases in corticospinal tract function by treadmill training after incomplete spinal cord injury. *J. Neurophysiol* 94:2844–2855, 2005.

Uozumi, Y., Tamagawa, A., Hashimoto, T., and Tsuji, S. Motor hand representation in cortical area 44. *Neurology* 62:757–761, 2004.

Spinal Cord Disorders

Bogdanov, E. I., Heiss, J. D., Mendelevich, M. D., et al. Clinical and neuroimaging features of "idiopathic" syringomyelia. *Neurology* 62:791–794, 2004.

Olivas, A. D., and Noble-Haeusslein, L. J. Phospholipase A_2 and spinal cord injury: A novel target for therapeutic intervention. *Ann Neurol* 59:577–579, 2006.

Spasticity

Ashworth, V. B. Preliminary trial of carisoprodol in multiple sclerosis. *Practitioner* 192:540–542, 1964.

Bohannon, R. W., and Smith, M. B. Interrater reliability of a modified Ashworth scale of muscle spasticity. *Phys Ther* 67:206–207, 1987.

Invanhoe, D. V., and Reistteter, T. A. Spasticity. The misunderstood part of the upper motor neuron syndrome. *Am J Phys Med Rehabil* 83(Suppl):S3–S9, 2004.

Malhotra, S., Pandyan, A. D., Day, C. R., Jones, P. W., and Hermens, H. Spasticity, an impairment that is poorly defined and poorly measured. *Clin Rehabil* 23:651, 2009.

Priori, A., Cogiamanian, F., and Mrakic-Sposta, S. Pathophysiology of spasticity. *Neurol Sci* 27:S307–S309, 2006.

Autonomic Nervous System

12

LEARNING OUTCOMES

This chapter prepares the reader to:

1. Compare and contrast somatic and autonomic systems with respect to the structures receiving afferent information and the origin of efferent information.

2. Explain the role of ganglia in the ANS and describe the location of important ganglia.

3. Compare and contrast the sympathetic and parasympathetic systems in terms of the following:

   a. Location of the sites of origin within the CNS.

   b. Location of the peripheral autonomic ganglia.

   c. Role of the neurotransmitters.

4. Describe the general pathway by which autonomic afferent information travels through the CNS and differentiate the origins from smooth muscles of the thorax, abdomen, and pelvis. Give examples of each.

5. Provide an anatomical explanation for the occurrence of referred pain associated with viscera.

6. Relate common sites of referred pain to their organ of origin.

7. Describe the various efferent innervations derived from the ANS.

8. Explain the concept of control centers for autonomic activity and identify the location of neurons that control the following: respiration, cardiovascular function, pupillary size and visual accommodation, micturition, and arousal/ejaculation.

9. Discuss how the sympathetic and parasympathetic systems work together to control bladder function.

10. Compare and contrast the consequences of spinal cord injury at different levels with respect to bladder dysfunction.

ACRONYMS

ACh Acetylcholine

ANS Autonomic nervous system

CNS Central nervous system

DC-ML Dorsal column–medial lemniscal system

LMN Lower motor neuron

NE Norepinephrine

PNS Peripheral nervous system

UMN Upper motor neuron

VPM Ventral posteromedial nucleus of the thalamus

Introduction

The previous two chapters considered motor regulation of skeletal muscle activity. This chapter focuses on the autonomic division of the nervous system (ANS) that regulates the activity related to viscera—the essential components of which are cardiac muscle, smooth muscle, and glandular tissue.

The first major section of this chapter provides an overview of the role of the ANS, compares the structural organization of the somatic and autonomic divisions of the nervous system, and describes the sympathetic and parasympathetic components of this system. The next major section describes the autonomic afferent system in more detail. The afferent system is made up of fibers originating in the viscera that travel in the sympathetic and parasympathetic divisions of the nerves to the CNS. The third major section describes the autonomic efferent system in detail. The fourth section introduces the autonomic innervation of specific organs. With several minor exceptions (sweat glands and smooth muscle associated with blood vessels and hairs in the skin), all visceral organs and tissues are innervated by both sympathetic and parasympathetic divisions so that all of the viscera are supplied by four types of fibers: sympathetic afferents and efferents and parasympathetic afferents and efferents. In the final section, several clinical conditions are presented involving the ANS.

OVERVIEW OF THE STRUCTURE AND FUNCTION OF THE ANS

The word *autonomic* comes from the term *autonomous*, meaning self-governing. Autonomic also has come to mean acting independently of volition. Neither meaning fully captures the reality of the ANS. The ANS is not self-governing at all. One's motivations and affects dictate not only the contractions of skeletal muscle from moment to moment, but simultaneous functional shifts in the status of the body's internal organs as well. Although convenient for teaching purposes, divorcing the activities of the ANS from those of the somatic division of the nervous system does not do justice to their fully integrated action. The ANS sometimes is considered as belonging only to the PNS. This is untrue, as just implied. As with the somatic division of the nervous system, the ANS has robust representation in the CNS.

With respect to volition—the act of willing, choosing, or deciding on a course of action—it may be stated that the activity of the autonomic nervous system is more involuntary than that of the somatic division of the nervous system. While autonomic activity is not divorced from volition, it is clear that certain stimuli and responses are important to the maintenance of life itself. A precipitous drop in blood pressure, for example, requires a response from the nervous system that is independent of all other aspects of the state of the body or mind. As derisively noted by Claude Bernard, a French physiologist of the 19th century, "nature thought it prudent to remove these important phenomena from the caprice of an ignorant will." Having to occupy our brains with the act of breathing, the regulation of heart rate and blood pressure, digestion, and the like, would seemingly preclude the very human mental activities of reflection, discursive thought and ethical judgment, as well as compromise attention, perception, and memory.

The preceding text implies that the ANS is exclusively a motor system—and this would be consistent with its earliest definition by John Newport Langley in the late 19th century. However, Langley's definition arbitrarily excluded afferent fibers arising from the viscera as playing any role in determining the activity of autonomic output. The fact is, visceral afferent fibers play just as important a role in regulating the activity of autonomic output as do somatic afferent fibers in regulating the activity of striated muscle. Clearly, afferent information from the structures being regulated is vital to their effective control by the brain.

Somatic and Autonomic Nervous Systems

Broad similarities as well as differences exist between the somatic and autonomic divisions of the nervous system (Table 12-1 ■). Both divisions involve specialized afferent

Table 12-1 Comparison of the Somatic and Autonomic Divisions of the Nervous System

FEATURE	SOMATIC	AUTONOMIC
Specialized afferent and efferent fibers with reflex connections within the CNS	Present	Present
Connections with higher levels of CNS via ascending and descending pathways	Present	Present
Major brain structure receiving afferent information	Thalamus	Hypothalamus
Major source of descending pathways	Cerebral cortex	Hypothalamus

and efferent fibers and reflex connections within the CNS. Likewise, both systems are connected with higher levels of the CNS by ascending and descending pathways.

In the case of the ANS, however, the major brain structure receiving afferent information is the hypothalamus, in contrast to the thalamus that receives somatic afferent information. The hypothalamus is also the single major source of descending pathways that regulate activity of the sympathetic and parasympathetic divisions of the ANS. In contrast, the cerebral cortex is the major source of descending pathways that regulate the activity of the somatic division of the nervous system.

An additional major difference between the autonomic and somatic divisions of the nervous system has to do with the route of transmission from the CNS to the target tissues. As a result, the anatomical location of major components of each system is different (Figure 12-1 ■).

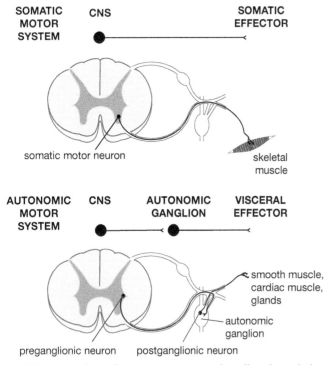

FIGURE 12-1 Somatic motor neurons project directly to their target skeletal muscle from the CNS. Autonomic sympathetic preganglionic motor neurons within the CNS project to an autonomic sympathetic ganglion located outside the CNS, where they synapse on autonomic postganglionic motor neurons. The postganglionic neuron then projects to its target viscera.

The myelinated axons of lower motor neurons of the somatic division exit the spinal cord in the ventral roots (or exit the brainstem via cranial nerves) and reach skeletal muscle directly. In contrast, the link between the CNS and viscera innervated by the autonomic division involves two neurons. An intervening synapse occurs in **autonomic ganglia** situated outside the CNS. Lightly myelinated **preganglionic** axons exit the CNS via the ventral roots and synapse on **postganglionic** neurons in autonomic ganglia. Unmyelinated postganglionic axons then project to smooth muscle, cardiac muscle, or glandular tissue of a visceral organ.

This difference means that the cell bodies of neurons making up a major part of the efferent component of the ANS are located outside of the CNS, in specialized peripheral ganglia. In contrast, the cell bodies of the efferent component of the somatic division are all positioned within the CNS.

The innervation of skeletal muscle, on the one hand, and cardiac and smooth muscle, on the other, is fundamentally different. The former is highly discrete, whereas the latter is specialized for the synchronous contraction of many muscle fibers. The fibers (cells) of smooth muscle of the viscera are in contact with one another through numerous gap junctions (see Figure 4-28). Consequently, when a single smooth muscle cell is stimulated by an action potential from the ANS, not only does it contract, but it also spreads the action potential to adjacent muscle cells. This ensures a steady wave of contraction necessary, for example, to push food through the digestive tract. The cells of cardiac muscle also are connected by gap junctions, which enable the almost instantaneous transmission of electrical activity from one cardiac cell to the next. This serves to synchronize cardiac muscle contractions. As a consequence of gap junction connections between muscle cells innervated by the ANS, it is not necessary that each muscle cell be innervated by its own efferent. As shown in Figure 12-2 ■, the autonomic efferent innervating smooth and cardiac muscle winds its way among the muscle cells,

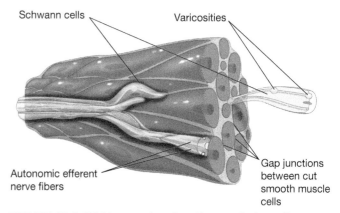

FIGURE 12-2 Within smooth and cardiac muscle (as well as glandular tissue), autonomic postganglionic neurons contain linear arrays of varicosities along their length that represent sites of transmitter release. In addition, not every muscle cell is innervated.

and not all muscle cells are innervated. Along its length, the axon contains swellings, or varicosities (called *boutons en passage*), that represent sites of transmitter release. This innervation contrasts with that of striated muscle by the somatic division of the nervous system. In striated muscle, each individual muscle cell is innervated by a single axon that terminates on the sarcolemma to form a neuromuscular junction (Chapter 10). This pattern of innervation enables the CNS to control voluntary muscle contraction in a discrete and finely graded manner.

Finally, the somatic and autonomic divisions differ in the mechanisms by which muscle contraction is inhibited. The ANS can directly inhibit smooth and cardiac muscle contraction. This is because autonomically innervated muscle cells contain different types of receptors—some of which cause contraction when stimulated by the appropriate transmitter, while others result in relaxation. In contrast, skeletal muscle cannot be directly inhibited because all the receptors on its cell membrane are excitatory, resulting in contraction. Thus, the relaxation of skeletal muscle can only be achieved by inhibiting the LMNs in the spinal cord or brainstem that excite the muscle.

Sympathetic and Parasympathetic Components of the ANS

Two distinct divisions of fibers are found within the ANS: the **sympathetic** and **parasympathetic** divisions. These two divisions differ anatomically from one another in a number of respects. To appreciate the anatomical differences, it is important to recall that the efferent component of fibers of the ANS synapse in a ganglion outside of the CNS.

One difference in the sympathetic and parasympathetic systems is that their sites of origin in the CNS differ markedly. Preganglionic *sympathetic* fibers originate from neurons located in the thoracic and upper two or three lumbar segments of the spinal cord (Figure 12-3 ■). Thus, the sympathetic division of the ANS is also referred to as the **thoracolumbar division**. Preganglionic *parasympathetic* fibers originate from neurons located in two widely separated parts of the CNS. The cranial part of the parasympathetic division originates from neurons located in the brainstem (the medulla, pons, and midbrain), whereas the spinal part originates from neurons in the sacral spinal cord, specifically, in segments S2, S3, and S4 (Figure 12-4 ■). Therefore, the parasympathetic component of the ANS is also referred to as the **craniosacral division**.

Secondly, the location of the peripheral ganglia belonging to the sympathetic and parasympathetic divisions is different. Some sympathetic ganglia are located adjacent to the CNS; others, called prevertebral or collateral ganglia, are more distally located (e.g., celiac ganglia, superior mesenteric ganglia, and inferior mesenteric ganglia). In contrast, parasympathetic ganglia are positioned close to or within the target organ they innervate. This results in the sympathetic division typically having short preganglionic axons and long postganglionic fibers, while the reverse is the case for the parasympathetic division (see Figure 12-3).

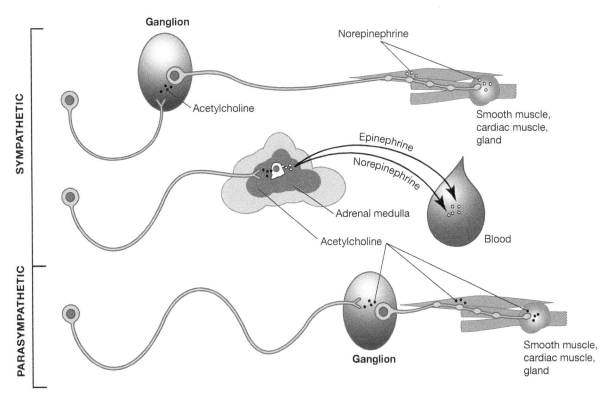

FIGURE 12-3 Comparison of the sympathetic and parasympathetic efferents of the autonomic nervous system.

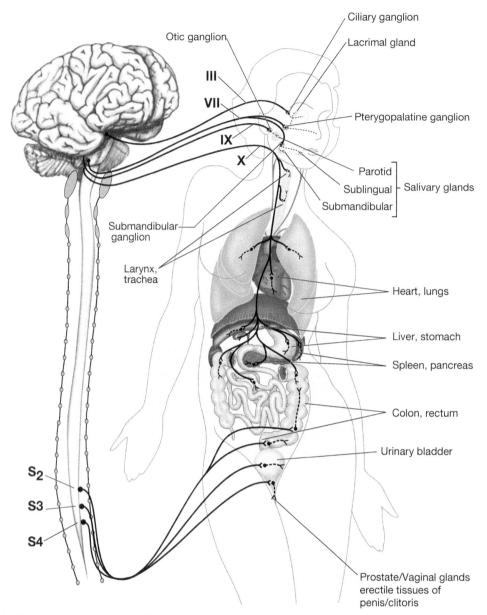

FIGURE 12-4 Distribution of the parasympathetic outflow via cranial nerves III, VII, IX, and X and spinal nerves S2–S4.

Thought Question

Describe the organization of the sympathetic and parasympathetic systems with respect to different segments of the spinal cord, identify the origin of neurons that relate to each part, and contrast the peripheral ganglia associated with each.

A third difference between the sympathetic and parasympathetic divisions is the ratio of preganglionic to postganglionic fibers. Much more divergence occurs in the sympathetic division, where the ratio of preganglionic to postganglionic fibers has been estimated to range from 1:10 to 1:196. The parasympathetic division, on the other hand, is less diffusely organized, having a ratio of preganglionic to postganglionic fibers of 1:3. This enables the parasympathetic division to exert more discrete, localized control over its target structures, whereas the effects of the sympathetic division are more widespread.

Lastly, while all autonomic activity is mediated through the release of chemical neurotransmitters, the chemicals utilized by the sympathetic and parasympathetic divisions differ. The transmitter acetylcholine (ACh) is released at the terminals of all preganglionic fibers in both the sympathetic and parasympathetic divisions. In addition, ACh is released at the terminals of all postganglionic parasympathetic fibers. In contrast, postganglionic sympathetic fibers release the transmitter norepinephrine (NE) at their terminals. Exceptions to this general rule are the postganglionic sympathetic fibers ending on sweat glands and blood vessels in muscles that release ACh. Acetylcholine is also released by the preganglionic sympathetic fibers onto the chromaffin cells of the adrenal medulla.

AUTONOMIC AFFERENTS

Clinical Preview ·················

You had successfully treated Maria Gonzales, who had a left rotator cuff tear. Today, she called because she has had left shoulder discomfort for the past three days. She commented that the discomfort worsens with exertion, even when she isn't doing any activities that put demands on the shoulder itself. As you read through this section, consider the following:

- Why would you be concerned that her pain worsens with exertion?

- What other explanations should you be aware of and rule out for her complaint of shoulder pain?

- What could be the ramifications of misunderstanding her shoulder pain?

Most of the afferent fibers conveying autonomic sensory impulses originate from free and encapsulated receptors in the viscera and walls of blood vessels. Afferent fibers from receptors of the thoracic and abdominal viscera reach the spinal cord via the sympathetic trunks and the brainstem via the glossopharyngeal and vagus nerves. The cell bodies of the visceral afferents of cranial nerves IX and X are located in the inferior ganglia of these nerves. From the thoracic viscera (heart, coronary vessels, bronchial tree and lungs), the primary visceral afferents travel to the sympathetic trunk in the cardiac and pulmonary nerves. From the abdominal viscera (stomach, intestines, liver, spleen, pancreas, kidneys, gall bladder, peritoneal cavity), afferents travel to the sympathetic trunk in the splanchnic nerves

(Figure 12-5 ■). They traverse the sympathetic trunk, enter white communicating rami (a nerve that connects two other nerves), and join the thoracic and upper lumbar spinal nerves. The cell bodies of these primary visceral afferents are located in the dorsal root ganglia of T1–L2.

From the pelvic viscera (urinary bladder, rectum, proximal part of the urethra, cervix of the uterus), autonomic afferents reach the spinal cord by two routes. One is through the lumbar splanchnic nerves, sympathetic trunk, and white communicating rami to the lower thoracic and upper lumbar spinal nerves. The other is by the pelvic splanchnic nerves to the second, third, and fourth sacral spinal nerves. These autonomic afferents also have their cell bodies in the appropriate dorsal root ganglia.

Visceral afferent fibers enter the spinal cord through the lateral division of the dorsal root. They synapse on neurons located in the dorsal horn and intermediate zone of the spinal gray matter. Most of these afferents carry information associated with the initiation of visceral reflexes. They make secondary connections with visceral or somatic motor neurons, or both, of the spinal gray. Visceral reflexes regulate blood pressure and blood chemistry by altering such functions as heart and respiratory rates and the resistance of blood vessels (discussed later). Afferent information that does reach consciousness ascends bilaterally in the anterolateral funiculi of the spinal cord. On reaching the brainstem, this information ascends through multisynaptic pathways in the reticular formation to higher centers. Sensations arising from the urethra indicating that urination is imminent ascend by a different route, the DC-ML system.

Visceral Sensations and Referred Pain

Those visceral sensations that reach consciousness tend to be vague, poorly localized, and predominantly of an affective nature. Examples are heartburn, hunger, and nausea.

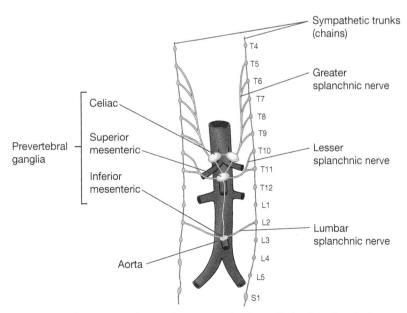

FIGURE 12-5 Preganglionic sympathetic axons project to the prevertebral ganglia in the splanchnic nerves.

Visceral organs themselves are insensitive to ordinary thermal and mechanical stimuli. Patients who are operated on under local anesthesia may have their viscera handled, cut, clamped, and even cauterized (burned) by a surgeon without evoking conscious sensations. On the other hand, sudden distensions and spasms of the muscular walls of hollow viscera may produce acute distress and severe pain. Acute pain also results from decreased blood supply (ischemia) to the viscera.

Pain that is experienced under these conditions may be felt in various locations. True, visceral pain may be experienced in the region of the organ itself. However, visceral pain may be referred to an area of the body surface; the patient may then assume that the pain is of cutaneous origin. This is called **referred pain**.

The neural basis of referred pain is related to the fact that visceral and somatic afferents converge on common spinal cord neurons. Visceral nociceptive afferents from a given organ project to specific segmental levels of the spinal cord. In the case of the heart, nociceptive afferents project to upper thoracic levels of the cord, as shown in Figure 12-6 ■ . These same segmental levels also receive somatic pain information from specific parts of the body surface. It is this specific body surface area to which the visceral pain is referred. It has been proposed that within the dorsal horn, visceral pain afferent impulses converge on neurons belonging to the somatic pain-mediating spinothalamic

> **Thought Question**
>
> Pain associated with kidney disorders can be referred to the low back, whereas pain associated with gall bladder or diaphragmatic dysfunction can be referred to the right shoulder. Provide a possible neuroanatomical explanation of this phenomenon.

tract, causing them to discharge. This information ultimately reaches the cerebral cortex, which has no way of knowing the actual source of the noxious stimulus. Thus, the brain mistakenly interprets the spinothalamic tract activity as cutaneous pain in a specific location, such as the chest and left arm in the case of a myocardial infarction or angina. Knowledge of the typical patterns of referred pain is important clinically. These patterns are summarized in Table 12-2 ■ and illustrated in Figure 12-7 ■ .

AUTONOMIC EFFERENTS

Efferent innervations derived from the ANS originate in a variety of CNS structures, eventually reaching their target organs. Their role is most often related to secretory functions of those organs. However, the functional role of the sympathetic and parasympathetic efferent systems is quite different.

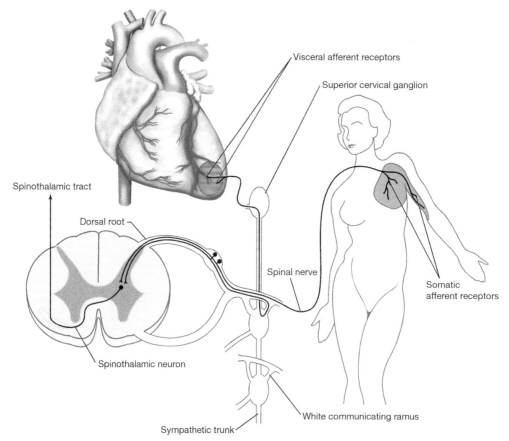

FIGURE 12-6 A hypothesized anatomical basis for visceral referred pain. In this case, pain originating in the heart (e.g., from angina pectoris) is referred to the upper thorax (T2–T4 dermatomes) or down the inside of the left arm (T1 dermatome).

Table 12-2 Patterns of Referred Pain

DAMAGED ORGAN	DERMATOMES IN WHICH PAIN IS FELT
Diaphragm	C3–C4
Heart	T1–T4 (left)
Stomach	T6–T9 (mainly left)
Gallbladder	T7–T8 (right)
Duodenum (small intestine)	T9–T10
Appendix (large intestine)	T10 (right)
Reproductive organs	T10–T12
Kidneys, ureters	L1–L2

Recall that autonomic efferent fibers originate in the hypothalamus. In this context, it is important to recall that not all efferent fibers reach the periphery. Efferent fibers from the hypothalamus form part of the descending supraspinal projections to preganglionic sympathetic neurons in T1–L2 and preganglionic parasympathetic neurons in the brainstem and S2–S4. Here, we focus on the spinal cord and brainstem components of these systems. It is important to recognize that most of the peripheral nerves carrying autonomic efferent fibers also carry afferent fibers and, hence, are mixed nerves.

Sympathetic Division

All activity in sympathetic nerve fibers originates exclusively from neurons in the spinal cord. The cell bodies of sympathetic preganglionic neurons are located in the intermediolateral cell column of spinal cord segments T1 to L2 or L3 (see Figure 5-4). The axons of these neurons are of small diameter and are lightly myelinated. They exit the spinal cord in the ventral roots of spinal nerves T1–L2. These preganglionic fibers synapse with the cell bodies of postganglionic neurons located either in the **paravertebral ganglia** of the sympathetic trunk or in **prevertebral ganglia** (also called collateral ganglia).

The paravertebral ganglia consist of 20 to 25 collections of cell bodies that form two large ganglionated chains on each side of the vertebral column (Figure 12-8 ■). The sympathetic trunks extend from the base of the skull to the coccyx. The lightly myelinated preganglionic axons reach the sympathetic trunk by exiting spinal nerves T1–L2 in the **white communicating rami**, which appear white

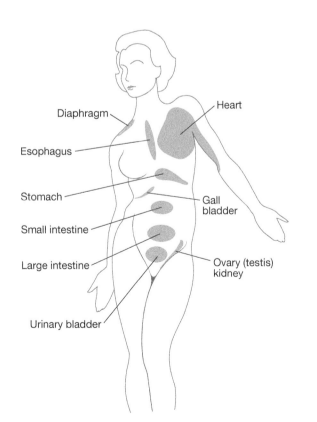

FIGURE 12-7 Typical cutaneous areas (dermatomes) to which pain from specific visceral organs is referred.

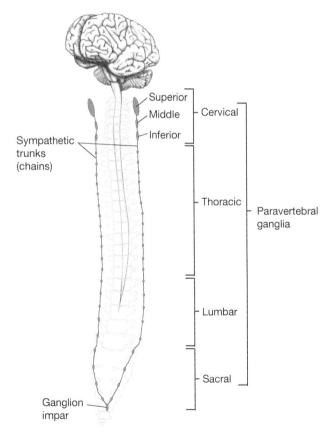

FIGURE 12-8 The paravertebral ganglia of the sympathetic nervous system are organized into interconnected chains on either side of the vertebral column. Paravertebral ganglia are associated with all spinal nerves, although at cervical levels, its eight spinal nerves share three autonomic ganglia: the superior, middle, and inferior.

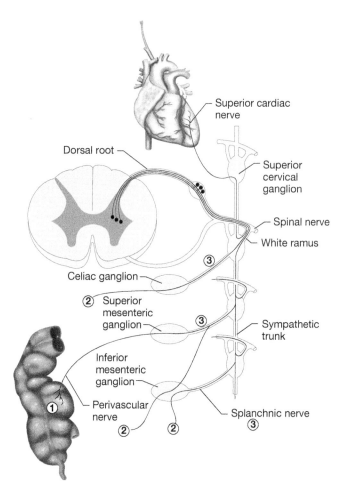

FIGURE 12-9 Visceral afferent fibers from the thoracic and abdominal viscera traverse the sympathetic trunk, enter white communicating rami, and join the thoracic and upper lumbar spinal nerves to reach the spinal cord.

because the axons are myelinated (Figure 12-9 ■). Within the sympathetic trunks, preganglionic axons follow one of three possible courses (Figure 12-10 ■). Some axons synapse immediately with postganglionic neurons at the same level as they entered; others ascend or descend in the sympathetic trunk to synapse in a more cranial or caudal paravertebral ganglion; still other preganglionic axons continue through the chain without synapsing and emerge from the trunk in the abdominopelvic splanchnic nerves in which they project to a prevertebral ganglion.

> **Thought Question**
>
> What specific nerve roots are associated with preganglionic sympathetic fibers?

Postganglionic axons from the sympathetic trunk are small in diameter and unmyelinated. Those destined to be distributed within the neck, body wall, and limbs exit the paravertebral ganglia in the **gray communicating rami**, which is gray-colored because the axons are unmyelinated.

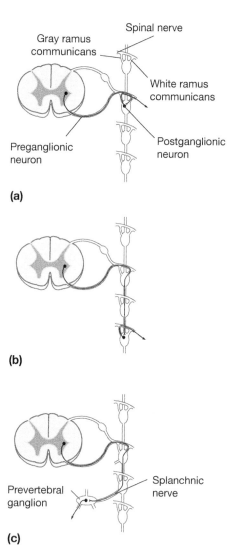

FIGURE 12-10 Courses pursued by preganglionic axons within the sympathetic trunk. (a) Some axons synapse immediately with postganglionic neurons at the same level as they entered the sympathetic chain. (b) Some descend (or ascend) in the sympathetic trunk to synapse in a more caudal (or cranial) paravertebral ganglion. (c) Still others continue through the chain without synapsing and exit the trunk in a splanchnic nerve in which they project to a prevertebral ganglion.

These postganglionic axons enter the ventral rami of adjacent spinal nerves through which they reach blood vessels, hair follicles, and sweat glands (Figure 12-11 ■). They stimulate the contraction of blood vessels (*vasomotion*) and arrector pili muscles associated with hairs (*pilomotion*, producing "goose bumps") and cause sweating (*sudomotion*). Postganglionic sympathetic fibers innervating smooth muscle and glands of the head (and the dilator muscle of the iris) arise from cells of the **superior cervical ganglion** at the superior end of the sympathetic trunk (see Figure 12-8). They form a perivascular plexus of nerves—the carotid plexus—and follow the branches of the carotid arteries to their destinations in the head. Postganglionic sympathetic axons that supply the viscera of the thoracic

Body wall and limbs | Viscera

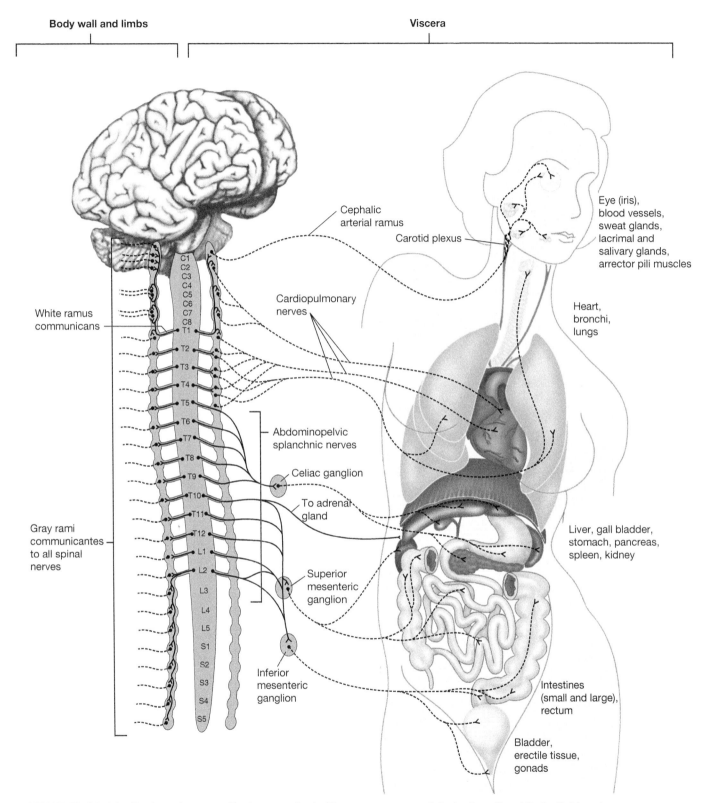

FIGURE 12-11 Distribution of postganglionic sympathetic fibers to structures of the body wall and limbs (left) and to the viscera (right).

Thought Question

What is the difference between white and gray communicating rami associated with the ANS?

cavity (e.g., the heart and lungs) reach plexuses in these structures via the cardiac and pulmonary nerves.

The prevertebral ganglia, collectively representing the second site of synapse of preganglionic sympathetic axons, are located along the abdominal aorta, particularly around the origins of the celiac and superior and inferior mesenteric arteries with the ganglia bearing the same names. These prevertebral ganglia receive their preganglionic fibers from the splanchnic nerves. The postganglionic fibers from the prevertebral ganglia form periarterial plexuses that follow branches of the abdominal aorta to reach smooth muscle, blood vessels, and glands of the abdominal and pelvic viscera. The abdominal viscera include the liver, gall bladder, stomach, pancreas, spleen, kidney, and small and large intestines. The pelvic viscera include the urinary bladder, sex organs, and prostate.

Visceral organs innervated by the autonomic nervous system receive only postganglionic fibers. Thus, the sympathetic innervation of the medullary cells of the **suprarenal gland** (the **adrenal medulla**) is unique (see Figure 12-3). The secretory cells of the adrenal medulla are postsynaptic sympathetic neurons that lack axons and dendrites. In other words, the adrenal medulla is really a modified autonomic ganglion. Rather than releasing their neurotransmitters (epinephrine and norepinephrine) onto the cells of a specific effector organ, adrenal medullary cells release them directly into the blood stream to circulate throughout the body. This results in a widespread response to activation of the sympathetic nervous system.

> **Thought Question**
>
> Where are the prevertebral ganglia? Can you compare and contrast the three main pathways that they follow?

Parasympathetic Division

In contrast to the sympathetic division of the ANS, the parasympathetic division involves both the spinal cord *and* brainstem structures. Furthermore, the spinal structures are only found in the portion of the cord not innervated by the sympathetic division—namely, the sacral regions.

The sacral part of the parasympathetic system originates in neurons located in the intermediate gray matter of spinal cord segments S2, S3, and S4 (see Figure 12-4). These axons do not enter the sympathetic chain. The preganglionic axons exit the spinal cord in the ventral roots of spinal nerves S2–S4 and synapse in terminal ganglia that lie within the walls of the colon, rectum, urinary bladder, prostate and vaginal glands, and erectile tissues of the penis and clitoris. The sacral part of the parasympathetic system controls urination, defecation, and erection.

The cranial component of the parasympathetic division is associated with the brainstem nuclei of four cranial nerves (III, VII, IX, and X) (see Figure 12-4). The **Edinger-Westphal nucleus** of the oculomotor nuclear complex in the midbrain contains the cell bodies of the preganglionic neurons that exit the brainstem in the oculomotor nerve (III) (see Figure 13-3). These preganglionic fibers synapse in the ciliary ganglion located toward the posterior limit of the bony orbit. The postganglionic parasympathetic axons (visceromotor) run in the short ciliary nerves to the sphincter muscle of the iris and smooth muscle of the ciliary body. The **superior salivatory nucleus** in the pons contains the cell bodies of the preganglionic neurons that exit the brainstem in the intermediate nerve, a branch of the facial nerve (VII) (see Figure 13-16). The preganglionic fibers synapse in two ganglia. The pterygopalatine ganglion, located in the pterygopalatine fossa of the skull, sends postganglionic axons (viscerosecretory) to the lacrimal glands and to the blood vessels and glands of the mucous membranes of the nose and palate. The second ganglion in which the preganglionic axons synapse is the submandibular ganglion, lying over the submandibular gland, which sends postganglionic axons (viscerosecretory) to the submandibular and sublingual salivary glands. The **inferior salivatory nucleus** in the medulla contains the cell bodies of the preganglionic neurons that exit the brainstem in the glossopharyngeal nerve (IX) (see Figure 13-21). These axons synapse in the otic ganglion, located in the foramen ovale, which send postganglionic axons (viscerosecretory) to the parotid gland, the largest of the salivary glands. It should be noted that these preganglionic parasympathetic neurons in cranial nerves VII and IX have overlapping brainstem origins. This has led some to question the appropriateness of distinguishing separate superior and inferior salivatory nuclei. The **dorsal motor nucleus of the vagus** in the medulla (see Figure 13-22) contains the cell bodies of preganglionic neurons that exit the brainstem in the vagus nerve (X) to innervate nearly all of the thoracic and abdominal viscera except those in the pelvic region (visceromotor and viscerosecretory). In the thoracic cavity, these axons synapse in the intrinsic ganglia of the heart and bronchial musculature, which send short postganglionic fibers to the muscles of the heart and bronchi. In the abdominal cavity, the preganglionic axons of the dorsal motor nucleus of the vagus synapse in terminal ganglia of the gastrointestinal tract (as far as the descending colon), liver, pancreas, and kidneys. Table 12-3 ■ summarizes the cranial component of the parasympathetic division of the ANS.

> **Thought Question**
>
> In Chapter 13, you will learn about the importance of the Edinger-Westphal nucleus with respect to brainstem injuries. For now, recall the cranial nerve associated with this nucleus.

> **Thought Question**
>
> Thinking ahead, and based on what you have learned so far, what might be the consequence of a large area of damage in the tegmentum of the medulla?

Table 12-3 Cranial Component of the Parasympathetic Division of the ANS

PREGANGLIONIC CELL BODIES	CRANIAL NERVE*	POSTGANGLIONIC CELL BODIES	POSTGANGLIONIC AXONS
Edinger-Westphal nucleus in midbrain	III	Ciliary ganglion	Ciliary nerves to sphincter of iris and ciliary body
Superior salivatory nucleus in pons	VII	Pterygopalatine ganglion	To lacrimal glands
		Submandibular ganglion	To submandibular and sublingual salivary glands
Inferior salivatory nucleus in medulla	IX	Otic ganglion	To parotid gland
Dorsal motor nucleus of vagus in medulla	X	Intrinsic and terminal ganglia	To heart, bronchi, gastrointestinal tract (as far as descending colon), liver, pancreas, kidneys

*Preganglionic axons

General Functions of Autonomic Efferents from the Sympathetic and Parasympathetic Systems

The overall function of the autonomic nervous system is to regulate and control those visceral activities that maintain a stable internal environment in response to changing internal conditions and external stresses. Most visceral organs are innervated by both sympathetic and parasympathetic divisions of the ANS. However, a number of structures—sweat glands, somatic blood vessels, and hair follicles—receive only sympathetic postganglionic fibers, and the adrenal medulla receives only preganglionic sympathetic fibers. In certain structures (e.g., the heart and digestive tract), the sympathetic and parasympathetic divisions have opposite effects; in others, one division is unopposed (sympathetic innervation of the sweat gland and limb blood vessels) or one is dominant (parasympathetic innervation of the bladder); in still others, the two divisions cooperate to fulfill a single function (innervation of male sex organ). Sympathetic and parasympathetic actions on visceral structures are summarized in Table 12-4 ■.

In general, the sympathetic system is catabolic, or energy expending, which enables the body to deal with stresses, such as preparing the body for fight or flight. Activation of the sympathetic division tends to produce widespread and relatively long-lasting effects. This is because of the wide divergence that occurs in sympathetic ganglia and because sympathetic stimulation causes the adrenal medulla to release epinephrine and norepinephrine into the systemic circulation. In contrast, the parasympathetic division is anabolic, or energy conserving, and promotes the maintenance and restoration of bodily reserves. Autonomic control of specific organs is discussed later.

Thought Question

Which system is involved with the so-called flight or fight response, and how does the metabolism of this system support its function?

AUTONOMIC INNERVATION AND CONTROL OF SPECIFIC ORGANS

Clinical Preview ....

Mohan Gupta is a 38-year-old attorney who sustained a C-6 spinal cord injury when he was in high school. You have treated him off and on since that time. Drawing on information you learned in Chapters 9, 10, and 11, consider the following:

• What motor and sensory losses will he have?

• What will be his muscle tone?

Now, as you read through this section, consider why he might have problems with the following:

• Blood pressure and heart rate.

• Control of bowel and bladder.

• Autonomic dysreflexia.

Autonomic Control Centers

Groups of rather imprecisely defined neurons in the brainstem regulate autonomic activities. In the midbrain, the regulation of pupillary size and visual accommodation is mediated by neurons in the pretectal area,

Table 12-4 Innervation of Selected Viscera

ORGAN	SYMPATHETIC			PARASYMPATHETIC		
	PREGANGLIONIC	POSTGANGLIONIC	FUNCTION	PREGANGLIONIC	POSTGANGLIONIC	FUNCTION
Iris	C8–T3	Superior cervical ganglion	Dilation of pupil	Edinger-Westphal nucleus in midbrain	Ciliary ganglion	Constriction of pupil
Parotid gland	T1–T3	Superior cervical ganglion	Secretion reduced and viscid	Inferior salivatory nucleus in medulla	Otic ganglion	Secretion increased and watery
Heart	T1–T5	Cervical and upper thoracic ganglia	Increased rate	Dorsal motor nucleus of vagus in medulla	Intracardiac ganglia	Decreased rate
Coronary vessels	T1–T5	Cervical and upper thoracic ganglia	Dilation or constriction	Dorsal motor nucleus of vagus in medulla	Intracardiac ganglia	Constriction
Bronchi	T2–T5	Upper thoracic ganglia	Dilation	Dorsal motor nucleus of vagus in medulla	Pulmonary ganglia	Constriction
Stomach	T6–T10	Celiac ganglion	Inhibition of peristalsis and secretion	Dorsal motor nucleus of vagus in medulla	Myenteric and submucosal ganglia	Increased peristalsis and secretion
Sex organs	T10–L2	Inferior mesenteric ganglion	Ejaculation	S2–S4	Ganglia along branches of aorta and int. iliac arteries	Produces engorgement (erection) of erectile tissues of external genitals
Urinary bladder	T12–L2	Inferior mesenteric ganglion	Contraction of internal urethral sphincter to maintain urinary continence	S2–S4	Vesicle ganglia	Contraction of detrusor causing urination (and inhibition of internal urethral sphincter)
Sweat glands of head and neck	T1–T3	Upper 3 cervical ganglia	Promotes sweating*			
Sweat glands and blood vessels of lower extremity	L1–L2	Lumbar and sacral ganglia	Promotes sweating* and vasoconstriction			

*With the exception of the sweat glands, glandular secretion is parasympathetically stimulated.

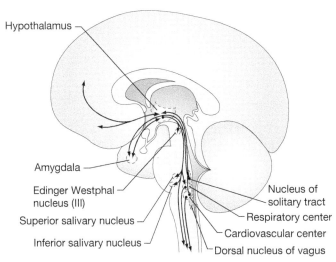

FIGURE 12-12 Central structures involved in the regulation of autonomic activities. The solitary nucleus projects directly to the hypothalamus and amygdala. Several regions of the hypothalamus project directly to autonomic centers in the brainstem and spinal cord.

Edinger-Westphal nucleus, and superior colliculus (see Chapter 18). In the tegmentum of the midbrain and pons are collections of neurons concerned with the regulation of micturition. In the tegmentum of the pons and medulla are sets of neurons involved with the regulation of respiration. Cardiovascular function is regulated by groups of neurons in the tegmentum of the medulla. Although these sets of neurons often are regarded as "centers," their distribution is more widespread than the concept would imply.

Many visceral afferents reach these so-called centers via the **solitary tract** and **nucleus**, both located in the dorsolateral medulla (Figure 12-12 ■). (Note that this does not pertain to those afferents that affect pupillary size or visual accommodation.) The solitary tract is formed by visceral afferent fibers of the facial (intermediate), glossopharyngeal, and vagus nerves. The afferents of each nerve terminate in different regions of the solitary nucleus. From the solitary nucleus, efferents synapse on the neurons of these various centers. In addition, neurons of the solitary nucleus project directly to the hypothalamus, a projection that reaffirms involvement of the hypothalamus in the regulation of autonomic homeostasis.

Thought Question

We will discuss the solitary tract and nucleus in the brainstem in Chapter 13. For now, identify the afferent fibers that form this tract, and indicate the destination of efferent fibers that arise from the tract.

Control of Respiration

One of the critical autonomic centers of the brainstem is that which controls respiration. This is accomplished through a network of complex circuitry, mostly located in the medulla. The respiratory system has a pacemaker, located in the medulla, analogous to the pacemaker for the cardiac system. The nucleus solitarius plays a role in this circuitry and receives inputs from many areas. Inputs to respiratory circuits come from many sources, including chemoreceptors for blood oxygen levels and pH as well as stretch receptors from the lungs. Efferents from the respiratory circuitry project to the cervical cord to excite the phrenic nerve, which supplies the diaphragm.

Damage to the respiratory centers can result in a variety of symptoms, depending on location and extent of the injury. Among possible consequences are ataxic respiration and hyperventilation. Cheyne-Stokes respiration can occur, in which breathing becomes progressively deeper with each breath and then progressively more shallow to the point of apnea. When severe (e.g., if the pacemaker is disrupted), such injury can result in respiratory arrest.

Heart

The heart is richly innervated by sympathetic, parasympathetic, and visceral afferent fibers. On the efferent side, it is necessary to differentiate the sympathetic and parasympathetic components. The preganglionic sympathetic neurons regulating cardiac function are located in the intermediolateral cell column of the upper five thoracic segments of the spinal cord (Figure 12-13 ■). Postganglionic fibers emerging from the three cervical and upper five thoracic ganglia of the sympathetic trunk travel to the heart in the cardiac nerves. These axons are distributed to the atria and ventricles, the sinoatrial and atrioventricular nodes, and the coronary arteries. Stimulation of this sympathetic innervation increases heart rate and the force of contraction, thereby increasing cardiac output. Parasympathetic innervation of the heart derives from the dorsal motor nucleus of the vagus, located in the medulla medial to the solitary tract and its nucleus (discussed later). Preganglionic parasympathetic axons exit the medulla in the vagus nerve (X) and travel to terminal ganglia located in the cardiac plexus and heart wall. Postganglionic parasympathetic axons terminate in the sinoatrial and atrioventricular nodes and musculature of the heart. Activation of this parasympathetic innervation decreases heart rate and the force of contraction. Thus, these two systems have opposite effects on heart rate and the force of contraction.

An important (but not the only) contingent of visceral afferent fibers arises from mechanoreceptors situated in

Thought Question

The sympathetic, parasympathetic, and visceral afferent fibers play very different roles with respect to regulation of heart rate and blood pressure. Explain how the different fibers work together to regulate these essential functions.

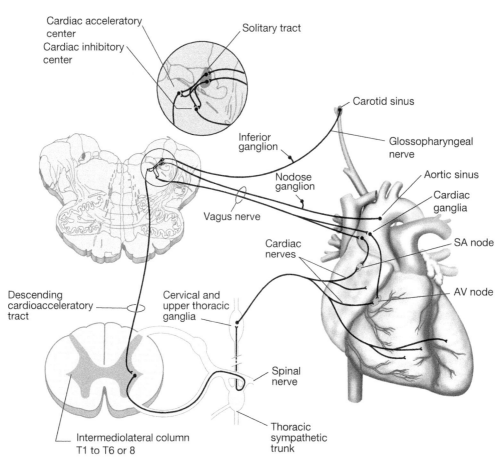

FIGURE 12-13 Innervation of the heart by the autonomic nervous system.

the aortic arch and carotid sinus, the latter being a slight dilation of the proximal part of the internal carotid artery. These receptors are **baroreceptors** that respond to changes in arterial blood pressure. Their primary afferents reach the medulla over the glossopharyngeal (IX) and vagus (X) nerves and have their cell bodies in the inferior and nodose ganglia, respectively (see Figure 12-13). These visceral afferents enter the solitary tract and synapse on neurons of the immediately adjacent nucleus of the solitary tract.

Blood pressure depends on a variety of factors, including the volume of intravascular blood, the resistance of systemic blood flow through the blood vessels, and the rate of blood output from the heart. The ANS regulates all of these factors, and its actions allow the reflex maintenance of blood pressure. A number of so-called centers located in the reticular formation of lateral medulla are involved in regulating the activity of the autonomic innervation that controls vascular resistance and cardiac output. The resistance of systemic arterioles is governed by changes in their diameter, resulting from contraction or relaxation of vascular smooth muscle, which receives sympathetic innervation; the parasympathetic system has little or no effect on vascular resistance. It is important to emphasize that ongoing tonic activity of this sympathetic innervation normally maintains systemic arterioles in a constricted state, at approximately half their maximal diameter. Therefore, a decrease in sympathetic activity leads to vasodilation, and an increase in sympathetic activities leads to further vasoconstriction. One of these medullary reticular formation centers governs vasoconstrictor tone. Another center is a cardioacceleratory center that influences the sympathetic innervation of the heart, whose preganglionic neurons are in the intermediolateral cell column of T1–T5. A third center is a cardioinhibitory center that influences the parasympathetic innervation of the heart via the dorsal motor nucleus of the vagus nerve.

Activation of baroreceptors in the carotid sinus and aortic arch signal an increase in blood pressure. Via the visceral afferents in cranial nerves IX and X, neurons of the nucleus solitarius are activated, and their output influences the three cardiovascular centers in the reticular formation (Figure 12-14 ■). The tonically active vasomotor neurons are inhibited. Neurons from this vasoconstrictor center descend in reticulospinal tracts to synapse on preganglionic sympathetic neurons over the full rostrocaudal extent of the intermediolateral column (T1 to L2 or L3). Axons of these preganglionic sympathetic neurons synapse on postganglionic neurons throughout the entire sympathetic trunk. Postganglionic axons enter all spinal nerves and terminate on systemic arterioles. Due to decreased sympathetic activity, the arterioles dilate and peripheral vascular resistance is reduced. Simultaneously,

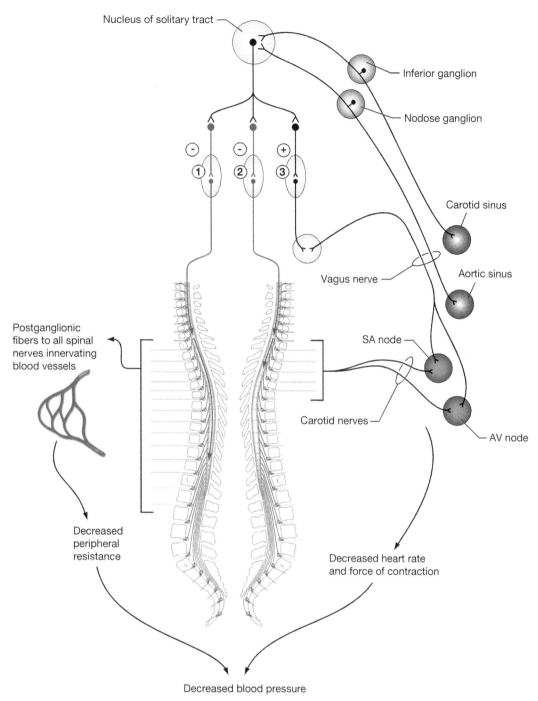

FIGURE 12-14 The baroreceptor reflex that reduces blood pressure.

the cardioacceleratory center is inhibited and the cardio-inhibitory center is excited, thereby reducing heart rate. Collectively, these actions combine to reduce blood pressure. The reflex has been termed the **baroreceptor reflex**.

Bladder

The urinary bladder is essentially a hollow bag of smooth muscle that collects urine from the **ureters** and stores it until it is eliminated from the body through the **urethra**. The innervation of the bladder and the control of urination (**micturition**)

are complex and not fully understood but are matters of great clinical importance. The urinary bladder and its sphincters are controlled by the interplay of parasympathetic, sympathetic, somatic motor, and visceral afferent fibers.

The smooth muscle of the bladder wall is arranged in three layers known collectively as the detrusor muscle (Figure 12-15 ■). A so-called internal urethral sphincter is located where the urethra leaves the bladder; however, it is not a distinct anatomical entity, but rather a continuation of fibers of the detrusor muscle. When the internal sphincter contracts, it prevents the bladder from emptying.

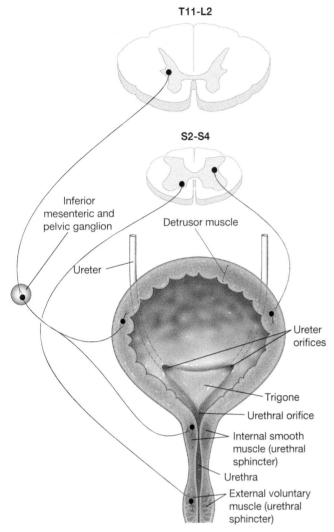

FIGURE 12-15 Frontal section through the urinary bladder. Note that the internal urethral sphincter is smooth muscle and the external urethral sphincter is voluntary muscle.

A true external urethral sphincter muscle occurs in the middle, membranous portion of the urethra. It is composed of voluntary skeletal muscle whose contraction also prevents bladder emptying.

Innervation of the Lower Urinary Tract (Bladder and Urethra)

The sympathetic innervation of the bladder originates from neurons of the intermediolateral cell column in spinal cord segments T11–L2 (see Figure 12-15). Preganglionic axons travel in the lumbar splanchnic nerves to the **inferior mesenteric ganglion**, where they synapse. Postganglionic sympathetic fibers traveling in the hypogastric plexus innervate the bladder wall (including parasympathetic ganglia in the bladder wall) and the internal urethral sphincter. This sympathetic innervation relaxes the detrusor muscle, allowing the bladder to distend, and simultaneously causes contraction of the

internal urethral sphincter which closes the urethra and prevents the bladder from emptying prematurely.

The parasympathetic innervation of the bladder originates from neurons of the intermediate gray matter in the second, third, and fourth sacral segments (see Figure 12-15). These preganglionic axons course in the pelvic nerve to reach vesical ganglion cells in the bladder wall. This parasympathetic innervation is excitatory and causes contraction of the detrusor muscle and emptying of the bladder.

Alpha lower motor neurons innervating the voluntary muscle of the external urethral sphincter are located in the ventral horn of spinal cord segments S2–S4, in a nucleus known as the **Onuf nucleus**. These LMN axons travel in the pudendal nerve. Activity in Onuf's nucleus causes the external urethral sphincter to contract, which holds back urine until micturition is convenient.

> **Thought Question**
>
> Collection and elimination of urine relies on a complex interplay of the sympathetic and parasympathetic systems and also requires voluntary control. Explain how these different control systems work together.

Micturition

Urine is first collected and stored over a relatively long time period and then briefly eliminated in the act of micturition. In the adult, this switch from a storage mode to an elimination mode is controlled consciously, and the person is said to be continent. The process of collection and storage is maintained by sympathetic activity and the absence of parasympathetic input. Sympathetic activity facilitates relaxation of the detrusor muscle, primarily by inhibiting postganglionic parasympathetic neurons in the vesical ganglia that cause contraction of the detrusor. Sympathetic activity also affects the detrusor muscle itself, but this is a minor influence. In addition, sympathetic activity excites the internal urethral sphincter. At the same time, the external urethral sphincter remains contracted by the tonic activity of alpha motor neurons in Onuf's nucleus.

During micturition, the conditions promoting bladder filling are reversed. Micturition occurs following high levels of bladder distension, during which reflex afferent activity generated by stretch receptors in the bladder wall is relayed to a micturition center in rostral pons (Figure 12-16 ■). This **pontine micturition center** integrates the function of the detrusor and sphincter muscles that, acting alone, would have opposite effects on the capacity to empty the bladder. The center sends excitatory impulses to sacral parasympathetic neurons and elicits contraction of the detrusor muscle. At the same time, the center inhibits alpha motor neurons in Onuf's nucleus and T11–L2 sympathetic neurons, thereby relaxing the external and internal urethral sphincters, respectively. The bladder then empties.

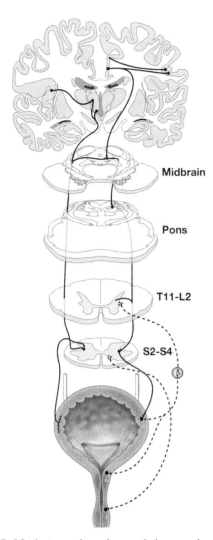

FIGURE 12-16 Autonomic and somatic innervation of the urinary bladder.

Voluntary control of micturition depends on the capacity to sense bladder fullness. The same information that feeds into the reflex circuitry mediating bladder control ascends bilaterally in axons of the lateral funiculus to the periaqueductal gray, hypothalamus, and the ventral posteromedial nucleus (VPM) of the thalamus (see Figure 12-16). The latter relays information to the insula, where bladder status is consciously perceived. When bladder fullness is sensed and micturition is perceived as imminent, the voluntary restraint of micturition until the time and place are appropriate depends on the frontal lobes (cingulate gyrus and prefrontal cortex). This information, along with that of bladder status, is integrated in the periaqueductal gray that activates the pontine micturition center; the elimination mode is then engaged.

Sex Organs

The sympathetic innervation of the pelvic viscera arises from spinal cord segments T10–L2. The preganglionic fibers synapse mainly in the inferior mesenteric ganglion.

In the female, postganglionic sympathetic fibers innervate the blood vessels and smooth muscle of the uterus and vagina. Sympathetic activation results in rhythmic contractions of the vagina. In the male, the postganglionic sympathetic fibers supply the prostate gland, ductus deferens, and seminal vesicle. Sympathetic activation is essential to ejaculation. Peristalsis of the ductus deferens and seminal vesicles move semen into the prostatic urethra, and the bladder neck constricts, preventing retrograde emission of semen into the bladder.

Parasympathetic preganglionic fibers originate in S2–S4 and enter the pelvic cavity in the pelvic nerve. Postganglionic axons innervate the vaginal glands and erectile tissue of the clitoris in the female. Parasympathetic activity causes secretion of the vaginal glands and engorgement of the clitoris. In the male, parasympathetic postganglionic fibers innervate arterial smooth muscle involved in producing penile erection. Parasympathetic activity opens vascular channels, allowing blood to flow into and dilate the cavernous spaces (erectile tissues) in the corpora of the penis.

CLINICAL CONNECTIONS

Primary (Idiopathic) Orthostatic Hypotension

In primary orthostatic hypotension, blood pressure falls suddenly upon standing from a recumbent position. Capacitance vessels (veins) in the legs fail to constrict, resulting in a lower venous return and diminished cardiac output. Several types of primary orthostatic hypotension are recognized, but the cause(s) are unknown. In one, there is a degeneration mainly of postganglionic sympathetic fibers, with a relative sparing of parasympathetic fibers and no CNS involvement. In another, there is degeneration of preganglionic intermediolateral cell column neurons in thoracic segments of the spinal cord. Later, other signs of CNS involvement appear. In both types, disturbances of sweating, bladder, and sexual functions usually occur.

It is important to note there are other common conditions that may cause low blood pressure, including pregnancy, dehydration, and endocrine problems (especially in people with diabetes). Likewise, hypotension can be a side effect of prescribed medication.

Bladder Dysfunction

The storage of urine and the complete emptying of the bladder depend on reciprocal reflex connections between the appropriate spinal cord segments and the pontine micturition centers, together with the intactness of the visceral afferent and efferent connections of the bladder with the spinal cord. Interruption of these reflex connections at any point produces a **neurogenic bladder** (Figure 12-17 ■).

Bilateral spinal cord lesions above T12 produce a UMN paralysis of the bladder. This is called a **reflex neurogenic**

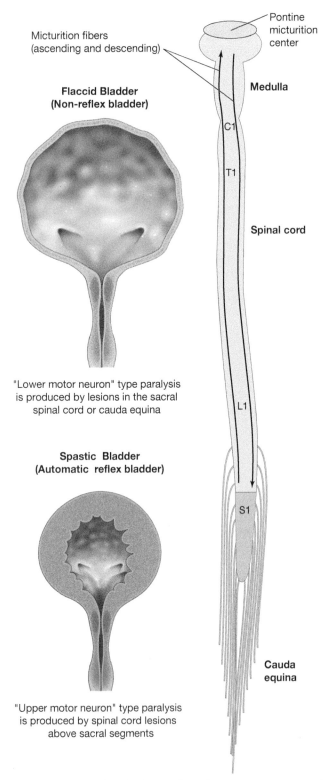

FIGURE 12-17 Lesions in the cauda equina or sacral segments of the spinal cord cause a flaccid neurogenic bladder (left), whereas spinal cord lesions rostral to sacral levels cause a spastic neurogenic bladder (right).

the reflex connections between the spinal cord and pontine micturition centers have been interrupted. Also, because the bladder is spastic, only a small volume of urine can be retained.

Bilateral lesions involving sacral levels of the spinal cord result in a **nonreflex neurogenic bladder**. This is an LMN paralysis of the bladder. The bladder is flaccid (the tonus of the detrusor muscle is lost) so that the bladder distends as urine accumulates until there is a continual dribbling incontinence. There is considerable urinary retention, with a high risk of infection. There is no awareness of bladder fullness, and the voluntary initiation of micturition is impossible. Lesions of the spinal nerve roots in the cauda equina also result in a nonreflex neurogenic bladder. In diseases such as multiple sclerosis and subacute combined degeneration, a mixed type of neurogenic bladder can occur, consisting of a combination of lower and upper motor neuron types of bladder paralysis.

Horner's Syndrome

Horner's syndrome consists of a combination of **miosis** (small pupil), **ptosis** (drooping eyelid), and apparent **enophthalmos** (retraction of the eyeball). The enophthalmos is probably an illusion due to narrowing of the palpebral fissure. In addition, depending on the site of the lesion, flushing and anhidrosis (absence of sweating) over one side of the face may occur. The syndrome occurs as a result of a lesion to certain fibers of the sympathetic division of the ANS (Figure 12-18 ■). The signs of the syndrome occur ipsilateral to the lesion.

Peripheral lesions resulting in Horner's syndrome involve preganglionic sympathetic fibers that emerge from T1 and T2, the superior cervical ganglion, or postganglionic sympathetic axons (at any point along their course) that emerge from the superior cervical ganglion. Lesions in the lower neck affect sweating over the entire face. Lesions above the superior cervical ganglion may not affect sweating because the main outflow to the facial blood vessels and sweat glands is below the superior cervical ganglion. Tumors or inflammatory involvement of cervical lymph nodes, surgical trauma to the sympathetic chain during procedures on the larynx or thyroid, and neoplasms of the brachial plexus or apex of the lung are examples of peripheral lesions.

Central lesions that produce Horner's syndrome involve preganglionic neurons of the intermediolateral cell column of C8–T2 (the ciliospinal center) or interruption of uncrossed fibers that descend to the ciliospinal center from the hypothalamus anywhere along their course in the tegmentum of the brainstem or cervical spinal cord. CNS involvement can result from tumor, syringomyelia, or traumatic lesions of the first and second thoracic segments of the spinal cord. Far more common causes of Horner's syndrome are brainstem strokes or other brainstem lesions.

(spastic) bladder. Bladder fullness is not appreciated, and voluntary control is lost (the person is incontinent). The bladder empties suddenly and reflexively (the so-called **automatic bladder**). But emptying is incomplete because

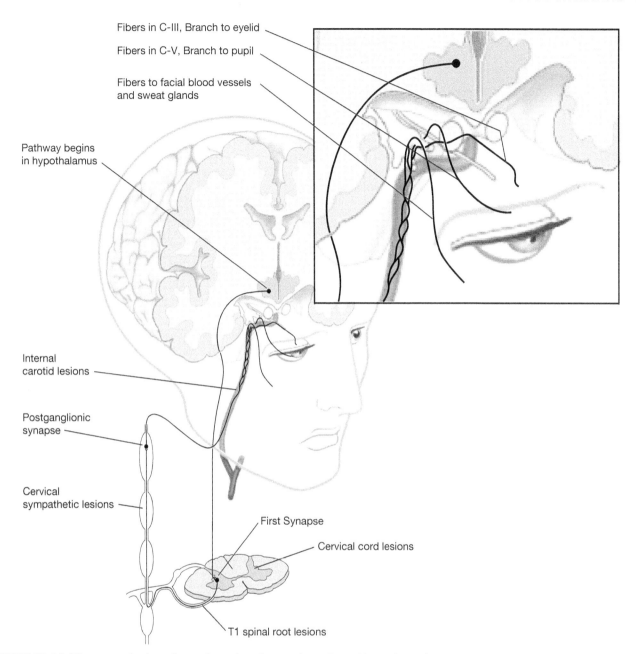

Fibers in C-III, Branch to eyelid

Fibers in C-V, Branch to pupil

Fibers to facial blood vessels and sweat glands

Pathway begins in hypothalamus

Internal carotid lesions

Postganglionic synapse

Cervical sympathetic lesions

First Synapse

Cervical cord lesions

T1 spinal root lesions

FIGURE 12-18 The sympathetic pathway that, when damaged, produces Horner's syndrome.

Acute Autonomic Paralysis

Complete lesions of the cervical spinal cord, due most often to trauma, interrupt all suprasegmental control of the sympathetic and sacral parasympathetic components of the ANS. Lesions involving lower thoracic segments of the spinal cord leave most of the descending sympathetic suprasegmental control intact, but interrupt descending control of the sacral parasympathetic system.

During the period of spinal shock, following spinal cord compression or transaction, somatic and autonomic functions are lost. The autonomic effects include paralysis of the bowel and bladder, anhidrosis, loss of piloerection and sexual function, and potentially severe hypotension. Within one to six weeks, spinal shock subsides and

autonomic function returns because the afferent and efferent connections of the viscera with the isolated spinal cord segments remain intact.

Autonomic Dysreflexia

A potentially life-threatening condition associated with lesions of the spinal cord is **autonomic dysreflexia**. This condition is more likely to occur in individuals with a complete lesion of the sixth thoracic cord level and above; it results because the normal regulatory control of heart rate and blood pressure is disrupted.

In the individual with a healthy nervous system, noxious sensory input typically excites the sympathetic portion of the autonomic nervous system via the splanchnic outflow. This sympathetic outflow causes vasoconstriction and increases cardiac output, with the result that blood pressure is elevated. The elevation of blood pressure is sensed by receptors in the aortic arch and carotid sinus, triggering a brainstem reflex response referred to as the baroreceptor reflex. This parasympathetic response serves to decrease the sympathetic drive to the blood vessels. Thus, in normal circumstances, activation of the sympathetic response to a noxious stimulus is balanced by the parasympathetic system. In people with spinal cord injury above the sixth thoracic level, the normal balance is disrupted because the descending parasympathetic signals cannot be transmitted below the level of the injury. Thus, blood pressure can continue to elevate, potentially with life-threatening consequences. Occurrences such as a kinked catheter, urinary retention, pressure ulcers, bowel distension,

restrictive clothing, or the use of electrical stimulation can all be perceived as noxious stimuli that may elicit the sympathetic-driven increase in blood pressure.

Autonomic dysreflexia is characterized by increased blood pressure, severe headache, goose bumps, and sweating. Initially, heart rate is elevated (mediated by the sympathetic system), followed soon thereafter by a reduced heart rate (mediated by the parasympathetic system). The individual may also report a feeling of anxiety or a sense that something is wrong. It is important to recognize symptoms associated with autonomic dysreflexia and respond quickly. The individual should be assisted to an upright position and any instigating noxious stimuli removed. If blood pressure does not decline, further medical attention is needed.

Summary

The autonomic nervous system is represented in both the central and peripheral nervous systems. Aspects of its general organization parallel those of the somatic division of the nervous system. Thus, for example, sensory inputs from the viscera modulate autonomic activity, just as sensory inputs from structures of the musculoskeletal system modulate somatic activity. But, in many important respects, the autonomic and somatic divisions of the nervous system are markedly different in terms of both structure and function. Nonetheless, activity in the two divisions is highly integrated.

Depending on the specific organ innervated, activity in the sympathetic and parasympathetic divisions can oppose one another, be collaborative, or one division may be dominant. In general, the sympathetic division is energy expending and mobilizes bodily functions to meet behavioral

needs depending on emotion and (potentially) demanding physical exertion (e.g., threat, aggression). Thus, sympathetic activity produces widespread and relatively long-lasting behavioral effects. In contrast, the parasympathetic division is energy conserving (anabolic) and facilitates the restoration and maintenance of bodily reserves. Its actions are more discrete and enable localized control of specific target structures.

The autonomic innervation and control of three structures was discussed in detail: the heart, bladder, and sex organs. In the case of the heart, the sympathetic and parasympathetic divisions have opposite effects, whereas in the case of male sexual function, they cooperate to fulfill a single function. In the case of autonomic innervation of the bladder, the parasympathetic division is dominant.

Applications

1. Patrick is a 19-year-old college student who dove into a shallow lake, hitting his head and fracturing his seventh cervical vertebra. This resulted in a complete spinal cord injury at the level of C8. Immediately after the injury, Patrick experienced spinal shock, which resolved one month later. He was actively involved in rehabilitation. Five weeks after his injury, the neurological examination revealed decreased sensation to all modalities in both of his legs, his trunk, and the most lateral aspect of his hands. Both of his legs were weak. He had heightened reflexes at both knees and ankles. One day in physical therapy, while practicing rolling from supine to prone, he developed a sudden pounding headache. His face was flushed and he was profusely sweating. The therapist recognized this as autonomic dysreflexia and immediately sat Patrick up, called for help, and assessed his vital signs. His blood pressure measured 210/98 and pulse rate was 50.

    a. Describe the causes and consequences of spinal shock.
    b. Drawing on information presented in Chapter 11, explain the spastic paresis that Patrick developed below the level of C8.
    c. What is autonomic dysreflexia and what are some common triggers?
    d. In what way is hyperreflexia analogous to autonomic dysrefleia?
    e. What are the symptoms of autonomic dysreflexia and how is this condition treated?

2. Lateral medullary syndrome (Wallenberg's syndrome) and cervical spinal cord injuries can both result in Horner's syndrome.

    a. Identify the constellation of findings that indicate Horner's syndrome.

b. What is the neuroanatomical site of dysfunction that results in Horner's syndrome?

c. Are the symptoms of Horner's syndrome contralateral or ipsilateral to the lesion?

d. Given what you know about the spinal cord, what other conditions can you think of that might cause Horner's syndrome?

References

Andersson, K. E., and Wagner, G. Physiology of penile erection. *Physiol Rev* 75:191, 1995.

Appenzeller, O., and Oribe, E. *The Autonomic Nervous System: An Introduction to Basic and Clinical Concepts*, 5th ed. Elsevier, Amsterdam, 1997.

Cervero, F., and Morrison, J. F. B., eds. Visceral sensation. *Prog Brain Res*, vol 67. Elsevier, Amsterdam, 1986.

deGroat, W. C., et al. Mechanisms underlying the recovery of urinary bladder function following spinal cord injury. *J Autonom Nerv Sys* 30:S71, 1990.

Janig, W., and McLachlan, E. M. Neurobiology of the autonomic nervous system. In: Mathias, C. J. and Bannister, R., eds. *Autonomic Failure*, 4th ed. Oxford University Press, Oxford, 1999.

Nathan, P. W., and Smith, M. C. The location of descending fibres to sympathetic preganglionic vasomotor and sudomotor neurons in man. *J Neurol Neursurg Psychiatry* 50:1253, 1987.

Nolte, J. *The Human Brain: An Introduction to Its Functional Anatomy*. Mosby Elsevier, Philadelphia, 2009.

Ropper, A. H., and Brown, R. H. Ch. 26. Disorders of the autonomic nervous system, respiration, and swallowing. In: *Adams and Victor's Principles of Neurology*, 8th ed. McGraw-Hill, New York, 2005.

Wang, F. B., Holst, M. C., and Powley, T. L. The ratio of pre- to postganglionic neurons and related issues in the autonomic nervous system. *Brain Res Rev* 21:93, 1995.

PEARSON

myhealthprofessionskit™

Use this address to access the Companion Website created for this textbook. Simply select "Physical Therapy" from the choice of disciplines. Find this book and log in using your username and password to access self-assessment questions, a glossary, and more.

PART IV

Somatosensory and Motor Systems of the Head and Neck

The nervous system provides the means by which somatosensory information is transmitted from the periphery via the spinal cord to the cerebral cortex for processing related to perceptual understanding of the somatosensory information. Likewise, information is transmitted from the cortex to the periphery to elicit contractions of muscles for movement and function. Because the brainstem lies between the spinal cord and cortex, all ascending and descending information traverses this important structure. One can infer that the brainstem is more than a simple conduit for information; otherwise, there would be no need for a brainstem separate from the spinal cord. Rather, the brainstem fulfills a number of important functions.

In terms of its role as a conduit, somatosensory pathways for touch, pressure, pain, and temperature ascend through the brainstem on the way to the cortex, while motor pathways, originating in the cortex, descend via the brainstem to the spinal cord and thence to the relevant muscles. Recall, however, that the pathways from the spinal cord only convey somatosensory information from the extremities and torso, while the motor pathways to the spinal cord innervate muscles of those same structures. Yet, important somatosensory information also arises from the head, face, and neck such that we can feel the soft touch of a baby's hand on our face as well as the harsh pain from an infected tooth. Likewise, motor pathways descend to innervate muscles of the head, face, and neck, allowing for a myriad of facial expressions—from the quizzical look of a student trying to master a difficult concept of neuroscience, to the excited expression when his basketball team wins, to grief at loss of a loved one. Thus, the brainstem plays an important role in processing somatosensory and motor information for the head, face, and neck.

Associated with these sensory and motor pathways of the brainstem are cranial nerves and their related nuclei. Furthermore, the brainstem, unlike the spinal cord, also is the origin of sensory information of a special nature—for example, hearing, equilibrium, and vision. These so-called special senses likewise have cranial nerves and associated cranial nuclei located within the brainstem. And finally, recall that the brainstem has large and important connections with the cerebellum, as well as an enlargement from the cerebral aqueduct at the level of those connections. Along with these structures is a diffuse network of cells and their processes, referred to as the reticular system. Taken together, all of these features convey a substantially different shape to the brainstem as compared with the spinal cord. In light of the complex structure and function of the brainstem, Part IV is divided into three chapters, each building systematically and deliberately on material presented in the previous chapter.

As fundamental background necessary for an understanding of the complex organization of the brainstem, it is first important to become familiar with the cranial nerves that enter and exit that structure, to know where within the brainstem they are located, and to learn the motor and sensory functions that they subserve. This is the focus of Chapter 13.

Chapter 14 builds on this foundational information by exploring the pathways associated with somatosensory information of the head, neck, and face as well as some of the important reflexes associated with these structures. Also in this chapter is an introduction to the reticular system, which plays a fundamental role in a number of integrative functions, including consciousness and pain. It should be noted that the special senses (e.g., auditory, visual) are only briefly addressed in this chapter because they are so important and so complex that an entire chapter is devoted to each in Part V of the text.

Finally, the structures and functions of the brainstem are synthesized in Chapter 15. Only through a working knowledge of the relevant structures of the brainstem and the associated blood supply can the rehabilitation professional relate lesions to resulting consequences. This chapter begins with a systematic approach to recognizing components of the brainstem in cross section, followed by discussions of the blood supply of this important part of the nervous system and examples of disorders that would occur in selected lesions from the medulla to the midbrain.

13

Brainstem I: Cranial Nerves

LEARNING OUTCOMES

This chapter prepares the reader to:

1. Name the 12 cranial nerves and identify where they attach to the brainstem.

2. Differentiate general sensory, special sensory, and visceral sensory functions.

3. Identify cranial nerves associated with each of the following: general sensory, special sensory, and visceral sensory functions.

4. Contrast somatic motor, branchial motor, and visceral motor functions.

5. Identify cranial nerves that are associated with each of the following: somatic motor, branchial motor, and visceral motor functions.

6. Discuss those cranial nerves that have both motor and sensory components.

7. Describe the clinical evaluation of each cranial nerve.

8. Relate lesions of each cranial nerve to the resulting consequences.

ACRONYMS

DC-ML Dorsal column–medial lemniscus

MLF Medial longitudinal fasciculus

PPRF Paramedian pontine reticular formation

STT Spinothalamic tract

V_1 Ophthalmic division for afferent fibers of the trigeminal nerve

V_2 Maxillary division for afferent fibers of the trigeminal nerve

V_3 Mandibular division for afferent fibers of the trigeminal nerve

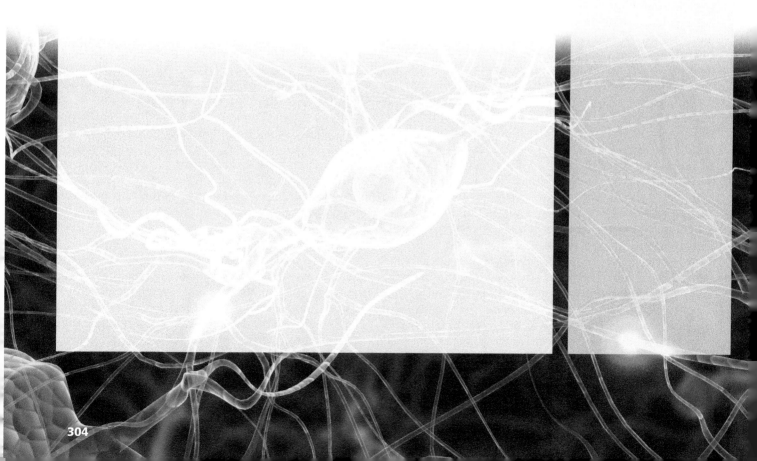

Introduction

As a first step to understanding the brainstem, we learn about the sensory and motor nerves of the head, face, and neck. These nerves and their related nuclei are responsible for general sensory and motor information, analogous to that which we learned about for the extremities and torso (e.g., touch, pain, temperature, and proprioception and activation of the muscles of the head, face and neck). However, in the brainstem, there are special functions that have no analogy to the extremities and torso. These relate to hearing, equilibrium, and vision. The term *cranial* derives from the fact that these peripheral nerves enter and exit the cranium (via the foramina and fissures presented in Chapter 1).

The fibers comprising the 12 pairs of cranial nerves subserve one or more of six functions. With regard to sensory functions, there are general sensory, special sensory, and visceral sensory axons. **General sensory axons** transmit afferent information from receptors distributed in the skin, mucous membranes, muscle, and joints, just as do afferent axons in spinal nerves. **Special sensory axons** transmit information from receptors that are not present in the trunk

and extremities, these being receptors for equilibrium, hearing, vision, smell, and taste. Finally, **visceral sensory axons** convey information from receptors distributed in smooth muscle, cardiac muscle, branchially derived muscle, and glands. With regard to the motor functions, there are somatic motor, branchial motor, and visceral motor axons. **Somatic motor axons** innervate striated muscles that are derived embryologically from somites (as are the striated muscles of the body). **Branchial motor axons** also innervate striated muscle, but in this case the muscles are derived embryologically from the branchial (pharyngeal) arches that are unique to the head and neck. Thus, they innervate muscles of mastication, facial expression, middle ear, pharynx, larynx, sternocleidomastoid, and the upper portion of the trapezius. **Visceral motor axons** supply smooth muscle and glands, just as they do in spinal nerves. Three of the cranial nerves are wholly sensory, five are wholly motor, and four are mixed. They are numbered from CN I to XII, based on the position of their nerve roots from anterior to posterior, beginning most rostrally.

OVERVIEW OF THE CRANIAL NERVES

Clinical Preview

Dr. Murphey is a physical therapist who works in the school system and annually runs a well-child screening clinic. Children are screened for height, weight, vital signs, fine and gross motor skill development, deep tendon reflexes, and assessment of cranial nerve function. As you read through this chapter, consider the following:

- What functions will Dr. Murphey learn about with each cranial nerve test?
- Why might it be important to assess cranial nerves in young children?

Similar to what we learned with respect to the spinal cord, cranial nerve sensory fibers synapse in cranial nerve sensory nuclei, while cranial nerve motor fibers are the axons of cell bodies residing in cranial nerve motor nuclei. Cranial nerve nuclei are distributed in the tegmentum of the three subdivisions of the brainstem, with two notable

exceptions: the olfactory (I) and optic (II) cranial nerves synapse on neurons of sensory tracts in the CNS that are not located in the brainstem.

This chapter's consideration of cranial nerves does not follow their numerical order. The reason for this is that three of the cranial nerves—the oculomotor (III), trochlear (IV), and abducens (VI)—have in common their innervation of striated muscles of the eye and control of the position of the eyeball in the orbit. In the neurological examination, these nerves are tested as a group; similarly they are presented together in this chapter. Also, not all of the nerves are discussed in similar detail. Three of the cranial nerves—the optic (II), trigeminal (V), and vestibulocochlear (VIII)—represent the origins of sensory systems whose connections have widespread distributions in the CNS and subserve unique and clinically important functions. They are introduced here but each has a separate chapter devoted to its distribution and function (Chapters 14, 17, and 18).

Two summary tables are provided. Table 13-1 ■ provides a comprehensive summary of all 12 cranial nerves. This table includes the functional components of each nerve, the location of the nerve's cell bodies, the cranial exit of the nerve, and its primary function. Table 13-4, at the end of the chapter, summarizes some of the important tests of the cranial nerves.

Thought Question

What is the difference between general sensory and special sensory nerves?

Thought Question

What are the origins of the terms *branchial motor* and *somatic motor* nerves? What differentiates the muscles that are innervated by each? Which are the *specific muscles* innervated by the branchial motor nerves?

Table 13-1 Summary of Cranial Nerves

NERVE	FUNCTIONAL COMPONENTS	LOCATION OF NEURONAL CELL BODIES	CRANIAL EXIT OR ENTRY	MAIN FUNCTION
Olfactory (I)	Special sensory	Olfactory epithelium	Foramina in cribriform plate of ethmoid bone	Smell from nasal mucosa of each nasal cavity
Optic (II)	Special sensory	Retina (ganglion neurons)	None*	Vision
Oculomotor (III)	Somatic motor	Midbrain	Superior orbital fissure	Motor to superior, inferior, and medial rectus, inferior oblique, and levator palpebrae superioris muscles
	Visceral motor	Presynaptic: midbrain; postsynaptic: ciliary ganglion		Parasympathetic innervation to sphincter pupillae and ciliary muscle; constricts pupil and accommodates lens of the eye
Trochlear (IV)	Somatic motor	Midbrain	Superior orbital fissure	Motor to superior oblique muscle
Trigeminal (V)	General sensory	Trigeminal ganglion	Superior orbital fissure	Sensation from cornea, skin of forehead, scalp eyelids, nose and mucosa of nasal cavity and paranasal sinuses; dura mater of anterior and middle cranial fossae
Ophthalmic division (V₁)	General sensory	Trigeminal ganglion	Foramen rotundum	Sensation from the skin of face over maxilla, including upper lip, maxillary teeth, mucosa of nose, maxillary sinuses, and palate; dura mater of anterior and middle cranial fossae
Maxillary division (V₂)	General sensory	Trigeminal ganglion	Foramen ovale	Sensation from the skin over mandible, including lower lip and side of head, mandibular teeth, temporomandibular joint, and mucosa of mouth and anterior two-thirds of tongue; dura mater of anterior and middle cranial fossae
Mandibular division (V₃)	Branchial motor	Pons	Foramen ovale	Motor to muscles of mastication, mylohyoid, anterior belly of digastric, tensor veli palatini, and tensor tympani
Abducens (VI)	Somatic motor	Pons	Superior orbital fissure	Motor to lateral rectus
Facial (VII)	Branchial motor	Pons	Internal acoustic meatus, facial canal, and stylomastoid foramen	Motor to muscles of facial expression and scalp, stapedius of middle ear, stylohyoid, and posterior belly of digastric
	General sensory	Geniculate ganglion		Sensation from skin of external auditory meatus
	Special sensory	Geniculate ganglion		Taste from anterior two-thirds of tongue
	Visceral motor	Presynaptic: pons; postsynaptic: pterygopalatine ganglion and submandibular ganglion		Parasympathetic innervation to submandibular and sublingual salivary glands, lacrimal gland, and glands of nose and palate

NERVE	FUNCTIONAL COMPONENTS	LOCATION OF NEURONAL CELL BODIES	CRANIAL EXIT OR ENTRY	MAIN FUNCTION
Vestibulocochlear (VIII) Vestibular	Special sensory	Vestibular ganglion	Internal acoustic meatus	Equilibrium from semicircular canals, utricle, and saccule related to position and movement of the head
Cochlear	Special sensory	Spiral ganglion		Hearing from organ of Corti
Glossopharyngeal (IX)	Branchial motor	Medulla	Jugular foramen	Motor to stylopharyngeus to assist swallowing
	Visceral motor	Presynaptic: medulla; postsynaptic: otic ganglion		Parasympathetic innervation of parotid gland
	General sensory	Inferior ganglion		Skin of external ear, somatosensory from posterior third of tongue
	Special sensory	Inferior ganglion		Taste from posterior third of tongue
	Visceral sensory	Superior ganglion		Visceral sensation from parotid gland, carotid body and sinus, pharynx, and middle ear
Vagus (X)	Branchial motor	Medulla	Jugular foramen	Motor to constrictor muscles of pharynx, intrinsic muscles of larynx, muscles of the palate, and upper esophagus
	Visceral motor	Presynaptic: medulla; postsynaptic: neurons in, on, or near viscera		Parasympathetic innervation to smooth muscle of trachea, bronchi, digestive tract, and cardiac muscle
	General sensory	Superior ganglion	Jugular foramen	Sensation from auricle, external auditory meatus, and dura mater of posterior cranial fossa
	Special sensory	Inferior ganglion		Taste from epiglottis and palate
	Visceral sensory	Superior ganglion		Visceral sensation from base of tongue, pharynx, larynx, trachea, bronchi, heart, esophagus, stomach, and intestine
Accessory (XI) Cranial root	Branchial motor	Medulla	Jugular foramen	Motor to striated muscles of soft palate, pharynx and larynx
Spinal root	Branchial motor	Spinal cord		Motor to sternocleidomastoid and trapezius muscles
Hypoglossal (XII)	Somatic motor	Medulla	Hypoglossal canal	Motor to intrinsic and extrinsic muscles of tongue

*The optic tract is composed of retinal ganglion cell axons, is a tract of the CNS, and exits the orbit in the optic canal

OLFACTORY NERVE (I)

The olfactory nerve is a special sensory nerve. It is unique in several respects. First, this nerve is the peripheral component of the only sensory system that does not first synapse in the thalamus before reaching the cerebral cortex. Second, this nerve (and one other, CN II) does not attach to the brainstem and does not have a dorsal root ganglion equivalent.

Axons of primary olfactory neurons comprise the olfactory nerve. These axons arise from bipolar neurons located in the olfactory epithelium, situated primarily in the roof of the nasal cavity (Figure 13-1 ■). Olfactory receptors are located on the terminals of the peripheral processes of these bipolar neurons. The olfactory epithelium is kept moist by secretions of the olfactory gland that provides the medium through which inhaled aromatic molecules (scents or odorants) are dissolved. These odorants bind to the surface of cilia projecting from the nerve terminal, which activates the transduction process.

The central processes of the bipolar olfactory neurons pass through tiny foramina in the cribriform plate of the ethmoid bone and synapse on mitral cells of the **olfactory bulb** that lies in contact with the orbital surface of the frontal bone. During development, the olfactory bulb forms as an outgrowth of the telencephalon, traveling directly to the cerebral hemisphere without relaying first in the thalamus, as noted earlier. In addition, the olfactory bulb contains the cell bodies of secondary sensory neurons that conduct olfactory sensations to other places in the brain. Axons from neurons of the olfactory bulb form the **olfactory tract**, which is a tract of the CNS. Sometimes the olfactory bulb and tract are considered to represent the olfactory "nerve."

Most of the axons of the olfactory tract synapse in the **primary olfactory cortex** and in the adjacent amygdala (Figure 13-2 ■). The primary olfactory cortex consists of the pyriform area in the anterior part of the medial temporal lobe, the cerebral cortex overlying the amygdala (periamygdaloid cortex), and a restricted area of the anterior parahippocampal gyrus (also called the **entorhinal area**). Olfaction thus differs from other exteroceptive sensory modalities (somatosensory, visual, auditory) that only reach cerebral cortex after first traversing a thalamic nucleus. Smaller contingents of olfactory tract axons terminate in the medial surface of the frontal lobe beneath the corpus callosum and in the posterior orbital surface of the frontal lobe extending onto the anterior insula. Axons issuing from neurons in these sites of termination project either directly or indirectly to the hypothalamus, to other limbic structures such as the hippocampus and rest of the amygdala, and to the thalamus (**dorsomedial nucleus**). From the hypothalamus, projections are sent to nuclei of the cranial component of the parasympathetic nervous system, to the **superior** and **inferior salivatory nuclei** responsible for salivation in response to pleasant cooking odors, and to the dorsal motor nucleus of the vagus responsible for nausea in response to unpleasant odors as well as increased peristalsis of the gastrointestinal tract and increased gastric secretion.

> **Thought Question**
>
> The olfactory nerve differs from most other nerves in several important ways. What are these differences?

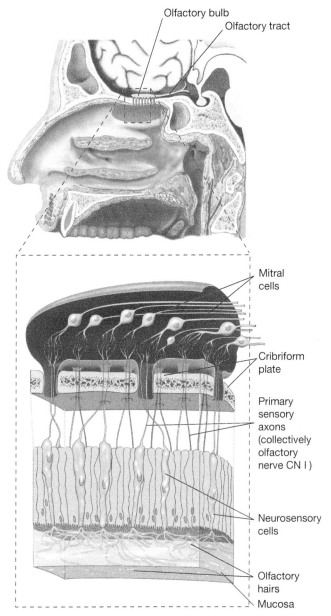

FIGURE 13-1 Primary olfactory neurons comprising the olfactory nerve pass through the cribriform plate and synapse upon mitral cells of the olfactory bulb.

Olfactory bulb
Olfactory tract

Mitral cells

Cribriform plate

Primary sensory axons (collectively olfactory nerve CN I)

Neurosensory cells

Olfactory hairs

Mucosa

CLINICAL CONNECTIONS

Clinical Evaluation of the Olfactory Nerve

Because olfactory loss may be unilateral, each nostril must be tested separately. Odoriferous substances, such as wintergreen and camphor, are used when testing olfactory sensation. With

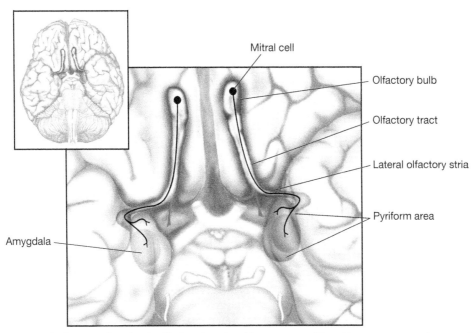

FIGURE 13-2 The olfactory bulbs contain mitral cells forming the olfactory tract. The olfactory tract projects to the amygdala and primary olfactory cortex, the pyriform area of the medial temporal lobe.

the person's eyes closed, the substance is placed near one nostril while the examiner closes the other nostril. The person is asked first to state whether he or she perceives an odor, and, if so, to identify it. Even though the individual may not be able to identify the odor, the ability to appreciate its presence is sufficient to rule out **anosmia** (inability to smell).

Olfaction, Emotion, and Memory

It is a common experience that an aroma can restore long-forgotten memories or elicit an emotional response. The idea is not new that olfaction may play a role in emotional experience and memory. In the early part of the 20th century, for example, it was suggested that olfaction, unlike other exteroceptive senses, may serve to link together anticipation and consumption into a single experience and thereby provide a "germ" for memory. The connections of the olfactory apparatus with medial temporal lobe limbic structures (such as the amygdala) and the medial temporal lobe memory system (see Chapter 22) strongly support roles for olfaction in emotion and in some types of memory.

Olfaction also is important for enjoyment of food. A progressive loss of neurosensory olfactory cells in the olfactory epithelium occurs with aging. Because the flavor of food depends on a normal olfactory system (to which everyone with a severe head cold can attest), a common complaint of older adults is that their food is tasteless.

Anosmia

The most frequent temporary cause of anosmia is the common cold, in which the mucus that filters the odorants is changed. Anosmia also may occur from a blow to the head that tears the delicate primary olfactory afferents as they pass through the foramina of the cribriform plate. Fractures of the base of the cranium may cause anosmia by tearing fibers of the olfactory tract. Compression of the olfactory bulb and/or tract resulting in anosmia may occur with a meningioma in the floor of the anterior cranial fossa or with masses (tumors or abscesses) of the frontal lobe. A significant proportion of people with degenerative diseases of the brain, such as Alzheimer's disease, Parkinson's disease, and Huntington's disease, exhibit anosmia or hyposmia. The reason is unclear.

OPTIC NERVE (II)

The optic nerve is a special sensory nerve that mediates vision and is discussed in detail in Chapter 18. Coverage there also details its clinical evaluation and disorders. The axons of ganglion cells in the retina project from the eyeball to the brain in the **optic tract**, where most synapse in the thalamus. The part of the optic tract that runs from the eyeball to the optic chiasm is called the **optic nerve**, even though it is a component of the CNS and not a peripheral nerve. As such, the optic nerve is subject to the same diseases (e.g., multiple sclerosis) and pathological processes (e.g., elevated intracranial pressure) that affect the CNS.

Thought Question

Is the optic nerve more similar to the olfactory nerve or to CNs III, IV, and VI? Explain your answer.

CRANIAL NERVES INNERVATING THE EXTRAOCULAR MUSCLES

Three cranial nerves participate in innervating the six extraocular muscles that control movements of the eyes. This innervation comprises the somatic motor component of each nerve. These three cranial nerves are the *oculomotor (III)*, *trochlear (IV)*, and *abducens (VI)*. The trochlear and abducens nerves consist exclusively of somatic motor fibers, while the oculomotor nerve contains, in addition, a visceral motor component consisting of the parasympathetic supply to the to the ciliary and pupillary constrictor muscles (see Chapter 12).

The somatic motor component of these three nerves innervates the six extraocular muscles in each eye that control the position of the eye in its orbit. We shall consider them as a group for a number of reasons. First, in order to change visual fixation or to maintain visual fixation on an object that is moving through space, the eyes must move with exceptional precision, and both must move together to precisely the same degree (referred to as conjugate movements). Thus, there must be exquisite coordination of the contractions of individual muscles in each eye as well as coordination of the action between the sets of muscle in each orbit. In principle, any given direction of eye movement could be specified by independently adjusting the activity of individual eye muscles, but this would be an extraordinarily complex task. Instead, coordinated conjugate movements of the eyes are generated by two centers located in the brainstem reticular formation, referred to as **gaze centers**. These two gaze centers regulate the activity of LMNs in the nuclei of cranial nerves III, IV, and VI in particular combinations or as an entire group, depending on the direction of eye movement needed. Gaze centers are discussed in Chapter 14. Second, the intracranial courses of the three nerves after they exit from and attain the ventral surface of the brainstem are long and virtually identical. Therefore, they are often affected by pathological processes as a group or in combination. Finally, a single clinical protocol is used to assess eye movements, and it applies to all three of the nerves. Table 13-2 ■ summarizes the terminology used to describe movements of one eye.

Because the actions of the extraocular muscles in the two eyes function in concert and because individual muscles in a single eye do not typically contract in isolation, the movements produced by the muscles innervated by a single cranial nerve are not presented with that nerve. Rather, the cardinal positions of the right and left eyes and the actions of the muscles primarily responsible for these movements of the eyes are illustrated in Figure 13-7, after the individual cranial nerves have been presented.

Oculomotor Nerve (III)

The axons of the somatic motor component of the oculomotor nerve originate from cells of the oculomotor nuclear complex situated in the midbrain, near the

Table 13-2 Monocular Ocular Movement Terminology

EYE MOVEMENT	TERM
Medial	Adduction
Lateral	Abduction
Up	Elevation, supraduction
Down	Depression, infraduction
Rotation of 12 o'clock position medially	Intorsion
Rotation of 12 o'clock position laterally	Extorsion
Anterior out of orbit	Protrusion or exophthalmos
Posterior into orbit	Retraction or enophthalmos

midline (Figure 13-3 ■). The axons exit from the brainstem in the interpeduncular fossa at the junction of the midbrain and pons to form the oculomotor nerve. The nerve passes between or though a number of structures whose pathology may damage axons of the nerve (see Clinical Connections). The nerve passes between the posterior cerebral and superior cerebellar arteries, pierces the dura, and enters the cavernous sinus. The nerve continues anteriorly through the superior orbital fissure and enters the orbit.

The oculomotor nerve innervates four of the six extraocular muscles that move the eyeball. The nerve on each side supplies the inferior rectus, inferior oblique, and medial and superior rectus muscles. Additionally, the oculomotor nerves innervate the levator palpebrae superioris.

The anatomy of the parasympathetic visceral motor component of the oculomotor nerve was presented in Chapter 12. The axons arise from cells of the **Edinger-Westphal nucleus** of the oculomotor complex (see Figure 13-3). In innervating smooth muscle of the pupillary sphincter and ciliary body, the postganglionic fibers control the size of the pupil and shape of the lens, respectively. This innervation functions in mediating the pupillary light reflex and accommodation reflex, both presented in Chapter 18.

Thought Question

What is the function of the axons that originate in the Edinger-Westphal nucleus?

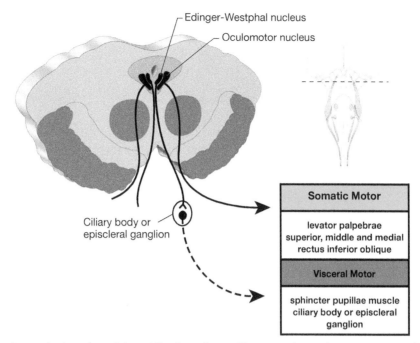

FIGURE 13-3 A cross section at the junction of the midbrain and pons illustrates the oculomotor nerve as it exits the brainstem. The oculomotor nerve has both somatic motor and parasympathetic visceral motor components. Somatic motor fibers leave the oculomotor nucleus to innervate extraocular muscles directly. The visceral motor fibers leave the Edinger-Westphal nucleus and synapse upon neurons of the ciliary body, whose neurons in turn control the size of the pupil and shape of the lens.

Trochlear Nerve (IV)

The trochlear nerve innervates a single extraocular muscle, the superior oblique. Its axons arise from the trochlear nucleus situated in the midbrain tegmentum near the midline (Figure 13-4 ■). Before exiting the midbrain, the axons of each side cross so that each superior oblique muscle is innervated by the *contralateral* trochlear nucleus. The trochlear nerve is the only cranial nerve to exit on the dorsal surface of the brainstem. After exiting the midbrain, the nerve decussates immediately, travels ventrally and rostrally to wrap around the cerebral peduncle, and passes between the posterior cerebral and superior cerebellar arteries along with the CN III. Like CN III, the trochlear nerve pierces the dura, enters the cavernous sinus, and exits via the superior orbital fissure into the bony orbit.

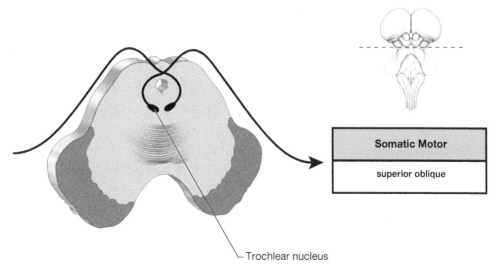

FIGURE 13-4 The trochlear nerve containing somatic motor fibers exits the brainstem at the level of the midbrain to innervate the superior oblique muscle. The trochlear nerve is unique in two ways: it is the only cranial nerve to exit the dorsal brainstem, and its fibers innervate the contralateral muscle.

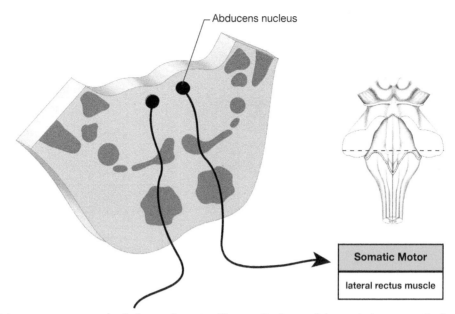

FIGURE 13-5 The abducens nerve, comprised of somatic motor fibers, exits the caudal pons to innervate the lateral rectus muscle.

Abducens Nerve (VI)

Like the trochlear nerve, the abducens nerve innervates just a single extraocular muscle, the lateral rectus muscle. The abducens nucleus is located in the dorsal tegmentum of caudal pons, near the midline (Figure 13-5 ■). The axons that form the nerve emerge from the ventral surface of the brainstem at the junction of the pons and medulla, relatively near the midline. The nerve runs anteriorly in the subarachnoid space of the posterior cranial fossa and pierces the dura that is lateral to the dorsum sella of the sphenoid bone (Figure 13-6 ■). At the approximate apex of the petrous portion of the temporal bone, the nerve runs dorsally, then makes a sharp bend over the ridge of the bone. It enters the cavernous sinus, where it

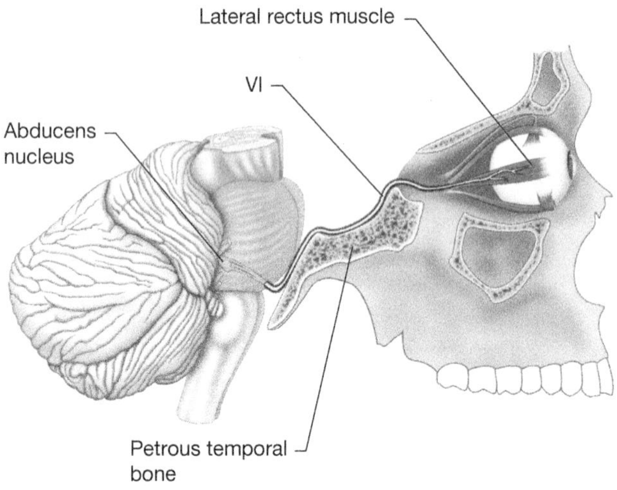

FIGURE 13-6 The abducens nerve leaves the caudal pons and runs anteriorly to innervate the lateral rectus muscle.

is lateral to the internal carotid artery and medial to III, IV, and two branches of the trigeminal nerve. The nerve enters the orbit via the superior orbital fissure and terminates in the ipsilateral lateral rectus muscle.

Combined Actions of Cranial Nerves III, IV, and VI

The primary and secondary actions of the six extraocular muscles and their innervations are summarized in Table 13-3 ■. Figure 13-7 ■ presents the cardinal positions of the right and left eyes and the actions of the oblique and rectus muscles primarily responsible for their movements.

Thought Question

CNs III, IV, and VI work together to control eye movement. What is the function of each of these three nerves? Which nerve innervates the most muscles? And what would be the consequence of loss of each of these nerves (either separately or together)?

CLINICAL CONNECTIONS

Clinical Evaluation of Eye Movement

The actions of the extraocular muscles are outlined in Table 13-3 and form the basis for the neurological examination of the integrity of cranial nerves III, IV, and VI. The medial rectus of one eye and the lateral rectus of

Table 13-3 **Functions and Innervations of the Extraocular Muscles**

MUSCLE	INNERVATION	PRIMARY ACTION	SECONDARY ACTION
Lateral rectus	Abducens (VI)	Abduction	None
Medial rectus	Oculomotor (III)	Adduction	None
Superior rectus	Oculomotor (III)	Elevation	Adduction, intorsion
Inferior rectus	Oculomotor (III)	Depression	Adduction, extorsion
Superior oblique	Trochlear (IV)	Intorsion	Depression, abduction
Inferior oblique	Oculomotor (III)	Extorsion	Elevation, abduction

the other function as a pair to produce lateral eye movements (Figure 13-8 ■). Thus, the individual is first asked to look to one side, then the other. The function of individual muscles is tested most easily when they are acting with maximal effectiveness. For example, the vertically acting recti muscles are most effective when the eye is *abducted* because then the line of pull of the muscles is along the vertical axis of the eye, with the superior rectus elevating the eye and the inferior rectus depressing

it. The oblique muscles are maximally effective when the eye is *adducted* because then the line of pull of the obliques is along the vertical axis of the eye, with the superior oblique rotating the eye downward and the inferior oblique rotating it upward. Thus, while looking to one side, the person is asked to rotate the eyes up and down. Then, the person is asked to look to the opposite side, and the procedure is repeated, testing the opposite pair of muscles.

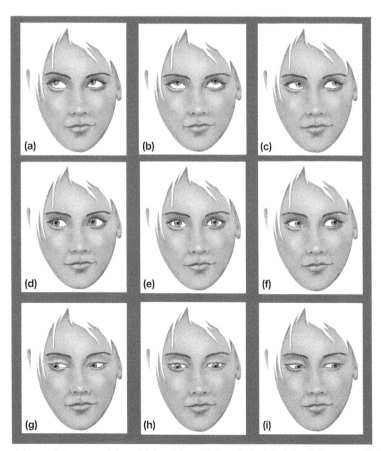

FIGURE 13-7 The cardinal positions of the eyes: (a) up/right; (b) up; (c) up/left; (d) right; (e) center; (f) left; (g) down/right; (h) down; (i) down/left.

A paralysis of one or more of the extraocular muscles is termed **ophthalmoplegia**. An inability to direct both eyes to the same object so that the visual axes of the two eyes are misaligned is termed **strabismus**. Strabismus results in **diplopia**, or double vision.

Disorders of Eye Movements

A number of disorders of eye movement occur, each depending on the nerve or combination of nerves affected. The single symptom that indicates damage to cranial nerve III, IV, or VI is diplopia. Diplopia occurs only with binocular vision. In normal binocular vision, the eyes are positioned such that the fixated image falls on exactly the same spot on the retina of each eye (i.e., the macula of each eye). Even the slightest displacement of either eye causes diplopia because the image shifts to a different spot on the retina of the displaced eye.

The collection of signs observed following damage to CN III (oculomotor ophthalmoplegia) is illustrated in Figure 13-9 ■ . **Lateral strabismus** is due to paralysis of CN III because of the unopposed action of the lateral rectus innervated by CN VI. **Ptosis** is due to weakness or paralysis of the levator palpebrae superioris muscle. The individual attempts to compensate for the drooping upper eyelid by contracting the frontalis muscle so that the forehead is

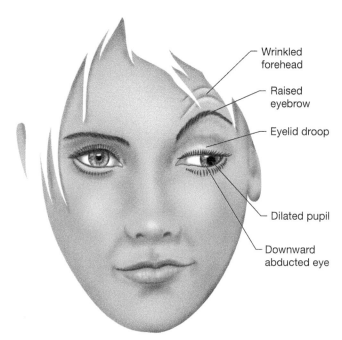

FIGURE 13-9 Oculomotor ophthalmoplegia following damage to CN III results in eyelid droop (ptosis), dilated pupil, and a downward abducted eye position (lateral strabismus).

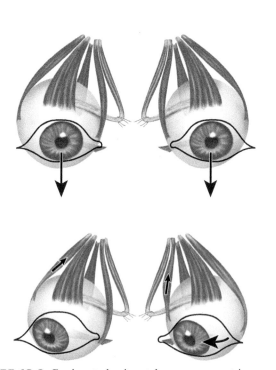

FIGURE 13-8 Conjugate horizontal eye movement is produced by the medial rectus of one eye and the lateral rectus of the other eye. Here, the horizontal movement of both eyes to the right is produced by activation of the left medial rectus and right lateral rectus. There is concurrent inhibition of the antagonistic muscles (in this case, right lateral rectus and left medial rectus).

wrinkled. Diplopia occurs only when the ptosed eyelid is held up. When the upper eyelid is lifted, the lateral deviation of the eye is apparent. The pupil will be dilated due to a loss of tone in the pupillary sphincter muscle. Recall that CN III has both a somatic and autonomic component. It is the parasympathetic loss that causes the unopposed sympathetic action to dilate the pupil; hence, no pupillary light reflex can be elicited in the affected eye. There is a paralysis of accommodation.

Paralysis of the superior oblique muscle with the eye in the primary position (looking straight ahead) results in outward rotation (**extortion**) of the affected eye attributed to the unopposed action of the inferior oblique muscle (trochlear ophthalmoplegia) (Figure 13-10 ■). Because the superior oblique muscle helps to move the eye downward and laterally, the person's chief complaint is diplopia with attempted movement in these directions, as in reading or descending a flight of stairs. Head tilt in a neurologically intact person results in the eyes reflexively rotating in the opposite direction in order to maintain a vertical image on the retina (see Chapter 17). People with trochlear nerve palsies compensate for the paralyzed superior oblique muscle by tilting their heads to the unaffected side. This causes the normal eye to intort so as to line up its visual axis with that of the extorted, affected eye, thereby restoring binocular vision.

Lesions of the abducens nerve (abducens ophthalmoplegia) result in weakness or paralysis of the lateral rectus muscle on the ipsilateral side. This causes an inability to abduct the affected eye beyond midline of gaze. The affected eye is pulled medially by the unopposed

NORMAL

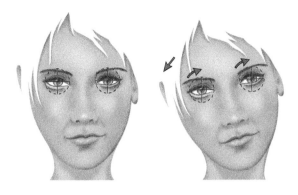

LEFT SUPERIOR OBLIQUE PARALYSIS

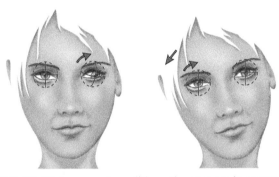

FIGURE 13-10 In normal conditions, the eyes are in center position, and when the head tilts, the eyes reflexively rotate in the opposite direction in order to maintain a vertical image on the retina. This maintains binocular vision. With left superior oblique paralysis, following damage to CN IV, the left eye is deviated up and left. This is also referred to as trochlear ophthalmoplegia. The person compensates by tilting his or her head to the unaffected side to restore binocular vision.

action of the medial rectus muscle. This is referred to as **medial strabismus**. The individual complains of diplopia, just as occurs with lateral strabismus. Binocular vision can be restored by rotating the head so that the affected eye is brought into line with the object of fixation (Figure 13-11 ■).

> **Thought Question**
>
> Explain how ophthalmoplegia, strabismus, and diplopia are related, and give an example that would result in these three conditions.

Lesions of Cranial Nerves III, IV, and VI

Pathological processes that affect the meninges lining the base of the skull can involve all three nerves. The meningeal inflammation can be from bacterial meningitis or other viral inflammations and from meningiomas. Dilation of the upper basilar artery by an aneurysm may result in multiple nerve palsies, especially bilateral oculomotor nerve lesions.

The oculomotor nerve may also be compressed in several other ways. An aneurysm of the posterior communicating artery may directly compress the nerve, as can trauma. Space-occupying processes such as tumor, abscess, or extradural hematoma affecting the temporal lobe may cause its undersurface to herniate through the tentorial incisure, displacing the cerebral peduncle to the opposite side and compressing the oculomotor nerve against the petrous part of the temporal bone.

A severe rise in intracranial pressure may result in the supratentorial parts of the brain trying to squeeze

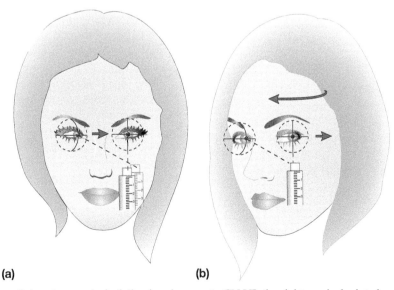

(a)   (b)

FIGURE 13-11 With right medial rectus paralysis, following damage to CN VI, the right eye is deviated medially. This is also referred to as abducens ophthalmoplegia. This results in diplopia. The person compensates by rotating his or her head so the affected eye is brought into line with the object of fixation. This restores binocular vision.

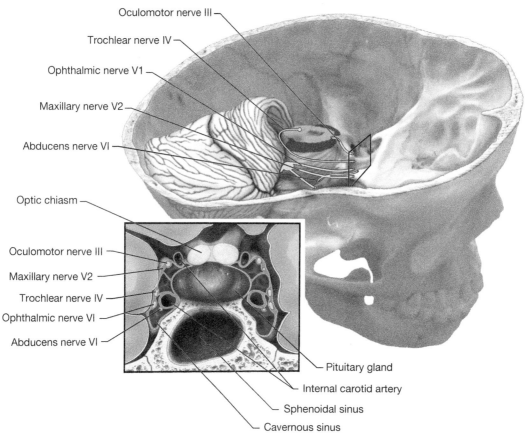

FIGURE 13-12 Relationship between temporal bone and cranial nerves III, IV, V, and VI. These nerves may be damaged as they course along bone through the cavernous sinus. Also note the relationship of the pituitary gland to the cranial nerves. In the event of pituitary tumor, these cranial nerves may be damaged.

through the tentorial incisure. This pushes the brainstem downward and stretches the abducens nerve as it angles over the ridge of petrous portion of the temporal bone (see Figure 13-6). Potentially, all three nerves may be involved as they course through the cavernous sinus (Figure 13-12 ■).

Infections of the skin of the upper face or in the paranasal sinuses may spread to the cavernous sinus, resulting in thrombosis in the sinus. Tumors may invade the sinus, compressing one or more of the nerves. Dilation of the intracavernous portion of the internal carotid artery by an aneurysm may compress one or more of the nerves. Aneurysms in a number of other nearby vessels may also compress one or more of these nerves.

Thought Question

A rise in intracranial pressure could cause a lesion to one of the cranial nerves that controls eye movement. Which nerve can be affected, and why?

TRIGEMINAL NERVE (V)

The trigeminal nerve is the largest sensory nerve innervating the head (general sensory fibers) and contains, in addition, a small motor branch that innervates the muscles derived from the first branchial arch (the branchial motor component innervating, in particular, the muscles of mastication). Accordingly, the sensory nucleus of the trigeminal nerve is the largest of the cranial nerve nuclei extending caudally as a continuous cell column from the level of the midbrain into the spinal cord as far as the second cervical segment. The sensory nucleus is subdivided into three subnuclei (Figure 13-13 ■). These three subnuclei are the **mesencephalic nucleus**, the **main sensory nucleus**, and the **spinal trigeminal nucleus**, all of which are discussed in more detail in Chapter 14. The **motor nucleus of the trigeminal** is located in mid-pons at the level at which the trigeminal nerve attaches to the brainstem (Figure 13-14 ■) and is composed of lower motor neurons. Axons of these LMNs join the mandibular division of the nerve. They innervate the following striated muscles: the muscles of mastication (temporalis, masseter, pterygoid), tensor tympani, tensor veli palatini,

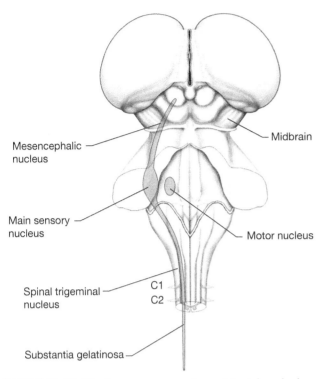

mylohyoid, and anterior belly of the digastric. The trigeminal nerve attaches to the brainstem in the ventrolateral aspect of the mid-pons.

CLINICAL CONNECTIONS

Clinical Evaluation of the Trigeminal Nerve

An early sign of trigeminal nerve damage could be an impaired or absent **corneal reflex**. The corneal reflex is tested in the clinical examination by having the person look to one side while the cornea is lightly touched with a wisp of cotton that has been drawn into a point (Figure 13-15 ■). The normal response to this stimulus is an immediate partial or complete closure of both eyelids. The input side (afferent

FIGURE 13-13 The large sensory nucleus of the trigeminal nerve spans the brainstem and upper cervical spinal cord. It is comprised of three subnuclei: the mesencephalic nucleus, the main sensory nucleus, and spinal trigeminal nucleus. The trigeminal nerve has a single, more medially located, motor nucleus.

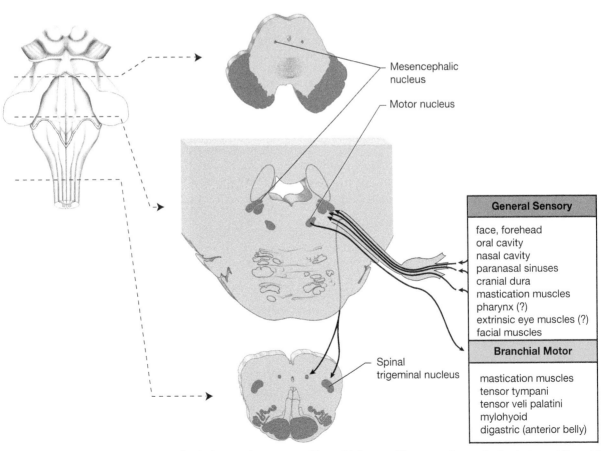

FIGURE 13-14 The trigeminal nerve, comprised of general sensory and branchial motor fibers, attaches to the brainstem at the mid-pons.

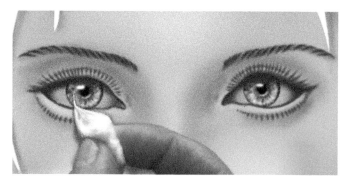

FIGURE 13-15 The corneal reflex is tested by lightly touching a wisp of cotton to the cornea.

limb) of this reflex arc is the ophthalmic division of V and the output side (the efferent limb) is the facial nerve (VII).

The same battery of sensory tests outlined for the DC-ML and STT tracts in Chapter 9 is applied to orofacial structures. The motor component of the trigeminal nerve also is examined. Specifically, the motor component is tested by having the person clamp his or her jaws together while the examiner palpates the temporal and masseter muscles and then attempts to separate the jaws by downward pressure with the thumb on the bony ledge of the individual's chin. Jaw opening is tested by placing a finger or fist under the person's chin and asking him or her to open the mouth against moderate resistance. The mouth must be allowed to open slowly. In unilateral weakness of the pterygoid muscle, the jaw deviates toward the side of the weakened muscle as it is opened slowly.

Lesions of the Trigeminal Nerve

Tumors in the middle fossa of the cranium and in the cerebellopontine angle may affect one or more divisions of the trigeminal nerve. A consistent early physical sign of cerebellopontine angle tumors is depression or loss of the corneal reflex on the same side.

Trigeminal neuralgia (*tic douloureux*) is the most frequent disorder affecting CN V. There are no demonstrable sensory or motor deficits in trigeminal neuralgia. Rather, the disorder is characterized by brief paroxysms of excruciating pain (usually lasting only seconds) localized to the peripheral area of one, occasionally more, of the three branches of the trigeminal nerve—most typically, the mandibular or maxillary divisions. The ophthalmic division is involved in only a small percentage of cases. The entire peripheral territory of a division is not involved. In most people, the paroxysms of pain occur in one of two zones. Attacks, varying in frequency from one every few minutes to one or two per day, are usually spontaneous, although even a light breeze can trigger them. Other stimuli also can be triggers. Examples include use of the jaw in chewing, smiling, or yawning; hot or cold fluids in the mouth; blowing the nose; or brushing the teeth. Not surprisingly, people with trigeminal neuralgia may be distraught because of the pain and have an unkempt appearance because of the

triggers associated with washing, applying makeup, shaving, or brushing the teeth.

Herpes zoster ophthalmicus accounts for 10 to 15 percent of all cases of herpes zoster and is the most common of the inflammatory and infectious diseases to affect the trigeminal nerve. The pathologic changes caused by the virus are in the semilunar ganglion. The usual history is that the person experiences two or three days of severe pain in the forehead, after which the rash erupts. At its height, the rash may cover the entire distribution of V_1. Permanent damage to the cornea can result from the herpetiform infection.

FACIAL NERVE (VII)

The facial nerve is the first nerve we have encountered that contains four functional components: general sensory afferent, special sensory afferent, branchial motor, and parasympathetic motor. These fibers synapse in a variety of nuclei as follows: pain, temperature, and crude touch of the face synapse in the spinal trigeminal nucleus; proprioception from muscles of mastication synapse in the mesencephalic nucleus; and fine touch and discriminative touch sensations of face synapse in the pontine nucleus. The special sensory afferents innervate taste buds in the anterior two-thirds of the tongue. The latter set of axons is bound in its own fascial sheath separate from that of other components of the facial nerve and is called the intermediate nerve, even though it is a component of the facial nerve. The special sensory afferents of the intermediate nerve synapse in the rostral portion of the **nucleus solitarius (nucleus of the tractus solitarius)**, called the gustatory division of the nucleus that is located in rostral medulla-caudal pons.

The branchial motor fibers are the largest contingent of axons in the nerve, innervating the voluntary muscles of facial expression. These motor fibers arise from the facial nucleus situated in caudal pons (Figure 13-16 ■). Additionally, the branchial motor fibers innervate the stapedius muscle of the middle ear. Contraction of the stapedius muscle stiffens the chain of middle ear ossicles so that less low-frequency sound energy is transferred along the ossicular chain. When loud sounds enter one ear, both stapedius muscles reflexively contract, reducing the effects of low-frequency noise.

Thought Question

Is the facial nerve a sensory nerve, a motor nerve, or both? Can you give examples of its main roles?

The remaining axons in the facial nerve are visceral motor, innervating the lacrimal, submandibular, and sublingual salivary glands. The parasympathetic visceral motor component (discussed in Chapter 12) arises from cell bodies in the superior salivatory nucleus, a scattered group of nuclei in the tegmentum of the pons (see Figure 13-16).

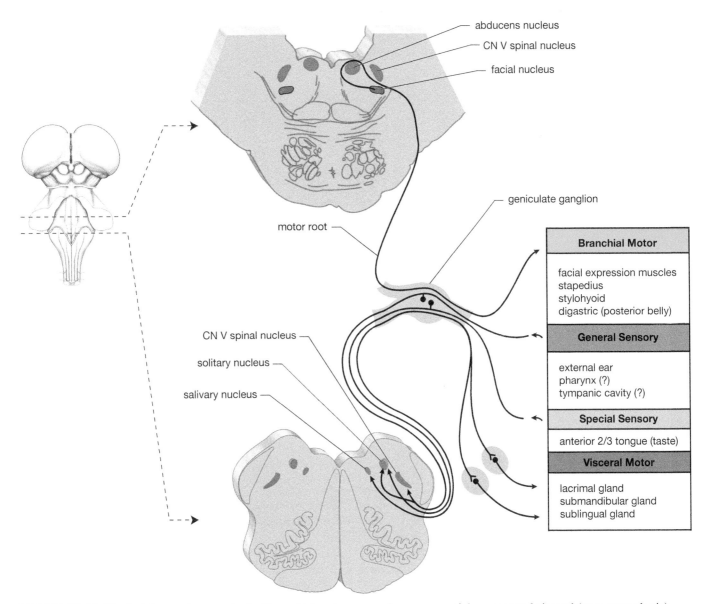

FIGURE 13-16 The facial nerve is comprised of branchial motor, general sensory, special sensory, and visceral (parasympathetic) motor fibers. Branchial motor fibers leave the facial nucleus to innervate muscles directly.

The facial nerve emerges from the ventrolateral surface of the brainstem at the caudal border of the pons (i.e., it emerges from the inferior pontine sulcus). It enters the internal auditory meatus, along with CN VIII, located in the petrous portion of the temporal bone. The internal auditory meatus leads into a canal, the facial canal (Figure 13-17 ■). Within the facial canal is the geniculate ganglion, a swelling in the nerve containing the cell bodies of the special sensory afferents carrying taste impulses from the anterior two-thirds of the tongue and general sensory afferents supplying portions of the skin of the external ear. Still within the canal, the facial nerve gives rise to the greater petrosal nerve that is parasympathetic and projects to the pterygopalatine ganglion. A branch containing branchial motor neurons is given off to innervate the stapedius muscle. The nerve then gives rise to the chorda tympani nerve that carries taste sensation from

the tongue and parasympathetic motor fibers out to the submandibular ganglion. The facial nerve exits from the skull via the stylomastoid foramen, the termination of the facial canal. The nerve passes through the parotid gland, within which it divides into branches that innervate the muscles of facial expression.

CLINICAL CONNECTIONS
Clinical Evaluation of the Facial Nerve

Only two of the functional components of the facial nerve are tested in the neurological evaluation. These are the special sensory afferent carrying taste from the tongue and the brachial motor innervating the muscles of facial expression.

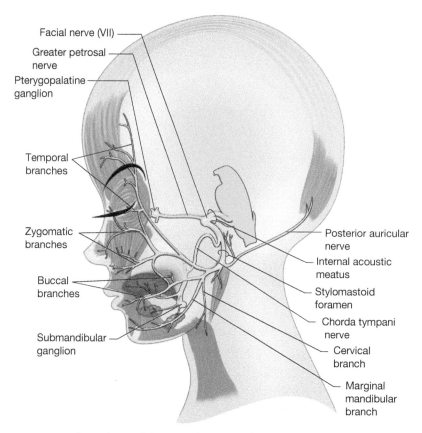

FIGURE 13-17 A facial nerve emerges from the caudal pons to innervate the muscles of facial expression.

Taste is tested with the use of sweet, salty, or sour flavors. The individual is instructed to protrude the tongue, and a cotton applicator on which a drop of the flavor has been placed is stroked along one side of the tip of the tongue. The individual is asked to signal his or her identification of the test substance before withdrawing the tongue back into the mouth. The latter action would obscure an accurate test result by permitting diffusion of the test substance to the opposite side of the tongue or to its posterior one-third, where taste is mediated by the glossopharyngeal nerve. A lesion of the facial nerve distal to its junction with the chorda tympani will not produce an impairment of taste.

The evaluation of motor function of the facial nerve function begins with observation of the person as he or she talks, smiles, or frowns, during which asymmetries or slowness of contraction are noted. It must be cautioned, however, that a degree of facial asymmetry is quite normal. The individual is instructed to wrinkle his or her forehead by looking upward. An individual's capacity to shut the eyelids tightly is tested against attempts by the examiner to pry them open. The individual is asked show his or her teeth, smile, to whistle, and to purse the lips against the pressure of the examiner's fingers. The person is asked to blow his or her cheeks out fully, and the examiner then presses against them, noting whether there is an escape of air from one side. The platysma muscle is tested, after demonstration by the examiner, by asking the person to make a maximal effort to draw the lower lip and angle of the mouth downward and outward while tensing the skin over the anterior surface of the neck.

Lesions of the Facial Nerve

The most common disease affecting the facial nerve is **Bell's palsy**, which has an incidence rate of 23 per 100,000 annually. Bell's palsy is often caused by the **herpes simplex virus**, although some cases are of unknown origin (idiopathic). The onset of Bell's palsy is acute, with about one-half of patients attaining maximum paralysis in 48 hours and virtually all patients within five days. Approximately 80 percent of patients recover in several months. However, if electromyography shows evidence of degeneration, the onset of recovery may not occur for several months because it depends on regeneration of facial nerve fibers. Recovery may then require several years and may not be complete.

All actions of the facial muscles are affected, whether voluntary, reflex, or in response to emotional input or states. Involvement of the nerve on one side results in a marked facial asymmetry (Figure 13-18 ■). The eyebrow droops, the nasolabial fold smoothes out, the corner of the mouth droops, and the palpebral fissure widens due to the unopposed action of the levator palpebrae superioris muscle. The lips cannot be pursed as in whistling nor can they be held together tightly enough during eating to keep food in the mouth. Food remains lodged in the cheek due to paralysis of the buccinator muscle. The corneal reflex is lost on the side of the lesion, and the patient may complain that sounds are too loud in the ipsilateral ear. This condition is called **hyperacusis** and is due to a paralysis of the stapedius

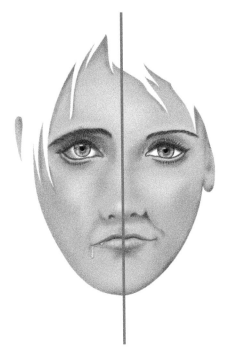

FIGURE 13-18 Bell's palsy results in marked facial asymmetry, with one half of the face affected. The eyebrow and corner of the mouth droop on the affected (right) side.

muscle. Impairment of taste is present to some degree in nearly all patients.

The herpes zoster virus also can damage the facial nerve (Ramsay Hunt syndrome), resulting in a facial palsy and a rash in or around the external auditory meatus or over the mastoid process. Another disorder, **hemifacial spasm**, consists of continual twitching movements most

severe around the mouth and eye. It is due to compression of the facial nerve caused by an aberrant blood vessel with a resultant segmental demyelination of axons.

VESTIBULOCOCHLEAR NERVE (VIII)

The vestibulocochlear nerve is a special sensory nerve that conveys vestibular (equilibrium) and auditory (hearing) information from highly specialized receptors (hair cells) in the inner ear to the brainstem. Because of their great functional and clinical importance, a separate chapter is devoted to the vestibular and auditory systems (see Chapter 17).

The nerve is made up of the peripheral and central processes of bipolar ganglion cells. The peripheral processes are short because the ganglia are positioned close to the sensory receptors. The vestibular nerve arises from bipolar cells in the **vestibular ganglion (ganglion of Scarpa)** at the outer end of the internal auditory meatus (Figure 13-19 ■). The cochlear nerve arises from bipolar cells in the **spiral ganglion of the cochlea**, situated near the inner edge of the osseous spiral lamina. The central processes of these bipolar neurons travel through the internal auditory meatus together with the facial nerve. The cochlear nerve is lateral to the vestibular nerve. Cranial nerve VIII enters the medulla at its junction with the pons, just lateral to the

> **Thought Question**
>
> What two sensory modalities are carried in CN VIII?

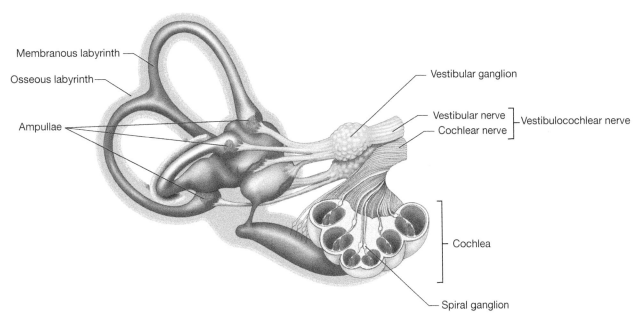

FIGURE 13-19 The vestibulocochlear nerve is a special sensory nerve comprised of afferents from the labyrinth, conveying information about equilibrium, and the cochlea, conveying auditory information. Primary afferent vestibular fibers synapse in the vestibular ganglion. These fibers then project as the vestibular nerve. Primary afferents from the cochlea synapse at the spiral ganglia. These fibers then project as the cochlear nerve. Together, the vestibular and cochlear nerves combine to form the vestibulocochlear nerve, CN VIII.

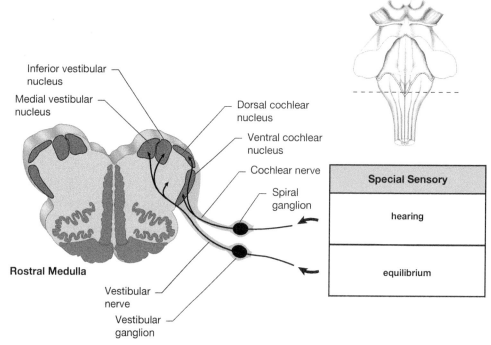

FIGURE 13-20 The vestibulocochlear nerve enters the brainstem at the rostral medulla. The vestibulocochear nerve is comprised of special sensory fibers for hearing and equilibrium.

attachment of CN VII. The central processes of vestibular ganglion cells synapse in four vestibular nuclei located throughout the medulla and caudal pons in the dorsolateral tegmentum (Figure 13-20 ■). The central processes of spiral ganglion cells synapse in the ventral and dorsal cochlear nuclei positioned on the dorsolateral surface of the rostral medulla.

Testing of the vestibulocochlear nerve includes testing both the ability to coordinate eye–head movements (vestibular component) and of hearing (audition). Because these tests are specialized, they are discussed in detail in Chapter 17.

GLOSSOPHARYNGEAL NERVE (IX)

The glossopharyngeal nerve subserves general sensation from the posterior one-third of the tongue, the skin of the external ear, and the internal surface of the tympanic membrane; special sensation for the sense of taste from the posterior one-third of the tongue; visceral sensation from the carotid body and carotid sinus; branchial motor to the striated stylopharyngeus muscle; and visceral motor parasympathetic fibers to the parotid gland via the otic ganglion.

The general sensory afferents terminate in the **spinal trigeminal nucleus**, as noted in Chapter 14. The special sensory afferents synapse in the rostral part of the nucleus solitarius (gustatory nucleus), along with similar fibers of the facial nerve (Figure 13-21 ■). The visceral sensory fibers terminate in the caudal part of the nucleus solitarius (nucleus of the tractus solitarius). The branchial motor component arises from LMNs in the rostral part of the **nucleus ambiguus**. The parasympathetic visceral

motor preganglionic fibers arise from the **inferior salivatory nucleus**, scattered cells in the tegmentum of the rostral medulla.

The role of the baroreceptors in the wall of the carotid sinus in regulating blood pressure was discussed in Chapter 12. The chemoreceptors in the carotid body monitor oxygen tension in the circulating blood and are responsible for respiratory responses to hypoxia.

The glossopharyngeal nerve emerges from the medulla as the most rostral of the series of rootlets to exit from the postolivary sulcus. The rootlets converge to form CN IX. Just before it exits the skull in the jugular foramen, the nerve gives rise to the tympanic nerve. The **superior** and **inferior glossopharyngeal ganglia** are located in the jugular foramen. General sensory axons for pain and temperature from the skin of part of the external ear, the inner surface of the tympanic membrane, the posterior one-third of the tongue, and the upper pharynx; visceral afferent fibers from the carotid body and carotid sinus; and special sensory afferents subserving taste from the posterior one-third of the tongue have their cell bodies in one of these two ganglia.

CLINICAL CONNECTIONS

Clinical Evaluation of the Glossopharyngeal Nerve

The integrity of the glossopharyngeal nerve is tested by gently touching the posterior wall of the pharynx with an applicator stick or wooden tongue depressor. A normal response consists

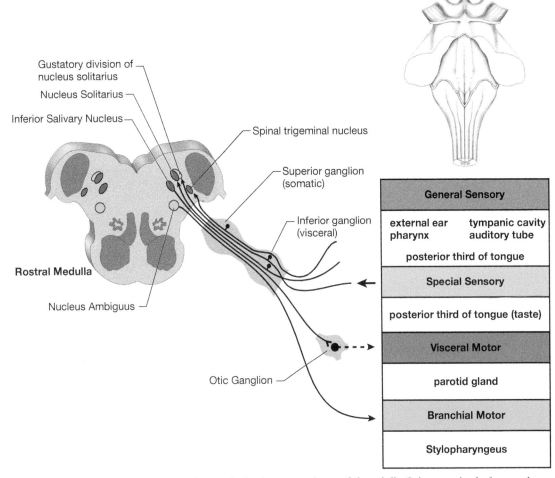

FIGURE 13-21 The glossopharyngeal nerve attaches to the brainstem at the caudal medulla. It is comprised of general sensory, special sensory, visceral motor, and branchial motor fibers. It shares some common functions and nuclei with the vagus nerve (see Figure 13-22).

of prompt contraction of the pharyngeal muscles, with or without a gag reflex. However, the gag reflex is an unreliable test of glossopharyngeal nerve function because the posterior pharyngeal wall is also innervated by the vagus nerve.

> **Thought Question**
>
> In what ways do CNs IX and X have similar functional roles? Which of the contributions are most likely to be important with respect to rehabilitation?

Lesions of the Glossopharyngeal Nerve

Isolated lesions of the glossopharyngeal nerve are rare, and the resulting deficits are not fully known. **Glossopharyngeal neuralgia** is an uncommon disorder that resembles trigeminal neuralgia except that the paroxysms of intense pain begin in the throat or root of the tongue. The pain may be triggered by coughing, swallowing, touching the palatine tonsil, or protruding the tongue.

VAGUS NERVE (X)

The vagus nerve contains general sensory fibers innervating cutaneous areas at the back of the ear and in the external auditory meatus; special sensory fibers innervating taste buds of the epiglottis; visceral sensory fibers from the pharynx, larynx, trachea, esophagus, and thoracic and abdominal viscera; branchial motor fibers innervating the striated muscles of the pharynx and larynx (except stylopharyngeus innervated by CN IX and tensor veli palatini innervated by V_3); and visceral motor fibers innervating parasympathetic ganglia located near the thoracic and abdominal viscera. The clinically most important component of the vagus nerve—the branchial motor fibers—arises from cell bodies of the nucleus ambiguus in the tegmentum of the medulla (Figure 13-22 ■). (The term *ambiguus* reflects the fact that the neuronal cell bodies are rather scattered so that a given section through the medulla may fail to capture the nucleus.) The parasympathetic visceral motor component arises from cells in the **dorsal motor nucleus of the vagus** in the dorsal tegmentum of mid-medulla. The general sensory afferents terminate in the spinal trigeminal nucleus. The visceral sensory fibers synapse in the caudal part of the nucleus of the tractus solitarius.

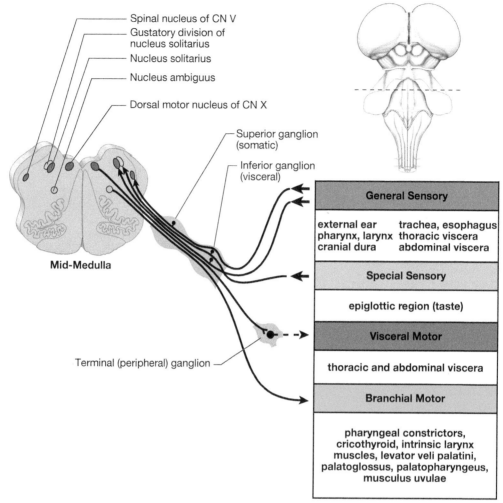

FIGURE 13-22 The vagus nerve attaches to the brainstem at the mid-medulla. It is comprised of general sensory, special sensory, visceral motor, and branchial motor fibers. It shares some common functions and nuclei with the glossopharyngeal nerve. (see Figure 13-21).

The vagus nerve emerges from the medulla as several rootlets that attach at the postolivary sulcus, immediately inferior to the rootlets of CN IX. These rootlets unite into a flat cord, and the nerve exits the cranial cavity via the jugular foramen. The **superior sensory ganglion (jugular ganglion)** of the vagus is located in the jugular foramen. The superior ganglion contains the unipolar cell bodies of the general sensory fibers from the skin at the back of the ear and in the external acoustic meatus. The swelling produced by the unipolar cells of the larger **inferior sensory ganglion (nodose ganglion)** is located on the vagus nerve after its exit from the jugular foramen. The cell bodies of the visceral sensory fibers from the thoracic and abdominal viscera are in the inferior ganglion. Just distal to the inferior ganglion, the cranial part of the accessory nerve (XI) joins the vagus nerve and is the source of the majority of fibers in the motor branches of the vagus distributed to the striated muscles of the pharynx and larynx. In the neck, the vagus nerve descends vertically in the carotid sheath, within which it is between the internal jugular vein and internal carotid artery. Numerous branches are given off in the neck. The nerves pass through the superior thoracic

aperture into the thoracic cavity, within which branches are given off to the esophagus, heart, bronchi, and lungs. The nerves pass through the esophageal hiatus in the diaphragm and enter the abdomen, within which branches are given off to the esophagus, stomach, and intestinal tract as far as the left colic flexure.

CLINICAL CONNECTIONS
Clinical Evaluation of the Vagus Nerve

In spite of its considerable size and diverse functions, clinical testing of the vagus nerve is difficult. Examination of the integrity of the nerve focuses on its branchial motor component. The examination should include examination of movements of the soft palate as the individual says "Ah." Normally, the median raphe of the soft palate rises in the midline, but if one side is weak, the soft palate and uvula will deviate toward the unaffected side (Figure 13-23 ■). Additionally, the person's voice should be analyzed as well as the ability to cough.

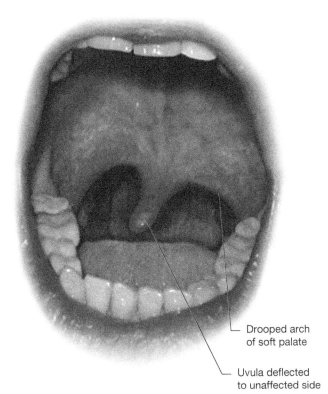

└ Drooped arch
of soft palate

└ Uvula deflected
to unaffected side

FIGURE 13-23 Clinical evaluation of the vagus nerve is performed by examination of the soft palate and uvula as the person opens the mouth and says "Ah." Illustrated here is a unilateral lesion, resulting in a drooped palate on the affected side and the uvula deviated to the unaffected side.

Lesions of the Vagus Nerve

Tumors and infections affecting the meninges may involve the vagus nerve. The **herpes zoster** virus may damage the nerve either alone or along with the glossopharyngeal nerve. An aneurysm of the carotid artery at the base of the skull may affect the vagus along with the glossopharyngeal nerve. Advanced alcoholic or diabetic neuropathy may affect the vagus nerve.

A characteristic paralysis results from the intracranial damage of the vagus nerve on one side. The voice is hoarse with **dysarthria** (difficulty speaking) as a consequence of the paralysis of the vocal cord on one side, which lies immobile, fixed midway between abduction and adduction. Speech is nasal because of paralysis of the muscles of the soft palate (levator palati) such that the oral resonating cavities cannot be effectively shut off from the nasal cavity. The soft palate droops on the ipsilateral side and does not rise on phonation; the uvula deviates to the unaffected side (see Figure 13-23). There may be a nasal regurgitation of liquids or food during swallowing, and swallowing may be impaired (**dysphagia**). Cutaneous sensation may be lost in the skin at the back of the ear and at the external auditory meatus. Typically, no change in visceral function can be demonstrated with a unilateral lesion.

The recurrent laryngeal nerve, innervating the intrinsic muscles of the larynx, merits special mention. The nerve is longer and pursues a different course on the left than on the right side. For one thing, the nerves may be severed or stretched during the course of thyroid surgery or a carotid endarterectomy. For another, when the recurrent laryngeal nerve is damaged by pathology in the thoracic cavity, there is no dysphagia because the branches of the vagus that innervate the pharynx already have been given off. Paralysis of both recurrent nerves results in **aphonia**, an inability to give voice, and **inspiratory stridor**, a harsh, high pitched (crowing) sound on the inspiratory phase of respiration.

ACCESSORY NERVE (XI)

The accessory nerve is exclusively motor, containing branchial motor fibers that innervate striated muscle. The nerve is traditionally considered to consist of cranial and spinal parts, a practice we will continue. The cranial

Neuropathology Box 13-1: The Sensory System and Taste

The sensation of taste is conveyed by several cranial nerves (CN V, VII, IX, and X), just as eye movements are controlled by a combination of cranial nerves. The tongue consists of an anterior (or buccal) portion and a posterior (or pharyngeal) part ,separated by the V-shaped sulcus terminalis. These two parts have separate embryological origins. As a result, the innervation of these two parts is different. General somatic sensation from the tongue is carried in two separate cranial nerves. From the anterior two-thirds of the tongue (the buccal part) it is carried in the lingual branch of the trigeminal nerve (V), whereas general sensation from the posterior one-third of the tongue (the pharyngeal part) is carried in the lingual branch of the glossopharyngeal nerve (IX).

The special visceral afferents mediating the sense of taste are also related to multiple cranial nerves (Figure 13-24 ■). Most taste receptors, the taste buds, are distributed in the tongue, and their afferents are associated with two cranial nerves. Again, the boundary separating their innervations is the sulcus terminalis. Thus, taste from the anterior two-thirds of the tongue is carried in the chorda tympani branch of the facial nerve (VII), whereas taste from the posterior one-third of the tongue is carried by the lingual branch of the glossopharyngeal nerve (IX). In addition to the tongue, some taste buds are distributed on the epiglottis and adjacent part of the pharynx. These are innervated by the vagus nerve (X).

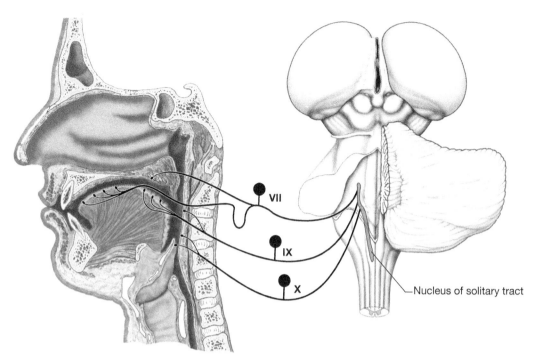

FIGURE 13-24 The special sense of taste mediated by cranial nerves VII, IX, and X. Primary afferent signals originating from the oral cavity project via these three cranial nerves to the nucleus of the solitary tract located in the brainstem.

root of the nerve is motor to the muscles of the soft palate and pharynx, and its course was described earlier in conjunction with the vagus nerve (Figure 13-25 ■). The spinal root innervates the sternocleidomastoid and trapezius muscles. The two roots are united only for a short distance.

The spinal root of the accessory nerve arises from LMNs of the anterior horn of the first five or six cervical segments of the spinal cord. These cells are called the **accessory** or **spinal nucleus**. The axons emerge as a series of rootlets from the lateral aspect of the spinal cord between the dorsal and ventral roots. The rootlets unite

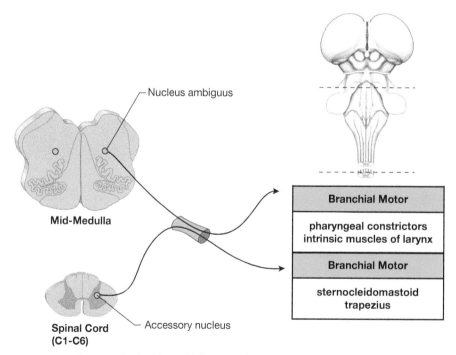

FIGURE 13-25 The accessory nerve is comprised of branchial motor fibers. From the nucleus ambiguus in the medulla, fibers forming the cranial root of this nerve exit to innervate muscle of the pharynx and larynx. From the accessory nucleus in the upper cervical cord, fibers forming the spinal root exit to innervate the upper trapezius and sternocleidomastiod muscles.

into a common trunk that ascends posterior to the denticulate ligaments. The nerve enters the posterior cranial fossa through the foramen magnum and exits the skull via the jugular foramen in association with the glossopharyngeal and vagus nerves. Upon exiting the foramen, the spinal root separates from these nerves and descends to innervate the sternocleidomastoid and upper part of the trapezius muscles. These muscles are at least partially of branchial arch origin.

The superior fibers of the trapezius muscle elevate the scapula. Contraction of the sternocleidomastoid muscle pulls the mastoid process toward the clavicle, which results in a rotation of the head and an upward tilting of the chin to the opposite side.

CLINICAL CONNECTIONS
Clinical Evaluation of the Accessory Nerve

The integrity of the accessory nerve is tested by having the person turn his or her head away from the muscle being tested against resistance of the examiner's hand while the sternocleidomastoid muscle is palpated. Then the person is asked to shrug (elevate) his or her shoulders while the examiner attempts to depress them and palpates both upper trapezii. Unilateral damage to the accessory nerve results in some dropping of the ipsilateral shoulder and winging of the scapula while the arms are at the sides due to weakness of the trapezius muscle. Turning of the head to the side opposite the lesion is weak due to weakness of the sternocleidomastoid muscle.

Thought Question

On protrusion, the tongue may deviate to the side of the inactive muscle. Explain this phenomenon, noting that the action of the genioglossus muscle is to push, not pull, the tongue.

Lesions of the Accessory Nerve

Because of its relatively long course across the posterior triangle of the neck, where it is closely related to superficial cervical lymph nodes, the accessory nerve is susceptible to damage during surgical procedures such as lymph node biopsy, cannulation of the internal jugular vein, and carotid endarterectomy. In its intracranial course, the accessory nerve may be affected, along with the glossopharyngeal and vagus nerves, by the herpes zoster virus or by tumors affecting the contents of the jugular foramen or tumors that invade the foramen. Of particular importance to the orthopedic rehabilitation specialist, whiplash also can cause damage to the accessory nerve.

HYPOGLOSSAL NERVE (XII)

The hypoglossal nerve is a somatic motor nerve that consists of general somatic efferent fibers that innervate all of the striated intrinsic and extrinsic muscles of the tongue, except the palatoglossus, which is innervated by the vagus nerve. The axons of the nerves arise from neurons of the hypoglossal nuclei situated in the dorsal tegmentum of the medulla close to the midline (Figure 13-26 ■). The nerve emerges from the preolivary sulcus of the medulla as a series of

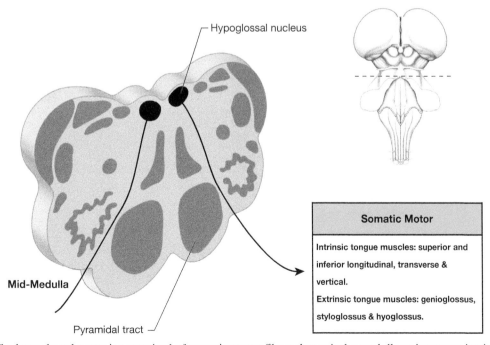

Hypoglossal nucleus

Mid-Medulla

Pyramidal tract

Somatic Motor

Intrinsic tongue muscles: superior and inferior longitudinal, transverse & vertical.

Extrinsic tongue muscles: genioglossus, styloglossus & hyoglossus.

FIGURE 13-26 The hypoglossal nerve is comprised of somatic motor fibers that exit the medulla to innervate intrinsic and extrinsic muscles of the tongue.

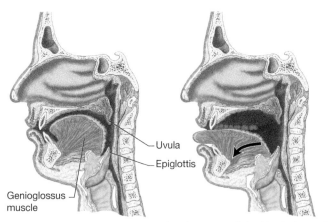

FIGURE 13-27 Tongue protrusion is accomplished by balanced contractions of the paired genioglossi muscles.

rootlets that unite to form the trunk of the nerve that exits the posterior cranial fossa via the hypoglossal foramen.

Balanced contractions of the paired genioglossi muscles are required in order to protrude the tongue straight out of the mouth (Figure 13-27 ■). When one genioglossus muscle is inactive, the action of the intact muscle is unopposed. On protrusion, the tongue will deviate toward the side of the inactive muscle.

CLINICAL CONNECTIONS
Clinical Evaluation of the Hypoglossal Nerve

The individual is asked to protrude the tongue straight out of the mouth. Then he or she is asked to execute rapid alternate movements of the tongue, such as moving it rapidly in and out of the mouth or wiggling it rapidly from side to side. The person is asked to push out the cheek on each side with his tongue while the examiner assesses the strength of the tongue by pushing against it through the bulging cheek. Additionally, speech articulation may be tested by asking the person to repeat, "Late night downtown." Unilateral damage to the hypoglossal nerve results in the tongue deviating toward the side of the lesion on protrusion. Atrophy is manifest by wrinkling of the surface of the tongue and loss of volume.

Lesions of the Hypoglossal Nerve

In its intracranial course, pathological processes affecting the basal meninges may affect the hypoglossal nerve. In its extracranial course, the nerve may be damaged in operations on the neck.

SUMMARY OF THE CLINICAL EXAMINATION OF THE CRANIAL NERVES

Clinical examination procedures were described for each cranial nerve. They are summarized in Table 13-4 ■.

Table 13-4 Tests of Cranial Nerves

CRANIAL NERVE	CLINICAL TESTS
Olfactory nerve (I)	Use familiar odors such as peppermint, coffee, vanilla, or a bar of soap, and avoid irritants such as ammonia or vinegar. The person must identify the substance with eyes shut and one nostril occluded.
Optic nerve (II)	**1.** Visual acuity test With best corrected vision, if needed, and one eye covered, each eye is tested separately using an eye chart (Snellen chart). **2.** Ophthalmoscopic examination Examine both retinas with an ophthalmoscope. Note the color, size, and shape of the optic disc; the characteristics of the physiologic cup; the distinctness of the edges of the optic disc; the size, shape, and configuration of retinal vessels; the presence of hemorrhage, exudates, or pigment. **3.** Visual field test Visual fields for each eye are tested (with the other eye covered) by confrontation. This test is described fully in Chapter 18. **4.** Pupillary responses The direct and consensual responses to illumination of one pupil are assessed in the swinging flashlight test described in Chapter 18.

(continued)

Table 13-4 Tests of Cranial Nerves (continued)

CRANIAL NERVE	CLINICAL TESTS
Oculomotor (III), trochlear (IV), and abducens (VI) nerves	Extraocular movements are assessed by having the person look in all directions without moving his or her head. 1. Smooth pursuit is tested by having the person follow an object across his or her full range of horizontal and vertical movements. 2. Convergence movements are tested by having the person fixate on an object as it is moved slowly toward a point between his or her eyes. 3. Saccades are tested by asking the person to look back and forth between two separated targets. 4. Note whether nystagmus is present. (See Chapter 17.)
Trigeminal nerve (V)	1. Sensation The ability to perceive a pinprick or light touch from a wisp of cotton is tested over the three divisions of the nerve and anterior half of the scalp. Corneal sensation is tested by evoking the corneal reflex. 2. Motor function Palpate the masseter muscles during jaw clench. Have the person open his or her mouth against resistance applied at the base of the the chin. Test the jaw-jerk reflex.
Facial nerve (VII)	1. Sensation Assess taste sensation in the anterior two-thirds of the tongue by applying sweet (sugar), salty (saline), bitter (quinine), and sour (vinegar) solutions to the protruded tongue with a cotton applicator. 2. Motor function Assess voluntary movements of the lower facial musculature by having the person smile, bare the teeth, whistle, puff out both cheeks, or pucker the lips. Closing the eyes, raising the eyebrows, and frowning are maneuvers that test voluntary control of the upper facial musculature.
Vestibulocochlear nerve (VIII)	1. Cochlear nerve The ability of the person to hear words whispered or the sound produced by rubbing the thumb and forefinger together just outside the pinna is tested. Using a tuning fork vibrating at 256 Hz, air and bone conduction are tested for each ear. This is the Rinne test. The Weber test is a test for lateralization. Pure tone audiometry may be used. (See Chapter 17.) 2. Vestibular nerve The caloric test may be used in people suspected of vestibular dysfunction. (See Chapter 17.)
Glossopharyngeal nerve (IX)	Touching the posterior wall of the pharynx with a tongue depressor elicits contraction of the pharyngeal muscles, with or without a gag reflex.
Vagus nerve (X)	The person is instructed to say "Ah" with the mouth open wide and tongue protruded. The median raphe of the soft palate should rise symmetrically, with the uvula remaining in the midline. The character, sound, and volume of his or her voice should be noted.
Accessory nerve (XI)	The individual is instructed to rotate his or her head against resistance of the examiner's hand while the sternocleidomastoid muscle is palpated. The trapezius muscle is tested by having the person shrug each shoulder against resistance of the examiner's hand.
Hypoglossal nerve (XII)	The individual is asked to "stick out his or her tongue" and move it rapidly from side to side.

Summary

This chapter presented some of the "hardware" that is unique to the brainstem—namely, the cranial nerves and their major nuclei. In addition, many of the typical clinical tests were presented that are used to establish whether or not specific nerves are intact. The information in this chapter provides a starting point for understanding the brainstem. However, much is left to be learned. In Chapter 14, we discuss how information is integrated in the brainstem. Then in Chapter 15, we summarize brainstem structure and function by considering vascular damage at different levels from the medulla to the midbrain.

Applications

1. Maria is 15 years old. During a school health screening, it was discovered she had a loss of hearing in her left ear. The school nurse advised the parents; the parents then took her to the pediatrician, who performed a thorough examination, including ordering an MRI. The MRI identified a tumor that was subsequently surgically removed. Following the surgery, Maria presented with the following signs and symptoms:

   - Hearing loss left ear.
   - Left facial droop.
   - Talkative, but with dysarthric speech.
   - Difficulty eating.
   - Drooling from left side of mouth.
   - Complaints of dizziness and feeling "off balance."
   - Difficulty going sit to stand.
   - Wide based, slow, and uncoordinated gait.
   - Normal discriminative touch, proprioception, and pain and temperature sensibility in the face and body.
   - Normal strength of her arms and legs.

   a. For each of these symptoms, identify which structure is implicated.
   b. Given Maria's symptoms, where is the location of the lesion?
   c. What findings would you anticipate when testing her corneal reflexes? What is the functional implication of these findings?
   d. Practice testing the cranial nerves that are involved in Maria's situation.
   e. Consider how Maria's signs and symptoms might affect her life at home and at school.

2. Review the structure and function of cranial nerve V.

   a. Describe its location within the central nervous system and within the peripheral nervous system.
   b. What are the functions of this cranial nerve, and how are these functions tested?

References

Brodal, A. *The Cranial Nerves: Anatomy and Anatomic-Clinical Correlations*, 2nd ed. Blackwell Scientific Publications, Oxford, 1965.

Katusic, S., Beard, C. M., Bergstralh, E., and Kurland, L. T. Incidence and clinical features of trigeminal neuralgia, Rochester, Minnesota, 1945–1984. *Ann Neurol* 27:89, 1990.

Leblanc, A. *The Cranial Nerves: Anatomy, Imaging, Vascularisation*, 2nd ed. Springer-Verlag, Berlin, 1995.

Maciewicz, R., Scrivani, S. Trigeminal neuralgia: gamma radiosurgery may provide new options for treatment. *Neurology* 48:565–566, 1997.

Murakami, S., Mizobuchi, M., Nakashiro, Y, et al. Bell palsy and herpes simplex virus: Identification of viral DNA in endoneurial fluid and muscle. *Ann Intern Med* 124:27, 1996.

Nolte, J. *The Human Brain: An Introduction to Its Functional Anatomy*. Mosby Elsevier, Philadelphia, 2009.

Wilson-Pauwels, L., Akesson, E. J., and Stewart, P. A. *Cranial Nerves: Anatomy and Clinical Comments*. B. C. Decker, Toronto, 1988.

Brainstem II: Systems and Pathways

LEARNING OUTCOMES

This chapter prepares the reader to:

① Discuss the main functions of the trigeminal system and the nerves that contribute to this system.

② Identify the three major divisions of the trigeminal nerve and describe the general distribution of the receptors for each and their entrance to the brainstem.

③ Identify three major nuclei associated with CN V, describe their location, and identify the modalities conveyed by each.

④ Identify the second-order neurons that arise from the following nuclei: spinal trigeminal nucleus, main sensory nucleus, and nucleus caudalis; compare and contrast the pathway associated with each.

⑤ Recall the third-order neuron(s) associated with the trigeminal system and describe their destinations.

⑥ Relate trigeminal neuralgia to the neural structures that are most likely involved.

⑦ Discuss the location and role of surgical interventions for people with trigeminal neuralgia.

⑧ Recall the components subserving the following brainstem reflexes: jaw-jerk, blink, corneal, and swallowing.

⑨ Describe the pathway of the corticobulbar tract.

⑩ Discuss symptoms that occur with damage to the corticobulbar tract.

⑪ Contrast the neurons of the reticular formation with those associated with major ascending and descending tracts (e.g., DC-ML, CST) and discuss the functional importance of the organization of the RF.

⑫ Relate symptoms associated with damage to the RF to symptoms associated with pain, vision, and autonomic activity.

⑬ Relate nuclei and major neurotransmitters to the control of consciousness.

⑭ Explain why extensive lesions of the brainstem can have catastrophic consequences.

⑮ Compare and contrast the role of two gaze centers of the brainstem reticular formation.

ACRONYMS

ARAS Ascending reticular activating system

DC-ML Dorsal column–medial lemniscus

DCN Dorsal column nulei

EEG Electroencephalography

EMG Electromyography

LMN Lower motor neuron

ML Medial lemniscus

MLF Medial longitudinal fasciculus

PPRF Paramedian pontine reticular formation

RF Reticular formation

riMLF Rostral interstitial nucleus of the medial longitudinal fasciculus

S1 Sensory area 1

UMN Upper motor neuron

V₁ Cranial nerve V, ophthalmic branch

V₂ Cranial nerve V, maxillary branch

V₃ Cranial nerve V, mandibular branch

VPM Ventral posterior medial nucleus of the thalamus

VPL Ventral posterior lateral nucleus of the thalamus

Introduction

Having defined the peripheral innervation of structures of the head and neck, we now are in a position to explore the anatomic substrates in the CNS that subserve the processing of somatosensory information from the head and neck and control the movements of their striated muscles. This chapter focuses on general somatosensory information and is organized into three major sections. The first section addresses somatosensory information for the head. This information is primarily conveyed into the nervous system by the trigeminal nerve (CN V), which carries the primary afferent fibers for two major mechanosensory pathways conveying: (1) touch and pressure and (2) pain and temperature. These pathways are analogous to the DC-ML system and spinothalamic tract that were introduced in Chapter 9. They are comprised of the ascending information that originates in the brainstem and terminates in the cerebral cortex after a relay in the thalamus. Note that special sensory information is addressed in later chapters (hearing and vestibular inputs in Chapter 17 and vision in Chapter 18).

The second major topic addresses some of the important somatic motor innervations of the head and neck. This information is presented in the same format as Chapter 11, the motor innervations of the body. Thus, we begin with the brainstem reflexes, using the same strategy as for the spinal cord. We first describe the reflex behaviorally and then discuss the components of the reflex arc. We next examine the major descending UMN pathway that controls cranial nerve LMNs residing in the cranial nerve motor nuclei of the brainstem. As with the somatosensory section, motor information related to the visual system and vestibular systems is addressed in later chapters (vestibular outputs in Chapter 17 and vision in Chapter 18).

The third major section of this chapter focuses on the major integrative system of the brainstem, the reticular formation. The reticular formation was first introduced in Chapter 5. Here, we explore its integrative function in more detail by first considering how the anatomical arrangement of reticular formation neurons enables them to subserve a diverse set of integrative functions related to consciousness, modulation of pain, and the regulation of motor and autonomic activity.

SOMATOSENSORY SYSTEMS FOR THE HEAD AND NECK

The Trigeminal Nerve and Associated Receptors

Somatic sensation in the head is subserved primarily by the **trigeminal system**, which comprises a set of brainstem nuclei and their secondary projections. This system is responsible for the transmission of tactile and proprioceptive information—as well as pain and temperature—from the head to the cerebral cortex for conscious recognition and discrimination. It possesses an organization paralleling that mediating somatic sensation from the body. Even though the system is named "trigeminal," somatosensory information enters the brainstem via the trigeminal system from several cranial nerves, including the trigeminal nerve (CN V) and CNs VII, IX, and X. The focus of this chapter is on the trigeminal nerve, which is the major nerve contributing to this system.

An array of receptors resides in somatic structures of the head and parallels the array of receptors feeding into the somatosensory systems of the body (see Chapter 9). The innervation of the skin of the head has been mapped out in detail. The trigeminal nerve, largest of the sensory nerves innervating the head, arises from three major peripheral routes, forming three divisions (hence, the name *trigeminal*). The three major divisions of the trigeminal nerve are the **ophthalmic (V$_1$)**, **maxillary (V$_2$)**, and **mandibular (V$_3$)**. These three branches join together at the brainstem and enter the brainstem from the lateral surface of the pons at about a mid-pontine level. The crescent-shaped sensory ganglion of the nerve is the **semilunar ganglion** (or **trigeminal ganglion**), which is analogous to the dorsal root ganglion of the spinal cord. The semilunar ganglion resides in a depression in the floor of the middle cranial fossa. The foraminae of the skull through which these three branches access the brainstem are illustrated in Chapter 13, Figure 13-14. The ophthalmic branch enters the skull via the superior orbital fissure, the maxillary via the foramen rotundum, and the mandibular via the foramen ovale.

Table 14-1 ■ summarizes the structures innervated by each branch. The ophthalmic branch (V_1) carries afferents from the skin of the forehead and head back to the vertex, upper eyelid, and nose; the cornea and periosteum of the orbit; and the mucous membrane of the nasal vestibule and frontal sinus. The maxillary branch (V_2) carries afferents from the skin of the face and lower eyelid; the mucous membrane of the cheek, nose, and paranasal sinuses; and the gums and teeth of the upper jaw. The mandibular branch (V_3) carries afferents from the skin of the lower jaw, side of the head, and part of the auricle; the mucous membrane of the cheek, floor of the mouth, and anterior two-thirds of the tongue; the gums and teeth of the lower jaw; the temporomandibular joint; and the muscles of mastication. All three divisions carry afferents from the dura mater. The sensory modalities subserved by these primary afferents are touch, proprioception, pain, and temperature.

Table 14-1 Distribution of the Trigeminal Nerve

Ophthalmic Division (V_1)
    Area of skin labeled in Figure 14-2
    Cornea, conjunctiva, and intraocular structures
    Mucosa of paranasal sinuses (frontal, sphenoid, and ethmoid)
    Mucosa of upper and anterior nasal septum and lateral wall of nasal cavity
    Lacrimal duct

Maxillary Division (V_2)
    Area of skin labeled in Figure 14-2
    Mucosa of maxillary sinus
    Mucosa of posterior part of nasal septum and lower part of nasal cavity
    Upper teeth and gum
    Hard palate
    Soft palate and tonsil

Mandibular Division (V_3)
    Area of skin labeled in Figure 14-2
    Mucosa of the cheek, lower jaw, floor of the mouth, and tongue
    Lower teeth and gum
    Proprioception from jaw muscles
    Mastoid cells
    Muscles of mastication

Thought Question

The trigeminal system is analogous to some of the somatosensory system(s) that convey information from the extremities and torso to the cortex. To what system(s) is the trigeminal system analogous? In what ways are these systems similar, and in what ways do they differ?

Primary afferents of the trigeminal system include fibers of all diameters and degrees of myelination and also include unmyelinated fibers. As discussed in Chapter 9, fibers of different diameters and degrees of myelination carry different types of peripheral receptor information and terminate in different components of the somatosensory system. Similarly, different subsets of trigeminal primary afferents synapse in different nuclei of the sensory trigeminal system.

First-order afferent neurons from the trigeminal nerve terminate in three major nuclei: the **main (chief or principal) trigeminal sensory nucleus**, the **spinal nucleus**, and the **mesencephalic nucleus**. Together, these three nuclei form a column of cells that extends all the way from the upper cervical spinal cord to the midbrain. The main sensory nucleus is located in the mid-pons, just lateral to the trigeminal motor nucleus. The spinal nucleus, in contrast, extends from the mid-pons caudally to the upper cervical spinal cord, while the mesencephalic nucleus extends rostrally from the mid-pons into the midbrain (Figure 14-1 ■).

Primary afferents terminating in the main sensory nucleus are large-diameter fibers conveying fine touch and dental pressure. The main sensory nucleus is similar to the dorsal column nuclei of the brainstem in structure and function, is a rostral continuation of the spinal trigeminal nucleus (the boundary is indistinct), and is located in mid-pons. The nucleus is somatotopically organized with ophthalmic division afferents terminating ventrally, mandibular division afferents dorsally, and maxillary division afferents in between.

Primary afferents from the trigeminal nerve also terminate in the spinal trigeminal nucleus. This nucleus extends caudally as a continuous cell column from the level of entrance of the root fibers in the pons into the upper cervical segments of the spinal cord, where it blends with the substantia gelatinosa of the dorsal horn. The afferent fibers likewise run caudally from the entrance point in the mid-pons, terminating in the spinal trigeminal nucleus at various points from the pons to the spinal cord. Thus, the

Thought Question

Where is the mesencephalic nucleus located? Which afferents terminate in this nucleus? What is unique about the cell bodies associated with those first-order afferent neurons?

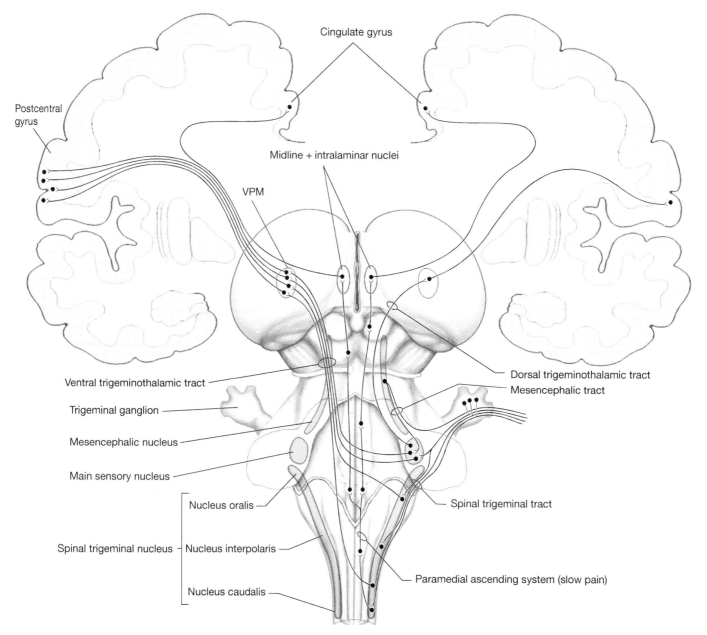

FIGURE 14-1 Primary afferents of the trigeminal system terminate in three nuclei: the main (chief or principal) trigeminal sensory nucleus, the spinal nucleus, and the mesencephalic nucleus. These nuclei, in turn, project mostly to the VPM thalamic nuclei. There are smaller projections to midline and intralaminar thalamic nuclei and to areas of the reticular formation and midbrain nuclei.

tract and nucleus are both visible in cross sections of the high cervical cord through the midbrain, as we will see in Chapter 15. The trigeminal nucleus is analogous to the dorsal horn, and the spinal trigeminal tract is analogous to Lissauer's tract.

Components of the spinal trigeminal complex occupy the upper three or four cervical segments. The spinal trigeminal tract is situated at the superficial margin of the spinal cord, in the area occupied more caudally by the dorsolateral fasciculus. The tract is smallest caudally because most of its fibers already have terminated within the nucleus.

The spinal trigeminal complex occupies a lateral position throughout the medulla. The spinal trigeminal tract is superficially positioned in the caudalmost medulla.

Progressing rostrally, the spinal trigeminal tract is bordered laterally, first, by the thin band of fibers of the dorsal spinocerebellar tract and, more rostrally, by the progressively thickening bundle of fibers of the inferior cerebellar peduncle (restiform body). The nucleus continues to be

Thought Question

The spinal trigeminal nucleus is unique in that it is clearly visible from the mid-pons to the high cervical area. Explain why this nucleus covers such an extensive area. Describe the relationship of the spinal trigeminal nucleus to the spinal trigeminal tract, both in terms of function and location.

medial to the spinal trigeminal tract, and both tract and nucleus increase in size as they progress rostrally through the medulla.

The spinal trigeminal nucleus is divisible into three regions, or subnuclei, on the basis of its cytoarchitecture (refer to Figure 14-1). The nucleus oralis is the most rostral subdivision and extends from the main sensory nucleus to about the pontomedullary junction. The nucleus caudalis is the most caudal subdivision and extends from the spinal cord to the level of the obex. The nucleus interpolaris is between these two nuclei and occupies mid to rostral levels of the medulla. Each subnucleus of the spinal trigeminal nucleus differs with respect to the afferent information it receives and the destination of the secondary projections arising from its cells. The nucleus caudalis is known to be associated with processing of pain and temperature information from the head. However, the somatosensory submodalities processed by the oral and interpolar nuclei are not completely understood.

Finally, cell bodies of a small contingent of primary afferent fibers are found within the central nervous system. The cell bodies of these fibers are found in the mesencephalic nucleus itself. This is the only example of sensory afferent fibers that do not have a ganglion in the peripheral nervous system. The main sensory nucleus of CN V also receives input from the mesencephalic nucleus of V composed of primary afferents from V_3. This input carries proprioceptive information from the muscles of mastication. It reaches consciousness via the secondary projection from main sensory nucleus of V. Some primary afferents terminate in the reticular formation, particularly on cells adjacent to the spinal trigeminal nucleus. Because this nucleus and the tracts that arise from it are not well described, they are not discussed further in this chapter.

So far, we have focused on the contributions of the trigeminal system from CN V. It is important to note that a number of cranial nerves besides the trigeminal contribute somatosensory information to the trigeminal system. The general sensory component of the facial nerve (VII) carries pain, touch, and temperature sensations from the concha of the external ear and a small area of skin behind the ear. The glossopharyngeal nerve (IX) provides general somatic sensation from the posterior one-third of the tongue and upper pharynx, the skin of the external ear, and the internal surface of the tympanic membrane. The general sensory component of the vagus nerve (X) carries pain, temperature, and touch sensations from the larynx, pharynx, skin of the external ear and external auditory canal, the external surface of the tympanic membrane, and the meninges of the posterior cranial fossa. The spinal trigeminal nucleus thus serves as a terminus for all general somatic afferent modalities (except proprioception) from cranial nerves innervating the head.

Furthermore, cutaneous branches of spinal cervical nerves (C2, C3) from the cervical plexus innervate skin of the jaw, external ear, and scalp over the vertex and top of

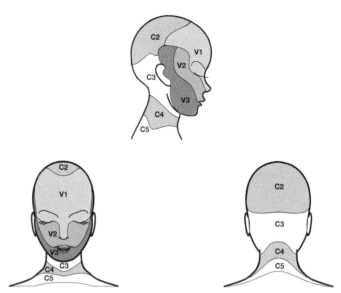

FIGURE 14-2 Somatic sensation of the face, head, and neck is mediated by the trigeminal system and spinal cervical nerves. The trigeminal system has three divisions: V_1, ophthalmic; V_2, maxillary; and V_3, mandibular.

the head. They overlap with areas of the skin innervated by the trigeminal and other general somatic afferent cranial nerves (Figure 14-2 ■).

> **Thought Question**
>
> Which cranial nerves, in addition to the trigeminal nerve, send afferent information into the CNS via the trigeminal system?

Second-Order Neurons

Second-order neurons arise from each of the three sensory nuclei of the trigeminal system. From these nuclei, the fibers travel rostrally to the thalamus, analogous to the pathways conveying somatosensory information from the extremities and torso.

Trigeminal Lemniscus for Fine Touch and Dental Pressure

The main sensory nucleus is similar to the dorsal column nuclei of the spinal cord in structure and function. The main sensory nucleus receives large-diameter fibers conveying fine touch and dental pressure via the trigeminal system. Similar to the DC-ML, the second-order neurons in the **trigeminal lemniscal** system decussate and travel contralaterally to the thalamus. However, the medial lemniscus terminates in the VPL, whereas the trigeminal lemniscus synapses in the contralateral VPM of the thalamus. Although projections from the main sensory nucleus to the VPM of the thalamus are predominantly contralateral (the *ventral trigeminal tract*), there is a smaller ipsilateral projection to the VPM that is termed the *dorsal trigeminal tract* (see Figure 14-1).

Thought Question

From which trigeminal nuclei do second-order neurons arise that are equivalent to the DC-ML system, and from which trigeminal nuclei do projections arise that are equivalent to the spinothalamic tract?

Trigeminal Thalamic Tract for Pain and Temperature as Well as Crude Touch

The spinal trigeminal nucleus receives first-order neurons that convey afferent information about pain and temperature as well as crudely localized touch (referred to as crude touch). Second-order neurons of the spinal trigeminal nucleus decussate and ascend as the trigeminal thalamic tract, joining the spinothalamic tract to synapse in the VPM of the thalamus. Recall that the spinal trigeminal nucleus is analogous to the dorsal horn while the spinal trigeminal tract is analogous to Lissauer's tract.

The contingent of descending primary afferents makes up the **spinal trigeminal tract**, a well-defined fiber bundle throughout its brainstem trajectory (see Figure 14-1). Projections of second-order neurons of the nucleus caudalis of the spinal trigeminal complex are different from those of other components of the nucleus. They enter the paramedial ascending system that mediates slow pain (see Chapter 16).

Only some of the second-order neurons from the spinal trigeminal nucleus project to the thalamus. These cross to the contralateral side of the brainstem and are the first fibers to form the **ventral trigeminal (trigeminothalamic) tract** (see Figure 14-1). This crossing takes place over a large caudorostral extent (due to the length of the nucleus) so that insufficient numbers of fibers aggregate at any given level to be readily observed in myelin-stained sections of the brainstem.

Other second-order neurons from the trigeminal nucleus travel to intralaminar thalamic nuclei, the reticular formation, and other areas where they mediate arousal and affective responses to facial pain. This arrangement is analogous to the pathways traveled by fibers conveying pain and temperature from the extremities and torso.

It is important to recognize that the spinal trigeminal system is made up of phylogenetically new and old parts, just as the spinothalamic tract (described in Chapter 9) is further divided into a neospinothalamic tract and a paleospinothalamic tract: each mediates unique aspects of

Thought Question

Many second-order neurons that convey pain and temperature travel to the thalamus. However, some travel to the reticular formation. What information do they convey, and what is the reason for their termination in the RF? What is a fundamental difference in function for those that terminate in the RF versus those that terminate in the thalamus?

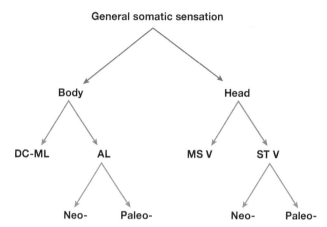

FIGURE 14-3 General somatic sensation is mediated by the dorsal column–medial lemniscal (DC-ML) and anterolateral (AL) systems for the body and the main sensory (MS V) and spinal trigeminal (ST V) systems for the head. Note that both the AL and ST, mediating information about pain and temperature, have an older and a newer subdivision. (See Chapter 16.)

Thought Question

Now is a good time to synthesize information. What are the three nuclei of the trigeminal system from which second-order neurons originate? How do these three nuclei compare with their counterparts for the somatosensory system of the extremities and torso?

somatic sensation (Figure 14-3 ■). In this chapter, we focus on the phylogenetically new component of the system that projects to the thalamus and from there to the primary somatosensory cortex. The phylogenetically old components of both the spinothalamic tract and spinal trigeminal systems are discussed in Chapter 16.

Third-Order Neurons of the Trigeminal System

The cell bodies of the third-order neurons of the trigeminal system that subserve conscious somatic sensation from the face are located primarily in the **ventral posteromedial nucleus (VPM)** of the thalamus. The VPM nucleus is crescent shaped and lies medial to the nucleus VPL and lateral to the curved boundary of the centromedian nucleus of the thalamus. It is important to recognize that the VPM receives input from a number of sources. These include fibers of the ventral trigeminal tract that originate from the main sensory and spinal trigeminal nuclei and ascend in association with the medial lemniscus as well as fibers of the dorsal trigeminal tract that originate from the dorsomedial part of main sensory nucleus of V. Additionally, fibers that descend from the face representations of the sensory and motor cortices also terminate on the VPM.

Thought Question

Where is the nucleus located in which third-order neurons of the trigeminal system arise? What is the name of this nucleus?

Third-order fibers from VPM are part of the thalamocortical radiation (see Figure 14-1). They ascend in the posterior limb of the internal capsule and terminate in the extensive facial representations in both the primary somatosensory cortex of the postcentral gyrus and the primary motor cortex of the precentral gyrus. The face representation in the primary somatosensory cortex (S1) approximately occupies the ventral one-third of the postcentral gyrus on the lateral hemispheral surface—as does the face representation in the primary motor cortex, but in the precentral gyrus (see Figure 7-7). The sensory and motor representations are organized in parallel (in register) across the central sulcus and are reciprocally interconnected by short association fibers. Recall that the VPM received predominantly contralateral information although it also receives some ipsilateral information. The VPM to S1 projection is entirely ipsilateral. As a consequence, the cortex receives bilateral representation from the face (see Figure 14-3).

Thought Question

By now you should be able to synthesize concepts related to somatosensory information from the extremities, torso, head, neck, and face. Compare the tract that carries touch and pressure from the face to the cortex to its counterpart for the extremities and torso, and then compare the tract that carries pain and temperature from these locations.
    In each case, be able to do the following:

1. Describe the location(s) of first-order neurons.
2. Name the nuclei in which the second-order neurons synapse.
3. Name the tract followed by the second-order neurons, and describe its pathway (including any decussation).
4. Name the nuclei for the third-order neurons and the pathway that that these neurons follow.

Functions of the Trigeminal System

The functions of the trigeminal system with respect to facial sensibility are broadly analogous to those subserved conjointly by the DC-ML and the spinothalamic tract for body sensation. Thus, the main sensory nucleus, its thalamic projection, and thalamocortical projection to the face area of the primary somatosensory cortex are considered to subserve functions in somatic facial sensation that are analogous to those subserved by the DCN, ML, and thalamocortical projection to the body area of the primary somatosensory cortex in body sensation. Examples of these functions include discriminative tactile sensations involving spatial and temporal analyses of incoming sensory data (graphesthesia, traced-figure identification, and oral stereognosis; the latter being a highly developed capacity); and position-movement sensibility (kinesthesia) in the jaw. Both systems focus on the innervation of single body parts: the hand in the case of the DC-ML system and the mouth in the case of the main sensory nucleus of V component of the trigeminal system. In fact, the anterior tip of the tongue is even more sensitive to tactile stimulation than are the fingertips (Figure 14-4 ■).

The main sensory nucleus of V, by virtue of its sending information to the face area of the primary motor cortex, subserves important indirect motor functions in the orofacial

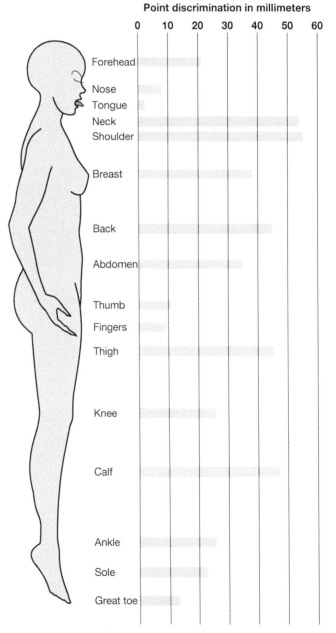

FIGURE 14-4 Regional variation in two-point discrimination over the face and body. Areas of the tongue and fingers discriminate the smallest increments.

musculature, in partial analogy with the indirect motor functions subserved by the DC-ML system. In particular, discriminate tactile sensibility is essential to active exploration of peri- and intraoral surfaces by the tongue. Such exploratory movement is vital to the evolution, refinement, and maintenance of oral perceptual and motor skills underlying eating and speech.

The rostralmost part of the spinal trigeminal nucleus (the subnucleus oralis) is considered to be the homologue of the neospinothalamic component of the AL system. The response properties of its cells suggest it could subserve a role in certain forms of discriminative tactile sensation as well as fast pain.

CLINICAL CONNECTIONS

Determination of the level of involvement of brainstem injury often can be inferred by the accompanying cranial nerve deficits (see Chapter 13). Lesions in the brainstem can affect the cranial nerves alone or can also affect the body, depending on where the lesion is located and how large it is. Therefore, it is necessary to know where the cranial nerves attach to the brainstem, the location of the cranial nerve nuclei, and the location of both ascending and descending tracts associated with the spinal cord and those that arise in the brainstem. In the brainstem, most pathways descending to the spinal cord from higher centers travel contralateral to the side of the body in which they will terminate. Likewise, most pathways ascending from the spinal cord travel contralateral to the side from which they originated. As a consequence, damage within the brainstem results in *contralateral* motor and sensory involvement of the body. However, damage to the motor cranial nerves themselves, associated with the head, neck, and face, results in *ipsilateral* motor loss. Hence, brainstem damage demonstrates the possibility of a crossed or alternating presentation of symptoms. This is best illustrated by Wallenberg's syndrome, as discussed later.

Trigeminal Neuralgia

Trigeminal neuralgia, also referred to as **tic douloureux**, is a disease of the PNS affecting the trigeminal ganglion and/or nerve (see Chapter 13). This condition is characterized by brief attacks of excruciating pain in one or more divisions of the trigeminal nerve. The pain typically lasts less than a minute. The mechanism for this condition is unknown, and the neurological examination is normal.

In severe cases of trigeminal neuralgia, in which pharmacological treatment is unsuccessful and the pain is intractable, surgical intervention can be used. In such

---

Thought Question

What are the symptoms of trigeminal neuralgia? What nuclei and tracts are implicated? And how can the symptoms be alleviated?

---

cases, secondary neurons of the trigeminal system may be sectioned (although other neurosurgical treatments are now preferred). Section of the spinal trigeminal tract slightly below the obex (a medullary tractotomy) relieves the pain attacks and produces a loss of pain and temperature sensibility in the skin and mucous membranes of the ipsilateral face. Given the somatotopic organization of the spinal trigeminal tract, an appropriately placed incision can produce analgesia confined almost entirely to one branch of the trigeminal nerve. Typically, there is also some loss of tactile sensation. The corneal reflex is preserved (as discussed later) and the complication of corneal ulceration avoided. By performing the tractotomy at this level, it is possible to avoid damage to the restiform body (preventing ataxia) and vagus nerve (preventing unilateral vocal cord palsy).

Thought Question

Occlusion of the posterior inferior cerebellar artery can damage the trigeminal system. Can you identify the artery both on the surface and in cross sections of the brainstem? What tract and nucleus is affected, and what symptoms would result from this occlusion? Note that this topic will be revisited in detail in Chapter 15.

Vascular Lesions

Vascular lesions can damage the spinal trigeminal tract and nucleus as well as the spinothalamic tract. These typically occur as a result of occlusion of the posterior inferior cerebellar artery in the lower medulla involving dorsolateral brainstem structures. Such occlusion produces loss of pain and thermal sense over the face ipsilaterally and loss of pain and thermal sense, as well as impairment of tactile sensation over the contralateral half of the body. These are important clinical signs of the **Wallenberg syndrome** (also known as the lateral medullary syndrome) (see Chapter 15).

Lesions involving ventral trigeminal tract projections in the upper pons and midbrain as well as in the nucleus VPM produce contralateral somatosensory deficits of fast pain, temperature, and tactile sensation (discriminative and nondiscriminative). Deficits in discriminative tactile sensation in structures subserved by mandibular division afferents (e.g., the tongue) would be less severe because of the uncrossed projection of the dorsal trigeminal tract.

Thought Question

Vascular lesions that produce loss of pain and temperature on one side of the face also produce loss of pain and temperature of the contralateral extremities. What accounts for the difference in the side on which symptoms are experienced?

SOMATIC MOTOR SYSTEMS OF THE HEAD AND NECK

Clinical Preview . . . .

In your inpatient rehabilitation practice, you frequently treat individuals who have combined spinal cord and traumatic brain injuries. Many of these individuals have exaggerated reflexes related to spinal reflexes. In addition, the traumatic brain injury can affect both the cerebrum and brainstem, with resulting altered brainstem reflexes. As you read through this section, and drawing from Chapter 13, consider the following:

- Which brainstem reflexes could be affected by such injury?
- Which of these reflexes can be functionally limiting, and which could be life-threatening?
- How would you test brainstem reflexes to localize damage to the brainstem?
- Consider why a person with altered brainstem reflexes associated with a traumatic injury could also have altered spinal reflexes, even if the spinal cord is not injured.

The somatic motor innervation of striated muscle in both the head and neck is via cranial nerves. Somatic motor innervations of the muscles of the neck are delivered to the trapezius and sternocleidomastoid muscles by cranial nerve XI. However, CN XI derives from LMNs whose cell bodies are in the upper five cervical segments of the spinal cord (see Chapter 13).

The somatic innervation of the striated muscle of the head and neck has been investigated far less intensively than that of the body, with the notable exception of the UMN vestibular control of eye movement. In part, this is due to the difficulty with experimentation—stemming from the anatomical proximity (crowding) of cranial nerve motor nuclei and brainstem UMN systems and the lack of well-defined fiber bundles (with the exception of the medial longitudinal fasciculus discussed in Chapter 17) relating brainstem UMN systems to cranial nerve motor nuclei. Additionally, the brainstem reticular formation centers that regulate vital and other functions present problems to the researcher attempting to untangle brainstem motor control systems.

Recall that there is an anatomical hierarchy in the CNS for control of musculature of the body. A similar hierarchy exists for the musculature of the head, neck, and face, except that there is no analogy to the brainstem component regulating the lower motor neurons of the torso and extremities as occurs through long descending pathways such as the reticulospinal and vestibulospinal pathways.

In this chapter, we consider brainstem reflexes first and follow this with a discussion of the corticobulbar tract (the functional equivalent of the corticospinal tract regulating spinal cord LMNs). Next, we consider several clinical disorders that focus on the innervations of cranial nerve motor nuclei. We address the vital roles that UMNs of the vestibular nuclei and reticular formation play in regulating the activity of the extraocular muscles in Chapter 17.

Brainstem Reflexes

Like the spinal cord, the brainstem participates in mediating a variety of reflexes. In some cases, brainstem reflexes exactly parallel those of the spinal cord in terms of general anatomical layout and function. However, it is more typical for brainstem reflexes to exhibit more complicated neuroanatomical arrangements, reflecting the more diversified and segregated structure (and function) of the brainstem. Only a few reflexes mediated by the brainstem are described in this chapter because many are best discussed in conjunction with the overall function of the system in which they act. Reflexes mediated by the vestibular system are discussed in Chapter 17, and those mediated by the visual system are discussed in Chapter 18.

The brainstem reflex arc, like that of the spinal cord, consists of five components:

1. A *receptor* that transduces the environmental stimulus.
2. An *afferent fiber* (the afferent limb of the arc) whose axon is in a cranial nerve and whose cell body (with the exception of the mesencephalic nucleus, see later discussion of the jaw-jerk reflex) is in a cranial nerve sensory ganglion.
3. A *reflex center* containing interneurons on which the central processes of the primary afferent synapse. In the case of brainstem reflexes, interneurons of the reflex center are located in a cranial nerve sensory nucleus, in the brainstem reticular formation, or both.
4. Axons from these sources that form synapses on cranial nerve motor nuclei, where the cell bodies of the *efferent fiber* (the efferent limb of the arc) of the reflex arc are located.
5. An *effector* that produces the response completes the reflex arc. The effector may be striated, smooth, or cardiac muscle or a gland, depending on the reflex.

A number of brainstem reflexes involve more than one cranial nerve motor nucleus, even though the afferent limb of the reflex arc involves fibers of just one cranial nerve. In some cases, the cranial nerve motor nuclei are located in different brainstem subdivisions. Thus, there must be a mechanism for distributing the reflex input entering at one level to other levels. This is accomplished by interneurons of the reflex center. In certain instances, a reflex response to a cranial nerve input includes the spinal cord. This was the case, for example, with the visceromotor baroreceptor reflex discussed in Chapter 12. In the baroreceptor reflex, CN IX and X input influences (via a brainstem reflex center) spinal cord autonomic neurons to reduce blood pressure.

Jaw-Jerk Reflex

The **jaw-jerk reflex** is the simplest of all brainstem reflexes and is the cranial nerve reflex most widely used in clinical neurology. Like the stretch myotatic reflex of the spinal cord, it is a monosynaptic stretch reflex. With the jaw relaxed and half open, the examiner's finger is placed over the middle of the individual's chin with a slight downward pressure. The examiner's finger is then tapped gently with a reflex hammer. The response consists of bilateral contraction of the masseter muscle. In healthy individuals, this reflex is not easily elicited. Thus, when it can be readily elicited, it is usually a sign of hyperreflexia, indicating neurological damage.

The tap stretches the masseter muscle (bilaterally) and synchronously activates its complement of muscle spindles. The muscle spindles are innervated by the peripheral processes of the mesencephalic nucleus of the trigeminal nerve (Figure 14-5 ■). As noted earlier, the mesencephalic nucleus is a sensory ganglion whose cell bodies are atypically located in the central nervous system, not the peripheral nervous system as is the case for all other sensory ganglia. The central processes of these primary afferents project to the motor trigeminal nucleus on each side

causing the lower motor neurons to discharge resulting in contraction of the masseter muscle. The jaw-jerk reflex is influenced by age, capacity of the individual to cooperate, position of the mandible, extent of muscle relaxation, and extent of contact between the upper and lower teeth.

The Blink and Corneal Reflexes

Two brainstem reflexes, the blink reflex and the corneal reflex, result in reflexive closure of both eyes (partial or complete) in response to a unilateral stimulus. Both reflexes involve the ophthalmic branch (V_1) of the trigeminal nerve as their afferent limb and the facial nerve as their efferent limb. However, the blink reflex and the corneal reflex do not utilize the same receptors or afferent fibers. The blink reflex is mediated primarily by large fiber non-nociceptive A-beta afferents in the supraorbital nerve that synapse in a portion of the spinal trigeminal nucleus different from that upon which corneal afferents synapse. In contrast, the corneal reflex is purely nociceptive and is mediated by small-diameter A-delta afferents in the ciliary nerves that synapse in a more caudal portion of the spinal trigeminal nucleus.

BLINK REFLEX The simplest neurophysiological technique for assessing the function of the brainstem and certain cranial nerves is the electromyographic (EMG) recording

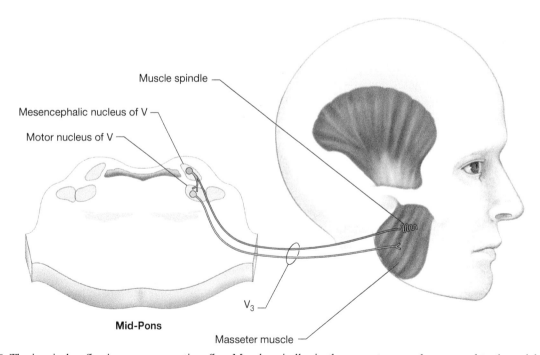

FIGURE 14-5 The jaw-jerk reflex is a monosynaptic reflex. Muscle spindles in the masseter muscles respond to the quick stretch elicited by tapping the jaw. The primary afferents synapse on lower motor neurons, which, in turn, project back to the masseter muscle. This is illustrated unilaterally; however, the tapping elicits the reflex bilaterally.

of muscle contractions elicited by brainstem reflexes. The technique is especially valuable in people who do not exhibit overt cranial nerve motor deficits. In the case of the **blink reflex**, the patient's supraorbital nerve is transcutaneously stimulated and the reflex contractions of both orbicularis oculi muscles (that close the eye lids) recorded with surface electrodes. Two bursts of EMG activity are recorded. The first, called R1, is observed only ipsilaterally and has a latency of approximately 10 msec after the stimulus. The second burst, called R2, is a bilateral response: it appears on the ipsilateral side with a latency of approximately 30 msec and on the contralateral side with a latency of approximately 35 msec. Although R1 can be recorded electromyographically, it does not generate a clinically observable blink.

R1 is mediated by a reflex circuit in the pons consisting of one to three interneurons located in the region of the trigeminal main sensory nucleus. The R2 reflex circuit is longer and involves the spinal trigeminal nucleus in the medulla. Interneurons in the spinal trigeminal nucleus project into the adjacent reticular formation whose neurons, in turn, project bilaterally onto lower motor neurons

Thought Question

In what ways are the blink and corneal reflexes anatomically similar, and in what ways do they differ?

of the facial nucleus. R1 and R2 engage the same facial motor neurons.

The blink reflex is elicited to assess the integrity of the afferent trigeminal nerve, the interneurons in the pons (R1) and medulla (R2), and the efferent facial nerve. Thus, it is valuable in diagnosing cases of demyelinating neuropathy and other local pathologies affecting the trigeminal or facial nerve, as well as certain pontine and medullary lesions (most often infarctions), especially when the extremities are relatively spared so that spinal nerve conduction studies are normal.

CORNEAL REFLEX As noted in Chapter 13, the corneal reflex consists of partial or complete closure of both eyelids in response to the stimulation of one cornea with a wisp of cotton. The receptors for this reflex arc are free nerve endings in the cornea. The afferent limb of the arc is a branch of the ophthalmic division of the trigeminal nerve. The central processes of the ganglion neurons synapse on neurons in the caudal part of the spinal trigeminal nucleus. Spinal trigeminal neurons project into the adjacent reticular formation whose neurons, in turn, project bilaterally to lower motor neurons of the facial nuclei. The reflex center consists of interneurons of the spinal trigeminal nucleus and interneurons of the reticular formation. Axons from lower motor neurons in the facial nuclei exit the brainstem in the facial nerve (efferent fibers) and cause contraction of the **orbicularis oculi** muscles (effectors) (Figure 14-6 ■).

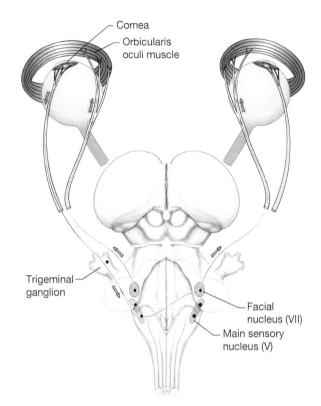

FIGURE 14-6 The afferent limb of the corneal reflex is a branch of the ophthalmic division of the trigeminal nerve (V). The central processes form synaptic connections within the main sensory nucleus of the brainstem. In turn, neurons project from the main sensory nucleus to the facial nuclei bilaterally, where they synapse upon motor neurons of the facial nerve.

Stapedius Reflex

A loud sound entering one ear causes stapedius muscles to contract bilaterally, thereby stiffening the ossicular chain transmitting sound from the outer to inner ear. This is the **stapedius reflex**. The stiffening reduces the transmission of low-frequency sound. The receptors for this reflex arc are hair cells of the cochlea. The primary afferents are axons of the cochlear division of the CN VIII. The peripheral processes of the bipolar spiral ganglion cells synapse with the auditory hair cells (Figure 14-7 ■). The central processes synapse on cells of the **ventral cochlear nucleus**. Axons from the ventral cochlear nucleus project bilaterally to the **superior olivary nuclei**, where they synapse. The superior olivary nuclei are relay nuclei with specific functions in the auditory system (see Chapter 17). Both the ventral cochlear nucleus and superior olivary nuclei represent the reflex center for the stapedius reflex. The superior olivary nucleus of each side projects to the ipsilateral facial nucleus. Axons of lower motor neurons of the facial nucleus exit the brainstem in the facial nerve and innervate the stapedius muscle.

Swallowing Reflex

Among the important reflexes for rehabilitation, one of the most complex is the **swallowing reflex**. Deglutition (swallowing) is initiated as solid food is masticated and

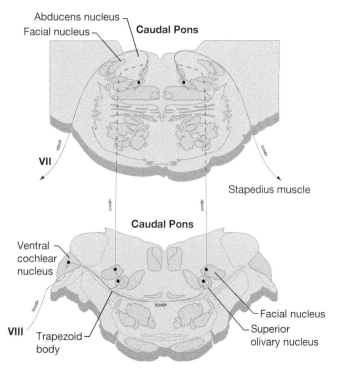

FIGURE 14-7 The stapedius reflex. Primary afferents of the cochlear division of cranial nerve VIII project to the ventral cochlear nucleus of the brainstem. Axons from the nucleus project bilaterally to the superior olivary nuclei, where interneurons project to the facial nuclei. Axons leaving the facial nuclei innervate the stapedius muscles.

Thought Question

The swallowing reflex involves three different cranial nerves. Name them. What is the relevant motion contributed by each?

mixed with saliva to form a soft bolus. The first phase of swallowing is voluntary. The soft bolus of food is compressed against the hard and soft palates and pushed from the mouth into the oropharynx, primarily by the movements of the tongue (innervated by XII) and elevation of the floor of the mouth by contraction of the mylohyoid (innervated by V_3). The reflex is then triggered as the bolus stimulates the walls of the oropharynx that extends from the soft palate to the superior border of the epiglottis and is innervated by sensory afferents of IX and X. The soft palate is elevated by contraction of the levator veli palatini (innervated by the cranial root of XI), and this action seals off the nasopharynx from the oropharynx to prevent the reflux of food into the nose during swallowing. To receive the bolus of food, the pharynx is simultaneously elevated and widened by contraction of the longitudinal pharyngeal muscles (innervated by IX and the cranial root of XI). The third phase of swallowing is also reflexive and

consists of the sequential contraction of the three overlapping pharyngeal constrictor muscles (innervated by the branchial motor fibers of X and the cranial root of XI). Their sequential contraction acts to squeeze the bolus of food down the pharynx into the esophagus.

Thus, the cranial nerves involved in this purely reflexive stage of swallowing are IX and X as the afferent limb of the reflex and IX, X, and the cranial root of XI as the efferent limb. Afferent neurons carrying information from mucous membranes of the oropharynx synapse in the nucleus of the solitary tract. Projections from the solitary nucleus, in turn, terminate in the midline reticular formation of the medulla. Neurons in this part of the reticular formation then project onto cells the cranial nerve motor nuclei involved in this stage of the swallowing reflex. The reflex center that controls this exquisitely orchestrated sequence of muscular contractions is located within the reticular formation (RF). Because the arrangement of the connections of these interneurons to the different motor nuclei must be so precise and because the timing of their initiation and cessation of discharge must be so exact in order to ensure that the bolus of food is transferred from the mouth through the pharynx and esophagus into the stomach, the set of reticular formation neurons is sometimes referred to as a pattern generator.

Corticobulbar Tract

Voluntary control of muscles of the head and neck are mediated in part by monosynaptic descending tracts from cerebral cortex to brainstem or "bulb," and hence is referred to as the *corticobulbar tract*, which subserves innervation of LMNs of cranial nerve motor nuclei. Like the corticospinal tract, the corticobulbar tract is responsible for mediating voluntary movement. Also noted earlier was the fact that the term *corticobulbar fibers* is generic because it can refer to any fibers that originate in the cerebral cortex and terminate in the brainstem. However, as used in this text, corticobulbar tract is specific to the preceding definition. UMN axons of the corticobulbar tract often are referred to as supranuclear fibers, whereas LMN axons are referred to as nuclear. Thus, clinical usage often refers to supranuclear and nuclear lesions.

The cortical origin of corticobulbar tract fibers is somewhat more complicated than that of corticospinal fibers. For one thing, the cranial nerve nuclei innervating the extraocular muscles—the oculomotor, trochlear, and abducens nuclei—present a special case. They receive their innervation from the visual association cortices, areas 18 and 19, and from the frontal eye field, located in the lower part of Brodmann's area 8 (and contiguous parts of area 6). The frontal eye field then projects to the vertical gaze center (rostral interstitial nucleus of the medial longitudinal fasciculus in the midbrain) and horizontal gaze center (paramedian pontine reticular formation). Corticobulbar fibers travel adjacent to corticospinal fibers. They descend via the posterior limb of the internal capsule and then travel through the cerebral peduncle.

Corticobulbar fibers projecting to the trigeminal, facial, and hypoglossal nuclei, as well as to the nucleus ambiguus, arise from cells within the multiple face representations of the motor cortices. Five motor face representations have been identified, and all are interconnected with one another via corticocortical association fibers. The representations are located in the ventral portion of the precentral gyrus, Brodmann's area 4 (M1); in the ventral lateral-premotor cortex, Brodmann's area 6v; in the supplementary motor cortex, Brodmann's area 6m on the medial hemispheral surface (M2); in the rostral cingulate motor cortex, Brodmann's area 24c on the medial hemispheral surface (M3); and in the caudal cingulate motor cortex, Brodmann's area 23c (M4) (see Figure 7-5). Fibers destined to supply cranial nerve motor nuclei exit from the corticobulbar tract when the latter has reached the brainstem level in which a motor nucleus resides. Such corticobulbar fibers sometimes aggregate into identifiable obliquely running fascicles (sometimes called aberrant pyramidal bundles), especially in the medulla and lower pons.

The termination of corticobulbar fibers parallels that of corticospinal fibers in that access to the LMN is effected either directly or, more commonly, indirectly via interneurons. The interneuronal pool for cranial nerve motor nuclei is represented by cells distributed in the reticular formation (discussed later) and, in the case of the facial, trigeminal, and hypoglossal nuclei, in a particular part of the reticular formation called the lateral tegmental field.

Frequently, the cranial nerve motor nuclei receive bilateral input from the cerebral cortex, although the proportion derived from one side or the other varies across nuclei (Figure 14-8 ■). The bilaterality of cortical input

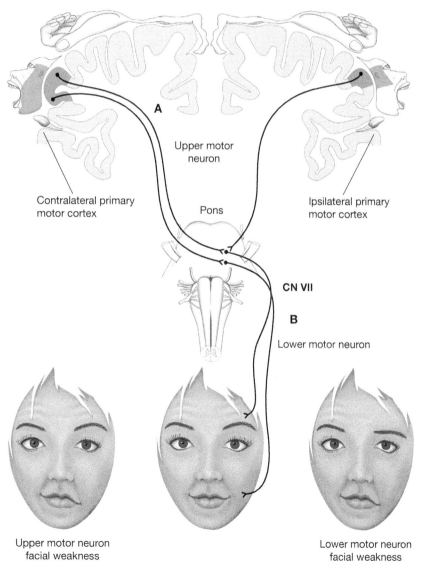

FIGURE 14-8 The motor nucleus of cranial nerve VII receives bilateral input from the cerebral cortex. Upper motor neuron facial weakness is more observable in the lower facial muscles, whereas lower motor neuron facial weakness is observable in both the upper and lower facial muscles. Although this understanding is useful, it is a simplification. As explained in text, the innervation of facial muscles is more complex.

means that to produce an upper motor neuron paralysis of the cranial nerve musculature, bilateral lesions must occur. Unilateral lesions may produce a mild paresis so that, for example, there may be a slight deviation of the tongue and jaw to the side opposite the lesion.

It is commonly accepted that the LMNs that innervate muscles of the upper face are innervated by bilateral cortical projections, whereas the LMNs that innervate muscles of the lower face are innervated purely through contralateral cortical projections. This implies that a unilateral cortical lesion could result in sparing of the upper face, but motor and/or somatosensory loss of the contralateral lower face. However, anatomical studies do not clearly support the notion that there is an anatomical supply from the cortex to the nucleus of the upper facial muscles.

CLINICAL CONNECTIONS

The corticobulbar innervation of the facial nucleus is important clinically, given the numerous alterations in facial expression that follow localized injury. Facial paralysis can be categorized as relating to upper or lower motor neuron lesions, with upper motor neuron lesions producing a "central paralysis" and lower motor neuron lesions referred to as "peripheral paralysis."

Frequently, a cortical stroke involving the face representation results in a paralysis of the muscles of facial expression for the lower half of the face, but it spares voluntary contraction of muscles of the upper face. This difference has been interpreted as implying that LMNs innervating muscles of the lower face receive innervation only from the contralateral M1, whereas the LMNs innervating muscles of the upper face receive bilateral cortical innervations (see Figure 14-8). However, as noted earlier, current evidence does not support this anatomical arrangement. An alternative explanation is that other innervations exist for facial muscles, outside of the middle cerebral artery distribution.

Thought Question

Can you think of disorders resulting in central versus peripheral paralysis that affect muscles of facial expression?

Dysarthria

The term **dysarthria** applies exclusively to motor deficits in the production of articulated speech. Dysarthria is defined as a disturbance in the execution of normal motor speech patterns due to abnormalities in the neuromuscular system subserving the muscles of articulation. Thus, dysarthria may follow damage to cell bodies or axons of UMNs and LMNs in the CNS, cranial nerves in the PNS, the neuromuscular junction, and the contractile machinery in muscle itself. The roster of clinical disorders resulting in dysarthria is legion. Stroke, trauma, or disease that affects the UMN orofacial representation in the precentral gyrus or their axonal projections to cranial nerve motor nuclei in the brainstem. This is referred to as pseudobulbar palsy. Other disorders resulting in dysarthria include involvement of LMNs in the cranial nerve motor nuclei or their axons in the brainstem (referred to as bulbar palsy), tumors or trauma affecting cranial nerves in their peripheral course toward the speech musculature, myasthenia gravis affecting neuromuscular transmission, and the muscular dystrophies affecting voluntary muscle contraction. Furthermore, disorders of the basal ganglia such as Parkinson's and Huntington's disease (see Chapter 19) may result in dysarthtria. Additionally, damage to the cerebellum may result in so-called "ataxic dysarthria" (see Chapter 19).

Dysarthria may manifest as dysfunction in any of the speech musculature: as **aphonia** (inability to generate speech sounds) or **dysphonia** if innervation to the larynx (vocal folds) is involved, as **nasality** if innervation to the soft palate is damaged, or as slurred consonant production if innervation to the tongue or lips is affected. Speech may become monotone, stuttered, or explosive. But the cardinal

---

Neuropathology Box 14-1: Dissociation between Voluntary and Emotional Facial Expression

It has long been recognized clinically that localized brain injury may result in a dissociation between voluntary and emotional facial expression. The most typical dissociation is where voluntary movement of the lower facial muscles on the contralateral side is impaired following a cortical lesion in M1, but during spontaneous laughter or after a humorous remark, for example, the muscles of the lower half of the face contract normally. A less common reciprocal dissociation occurs in emotional facial paralysis. Here, there is an inability to spontaneously smile on one side of the face, but voluntary control over the same muscles is largely unaffected. Emotional facial paralysis may follow lesions of the midline cortex, insula, thalamus, and region of the internal capsule and striatum. These clinical findings indicate that separate neural systems mediate voluntary and emotional facial expression. This difference is reflected in the cortical innervation of the facial nucleus. M3, the rostral anterior cingulate face representation (Brodmann's area 24c), controls emotional facial expression, while voluntary facial expression is mediated by the lateral hemispheral face representations (M1 and Brodmann's area 6v).

feature of the deficit causing dysarthria is that the abnormal motorics are not confined exclusively to speech. Thus, if a person is asked to blow out a match, purse his lips, wiggle his tongue back and forth, and say "ah," performance is defective—just as it is in speech production. This contrasts with disorders of language, known as *aphasias*, in which each of these motor actions occurs normally (e.g., pursing the lips, blowing out) but the movements cannot be used in coordinated output for speech.

Progressive Bulbar Palsy

Progressive bulbar palsy is a motor system disease in which the first and dominant clinical signs relate to weakness in the orofacial muscles. The term *motor system disease* was defined in Chapter 10. Its distinguishing feature is that it is characterized by a *combination* of LMN and UMN signs. Dysarthria results, the pharyngeal (gag) reflex is lost, swallowing and chewing are impaired, and the facial muscles sag. Atrophy and fasciculations of the tongue are present and the twitching tongue lies uselessly on the floor of the mouth. Even though the jaw muscles are weak, the jaw jerk reflex may be exaggerated, and the jaws may snap shut involuntarily (the "bulldog" reflex). The presence of both weakness (paresis) and spasticity is a reflection of UMN damage and is distinct from the weakness resulting from LMN damage. The extraocular muscles are never impaired in progressive bulbar palsy (an observation likely related to the fact that they are the first affected in myasthenia gravis). Pathologic laughter and crying, signs of pseudobulbar palsy defined in the next section, are present, presumably due to limbic system involvement.

Pseudobulbar Palsy

Pseudobulbar palsy, also called **spastic bulbar paralysis**, is most often caused by bilateral lesions of the internal capsule affecting the corticobulbar tracts. The syndrome is discussed in Chapter 24 because it results from cerebrovascular disease.

> **Thought Question**
>
> Name five signs of progressive bulbar palsy. Which of these signs are associated with LMN and which with UMN damage? Based on what you know about the location of the internal capsule, what is a main feature that differentiates progressive bulbar palsy from pseudobulbar palsy?

Conditions Affecting the Blink Reflex

A variety of clinical conditions adversely affect the blink reflex. In Bell's palsy, R1 and R2 blink reflex EMG activity may be delayed or lost on the affected side. Acoustic neuromas in the cerebellopontine angle compress the trigeminal nerve, resulting in abnormal responses on the involved side. R2 is absent in Parkinson's disease and exaggerated

in pseudobulbar palsy (see Chapter 24). A significant percentage of people with multiple sclerosis will manifest impaired blink reflexes.

RETICULAR FORMATION

Clinical Preview

You are a member of the team that treats patients in the medical intensive care unit (MICU) of a major trauma center. Frequently, you are called on to evaluate patients who are in coma. As you read through this section, and drawing from information in Chapter 13 about vital functions, consider the following:

- How is the brainstem involved in control of consciousness?
- How is the brainstem involved in the control of autonomic activities such as heart rate and respiration?
- When would injuries to the brainstem that result in deep coma most likely also be fatal?

The brainstem reticular formation was introduced in Chapter 5 in terms of its anatomicofunctional zones, projections, and role in regulating consciousness. In this chapter, we focus on the integrative aspects of reticular formation function whose basis resides in the anatomical characteristic of its resident neurons.

Anatomical Characteristics of Reticular Formation Neurons

Neurons of the reticular formation function to integrate diverse information from a variety of sources and to organize generalized responses. Therefore, reticular formation neurons have structural features that subserve these functions. First, many neurons have simple, relatively large dendritic trees that are oriented in a plane perpendicular to the long axis of the brainstem. Second, the dendritic trees of neurons adjacent to one another in the reticular formation overlap extensively so that overlapping dendritic fields extend across the long axis of the brainstem (Figure 14-9 ■). Third, as the axons of the long ascending and descending tracts traverse the brainstem, they give off collateral branches that intermingle with the dendrites of reticular formation neurons. Fourth, individual cells of the reticular formation receive information from a wide variety of sources (Figure 14-10 ■), even though one category of input may dominate. Thus, any given neuron may receive sensory and motor information, visceral and somatic information, and information from ascending and descending tracts, as well as from other reticular formation neurons. Finally, axons of cells of the effector

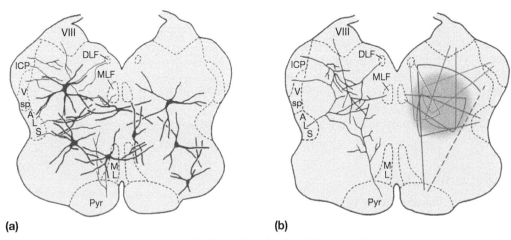

(a)   **(b)**

FIGURE 14-9 Cross section at the level of the medulla illustrating the dendritic trees of reticular formation neurons. (a) large dendritic trees; (b) adjacent neurons with extensive overlap.

Pyr: pyramids, ML: medial lemniscus, MLF: medial longitudinal fasciculus, ICP: inferior cerebellar peduncle, ALS: anterolateral system, DLF: dorsal longitudinal fasciculus, VSP: spinal trigeminal tract, VIII: vestibular nuclei.

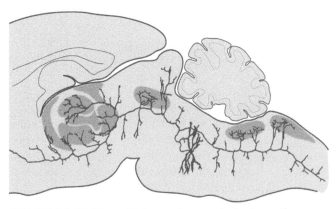

FIGURE 14-10 Dendritic trees of one reticular formation neuron within a rat brainstem.

zone of the reticular formation have a widespread output. By means of a long axon with numerous collaterals, a single reticular formation neuron may synapse on 25,000 other neurons distributed from the spinal cord to the diencephalon.

> **Thought Question**
>
> Neurons of the RF are very different anatomically from neurons of the ascending DC-ML and descending corticospinal and corticobulbar tracts. Describe three features that distinguish neurons of the RF, and relate the structure difference to the functional role of the RF.

Functional Characteristics of Reticular Formation Neurons

The generalized thalamocortical system is also concerned with maintaining an appropriate level of cortical activity that, in turn, can be modulated by specific sensory inputs.

Specific sensory inputs reach the cerebral cortex via a different set of thalamic nuclei, the specific relay nuclei (see Chapter 6). The latter nuclei comprise the **specific thalamocortical system**. Sensations can only be accurately experienced against an optimum level of background activity in a population of cortical neurons. Thus, cortical inputs from both the generalized and specific thalamocortical systems have to converge on the same sets of cortical neurons in each of the primary sensory cortical areas. The reticular formation plays a key role in setting up the brain to pay attention and in modulation of sensory experiences related to pain.

The functional characteristics of many reticular formation neurons follow logically from these anatomic features. First, reticular formation neurons are able to monitor the nerve impulse activity occurring in the ascending and descending tracts that pass through the brainstem tegmentum or systems that surround the tegmentum. A given dendritic shaft of a reticular neuron receives most of its input from a particular ascending or descending system, depending on the tract it is closest to. Other dendrites of the same neuron may have a dominant input from a different source. Second, reticular formation neurons subserve integrative functions individually as well as collectively. This capacity derives from the fact that the input to individual neurons is diverse and from the fact that no two neurons receive exactly the same array of input (owing, in part, to their different positions in the reticular formation). The latter dictates that groups of reticular formation neurons work together to attain a desired functional end. Finally, in integrating all of the diverse input onto the cell, it is unlikely that reticular formation neurons respond to the specific information content in a given input, but rather to the degree and pattern of activity in the input. But this is sufficient for regulating such functions as the level of consciousness.

Functions of the Reticular Formation

Control of the Level of Consciousness

Regulation of the level of consciousness depends on widespread, diffuse modulation of cerebrocortical activity such as that reflected in an electroencephalogram (EEG). The EEG in an alert state is characterized by low-voltage, desynchronized electrical activity, whereas, for example, in sleep it may be characterized by high-voltage, synchronized activity. Systems of reticular formation neurons accomplish such widespread modulation of cortical activity via two routes: **noradrenergic neurons**, from reticular formation neurons in the **locus coeruleus**, and **serotonergic neurons**, from reticular formation in the **midbrain raphe nuclei**, access cortical neurons directly (i.e., without first synapsing in the thalamus). They have a global distribution in the cerebral cortex.

The second route depends on reticular formation neurons influencing the cerebral cortex via a specific set of nuclei in the thalamus making up the **generalized thalamocortical system**. As noted earlier, the hallmark of the generalized thalamocortical system is its widespread distribution throughout the cerebral cortex. The intralaminar thalamic nuclei (see Chapter 6) are prominent members of the generalized thalamocortical system. A massive input to the intralaminar nuclei derives from the **pedunculopontine tegmental nucleus** of the pontine reticular formation whose neurons are **cholinergic**. The interplay of these three transmitters modulates the level of cortical activity acting to increase wakefulness and vigilance. Bilateral damage to the midbrain reticular formation and the projections traversing it results in a comatose state. The portion of the reticular formation producing this general arousing effect is the **ascending reticular activating system (ARAS)**. It is an important component of the more widely distributed system of neurons having the same effect, the ascending arousal system. The ascending arousal system has additional components in the basal forebrain and hypothalamus.

Modulation of Pain

Particular nuclei of the brainstem reticular formation play a vital role in the modulation of pain. These are the **locus coeruleus** located in the pons and the **raphe nuclei** in the rostral medulla. Neurons of the locus coeruleus release norepinephrine onto neurons of the dorsal horn

> **Thought Question**
>
> What three neurotransmitters mediate control of wakefulness and vigilance? From what specific nuclei do these neurotransmitters arise? Describe the location of damage (both the general brainstem location and the specific nuclei) that can affect wakefulness and vigilance.

> **Thought Question**
>
> Which neurotransmitters are of particular importance in the mediation of pain? From what nuclei are these neurotransmitters released? How do the nuclei that produce these neurotransmitters relate to the nuclei that produce neurotransmitters associated with levels of consciousness? Note that Chapter 16 discusses modulation and mediation of pain in much greater detail.

of the spinal cord, while raphe nuclei release serotonin onto these neurons. Pain modulation is further discussed in Chapter 16.

Regulation of Motor Activity

Voluntary motor activity can be modulated by descending inputs from the reticular activating system. The medial and lateral reticulospinal tracts terminate on the cell bodies and dendrites of interneurons of the spinal gray. Some lateral reticulospinal neurons end directly on lower motor neurons of the ventral horn. Gamma motor neurons, innervating the contractile portions of muscle spindle intrafusal fibers, also receive reticulospinal innervation. These tracts influence motor activity bidirectionally, either facilitating or inhibiting voluntary movement and reflex activity. Muscle tone is influenced by reticulospinal regulation of the activity of the gamma system. Many structures involved in regulating motor function (see, e.g., Chapters 17 and 19) project to the reticular formation in addition to the corticoreticular projections arising primarily from the motor cortex. The reticulospinal tracts, in addition to the pyramidal (corticospinal) tract, thus represent a major route by which spinal motor neurons are regulated. Inputs from cerebellar, vestibular, and cortical sources are integrated within the reticular formation; single neurons of the reticular formation then may project integrated cerebellar, vestibular, and cortical influences onto spinal cord motor neurons.

Coordination of Vision (the Gaze Centers)

There are two gaze centers in the brainstem reticular formation, each being responsible for generating eye movements along a particular axis. The neural circuitry for generating rapid horizontal eye movements resides in a set of neurons located in the medial reticular formation of the pons near the abducens nucleus, referred to as the **paramedian pontine reticular formation (PPRF)**. This is the **lateral**, or **horizontal**, **gaze center**. The circuitry for generating rapid

> **Thought Question**
>
> The RF plays a key role in modulation of muscle tone. How is this accomplished?

vertical movements resides in a set of neurons located in the reticular formation dorsomedial to the red nucleus at the junction of the midbrain and diencephalon referred to by the cumbersome name **rostral interstitial nucleus of the medial longitudinal fasciculus (riMLF)**. This is the **vertical gaze center**.

The lateral gaze center is discussed to illustrate the principles of operation of the gaze centers (Figure 14-11 ■). Neurons in the PPRF project to cells in the abducens nucleus on the same side of the brain. There are two types of neurons in the abducens nucleus. The first are LMNs that innervate the ipsilateral lateral rectus muscle. The second are called internuclear neurons. Internuclear neurons cross the midline and enter a tract named the **medial longitudinal fasciculus (MLF)**, in which they ascend to the portion of the oculomotor nucleus containing LMNs that innervate the medial rectus muscle. This tract is critical for coordinating the medial and lateral recti muscles in all lateral gaze functions. Its length renders it vulnerable to pathological processes affecting the brainstem. Thus, the PPRF of one side controls the ipsilateral lateral rectus muscle and the contralateral medial rectus muscle. Activation of the PPRF on the right side of the brainstem generates horizontal movement of both eyes to the right. PPRF neurons in the left half of the brainstem generate conjugate horizontal

movement to the left. PPRF neurons also project to the medullary reticular formation, where they terminate on inhibitory interneurons. These inhibitory interneurons, in turn, terminate on LMNs and internuclear neuron of the contralateral abducens nucleus. Thus, activation of PPRF neurons on the right side inhibits activity in the left abducens nucleus, resulting in relaxation of the left lateral rectus and right medial rectus muscles (i.e., the muscles that would oppose movements of the eyes to the right). This is the principle of reciprocal innervation, first introduced in Chapter 8.

The vertical gaze center in the MLF contains neurons that project to the portions of the oculomotor nucleus whose LMNs innervate the superior and inferior rectus and inferior oblique muscles and to the trochlear nucleus, whose LMNs innervate the superior oblique muscle. Simultaneous activation of the vertical and horizontal

> **Thought Question**
>
> Explain the important role of the medial longitudinal fasciculus (MLF) in the control of eye movement.

gaze centers generates oblique movements whose trajectories are determined by the relative contributions of each center. CNS demyelinating disorders such as multiple sclerosis (MS) can affect the MLF and therefore disrupt the gaze centers. Resulting symptoms include altered vestibulo-ocular reflexes, diplopia, and nystagmus. Gaze centers and visual symptoms are discussed further in Chapter 18.

Control of Autonomic Activity

A number of groups of reticular formation neurons are specialized to carry out vital functions. Centers controlling heart rate and blood pressure, as discussed in Chapter 12, are present in the medullary reticular formation, as are respiratory centers (inspiratory and expiratory). These centers project locally to parasympathetic nuclei of the brainstem and to the intermediolateral and sacral preganglionic neurons of the spinal cord via reticulospinal tracts.

CLINICAL CONNECTIONS

Widespread and bilateral damage involving the RF can occur as a consequence of traumatic brain injury (TBI) and/or massive strokes. Such widespread damage to the RF has catastrophic consequences. Individuals with such damage are typically in a coma (due to involvement of the arousal system) or do not survive (due to involvement of the vital centers that control heart rate and blood pressure).

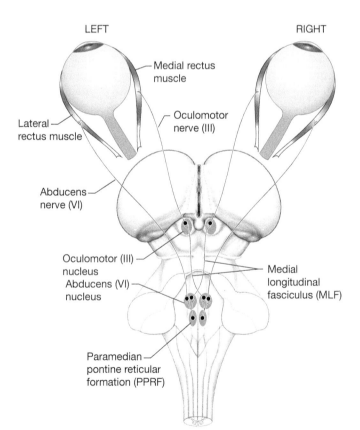

FIGURE 14-11 A simplified diagram illustrating that the lateral gaze center originates in the paramedian pontine reticular formation (PPRF). This circuitry is responsible for generating lateral, or horizontal, eye movements.

Summary

This chapter drew broad parallels between the organizations and functions of somatosensory and motor systems that innervate structures supplied by the spinal cord and cranial nerves. On the somatosensory side, there are "lemniscal" and "anterolateral" components in both innervations, with the tracts from the main sensory nucleus of V being the "lemniscal" component of the trigeminal system and the spinal trigeminal nucleus being the "anterolateral" component. And, as we shall see in Chapter 16, the organizations of the somatic systems mediating slow pain also are similar for spinal cord and cranial nerves. In general, although composed of the same five neural components, somatic reflexes mediated by cranial nerves are more complex than those mediated by the spinal cord, with the notable exception of the monosynaptic stretch reflex. With the exception of laterality, the pyramidal tract and the corticobulbar tract exhibit similar organizations in that both tracts have polysynaptic (via interneurons) as well as monosynaptic terminations on alpha LMNs. With regard to laterality, most pyramidal tract axons control LMNs on the side of the spinal cord contralateral to their cortical origin, whereas most corticobulbar tract axons control LMNs on both sides of the brainstem. Corticobulbar tract innervation of LMNs of the facial nucleus is unique and of clinical significance.

The reticular formation is the major integrative structure of the brainstem. It is the major structural component of the tegmentum and extends through all three brainstem subdivisions. Its neurons are organized anatomically to "capture" information traversing the brainstem in ascending somatosensory and descending motor tracts, and they respond more to the patterns of incoming information than to its specific modality content. The reticular formation plays a vital role in regulating the level of consciousness via the ascending activating system. The reticular formation also is involved in the regulation of motor and autonomic activity and in the modulation of pain.

Applications

1. Chapter 13 discussed the presentation of trigeminal neuralgia, and Chapter 14 discussed the surgical treatment thereof. Investigate this diagnosis further to answer the following questions:
   a. What is this condition, and what are the proposed causes of trigeminal neuralgia?
   b. Identify the medical and alternative treatments available.
   c. What is the prognosis for an individual diagnosed with trigeminal neuralgia?

2. Franco is 68 years old. He has recently developed some curious problems. His family reports he has been laughing inappropriately, and he sometimes cries for no apparent reason. He speaks with dysarthria. You wonder whether Franco has progressive or pseudobulbar palsy. What further information would you need to discern whether Franco is presenting with progressive bulbar palsy or pseudobulbar palsy? How could you obtain this information?

References

Somatosensory Systems

Bowman, J. P. *The Muscle Spindle and Neural Control of the Tongue.* Charles C. Thomas, Springfield, IL, 1971.

Bowman J. P. Lingual mechanoreceptive information II: An evoked-potential study of the central projections of low-threshold lingual nerve afferent information. *J Speech Hearing Res*, 25:357–363, 1982.

Dubner, R., Sessle, B. J., and Storey, A. T. *The Neural Basis of Oral and Facial Function.* Plenum, New York, 1978.

Kruger, L. Functional subdivision of the brainstem sensory trigeminal nuclear complex. In: Bonica, J. J., et al., eds. *Advances in Pain Research and Therapy*, Vol 3. Raven Press, New York, 1979.

Nolte, J. *The Human Brain: An Introduction to Its Functional Anatomy.* Mosby Elsevier, Philadelphia, 2009.

Ohya, A. Responses of trigeminal subnucleus interpolaris neurons to afferent inputs from deep oral structures. *Brain Res Bull* 29:773, 1992.

Olszewski, J. On the anatomical and functional organization of the spinal trigeminal nucleus. *J Comp Neurol* 92:401, 1950.

Rovit, R. J. Murali, R., and Jannetta, P. J., eds. *Trigeminal Neuralgia.* Williams & Wilkins, Baltimore, 1990.

Stewart, W. A., and King, R. B. Fiber projections from the nucleus caudalis of the spinal trigeminal nucleus. *J Comp Neurol* 121:271, 1963.

Torvik, A. The ascending fibers from the main trigeminal sensory nucleus. *Am J Anat* 100:1, 1957.

Young, R. F. Effect of trigeminal tractotomy on dental sensation in humans. *J Neurosurg* 56:812, 1982

Brainstem Reflexes and Corticobulbar Tract

Cruccu, G., Iannetti, J. J., Marx, F., et al. Brainstem reflex circuits revisited. *Brain* 128:386–394, 2005.

Illingworth, R. D., Porter, D. G., and Jakubowski, J. Hemifacial spasm: A prospective long-term follow up of 83 patients treated by microvascular decompression. *J Neurol Neurosurg Psychiatry*, 60:73, 1996.

Jean, A. Brainstem control of swallowing: neuronal network and cellular mechanisms. *Physiol Rev* 81:871, 2001.

Morecraft, R. J., Louie, J. L., Herrick, J. L., and Stilwell-Morecraft, K. S. Cortical innervation of the facial nucleus in the non-human primate. A new interpretation of the effects of stroke and related subtotal brain trauma on the muscles of facial expression. *Brain* 124:176–208, 2001.

Ropper, A. H., and Brown, R. H. *Adams and Victor's Principles of Neurology*, 8th ed. McGraw-Hill, New York, 2005.

Urban, P. P., Hopf, H. C., Connemann, B., Hundemer, H. P., and Koehler, J. The course of cortico-hypoglossal projections in the human brainstem. *Brain* 119:1031–1038, 1996.

Reticular Formation

Brodal, A. *The Reticular Formation of the Brainstem. Anatomical Aspects and Functional Correlations.* Charles C. Thomas, Springfield, IL, 1957.

Hobson, J. A., and Brazier M. A. B., eds. *The Reticular Formation Revisited: Specifying Function for a Nonspecific System.* International Brain Research Organization monograph series, vol 6. Raven Press, New York, 1980.

Huang, X-F., and Paxinos, G. Human intermediate reticular zone: A cyto- and chemoarchitectonic study. *J Comp Neurol* 360:571, 1995.

Kinomura, S., et al. Activation by attention of the human reticular formation and thalamic intralaminar nuclei. *Science*, 271:512, 1996.

Mesulam, M.-M., et al. Human reticular formation: Cholinergic neurons of the pedunculopontine and laterodorsal tegmental nuclei and some cytochemical comparisons to forebrain cholinergic neurons. *J Comp Neurol*, 281:611, 1989.

Scheibel, M. E., and Scheibel, A. E. Structural substrates for integrative patterns in the brainstem reticular core. In: Jasper, H. H., et al., eds. *Reticular Formation of the Brain*. Little Brown, Boston, 1958.

PEARSON
myhealthprofessionskit

Use this address to access the Companion Website created for this textbook. Simply select "Physical Therapy" from the choice of disciplines. Find this book and log in using your username and password to access self-assessment questions, a glossary, and more.

Brainstem III: Organization, Blood Supply, and Clinical Correlates

LEARNING OUTCOMES

This chapter prepares the reader to:

1. Identify specific levels of the brainstem from which typical cross sections are derived.

2. Compare the appearance of cross sections from the medulla, pons, and midbrain in terms of major distinguishing features of each.

3. In representative cross sections through the brainstem from medulla to pons, identify the following structures: ascending through tracts (DC-ML, STT), descending through tracts (CST), cranial nerve nuclei and nerves, and cerebellar peduncles.

4. Contrast the shape of the ventricles from the medulla to midbrain and explain the reasons for the changing shape.

5. Predict the classic symptoms associated with occlusion of the main blood vessels of the brainstem.

6. In representative cross sections of the brainstem, depict the area that would be damaged with occlusion of specific blood vessels.

7. Relate symptoms to the specific structures that are affected for specific brainstem syndromes.

8. Compare and contrast the impairments that would be expected with the classic syndromes of the brainstem from medulla to midbrain.

ACRONYMS

AICA Anterior inferior cerebellar artery

AL Anterolateral system

ARAS Ascending reticular activating system

CST Corticospinal tract

DC-ML Dorsal column–medial lemniscus system

ML Medial lemniscus

PICA Posterior inferior cerebellar artery

PCA Posterior cerebral artery

PSA Posterior spinal artery

SCA Superior cerebellar artery

STT Spinothalamic tract

VPL Ventral posterolateral nucleus

Introduction

Application of brainstem anatomy in clinical practice requires a mastery of three-dimensional relationships of the brainstem's internal structures from medulla to midbrain. This mastery is necessary in order to relate (and predict) the occurrence of specific symptoms to the structures affected by specific disorders (e.g., strokes associated with particular blood vessels, tumors in specific locations, traumatic injuries). For example, the posterior inferior cerebellar artery supplies a wedge-shaped region of lateral medulla. By knowing the internal structures that reside in that region, we can predict the symptoms that likely will occur and their laterality. More specifically, by knowing the location of cranial nerve nuclei, we can predict the symptoms and their laterality that should be manifest in the head and neck. By knowing the location of the long ascending and descending pathways that traverse the entirety of the brainstem connecting the spinal cord and cerebral cortex, we can anticipate whether sensory or motor loss will occur in the extremities and trunk. And by knowing where decussations in fiber tracts occur in relation to the brainstem, it is possible to anticipate whether symptoms will occur ipsilateral or contralateral to the lesion site. Furthermore, a working knowledge of three-dimensional neuroanatomy is needed to recognize the locations of specific brainstem structures in sectional slices obtained by CT or MRI scans.

This chapter draws on information presented in previous chapters. However, in this chapter, the information is synthesized to assist in developing a three-dimensional appreciation of brainstem anatomy in relation to function.

The first major section of this chapter provides an overview of several level-determining brainstem features. In the second major section, images are presented, depicting transverse sections through each of the three brainstem subdivisions. The major structures in each section are labeled in accompanying line drawings of the section. By utilizing information presented in the first section of the chapter and the related figures, we can begin to recognize key features in cross section. The third major section of this chapter applies the preceding information to predict impairments associated with disorders of specific blood vessels. The different arteries that nourish the brainstem are described, along with their regionally specific vascular territories. Occlusion of four vessels and the resulting vascular syndromes are then presented. Although these syndromes are not often encountered in pure form in clinical practice, they are excellent instructional cases by which learners can appreciate the relationship of vascular supply to resulting impairments, which facilitates an understanding of the three-dimensional organization of the brainstem.

ORGANIZATIONAL PRINCIPLES FOR AN UNDERSTANDING OF INTERNAL BRAINSTEM STRUCTURE

An understanding of internal brainstem structure is readily appreciated by studying its cross-sectional anatomy. In Chapter 5, we learned how to differentiate the three brainstem subdivisions from one another in cross sections by looking at specific external features that are present throughout the caudorostral extent of that subdivision. We

then learned to determine whether the section was taken through a caudal or rostral level of that particular subdivision by considering additional external features that are specific to that level. The criteria for these differentiations are summarized in Table 15-1 ■ and were described in Chapter 2.

In this chapter, we examine additional internal anatomical features that assist us in understanding the brainstem's internal structure and recognizing brainstem level. We shall organize these features in terms of four

Table 15-1 Defining Brainstem Level by External Features

SUBDIVISION	DETERMINING FEATURE	CAUDAL TO ROSTRAL
Medulla	Pyramids	Configuration of the fourth ventricle
		Configuration of inferior cerebellar peduncle
		Configuration of the olivary eminence
Pons	Basilar pons	Configuration of the fourth ventricle
	Transverse fibers of the pons	Configuration of basilar pons
		Superior cerebellar peduncle
Midbrain	Cerebral peduncles	Inferior colliculi
	Interpeduncular fossa	Superior colliculi

organizational principles, understanding that their order of discussion is not a reflection of their importance. The first principle involves the distribution of the cranial nerves and their nuclei across the three brainstem subdivisions. In general, these nuclei are located at longitudinal levels in the brainstem interior that correspond approximately to the exterior (surface) attachment sites of the cranial nerves. The second principle concerns the long ascending sensory and descending motor tracts that traverse the entire brainstem without synaptic interruption. These are considered the "through tracts" and include the ascending somatosensory tracts (dorsal column–medial lemniscal system, spinothalamic tract) and the descending pyramidal tract (corticospinal tract). The third organizational principle involves the distinctive shape of the ventricular system in the different brainstem subdivisions. The fourth principle applies to the disposition of the cerebellar peduncles within the three brainstem subdivisions. The inferior and superior cerebellar peduncles frame the outlines of the fourth ventricle, contributing to the shape (as noted in the third principle).

The first principle involving the cranial nerves was addressed, initially, in Chapter 1 and again in Chapters 2 and 13. Recall that each subdivision of the brainstem bears the attachments of a unique set of cranial nerves. Although the correspondence is not exact, each subdivision will house the sensory and/or motor nuclei of those nerves. But, as discussed in Chapter 14, one cranial nerve dramatically violates this principle—the trigeminal nerve. While the nerve attaches to the brainstem at a midpontine level, its sensory nuclei are spread throughout the *entire* brainstem as well as the upper cervical cord. This is because the somatic sensory component of the trigeminal nerve subserves the entire head, as well as being somatic sensory relay nuclei of other cranial nerves (see Chapter 14). In contrast, the much smaller motor component of the trigeminal nerve has its nucleus only at a midpontine level. The vestibular nuclei also have a widespread brainstem distribution, extending throughout most of the pons and medulla, even though cranial nerve (CN) VIII itself attaches at the ventrolateral aspect of caudal pons. The cranial nerve nuclei residing in each of the brainstem subdivisions are indicated in Figure 15-1 ■.

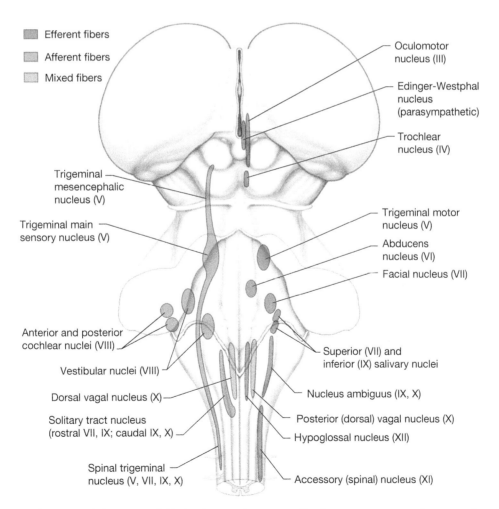

FIGURE 15-1 Distribution of cranial nerve nuclei in brainstem. As a generalized pattern, sensory columns are located laterally and motor columns more medially. Nuclei are also generally located within the brainstem level at which their associated nerve fibers emerge. A notable exception is the trigeminal nuclei, which span the entire length of the brainstem and upper cervical spinal cord.

Thought Question

What anatomic features of the brainstem frame the fourth ventricle?

Moreover, there is a generalized pattern of arrangement of cranial nerve sensory and motor nuclei within the brainstem. This arrangement results from their repositioning (relative to the spinal cord) in the developing embryo. The four cell columns in the developing spinal cord are arranged dorsoventrally in reference to the **sulcus limitans**, with sensory columns dorsal, motor columns ventral, and visceral sensory and visceral motor columns immediately flanking the sulcus limitans (see Figure 1-22). But because of the pontine flexure (refer back to Chapter 1), the ventricular system flattens out into the large fourth ventricle and rhomboid fossa so that these cell columns are now dorsally located and oriented mediolaterally, with the motor columns medial, the sensory columns lateral, and the visceral columns in between, closest to the sulcus limitans (see Figure 1-23). In addition to these general cell columns and nuclei present in both the spinal cord and brainstem, the brainstem contains special sensory and branchial motor nuclei not found in the spinal cord. Thus, as stated in Chapter 13, there are six functional categories of cranial nerve fibers and nuclei, but it is important to emphasize that all six cranial nerves do not simultaneously reside in any of the three brainstem subdivisions. The medulla is unique among the three brainstem subdivisions in that cross sections through rostral levels do reveal the simultaneous presence of all six categories of cranial nerve nuclei, although the branchial motor and general somatic afferent nuclei have migrated ventrally from their embryologically predicted dorsal locations. Although the pons also contains the nuclei of all six functional categories, they are differentially distributed over its caudorostral extent such that all six are not captured in a single cross section. The midbrain contains only three of the six categories.

There are caveats related to this principle. First, with a few notable exceptions that will be pointed out later, the rostrocaudal extents of many cranial nerve nuclei do not confine themselves just to caudal or rostral levels of that subdivision. Second, in order to clearly delineate the positions of the cranial nerve nuclei, one needs to examine Nissl stained sections that reveal the location of their cell bodies—and these are not used in this text. Third, in this text, only six representative transverse brainstem sections are included, and their spacing is not sufficiently close to reveal all of the cranial nerve nuclei.

The nuclei that help identify the brainstem level in cross sections are as follows: the medially located abducens

nucleus (somatic motor) and laterally positioned facial nucleus (branchial motor) are at a caudal pontine level; the laterally located main sensory (general sensory afferent) and motor (branchial motor) trigeminal nuclei are at a midpontine level; the medially located trochlear nucleus (somatic motor) resides in caudal midbrain, while the medially located oculomotor nucleus (somatic motor) resides predominantly in rostral midbrain.

The second principle involves the disposition of the through tracts that are present in all transverse sections taken at any level of the brainstem. These tracts reposition themselves as they approach the target structures in which they will terminate. This is easiest to visualize in the mediolateral dimension but occurs in other dimensions as well. Note in Figure 1-13 that in moving rostrally from the spinal cord through the brainstem to the thalamus and then cerebral cortex, there is a progressive increase in the width of the CNS. Reciprocally, in moving caudally from the cerebral cortex to the thalamus through the brainstem and then to the spinal cord, there is a progressive constriction in the mediolateral dimension.

Thought Question

The DC-ML migrates laterally as it progresses rostrally from the spinal cord. Considering both the configuration of the brainstem and the location of the thalamus, explain this migration.

One of the two ascending somatosensory through tracts of the brainstem, the medial lemniscus, begins in the caudal medulla in the midline as the decussation of the medial lemniscus (Figure 15-2 ■). Then, in ascending through the medulla, the medial lemnisci abut one another on either side of the midline. The medial lemniscus must reposition itself in ascending through the brainstem in order to be properly positioned to terminate in the laterally placed VPL nucleus of the thalamus. It does this, first, by changing its orientation from a dorsoventrally oriented ribbon (the term *lemniscus* means ribbon) in the medulla to a transversely oriented ribbon in the pons. One way to visualize this change in orientation is that areas related to the "feet" of the somatotopically organized medial lemniscus in the medulla kick upward and outward as they enter the pons to avoid hitting the bridge (the term *pons* means bridge) consisting of the transverse fibers of the pons (i.e., the middle cerebellar peduncle). The dorsally and medially located abducens nucleus and the ventrally and laterally located facial nucleus are both visible as the transition occurs to a mediolaterally oriented medial lemniscus. By a midpontine level, this shift brings the "feet" of the ML immediately

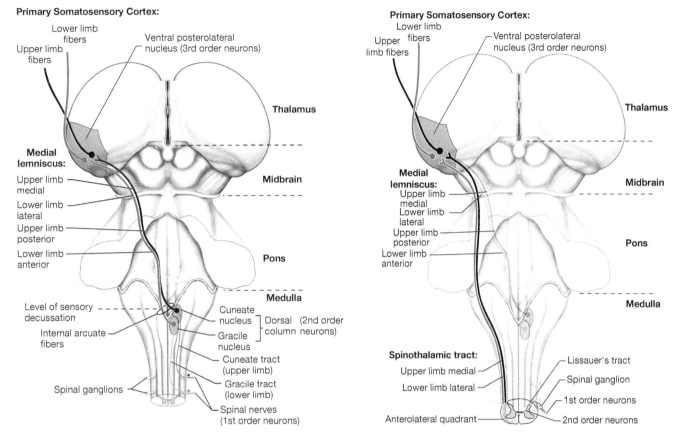

FIGURE 15-2 Decussation of medial lemniscus. Fibers leaving the cuneate and gracile nuclei decussate in the medulla as the internal arcuate fibers. As they ascend the brainstem, they begin medially and project superiorly and laterally to reach the ventral posterior lateral nucleus of the thalamus.

adjacent to the second of the through ascending somatosensory systems—the neospinothalamic component of the anterolateral system. When this occurs, the laterally located motor and main sensory trigeminal nuclei can be seen.

The AL system, containing the spinothalamic tract (STT), has maintained a lateral position throughout the medulla. Beginning at a midpontine level and extending throughout the midbrain, the ML and AL systems form a continuous band of somatosensory fibers, those of the AL being immediately lateral to those of the ML. The second positional change of the through sensory systems is that they must continue to shift laterally and bend dorsally in order to be properly positioned to synapse in the somatotopically organized VPL nucleus of the thalamus. As these tracts shift laterally and dorsally, the medially located trochlear nucleus can be seen and then the medially located oculomotor nucleus; both are situated immediately ventral to the periaqueductal gray. In the VPL nucleus of the thalamus, the arm is represented medially and the leg laterally. Fibers of the AL and DC-ML systems merge into a common somatotopic

pattern with the arm medial and leg (foot) lateral as they enter the VPL nucleus.

> **Thought Question**
>
> Do you remember where the trigeminal thalamic tract joins with the medial lemniscus?

A reverse positional shift occurs in the corticospinal tract—the single through descending motor tract of the brainstem. Rather than diverging, as in the case of the somatosensory through tracts as they approach their thalamic termination, the corticospinal projections converge in the posterior limb of the internal capsule and then travel in a relatively tight bundle. From the posterior limbs of the internal capsules, they enter the cerebral peduncles of the midbrain and descend through the pons. Within the medulla, each corticospinal tract (CST) flanks the midline anterior median fissure as a medullary pyramid (Figure 15-3 ■). Fibers of the medullary

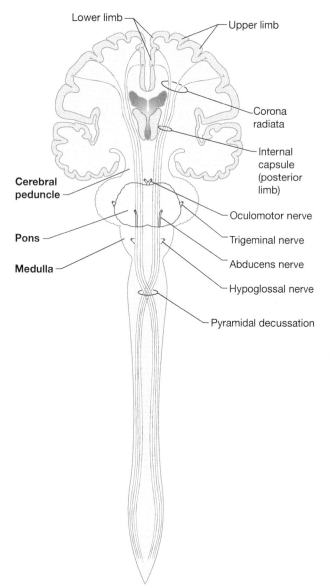

FIGURE 15-3 Descending corticospinal tract fibers converge in the posterior limb of the internal capsule. They continue to project inferiorly and medially to their decussation in the caudal medulla.

pyramids then attain the midline in the caudalmost medulla, where most axons decussate in the pyramidal decussation and then enter the cervical spinal cord. The pyramidal decussation is situated caudal to the decussation of the medial lemniscus.

Thought Question

Which tract decussates most rostrally—the DC-ML or the CST?

In the third organizational principle, consideration is given to the essential shape of the ventricular system

as we progress rostrally through the three brainstem subdivisions. The system forms as a narrow canal in the caudal medulla and ends as another narrow canal in the midbrain; in between, however, it expands dramatically then contracts, giving it a rhomboid shape (see Figure 2-10). Remember that the term *rhomboid*, while literally meaning an equilateral parallelogram, can be applied to the shape of a diamond. The rhomboid fossa represents the floor of the fourth ventricle so that the fourth ventricle is shaped like a diamond with an expanded lateral recess on either side. Thus, the fourth ventricle overlying the dorsal surfaces of both the medulla and pons begins in the caudal medulla (called the "closed" medulla) as a continuation of the narrow central canal of the spinal cord surrounded by central gray substance, expands progressively over the extent of the medulla (called the "open" medulla because there are no structures of the medulla forming the roof), has its widest mediolateral expanse with lateral recesses at approximately the junction of the medulla and pons, then begins to narrow in the caudal pons (see Figure 5-24). The narrowing continues progressively so that the fourth ventricle narrows rostrally to form the cerebral aqueduct at the level of the midbrain, located in the center of the periaqueductal gray. Thus, the shape of the ventricular system is a key to recognizing where you are in a section of the brainstem.

Thought Question

Which of the cerebellar peduncles decussate, and where?

In the fourth organizational principle, consideration is given to the three pairs of cerebellar peduncles because their presence and spatial separation also help us in recognizing brainstem level. The inferior and superior cerebellar peduncles frame the fourth ventricle, with the inferior peduncles exhibiting the characteristic of divergence and the superior peduncles the characteristic of convergence, again repositioning themselves in preparation for their terminations (Figure 15-4 ■). The inferior cerebellar peduncles begin in the caudal medulla and progressively expand in size as they ascend through the medulla, where they form the lateral aspect of the caudal portion of the fourth ventricle. As they do so, they are diverging laterally as the rhomboid fossa expands. One of the most conspicuous features of the pons is the massive middle cerebellar peduncles that seem to suspend the pons in a sling from the cerebellum. Note that in the caudal pons, the middle cerebellar peduncles are lateral to the inferior cerebellar peduncles. In rostral pons, as the fourth ventricle is narrowing, the superior cerebellar peduncles make their appearance and frame the lateral walls of the remaining rostral portion of the fourth

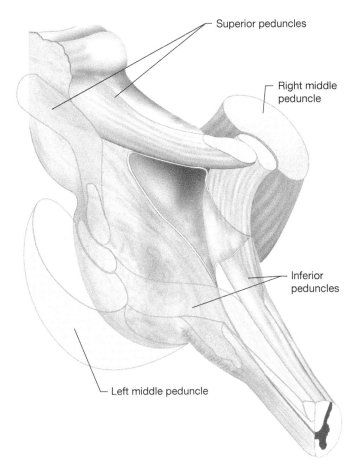

FIGURE 15-4 Three pairs of cerebellar peduncles frame the fourth ventricle. The superior cerebellar peduncles are located in the caudal midbrain, the middle cerebellar peduncle in the pons, and the inferior cerebellar peduncles in the rostral medulla.

ventricle. As the fourth ventricle narrows, the two superior cerebellar peduncles converge. Upon reaching the midbrain, the superior cerebellar peduncles dip deeply into the midbrain tegmentum and bear no immediate relation to the cerebral aqueduct. Their convergence, however, "prepares" them to cross in the midline of caudal midbrain as the **decussation of the superior cerebellar peduncle**. The decussation occurs at the level of the trochlear nucleus and is completed just caudal to the red nucleus in the midbrain, at the level of the oculomotor nucleus.

Thought Question

What do you recall about the attachments to the brainstem of the cranial nerves, the medial lateral arrangement of cranial nerve nuclei within the brainstem, and the relative position of the ascending and descending long tracts through the brainstem?

REPRESENTATIVE CROSS SECTIONS THROUGH THE BRAINSTEM

In this section, we present cross sections of the brainstem with some of the major structures of importance to rehabilitation highlighted. We begin with a lateral view of the brainstem (Figure 15-5 ■), showing the levels at which six Weigert stained cross sections are taken (Figures 15-6 ■ through 15-11 ■). Finally, the major structures, presented at the different levels of the brainstem, are identified schematically in (Figure 15-12 ■).

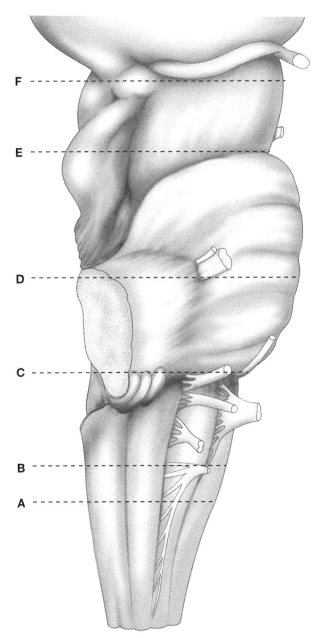

FIGURE 15-5 Lateral view of the brainstem. Cross sections that follow are of the (a) caudal medulla, (b) rostral medulla, (c) caudal pons, (d) rostral pons, (e) caudal midbrain, and (f) rostral midbrain.

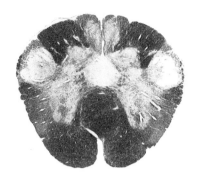

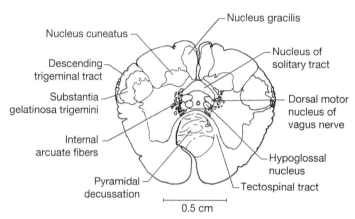

FIGURE 15-6 Caudal medulla with presence of nucleus gracilis and nucleus cuneatus dorsally and the pyramidal decussation ventrally.

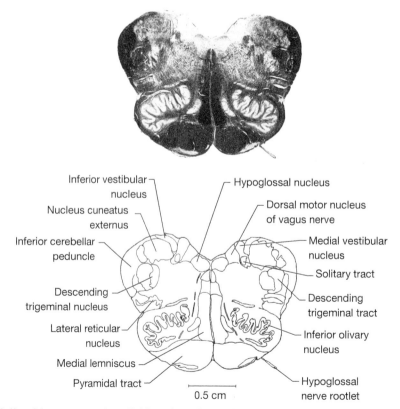

FIGURE 15-7 Rostral medulla with presence of medial lemniscus located near midline and the pyramids located ventrally.

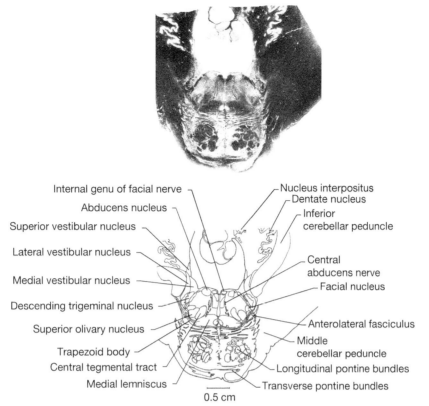

FIGURE 15-8 Caudal pons with medial lemniscus moving posterolaterally and the descending corticospinal tract in the longitudinal pontine bundles.

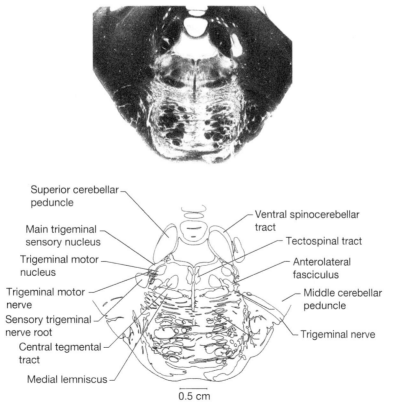

FIGURE 15-9 Rostral pons with the medial lemniscus and anterolateral fasciculus approximating as they ascend the brainstem.

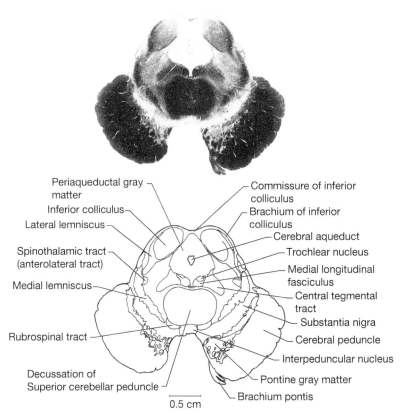

FIGURE 15-10 Caudal midbrain with the medial lemniscus and anterolateral tract in close proximity. Note the presence of the large cerebral peduncles ventrally and the inferior colliculi posteriorly.

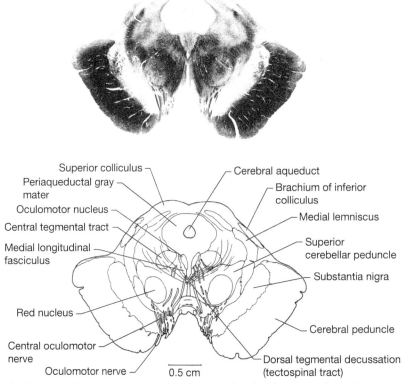

FIGURE 15-11 Rostral midbrain. Note the presence of the large cerebral peduncles ventrally and the superior colliculi posteriorly.

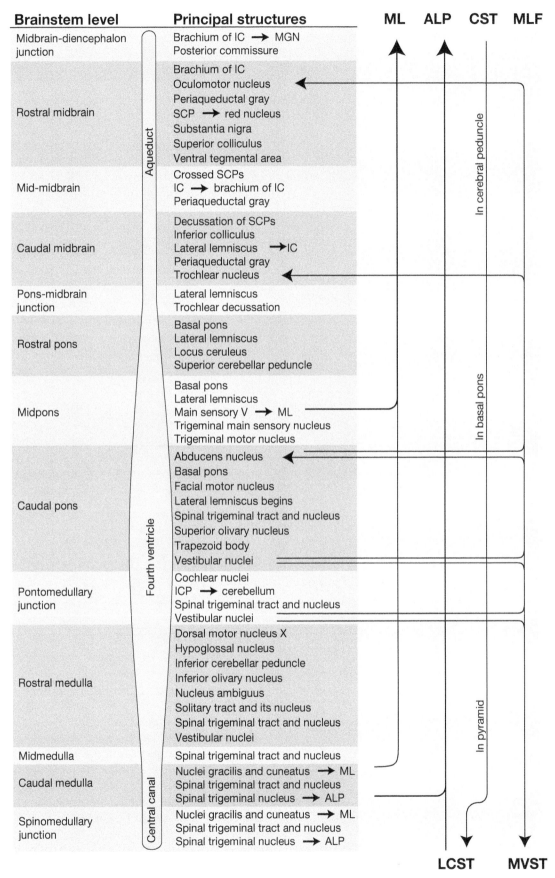

FIGURE 15-12 Schematic of the major structures present in the brainstem. ALP, anterolateral pathway; CST, corticospinal tract; MLF, medial longitudinal fasciculus; LCST, lateral cortical spinal tract; ML, medial lemniscus; MVST, medial vestibulospinal tract; IC, inferior colliculi; MGN, medial geniculate nucleus; SCP, superior cerebellar peduncles; SCTs, spinocerebellar tracts; ICP, inferior cerebellar peduncles

Table 15-2 Focal Vascular Syndromes of the Medulla

REGION	SYNDROME NAMES	VASCULAR SUPPLY	ANATOMICAL STRUCTURES	CLINICAL FEATURES
Lateral medulla	Wallenberg's syndrome, lateral medullary syndrome	Vertebral artery or PICA	Spinal trigeminal nucleus and tract	Ipsilateral facial decreased pain and temperature sense
			Spinothalamic tract	Contralateral body decreased pain and temperature sense
			Descending sympathetic fibers	Ipsilateral Horner's syndrome
			Nucleus ambiguus, fibers of CNs IX, X, XI	Dysphonia, dysphagia, dysarthria, diminished gag reflex, hiccups
			Vestibular nuclei	Nystagmus, diplopia, oscillopsia, vertigo, nausea and vomiting, lateropulsion
			Inferior cerebellar peduncle	Ipsilateral ataxia
Medial medulla	Medial medullary syndrome, inferior alternating hemiplegia	Paramedian branches of vertebral and anterior spinal arteries	Hypoglossal nucleus and/or exiting CN XII fibers	LMN paralysis of ipsilateral half of tongue
			Corticospinal tract	UMN paralysis of contralateral arm and leg
			Medial lemniscus	Contralateral decreased position, vibration, and discriminative touch sense

BLOOD SUPPLY OF THE BRAINSTEM AND NEUROVASCULAR SYNDROMES

Clinical Preview ················

Joe Garcia and Martin Chen both are residents in the skilled nursing facility where you work. Both were diagnosed with brainstem strokes at the level of the medulla; however, their symptoms differ greatly. For example, Joe has severe dizziness, whereas Martin is more bothered by difficulty eating and articulation of speech. As you read through this section, consider the following:

• Why do these two gentleman report being bothered by very different symptoms, given that both of them had a stroke affecting the medulla?

• Where in the medulla could these two strokes be located, and what blood supply might be involved?

• What other symptoms might each of them have?

Review of the Blood Supply

Thought Question

How do the PICA and the PCA differ in terms of their origins and the territories that they supply?

Recall from Chapter 2 that the blood supply of the brainstem is derived from the vertebrobasilar system and is part of the posterior circulation of the brain. The paired **vertebral arteries** arise from the subclavian arteries at the base of the neck and ascend through the transverse foramina of the upper six cervical vertebrae (see Figure 2-28). They then pierce the dura mater and enter the cranial cavity through the foramen magnum. Each ascends along the ventral surface of the medulla and unites with its counterpart from the opposite side at the caudal border of the pons to form the unpaired **basilar artery** (Figure 15-13 ■). The basilar artery ascends on the ventral pontine surface in the basilar sulcus to the level of the midbrain, where it bifurcates into the two **posterior cerebral arteries (PCAs)**. Thus, the three major components of the

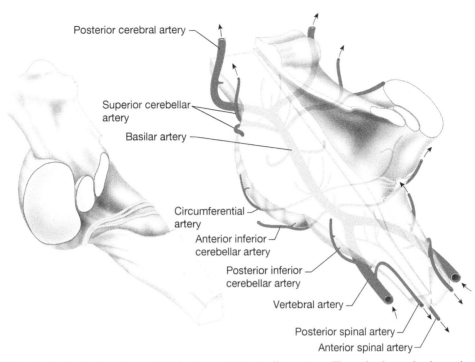

Posterior cerebral artery

Superior cerebellar artery

Basilar artery

Circumferential artery

Anterior inferior cerebellar artery

Posterior inferior cerebellar artery

Vertebral artery

Posterior spinal artery

Anterior spinal artery

FIGURE 15-13 Blood flow to the brainstem is provided by the vertebrobasilar system. The paired vertebral arteries join the caudal pons to form the single basilar artery. Many paired arteries arise from the basilar artery as it ascends the brainstem. At the level of the midbrain, the basilar artery bifurcates to form the paired posterior cerebral arteries.

vertebrobasilar system are the vertebral arteries, the basilar artery, and the PCAs. Each component supplies structures other than the brainstem, including the cerebellum (Chapter 6), diencephalon (Chapter 6), internal capsule, occipital lobes, and inferior and medial portions of the temporal lobes (Chapter 7).

Four main branches arise from the vertebral and basilar arteries. In caudal to rostral sequence, these are the **posterior inferior cerebellar artery (PICA)** that arises from each vertebral artery, the **anterior inferior cerebellar artery (AICA)** and the **superior cerebellar artery (SCA)**, both of which arise from the basilar artery, and finally the PCA that arises from the terminal splitting of the basilar artery as already noted (see Figure 15-13). The PICA usually is the largest of the three cerebellar arteries; it wraps around the lateral medulla and pursues a rather tortuous course as it does so. The AICA is the smallest of the three and arises from the proximal basilar artery just rostral to where the vertebral arteries fuse, at the level of caudal pons. The SCA arises from the most distal basilar artery at the level of rostral pons. The PCA wraps around the midbrain en route to the infero-medial surfaces of the temporal and occipital lobes. The oculomotor nerves pass between the SCA and PCA (see Figure 6-20).

The PICA, AICA, and SCA are referred to as **long circumferential arteries** because they wrap around the lateral surface of the brainstem to attain its dorsal surface. There also are numerous and unnamed **short circumferential arteries** that emerge from the basilar artery to supply the pons and midbrain. Penetrating branches are given off from these circumferential arteries that extend deeply into the lateral and dorsal brainstem. Penetrating branches are likewise given off from the proximal portion of the PCA that supplies the midbrain. Yet another set of penetrating branches are given off the vertebral and basilar arteries to supply the midline regions of all three subdivisions of the brainstem and are called **paramedian branches** (see Figure 15-13).

> **Thought Question**
>
> Which arteries that perfuse the brainstem arise from the vertebral artery, and which arise from the basilar artery? Describe the specific territory supplied by each.

CLINICAL CONNECTIONS

> **Thought Question**
>
> In preparation for the material in this section,
>
> 1. Recall the medial lateral arrangement of cranial nerves (refer back to development in Chapter 1).
> 2. Then review the position of the ascending and descending through tracts in the brainstem (Chapters 8–11).
> 3. Review the attachments of the cranial nerves and the location of their first-order neurons (Chapters 13 and 14).

The syndromes described here will help you synthesize information, although you will most likely not see them clinically in their pure form.

Medulla

As each vertebral artery ascends on the ventral surface of the medulla, it gives rise to an orderly sequence of arteries. From caudal to rostral these are the **posterior spinal artery (PSA)**, the posterior inferior cerebellar artery (PICA), and the **anterior spinal artery**. The posterior spinal artery is not a clinically significant source of blood to the medulla. However, the other two arteries are. The PICA is the largest branch of the vertebral artery. It winds posteriorly around the medulla and over the inferior cerebellar peduncle. As it does so, it gives off penetrating branches that supply structures in lateral medulla. Occlusion or bleeds in these arteries result in the lateral or medial medullary syndromes, as described next.

Lateral Medullary Syndrome (Wallenberg's Syndrome)

The lateral medullary syndrome, or **Wallenberg's syndrome**, is the most common vascular syndrome of the entire brainstem. It can occur in either a complete or modified form and is most often attributed to occlusion of the PICA. However, because of the variability of the brainstem's blood supply, it is incorrect to regard Wallenberg's syndrome as synonymous with PICA occlusion. Most cases actually may be due to occlusion of the parent vertebral artery. In either situation, a wedge-shaped region of the lateral medulla is infarcted (Figure 15-14a ■). Full-blown Wallenberg's syndrome includes involvement of a number of tracts and nuclei with characteristic signs and symptoms.

Note that this damage affects the sense of equilibrium and the control of eye movement. For now, it is important to learn the expected signs and symptoms. However, the vestibular and visual systems, and the consequences of damage to these systems, are discussed in detail in Chapters 17 and 18, respectively.

Structures damaged in Wallenberg's syndrome include the ascending spinothalamic tract; the spinal trigeminal system; the descending sympathetic fibers; and nuclei for cranial nerves VIII, IX, X, and XI. Damage to the ascending spinothalamic tract (STT) results in impaired pain and temperature sensibility over the *contralateral* half of the body. (Recall from Chapter 9 that tracts carrying this information decussated in the spinal cord.) There is a concurrent loss of pain and temperature sensation over all or part of the *ipsilateral* half of the face due to involvement of the spinal trigeminal system, sometimes with pain in the face. Damage to the descending sympathetic tract results in a triad of symptoms referred to as an ipsilateral **Horner's syndrome** in which the patient will have a small pupil (**meiosis**), drooping of the upper eyelid (**ptosis**), and decreased sweating on one side of the face (**anhydrosis**). Damage to the laterally located nucleus ambiguus and fibers of cranial nerves IX, X, and XI results in a constellation of symptoms including hoarseness (**dysphonia**), difficulty swallowing (**dysphagia**), difficulty speaking (**dysarthria**), diminished **gag reflex**, and the presence of hiccups.

> **Thought Question**
>
> What is Horner's syndrome? What tract must have been damaged in order for this syndrome to occur?

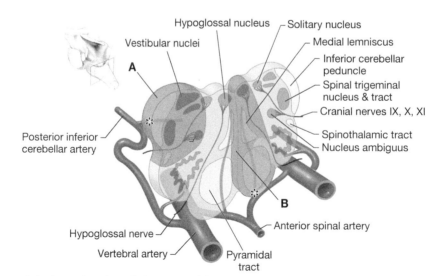

FIGURE 15-14 Infarcts of the lateral and medial medulla. (a) Occlusion of the PICA results in lateral medullary syndrome (Wallenberg's syndrome). (b) Occlusion of the paramedian branches of the anterior spinal artery results in medial medullary syndrome (alternating hypoglossal hemiplegia or inferior alternating hemiplegia).

Damage to the vestibular nuclei, which also reside in the lateral medulla, results in problems related to the control of eye movement, affecting visual acuity and balance because of the vestibular system's role in the vestibular ocular reflex (VOR) (see Chapter 17). There may be observable involuntary rhythmic movements of the eyes, referred to as **nystagmus**. Patients may report double vision (**diplopia**) and may report a sensation that objects are oscillating when looking at them (**oscillopsia**). Likewise, they may report the sensation that they are turning or that external objects are whirling. This is referred to as **vertigo** and may be accompanied by nausea and vomiting. There may be a tendency to fall sideways without accompanying vertigo. This is known as *lateralpulsion*, and it occurs toward the side of the lesion (ipsiversive). Damage to the fibers projecting to the cerebellum (olivocerebellar, spinocerebellar, and/or inferior cerebellar peduncle) results in incoordination of movements (**ataxia**) on the side of the body ipsilateral to the lesion.

Thought Question

In this chapter, you should begin to relate anatomical lesions to functional consequences. Consider the following in relation to Wallenberg's syndrome:

1. Based on your knowledge to this point, what nuclei or tract(s) may be involved when a person has nystagmus and vertigo?
2. Explain why pain and temperature are diminished ipsilaterally in the face but contralaterally in the body.
3. A number of different nerves or nuclei are affected in this syndrome. Which symptoms relate to which cranial nerves or nuclei? What is the commonality in location of these structures, explaining their involvement in this syndrome?

Medial Medullary Syndrome (Alternating Hypoglossal Hemiplegia)

The **medial medullary syndrome** is a less common syndrome, resulting from occlusion of the proximal anterior spinal artery. The anterior spinal artery arises near the termination of each vertebral artery, descends on the anterior surface of the medulla, and unites with its fellow of the opposite side at the level of the foramen magnum. As

it descends, each anterior spinal artery gives rise to paramedian penetrating branches that supply a vertical strip of the medulla adjacent to the midline. This strip may extend as far dorsally as the floor of the fourth ventricle (Figure 15-14b). Infarction of the paramedian territory supplied by these vessels results in the medial medullary syndrome. The full-blown medial medullary syndrome includes involvement of a number of tracts and nuclei with characteristic signs and symptoms as outlined below.

Damage to the ascending medial lemniscus results in loss of discriminative touch and kinesthetic sense of the contralateral one-half of the body. Damage to the medullary pyramid, containing descending fibers of the corticospinal tract, results in weakness of the contralateral arm, trunk and leg.

Damage to the hypoglossal nucleus, or cranial nerve XII, results in LMN paralysis and atrophy of the ipsilateral one-half of the tongue. This syndrome also is called **alternating hypoglossal hemiplegia**, or **inferior alternating hemiplegia**. The term derives from the fact that there is an LMN paralysis of the *ipsilateral* half of the tongue and an UMN paralysis of the *contralateral* arm, trunk, and leg. Table 15-2 ■ on page 362 summarizes focal vascular syndromes of the medulla.

Pons

The pons is nourished by arterial branches of the basilar artery. Ascending in the basilar sulcus of the pons, the major branches given off from the basilar artery are the AICA and the SCA, the latter arising near the termination of the basilar artery. Both wrap around the lateral surface of the pons and, as they do so, give off penetrating branches. However, the basilar artery gives off other clinically relevant arteries. First, paramedial arteries nourish structures in vertical strips of the pons adjacent to the midline. Second, there are short and long circumferential branches given off from the basilar artery as it ascends between the AICA and SCA. These supply structures in lateral pons.

Medial (Paramedian) Inferior Pontine Syndrome

Medial (paramedian) inferior pontine syndrome, also called **middle alternating hemiplegia**, results from occlusion of the paramedian branches of the basilar artery that supply a wedge of pons on either side of the midline

---

Disorders 15-1: Nystagmus

Nystagmus refers to involuntary conjugate eye deviations in response to activation of the semicircular canals, wherein the eyes rhythmically move rapidly back and forth. Nystagmus occurs in healthy individuals when head rotations are too large to be compensated for by the visual ocular reflex or

when visual stimuli move too rapidly to be fixed on the retina. Nystagmus can also occur due to a variety of pathological conditions affecting the PNS or CNS. Nystagmus is discussed in detail in Chapter 17.

Table 15-3 Focal Vascular Syndromes of the Pons

REGION	SYNDROME NAMES	VASCULAR SUPPLY	ANATOMICAL STRUCTURES	CLINICAL FEATURES
Medial inferior pontine basis and tegmentum	Medial (paramedian) inferior pontine syndrome, middle alternating hemiplegia	Paramedian branches of basilar artery	Exiting fibers of CN VI	LMN paralysis of ipsilateral lateral rectus muscle causing medial deviation of ipsilateral eye
			Paramedian pontine reticular formation	Ipsilateral horizontal gaze palsy
			Corticospinal and corticobulbar tracts	UMN spastic paralysis of contralateral lower face, arm, and leg
			Medial lemniscus	Contralateral body decreased position, vibration, and discriminative touch sense
			Axons forming the middle cerebellar peduncle	Limb and gait ataxia
Dorsolateral rostral pons	Lateral superior pontine syndrome, syndrome of the SCA	SCA	Superior cerebellar peduncle	Ipsilateral limb and gait ataxia, intention tremor
			Spinothalamic and trigeminothalamic tracts	Contralateral decreased body and face pain and temperature sense
			Medial lemniscus	Contralateral leg decreased position, vibration, and discriminative touch sense
			Descending sympathetic fibers	Ipsilateral Horner's syndrome

(Figure 15-15 ■). Occlusion of these branches on one side damages ascending and descending structures as well as cranial nerves and the lateral gaze center. Involvement of the medial lemniscus causes impaired tactile (touch), vibration, and proprioceptive (position) sense on the opposite half of the body. Involvement of the corticobulbar and corticospinal tracts results in contralateral spastic

paralysis of the lower face, arm, and leg. Infarction of the fibers of CN VI (abducens) results in medial deviation of the ipsilateral eye due to a weakness of the lateral rectus muscle (**medial strabismus**). This also causes double vision when looking to the side. There is also an inability to look laterally toward the side of the lesion (paralysis of conjugate gaze) due to involvement of the pontine center for

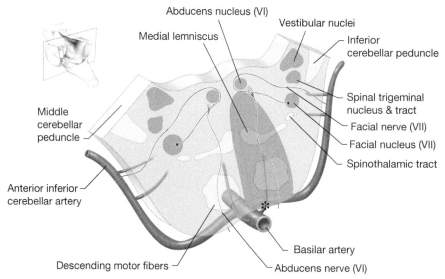

Abducens nucleus (VI)
Medial lemniscus
Vestibular nuclei
Inferior cerebellar peduncle
Spinal trigeminal nucleus & tract
Facial nerve (VII)
Facial nucleus (VII)
Spinothalamic tract
Middle cerebellar peduncle
Anterior inferior cerebellar artery
Basilar artery
Descending motor fibers
Abducens nerve (VI)

FIGURE 15-15 Occlusion of the paramedian branch of the basilar artery results in medial (paramedian) inferior pontine syndrome.

lateral gaze. Furthermore, because of involvement of fibers projecting to the cerebellum within the middle cerebellar peduncle, there may be uncoordinated movements of the limbs and gait (ataxia).

Lateral Superior Pontine Syndrome (Syndrome of the Superior Cerebellar Artery)

The **lateral superior pontine syndrome** results from occlusion of the SCA, the last long circumferential branch of the basilar artery (Figure 15-16 ■) that supplies the lateral pons. As such, it results in damage to ascending and descending tracts of the lateral pons. Somatosensory deficits occur due to involvement of the medial lemniscus, spinothalamic, and trigeminothalamic (face) tracts. These include contralateral loss of discriminative touch, vibration, and position sense more in the leg than in the arm and a contralateral loss of pain and temperature sensation from the trunk, leg, arm, and face. As also seen with damage to the lateral medulla, damage to the lateral pons results in an ipsilateral Horner's syndrome due to involvement of the descending sympathetic tract. Due to involvement of fibers projecting to or coming from the cerebellum in the middle and superior cerebellar peduncles, ataxia of the limbs and gait on the side of the lesion, falling to the side of the lesion, and **intention tremor** on the side of the lesion are also characteristic of this syndrome.

Complete Basilar Syndrome

The **complete basilar syndrome** results from bilateral occlusion that affects both paramedian and circumferential arteries. Such bilateral occlusion produces an incomplete ischemic transection of the brainstem. Usually, the patient is in a coma and shows pinpoint, irregular, or unequal pupils; bilateral conjugate gaze paralysis; or internuclear opthalmoplegia and paralysis of all limbs. Few patients survive for more than a few days with this syndrome.

Locked-In Syndrome

The **locked-in syndrome** may follow occlusion of the basilar artery. This syndrome is quite distinct from syndromes in which consciousness is disturbed, as in the complete basilar syndrome discussed earlier in which coma occurs. An infarct confined to the ventral pons spares both the ascending somatosensory pathways responsible for the perception of bodily sensations, as well as the ascending system of neurons that is responsible for maintaining arousal and wakefulness (ARAS, see Chapter 5). As a result, the patient is conscious—he or she is alert, aware of the environment, and understands what is said. However, the lesion interrupts the corticospinal and corticobulbar tracts located in the ventral pons, leaving the individual in a state of near-total motor paralysis, including an inability to speak and eat. Thus, although consciousness is retained, it is virtually inexpressible. In the full-blown locked-in syndrome, only vertical eye movements and convergence remain. The vertical eye movements are intact because the vertical gaze center is in the midbrain. In contrast, the horizontal eye movements are lost because the horizontal gaze center is in the pons. Thus, horizontal eye movement is damaged in this syndrome, but vertical eye movement is unscathed. Furthermore, somatosensory sensations can be intact or disrupted in this syndrome.

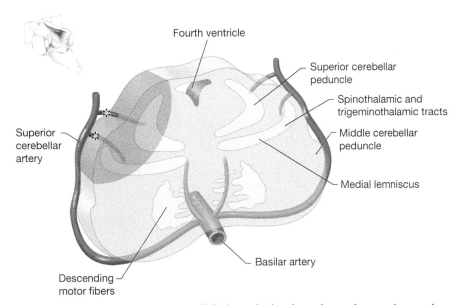

FIGURE 15-16 Occlusion of the superior cerebellar artery (SCA) results in a lateral superior pontine syndrome.

Neuropathology Box 15-1: Experience of the Locked-In Syndrome

None of us are likely to relate, even remotely, to the experience of enduring what certainly must be the ultimate in agonizing frustration. However, the late Jean-Dominique Bauby, in a most remarkable autobiography painstakingly put to paper by an assistant transcribing Bauby's eye blinks, described his "locked-in experience" in *The Diving Bell and the Butterfly*.

Table 15-3 ■ summarizes several of the many focal vascular syndromes of the pons.

Midbrain

The midbrain is nourished by penetrating branches from the top of the basilar artery as well as by branches from the proximal portions of the PCA. Arising from the bifurcation of the basilar artery, each PCA passes laterally, parallel to the SCA, and winds around the cerebral peduncle. Like arteries supplying the pons, branches of these arteries can be grouped into paramedian arteries that supply structures on either side of the midline and short and long circumferential arteries that nourish lateral and dorsal regions of the midbrain.

> ### Thought Question
>
> You are working with a person who has Horner's syndrome. Name two possible lesions that could cause this syndrome. What other symptoms would you look for to determine where the lesion most likely is located?

Weber's Syndrome

Weber's syndrome is a paramedian syndrome also referred to as **superior alternating hemiplegia**. It is caused by infarction in the territory of the midbrain supplied by the paramedian penetrating branches of the PCA. These branches are sometimes called the interpeduncular branches (Figure 15-17a ■). This syndrome is characterized by deficits of the motor system. Involvement of the descending tracts within the cerebral peduncle results in contralateral UMN hemiparesis of the trunk and extremities (due to involvement of the corticospinal tract) and an UMN weakness of the contralateral lower half of the face, tongue, and palate (due to involvement of the corticobulbar tract). Because of the involvement of CN III (the oculomotor nerve), a complete LMN paralysis of specific muscles that move the eyes occurs. This is referred to as an oculomotor nerve paralysis, third-nerve palsy, or oculomotor ophthalmoplegia. The eye on the side of the damage (the ipsilateral side) is deviated laterally (abducted) and depressed. The upper eyelid droops (ptosis), the pupil is dilated (**mydriatic**), and it will not constrict properly when a light is shone in that eye (**fixed pupil**) due to loss of the pupillary light reflex. The ascending DC-ML and STT are more laterally located and thus are spared in this syndrome.

Benedikt's Syndrome

Benedikt's syndrome results from occlusion of penetrating branches of the PCA that supply the tegmentum of the midbrain (Figure 15-17b). With damage to the oculomotor nuclei and nerve, there is a complete oculomotor nerve paralysis (see discussion of Weber's syndrome). Due to involvement of the cerebellothalamic tract that connects the cerebellum with the thalamus (see Chapter 19), there

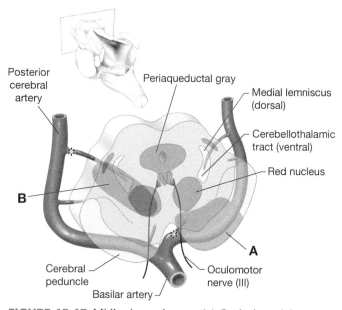

FIGURE 15-17 Midbrain syndromes. (a) Occlusion of the paramedian penetrating branches of the PCA results in superior alternating hemiplegia (Weber's syndrome). (b) Occlusion of the penetrating branches of the PCA that supply the tegmentum results in Benedikt's syndrome.

Table 15-4 Focal Vascular Syndromes of the Midbrain

REGION	SYNDROME NAMES	VASCULAR SUPPLY	ANATOMICAL STRUCTURES	CLINICAL FEATURES
Medial midbrain cerebral peduncle (basis pedunculi)	Weber's syndrome, superior alternating hemiplegia	Paramedian branches of PCA and top of basilar artery	Exiting fibers of CN III Corticobulbar and corticospinal tracts in cerebral peduncle	Ipsilateral LMN third-nerve palsy Contralateral UMN spastic paralysis of the lower half of the face, tongue, palate, arm, and leg
Midbrain tegmentum	Benedikt's syndrome	Branches of PCA	Exiting fibers of CN III Fibers of superior cerebellar peduncle	Ipsilateral LMN third-nerve palsy Contralateral ataxia and intention tremor

is an associated tremor in the contralateral extremities. Movements of the extremities may also be uncoordinated (ataxia).

Associated Signs

The syndromes described in the preceding sections may occur in combination with other deficits such as hemiballism and apathetic akinetic mutism. **Hemiballism** has a variety of causes, but one of the most common is involvement of a penetrating small branch of the PCA. The disorder consists of violent, forceful, flinging involuntary movements of the contralateral extremities. **Apathetic akinetic mutism** results from an infarction in

Thought Question

What differentiates apathetic akinetic mutism from locked-in syndrome?

the territory of the midbrain periaqueductal gray matter. In this condition, the patient is in a drowsy, relatively immobile state and can only be aroused with strong stimulation.

Table 15-4 ■ summarizes several of the many focal vascular syndromes of the midbrain.

Summary

The first section of this chapter discussed the principles by which the brainstem is organized. In the second major section, transverse sections were presented, showing the principal structural contents at each of six levels. This information was followed by a discussion of the blood supply of each of the three brainstem subdivisions,

derived from penetrating branches of the vertebrobasilar system. Representative neurovascular syndromes were presented, each of which follows occlusion of specific vessels. These syndromes illustrate the clinical relevance of regional anatomy of the brainstem and assist in learning relationships between structure and function.

Applications

1. Revisit your work from Chapter 1. Identify the presence of the sulcus limitans in a cross section of the adult brainstem. Differentiate the locations of motor and sensory nuclei in relationship to the sulcus limitans.

2. Now is an excellent time to solidify your understanding of the blood supply of the brainstem, brainstem anatomy, and functional consequences of lesions. For each of the major syndromes identified in the chapter, list the symptoms and use sketches of the

whole brainstem and cross sections to locate the specific components that account for each of the symptoms.

3. For the following six representative levels of the brainstem, sketch out a cross section: caudal medulla, rostral medulla, caudal pons, rostral pons, caudal midbrain, and rostral midbrain. Then identify and locate the positions in each of the six representations of the following structures:

a. Medial lemniscus.

b. Spinothalamic tract.

c. Corticospinal tract.

4. Now analyze how these sensory tracts change in the relative locations as they ascend or descend the brainstem, and contrast their position to that of the corticospinal tracts. Consider the relationship of each level to the ventricles, the cerebellum, and the cranial nerve nuclei.

References

Blumenfeld, H. *Neuroanatomy through Clinical Cases.* Sinauer Associates, Sunderland, Massachusetts, 2002.

Bowman, J. P., and Giddings, F. D. *Strokes: An Illustrated Guide to Brain Structure, Blood Supply, and Clinical Signs.* Prentice-Hall, New Jersey, 2003.

Bauby, J-D. *The Diving Bell and the Butterfly.* Éditions Robert Laffont, S.A., Paris, 1997.

Duvernoy, H. M. *Human Brainstem Vessels,* 2nd ed. Springer-Verlag, Heidelberg, 1999.

Nolte, J. *The Human Brain: An Introduction to Its Functional Anatomy.* Mosby Elsevier, Philadelphia, 2009.

Tatu, L. et al. Arterial territories of human brain: Brainstem and cerebellum. *Neurol.* 47:1125, 1996.

PEARSON
myhealthprofessionskit™

Use this address to access the Companion Website created for this textbook. Simply select "Physical Therapy" from the choice of disciplines. Find this book and log in using your username and password to access self-assessment questions, a glossary, and more.

PART V

Special Functional Systems of the CNS: Motor and Sensory Systems

The first four parts of this text focused on the physiological and structural basis by which the nervous system operates. Examples were provided that are of importance for rehabilitation to illustrate how the nervous system conveys and processes somatosensory and motor information. By now, you should be developing confidence in your ability to link these basic concepts to an appreciation of how the nervous system utilizes such information to orchestrate function. For the rehabilitation professional to utilize knowledge of the nervous system when making clinical decisions related to people with neuromusculoskeletal disorders, a further level of understanding is still required. Specifically, the rehabilitation professional also needs to understand how sensory and motor *systems* are organized, the functional implications of damage to specific parts of those systems, and how rehabilitation strategies are developed based on that understanding. With the basic foundations of sensory and motor structures and pathways, it is now possible to explore these key concepts.

The first three chapters in Part V of this text address specific sensory systems. Pain, the focus of Chapter 16, is addressed as a distinct topic for two reasons: (1) pain is integral to many of the problems of people who seek assistance from the rehabilitation professional, and (2) the mechanisms that underlie perception of pain, and interventions related to pain, are exquisitely complex and therefore require special consideration.

Chapter 17 addresses two related sensory systems: the auditory and vestibular systems. Without the auditory system, it would be impossible to communicate verbally, appreciate music, or listen to crickets on a summer evening and birds awakening at dawn. The vestibular system, which relies on some of the same structural components as the auditory system, plays a very different role. Through its role in balance and postural control, it is possible for a person to walk through the park, adjust to elevators and escalators, play soccer, dance, ice skate, and even dive. The importance of the vestibular system only becomes evident when it is injured; hence, we draw on specific conditions to illustrate both its function and malfunction.

The last of the sensory systems in this part of the text is the visual system, the topic of Chapter 18. This is the system that allows us to interpret the mood from a loved one's facial expression and carriage, appreciate the grandeur of a 17th-century cathedral, and read the schedule board at an airport.

The last two chapters in this part of the text address the coordinated actions of the motor system. Chapter 19 explores the specific roles of the cerebellum and basal ganglia in the control of movement. Their important functions are most evident when one or the other is damaged. Hence, much of this chapter focuses on disorders first of the cerebellum and then of the basal ganglia. Finally, in Chapter 20, the functions of all parts of the motor system are synthesized as they relate to the control of movement. This chapter ends with an analysis of pitching a baseball—a familiar action that nevertheless requires specific and sophisticated integrated action across the vast array of structures that together form the motor system.

Pain and Its Modulation

LEARNING OUTCOMES

This chapter prepares the reader to:

1 Recall the meaning of the following terms: allodynia; hyperalgesia; and neuropathic, and nociceptive pain.

2 Differentiate acute from chronic pain and nociceptive from neuropathic pain, both in terms of the origin and quality of the pain and the responsiveness to pharmacologic and physical interventions.

3 Differentiate fast and slow pain in terms of their clinical relevance as well as the receptors and fibers that transmit the information.

4 Explain the role of receptors and afferent fibers in setting up the dual nature of pain.

5 Discuss the role of the following mediators of pain, their origin, and their site of action: histamine, serotonin, prostaglandins, bradykinin, substance P, leukotrines, and potassium.

6 Discuss the role of the following molecules in the transmission and modulation of pain: serotonin, norepinephrine, enkephalin, GABA, substance P, NMDA, and AMPA.

7 Describe the sequence of events by interpreting which WDR neurons elicit allodynia.

8 Differentiate peripheral from central sensitization and discuss the functional importance of each.

9 Explain how peripheral sensitization relates to the inflammatory process and related pain.

10 Explain the role of antidromic action potentials in release of substance P.

11 Explain why peripheral nerve damage can cause intractable pain and provide examples.

12 Discuss processes of the spinal cord that produce and sustain allodynia.

13 Differentiate the paleospinal and neospinal contributions to pain, including the receptors or origin, pathways, and ultimate destination of the painful afferent information.

14 Explain the relationship of nuclei in which the paleospinothalamic pain system synapses to the functional roles of that system.

15 Discuss the role of opiates in the experience of pain, including the relationship of endogenous opiates to descending modulation pathways.

16 Apply the gate-control theory of pain modulation to approaches used in management of pain and discuss the limitations.

17 Analyze the use of the following modalities in pain management: massage, heat and cold, electrical stimulation, and acupuncture.

18 Apply knowledge of the neuroanatomical and neurophysiological bases of pain to interpreting conditions including the following: thalamic pain, complex regional pain syndrome, phantom limb pain, and migraine headache.

19 Compare and contrast the types of neurotransmitters that affect pain through the dorsal horn versus the brainstem.

ACRONYMS

AMPA α-amino-3-hydroxyl-5-methyl-4-isoxazole-propionate

CRPS Complex regional pain syndrome

DC-ML Dorsal column-medial lemniscus system

EPSP Excitatory post-synaptic potential

GABA Gamma-amino butyric acid

NMDA N-methyl-D-aspartate

PAS Paramedial ascending system

PKA Protein kinase A

RSD Reflex sympathetic dystrophy

STT Spinothalamic tract

TENS Transcutaneous electrical nerve stimulation

VPL Ventral posterior lateral nucleus of the thalamus

VPM Ventral posterior medial nucleus of the thalamus

WDR Wide, dynamic-range neurons

Introduction

Pain is a vital perceptual experience. The experience of pain teaches us to avoid potentially harmful situations. It elicits protective withdrawal reflexes from noxious stimuli. Pain encourages us to protect and rest injured parts of our body. Pain is also one of the most common complaints causing individuals to seek physical intervention. Pain can be associated with a wide variety of circumstances from acute conditions (e.g., ankle sprain) to chronic pain (e.g., associated with arthritic conditions). Pain can be associated with disorders of a variety of tissues from muscle (e.g., tears, strains and sprains) to bone (e.g., fractures, certain cancers) to nerve (neurogenic) pain. Conditions of chronic pain (e.g., fibromyalgia, complex regional pain syndrome [also called reflex sympathetic dystrophy], and associated with stroke) are quite different than acute conditions. Differences in mechanisms of pain lead to differences in pharmacological or surgical interventions, as well as distinct approaches to physical intervention. A working knowledge of the mechanisms underlying pain is needed in order for the clinician to make appropriate decisions regarding intervention. This chapter lays the groundwork for understanding the rationale for different pharmacological, surgical, and physical intervention strategies.

This chapter builds on information that was introduced in Chapters 9 and 14. In those earlier chapters, pathways related to the perception of pain were introduced and discussed. However, transmission of information from spinal cord to cortex is only one small component of the overall pain system. Perception of pain can be guided by many factors, including cultural rules, ethnicity, motivation, beliefs, and personal values. Pain can become persistent and chronic, even after all stimuli causing pain have resolved, and likewise situations that should be excruciatingly painful can be entirely ignored by an individual. Hence, much more is to be learned than just the spinothalamic system and its pathways in order to fully appreciate the pain system.

The first section of this chapter considers the important issue that pain is such a unique perceptual experience that it cannot be regarded simply as a submodality of somatic sensation along with touch, temperature, and proprioception. In the second major section, we address the neural substrates involved in mediating the sensation of pain. We begin our inquiry in the periphery, specifically, with nociceptors themselves and the normal factors that condition their sensitivity to noxious stimuli. We then progress into the CNS, beginning with the spinal cord, and examine how dorsal horn neurons change their behavior in response to factors that have occurred in the periphery. We next delineate the organization of the pathways in the CNS that mediate the pain experience, culminating with an analysis of the role played by the cerebral cortex in pain perception.

The third major section considers theories of pain modulation, including a discussion of the descending system that begins in the cerebral cortex and ends on spinal cord dorsal horn neurons whose function it is to modulate the intensity of the pain experience. Therapeutic approaches then are considered, including both physical approaches (such as heat, cold, and transcutaneous electrical stimulation) and pharmacologic approaches. The role of acupuncture is also discussed.

The fourth section focuses on chronic pain. Examples discussed include phantom limb pain and complex regional pain syndromes. After a presentation of some common drugs used in the medical management of chronic pain, the final section of this chapter discusses the mechanisms thought to mediate migraine headache and its treatment.

FOUNDATIONAL INFORMATION

Clinical Preview

Alphonso Gutierrez fell hard on his right arm. He did not sustain any fractures or lasting musculoskeletal damage during the fall, but he has had severe pain in his right arm ever since. The pain has become debilitating. He was referred to the chronic pain clinic where you work. In your initial evaluation, he describes two different events. The first event is the initial fall and the pain that developed at that time; the second is unremitting dull, aching pain that developed over the next few weeks and that has not resolved over the year since the initial injury. As you read through this section, consider the following:

- What differentiates the initial pain immediately following the fall and the subsequent pain?
- How does the purpose of these two types of pain compare?

This chapter builds on the basic anatomical information presented in Chapters 9 and 14. In Chapter 9, it was pointed out that the **anterolateral system** consists of two components: a **neospinothalamic** component and a **paleospinothalamic** component. The former mediates fast pain (as well as temperature and touch), and the latter mediates **slow pain**, a more enduring, aching, and intense pain that has a strong emotional (affective) component. The term *anterolateral system* is derived from the fact that the ascending axons of both components intermingle in the anterior and lateral funiculi of the spinal cord. In fact, the two components are distinct both functionally and anatomically; they represent separate pathways in the pain system. Once attaining the level of the brainstem, the two pathways segregate themselves positionally into lateral (neospinothalamic) and medial (paleospinothalamic) projections, each having a unique synaptic organization. Chapters 9 and 14 focused on a specific neospinothalamic pathway—the spinothalamic tract—and its counterparts in the brainstem. However, this tract does not explain the multifaceted experience of pain. Here, we draw on that information but expand it to discuss the system by which pain is mediated and modulated. To this end, we consider both the neospinothalamic and paleospinothalamic components of pain.

For years, pain was regarded as a submodality of somatic sensation along with touch, pressure, vibration, and position sense. This concept was a product of the neurological evaluation of somatic sensation, which focuses on the discrimination of stimulus quality, intensity, and localization. As we shall see, this concept could apply only to fast pain that can be topographically precisely localized on the body surface, scaled in intensity, and tested in the neurologic examination by pinprick. But it is wholly unnatural to separate fast pain from slow pain. This is because the two pain-mediating projections are usually activated simultaneously. Even in the latter, it is uncertain that pain is actually being assessed. Rather, naturally occurring stimuli that elicit the perception of pain activate the slow and fast pain pathways in parallel.

Moreover, compelling reasons exist to *not* classify pain as a submodality of somatic sensation. Pain should be considered as being mediated by a conceptually and functionally unique kind of sensory system. For one thing, alerting the brain to potential dangers implied by the presence of noxious stimuli is quite distinct from informing it about, for example, touch. Therefore, pain mediation required the evolution of a special sensory system dedicated to the perception of potentially threatening circumstances. For another thing, the perception of pain is not the direct result of activity in nociceptive afferent fibers but is regulated by concurrent activity in myelinated afferents that themselves are not directly involved with the transmission of nociceptive information (see gate control). Moreover, pain differs markedly from somatosensory perceptions such as touch or vibration where the neurons in the somatic sensory system obey predictable rules. Under appropriate circumstances, for example, pain can be elicited by a light touch stimulus mediated by low-threshold, A-beta afferent fibers. Finally, pain is overtly manifest by aversive behavior and signs of autonomic system activity such as alterations in blood pressure, heart rate, and respiration.

The relationship of pain to affect and motivation is of particular importance. **Affect** refers to the vital feelings engendered in us by our internal and external environments. It is the emotional feeling, tone, or mood attached to a thought elicited by conditions and circumstances in these environments. **Motivation** designates a state of need in us

that arouses, maintains, and directs behavior toward a goal. Affect and motivation are frequently related because an affect can be the source of a motivation. Pain is a subjective experience, known only to its perceiver, which requires the presence of a mental state to be experienced and evaluated. As such, pain is subject to considerable variation over time in the same individual, depending on affect. It is a commonplace observation that the perception of pain increases when attention is directed to it (or when we are anxious) and decreases when attention is diverted from it. Additionally, cultural factors play a significant role in the perception of pain. Most significantly, acute pain nearly always motivates its possessor to seek relief.

A distinction is made between acute and chronic pain. **Acute pain** that occurs as a result of tissue damage has a well-defined onset with a well-defined pathology and is protective in nature. In contrast, **chronic pain** has no protective function, outlasts the time expected for tissue healing, is of greater magnitude than would be expected based on the initial tissue damage, and may occur without a clearly defined tissue pathology. It should be noted that terminology here is somewhat confusing from the standpoint that acute pain can be persistent. When persistent, acute pain can be the primary reason for the individual to seek medical and therapeutic attention.

> **Thought Question**
>
> Acute and chronic pain share some commonalities, but are also very different in terms of origin, consequence, and treatment. What are the relevant issues to consider?

The biologic role of acute pain is apparent. For example, when damage to skin, muscle, joints, or bone has occurred, acute pain resulting from movement encourages an injured person to rest and recuperate. In addition, acute pain is subject to modulation by systems in the brain. In contrast, chronic pain typically results from severe, long-term disease or psychiatric disturbance, and its biological role, other than causing a person to suffer, is difficult to determine. Nonetheless, chronic pain is subject to modulation of its intensity by the system evolved for the modulation of acute pain.

Clinical Application Box 16-1: Pain Assessment in the Neurological Examination

We can question to what extent the pain system is assessed in the neurological examination of pain. The neurological evaluation of pain involves instructing the patient to say "sharp" when they feel a pinprick on the skin. The patient is shown the pin that will be used *to alleviate any fear of being hurt* during the examination. Any medical definition of pain states that the perception includes physical discomfort, hurt, or suffering resulting from actual or potential tissue damage. As such, pain is not inflicted on a patient undergoing a neurological evaluation. The distinction between "sharp" and "dull" may, in part, be a quality of somatic sensory discrimination.

Persistent acute pain is classified as being either **nociceptive** or **neuropathic (neurogenic)**. Nociceptive pain is due to the activation of peripheral nociceptors in skin and other soft tissues in response to tissue injury and inflammation. A common cause of nociceptive pain is arthritis. Invasion of tissue by tumors provides another example. Neuropathic pain is the presence of pain due to nervous system pathology in the absence of peripheral nociceptor activation. Neuropathic pain results most commonly from injury or inflammation of peripheral nerves and far less often from pathological involvement of neurons of the CNS. A wide variety of disorders of the PNS cause neuropathic pain, including herpes zoster, diabetes, trigeminal neuralgia, and trauma resulting in complex regional pain syndrome (discussed in Clinical Connections). The **thalamic syndrome** (also referred to as **central post-stroke pain, or Dejerine-Roussy syndrome**) is a condition in which damage to the thalamus elicits intractable pain, without noxious stimulation, by causing firing of thalamic neurons that normally transmit information about painful stimuli to the cerebral cortex. This syndrome "...is *par excellence* the exemplar of central pain—for it is due not to anything affecting peripheral nerves or their terminals, but to a hole in the head" (Bowsher, 1996). The distinction between nociceptive and neuropathic pain is important because the symptoms and effectiveness of treatment differ significantly. For example, neuropathic pain is importantly dependent upon on the presence of Na^+ channels and action potential conduction (discussed later) so that systemically administered Na^+ channel blockers (e.g., lidocaine, carbamazepine, gabapentin-like drugs) are used in its management. In contrast, nociceptive pain is not responsive to Na^+ channel blockers.

ANATOMY AND FUNCTION

Clinical Preview ················

Recall Alphonso Gutierrez, who you met in the last section. He fell on his right arm and has had severe persistent pain ever since. As you read through this section, consider the following:

- What mechanisms contributed to the initial awareness of pain?
- What mechanisms contribute to his chronic condition of pain?
- How does the concept of "sensitization" relate, and what is the underlying mechanism?

The Periphery

The perception of pain results from appropriate stimulation of superficial and deep tissues or visceral organs of the body. Stimuli that depolarize nociceptors are different depending on the tissue in which the pain receptors are embedded, with the exception of inflammation that activates polymodal nociceptors in all tissue types. Damage to the periosteum (as in a fracture or with bone cancer) causes bone pain. Pain-producing stimuli for the skin are those that damage tissue: cutting, burning, pricking, crushing, and freezing. Note, however, that such stimuli do not result in pain in the viscera, where pain is generated by distension of the walls of hollow viscera or spasm of smooth muscle. Ischemia or damage to investing connective tissue sheaths causes skeletal muscle pain. Ischemia is also the primary cause of pain in cardiac muscle.

Thought Question

Where is the dual nature of pain established, and what does this dual nature imply?

Recall from Chapter 9 that four major classes of nociceptors are widely distributed in skin and subcutaneous tissues. **Mechanical nociceptors** are activated by intense pressure applied to the skin and represent the peripheral terminals of small diameter, thinly myelinated A-delta fibers with a conduction velocity of 5 to 30 m/sec. **Thermal nociceptors** are activated by extreme temperatures, greater than 45°C or less than 5°C. They also represent the peripheral terminals of A-delta fibers. **Chemically sensitive nociceptors** and **polymodal nociceptors** (responding to intense mechanical, thermal, and chemical stimuli) represent the peripheral terminals of unmyelinated C fibers that conduct information at the slow velocity of 0.5 to 2 m/sec.

When these nociceptors and their afferents work together to generate a pain response, the initial pain experience is dual in nature (Figure 16-1 ■). When, for example, the skin is penetrated by a needle, there is an immediate pricking pain (fast pain), followed 1 or 2 seconds later by a more prolonged stinging or burning pain (slow pain). The sharp first pain is mediated by A-delta fibers that transmit information from the mechanical and thermal nociceptors. In contrast, the duller, more aching pain is carried by unmyelinated, slower-conducting C fibers that are activated by chemical and polymodal nociceptors. Thus, the dual nature of the pain experience is established in the periphery by the types of nociceptors activated and differences in the conduction velocity of their respective nerve fibers.

Sensitization of the Pain System, Hyperalgesia, and Allodynia

The pain generated during the initial noxious event results from the activation of normally functioning nociceptors, as delineated earlier. However, spontaneous pain beyond the first few seconds (i.e., ongoing pain experienced as

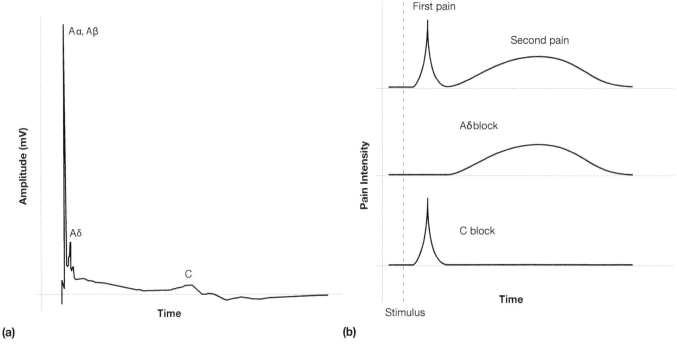

(a)   **(b)**

FIGURE 16-1 The dual nature of the pain response. (a) An electrical recording illustrating a compound action potential traveling in a peripheral nerve in response to electrical stimulation of nerve fibers. Faster conducting fibers have shorter latency, depicted on the left in the graph. (b) The first and second pain signals are carried by different afferent axons and A-delta and C fibers. By selectively blocking A-delta myelinated fibers, the first pain (sharp sensation, well localized) is abolished. Likewise, by selectively blocking the C fibers, the second pain (dull sensation, poorly localized) is abolished.

tenderness, burning, stinging, aching) results from processes that increase the sensitivity of the pain system itself. This is a normal function of the pain system and not a reflection of pathology. It is an adaptive response to tissue injury thought to have evolved to minimize the use of injured tissue until the inflammatory response has subsided and tissue repair occurred.

> **Thought Question**
>
> What is meant by sensitization? When is this occurrence normal, and when does it become a pathological phenomenon?

The responsiveness of nociceptors to painful stimuli can be modified such that the response is lessened or heightened (sensitization). **Sensitization** of the pain system involves changes in the function of receptors in the PNS, as well as alteration in the function of dorsal horn neurons in the CNS, referred to as peripheral sensitization and central sensitization (discussed later), respectively. Both peripheral and central sensitization reflect themselves in hyperalgesia and allodynia. **Hyperalgesia** is an exaggerated sensitivity to a noxious stimulus; for example, a normally uncomfortable slap on a sunburned back becomes painful. Peripheral sensitization is said to cause primary hyperalgesia, whereas central sensitization is said to cause secondary hyperalgesia. **Allodynia** refers to the situation in which

a normally innocuous stimulus mediated by A-beta fibers evokes the perception of pain.

> **Thought Question**
>
> How do hyperalgesia and allodynia differ, and why is this difference important to the rehabilitation specialist?

PERIPHERAL SENSITIZATION The term **peripheral sensitization** refers to a decreased threshold and increased responsiveness of the nociceptor to stimulation of the receptive field. Peripheral sensitization results from the release of a large number of chemical mediators into the environment of the inflammatory response—which includes the area of the tissue injury itself, as well as a surrounding area of noninjured tissue—within the area of inflammation. Some of these mediators are released by cells in the area of injury. Included are histamine and serotonin that are released by mast cells and prostaglandins that are released by fibroblasts. These mediators (but only some of the prostaglandins) act directly on the receptive membrane of nociceptors. Other mediators are released by cells of the immune system, such as macrophages, that invade injured tissue. Some of these mediators act indirectly by causing the release of direct-acting mediators from other cells. Macrophages, for example, release leukotrines (interleukin-1) that activate fibroblasts to release prostaglandins. Still others, such as bradykinin, are derived from blood plasma, an event made possible by the fact that

Table 16-1 Naturally Occurring Chemicals That Activate or Sensitize Nociceptors

AGENT	SOURCE	EFFECT ON PRIMARY AFFERENT FIBERS
Potassium	Resident and damaged cells	Activation
Serotonin	Platelets and mast cells	Activation
Bradykinin	Plasma	Activation
Histamine	Mast cells	Activation
Prostaglandins	Resident and damaged cells	Sensitization
Leukotrines	Macrophages and damaged cells	Sensitization
Substance P	Primary afferent fibers	Sensitization

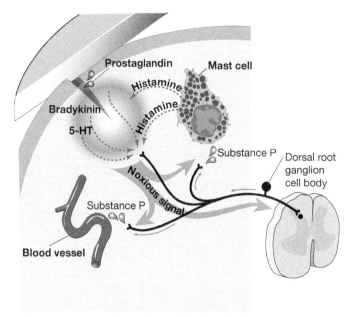

FIGURE 16-2 Peripheral chemical mediators of pain and hyperalgesia. Substance P is synthesized in the cell body of primary C fiber afferents and released during the axon reflex. Substance P is vasoactive and induces neurogenic inflammation.

capillaries in the area of inflammation are dilated and leaky. Finally, mediators such as substance P are released from the nociceptor terminals themselves (discussed later). All of these chemicals act to decrease the threshold (sensitization) for the activation of nociceptors. However, as summarized in Table 16-1 ■, some of these chemicals directly activate nociceptors. It is thought that there is a significant population of silent nociceptors that are activated only in the presence of these chemical mediators.

One of the prostaglandins (E2) is noteworthy because aspirin and COX inhibitors, which are nonsteroidal anti-inflammatory analgesics, inhibit prostaglandin synthesis, which accounts for their effectiveness in controlling pain. Bradykinin is a particularly active pain-producing chemical: not only does it directly activate both A-delta and C nociceptors, but it also increases the synthesis and release of prostaglandins.

> **Thought Question**
>
> What is substance P, what is its role with respect to pain, and what is the purpose of antidromic release of this substance?

Substance P is synthesized in the cell body (located in dorsal root ganglia or the trigeminal ganglion) of primary C fiber afferents. Not only is it transported centrally and released onto second-order dorsal horn neurons, but it is also transported to the *peripheral* terminals of the primary afferent—that is, to the nociceptor, where it is released into the microenvironment of the nociceptor. This peripheral release is generated by an axon reflex. Afferent impulses in the primary afferent generate the axon reflex, whereby action potentials travel antidromically to the terminal to

release the substance P (Figure 16-2 ■). Thus, different branches of a single primary afferent neuron form both the afferent and efferent limbs of the axon reflex.

Released substance P is vasoactive and is involved in the generation of the four cardinal signs of inflammation: dolor (pain), heat, erythema (redness), and swelling as a result of its direct action on capillaries. Heat and redness result from the dilation of blood vessels. Swelling is due to increased permeability of capillaries resulting in plasma extravasation, wherein proteins and fluid leak out of the capillaries into the extracellular fluid. This process is called **neurogenic inflammation** and is discussed later in conjunction with migraine headache. As noted earlier, released substance P also contributes to primary hyperalgesia by causing mast cells to degranulate and release histamine, which decreases the threshold for activation of nociceptors.

PERIPHERAL NERVE INJURY AND PAIN With peripheral nerve damage, the afferent pathway conducting pain information to the spinal cord is compromised so that one would expect pain to be depressed, not augmented. Yet, seemingly paradoxically, damage to peripheral nerves often results in many intractable pain states, including those associated with diabetic neuropathy, causalgia, phantom limb pain, trigeminal neuralgia, complex regional pain syndrome, and others. After being injured by axotomy or undergoing segmental demyelination, many afferent axons become hyperexcitable and generate an ongoing spontaneous discharge that originates from the site of the injury. Because the impulse activity originates from the site of injury and not at the initial segment of the axon, it is called **ectopic** (out-of-place) discharge. In people with peripheral neuropathies (see Chapter 10), there is a direct correlation between ectopic discharge and experienced pain and paresthesias.

Thought Question

People with diabetic neuropathy often develop pain, especially in the feet and lower extremities. Yet this is a neuropathic process. What is the mechanism accounting for pain as opposed to loss of pain sensation?

Ectopic discharge results from a remodeling of the nerve cell's membrane at the site of nerve injury or demyelination. Excessive numbers of voltage-sensitive Na^+ channels accumulate in regions of injury or denuded membrane and render the axon hyperexcitable. However, in order to generate ectopic firing, there must be an adequate generator current analogous to the receptor potential in the peripheral terminal that generates action potentials. Not only are Na^+ channels synthesized in dorsal root ganglia, but membrane leak channels and transducer receptors and channels are also synthesized. All of these channels are transported distally to the site of nerve injury and inserted into the membrane, where they reduplicate the membrane characteristics formerly residing at the normal transducer terminal before axotomy or demyelination. This is reflected in the fact that sites of ectopic discharge respond to temperature changes, chemical mediators, and mechanical displacement. The latter is exemplified by the **Tinel sign**. Lightly tapping on the skin of the forearm over the site of a median nerve injury evokes a burst of impulse activity, and the individual experiences paresthesia and pain in the medial part of his or her hand. However, in normal nerve, Na^+ channel density is too low to result in repetitive discharge to such naturally occurring stimuli. Thus, when skin over normal median nerve is lightly tapped, the subject experiences only local tapping, not painful sensations in the territory of distribution of the median nerve.

The Spinal Cord

Within the spinal cord, afferent neurons conveying nociceptive input synapse on neurons located in a number of Rexed's lamina of the dorsal horn. The most important of these are laminae I, II, and V, although other laminae (e.g., VII and VIII) also are involved. Recall from Chapter 9 that the somatosensory systems synapse on different types of neurons in the dorsal horns. Those afferents on which nociceptive and low-threshold touch converge are called **wide, dynamic-range (WDR) neurons**, which may monitor the precise location of a noxious stimulus on the body surface. Typically, the WDR neurons are found in lamina V. In contrast, neurons that respond only to nociceptive stimuli (nociceptive specific) may monitor the extent of injury as opposed to the exact location of a noxious stimulus and are located primarily in laminae I and II.

Nociceptive afferents have definable terminations on neurons in different Rexed lamina of the dorsal horn

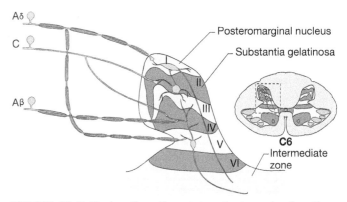

FIGURE 16-3 Nociceptive afferents terminate predominantly on neurons within laminae I, II, and V of the dorsal horn.

(Figure 16-3 ■). As examples, neurons in lamina I receive direct input from myelinated A-delta nociceptive fibers and also receive indirect input from unmyelinated C nociceptive afferents via interneurons of lamina II. Lamina II interneurons receive direct input from C nociceptive afferents. Neurons of lamina V are primarily wide, dynamic-range neurons. Lamina V projection neurons have dendrites that extend dorsally into lamina III. This enables lamina V neurons to receive direct, monosynaptic input from low-threshold, large-diameter myelinated A-beta mechanoreceptor fibers, as well as from nociceptive A-delta fibers, and indirect input from C fibers via interneurons in lamina II.

Two different neurotransmitters, glutamate and substance P, are released onto the neurons of the dorsal horn by axon terminals of A-delta and C fibers. Both A-delta and C nociceptive afferents release the excitatory neurotransmitter glutamate. Glutamate elicits *fast* excitatory postsynaptic potentials (EPSPs) in dorsal horn neurons via α-amino-3-hydroxyl-5-methyl-4-isoxazole-propionate (AMPA)-type glutamate receptors. Substance P, a neuropeptide, is co-released onto dorsal horn neurons by nociceptive afferent terminals. Substance P release elicits *slow* EPSPs in dorsal horn neurons. Substance P is released, in particular, from the terminals of C fiber afferents onto neurons of lamina I and parts of lamina II (Figure 16-4 ■). It is significant that dorsal horn substance P is markedly depleted in people with congenital neuropathy and insensitivity to pain and increased in people who experience persistent pain.

In addition to glutamate and substance P, other neurotransmitters released in the dorsal horn of the spinal cord mediate pain. Included are adenosine, gamma-amino butyric acid (GABA), and protein kinase A (PKA). Adenosine and GABA both have inhibitory effects on pain transmission, resulting in analgesia or reduction in hyperalgesia. In contrast, PKA is released during mechanical stimulation, and produces hyperalgesia by sensitizing the spinothalamic tract (STT) neurons. Furthermore, a number of descending supraspinal projections release neurotransmitters in the spinal cord dorsal horn that are involved in mediating central pain processing, including endorphins, serotonin, and norepenipherine. Their roles and actions are discussed later in the pain modulation discussion.

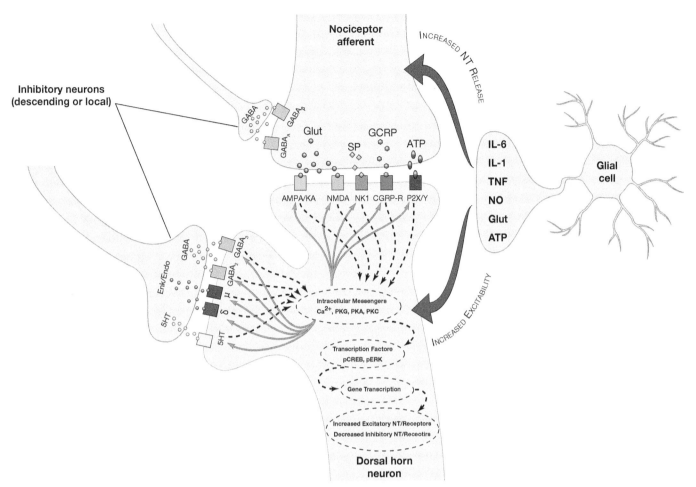

FIGURE 16-4 Inputs to dorsal horn neurons involved in pain mediation. When activated by noxious stimuli, glial cells release mediators that increase excitability of dorsal horn neurons. Descending and local neurons inhibit pain transmission presynaptically and postsynaptically. ATP, adenosine triphosphate; Enk/Endo, enkaphalin/endomorphine; GABA, gamma-amino butyric acid; Glut, glutamate; SP, substance P; NO, nitric oxide. Other neurotransmitters of importance, depicted in the figure, are not discussed in this text but are included for completeness.

Glial cells also play a particularly important role in processing nociceptive information, particularly in the spinal cord. Specifically, they express receptors for many of the relevant neurotransmitters and are also involved in clearing neurotransmitters from the synaptic cleft.

Central Sensitization

> **Thought Question**
>
> In preparation for the material that you are about to read, review Chapter 4 with reference to NMDA receptors. First, what is NMDA? With what neurotransmitter is NMDA important, and what is its role? Finally, how do NMDA-gated channels relate to AMPA-gated channels?

Following localized injury, allodynia may develop in a cutaneous area where there is no apparent inflammation to cause the discomfort, such that an ordinarily painless tactile stimulus is experienced as being painful. This phenomenon is due to **central sensitization**. Central sensitization is both

triggered and maintained by the abnormal noxious input resulting from peripheral sensitization. Central sensitization results from altered processing by dorsal horn WDR neurons of impulses entering the spinal cord over A-beta touch afferents and occurs as follows: A-beta afferents acquire the capacity to drive WDR neurons that they were previously ineffective at driving. In the absence of noxious stimuli, A-beta touch afferents release glutamate, which activates the WDR neurons. Normally, this activation is modest and is mediated only by non-NMDA receptors such as the AMPA receptors. At normal membrane potentials, N-methyl-D-aspartate (NMDA) is blocked within the pore of the channel by extracellular Mg^{2+} ions, and the activation of WDR neurons by A-beta touch afferents is insufficient to remove this block. However, when nociceptive receptors are stimulated, C nociceptor afferents release both glutamate and substance P. Intense C fiber input produces prolonged substance P–evoked depolarization of WDR neurons. The Mg^{2+} block is displaced, rendering NMDA receptors responsive to the glutamate released by A-beta touch afferents. The latter afferents now more effectively elicit action potentials from postsynaptic WDR neurons by both NMDA and AMPA receptors, thereby activating central synaptic circuits that produce allodynia.

Differentiate WDR neurons in the dorsal horn from other neurons associated with pain in terms of location, purpose, and destination of projections from these neurons.

Recall from Chapter 4 that glutamate NMDA receptor/channel complexes are unique in that they do admit Na^+, like AMPA channels, and in addition permit the entry of Ca^{2+}. Central sensitization persists beyond the duration of the substance P depolarization and results from the entry of Ca^{2+} through the NMDA channels. This activates a Ca^{2+}-dependent protein kinases that, in turn, phosphorylate ion channels, thereby sustaining central sensitization.

Thought Question

In the somatosensory system, damage to a peripheral nerve results in diminished perception (e.g., of proprioception, touch, or pressure). Yet damage to a peripheral nerve may also result in enhancement of pain. What accounts for this difference in response to nerve damage?

Ascending Systems

Projections to the Brainstem and Thalamus
In the previous section, we focused on the role of the peripheral somatosensory system in processing painful stimuli. However, to consciously experience pain, it is necessary for information to be transmitted to the cerebral cortex. The duality of the pain experience, first established in the periphery by A-delta and C fibers and their nociceptors as noted earlier, is preserved in the ascending projections. This is accomplished by virtue of the fact that each input preferentially engages an anatomically and functionally distinct projection system. Both systems access the thalamus, but they do so in ascending systems that have markedly different synaptic and biochemical organizations, and each synapses in distinct thalamic nuclei. A-delta nociceptive input engages projection neurons in lamina I of the dorsal horn, whose axons enter the **neospinothalamic component** of the anterolateral system and travel to the thalamus where they synapse in the VPL nucleus (refer to Chapter 9). The neospinothalamic component mediates sharp, well-localized, rapidly perceived pain. Fast pain is tested by pinprick in the neurological evaluation. This variant of pain is not associated with a strong emotional component. In contrast, C fibers preferentially engage a different set of dorsal horn neurons whose axons feed into the **paleospinothalamic component** of the anterolateral

system. This system mediates slowly perceived pain that is diffuse (poorly localized or *crude*) with an aching or burning quality. It is associated with a strong emotional component and may be the reason some people seek medical attention for pain. The axons of these dorsal horn neurons ascend in the lateral and anterior funiculi of the spinal cord, as do axons of the neospinothalamic tract. However, upon attaining the brainstem, axons of the paleospinothalamic tract assume a more medial position than neospinothalamic tract axons that remain laterally positioned (Figure 16-5 ■). For this reason, the paleospinothalamic tract is also referred to as the medial or, more accurately, the **paramedial ascending system (PAS)**. Like the neospinothalamic tract, the PAS reaches the diencephalon, but it gives off axon collaterals at, and has distinct projections to, a number of brainstem sites, including the raphe nuclei of midline reticular formation of the medulla and pons (via the *spinoreticular tract*) and the periaqueductal gray of the midbrain (via the *spinomesencephalic tract*). Upon reaching the diencephalon, axons of the PAS terminate in the hypothalamus—a structure immediately adjacent to the midline (via the *spinohypothalamic tract*)—and in the midline and intralaminar nuclei of the thalamus (*spinothalamic tract*). Axons arising from cells of these thalamic nuclei project to structures of the limbic system such as the prefrontal cortex, anterior cingulate gyrus, and subcortically located amygdala.

Thought Question

How does the PAS differ from the STT? Discuss the destinations of PAS fibers, and relate the specific nuclei in which these fibers terminate to their role in pain perception.

Nociceptive input to the hypothalamus activates the complex autonomic and endocrine responses to pain. Neurons from the midline and intralaminar thalamic nuclei project into the limbic system that mediates the affective and motivational responses to pain.

Thought Question

The neospinothalamic and paleospinothalamic systems are similar in some important ways and different in others. Compare and contrast the two systems in terms of origin of the stimulus, purpose, location in the spinal cord, and ultimate destination.

Cerebral Cortex
Beyond doubt, the pain experience requires participation of the cerebral cortex. Recall that cortical processing is necessary for the interpretation of incoming stimuli. Needless to say, this is true of painful stimuli as well. Indeed, there is

of the cerebral cortex through three major thalamocortical pathways.

One pathway, originating in lamina I of the spinal cord (part of the neospinothalamic component of the ALS), synapses in the VPL/VPM nuclei of the thalamus whose neurons project to the postcentral gyrus (primary somato-sensory cortex), ending mainly in Brodmann's area 1 (refer to Chapter 7). This is one component of the lateral pain system. This system is in somatotopic register with mecha-noreceptive input projecting to the postcentral gyrus via the DC-ML system. Pain neurons in VPL/VPM and the postcentral gyrus respond to the intensity of noxious stim-uli and have small contralateral receptive fields. This thala-mocortical projection is responsible for the sensory aspects of the pain experience—namely, intensity and location. Lesions of the postcentral gyrus may result in elevations in the threshold for detecting noxious stimuli and a reduced capacity to discriminate between noxious stimuli of differ-ent intensities. Note that there is only a reduced awareness of different intensities of pain, meaning that other cortical components of the pain system also have intensity coding functions.

A second part of the neospinothalamic system receives input from the small-fibered components of the spinotha-lamic (STT) and spinal trigeminothalamic systems and re-lays to part of the ventral posterior group of the thalamic nuclei. This projection is a second component of the lat-eral pain system whose neurons originate in lamina I. It terminates in the cortex of the dorsal and posterior parts of the insula and superior bank of the lateral (Sylvian) fis-sure, representing the second somatic sensory area (SII). SII also is somatotopically organized. Neurons in SII and the insular cortex code for the intensity of the noxious stimulus.

A third thalamocortical pathway of the STT and spinal trigeminothalamic small-fibered systems synapses in the intralaminar nuclei of the thalamus. These neurons, which are part of the paleospinothalamic component of the ALS, originate in laminae V and VI of the dorsal horn and proj-ect via the medial pain system to the intralaminar nuclei of the thalamus. They project diffusely to the frontal lobe and, in particular, to the cingulate gyrus. This pathway is essen-tial for the affective and motivation-evoking (cognitive) aspects of the pain experience and does not deal directly with its sensory aspects. Stereotaxic lesions placed in the intralaminar nuclei and cingulate gyrus may be successful in relieving intractable pain. In some cases, patients report that they still are aware of their pain, but it no longer is of any consequence to them.

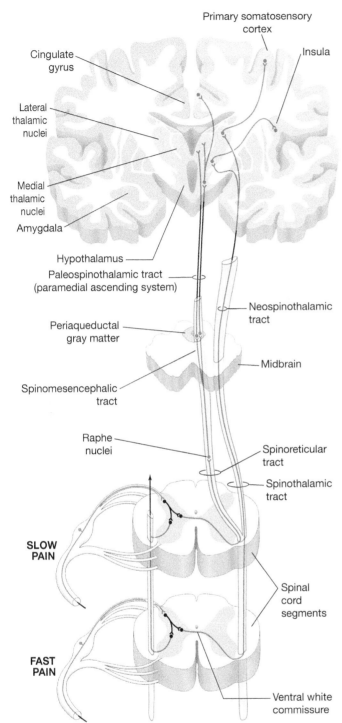

FIGURE 16-5 The duality of the pain experience, first established in the periphery by A-delta and C fibers and their nociceptors, as noted earlier, is preserved in the ascending projections. The neospi-nothalamic tract mediates fast pain and terminates in the cerebral cortex by way of the thalamus. The paleospinothalamic tract medi-ates slow pain and projects to the hypothalamus and thalamus.

a distributed cortical system involved in overall pain per-ception, and no single cortical area appears to be uniquely essential for it. The A-delta and C fiber systems of the spinal cord and trigeminal systems terminate in multiple targets in the brainstem and thalamus and engage multiple areas

Thought Question

A number of cortical areas are involved in the experience of pain. Contrast the areas that are involved with localiza-tion of pain with those involved with the emotional re-sponse to pain.

PAIN MODULATION

Clinical Preview ·················

Zunaira Ahmed was referred to you for rehabilitation following an unsuccessful lumbar fusion. This led to severe pain. During the healing process, you used TENS (transcutaneous electrical stimulation) to help with control of the pain. Eventually, the pain became so severe that Zunaira was given a prescription for a mild opiate. As you read through this section, consider the following:

- How does the use of TENS relate to the gate-control theory of pain?

- How does the mechanism of action of opiates compare with the mechanism of action of TENS?

- Why would TENS be of limited value for Alphonso Gutierrez (whom you met earlier in this chapter)?

- Would use of heat or cold likely be a good substitute for TENS? For opiates? Why or why not?

- What are the concerns associated with prolonged use of opiates, and what is the physiological basis for those concerns?

Theories of Pain Modulation

It is intuitively logical that the brain should evolve systems for modulating pain responses. In times of stress and emergency, suppressing a pain response can confer a biologic advantage on the organism. For example, a severe bodily response to pain and the associated fear and distress could impair the capacity of the organism to perform successfully, such as fighting off an intruder. Also, excessive autonomic and emotional responses could worsen bodily damage. Finally, the experience of inescapable and uncontrollable pain might make the organism unable to cope with a future encounter involving the same situation (learned helplessness).

The fundamental concept that pain is subject to modulation by the CNS (both pain facilitation and pain inhibition) was first put forward in 1965 in the *gate-control* theory of pain. The proposed gate was in the spinal cord, at the very entry where nociceptive input encounters its first central synapse on dorsal horn neurons. The idea was based on the commonplace observation that pain is reduced by gently rubbing the skin of an acutely injured area or shaking the hand when a finger is burned. It was proposed that nociceptive input is inhibited by concurrent activity in low-threshold, A-beta afferents. Thus, concurrent activity in low-threshold touch afferents "closed the gate." The gate-control hypothesis gave rise to sometimes successful (but temporary) attempts to relieve pain through high-frequency, low-intensity transcutaneous electrical stimulation of peripheral nerves. The stimulus parameters used were designed to preferentially activate A-beta fibers, which would simulate the "rubbing where it hurts" mode of pain gating. The large-diameter A-beta fibers activate

inhibitory interneurons in the dorsal horn. These inhibitory neurons, in turn, act both presynaptically (on nociceptor primary afferents) and postsynaptically (on second-order pain neurons in the dorsal horn). The net effect is reduced excitation of second-order nociceptive dorsal horn neurons.

It is now known that pain modulation is more complex than a simple gate operating at the first synapse in the pain pathways. Specifically, this gating only occurs for as long as the A-beta fibers are activated. As we shall see, this contrasts with the supraspinal gating mechanisms, which have longer-acting gating. This distinction is of particular importance with respect to modulation of chronic pain.

Pain modulation also occurs via a descending system that begins in the cerebral cortex and hypothalamus (Figure 16-6 ■). Projections from these structures

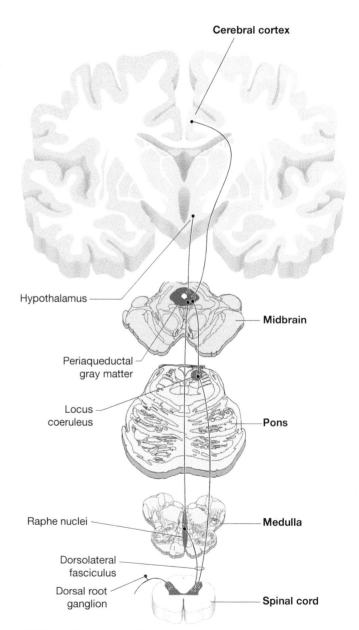

FIGURE 16-6 Descending pain modulation system. Projections from the cerebral cortex and hypothalamus influence nuclei in the brainstem and spinal cord to modulate the pain response.

terminate on neurons in the periaqueductal gray. The periaqueductal gray is pivotally positioned to transmit cortical and hypothalamic inputs to the lower brainstem. Cortical inputs from the frontal cortex represent the anatomic substrate for the cognitive activation of the pain modulating system. Input from the insular cortex modulates the autonomic response to pain that reciprocally influences the emotional response. From neurons of the **periaqueductal gray** of the midbrain, projections descend to serotonergic neurons of the raphe nuclei of the rostroventral medulla. Axons of the raphe nuclei descend in the dorsolateral funiculus of the spinal cord to synapse on cells of the dorsal horn. An additional brainstem projection to the spinal cord originates from noradrenergic cell groups in the pons and medulla, including the locus coeruleus. These descending projections inhibit nociceptive projection neurons in the dorsal horn both directly and indirectly through interneurons in the substantia gelatinosa (discussed later).

One of the major differences between the neospinothalamic tract and the PAS is that neurons of the PAS contain receptors for endogenous opiate neurotransmitters, whereas neospinothalamic tract neurons do not. This applies to neurons at all levels of the PAS: the spinal cord, brainstem, and cerebral cortex. Three endogenous opioid peptide transmitters are differentially distributed in the paramedial system. These are represented by beta-endorphin, met-enkephalin, and dynorphin, collectively referred to as **endorphins**, meaning *morphines within*. These endogenous opioid peptides modulate our response to pain. Such modulation applies to the extent to which pain is perceived in different contexts, as well to one's emotional response to a pain experience including its affective and motivational components. Given this differential distribution of opiate receptors in neurons of the neospinothalamic tract and those of the PAS, it should not be surprising that narcotic analgesics are most effective in relieving pain mediated by the PAS or by the spinal cord–mediated pain control achieved by rubbing where it hurts.

Thought Question

Compare the neurotransmitters that act at the dorsal horn with those that act in the brainstem.

In experimental animals, a potent analgesia has been induced by two techniques: electrical stimulation of specific targets in the brainstem and microinjection of opiates such as morphine into these same neuronal groups. Electrical stimulation of the following structures produces analgesia without altering behavior or motor activity: the periaqueductal gray of the midbrain, the dorsolateral pontine tegmentum, the nucleus raphe magnus, and the paragigantocellularis nuclei of rostroventral medulla. Stimulation-produced analgesia is so profound that animals can undergo surgical procedures without anesthesia. The microinjection of low doses of morphine into these same structures also induces a potent analgesia. Both

procedures act by inhibiting the discharge of nociceptive neurons in the dorsal horn. The opiate receptor antagonist naloxone blocks both stimulation-produced analgesia and morphine-induced analgesia. This suggests that both stimulation-produced and morphine-induced analgesia activate the same descending inhibitory projections.

The action of naloxone in inhibiting analgesia stimulated the search for naturally occurring (endogenous) opioid receptors in the CNS. Three different types of opioid receptors have been found differentially distributed in the pain-modulating system. Receptors for opiates are present in high densities on the terminals of A-delta and C afferents and on dorsal horn neurons of the spinal cord as well as on neurons of the medullary reticular formation, periaqueductal gray, hypothalamus, medial thalamus, amygdala, and cingulate gyrus. Subsequent research identified the three naturally occurring (endogenous) opioid transmitters mentioned earlier: beta-endorphin, met-enkephalin, and dynorphin. Collectively, their distribution parallels that of their corresponding receptors.

How is this extensive pain-modulating system activated? Noxious stimulation itself can activate the system via tracts of the PAS to the brainstem structures whose neurons represent the source of the descending modulating network. But noxious stimulation is not a prerequisite for activation of the descending opioid systems. Non-noxious stressors are effective in a variety of circumstances. Soldiers wounded while in battle sometimes experience little or no pain. Athletes injured while in the heat of a game may not experience pain until the contest is over. Non-noxious stressors are also represented by situations wherein noxious stimuli may be potentially experienced as when a person is confronted by a potentially hostile intruder. Anxiety can depress the modulating system, leading to an exacerbation of pain. Conditioning resulting from prior experience can affect the system, as can the expectation of relief as in the **placebo effect**. The latter is underscored by the fact that people suffering from postoperative pain experience relief when given a placebo. Significantly, the placebo effect can be blocked by naloxone, indicating that the pain-modulating system is involved in the mediation of a pain-related placebo.

Thought Question

Explain why the placebo effect is not just in the mind.

CLINICAL CONNECTIONS

A number of different approaches used for management of pain are discussed in this section. Some of these approaches manage pain through the peripheral nervous system. Examples include use of touch, massage, heat, cold, and peripheral electrical stimulation of nerves, referred to as transcutaneous electrical stimulation (TENS). Other intervention approaches are specifically directed to the central mechanisms of pain. Included are both allopathic and complementary approaches to pain management. Allopathic approaches are based on use of pharmacologic agents, whereas acupuncture is a common complementary approach.

Pain Management from the Periphery

Touch and Massage

We have all experienced the use of touch and massage to decrease pain. As discussed earlier, it is apparent that pain can be reduced by gently rubbing the skin of an injured area. Additionally, touch and massage often are used in rehabilitation. These techniques reduce pain by increasing local blood circulation and through sensory stimulation of low-threshold, A-beta afferents. These fibers, in turn, inhibit nociceptive input to the central nervous system at the level of the spinal cord.

Heat and Cold

It has been known for centuries that changing the local temperature of the body through use of heat and cold can alleviate pain. Modalities that rely on heat and cold decrease the activation of nociceptors in the periphery; hence, they are used to treat the injury at peripheral sites. Heat can be achieved via hot packs but also by using electrophysiological methods such as short-wave diathermy. Heat and cold are typically applied via conduction (hot and cold packs), convection (whirlpool baths), and conversion of another form of energy to heat (e.g., ultrasound, short-wave diathermy).

Heat is used to increase local circulation and remove the mechanical irritants from the nervous system, thereby reducing nociceptive input to the CNS. Even a modest reduction in temperature (less than 5°C) can have a substantial impact on both blood flow and nerve conduction velocity. Thus, the use of cold can affect pain through reduction of inflammation (via reduced blood flow) and the slowing of conduction of nerve impulses.

Electrophysiological approaches such as ultrasound and short-wave diathermy can provide significant heating of deeper tissues via energy absorption mechanisms.

Transcutaneous Electrical Nerve Stimulation

Transcutaneous electrical nerve stimulation (TENS) is an approach to pain management that grew out of the gate-control theory of pain. Applied to the skin, *high-frequency, low-intensity TENS* is used to preferentially stimulate large-diameter afferent fibers, which in turn inhibit the responses in the dorsal horn evoked by nociceptive inputs, as discussed with respect to the simple gate-control theory of pain. In contrast, the application of low-frequency, high-intensity TENS activates smaller C fibers in addition to the larger-diameter fibers. Because low-frequency, high-intensity TENS stimulates C fibers, this stimulation actually activates the pain pathway via the primary pain afferents, which paradoxically assists in control of the overall experience of pain. (Note that this mechanism is reminiscent of the mechanisms underlying acupuncture, discussed later.) Furthermore, this latter type of TENS activates descending

brainstem pathways, thereby activating the descending inhibitory systems involved in reduction of hyperalgesia. These supraspinal mechanisms provide longer-lasting pain control. Specific locations that have been implicated include the ventrolateral periaqueductal gray (PAG), rostral ventromedial medulla (RVM), and spinal cord. A number of neurotransmitters and receptors have been implicated in the response, including release of opioids, serotonin, and GABA in the spinal cord and activation of the adrenergic receptors in the periphery. In addition, opioids may act in the rostral ventral medulla.

Thought Question

What is the commonality in use of opioids to control pain and use of TENS? How do these two approaches differ?

Common Drugs for the Management of Pain

Dozens of different drugs have been prescribed for the management of chronic pain. These fall into four classes: (1) nonopioid analgesics, (2) tricyclic antidepressants, (3) anticonvulsants, and (4) narcotic (opioid) analgesics. The first three classes of drugs are considered milder therapeutic measures and are administered before resorting to narcotics.

One of the non-opioid analgesics, aspirin, has already been mentioned. Aspirin (acetylsalicylic acid) blocks the synthesis of prostaglandin, a chemical mediator released by damaged cells that sensitizes peripheral nociceptors. Other non-opioid analgesics include agents such as acetaminophen and ibuprofen. Acetaminophen acts centrally by elevating the pain threshold, although the exact mechanism by which this happens is not clear. Ibuprofen is a nonsteriodal anti-inflammatory drug that works by reversibly inhibiting a cyclooxygenase enzyme (COX), thereby inhibiting inflammation and the pain pathway.

Serotonin and norepinephrine can activate the pain-inhibiting enkephalinergic interneurons; hence, it is understandable that antidepressant drugs can be administered in the management of chronic pain. The tricyclic antidepressants used in pain management (imipramine, amitriptyline, and doxepin) block the reuptake (the inactivation mechanism) of *both* serotonergic and noradrenergic transmitters.

Anticonvulsant medications are widely used in the management of many pain syndromes. Phenytoin and carbamazepine act by reducing the repetitive firing of neurons by producing a use-dependent blockade of sodium channels on neuronal cell membranes, as mentioned earlier. The drugs allow neurons to fire at normal rates, but inhibit abnormally fast rates of discharge. The mechanism of action of gabapentin is not clear. Gabapentin, although it chemically appears similar to GABA, does not bind to GABA receptors. Gabapentin promotes the release of GABA by some unknown mechanism, but it does not consistently reduce the repetitive firing of action potentials.

The narcotic analgesics bind to one or more of the three classes of opiate receptors distributed in neurons of the pain-modulating network. Neurons always contain more receptors than are occupied by molecules of a given transmitter at a particular time. Thus, there is always a *receptor reserve*. The mechanism of action of the narcotic analgesics is that they potentiate the action of the endogenous opioid peptides by mobilizing this receptor reserve. This results in heightened activation of the pain-inhibiting network at spinal as well as higher levels. It should be noted that opioids also relieve anxiety by affecting neurons within the limbic system such as the cingulate gyrus. This is an important component of the anti-nociceptive action of opioid analgesics.

> **Thought Question**
>
> What is the neural mechanism that makes opioids the last choice for pain management, given their exceptional effectiveness?

Systemically administered opioid analgesics like morphine produce a variety of undesirable side effects such as respiratory depression, cardiovascular changes, and constipation. To avoid such side effects, morphine may be administered locally. For example, in the treatment of postoperative pain following a Caesarian section, or to relieve labor pain, morphine may be injected intrathecally into the cerebrospinal fluid of the subarachnoid space. Because there is no significant diffusion of the drug from the site of injection, side effects are avoided.

Interactions between nociceptive afferents, local interneurons, and descending pain-modulating fibers in the dorsal horn are depicted in Figure 16-7 ■. Many interneurons of the substantia gelatinosa release enkephalin and dynorphin. The terminals of these interneurons are in proximity to the synapses between primary nociceptive

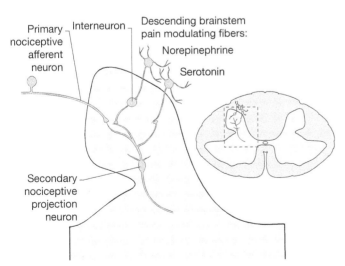

FIGURE 16-7 Primary nociceptive afferents, local interneurons, and descending inputs converge upon second-order projection neurons within the dorsal horn.

afferents and second-order projection neurons of the dorsal horn that enter the PAS. The terminals of these interneurons are thus in a position to influence the terminal of the primary afferent (a presynaptic influence), as well as the terminal of the dorsal horn projection neuron (a postsynaptic influence).

When the primary nociceptive afferent discharges, it releases glutamate and substance P onto the spinal cord projection neuron, depolarizing it and producing action potentials. Thus, the nociceptive message is transmitted to higher centers. The enkephalin-containing spinal cord interneurons are part of the pain-modulating system and are activated by descending serotonin projections from the raphe nuclei and descending norepinephrine projections from the locus coeruleus. Opiate receptors are present in the membranes of both the presynaptic primary afferent and the postsynaptic dorsal horn projection neuron. Activation of enkephalin-containing interneurons by the descending serotoninergic or norepinephrinergic fibers releases enkephalin onto presynaptic primary afferent terminals and postsynaptic projection neurons. In the presynaptic terminal, enkephalin acts to decrease Ca^{2+} influx into the terminal so that the amount of glutamate and substance P released is decreased and the postsynaptic neuron ineffectively depolarized. This action is called **presynaptic inhibition**, mediated by these axo-axonic synapses. In the postsynaptic projection neuron, enkephalin acts to hyperpolarize the membrane (**postsynaptic inhibition**).

The role of narcotic analgesics (opioids) in the therapy of chronic pain is problematic because clinical decision making is sometimes biased by concerns of addiction. Thus, people with persistent pain who might genuinely benefit from opioid medications may not receive them. The narcotic analgesics include the opium derivatives morphine and codeine and the synthetic opiates such as meperidine (Demerol) and propoxyphene (Darvon). Nociceptive pain is typically responsive to opioid analgesics, whereas neuropathic pain is usually poorly responsive and may necessitate higher doses of the drug.

> **Thought Question**
>
> A number of different agents play roles in either enhancing or diminishing the pain response. Some were introduced previously, and others are yet to come. Now is a good time to begin to tabulate these agents in terms of the following: location at which the agent is produced, location of action (e.g., receptor, specific location in the spinal cord, cortex), specific action (activation, sensitization, or reduction of pain response), and related pharmacologic agents (if known).

With respect to use of narcotic analgesics, along with addiction, is the potential for development of cellular tolerance. When morphine binds to normally unoccupied postsynaptic opioid receptors, an abnormal condition of receptor overload is created. The postsynaptic dorsal horn neuron then signals the presynaptic enkephalin neuron to decrease the release and eventually the synthesis of enkephalin, a response designed to return the system to normal. Faced with the reduction of enkephalin release, more exogenous morphine must now be administered to achieve the same pain-reducing effect that was formerly achieved by a lower dose of morphine. In other words, cellular tolerance has developed. If the administration of exogenous morphine is terminated, projection neurons are *devoid* of opiate influence and pain returns—a symptom of opiate withdrawal. The phenomena of cellular tolerance and withdrawal as discussed are to be distinguished from those characterizing addiction because there is no psychological craving that dominates the existence of an addict.

Acupuncture

Acupuncture is the ancient Chinese medical procedure in which long, fine needles are inserted into specific points at the skin, then twirled. Anesthesia sufficient to permit abdominal, thoracic, and head and neck surgery can be produced by the use of acupuncture alone, and indeed, surgery frequently is performed in China under acupuncture alone. The patient remains fully conscious during the surgery. The practice received little attention in Western cultures until the early 1970s.

The historical Chinese explanation is that Yin and Yang flow through hypothetic tubules called meridians and that the needles bring Yin and Yang into harmony with one another. It has been discovered that some insertion points correspond to myofascial trigger points. These are points over muscles, tendons, or bone where digital pressure produces a focal area of pain and are well known in Western medicine. Acupuncture may be effective in relieving low back pain and pain that is due to peripheral nerve injury. The neural mechanism underlying this relief appears to be that acupuncture activates the descending inhibitory pain-modulating system. This belief is strengthened by the claim that naloxone (a drug that blocks opioid receptors) abolishes the pain-relieving action of acupuncture.

CHRONIC PAIN

Clinical Preview

Renee Petzinger was referred to a rehabilitation professional by her primary care physician in hopes that he could assist her with control of her migraines. As you read through this section, consider the following:

- What is the current theory of the cause of migraines?
- What is the likelihood that physical intervention can assist with the migraine itself?
- Is there a potential role for a rehabilitation professional in treatment of this woman's migraines?

Chronic pain conditions are particularly problematic for the person and are difficult to manage by the rehabilitation specialist. Oftentimes, these conditions do not respond well to standard pharmacological and physical interventions. While these conditions are not totally understood, it is clear that their impact extends beyond the pain pathways discussed in this chapter. In some cases, chronic pain begins without a clear injury. In other cases, an acute condition goes on to become a chronic condition. For example, complex regional pain syndrome may arise as a result of a specific injury involving the pain pathways and physiology that are discussed in this chapter. However, if the acute condition transitions into a complex regional pain syndrome, other factors in addition to the pain pathways become important. Of particular importance is the person's psychological/emotional response to the condition, which in turn may be colored by cultural responses to pain. These critical aspects of the pain experience are of central importance when developing intervention strategies. The biology of this response is, however, beyond the scope of this text. Furthermore, evidence is growing to suggest that maladaptive plasticity—peripherally, centrally, or both—may contribute to chronic pain conditions. This maladaptive plasticity is discussed in Chapter 26.

CLINICAL CONNECTIONS

Phantom Limb Pain

Phantom limb pain refers to pain resulting from two different conditions involving the PNS. The first follows amputation of a limb either accidentally or surgically. The person continues to feel as though some (or all) of the nonexistent limb is still present, with 60 to 80 percent of people with these amputations complaining of the perception of pain in the missing limb. The second situation most frequently follows extensive denervation of a still-present living limb such as occurs with avulsion of nerve rootlets from the spinal cord with brachial plexus injuries.

The intensities and durations of phantom pain vary among people who have amputations. The usual condition for such indivuals is to experience phantom pain that causes considerable discomfort and disruption of normal life. The pain is permanent for a significant number. The treatment of phantom limb pain poses a great challenge, with more than four dozen treatment methods attempted, ranging from surgical ablation of pain pathways to hypnosis. Only about 1 percent of those treated report permanent relief. Phantom limb pain is discussed more fully in Chapter 26. V. S. Ramachandran has led many investigations about the experience, perceptions, and treatment of phantom-limb pain, illustrating the reorganization of the CNS with this condition.

Pain after Thalamic Stroke

In Chapter 6, the **thalamic syndrome** was introduced in which thalamic pain is a manifestation. In fact, pain is the cardinal symptom of the syndrome; hence, a better term for the syndrome is **central poststroke pain**. Thalamic pain is intractable because it is above the level at which modulation occurs. Thalamic pain is spontaneous, severe, paroxysmal, and burning. People with central poststroke pain also experience hyperalgesia (overreaction to noxious stimuli) as well as allodynia (painful sensation in response to non-noxious stimuli).

Thought Question

To fully understand thalamic pain syndrome, this is a good time to recall all levels at which pain is modulated and the pathways of pain from the periphery to the cortex. Using this information, explain in your own words why thalamic pain might occur and why it would be intractable.

Complex Regional Pain Syndromes

Following physical trauma, two clinical conditions sometimes occur, referred to under the heading of **complex regional pain syndromes (CRPS)**. The first (CRPS-I) is also referred to as **reflex sympathetic dystrophy (RSD)**, the second (CRPS-II) is referred to as **causalgia**. Although these conditions do not typically occur following injury, they have profound consequences when they do occur. CRPS is not manifest immediately following injury. CRPS-I occurs most commonly after trauma to the distal extremity, whereas CRPS-II occurs when trauma is to the nerve itself. The hallmark in both conditions is dysfunction of the sympathetic division of the ANS (discussed later). Autonomic changes are accompanied by a persistent, severe, burning pain in the affected extremity. They are due to a common mechanism: namely, partial interruption of nerves in the arm, shoulder, or leg. The pathogenesis of these signs and symptoms is commonly thought to be ectopic nerve impulse generation along the damaged (and denuded) axons, although the exact mechanisms and consequences have not been well established.

In complex regional pain syndromes, post-traumatic pain is disproportionate to the severity of the injury and spreads beyond the distribution of any single peripheral nerve, often (mysteriously) spreading to the opposite limb or the other ipsilateral limb—neither of which were themselves traumatized. The painful extremity is overly sensitive to stimuli such that even the pressure of clothing or drafts of air cannot be tolerated due to perceived pain by the individual, who then avoids moving the affected part. In addition to the persistent, burning, severe pain and allodynia in the affected limb(s), manifestations include signs of dysfunction of the sympathetic division of the ANS such as pallor or cyanosis and changes in the temperature (warmth or coldness) of the skin (vasomotor) and skin moistness (sudomotor). CRPS was first thought to be due to increased sympathetic nervous system discharge so that medications that block transmission in sympathetic ganglia (procaine) or surgical sympathectomy were attempted. However, such procedures lead to inconsistent and disappointing results. Although the precise pathogenetic mechanism underlying CRPS remains unknown, contemporary belief is that it is sympathetic denervation, not excessive outflow, that enhances pain transmission. Stimulation of the dorsal spinal cord with an electrode placed in the epidural space may prove to be a successful treatment. Whatever neuronal changes prove to be the cause of CRPS, those changes are regarded as an example of nonproductive (maladaptive) plasticity—that is, changes in neuronal function that mediate pathology and not recovery.

Migraine Headache

Migraine is a familial disorder characterized by paroxysmal, pulsatile, usually unilateral headaches. Migraine affects approximately 15 percent of the world's population and is more common in women (3:1), particularly during their reproductive years. Peak onset is before 30 years of age. Migraine degrades the general well-being of patients and represents a significant cost to society in terms of health care resource use and lost work productivity. Two major clinical syndromes are recognized: migraine with aura (also called classic, or neurologic) and migraine without aura (also called common migraine), which is about five times as common as migraine with aura.

Phases of Migraine

There are four distinct phases for migraine with aura. Days or hours before the onset of either type of migraine, the patient may have a *prodrome phase*. The patient is aware of affective or vegetative symptoms consisting of euphoria, depression, irritability, food cravings, constipation, neck stiffness, and increased yawning.

The second phase of the migraine is the *aura phase*. This consists of focal neurologic deficits preceding the onset of a migraine by 20 to 40 minutes. Such focal deficits usually consist of a homonymous visual hallucination or, much less commonly, other disturbances such as tingling and numbness of the lips, face, arm, and hand on one side, or even transient aphasia. The visual hallucinations take the form of flashing white, sometimes colored, lights, zigzag lines, or distortions of visual perceptions that move slowly across the visual field ("fortification spectrum"), sometimes leaving in their wake areas of blindness (scotomas).

The *headache phase* is the third phase of a migraine. The throbbing headache is often accompanied by autonomic symptoms such as nausea, vomiting, diaphoresis, piloerection, and tachycardia. Also during the headache phase, the person is very sensitive to all types of environmental stimuli, resulting in aversion to light, sounds, smells, and even movement. Migraine without aura presents with the same features and has the autonomic symptoms and sensitivity to environmental stimuli, but it does not have the antecedent focal neurological deficits.

A characteristic of people with migraines is that they can get relief by being in a dark, quiet, restful condition. Sleep often provides relief. The headache lasts for hours or days, but recovery is invariably complete.

Some people will evolve into a fourth phase, a *postdromal syndrome* of fatigue, poor concentration, and depression. Some patients will have continued migraine, lasting over days; this is referred to as *status migrainosus*.

Migraine attacks can be precipitated by a variety of factors. One is nonspecific stress, such as in the case of loss of sleep or overwork. Strong visual stimuli such as a glare or flashing lights may trigger an attack. Approximately 20 percent of people link their attacks to certain foods—in particular, chocolate, cheese, citrus fruits, foods with aspartame, or alcohol (especially red wine). Changes in the weather can precipitate migraine in some people. Attacks are associated with ovulation or the menstrual period in about 15 percent of women who experience migraines. Some women can date the onset of the headaches with menarche, and some will have a flurry of headaches as they enter menopause.

Anatomical Substrate, Mechanism, and Treatment of Migraine Headache

The neuronal mechanism that causes migraine headache remains unknown. However, the anatomical substrate that mediates the generation of migraine-associated pain is known. This anatomical substrate includes the meninges (in particular, meningeal blood vessels), the trigeminal nerve, the subnucleus caudalis of the spinal trigeminal nucleus, and the autonomic nuclei in the brainstem.

The peripheral terminals of primary trigeminal afferent fibers innervate most of the dura mater, including arteries embedded within it. The dura mater is a primary source of intracranial pain, given the fact that the brain itself does not contain pain receptors. Trigeminal afferents from perivascular free nerve endings enter the spinal trigeminal tract and synapse on cells of the subnucleus caudalis of the spinal trigeminal nuclear complex. Secondary projections from cells of the subnucleus caudalis enter the PAS to synapse in the structures previously delineated for this projection system (see Chapter 14).

It was formerly believed that the pain of migraine was due to abnormally dilated and stretched cerebral blood vessels, especially those in the dura mater, and that the mechanism of action in antimigraine drugs (such as ergotamine, a smooth muscle constrictor) was vasoconstriction. This view has changed. The mechanism that generates migraine pain is now thought to be neurogenic inflammation, and the action of antimigraine drugs is to selectively inhibit neurogenic inflammation.

Perivascular free nerve endings arising from the trigeminal ganglion surround meningeal blood vessels (Figure 16-8 ■). These afferent terminals contain substance P and other vasoactive neuropeptides. The membranes of these afferent terminals also have autoreceptors for both opiates and serotonin that regulate the release of these vasoactive peptides. When trigeminal C fibers are activated, substance P is released not only from the central processes of trigeminal ganglion cells onto neurons of the subnucleus caudalis of the spinal trigeminal nucleus, but also from the peripheral processes of ganglion cells onto the wall of meningeal blood vessels via an axon reflex, as shown in Figure 16-2. Peripherally released substance P causes vasodilation, increased permeability of the vessel wall, and plasma extravasation (edema). Bradykinins circulating in the plasma are released from blood vessels and activate the perivascular pain afferents directly. Substance P also causes nearby mast cells to degranulate and release histamine that likewise activates perivascular pain afferents. As a result of nociceptive activation by these mediators, more substance P is released from the afferent terminals—and a vicious cycle is established.

Drugs used to treat migraine include standard anti-inflammatory medications such as sumatriptan and ergot alkaloids such as ergotamine. The latter drugs act to block neurogenic inflammation. The mechanism of action in sumatriptan for blocking the development of neurogenic inflammation is to bind to serotonin receptors on the peripheral nociceptive terminals that surround meningeal vessels. This binding prevents the release of substance P and other vasoactive peptides from the terminals. However, this may not be the only site of action of sumatriptan as serotonin receptors are distributed throughout the pain-modulating network. The best clinical response to sumatriptan occurs in those people with the most severe migraines.

If an individual is debilitated by migraines for more than 15 days a month, he or she is said to have chronic migraine. It is recommended that these individuals be placed on prophylactic daily medications. Several families of medications have been used in this manner, including beta-blockers, barbiturates, and anti-epileptic agents. If the individual takes pain-blocking medications (such as opioids) in excess, he or she may sensitize the pain system and develop refractory continuous headaches.

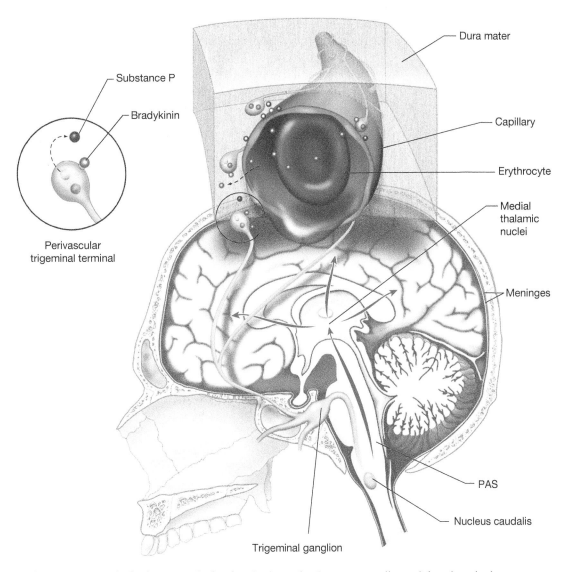

Substance P

Bradykinin

Perivascular
trigeminal terminal

Dura mater

Capillary

Erythrocyte

Medial
thalamic
nuclei

Meninges

PAS

Nucleus caudalis

Trigeminal ganglion

FIGURE 16-8 The neuroanatomical substrates of migraine. Perivascular free nerve endings of the trigeminal nerve surround the meningeal blood vessels. The activation of these terminals induces the release of substance P and initiates neurogenic inflammation. PAS, paramedical ascending system

Summary

Pain differs markedly from other somatic sensory modalities, and reasons were advanced as to why pain should not be considered as a submodality of somatic sensation. One focus of this chapter was on the duality of the pain experience and the projections that mediate it, with special emphasis on the paramedial ascending system (PAS), or paleospinothalamic tract. The neural bases of peripheral and central sensitization as manifest by hyperalgesia and allodynia were discussed, whereby the pain system possesses mechanisms whose purpose is to minimize the use of injured tissue to facilitate its repair. Neurons at all levels of the PAS contain

receptors for endogenous opioid neurotransmitters, collectively referred to as endorphins. This accounts for the effectiveness of narcotic analgesics in relieving enduring pain and altering the emotional response to it. Additionally, we discussed the descending pain modulating system that controls the intensity, as well as affective components, of the pain experience. This system originates in the cerebral cortex and ultimately influences synaptic transmission in neurons at the lowest level of the CNS—namely, those that link peripheral nociceptors with the transmission neurons of the PAS. The pain-modulating network may be activated by cognitions as well as by noxious stimuli themselves. Four classes of drugs are used in the management of enduring pain states: nonopioid analgesics, tricyclic antidepressants, anticonvulsants, and narcotic (opioid) analgesics. The mode of action of each class was discussed.

Migraine headache is mediated by the trigeminal component of the PAS that begins in perivascular primary afferents surrounding dural blood vessels. These primary afferents synapse in the subnucleus caudalis of the spinal trigeminal nucleus. The process of neurogenic inflammation, caused by a peripheral release of vasoactive neuropeptides from perivascular trigeminal terminals, is thought to be a substrate for migraine headache. Antimigraine drugs appear to block neurogenic inflammation.

Applications

1. Samuel is a 24-year-old college student who fell while skiing. He fractured his right distal tibia and fibula. The damage was repaired surgically with an open-reduction-internal fixation (ORIF). Three months later, he began to experience severe pain in his right lower leg. Samuel took a leave of absence from college because he was falling behind in his coursework. His orthopedic surgeon referred him for rehabilitation, with a diagnosis of complex regional pain syndrome. Samuel walked into the rehabilitation clinic with an antalgic gait and a single-point cane. On interview, he described his pain as burning and aching and indicated that it was constant in nature. He reported having trouble sleeping because even the weight of the bed sheets seemed to hurt his foot. Upon inspection, his right ankle appeared swollen and reddened. His right lower limb was warm to the touch.

   a. Differentiate nociceptive and neuropathic pain. What kind of pain was Samuel experiencing?
   b. Review the wide, dynamic-range neurons of the dorsal horn. Use this knowledge to explain how ordinarily painless stimuli can be perceived as painful.
   c. Explain ectopic discharge. How does this relate to Samuel's situation?
   d. Is all plasticity productive?
   e. Which of Samuel's symptoms are associated with autonomic nervous system dysfunction?

2. In rehabilitation, physical agents are often used to treat people who are experiencing pain. Identify commonly used physical agents and their mechanism of action in decreasing pain.

References

Apkarian, V., Thomas, P. S., Krauss, B. R., and Szevernyi, N. M. Prefrontal cortical hyperactivity in patients with sympatheticlly mediated chronic pain. *Neurosci Lett* 311:193–197, 2001.

Ballantyne, J. C., and LaForge, K. S. Opioid dependence and addiction during opioid treatment of chronic pain. *Pain* 129(3):235–255, 2007.

Bartsch, T., Knight, Y. E., and Goadsby, P. J. Activation of 5-HT$_{1B/1D}$ receptor in the periaqueductal gray inhibits nociception. *Ann Neurol* 56:371–381, 2004.

Beecher, H. K. Pain in men wounded in battle. *Ann. Surg* 123:96, 1946.

Birklein, F., and Rowbotham, M. C. Does pain change the brain? *Neurology*, 65:666–667, 2005.

Bowsher, D. Central pain of spinal origin. *Spinal Cord* 34:707–710, 1996.

Casey, K.L. Resolving a paradox of pain. *Nature* 384:217–218, 1996.

Craig, A. D., Reiman, E. M., Evans, A., and Bushnell, M. C. Functional imaging of an illusion of pain. *Nature* 384:258, 1996.

Devor, M. Pain mechanisms. *Neuroscientist* 2:233–244, 1996.

Edwards, R. R. Individual differences in endogenous pain modulation as a risk factor for chronic pain. *Neurology* 65:437–443, 2005.

Elkind, M. S. V., and Scher, A. I. Migraine and cognitive function. *Neurology* 64:590–591, 2005.

Goldstein, D. S., Tack, C., and Li, S.-T. Sympathetic innervation and function in reflex sympathetic dystrophy. *Ann Neurol* 48:49–59, 2000.

Hughes, J., Smith, T. W., Kosterlitz, H. W., et al. Identification of two related pentapeptides from the brain with potent opiate agonist activity. *Nature* 258:577, 1975.

Iadrola, M. J., Max, M. B., Berman, K. F., et al. Unilateral decrease in thalamic activity observed with positron emission tomography in patient with chronic neuropathic pain. *Pain* 63:55–64, 1995.

Kelman, L. The premonitory symptoms (prodrome): A tertiary care study of 893 migraineurs. *Headache* 44:865, 2004.

Kemler, M. A., DeVer, H. C. W., Berendse, G. A. M., et al. The effect of spinal cord stimulation in patients with chronic reflex synmpathetic dystrophy: Two years follow-up of the randomized control trial. *Ann Neurol* 55:13–18, 2004.

Lipton, R. B. Fair winds and foul headaches. Risk factors and triggers of migraine. *Neurol* 54:280–281, 2000.

Liu, H., Mantyh, P. W., and Basbaum, A. I. NMDA-receptor regulation of substance P release from primary afferent nociceptors. *Nature* 386:721–724, 1997.

McQuay, H. J. Pharmacological treatment of neuralgic and neuropathic pain. *Cancer Surv* 7:141–159, 1988.

Melzack, R., and Wall, P. D. Pain mechanisms: A new theory. *Science* 150: 971–979, 1965.

Merskey, H., and Bogduk, N. Classification of chronic pain. Description of chronic pain syndromes and definitions of pain terms. *Task Force on Taxonomy, International Association for the Study of Pain*, 2nd ed. IASP Press, Seattle, 1994.

Morris, R., Cheunsuang, O., Stewart, A., and Maxwell, D. Spinal dorsal horn neurone targets for nociceptive primary afferents: Do single neurone morphological characteristics suggest how nociceptive information is processed at the spinal level? *Brain Res Rev* 46:173–190, 2004.

Moskowitz, M. A., and Waeber, C. Migraine enters the molecular era. *Neuroscientist* 2:191–200, 1996.

Nathan, P. W. The gate-control theory of pain: A critical review. *Brain* 99:i23, 1976.

Ramachandran, V. S., Brang, D., and McGeoch, P.D. Dynamic reorganization of referred sensations by movements of phantom limbs. *Neuro Report* 21: 727–730, 2010.

Reynolds, D. V. Surgery in the rat during electrical analgesia induced by focal brain stimulation. *Science* 164:444, 1969.

Ron, M. A. Explaining the unexplained: Understanding hysteria. *Brain* 124:1065–1066, 2001.

Ropper, A. H., and Brown, R. H. *Adams and Victor's Principles of Neurology*, 8th ed. McGraw-Hill, New York, 2005.

Saito, K., Markowitz, M. D., and Moskowitz, M. A. Ergot alkaloids block neurogenic extravasation in dura mater: Proposed action in vascular headaches. *Ann Neurol* 24:732–737, 1988.

Sloka K. A., ed. *Mechanisms and Management of Pain for the Physical Therapist*. IASP Press, Seattle, 2009.

Snyder, S. H. Opiate receptors and internal opiates. *Sci. Am.* 236(3):44–56. 1977

Strassman, A. M., Raymond, S. A., and Burstein, R. Sensitization of meningeal sensory neurons and the origin of headaches. *Nature* 384:560–564, 1996.

Strassman, A. M., and Levy, D. Response properties of dual nociceptors in relation to headache. *J Neurophysiol* 95:1298–1306, 2006.

Vanegas, H., and Schaible, H.-G. Descending control of persistent pain: Inhibitory or facilitatory? *Brain Research Reviews* 46:295–309, 2004.

Verdugo, R. J., Bell, L. A., Campero, M., et al. Spectrum of cutaneous hyperalgesias/allodynaias in neuropathic pain patients. *Acta Neurol Scand* 110:368–376, 2004.

Wall, P, D. The placebo effect: An unpopular topic. *Pain* 51:1–3, 1992.

Wall, P. D., and Melzack, R., eds. *Textbook of Pain*, 3rd ed. Churchill-Livingston, London, 1994.

Waxman, S. G. $Na_v1.7$, its mutations, and the syndromes that they cause. *Neurology* 69:505–507, 2007.

Welch, K. M. A., and Levine, S. R. Migraine-related stroke in the context of the international hcadache society classification of head pain. *Arch Neurol* 47: 458–462, 1990.

Zubieta, J.-K., Bueller, J. A., Jackson, L. R., et al. Placebo effects mediated by endogenous opioid activity on mu-opioid receptors. *J Neurosci* 25:7754–7762, 2005.

PEARSON
myhealthprofessionskit™

Use this address to access the Companion Website created for this textbook. Simply select "Physical Therapy" from the choice of disciplines. Find this book and log in using your username and password to access self-assessment questions, a glossary, and more.

Auditory and Vestibular Systems

LEARNING OUTCOMES

This chapter prepares the reader to:

1. Recall the meaning of the following terms related to the structure of the inner ear: labyrinth, endolymph, perilymph, kinocilium, stereocilium, and tip links.

2. Discuss the role of K$^+$ in both polarization and depolarization of hair cells.

3. Describe the sequence of events leading to polarization and hyperpolarization of auditory and vestibular and bipolar neurons whose axons give rise to cranial nerve VIII.

4. Identify structures of the outer, middle, and inner ear and explain the purpose of the following: tympanic membrane, maleus, incus, stapes, oval window, round window, and organ of Corti.

5. Analyze the functions of the middle and inner ear and explain the structures that mediate each function.

6. Compare and contrast the structure and function of the outer and inner hair cells of the organ of Corti.

7. Describe the pathway from the sensory receptors (hair cells) to the cerebral cortex by which sounds are conveyed into the CNS for interpretation.

8. Recall the anatomical location and role of the following structures that are associated with the pathway for auditory afferent fibers: trapezoid body, superior olivary nucleus, lateral lemniscus, and planum temporal.

9. Compare conductive, sensorineural, and mixed hearing loss in terms of causes, consequences, and ease of correction.

10. Compare and contrast the role of the components of the vestibular labyrinth with respect to identifying angular velocity, linear acceleration, and rotational acceleration.

11. Analyze the orientation of the saccule, macula, utricle, and semicircular canals and explain the functional importance of each structure.

12. Discuss the anatomical location and role of the four vestibular nuclei associated with the vestibular sensory pathways.

13. Describe the destination and laterality of the second- and third-order neurons of the vestibular system.

14. Compare and contrast the anatomical location and roles of the following structures associated with the vestibular motor pathways: lateral vestibulospinal tract, medial vestibulospinal tract, reticular formation, medial longitudinal fasciculus, and juxtarestiform body.

15. Analyze the vestibulomotor pathways with respect to their functional relevance.

16. Discuss the following reflexes associated with the vestibular system and relate each to their relevant pathways: vestibulocollic, vestibulospinal, and vestibulo-ocular.

17. Explain how information from the semicircular canals and their afferent projections is integrated with information from the oculomotor, trochlear, and abducens nerves to produce the VOR.

18. Compare the tonic neck reflexes with the vestibular reflexes and explain the function of each reflex.

19. Relate clinical examination approaches to the structure and function of the vestibular system.

ACRONYMS

BAER Brainstem auditory evoked responses

BPPV Benign paroxysmal positional vertigo

BPV Benign positional vertigo

CNS Central nervous system

CSF Cerebrospinal fluid

CT Computed tomography

LMN Lower motor neuron

LVST Lateral vestibulospinal tract

MGB Medial geniculate body

MLF Medial longitudinal fasciculus

MRI Magnetic resonance imaging

MVST Medial vestibulospinal tract

OKN Optokinetic nystagmus

PET Positron emission tomography

PIVC Parieto-insular-vestibular cortex

PPRF Paramedian pontine reticular formation

RF Reticular formation

SCC Semicircular canal

SVV Subjective visual vertical

UMN Upper motor neuron

VOR Vestibulo-ocular reflex

VPI Ventral posterior inferior nucleus

VPL Ventral posterolateral nucleus

Introduction

The perception of sound is so markedly different from the perception of head movement and position that it seems counterintuitive to think that these two special sensory systems have much in common. Nonetheless, there is a commonality in the peripheral anatomy of these two systems. Both are components of the eighth cranial nerve (CN VIII), head position-movement sensation being mediated by its vestibular division and sound perception by its cochlear division. Both systems begin in similar sensory end organs, the hair cells.

The first major section of this chapter considers the inner ear, in which both the cochlear and vestibular nerves originate. We begin with the osseous and membranous labyrinths and the fluids they contain. We then discuss the structure and function of the labyrinthine hair cells that are common to both systems. The hair cells consist of a bundle of about 100 specialized microvilli (stereocilia) projecting from their superior surface—situated in the membranous labyrinth of the inner ear. The transduction mechanism is the same in all hair cells: bending of the stereocilia in one direction causes depolarization (and a receptor potential), whereas bending the stereocilia in the opposite direction causes a hyperpolarization. However, in the final analysis, these are commonalties possessing little, if any, significance. What is truly remarkable about comparing the auditory and vestibular systems is how such dramatically different perceptions as sound and position-movement of the head can result from a single receptor type residing in unique and highly specialized environments. Therefore, it is the environment in which the receptor finds itself embedded that determines whether it responds to sound or to movement or position of the head. These are not subtle differences. Rather, they are fundamental differences on a microscopic scale. They reflect how minute structural differences in the PNS can condition perceptions engendered in the brain.

In the second major section of this chapter, we consider the auditory system. We begin with the apparatus of the ear, starting with the outer ear and moving to the inner ear. We next consider the pathways by which sound travels through the nervous system to the cortex for interpretation. We end this section with a discussion of clinical consequences of damage within the auditory system.

In the third section, we consider the vestibular system. As with the auditory system, we begin with the sensory end organs and then consider projections within the nervous system. We end this section with a discussion of clinical consequences of damage within the vestibular system, including testing of the system.

Content is presented in this order because the auditory system follows the organizational principles already presented for other sensory systems in terms of having a robust projection to the cerebral cortex for the conscious discrimination of sound features. The vestibular system, on the other hand, is more complicated in several respects. First, many of the neurons are multimodal because balance is subserved not just by labyrinthine receptors in the inner ear, but also by vision and proprioception. Thus, there is a marked degree of convergence of visual and proprioceptive information on sensory neurons of the vestibular system. Second, the vestibular system is not only a sensory system, but also a motor system. On the sensory side, the nuclei of the vestibular system project to the cerebral cortex. However, in addition, as we noted in Chapters 8 and 11, the nuclei of the vestibular system contain UMNs as well. Axons of these upper motor neurons (UMNs) descend to the spinal cord in the vestibulospinal tracts and also ascend to control lower motor neurons (LMNs) innervating the extraocular muscles. Finally, just as the vestibular system is a multimodal sensory system, it also is an integrative motor system. UMNs of the vestibular system are important mediators of cerebellar influences on motor function. In addition, the reflexes mediated by the vestibular system function in inextricable collaboration with reflexes elicited by neck proprioceptors.

INNER EAR

Labyrinth

The inner ear is called the **labyrinth** owing to the complexity of its shape (Figure 17-1 ■). The labyrinth has two major divisions: a cochlear labyrinth and a vestibular labyrinth. Each division consists of two parts: an **osseous labyrinth**, which is a series of cavities and channels within the petrous part of the temporal bone, and a **membranous labyrinth**, which is a system of communicating membranous sacs and ducts, moored within the osseous labyrinth by fibrous bands. While preserving the general form of the osseous labyrinth, the membranous labyrinth is considerably smaller and is separated from the bony walls by a fluid called **perilymph**. Perilymph is secreted by arterioles of the periosteum lining the bony labyrinth. It has an ionic composition similar to that of the cerebrospinal fluid (CSF) and extracellular fluid of the CNS. Perilymph is in communication with the CSF-filled subarachnoid space via the **perilymphatic duct** (*cochlear aqueduct*).

> **Thought Question**
>
> Describe the components of the inner ear. Are any of these components important only for the auditory system and not for the vestibular system?

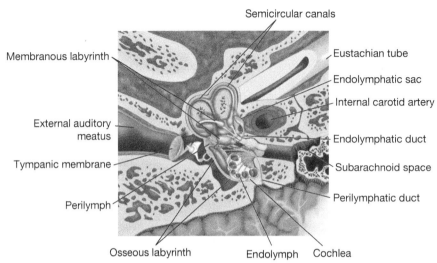

FIGURE 17-1 The osseous labyrinth is set in the petrous portion of the temporal bone. Within the general form of the osseous labyrinth is the membranous labyrinth.

The membranous labyrinth also contains a fluid, the **endolymph**. Endolymph is produced by secretory cells surrounding the sensory epithelia of the vestibular labyrinth and by cells of the stria vascularis of the cochlea (discussed later). Endolymph has an ionic composition similar to that of intracellular fluid. From the posterior wall of the saccule (see Figure 17-1), a canal—the **endolymphatic duct**—is given off that is joined in a Y-shaped configuration by a duct interconnecting the utricle and saccule. Endolymph leaves the labyrinth in the endolymphatic duct. The endolymphatic duct ends in a blind pouch—the **endolymphatic sac**—located on the posterior surface of the petrous portion of the temporal bone, where it is in contact with the dura mater. Endolymph circulates through the membranous labyrinth and then enters the endolymphatic duct and endolymphatic sac. Specialized epithelial cells of the sac remove endolymph via a pinocytotic mechanism, where it enters a dense vascular plexus surrounding the sac. An imbalance in the production and drainage of endolymph is related to Meniere's disease (see Clinical Connections).

Hair Cells

Auditory and vestibular receptors—the hair cells—are positioned at specific sites along the inner walls of the membranous labyrinth. These neurons are unique mechanoreceptors in that they are specialized non-neural cells that synapse with primary afferents of CN VIII. As noted in Chapter 9, hair cells represent independent transduction entities rather than the peripheral terminals of cranial nerve sensory fibers (Figure 17-2 ■). In essence, the hair cell is a synaptic terminal whose release of a chemical neurotransmitter excites a response in primary afferents of CN VIII. Thus, the hair cell is a specialized cell that can create a generator potential that then has a synaptic terminal to a primary afferent neuron. This is the first pathway that we will discuss in detail in which the first-order structure is not a nerve cell.

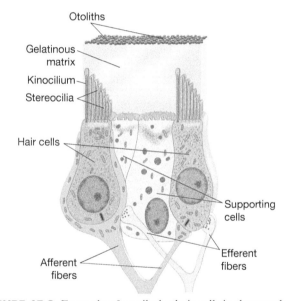

FIGURE 17-2 Example of vestibular hair cells in the membranous labyrinth with a single, large kinocilium and many smaller stereocilia.

Hair cells are structurally polarized. Each hair cell in the membranous labyrinth has a single, large **kinocilium** projecting from one edge of the cell surface, and a group of 60 to 100 smaller **stereocilia** ordered in ranks of increasing length toward the kinocilium that heads the *organpipe* array (see Figure 17-2). Hair cells in the cochlear labyrinth have kinocilia, but they degenerate during fetal development, leaving only stereocilia. The **adequate stimulus** for hair cells is a bending of the cilia.

Thought Question

Identify the components of the hair cell and explain the role of each component in the transduction of sensory information.

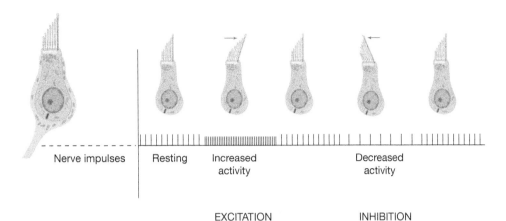

Nerve impulses   Resting   Increased
                                activity

                                            Decreased
                                            activity

EXCITATION   INHIBITION

FIGURE 17-3 Bending of the stereocilia toward the kinocilium depolarizes the hair cell, while bending of the stereocilia away from the kinocilium hyperpolarizes the hair cell. This leads to excitation or inhibition of the primary afferent.

The hair cell's structural polarization results in a functional polarization (Figure 17-3 ■). Bending the stereocilia *toward* the kinocilium depolarizes the hair cell, resulting in an increase in the release of neurotransmitter from the hair cell, while bending the stereocilia *away* from the kinocilium hyperpolarizes the cell, resulting in a decrease in the release of neurotransmitter.

Bending is not the best word to describe movements of stereocilia, which are packed with actin filaments that make them rigid. Thus, they do not really bend in response to mechanical displacement but pivot at their bases where they are attached to the surface of the hair cell. Because all stereocilia in a given hair cell are linked, the entire bundle is displaced as a unit. Elastic filamentous structures link the tip of each stereocilium to its adjacent tallest neighbor and are called **tip links** (Figure 17-4 ■). Tip links are coupled to mechanically gated cation channels. When the stereocilia are straight, tension on the tip link holds the channel in a partially opened state. This allows cations to flow from the endolymph into the hair cell in a manner analogous to leak channels in a neuron

establishing the resting membrane potential (see Chapter 4). Deflecting the stereocilia toward the kinocilium stretches the tip links and fully opens the cation channels, whereas deflecting the stereocilia in the opposite direction closes the channels.

What happens next in the transduction process is unusual in terms of its ionic basis. Potassium serves to both depolarize the hair cell as well as to repolarize it. This is because the ionic composition of the endolymph in which the surface of the hair cell and stereocilia are bathed has a high concentration of K^+. In contrast, the ionic composition of the perilymph in which the rest of the hair cell is bathed has a high concentration of Na^+. The ionic composition difference between endolymph and perilymph is maintained by tight junctions at the surface of hair cells and their supporting cells (Figure 17-5 ■). The hair cell exploits the different ionic environments at its apical and basal surfaces.

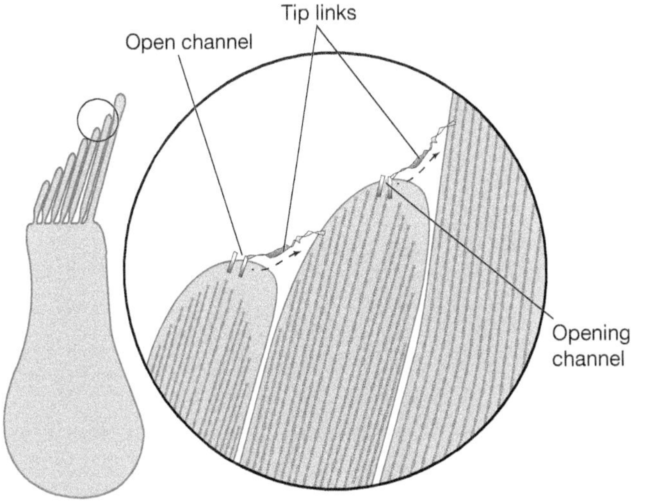

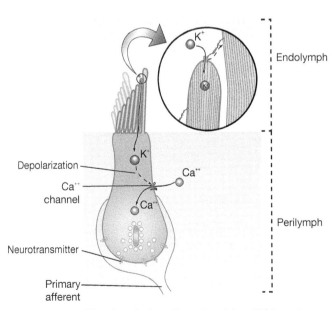

FIGURE 17-5 The electrical gradient that drives K^+ into the cell depolarizes the hair cell, causing opening of voltage-gated Ca^{2+} ion channels. In turn, this causes increased transmitter release by the hair cell and increased firing frequency of the primary afferent neuron.

FIGURE 17-4 Stereocilia are linked by elastic filaments called tip links. The entire hair bundle bends or pivots as a unit.

Thought Question

Tip links play a key role in the transduction of information into the nervous system because they are coupled to mechanically gated cation channels. Explain the significance of this coupling with regard to depolarization and repolarization.

Endolymph is an extracellular fluid (outside the hair cell) but is K^+ rich and Na^+ poor like intracellular fluid. Thus, the K^+ concentration in endolymph is about the same as that inside the stereocilia. But because the endolymph has a net positive charge, it combines with the net negative charge of the hair cell's membrane potential to form a powerful electrical gradient that drives K^+ ions into the hair cell through the open tip link–associated channels, thereby depolarizing the hair cell. This causes voltage-gated Ca^{2+} ion channels to open, triggering increased transmitter release onto the terminals of primary afferent neurons of CN VIII and an increased firing frequency (Figure 17-5). Transmitter release by hair cells is graded because there is a graded opening of voltage-gated Ca^{2+} channels according to membrane potential.

When the stereocilia are deflected in the opposite direction, away from the kinocilium, tension on the tip links is decreased, and the cation channels close. The baseline inward K^+ current stops, and the hair cell hyperpolarizes. Transmitter release by hair cells diminishes, as does the firing frequency of the postsynaptic primary afferents in CN VIII. The hair cells of the auditory system do not have kinocilia. This difference is discussed in the next section on the auditory system.

Thought Question

The ionic composition of the endolymph and perilymph differs. Explain how this difference is exploited in the transduction process.

AUDITORY SYSTEM

Clinical Preview ·················

In your clinical practice as a rehabilitation specialist, you frequently treat older individuals who have generalized loss of ability to perceive or discriminate sounds. You also treat young children with sensorineural hearing loss and those with conductive hearing loss. As you read through this section, consider the following:

- In both children and adults, damage can occur in components of the outer ear, middle ear, or inner ear. Which clinical conditions relate to which of these structures?

- What are the major differences between peripheral and central mechanisms of hearing loss?

Foundational Information

The auditory system detects and analyzes sounds in the environment in order to provide the brain with information on sound features (pitch, loudness, pattern) and localization. The auditory system is composed of a peripheral and a central apparatus. The elaborately organized peripheral apparatus consists of outer, middle, and inner ear structures for the registration and transduction of airborne vibrations. Transduction is dependent on hair cells. The central apparatus is composed of neurons, in serial and parallel arrangements, responsible for the discrimination and interpretation of sound. Within the cerebral cortex, this auditory information is transmitted to other cortical areas that decode the information into auditory perceptions such as music and sound recognition—and speech and language.

The auditory system is extraordinary in terms of the range of sound frequencies and intensities it can detect and with respect to the small differences in these parameters it can discriminate. A young, normal listener can hear sounds in the frequency range from 20 to 20,000 Hz and can detect displacements of the eardrum two orders of magnitude smaller than a hydrogen atom. Each ear has bilateral projections to all portions of the auditory system rostral to the lower brainstem so that damage to the central auditory apparatus rarely produces deficits that can be localized just to one ear. Peripheral auditory receptors are also subject to efferent control by the CNS.

Behavioral audiometric testing requires a response from the subject. It provides information relating largely to the effects of lesions at the two extremes of the auditory system: the peripheral apparatus and the neocortical end station. Relatively little is known about the pathophysiology of auditory brainstem disorders. Brainstem lesions affecting the auditory system almost invariably damage contiguous structures and produce a clinical picture in which auditory dysfunction is of less importance than other deficits.

The Peripheral Apparatus

Outer Ear

The outer (external) ear is essentially a complicated funnel, consisting of the **pinna** (or *auricle*) and the **external auditory meatus (canal)** (Figure 17-6 ■). These structures play major roles in the filtering (spectral shaping) of sounds that enter the ear. The external auditory meatus conducts sound to the tympanic membrane that represents the boundary between the outer and middle ear.

Middle Ear (Tympanic Cavity)

The **middle ear** or **tympanic cavity** resides within the temporal bone. It is filled with air, which is conveyed to it through the eustacian (auditory) tube from the nasal part of the pharynx (Figure 17-6). The air-filled middle ear is kept at atmospheric pressure by the periodic opening of the eustachian tube. The tympanic cavity contains a chain of movable bones, the **ossicles**, which form a bony

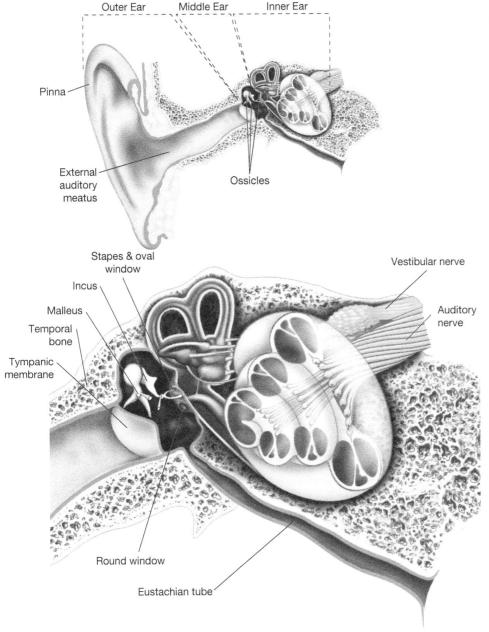

Outer Ear   Middle Ear   Inner Ear

Pinna

External
auditory
meatus

Ossicles

Stapes & oval
window

Incus

Malleus

Temporal
bone

Tympanic
membrane

Vestibular nerve

Auditory
nerve

Round window

Eustachian tube

FIGURE 17-6 The peripheral hearing apparatus includes the outer, middle, and inner ear. The outer ear consists of the pinna and external auditory meatus. The tympanic membrane separates the outer and middle ear. The middle ear resides within the temporal bone, is air-filled, and contains the three ossicles: malleus, incus, and stapes. The oval window separates the middle and inner ear.

connection between the tympanic membrane and the cochlea and serve to convey the airborne vibrations of the tympanic membrane across the cavity to the inner ear.

The task faced by the auditory system is to detect airborne sound vibrations by means of a set of receptor cells residing in a fluid-filled environment. In such an air-to-fluid interface, most of the sound energy would be reflected back because fluid has a higher acoustic impedance than does air. However, several structures in the middle ear make the transmission of sound from air in the outer ear to perilymphatic fluid motion in the inner ear as efficient as possible. These include the **tympanic membrane** and the set of three tiny bones called the ossicles. The tympanic membrane and ossicles establish an impedance match between the vibrations in air and fluid motion in the inner ear.

The tympanic membrane is a pearl gray translucent oval structure about 1 cm in diameter. It forms the lateral wall of the tympanic cavity. It is set at an oblique angle at the medial end of the external auditory meatus (Figure 17-6). The lateral surface receives innervation from the auriculotemporal branch of the trigeminal nerve (V) and the auricular branch of the vagus nerve (X), while its medial surface is innervated by the tympanic branch of the glossopharyngeal nerve (IX). The tympanic membrane acts somewhat as a loudspeaker, or microphone cone, that vibrates in response to sound waves striking its lateral surface.

Attached to the medial surface of the tympanic membrane is the first of the three ossicles, the **malleus**. Movements of the membrane are transferred directly to the malleus. Sound vibrations are then transferred to the

incus, the second of the ossicles, which bridges the malleus and the innermost of the three ossicles, the **stapes**.

The bony medial wall of the tympanic cavity contains two openings, one of which is the **oval window**. The oval-shaped footplate of the stapes fits into the opening of the oval window. The footplate of the stapes is anchored to the walls of the oval window by an elastic ring. The oval window separates the air-filled middle ear from the perilymphatic fluid of the inner ear (Figure 17-7 ■). Inward movement of the footplate presses on perilymph of the vestibule. The second opening in the bony medial wall of the tympanic cavity is the **round window**, which is covered by an elastic membrane and separates perilymph of the inner ear from the air-filled tympanic cavity.

The air-to-fluid impedance match is achieved because vibrations of the stapes have a much greater force per unit area (about 25 times) than vibrations of the tympanic membrane. This results from (1) a small mechanical advantage derived from the fact that the chain of middle ear ossicles acts as a lever system and (2) a large mechanical advantage derived from the fact that the area of the tympanic membrane is about 15 times larger than the area of the footplate of the stapes. The impedance match means that in intermediate ranges, nearly all sound energy incident on the tympanic membrane moves the perilymphatic fluid of the inner ear. The efficiency diminishes progressively at both higher and lower frequencies. For example, around 1,000 Hz, the system is only about 40 percent efficient.

> **Thought Question**
>
> What are the ossicles of the middle ear and what is their fundamental importance?

Two small muscles attach to the ossicles: the *tensor tympani* attaches to the malleus and is innervated by a branch of the trigeminal nerve; the *stapedius muscle* attaches to the stapes and is supplied by a branch of the facial nerve. The tensor tympani and stapedius muscles usually contract together and act to change the transmission of sound vibrations through the ossicular chain (see function and auditory reflexes discussed later, as well as Chapter 15).

Inner Ear

The structure of the auditory portion of the inner ear consists of a perilymph-filled bony labyrinth within which is suspended an endolymph-filled membranous labyrinth. The **cochlea** (L., snail) is the bony part of the auditory labyrinth (see Figure 17-7). It consists of a two-and-five-eighths-turn spiral wound around a central pillar called the **modiolus** (L., pillar, hub). The modiolus contains cavities within which reside bipolar neurons of the **spiral ganglion** that contain the cell bodies of primary auditory afferents. An osseous **spiral lamina** projects from the modiolus like the threads of a screw. The **cochlear duct** (*scala media*) forms the auditory portion of the membranous labyrinth. It is a membranous tube within the bony cochlea that ends blindly at the dome

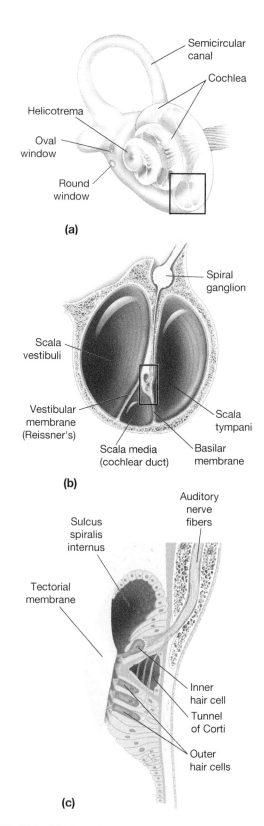

FIGURE 17-7 (a) The spiral-wound cochlea of the bony labyrinth contains the primary auditory afferent fibers. Note two openings: the oval window and the round window. (b) A segment of the cochlear duct, expanded to illustrate three compartments: the scala vestibuli, scala tympani, and scala media. (c) The inner portion of the cochlear duct, expanded to illustrate how the hair cells (receptors) embed into the tectorial membrane and connect with the primary afferent fibers.

of the cochlea. The cochlear duct is triangular in cross section and firmly anchored to the bony cochlea: one edge (the apex) attaches to the osseous spiral lamina, the other (the base) to the outer wall of the bony cochlea.

> ### Thought Question
>
> What is the cochlea, where is it located, and why is it essential to a person's ability to hear and interpret sounds?

Each wall of the cochlear duct has a unique structure and name. The delicate dorsal wall is called the **vestibular (Reissner's) membrane** and serves as a diffusion barrier between the perilymph in the scala vestibule and the endolymph within the duct. The lateral wall contains the **spiral ligament** that consists of thickened periosteal tissue attached to the outer wall of the bony cochlea. On the endolymph-facing surface of the spiral ligament is the **stria vascularis**, which is richly supplied with small blood vessels and produces the bulk of the endolymph within the entire membranous labyrinth. The floor of the duct is called the **basilar membrane**, upon which rests the **organ of Corti**. The organ of Corti contains the receptor (hair) cells of the auditory system.

Together with the osseous spiral lamina, the cochlear duct partitions the bony cochlea into three compartments: (1) a **scala vestibuli**, dorsal to the duct that contains perilymph; (2) a **scala tympani** below the cochlear duct that also contains perilymph; and (3) a **scala media** (the cochlear duct itself) that contains endolymph. The perilymph of the scala vestibuli and scala tympani communicate at the **helicotrema**, which is a narrow gap at the apex of the cochlea. Such communication results from the fact that the cochlear duct ends as a blind sac that leaves a small space between the duct and bony wall of the cochlea. The footplate of the stapes and oval window "look into" the perilymph-containing vestibule with which the scala vestibuli communicates. The scala tympani and elastic round window "look out" from the scala tympani into the air-filled middle ear cavity.

The function of the auditory inner ear is such that the three compartments of the cochlea convert differential pressure between the scala vestibuli and scala tympani into oscillations of the basilar membrane of the cochlear duct. This conversion derives from the arrangement of the three compartments and the fluid motion allowed by the elastic round window (Figure 17-8 ■). When the stapes vibrates, it pushes into and out of the perilymph of the scala vestibuli, setting up pressure waves (fluid shifts) in the vestibule's perilymph. Such fluid shifts are possible even though the perilymph itself is incompressible. This is the case because the perilymph of the scala vestibuli communicates with that of the scala tympani via the helicotrema, and the elastic membrane covering the round window of the scala tympani is free to bulge in and out. However, only a small amount of fluid can pass through the helicotrema because of its small size. This means

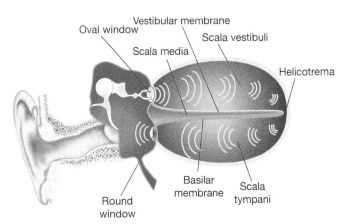

FIGURE 17-8 The stapes vibrates oval window pressure waves (fluid shifts) that are set up in the scala vestibule. Small amounts of fluid pass through the small helicotrema, causing pressure waves in the scala tympani, further causing movement of the round window.

that pressure waves set up in the scala vestibuli by vibration of the stapes will be transferred largely to the scala media because it effectively separates the two compartments. As the scala media is displaced, the basilar membrane is distorted, which activates the receptors resting on it.

The portion of the basilar membrane that moves in response to a sound stimulus depends on the frequency of the sound waves. The osseous spiral lamina of the cochlea becomes progressively narrower and the basilar membrane progressively wider in moving from the base to the apex of the cochlea (Figure 17-9 ■). The resultant systematic variation in the mechanical properties (stiffness) of the basilar membrane means that different sound frequencies cause different sectors of the basilar membrane to vibrate: low frequencies maximally distort the basilar membrane near the apex of the cochlea, while progressively higher frequencies cause the peak amplitude of distortion to move toward the base of the cochlea. This is an example of place coding, and it constitutes the initial processing of sound frequencies by the auditory system. The logarithmic

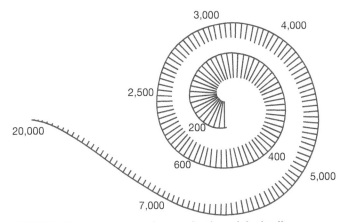

FIGURE 17-9 The tonotopic organization of the basilar membrane. Different sound frequencies cause different portions of the basilar membrane to vibrate. Higher frequencies (20,000 Hz) cause peak distortion toward the base of the cochlea, whereas lower frequencies (200 Hz) cause peak distortion toward the apex of the cochlea.

Neuropathology Box 17-1: Semicircular Canal Dehiscence

Perilymphatic fluid oscillations, set up by movement of the stapes, are ordinarily directed only into the cochlear portion of the membranous labyrinth. This is because it is only the cochlear portion of the bony labyrinth that contains flexible elastic membranes (the oval and round window membranes) that allow the incompressible perilymph to move. Because there are no such membranous-covered openings in the vestibule or osseous semicircular canals, the vestibular part of the membranous labyrinth is not affected by sound or pressure changes in the middle ear or CSF. However, chronic middle ear infection can erode bone and create an opening (called a *perilymph fistula*), typically in the horizontal osseous semicircular canal. Because a fistula then allows fluid movement, patients experience sound- and pressure-induced vertigo attacks and horizontal nystagmus following sustained positive or negative pressure changes in the external auditory meatus. The condition is called semicircular canal dehiscence (see Figure 17-10 ■ at the bottom of the page).

representation of frequencies along the length of the basilar membrane is called **tonotopic organization**.

Sensory End Organs

Auditory sensory transduction occurs in the hair cells of the organ of Corti. Resting on the basilar membrane of the inner ear, the organ of Corti is made up of hair cells and a variety of supporting cells. The hair cells, more than 18,000 in number in each cochlea, rest on the shoulders of supporting cells and are either flask or cylindrical in shape. They are arrayed along the length of the basilar membrane. Hair cells are arranged in two groups: flask-shaped *inner hair cells* (about 3,500) are arranged in a single row, while cylindrical-shaped *outer hair cells* (about 15,000) are arranged in three to four parallel rows (Figure 17-11 ■).

Inner and outer hair cells are separated by a perilymph-filled space called the **tunnel of Corti**. On either side of the

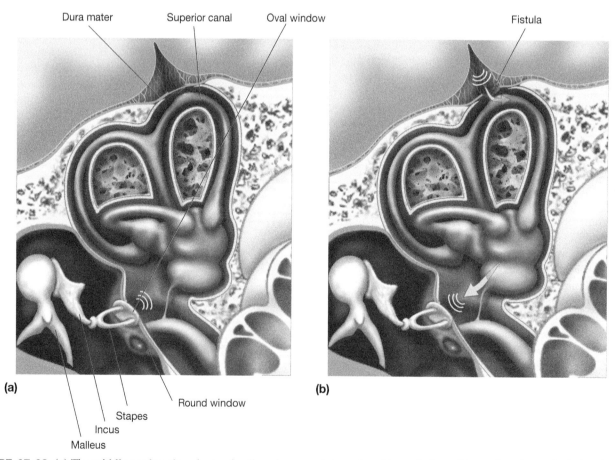

(a)

Dura mater   Superior canal   Oval window

Round window
Stapes
Incus
Malleus

(b)

Fistula

FIGURE 17-10 (a) The middle ear has three bones (malleus, incus, and stapes) and two windows (the oval and round windows). Sound is not transmitted to the vestibular portion of the labyrinth. (b) A fistula results in a third opening such that sound can be transmitted to the vestibular portion of the labyrinth. The presence of a perilymph fistula allows fluid movement with sound or pressure change in the middle ear or in the CSF. This movement can induce vertigo and nystagmus.

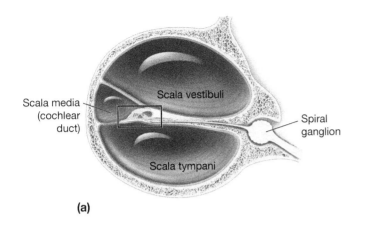

(a)

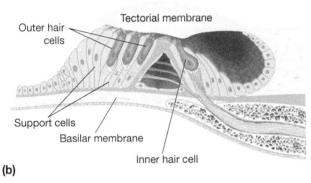

(b)

FIGURE 17-11 (a) Within the cochlea, hair cells are arranged on the basilar membrane. (b) A single row of inner hair cells and multiple rows of outer hair cells are arranged with the tips of their stereocilia embedded in the tectorial membrane.

tunnel of Corti are supporting pillar cells (also called *rods of Corti*) that contribute importantly to the mechanical stability of the organ of Corti. Outer hair cells are supported at their bases by cup-shaped phalangeal cells. Thin processes of the phalangeal cells extend to the top of the outer hair cells and end as plate-like expansions that fill the spaces between outer hair cells and form the reticular lamina. The reticular lamina imparts mechanical stability to this part of the organ of Corti. The cell bodies of hair cells are situated between the basilar membrane and the reticular lamina, with the reticular lamina forming the fluid barrier between the perilymph of the scala tympani and the endolymph of the scala media. As a result, the cell body of each auditory hair cell is bathed in perilymph, and the stereocilia are bathed in endolymph. Overlying the organ of Corti is the **tectorial membrane**, a cantilevered gelatinous shelf.

Several functionally critical differences exist in the relationships of inner and outer hair cells to surrounding structures. First, outer hair cells reside on the most flexible portion of the basilar membrane—being located midway between its attachments to the spiral lamina medially and spiral ligament laterally. In contrast, inner hair cells are

Thought Question

Within the organ of Corti, there are inner and outer hair cells. Identify the functional significance of each and their relationship to one another.

located above a less flexible part of the basilar membrane, adjacent to the spiral lamina.

Second, the tips of stereocilia of outer hair cells are embedded in the overlying tectorial membrane, whereas those of the inner hair cells are not. The stereocilia of inner hair cells reside in the endolymph of the internal tunnel of Corti.

Outer hair cells move as a unit toward or away from the tectorial membrane when the basilar membrane moves because of the rigid interconnections they have with surrounding structures. Because outer hair cells are distributed on the most flexible part of the basilar membrane, they move most in response to sound vibrations. Because the tectorial membrane holds the tips of outer (but not inner) hair cell stereocilia, lateral motion of the basilar membrane *relative to the tectorial membrane* bends their stereocilia one way or the other (Figure 17-12 ■). Outer hair cells then generate

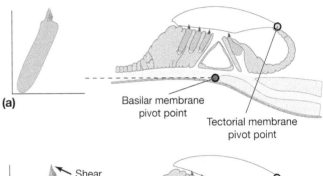

(a)

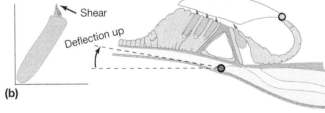

(b)

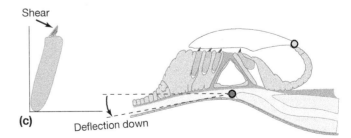

(c)

FIGURE 17-12 (a) The tips of the stereocilia of outer hair cells are embedded in the tectorial membrane, whereas those of the inner hair cells are not. (b) An upward deflection of the basilar membrane relative to the tectorial membrane stimulates the hair cells and results in depolarization. (c) A downward deflection of the basilar membrane relative to the tectorial membrane stimulates the hair cells and results in hyperpolarization.

receptor potentials that alternately depolarize and hyper-polarize from the resting membrane potential. In contrast to the outer hair cells, which are stimulated by movement of the membrane, the stereocilia of inner hair cells are stimulated by the back-and-forth movement of endolymph from the internal spiral tunnel through the narrow space between their tips and the tectorial membrane.

Another critical difference between inner and outer hair cells concerns their innervation. First, approximately 95 percent of all primary afferents in the cochlear division of CN VIII receive their input only from inner hair cells. Only about 5 percent receive their innervation from the far more numerous outer hair cells (Figure 17-13 ▣). This means that auditory sensation is dependent on the relatively few inner hair cells. Second, the predominant innervation of outer hair cells is efferent, being derived from neurons in the brainstem that project to outer hair cells in CN VIII. So what role, then, do outer hair cells play in mediating auditory sensation? A very significant one because their activity influences the transduction process in inner hair cells, as described next.

Outer hair cells amplify the movement of the basilar membrane (by as much as 100-fold) in response to low-intensity sound stimulation. For this reason, outer hair cells are referred to as the cochlear amplifier. They accomplish this function by changing their lengths via motor proteins located in their membranes. Such motor proteins are activated by depolarizing receptor potentials and result in a shortening of the outer hair cell (Figure 17-14 ▣). Shortening draws the basilar membrane toward the reticular lamina and tectorial membrane. When the receptor potential becomes hyperpolarizing, the motor proteins are inactivated. Outer hair cells lengthen, and the basilar membrane shifts further away from the reticular lamina and tectorial membrane. This shortening and lengthening of outer hair cells amplify the flexing of the basilar membrane in response to that particular sound frequency.

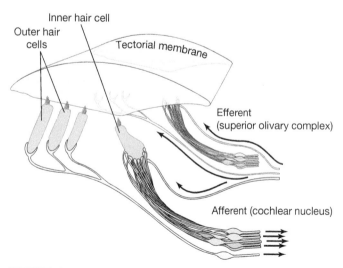

FIGURE 17-13 The vast majority (95 percent) of all primary afferents in the cochlear division of CN VIII receive their input from inner hair cells. A small contingent (5 percent) receive their input from outer hair cells.

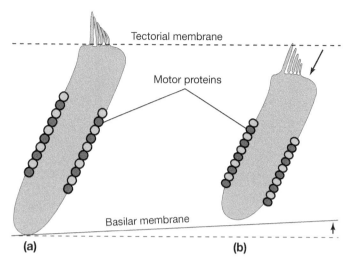

FIGURE 17-14 The activation of motor proteins induces the shortening of outer hair cells, thereby amplifying the flexing of the basilar membrane in response to low-intensity sound stimulation.

This amplified flexing of the basilar membrane, in turn, increases the oscillation of endolymph in the internal spiral tunnel, where the stereocilia of the inner hair cells reside. Their stereocilia thus bend more, thereby increasing the magnitude of their receptor potentials and causing enhanced responses in the auditory nerve. The sensitivity of individual cochlear nerve fibers at their preferred frequency is much greater—up to a thousand-fold in some fibers.

The cochlear amplifier functions not only in response to the receptor potentials generated by sound waves, but also in response to activation of cochlear efferents from the brainstem. As noted earlier, these synapse on outer hair cells. Stimulation of this efferent cochlear bundle activates its motor proteins, causing outer hair cells to shorten. Via this mechanism, the brain is able to regulate auditory sensitivity.

Primary Afferents

The cochlear nerve contains approximately 32,000 primary afferent fibers that arise from the inner and outer hair cells of the cochlea. These fibers enter the brainstem at the lower border of the pons, on its lateral aspect, posterior to the facial nerve. Each afferent arises from a bipolar neuron with its cell body in the spiral ganglion. Peripheral processes enter the organ of Corti to synapse on hair cells, while central processes form the cochlear nerve. Recall that the number of primary afferents innervating inner hair cells is much greater than the number innervating the outer hair cells.

Thought Question

Compare the first-order neurons associated with the auditory system to first-order neurons associated with the somatosensory systems. Then relate the spiral ganglion to analogous structures in the somatosensory systems.

The cochlear and vestibular divisions of CN VIII pursue distinctive courses upon entering the brainstem (see Figure 13-20). The larger cochlear division enters the brainstem lateral and slightly caudal to the vestibular division. Its axons pursue a trajectory directed lateral to the inferior cerebellar peduncle, whereas those of the vestibular division are directed medial to the peduncle. The brainstem trajectory of cochlear primary afferents accounts for the fact that the ventral and dorsal cochlear nuclei within which the primary afferent terminates reside on the lateral and dorsal surfaces of the inferior cerebellar peduncle.

Projections

Second-Order Neurons

The cell bodies of second-order auditory neurons reside in the cochlear nuclear complex situated at the junction of the medulla and pons. The cochlear nuclear complex consists of a **dorsal cochlear nucleus** and a **ventral cochlear nucleus**. The ventral cochlear nucleus, in turn, is subdivided into anterior and posterior parts. Upon entering the brainstem, primary afferents bifurcate and terminate in an orderly dorsoventral sequence throughout the nuclear complex. The tonotopic organization present in the cochlea is preserved in all three subdivisions of the nuclear complex; neurons responding to higher frequencies are dorsal, while those responding to lower frequencies are ventral.

Second-order axons arising from the cochlear nuclei pursue one of three trajectories (Figure 17-15 ■). Most enter the *ventral acoustic stria* that runs ventral to the inferior cerebellar peduncle and then forms the **trapezoid body**, a conspicuous bundle of transversely running fibers in the ventral part of the pontine tegmentum. Others enter the smaller *dorsal acoustic stria* or the still smaller *intermediate acoustic stria*, both of which arch over the superior surface of the inferior cerebellar peduncle to enter the pontine tegmentum. Auditory relay nuclei are distributed in the pontine tegmentum. Most obvious is the **superior olivary nucleus**. It is situated in the ventrolateral corner of the caudal pontine tegmentum, medial to the rostral end of the facial nucleus. There also are small poorly defined cell groups scattered among fibers of the trapezoid body forming the so-called **nucleus of the trapezoid body**. Axons of the three acoustic striae may terminate in any of the auditory relay nuclei on one or both sides. Thus, for example, the superior olivary nucleus processes information from both ears

The **lateral lemniscus** represents the principal ascending auditory pathway in the brainstem. It consists primarily of second-order fibers from the three acoustic striae that have crossed from the opposite side. It also contains uncrossed second-order fibers from the striae as well as third-order fibers that have arisen from cells in the superior olivary nuclei or trapezoid body. It carries information from both ears, but that from the contralateral ear is greater. Two nuclei of the lateral lemniscus reside along the course of this fiber bundle. They receive some fibers from the cochlear nuclei as well as collaterals and terminals of other afferents ascending in the lateral lemniscus. The nuclei also contribute fibers to the lateral lemniscus.

Throughout its extent, the lateral lemniscus ascends in proximity to the neospinothalamic tract. The lateral lemniscus is, at first, an ovoid-shaped group of fibers that shifts progressively laterally as it ascends through the pons. At rostral pontine levels, in preparation for its entry into the midbrain, the lateral lemniscus flattens out into a conspicuous band (L., *lemniscus*, ribbon) and curves steeply dorsalward. The lateral lemniscus is a distinct band of fibers positioned ventral to the inferior colliculus.

> **Thought Question**
>
> In what ways are the auditory pathways similar to and in what ways are they different from the spinothalamic tract?

Third-Order Neurons

Most axons of the lateral lemniscus terminate on third-order neurons of the inferior colliculus (see Figure 17-15). The inferior colliculi occupy the caudal tectum of the midbrain, where they form prominent bumps on the dorsal surface of the midbrain (see Figures 2-10 and 2-12). Axons from the inferior colliculus as well as the few from the lateral lemniscus form the **brachium of the inferior colliculus** that carries axons to the thalamus. The brachium of the inferior colliculus forms a conspicuous and readily identifiable surface feature of the midbrain.

Fourth-Order Neurons

Cell bodies of fourth-order neurons are situated in the **medial geniculate body (MGB)** of the thalamus. Each MGB is situated on the caudal aspect of the ventral tier of the thalamus and is a readily identifiable surface feature. Axons from the MGB give rise to the **auditory (geniculotemporal) radiation**. The auditory radiation runs in the posterior limb of the internal capsule. Specifically, it runs in the sublenticular portion, so named because the fibers run beneath the lentiform nucleus en route to the temporal lobe. Fibers of the auditory radiation terminate in the primary auditory cortex.

The **primary auditory cortex** is located in a region on the upper bank of the temporal lobe, buried in the Sylvian fissure (see Figure 7-6). This area corresponds to Brodmann's area 41 (refer to Chapter 7). The auditory cortex occupies the transverse temporal gyrus, or Heschl's gyrus, and a variable amount of the **planum temporale** posterior to Heschl's gyrus. The planum temporale is usually larger on the left than on the right side. Both of these hemispheral asymmetries are related to the typical left-hemisphere dominance for speech and language.

FIGURE 17-15 Acoustic central pathways. Primary afferents arise from bipolar neurons of spiral ganglion of the cochlea and enter the brainstem at the level of the posterolateral pons, where most will synapse in the cochlear nuclei. Second-order projections ascend the brainstem trajectories (see text) and terminate in the inferior colliculi. Third-order axons from the inferior colliculi project to the medial geniculate nucleus (MGN) and synapse on fourth-order neurons. These fourth-order neurons leave the MGN and project to the primary auditory cortex of the temporal lobes.

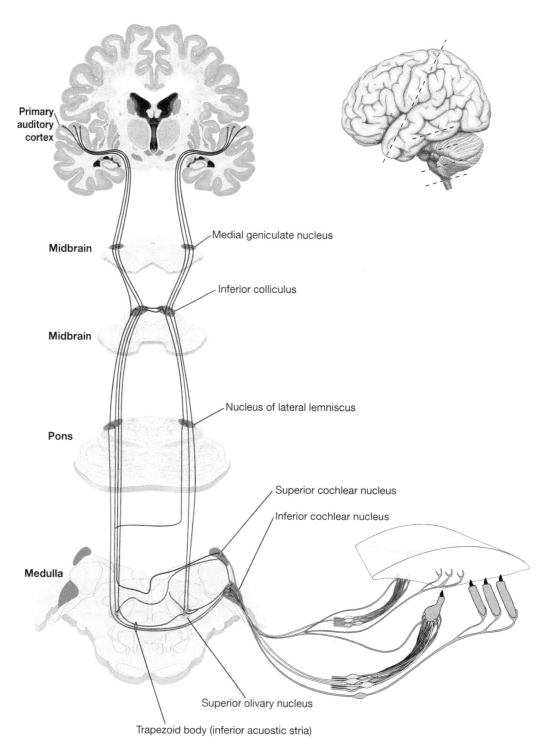

Decussations

The auditory relay nuclei of the brainstem all are interconnected by an extensive commissural fiber system (see Figure 17-15). Nuclei of the superior olivary complex are interconnected by fibers running in the trapezoid body. Nuclei of the lateral lemniscus give rise to fibers that decussate and end in the contralateral inferior colliculi. The two inferior colliculi are interconnected by the commissure of the inferior colliculus.

The commissural connections form the anatomical substrate for comparisons between the two ears (interaural) performed within each relay nucleus. Additionally, they are important determinants of the nature of the hearing loss following lesions of the auditory system. Unilateral brainstem lesions central to the cochlear nuclei still allow auditory information to reach both hemispheres. Such lesions result not in complete deafness in either ear, but rather in diminished hearing, particularly on the contralateral side.

Function

Relatively little is known of the function of the central auditory pathways and relay nuclei in humans. For one thing, naturally occurring brainstem lesions invariably damage contiguous structures that have a much greater impact on behavior than do auditory deficits. What is known of function has been derived from animal experimentation where, in principle at least, it is assumed similar organizations prevail.

Individual binaural neurons in the superior olivary complex are sensitive to differences in sounds at the two ears. Some of these cells are sensitive to differences in the time of arrival of sounds at the two ears. Such differences are one of the cues used in sound localization: that is, a sound originating on one side will reach that ear first and the contralateral ear a short time later. Others of these binaural cells are sensitive to differences in sound intensity at the two ears. Intensity difference is a second cue used to localize sound: a certain amount of sound energy, particularly high frequency, is reflected by the head so that sound arriving at the ear contralateral to its source is of lower intensity.

Like other nuclei in the auditory system, the **inferior colliculus** has a tonotopic organization. Some neurons respond to differences in the time of arrival of sound at the two ears and may exhibit sensitivity to a sound moving in space, toward or away from the midline.

The **primary auditory cortex** of the monkey has a precise tonotopic organization and a similar organization seems to be present in the human. Electrical stimulation of the primary auditory cortex (Brodmann's area 41) in humans is virtually impossible because of its position within the depths of the Sylvian fissure. Electrical stimulation in the region of areas 42 and 22 elicits responses that are most often referred to the contralateral ear. The sounds heard by the individual are elementary tones (clicking, buzzing, humming, ringing) devoid of complicated or changing qualities.

Auditory Reflexes

Two reflexes change the transmission of sound through the middle ear ossicles. These are the **stapedius reflex** (see Chapter 13) and the **tympanic reflex**. A contingent of fibers from the cochlear nuclei, superior olivary complex, and nuclei of the trapezoid body terminate bilaterally in the facial motor nucleus and the trigeminal motor nucleus. LMNs of the facial nucleus innervate the stapedius muscle and represent the efferent limb of the stapedius reflex (Figure 17-16 ■). Contraction of the stapedius muscle limits the sound-induced excursions of the stapes so that less sound energy incident on the eardrum is transferred to the oval window. LMNs of the trigeminal motor nucleus innervate the tensor tympani muscle and represent the efferent limb of a tympanic reflex. Contraction of the tensor tympani limits the amplitude of sound-induced excursions of the eardrum. Loud sounds usually lead to reflex contraction of the stapedius muscle alone, whereas the tensor tympani contracts with very high intensity sounds that elicit a startle defense response.

The major function of middle ear reflexes is to filter out disturbing low-frequency noise arising from the head region itself—for example, the noise generated by jaw movement. In chronic noise, they help protect the organ of Corti against excessive stimulation that is potentially damaging to the hair cells. The reflexes are subject to central

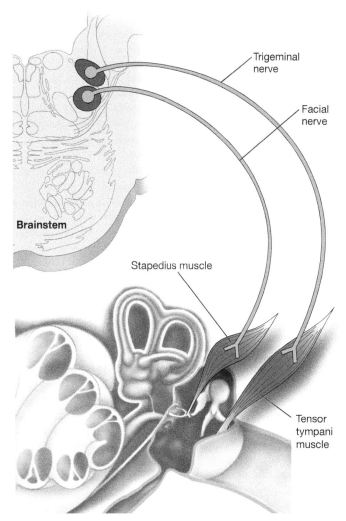

FIGURE 17-16 The stapedius reflex and the tympanic reflex change the transmission of sound by causing contraction of muscles that attach to the middle ear ossicles.

control. For example, middle ear muscles contract in advance of vocalization.

CLINICAL CONNECTIONS

Considerable information is available about the pathophysiology and etiology of disorders affecting the outer, middle, and inner ear. However, comparatively little is known about the consequences of damage to specific structures of the central auditory pathways.

Clinical Evaluation

There are two pathways for conducting sound to the inner ear (Figure 17-17 ■). One is by **air conduction** and involves sound coursing from the air through the outer and middle ears to the inner ear. The other is by **bone conduction** and involves vibrating the skull, which stimulates the inner ear directly and bypasses the outer and middle ears. Thus, hearing by bone conduction depends just on the inner ear and neural pathways.

In the normal ear, air conduction is greater than bone conduction. The **Rinne test** compares hearing by bone conduction and air conduction. The butt of a vibrating tuning fork is placed firmly against the mastoid process, and the person is instructed to indicate when he or she no longer hears the vibration. The U of the tuning fork is then placed beside the external auditory meatus (without touching it), and the person again indicates when the vibration is no longer heard. Normally, the tuning fork is heard about twice as long by air conduction as by bone conduction.

The **Weber test** is a test for lateralization. The butt of a vibrating tuning fork is placed on the vertex of the skull, and the person is asked to indicate where they hear the sound. Normally, the sound will be heard equally in both ears—that is, the sound is not lateralized.

A sophisticated battery of behavioral audiometric tests is required to establish the effects of auditory system

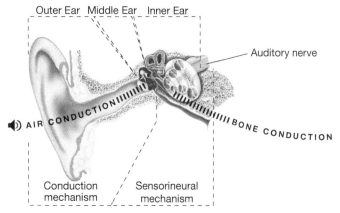

FIGURE 17-17 The conduction of sound occurs through two pathways. Air conduction involves sound moving through air of the outer and middle ears to the inner ear. Bone conduction bypasses the outer and middle ears and occurs through vibration of the skull, stimulating the inner ear directly.

disorders on an individual's capacity to function in everyday communication. The simplest tests generate an **audiogram**, a graphic record that charts the threshold of hearing at various frequencies against sound intensity in decibel. The subject's threshold for any given sound frequency is the lowest sound intensity that can be heard. Pure tones of different frequencies are presented either through earphones or by way of a vibrator applied to the mastoid process.

Signs and Symptoms

Lesions involving the middle and inner ears as well as the cochlear nerve are classified as peripheral lesions. Peripheral lesions result in three different categories of hearing loss: conductive, sensorineural, and mixed. The conductive mechanism consists of the outer and middle ears, while the sensorineural mechanism consists of the inner ear and cochlear nerve (see Figure 17-17).

Conductive Hearing Loss

A conductive hearing loss occurs with a lesion involving the middle ear. (Damage to the outer ear would produce the same result.) Pathologies of the middle ear may result from physical causes, disease processes such as **otitis media**, and the bone proliferation that characterizes **otosclerosis**. Otitis media is an inflammation of the middle ear resulting in fluid accumulation; otosclerosis involves the formation of spongy bone around the oval window that immobilizes the stapes. In both situations, there is impairment in the capacity of the ossicular chain to transmit vibrations from the tympanic membrane to the oval window. Another common cause of conductive hearing loss is excessive buildup of ear wax in the external auditory meatus, which muffles sound.

Such impairment results in the so-called air–bone gap with pure tone audiometry. The air-bone gap is revealed as follows. Sound delivered by vibration applied to the mastoid process bypasses the outer and middle ears and is registered directly by the inner ear. An audiogram taken via bone conduction is generated and compared with the audiogram generated by air conduction (from ear phones or a speaker). In cases of outer and middle ear pathology, the comparison shows normal hearing (inner ear function) with bone conduction, but a hearing loss with air conduction—hence, an air–bone gap.

Sensorineural Hearing Loss

A sensorineural hearing loss results when the pathology producing the loss is in the inner ear or cochlear nerve. An equivalent hearing loss occurs by both air conduction and bone conduction because the inner ear is involved in both transmission pathways. The conductive mechanism is thus eliminated as a possible cause of the hearing loss. Inner ear damage may result from a variety of causes such as trauma; anoxia; infections such as mumps, measles, or meningitis; and exposure to high levels of noise. A sensorineural hearing loss is characterized by three symptoms: selective loss of the higher frequencies by both air and bone conduction;

recruitment; and occasionally **tinnitus**, meaning any abnormal sound such as a ringing, buzzing, or hissing in the ears. Recruitment is an abnormal growth in loudness perception as sound intensity is increased.

Certain antibiotics (aminoglycosides such as kanamycin, gentamicin, and neomycin) can lead to deafness with excessive or prolonged administration. This is because such ototoxic drugs accumulate progressively in the perilymph and endolymph where they directly damage hair cells. However, the cellular damage seems confined almost exclusively to outer, not inner, hair cells. Thus, loss of or damage to the cochlear amplifier accounts for the sometimes dramatic increase in the auditory threshold that measures inner hair cell function. Ototoxicity is largely irreversible.

Involvement of the cochlear nerve most commonly is due to the so-called acoustic tumor (neurinoma, or Schwannoma of CN VIII). The tumor originates from Schwann cells, is slow growing, and can be removed surgically. The tumor begins in the internal auditory meatus, but as it grows, it extends into the posterior cranial fossa to occupy the angle between the cerebellum and pons. The tumor may press on CNs VII and V as well as on the cerebellum, leading to a variety of symptoms besides those attributable to CN VIII. Differentiating cochlear damage from cochlear nerve damage is difficult and, in some cases, impossible.

Thought Question

What differentiates conductive from sensorineural hearing loss?

Mixed Hearing Loss

A mixed hearing loss results when the pathology involves both the conductive and sensorineural mechanisms (see Figure 17-17). There is a hearing loss by bone conduction but an even greater loss by air conduction. This is because sound traveling to the inner ear by bone conduction is attenuated only by the sensorineural defect in the inner ear, whereas sound traveling via the air conduction pathway is attenuated by both the middle and inner ear pathologies.

Presbyacusis

Age-related metabolic changes may result in physical alterations of the inner ear, such as a loss of elasticity of the basilar membrane, and may contribute to **presbyacusis**, an age-dependent loss in the ability to perceive or discriminate sounds. The age of onset is variable, and the hearing loss is progressive and differentially impairs high-frequency hearing. However, presbyacusis yields a sensorineural type of audiogram, indicating an additional loss of hair cells and spiral ganglion neurons.

Central Auditory Pathway Disorders

Damage to components of the ascending auditory pathways is categorized as central lesions and may result from a variety of causes, most commonly vascular disorders or

tumors. Restricted lesions central to the cochlear nuclei will yield few, if any, overt symptoms because of binaural representation in the central projection. Damage to lower brainstem structures may reveal itself in **brainstem auditory evoked responses (BAERs)** in which a computer-averaged series of seven waves are recorded from the scalp in response to auditory click stimuli. The entire series of waves occurs within 10 msec after the stimulus. Each of the first five waves is supposedly generated in a specific brainstem structure, but this has not been conclusively determined in people. The amplitude and latency of individual waves are measured. BAER is useful for examination of people who are difficult to test (e.g., those who are not able to understand directions and/or easily communicate their perceptions).

Lesions of the MGB and auditory cortex do not lead to complete deafness unless they are bilateral, although deficits may occur in the capacity to localize sounds with cortical lesions. Temporal lobe damage will result in deficits in tests in which the listener must separate competing signals at the two ears. Impairment is greatest in the ear contralateral to the side of the damage. Additionally, subjective acoustic sensations may occur with temporal lobe lesions. The decoding into language of auditory information that is transmitted in the form of speech sounds is discussed in Chapter 22.

VESTIBULAR SYSTEM

Clinical Preview ················

Marcia Lamb was in a minor motorcycle accident that left her with cervical neck pain. She was referred to the outpatient orthopedic clinic at which you work. During the intake questions, you learned that she has also had intermittent vertigo since the accident. You performed specific tests and determined that she had benign positional vertigo (BPV). As you read through this section, consider the following:

- What structures are involved in BPV, and why might these structures have been affected by the motorcycle accident?

- How do the cause and symptoms of BPV compare with those associated with disorders such as Meniere's disease?

- Which of these conditions, if either, is likely to be more responsive to physical intervention?

Foundational Information

The vestibular system consists of those inner ear receptors that detect position and movement of the head and the set of CNS neurons that (1) contribute to conscious orientation in space and (2) mediate reflex adjustments for the maintenance of equilibrium and visual acuity during head movement. The vestibular system represents the most primitive neurologic mechanism by which we orient to the stable and permanent features of our environment—an essential prerequisite to all normal sensory and perceptual experience of posture and movement. It represents the major system governing the reflex muscular adjustments that compensate for the continuous changes in head position that occur during wakefulness and sleep.

As a group, cells of the vestibular nuclei within the CNS not only have a sensory function in processing and relaying afferent information from the periphery, they also have a motor function in regulating the activity of lower motor neurons. The vestibular nuclei are a major source of brainstem UMNs (see Chapter 11). Similar to the auditory system, the vestibular receptors also are subject to efferent control by the CNS (see Chapter 9). The vestibular system is one of the most widely distributed neural systems in the CNS: it influences all levels of the neuraxis, from the spinal cord to the cerebral cortex. Although the vestibular system is constantly active, vestibular sensations normally do not form part of our conscious experience of the real world.

A clinical distinction can be made between vestibular system dysfunction that results from damage to the peripheral vestibular apparatus and that which follows CNS damage. Nevertheless, clinical signs of vestibular system dysfunction that result from lesions of the CNS are of comparatively little localizing value to the neurologist because of the vestibular system's widespread CNS distribution. Despite its importance to motor activity, vestibular system damage produces surprisingly slight permanent motor deficits due to the nervous system's capacity to compensate by sensory substitution. However, the functional consequences are substantial. The vestibular system, not vision, determines our perception of being right side up. When damage occurs to the vestibular system, it can have a profound effect on a person's ability to remain stable and to feel comfortable during movement.

Sensory End Organs

Each membranous vestibular labyrinth consists of a utricle, a saccule, and three semicircular canals (SCCs). In each, hair cells occur in discrete patches in specific locations and have precise organizations (Figure 17-18 ■). Also, the stereocilia of hair cells of the semicircular canals always are embedded in an overlying gelatinous membrane that plays a critical role in determining the nature of the stimuli to which the hair cells respond.

Utricular and Saccular Maculae (Otolith Organs)

The kidney-shaped utricular and hook-shaped saccular maculae are specialized spots (L., *macula*, a spot) within the **utricle** and **saccule** containing hair cells, supporting cells, and other components of the receptor organ (see Figure 17-18). The cilia of a single layer of hair cells project upward into an overlying gelatinous membrane whose superior surface is weighted with crystals of calcium carbonate. These crystals are called **otoconia** (ear dust) or **otoliths** (ear stones) so that the membrane is referred to as the **otolithic membrane**. The otoliths render the otolithic

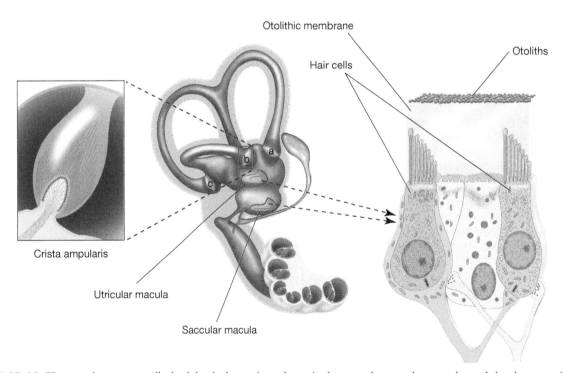

Otolithic membrane

Otoliths

Hair cells

Crista ampularis

Utricular macula

Saccular macula

FIGURE 17-18 The membranous vestibular labyrinth consists of a utricular macula, saccular macula, and the three semicircular canals. The maculae contain hair cells embedded in an overlaying gelatinous otolithic membrane whose surface is weighted with otoliths. Each canal is associated with an ampulla containing hair cells, called the crista ampullaris.

membrane, and stereocilia projecting into it, subject to the forces of gravity. Both maculae are divided into two portions by a curved line known as the **striola**. The hair cells of the utricular macula *all* have their kinocilia facing *toward* the striola, whereas hair cells of the saccular macula *all* have their kinocilia facing *away* from the striola. Thus, hair cells on opposite sides of the striola have opposite polarizations so that the otolith organs themselves are polarized. This feature enables each individual otolith organ to generate a differential signal when stimulated by the forces of gravity or acceleration/deceleration.

> **Thought Question**
>
> How are the utricle and macula similar and how do they differ? Explain the functional significance of their respective structures.

Two additional anatomical features are important in understanding the functions of the otolith organs. First, the planes of orientation of the two organs are different. The saccular macula has a vertical orientation, whereas the utricular macula has a horizontal orientation (parallel to the ground) when the head is in its normal upright position. Both maculae respond to changes in gravitational forces that occur with head tilt and transient linear (straight ahead) acceleration. But the horizontal orientation of the utricular macula tailors its response to linear acceleration in the horizontal plane (e.g., riding in a car), whereas the vertical orientation of the saccular macula tailors its optimum response to linear acceleration in the vertical plane (e.g., riding in an elevator). The second important structural feature of the maculae is that the striola of both otolith organs are curved. Thus, no matter how the head is turned or tilted, a given population of hair cells on opposite sides of the striola will be in an optimal position to have their cilia bent by the forces of gravity or linear acceleration.

The crystals of calcium carbonate embedded superficially in the otolithic membrane have a density about three times that of water (see Figure 17-18). As such, the otolithic membrane will be displaced preferentially by the pull of gravity on the head (static) and linear acceleration and deceleration (kinetic) of the head. That is, because of inertia, the otoconia tend to stay (for a short time) in their preexistent state. If at rest, the otoliths tend to stay at rest, thereby keeping the gelatinous membrane stationary. If in motion, the otoliths tend to stay in motion, thereby maintaining the motion of the gelatinous membrane. Thus, in response to the onset of a transient linear acceleration, the crystals tend to stand still while the patch of hair cells slides under the gelatinous membrane, bending the cilia of the hair cells backward (Figure 17-19 ■). In response to head tilt, the heavy crystals cause the gelatinous membrane to sag and pull on the patch of hair cells. Because of their opposite polarizations, hair cells on one side of the striola will be depolarized, while those on the opposite side

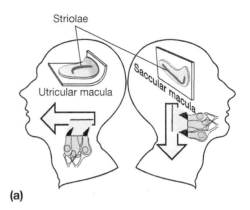

(a)

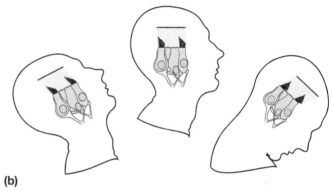

(b)

FIGURE 17-19 The planes of orientation of the maculae. (a) The utricular maculae are oriented horizontally and respond preferentially to linear acceleration in a horizontal plane. The saccular maculae are oriented vertically and respond preferentially to linear acceleration in a vertical plane. (b) Both otolith organs respond to head tilt due to the curved shape of the striola.

will be hyperpolarized. Thus, a single macula is capable of signaling the direction of head tilt owing to the differential discharge pattern coming from the primary afferents innervating cells on opposite sides of the striola.

The response to acceleration and tilt of the head is complex, relying on different end organs depending on the movement and direction of movement. Table 17-1 ■ summarizes these relationships.

Semicircular Canals

Three semicircular canals are present on each side of the head, oriented at approximate right angles to one another (see Figure 17-18): a **horizontal**, or **lateral**, **canal**; an **anterior**

> **Thought Question**
>
> The vestibular system is designed to respond differentially to motions such as forward motion of a moving car (forward linear), fast acceleration in an elevator (vertical), and figure skating or dancing (rotational). Which part of the vestibular system responds to forward linear, vertical, and rotational acceleration, respectively?

Table 17-1 Movements and Related Responses of Vestibular End Organs

MOVEMENT	UTRICLE	SACCULE	HORIZONTAL SCC	POSTERIOR SCC	ANTERIOR SCC
Acceleration in the anterior–posterior plane	Excitation				
Acceleration in the lateral or horizontal plane	Excitation				
Acceleration in the occipito–caudal plane		Excitation			
Tilt of head—static/upright	Tonic activity	Tonic activity			
Tilt of head—lateral (roll)	Excitation	Inhibition			
Tilt of head—fore (pitch)	Excitation	Inhibition			
Rotation to the right horizontal plane			Excitation right; inhibition left		
Rotation to the left horizontal plane			Excitation left; inhibition right		
Rotation to the right and posterior plane				Excitation right; inhibition left	Excitation left; inhibition right
Rotation to the left and posterior plane				Excitation left; inhibition right	Excitation right; inhibition left

vertical, or **superior**, **canal**; and a **posterior vertical canal**. In natural upright postures of the head, the horizontal and vertical canals tend to be oriented close to the true horizontal and vertical planes, although the horizontal canal is approximately 20 to 30 degrees off horizontal of the earth. Each canal has a dilatation at one end—the **ampulla**—containing a transversely oriented ridge of hair cells and supporting cells—the **crista (crista ampularis)** (Figure 17-20 ■). The **cupula** is a gelatinous structure surmounting each crista into which the cilia of the underlying hair cells project. The cupula completely closes off the lumen of the ampulla so that endolymph does not actually flow through the semicircular canal. Rather, the cupula functions as an elastic diaphragm responsive to displacement of the endolymphatic fluid within the canal. The hair cells of each crista ampullaris all have the same orientation. In the horizontal canals, the kinocilia all face toward the utricle, while in the vertical canals, the kinocilia all face away from the utricle.

The semicircular canals respond to angular acceleration and deceleration of the head—that is, to a change in the velocity of angular motion (Table 17-1). Given the head's attachment to the neck, head movement independent of body movement always has an angular component.

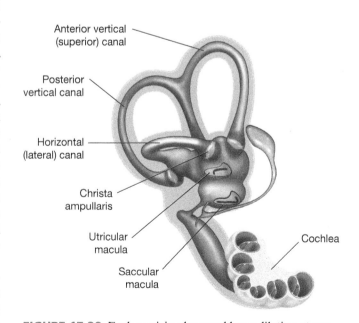

FIGURE 17-20 Each semicircular canal has a dilation at one end, the crista ampullaris.

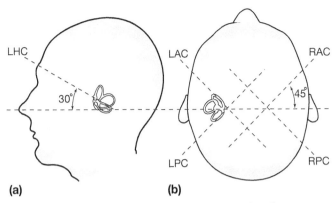

FIGURE 17-21 The three semicircular canals of each ear respond to angular acceleration and deceleration of the head. (a) The horizontal canals are oriented approximately 20 to 30 degrees off horizontal to the earth. (b) Sets of canals from opposite ears work in complementary co-planar pairs.

LAC, left anterior canal; LHC, left horizontal canal; LPC, left posterior canal; RAC, right anterior canal; RPC, right posterior canal

The canal, or canals, stimulated most effectively by head rotation lies in the plane closest to the plane of rotation. Sets of canals on either side of the head represent approximate mirror images of one another, and specific canals on opposite sides of the head operate in complementary pairs (Figure 17-21 ■). Rotation of the head in a given plane produces endolymph movements that are oppositely directed (relative to the ampullae) in complementary canal pairs on the right and left sides.

The inertial lag in the semicircular canals is provided by the endolymph. When the head starts to rotate, the endolymph tends to remain at rest, and the cupula, along with the cilia projecting into it, is displaced in a direction opposite the rotation (Figure 17-22 ■). As the head continues to rotate,

frictional forces eventually cause the endolymph to catch up with the head rotation, the cupula returns to its upright position, and the stimulation stops. When, after a period of rotation, the head stops rotating, the endolymph tends to keep moving, displacing the cupula and cilia in the direction of the preceding rotation. The hair cells of a given crista are all either depolarized or hyperpolarized because the stereocilia and kinocilia of each hair cell have the same orientation. Thus, under normal circumstances, signals must come from a complementary canal pair, not just a single canal on one side of the head, in order for the brain to determine the direction of head rotation. As discussed in the Clinical Connections, individuals can learn to compensate when they lack this redundant and confirmatory information.

Canal function is easiest to visualize for the horizontal canals (Figure 17-23 ■). All kinocilia in the horizontal canals face toward the utricle. Rotation (horizontal angular acceleration) of the head to the right produces displacement of the endolymph toward the ampulla in the right canal but away from the ampulla in the left canal. Thus, the hair cells in the right horizontal canal are depolarized, whereas those in the left horizontal canal are hyperpolarized. The result is that the associated primary afferents in the right CN VIII increase their discharge, while those in the left nerve decrease their basal discharge rate. Again, note that unlike the otolith organs, both right and left canals must be operative for the generation of a differential signal.

Thought Question

How does each member of a pair of semicircular canals respond to head movement? Thinking ahead, what do you suppose would happen if one of the pairs (or the afferent pathway from that canal) was not able to respond?

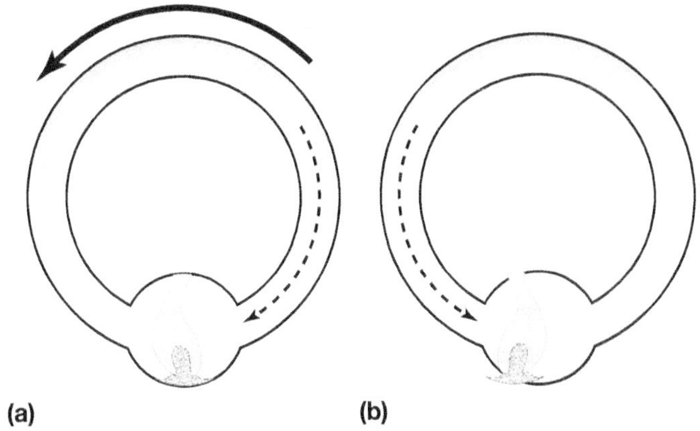

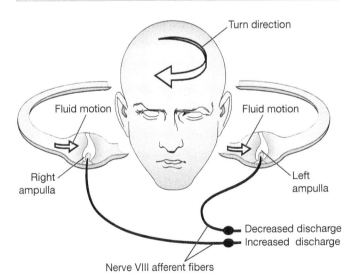

FIGURE 17-23 Horizontal rotation of the head to the right displaces the endolymph in the right horizontal canal toward the ampulla and away from the ampulla in the left horizontal canal. This results in increased discharge of the right afferent fibers and decreased discharge of the left afferent fibers.

FIGURE 17-22 As the head starts to rotate, the endolymph remains at rest due to inertia and, therefore, moves in the same direction as the head. (a) As the head continues to rotate, the endolymph begins to move in the opposite direction; the cupula, therefore, is displaced in the opposite direction. (b) When the head stops rotating, the endolymph continues to move, displacing the cupula in the direction of the preceding rotation. Bold solid lines represent direction of head movement; dashed lines represent direction of endolymph movement.

Primary Afferents

Primary afferents project toward the brainstem in the vestibular division of CN VIII, which enters the brainstem at the lower border of the pons, on its lateral aspect, posterior to the facial nerve. This region of the brainstem is referred to as the cerebellopontine angle. Primary vestibular afferents are bipolar neurons that have their cell bodies located in the two **vestibular ganglia**, or *ganglia of Scarpa*, aggregations of approximately 20,000 cell bodies located within the internal auditory meatus. The peripheral processes of the bipolar neurons synapse on hair cells, while most central processes within the brainstem divide into ascending and descending branches. Some of the descending fibers form a distinct bundle, the descending or spinal vestibular root. Most of the central processes of primary afferents terminate in the vestibular nuclei, but some terminate in a specific part of the cerebellum known as the **vestibulocerebellum** (see Chapters 6 and 19).

> **Thought Question**
>
> Where are the receptors, the peripheral processes (first order neuron), ganglia, and second-order neurons for vestibular inputs? How does this organization relate to the somatosensory systems?

Vestibular Nuclei

On each side of the brainstem, four major nuclei make up the vestibular nuclear complex and contain the cell bodies of second-order neurons (Figure 17-24 ■). These vestibular nuclei are located in the medulla and caudal pons: the **superior vestibular nucleus**, the **lateral vestibular nucleus**, the **medial vestibular nucleus**, and the **inferior** (spinal, descending) **vestibular nucleus**. Primary vestibular afferents project to all four nuclei, but fibers from the canals and maculae are distributed differentially within the nuclei. These, in turn, are further segregated within each nucleus according to specific semicircular canals, utricle, and saccule. Such segregation enables the vestibular nuclei to relay specific information to other parts of the CNS. However, some convergence of different labyrinthine inputs onto single nuclear neurons does occur.

Not all neurons in rather extensive regions of each vestibular nucleus receive the terminals of primary afferents. Some of these neurons receive labyrinthine information from nuclei of other vestibular neurons so that they are polysynaptically linked with labyrinthine receptors. Other neurons do not respond to labyrinthine input at all but receive input from other sources, such as the cerebellum. Finally, some neurons in the brainstem vestibular nuclei receive converging inputs from labyrinthine and nonlabyrinthine sources. Because nuclear output is functionally heterogeneous, it is clear that the vestibular nuclei represent

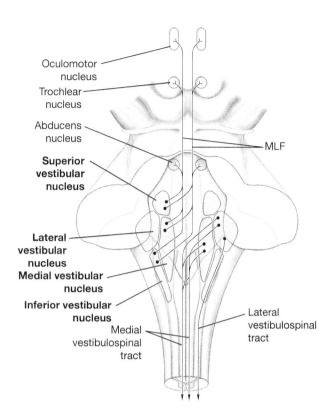

FIGURE 17-24 Four major nuclei make up the paired vestibular complex: the superior, lateral, medial, and inferior nuclei. Second-order projections ascend in the MLF to the three nuclei associated with eye movement (oculomotor, trochlear, and abducens). Second-order projections descend to the spinal cord as the medial and lateral vestibulospinal tracts. Note that the ascending and descending tracts are both ipsilateral and contralateral to the nuclei of origin.

more than aggregations of relay elements conveying labyrinthine information to the target structures they influence.

Commissural Inhibitory System

The vestibular nuclei of the right and left sides reciprocally interact by means of a commissural fiber system. The system is *inhibitory* so that increased activity of nuclear neurons on one side results in an inhibitory influence on neurons of the opposite side. Conversely, decreased activity on one side results in reduced inhibition of neurons on the opposite side. Thus, there are two mechanisms for enhancing the spontaneous activity of nuclear neurons: one is by increasing excitatory labyrinthine input and the second is by decreasing a tonic inhibitory input. The latter is known as **disinhibition** (Figure 17-25 ■).

Labyrinthine and inhibitory commissural influences normally interact to enhance the responsiveness of nuclear

> **Thought Question**
>
> Thinking ahead, why do you think disinhibition is key to the function of the vestibular system?

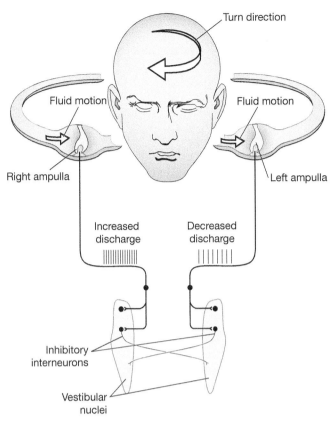

FIGURE 17-25 The vestibular nuclei of the right and left sides interact by way of inhibitory commissural fibers.

neurons. This is best illustrated by considering canal inputs resulting from horizontal angular acceleration of the head. As shown in Figure 17-25, when the head is accelerated to the right, canal input from the right side is increased, whereas that from the left horizontal canal is decreased. Nuclear neurons on the right side, then, will receive increased excitation from the ipsilateral labyrinth and decreased commissural inhibition from the contralateral vestibular nuclei. Both influences augment nuclear discharge on the right side. Further, neurons on the left side will receive, in addition to a suppressed excitatory drive from the left horizontal canal, an increased inhibitory drive via the commissural system. This interaction between labyrinthine and commissural inputs acts to enhance the differential nature of canal signals from the two ears. Nuclear neurons receiving otolith input may not be subject to commissural inhibition and, if true, this may be related to the fact that, unlike canal signals, otolithic macular signals from just one ear are differentially organized. The inhibitory commissural system also plays an important role in producing the clinical signs observed with peripheral vestibular lesions.

The Vestibular Sensory System

Projections

Projections of the vestibular system differ from those of the auditory system in a number of respects; projections to the cerebral cortex are less robust. However, there are more projections to the cerebellum, and there are many more reflex connections.

Axons from the vestibular nuclei ascend in a brainstem region between the lateral and medial lemnisci to the thalamus (Figure 17-26 ■). The projection on each side carries information originating from nuclei of both the right and left sides. Fibers originating from nuclei of the vestibular complex terminate in several thalamic nuclei that contain the cell bodies of third-order neurons. Most secondary vestibular afferents terminate in the ventral part of the **ventral posterolateral nucleus (VPL)** and in the dorsal part of the

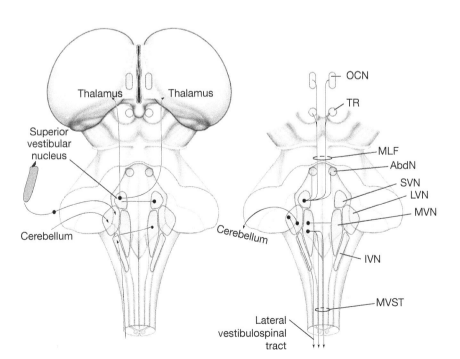

FIGURE 17-26 Some projections from the second-order neurons ascend while others descend. Some second-order neurons from the vestibular nuclei project directly to the thalamus. Ascending projections from the superior nuclei also terminate in the three pairs of oculomotor nuclei (occulomotor, trochlear, and abducens) as the afferent portion of the vestibulo-ocular reflex. Projections that descend from the vestibular nuclei travel in the medial and lateral vestibulospinal tracts.

AbdN, abducens nucleus; IVN, inferior vestibular nucleus; LVN, lateral vestibular nucleus; MLF, medial longitudinal fasciculus; MVN, medial vestibular nucleus; MVST, medial vestibulospinal tract; OCN, oculomotor nucleus; SVN, superior vestibular nucleus; TR, trochlear nucleus.

contiguous **ventral posterior inferior nucleus (VPI)** (see Figure 6-2). As revealed by MRI and CT Scans, thalamic infarctions involving parts of the ventral lateral thalamic nuclei (VL), VPL, and VPI cause pathological tilts of the patient's **subjective visual vertical (SVV)**, along with, in some patients, considerable postural instability. The SVV is measured by the patient's ability to adjust a black line from a random offset position to the subjective vertical. The tilt may be either ipsiversive (toward the side of the lesion) or contraversive (away from the side of the lesion) as a consequence of the fact that vestibular input to the thalamus is bilateral. Electrical stimulation of this same region during stereotaxic exploration of the human thalamus elicits vestibular sensations.

CEREBRAL CORTEX Vestibular projections to the cerebral cortex are bilateral so that activation of the labyrinth of one side generates activity in both cerebral hemispheres. However, activity is maximal in only one hemisphere, meaning that there is a cerebral dominance for vestibular cortical function. Which hemisphere is maximally activated depends on the handedness of the person and on which ear is stimulated. Interestingly, the dominance pattern for vestibular function is the opposite of that for handedness. Because a mature vestibular system (i.e., the accurate perception of gravity and motion and the maintenance of equilibrium) underlies the development of all motor function, it is possible that the side of dominance of the vestibular system determines the later development of handedness in the execution of motor skills.

The cerebral cortex contains multiple representations of the vestibular system. This possibility first suggested itself many years ago as a result of electrical stimulation of the human cerebral cortex in conscious patients undergoing neurosurgery. Two separate cortical areas were reported to elicit typical vestibular sensations when stimulated. One was located in the region of the intraparietal sulcus; when stimulated, this region evoked sensations of being rolled with apparent motion of the visual surroundings. The second area was situated in the depths of the Sylvian fissure; when stimulated, this region evoked subjective sensations of dizziness (vertigo). This area was incorrectly localized to the superior temporal gyrus close to the primary auditory cortex. In support of both areas were small groups of people suffering from so-called vestibular epilepsy, in which the onset of the seizure was heralded by an aura of vertigo. Such people had focal epileptogenic lesions either in the superior posterior part of the temporal lobe, near the temporoparietal border, or in the region of the intraparietal sulcus.

The preceding observations were of importance for several reasons. For one thing, identification of these areas in the human cortex guided the search for analogous areas in the monkey cortex, where more rigorous experimentation could be carried out. Even today, the human vestibular cortical areas are referenced to those previously identified in the monkey. The monkey cerebral cortex possesses at least

four distinct cortical areas that receive vestibular input. It should be noted that the monkey brain contains no equivalent of the human inferior parietal lobule, Brodmann's areas 40 and 39 (the supramarginal and angular gyri, respectively). In the monkey, Brodmann's area 7 makes up the cortex inferior to the intraparietal sulcus.

Three parietal projection fields have been identified in the monkey. The first corresponds to the area of the intraparietal sulcus identified in the human. This is area 2v at the tip of the intraparietal sulcus and is immediately caudal to the face (mouth) representation on the postcentral gyrus. The cells in this region possess a cytoarchitecture distinct from that of area 2;—hence, the designation area 2v. Specifically, area 2v, as well as the other cortical vestibular areas, contains cells characteristic of multisensory cortex as opposed to primary sensory cortex. A second focal representation is located in the anterior bank of the central fissure, within area 3a (which contains the somatosensory arm representation). The third parietal area receiving vestibular input is located in area 7 of the monkey cortex. Area 7 in the monkey has been shown experimentally to be a multisensory integration center for visuomotor function and spatial orientation. This area is thought to correspond functionally to areas 40 and 39 in the human.

The fourth cortical vestibular area is situated in the posterior insula and parietal operculum and is referred to as the **parieto-insular vestibular cortex (PIVC)**. Focal infarctions (as determined by CT and MRI scans) involving this area can occur following occlusion of specific branches of the middle cerebral artery. Such lesions result in an apparent tilt in the person's internal representation of gravity that can be measured in a test of the person's subjective visual vertical (SVV). Our perception of verticality is dominated by tonic (continuous, but variable activity) bilateral vestibular inputs from the otoliths and vertical semicircular canals. Such input stabilizes the eyes and head in a normal upright position in the roll plane (head rotation about the line of sight). It should be emphasized that infarctions in the territory of the posterior cerebral artery supplying the occipital lobe, while causing a visual field defect, do not affect perception of the visual vertical. Thus, it is not the visual system that determines what is up and down. In a normal individual, the SVV is aligned with the gravitational vertical, and the axes of the eyes and head are horizontal and directed straight ahead. However, in people with lesions centered in the PIVC, the SVV is tilted away from the side of the lesion. Such tilts may follow damage to the PIVC in either hemisphere. The tilts are most pronounced during the acute state of the infarction and show spontaneous recovery within weeks to months in most patients. Deviations of SVV are the perceptual correlate of a vestibular tone imbalance in the roll plane. The PIVC represents the cortical area showing an increase in regional cerebral blood flow during caloric vestibular stimulation (see Clinical Connections) in humans. The PIVC, rather than the superior temporal gyrus, also likely is the area referred to above that was activated by electrical stimulation with electrodes positioned in the depths of the Sylvian fissure.

Function

Gravity is the first sensory experience and is responded to even before birth. Postnatally, vestibular sensory input continues to occupy a unique position among our senses. Even though it plays a part in every perception, vestibular input does not form part of our normal conscious awareness. Only when the vestibular system malfunctions, or when we are subjected to unnatural passive motion, do we become acutely aware of its presence. A number of reasons have been advanced as to why we typically lack awareness of vestibular sensory input. First, vestibular input is not usually the topic of perceptual interest even when the head moves—as, for example, when localizing the source of a sound. Whenever we perceive an object, we already have the basic information about our spatial orientation and the relationship of our body to the object. Second, vestibular input is not topographically directed for the objects in the environment. As such, it differs fundamentally from other sensory modalities such as touch (both active and passive), vision, and audition.

The vestibular cortex mediates complex multimodal perceptions that allow us to perceive our own bodies as a standard, spatially oriented referent. Vestibular stimulation always results in the perception of body motion, but such stimulation is generated only by acceleration or deceleration. When the cupulae of the semicircular canals or the otolithic membranes have returned to their resting positions, information about change in motion ceases. This obviously occurs at rest, but it also occurs during constant velocity motion so that the perception of motion then depends entirely on visual input. It should be noted that otolith responses, discussed later, are gravity dependent and persist as long as a given head position is maintained.

However, input about visual motion can be perceived either as self-motion (a moving observer of a stationary environment) or object-motion (a stationary observer of a moving surround). A familiar example of visually induced apparent self-motion is the feeling of movement we have while sitting in a stationary train when we see a train on the next track move. During a constant velocity drive in a car, our perception of the horizontal direction and speed of motion (i.e., self-motion) is determined entirely by visual input. In order to properly steer the car, it is essential that this visual input be maintained undisturbed by competing input indicating another direction of movement. Thus, for example, involuntary head movements in a vertical direction resulting from sudden bumps in the road potentially could detract from the visual signal indicating the main direction of travel used to guide the vehicle.

How does the cerebral cortex prevent this visual-vestibular mismatch of self-motion information from degrading the ability to adequately steer the vehicle? This is accomplished by a reciprocal inhibitory interaction between the visual and vestibular cortices (as revealed by PET scanning). In the case of visually induced apparent self-motion, the activated visual cortex deactivates the vestibular cortex so that the sensitivity of the vestibular system to head acceleration is decreased. This negates the visual-vestibular input mismatch caused by head movement in a plane other than the main direction of travel. The deactivated vestibular area is the PIVC.

Thought Question

Here's a question to challenge you. When sitting in a stationary car, if the car next to you moves forward, you may experience a sensation of moving. Thinking ahead, what information would the brain require to resolve whether you are moving, the environment is moving, or both?

Two terms have evolved to depict the spatial relationships existing within the self, and between the self and extrapersonal space. The term **body schema** refers to our perception of the portion of space occupied by our bodies and of the relationship of the parts of the body to one another as noted in Chapter 9. The term **environmental schema** refers to the perception of the space around our body. As mentioned earlier, the vestibular system is an important contributor to both schemata, and both are learned phenomena that can be disrupted by brain disorders. The body and environmental schemata enable us to discriminate between movement of the head, movement of the eyes, and the movement of external objects. The two schemata continuously interact, forming a "space constancy mechanism" by which the ever-changing relationships between ourselves and the external environment are matched. This match yields the continuous perception of a distinction between the self and the outside world, between the ego and the object, and between the psychic world within and the real world without.

The Vestibular Motor System

As noted, in addition to its role as a motion-detecting system, the vestibular system plays a major role in the control of movement. This is accomplished through a variety of tracts, including the projections to the spinal cord, the reticular formation, the medial longitudinal fasciculus (MLF), and the cerebellum.

Spinal Cord Projections

Vestibular nuclei of each side give rise to two segmentally projecting upper motor neuron (UMN) tracts: a **lateral vestibulospinal tract (LVST)** and a **medial vestibulospinal tract (MVST)** (Figure 17-27 ■).

Axons of the LVST arise predominantly from neurons of the lateral vestibular nucleus (see Figure 17-24). The tract is entirely ipsilateral and descends in the anterolateral

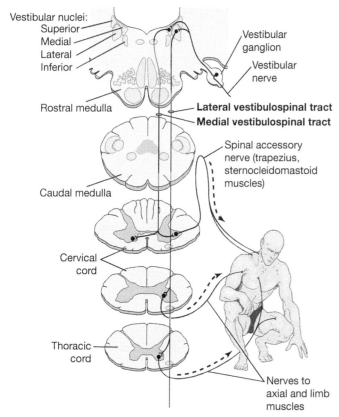

FIGURE 17-27 The vestibular motor system. Upper motor neurons project from the vestibular nuclei forming the lateral and medial vestibulospinal tracts. The lateral vestibulospinal tract descends ipsilaterally in the anterolateral spinal cord and terminates in the ventral gray of all levels of the spinal cord. The medial vestibulospinal tract descends in the medial longitudinal fasciculus and has bilateral connections cervical and rostral thoracic levels of the spinal cord.

The LVST conducts utricular, saccular, and semicircular canal information to the spinal cord. Its excitatory actions are exerted on ipsilateral neck and limb extensor motor neurons. Ipsilateral flexor motor neurons are simultaneously inhibited via segmental inhibitory interneurons. While the LVST is ipsilateral, it also influences contralateral motor neurons. Contralateral effects, which generally resemble those on the ipsilateral side, are mediated by interneurons that cross to the opposite side of the cord. Acting in concert with segmental myotatic reflexes, the LVST facilitates and maintains extensor muscle tone in the trunk and limbs that is essential to the support of the body against gravity—that is, for the maintenance of upright posture.

The MVST has not been investigated as thoroughly as the LVST, and most of the work has been concerned with the regulation of neck motor neurons. While MVST connections with the latter are not known in their entirety, many are monosynaptic. It is known that the MVST has predominantly ipsilateral effects in spinal cord, receives input from semicircular canals, and serves to stabilize the head and neck during rotation of the body on head. Axons of the MVST originate in the medial vestibular nucleus and descend in the **medial longitudinal fasciculus (MLF)**. In the spinal cord, the descending MLF is located in the sulcomarginal region of the anterior funiculus. The bulk of its fibers end at cervical levels, with some projecting to more rostral thoracic segments concerned with the innervation of upper back (axial) muscles.

Besides its predominantly cervical termination, the MVST differs from the LVST in several other ways. Importantly, the MVST inhibits cervical LMNs bilaterally. MVST inhibitory fibers are of vestibular nuclear origin so that inhibitory actions are exerted directly on neck motor neurons; that is, unlike the arrangement in other descending systems, MVST inhibition is not mediated by descending excitatory fibers that synapse with segmental inhibitory interneurons. The MVST participates in stabilizing and regulating head movements to ensure their appropriateness for maintaining equilibrium and fixation of gaze.

funiculus of the spinal cord, gradually assuming a more medial position in its descent. Its axons terminate at all cord levels—cervical through sacral—and influence alpha and gamma motor neurons. The lateral vestibular nucleus possesses a certain degree of somatotopic organization.

All LVST axons are excitatory and influence motor neurons either directly (monosynaptically) or via spinal cord interneurons (polysynaptically), depending on the muscle group innervated by the motor neuron. Motor neurons supplying the neck musculature receive the bulk of monosynaptic LVST input, whereas the majority of motor neurons supplying the limb musculature receive polysynaptic input. This difference in connectivity pattern has a significant functional correlate. Because a spinal interneuron mediates LVST-limb motor neuron interaction, the effectiveness of the interaction can be increased or diminished by altering the excitability of the interneuron. The latter can be brought about by segmental reflex input and/or by input from other descending pathways. By contrast, the monosynaptic pathway to neck (and some back) motor neurons is not subject to such regulation and thus reflects a more secure vestibular control over the neck musculature.

Reticular Formation

All four vestibular nuclei send fibers to the brainstem reticular formation (RF). The projections are bilateral and prominently related to the medial RF of the pons and medulla. Some of the connections are direct, but most are by complex pathways involving unknown numbers of neurons. Both semicircular canal and utricular input influence reticular neurons.

The pontomedullary sites to which vestibular information projects represent RF areas that give rise to long ascending and descending reticular fiber systems. The latter make up the UMN **reticulospinal tracts**, one of which originates in the pontine RF, the other in the medullary RF (see Chapter 5). These maintain separate positions in their descent through the spinal cord. Axons of both tracts project to all spinal cord levels and may end directly on LMNs or on interneurons. Flexor as well as extensor motor neurons are influenced, and the effects may be excitatory or inhibitory.

Vestibuloreticulospinal projections play a major role in transmitting labyrinthine information to the segmental motor apparatus and contribute importantly to vestibular reflexes. The precise nature of this function is not known, but it is clear that the contribution made by reticulospinal information is not redundant with MVST and LVST information. Considerable information processing occurs within the RF prior to spinal cord distribution; it seems likely that such integrated information is, in part, responsible for certain dynamic properties of vestibular reflexes that cannot be explained by relatively direct labyrinth-motor neuron linkages such as those that characterize the vestibulospinal tracts.

Labyrinthine information carried rostrally in the ascending reticular projections would appear to make an analogous contribution to vestibulo-ocular reflexes. Ascending projections may also contribute to vestibular sensations. Lastly, interactions between the vestibular nuclei and brainstem RF underlie the autonomic effects (nausea, vomiting, pallor, perspiration) evoked by excessive labyrinthine stimulation as well as by irritative lesions.

Thought Question

How is vestibular information integrated with information from the reticular formation?

Extraocular Projections

Eye movements are regulated by contractions of the six extraocular muscles in each eye innervated by LMNs of CNs III, IV, and VI (see Chapter 13). Connections between the vestibular nuclei and extraocular motor neurons represent a UMN system. They originate primarily in the superior and medial vestibular nuclei and ascend in the **medial longitudinal fasciculus** (MLF, ascending component) (Figure 17-28 ■).

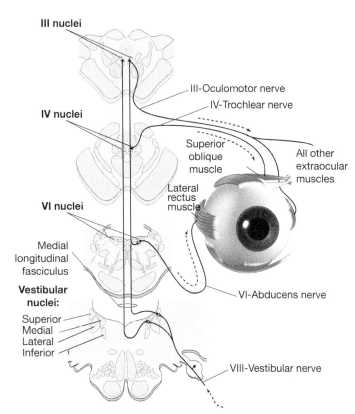

FIGURE 17-28 Neurons projecting from the vestibular nuclei ascend in the MLF to synapse on extraocular motor neurons. Illustrated here are the connections to the ipsilateral extraocular muscles. In reality, however, the MLF has bilateral connections to the extraocular nuclei—and, therefore, mediate bilateral control of extraocular eye muscles.

Although the projections to motor neurons supplying given muscles have specific laterality patterns, an acceptable operational statement is that the MLF of each side influences the extraocular nuclei bilaterally. Semicircular canal and otolith-dependent influences are both mediated by the MLF, the former being responsible for phasic, short-term adjustments of eye position in response to angular acceleration of the head; the latter for tonic, long-term position maintenance. MLF actions on extraocular motor neurons may be excitatory or inhibitory. As with the MVST, the inhibitory neurons are located within the vestibular nuclei (see the vestibulo-ocular reflex).

Eye movements of vestibular origin also are governed by ascending reticular projections, as noted in the previous section. Among other functions, it would appear these are importantly involved in nystagmus (discussed later) because nystagmus persists following transection of the MLF.

Thought Question

Thinking ahead, why would the vestibular system have connections with the oculomotor system?

Cerebellum

Thought Question

Thinking ahead, and given what you learned about the functions of lobes of the cerebellum in Chapter 6, with which lobe(s) would the vestibular system most likely have connections?

Primary vestibular fibers terminate in the vestibulocerebellum that consists primarily of the *flocculonodular lobe* (see Chapter 6). The vestibulocerebellum receives, in addition, secondary projections from all four vestibular nuclei. Both primary and secondary vestibulocerebellar fibers reach the cerebellum via the **juxtarestiform body**, a bundle of fibers medial to the inferior cerebellar peduncle. Semicircular canal as well as otolith-dependent information is carried by the secondary projections. Although parallel first- and second-order pathways conduct labyrinthine information to the vestibulocerebellum, their information content is different. The former are not subject to precerebellar modulation, whereas the latter carry information that reflects interactions with the commissural fiber system, as well as other converging inputs that influence vestibular nuclear neurons. Besides the vestibulocerebellum, primary and secondary vestibular fibers are distributed to other areas of the cerebellum. This widespread cerebellar distribution of labyrinthine information contradicts the classical notion of cerebellar functional subdivisions in which fibers of vestibular, spinal, and cerebrocortical origin distribute to separate cerebellar areas.

Direct and indirect labyrinthine inputs condition the discharge patterns of specific cerebellar output neurons. The outputs, in turn, project back to vestibular nuclear neurons to shape their discharge patterns and, thereby, the activity of extraocular and segmental LMNs.

Vestibular reflexes also are influenced by the cerebellum. However, the extent to which vestibulo-ocular, vestibulocollic (neck), and vestibulospinal reflexes are governed by cerebellar activity depends on whether the labyrinths detect the altered muscle position occasioned by the reflex—for example, whether the output (movement) is registered by the input signal generator (the labyrinths). Both vestibulo-ocular and vestibulospinal limb reflexes are **open loop** in that neither eye nor limb movements modify the peripheral vestibular stimulus. Open-loop reflexes are closely regulated by the cerebellum. Limb movements resulting from head displacement generate somatosensory input to vestibular nuclear neurons that is not detected by the labyrinths. Corrections of this open-loop reflex are executed by the cerebellar anterior lobe, which receives movement-related somatosensory information over the spinocerebellar tracts as well as information from vestibular nuclear cells activated by the initial vestibular stimulus. Accuracy of the open-loop vestibulo-ocular reflex is maintained by the vestibulocerebellum. In this case, the error

signals are in the form of retinally generated visual input (e.g., image blurring) that projects to the flocculonodular lobe. In contrast, vestibulocollic (neck) reflexes are **closed loop** in that head movement produced by neck muscle contraction inevitably alters the labyrinthine signal.

Reflexes

The earliest motor responses of the infant to the mother are vestibularly mediated and consist of the setting and adjusting of body tone in response to being lifted and positioned. A host of interactive reflexes, of labyrinthine as well as nonlabyrinthine origin, are involved in the maintenance of posture. Those of labyrinthine origin act on three muscle systems—eye, neck, and body—and may be grouped into two broad functional categories. Static (tonic, or *positional*) responses are elicited by the position of the head in space and are tonic in the sense that they persist so long as the head position is maintained. These responses are mediated by the otolith organs. Acceleratory (*statokinetic*) reflexes are elicited by acceleration and are phasic in the sense that they are short acting. Reflexes elicited by angular acceleration are mediated by the semicircular canals, and those elicited by linear acceleration are mediated by the otolith organs. Canal-dependent and otolith-dependent influences are brought to bear on each of the three muscle systems.

Thought Question

What three muscle systems are important in production of the labyrinthine reflexes? Compare and contrast the resulting static and acceleratory reflexes in terms of the following: source of the sensory input, components of the vestibular system involved, termination of the first-order neurons, and type of resulting muscle contraction.

Irrespective of type, labyrinthine reflexes result in adjustments that oppose a perturbing force, thus they represent compensatory muscular adjustments. They act to restore head and body to their normal upright positions. However, because abnormal head and body postures can be voluntarily assumed and maintained, it is clear that central gating mechanisms exist that are capable of overriding these reflexes, in animals as well as people. Indeed, vestibular reflexes acting on the body and neck musculature, as well as certain of those acting on the extraocular musculature, are brought under cortical control with maturation of the motor system. Thus, obligatory vestibular reflexes are most clearly demonstrable in human infants. Normally, canal- and otolith-elicited reflexes act simultaneously. Further, when the head moves relative to the body, neck reflexes combine with and modify vestibular reflex patterns.

Postural reflexes are difficult to analyze for a number of reasons. Some of these reflexes are interactive, and their functional meaning resides in their co-occurrence with other reflexes. Some of the reflexes are impossible to elicit in isolation from one another without a degree of experimental control unattainable in the neurologic examination. Lastly, the time at which some of the reflexes come under cortical control is so variable that the continued presence of a reflex is difficult to assess.

As mentioned earlier, primary vestibular afferents terminate on neurons of the brainstem vestibular nuclei, whose axons project to the spinal cord to influence the excitability of lower motor neurons either directly or indirectly. It also was noted that the brainstem reticular formation serves as a major distributing center for labyrinthine-mediated effects on motor neurons. Reflex actions exerted on neck and limb motor neurons are carried by vestibulospinal and reticulospinal tracts, while those on extraocular motor neurons are conveyed by the ascending component of the MLF plus ascending reticular projections. The cerebellum represents a regulatory mechanism superimposed on this reflex substrate: the spinocerebellum of the anterior lobe participates in governing vestibulospinal reflexes involving the limbs, while the vestibulocerebellum regulates reflexes of the extraocular muscles. In contrast, neck reflexes (closed loop) are not closely regulated by the cerebellum.

VESTIBULOCOLLIC (NECK) REFLEXES Labyrinthine reflexes acting on the neck musculature are termed **vestibulocollic** reflexes to distinguish them from vestibulospinal reflexes influencing the limbs. The neck musculature is subject to both semicircular canal- and otolith-evoked reflex inputs. However, because the semicircular canals respond only to short-term angular acceleration and deceleration of the head, canal-dependent vestibulocollic reflexes participate only in short-term compensatory adjustments of head position. The canals most effectively stimulated by any rotational head movement are those lying in or closest to the plane of rotation. While all rotational movement stimulates multiple canals (the pattern of the reflex response depends on which are excited), the resulting muscular contractions may be viewed as producing a reflex response that opposes the rotation causing ampullary excitation. Consequently, the pattern of neck muscle activation tends to stabilize head position by counteracting the disturbing force. The long-term maintenance of normal head position is a function of otolith-mediated vestibulocollic reflexes. Otolith responses are gravity dependent and persist as long as a given head position is maintained.

> **Thought Question**
>
> What is the functional importance of the vestibulocollic reflexes? Compare and contrast the reflexes that arise from the otolith organs versus those from the semicircular canals.

Vestibulocollic reflexes are unique among labyrinthine reflexes. Any reflex contraction of the neck muscles must alter head position and thus the vestibular signal to the CNS. Therefore, the compensatory head response tends to null the initial vestibular signal that produced it through mechanical negative feedback.

VESTIBULOSPINAL REFLEXES Vestibulospinal reflexes act to restore the head to its normal horizontal position by eliciting compensatory adjustments of the limb muscles. Like vestibulocollic reflexes, vestibulospinal reflexes oppose head displacement. However, unlike vestibulocollic reflexes, vestibulospinal reflexes influence muscle groups whose alignment with the head can vary. An unlimited variety of head–body alignments can exist because the head can move independent of the body. Although there is some plasticity to vestibulospinal reflexes, they nonetheless elicit stereotyped influences on limb motor neurons in response to head displacement in a given direction. Thus, drives that are appropriate to a particular head–body alignment might be inappropriate when the alignment is changed. In order to prevent destabilizing vestibulospinal reflexes, it is a functional necessity that vestibular signals to the limb muscles be adjusted to match changing needs. This matching is accomplished by collaboration with reflexes originating in neck receptors. Vestibulospinal and neck reflexes always act together, and the contributions of each to limb posture can be studied only in the experimental setting.

VESTIBULO-OCULAR REFLEXES Vestibulo-ocular reflexes function to maintain the stability of the visual image on the retina during head movement. These reflexes do so by evoking eye adjustments in a direction opposite to that of head displacement. Again, both canal- and otolith-mediated responses participate in such adjustments. The compensatory nature of these reflexes is exemplified by so-called **doll's eye movements**: horizontal rotation of the head to the right deviates both eyes to the left; downward tilt results in upward deviation, and so on. It should be noted that in the human infant, such doll's eye movements gradually disappear during the first postnatal month. This is because eye control comes to be increasingly dominated by visual input. Prolonged rotation in a given direction produces a repetitive repositioning of the eyes known as vestibular nystagmus. **Nystagmus** comprises a rhythmic series of conjugate eye deviations and is a normal response due to activation of the semicircular canals. Its direction varies depending on which canals, or combination of canals, are stimulated.

Both the visual and vestibular systems are involved in regulating eye position and thus in maintaining stability of the retinal image. However, visual tracking of a moving target remains accurate only for low-movement frequencies. When the head is held stationary, successful visual tracking (foveal pursuit) of a sinusoidally oscillating target is limited to frequencies below approximately 1.0 Hz. This can be demonstrated by holding your hand in front of you and focusing on the lines on your palm. While holding your head stationary, oscillate your hand to the right and left with increasing rapidity. You quickly will reach a frequency of hand movement at which you

Neuropathology Box 17-2: Role of Reflexes in Postural Adjustments

The role of visual, neck, and vestibulospinal reflexes in postural adjustments was described early in the 20th century by Rademaker, Twitchell, and others. These reflexes ensure that the head maintains an appropriate orientation with respect to gravity, irrespective of movements of the rest of the body, and that the head and neck follow body movements appropriately. Experiments in which monkeys were labyrinthectomized, blindfolded, or both illustrate these reflexes.

Head righting is illustrated by holding a monkey upside-down, so that the head would be facing the floor (Figure 17-29a ■). Reflexively, the head will right such that it is in a horizontal plane relative to the ground. Righting occurs even if the animal is blindfolded (Figure 17-29b) or has been labrynthectomized (Figure 17-29c). When the animal is blindfolded, the intact labyrinthine reflexes cause the head righting; when the animal is labrynthectomized, vision is the stimulus for head righting.

Reflexive righting responses of the body are illustrated in a monkey that has been labyrinthectomzied and is blindfolded. When the head is passively righted, the body automatically follows (Figure 17-29d). This response is thought to be subserved by neck reflexes because the animal has neither vision nor labyrinthine inputs to initiate the reflexes.

These reflexes are present in young infants and are an important component of developmental testing.

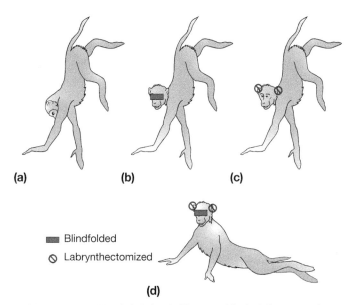

(a)　　　(b)　　　(c)

■ Blindfolded
⊘ Labrynthectomized

(d)

FIGURE 17-29 Head righting is illustrated by holding a monkey upside down so that the head would be facing the floor. Refer to Neuropathology Box 17-2.

will be unable to retain focus. At these higher frequencies, visual tracking cannot prevent retinal blurring and loss of acuity. Because, in everyday experience, active as well as passively induced head movements (running, jumping, etc.) routinely occur at frequencies well above this value, retinal image stability during such movements is maintained exclusively by vestibularly driven extraocular reflexes. This is easily demonstrated by reversing the maneuver just described. Again focus on the lines on the palm of your hand. But this time keep your hand stationary, and oscillate your head to the right and left. Unless you move your head rapidly enough (after about 5 Hz), you will not lose focus. Vestibulo-ocular reflexes achieve an almost perfect compensation of head displacement; that is, the velocity of vestibularly driven eye movement is nearly equal but opposite to head angular velocity. Long-term maintenance of vestibulo-ocular reflex accuracy as well as periodic tuning to accommodate changing needs apparently is accomplished by visual as well as centrally derived influences. As we shall see in Chapter 19, the vestibulo-ocular reflex is highly plastic and, under the right experimental conditions, can be made to completely reverse its normal direction.

Thought Question

Here's a question to stretch your mind. Think of functional situations in which it is necessary for the vestibulosinal, vestibulo-ocular, and vestibulocollic reflexes to all work together. Now identify as many pathways as possible that might mediate the action of these reflexes. And finally, what examples can you think of in which the person performs a task that requires overriding one of more of these reflexes?

The vestibulo-ocular reflex (VOR) pathway that maintains the stability of the retinal image during head movement involves the semicircular canals; secondary projections of vestibular nuclear neurons that function as interneurons in the reflex arc; and the oculomotor, trochlear, and abducens nuclei and their cranial nerves. Each semicircular canal has reflex connections appropriate to mediate eye deviations in its own plane. Depending on the nature of the head's angular motion, any combination of semicircular canals and extraocular muscle contractions may be involved in mediating the compensatory eye movements. This is easiest to visualize with activation of the horizontal semicircular canal.

When the head is turned to the left, the eyes must deviate to the right by contraction of the right lateral and left medial recti muscles and concomitant relaxation of

Head rotation

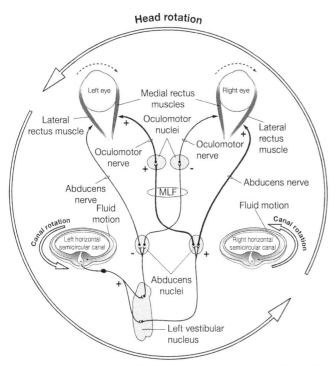

FIGURE 17-30 The vestibuloocular reflex maintains the stability of the retinal image during head movement, by moving the eyes in the opposite direction of head movement.

the antagonistic right medial and left lateral recti muscles (Figure 17-30 ■). With head rotation to the left, the cupula of the left horizontal canal is deflected to the right, *toward* the utricle, by the inertia of the endolymph, which depolarizes its hair cells resulting in increased firing of the CN VIII fibers that innervate them. From the left vestibular nuclei, secondary projections (interneurons) cross the midline to excite the right abducens nucleus. There are two populations of neurons in the right abducens nucleus that are excited by this vestibular input: motor neurons that project in the abducens nerve and excite the right lateral rectus muscle and neurons whose axons cross the midline and ascend in the left medial longitudinal fasciculus to the oculomotor nucleus, where they excite motor neurons that project to the left medial rectus muscle. These connections mediate rightward horizontal eye movement in both eyes that compensate for head rotation to the left. Simultaneously, inhibitory neurons in the left vestibular nuclei inhibit both populations of abducens neurons in the left abducens nucleus, resulting in motor neurons for the left lateral rectus and right medial rectus (the antagonistic muscles) becoming inhibited. Thus, the principle of reciprocal innervation applies to the VOR just as it does for spinal reflexes. Note that the same head movement to the left also causes a deflection of the right horizontal canal cupula to the right, *away* from the utricle, which hyperpolarizes its constituent hair cells. These connections are not shown in Figure 17-30 but would have a complementary effect in that there would be less inhibition of motor neurons innervating the right lateral rectus and left medial rectus and

Thought Question

How do reflexes mediated by the otolith organs differ from those mediated by the semicircular canals?

less excitation of motor neurons innervating the left lateral rectus and right medial rectus muscles.

Integration in the Vestibular System

Role in Postural Control

The regulation of postural activities such as standing (the maintenance of an upright stance) depends on three sensory modalities: proprioception, vision, and vestibular. The vestibular system provides information about head position in space, both when stationary and during movement. Vision is necessary for stabilization of gaze as the head moves. The role of vision in standing is readily apparent when we stand on a single foot and compare the amount of body sway with the eyes closed and with them open. Proprioception, especially of the lower extremities and neck, provides critical information about relationships of body segments in space. These three neurophysiologic systems work cooperatively to ensure stability, both when a person is stationary and during movements. To work effectively, a number of non-neurophysiologic systems also are involved. These systems work against a background of sufficient muscle strength in relevant muscle groups (e.g., those of the lower extremity and torso) as well as alignment and sufficient muscle length to permit appropriate postural adjustments. The complete system of balance and postural control, integrating neurophysiologic with non-neurophysiological systems, is beyond the scope of this text. The mechanisms by which vestibular and visual inputs are integrated, and the resulting outputs, are the subject of the information in this section.

Convergence onto Neurons of the Vestibular Nuclei

Because visual and somatosensory inputs both contribute to the maintenance of body orientation in space, vestibularly mediated reflexes are influenced by visual and somatosensory information. Interaction between these modalities occurs in neurons of the vestibular nuclei, although the latter are not the only loci for this integration.

Visual input to the vestibular nuclei functions in particular relevance to the vestibulo-ocular system. It is important not only to harmonizing actions of the two major reflex drives that control eye position, but it also maintains the accuracy of the vestibulo-ocular reflex by adjusting its gain to changing needs. Vision plays a less obvious role in postural responses of the limbs. However, contributions to postural stabilization are a consequence of vision's role in evaluating and maintaining proper body orientation. Visual information exerts a significant influence on leg adjustments to induced postural sway and on vestibularly mediated responses of the antigravity muscles in landing from a fall.

Somatosensory input to vestibular neurons is broad and is not somatotopically organized. It presumably provides a diffuse background facilitatory drive upon which more specific labyrinthine inputs act. Its functional utility lies in the fact that it helps to ensure a vestibular influence on motor neurons that is appropriate to prevailing peripheral conditions. The dominant input derives from muscle and joint receptors (with the somewhat surprising exception of group Ia spindle afferents), but cutaneous receptors also are involved. Most of the deep somatic proprioceptive input originates in receptors of neck and proximal limb joints and is related to both sides of the body. Spinal cord information reaches the vestibular nuclei directly, as well as by way of the brainstem reticular formation. Additionally, somatosensory information can influence vestibular neurons indirectly via transcerebellar pathways.

The important action of convergent somatosensory input on vestibular neurons is well illustrated by the behavioral effects resulting from electrical stimulation, section, or anesthetization in experimental animals of the upper cervical dorsal roots, which carry information from neck receptors. Anesthesia of the upper three cervical roots on one side results in disorientation, imbalance, and incoordination, resembling the deficits seen with unilateral labyrinthectomy. In contrast, electrical stimulation of these cervical roots may produce nystagmus and vertigo, resembling signs seen with unilateral irritative labyrinthine lesions. Both these experimental manipulations alter the output of vestibular projection systems, and both create an asymmetry between the outputs from the two sides. Asymmetrical nuclear discharge is a prerequisite to the display of clear vestibular signs. Although the experimental manipulation directly influences only ipsilateral nuclear output, the commissural inhibitory system exerts a reciprocal effect on the contralateral side.

Convergence onto Neurons of the Cerebral Cortex

Microelectrode recordings from cortical vestibular areas in the monkey show that their neurons are all multisensory, responding not only to vestibular, but also to somatosensory and visual stimuli. As noted previously, the neuronal cytoarchitecture supports this finding. That somatosensory and visual input should converge on vestibular neurons is understandable, given that natural stimulation of the vestibular system is the result of head motion and locomotion: the input to the brain is unavoidably polysensory. Because all of the vestibular cortical areas are multisensory, there is no primary vestibular cortex in that cortical vestibular neurons do not share a key characteristic of other primary sensory cortical areas—namely, neurons with unique response characteristics to modality-specific peripheral stimuli.

Vestibular and Neck Reflexes

As noted earlier, vestibulospinal and neck reflexes act together to ensure that reflex drives are appropriate to a particular head–body alignment. In order to study

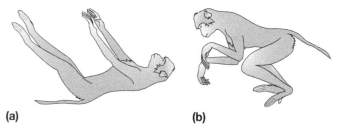

FIGURE 17-31 The tonic labrynthine reflexes are obligatory in an animal that does not have input from cervical (neck) receptors. When supine (a), the animal's limbs are in extension; when prone (b), the limbs are in flexion.

labyrinthine–limb (vestibulospinal) reflexes, it is necessary to eliminate input from neck receptors by immobilizing the neck or by sectioning the upper cervical dorsal roots. When this is done in an experimental animal, it is seen that both phasic canal-dependent and tonic otolith-dependent vestibulospinal reflexes act on the antigravity limb muscles. For example, tilting the animal's head upward and holding it in that position induces forelimb flexion and hind limb extension, which act to restore the head to a horizontal position. When the animal is placed supine, all four limbs will extend, whereas, if the animal is placed in prone, all four limbs will flex (Figure 17-31 ■). These are referred to as the **tonic labyrinthine reflexes**.

In order to study the neck reflexes, it is necessary to remove labyrinthine inputs. In labyrinthectomized animals, if the head is tilted downward relative to the horizontal plane, the upper limbs flex while the lower limbs are in extension. Conversely, when the head is tilted upward, the upper limbs are in extension and the lower limbs are in flexion. Figure 17-32 ■ illustrates these responses, which are referred to as the **tonic neck reflexes**. Furthermore, if the head is rotated so that the face is turned toward the right or left side, the limbs toward which the face is rotated extend while the contralateral limbs flex. These postures are referred to as the **asymmetrical tonic neck reflexes**.

Thought Question

The vestibular reflexes are adaptable, depending on the circumstances and the coordination with neck (among other) reflexes. Is this adaptability similar or different from other reflexes (e.g., somatic motor reflexes and auditory reflexes)?

Labyrinthine and neck afferent information must be centrally integrated to ensure appropriate head-to-body postural adjustments. The two interact summatively—in some cases canceling and in others reinforcing one another. Figure 17-33 ■ illustrates a range of head and limb relationships that can occur in a healthy animal. Were the CNS to consider only labyrinthine information, none of these positions would be possible. Similarly, if the CNS were only to consider neck proprioceptive information, these

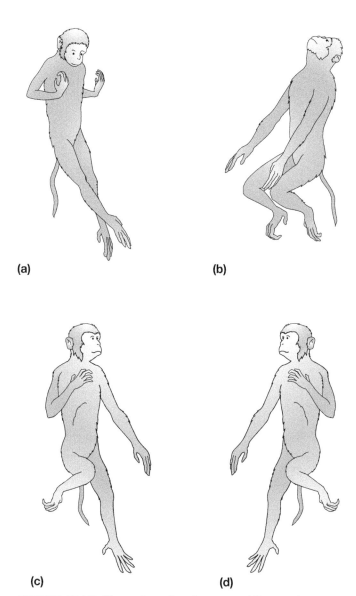

FIGURE 17-32 The tonic neck reflexes are obligatory in an animal that does not have input from labyrinthine receptors. When the head is flexed (a), the animal's upper limbs are in flexion, while the lower limbs are in extension; when the head is extended (b), the upper limbs are in extension, and the lower limbs are in flexion. These are the symmetrical tonic neck reflexes. When the head is rotated, an asymmetrical reflex occurs (c, d). The limbs on the side to which the head is turned are in extension, while the limbs on the contralateral side are in flexion.

Neck	Labyrinth		
	Head up	Head normal	Head down
Dorsiflexion			
Normal			
Ventriflexion			

FIGURE 17-33 The labyrinthine receptors control the orientation of the head relative to gravity, while the cervical receptors control the neck relative to the body. Acting together in the intact animal, the head and neck receptors work in concert to permit a wide range of positions. Thus, for example, the animal can maintain a neutral head position with respect to gravity, while either bucking or jumping (center column), by relying on the labyrinthine receptors and overriding the neck receptors. Similarly, the animal can maintain a neutral alignment of neck to body by relying on the neck receptors (middle row) while on hind legs or walking down hill. And finally, the animal can override these reflexes to assume a variety of other relative orientations of head, neck, and body.

positions would not be possible. However, each response is modulated by the reflex consequences of both vestibular and neck reflexes so that, in actuality, limb postures can vary, irrespective of the alteration in head attitude. Such interaction permits head movement on the body without affecting stability of the trunk.

While the CNS considers both inputs simultaneously, there are situations where one reflex system is dominant. Provided that the orientation of the head with respect to gravity is normal but body position is not, then neck reflexes acting alone function to realign the body with respect

to the head (see Figure 17-33, center column). Conversely, when head and body are normally aligned with one another but *whole* head–body position is not properly oriented with respect to gravity, then vestibulospinal reflexes alone act to restore the body–head back to a normal, upright position (see Figure 17-33, middle row).

Lastly, otolith-mediated vestibulospinal reflexes participate importantly in the motor adjustments associated with falling from a height. Contractions of the antigravity muscles that oppose landing forces occur prior to surface contact, thus eliminating segmental stretch reflexes as initiators of the landing response. The vestibular drive that prepares the muscular system for landing most likely originates from the saccular macula. This is, in part, predictable from the vertical orientation of the saccule and the fact that maculae respond best to shearing forces tangential to the macular surface, and not to perpendicularly directed forces.

CLINICAL CONNECTIONS

Clinical evaluation of the vestibular system is key to identifying causes of dysfunction in people who are dizzy or have vertigo and is also important when working with anyone who has postural instability, with or without falls.

These tests are of particular relevance when working with people who have brainstem injuries (e.g., from stroke or traumatic brain injury) as well as people with multiple sclerosis, because each of these conditions can affect the brainstem and, hence, vestibular/visual connections.

Understanding of vestibular system dysfunction is increasing, with great strides made in the past two decades with respect to rehabilitation. In part, current management of these conditions reflects an appreciation of the remarkable ability of this system for adaptation. Furthermore, current interventions reflect the growing ability of rehabilitation specialists to utilize knowledge of the neuroanatomy, neurophysiology, and plasticity of this system in designing evaluations; to predict the extent and nature of improvement that can occur; and to implement the most appropriate interventions accordingly.

Signs and symptoms of vestibular dysfunction vary but include some combination of the following: nystagmus; impaired VOR; nausea, vomiting, and/or vertigo. Postural instability can also occur, as can changes in gait (e.g., greater variability and a wide base of support, sometimes with drifting to one side). Nausea, vomiting, and vertigo are indicative of disruption of the vestibular/reticular formation connections, with resulting autonomic effects. The wide base of support during gait may be a compensation for instability associated with many vestibular disorders. The specific group of symptoms depends on the nature and location of the lesion.

The vestibular system has a remarkable ability for adaptation through central changes that permit the system to compensate for damage. However, such adaptations are likely to be most successful when injury is localized to the periphery. For example, adaptation can occur following vestibular neuritis, even if permanent damage occurs. On the other hand, damage to central structures, compounded by damage to other systems (as occurs in traumatic head injury), can be much more resistant to physical intervention. Furthermore, people with vestibular dysfunction compounded by premorbid conditions of depression or substance abuse (both of which may involve the reticular system with which the vestibular system connects) can be highly resistant to physical remediation. Resolution of symptoms is likely to be prolonged and may not be complete if damage to peripheral components of the vestibular system is coupled with damage to its central connections, making it impossible for the vestibular system to recalibrate fully and effectively. Successful intervention, therefore, depends on a careful examination and interpretation of findings, including both the findings from the current disorder or injury as well as implications for premorbid or co-morbid conditions.

Disturbances in vestibular function are often seen in people with nervous system pathology, but vestibular deficits play a more important role in otology than they do in neurology. Techniques for clinical analysis of labyrinthine influences on the spinal motor apparatus are imperfect and limited. However, precise methods are available for the clinical evaluation of vestibular influences on the oculomotor apparatus. These are based on the examination of nystagmus.

Nystagmus

Labyrinthine (Vestibular) Nystagmus

During a continuous head rotation that is too large to be compensated for by the VOR, the reflex is regularly interrupted by rapid eye movements that snap the eyes back to a midline position. For example, in Figure 17-34 ■, the eye movements engaged by the VOR with rotation of the head to the left have reached their physical limit. That is, the mechanical constraints of the eyes moving in their orbits preclude the continued operation of the VOR to compensate for a continued left rotation. Therefore, the slow compensatory movements of the eyes to the right (driven by the VOR) are interrupted by fast movements in the leftward direction of the rotation that return the eyes to the midline. This series of rhythmic, conjugate deviations of the eyes consisting of a slow phase in one direction and a fast phase in the other is **nystagmus** (Gr., *a nodding*, refers to the head movements of a sleepy person trying to stay awake wherein the head slowly sags then snaps back upright). Technically this is called *jerk nystagmus* and is the most common form of nystagmus. Jerk nystagmus may be horizontal, vertical, or torsional, depending on which semicircular canal (or combination of canals) is being stimulated by the plane of head rotation. The direction of nystagmus is named after the direction of its fast component. In a way, this is unfortunate terminology because the return to the midline is not mediated by the vestibular system and VOR. This is unfortunate because, as we shall see, continued rotation in one direction elicits signs in the limbs when the rotation is stopped. These are actively mediated by the

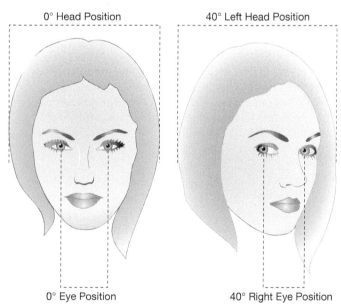

FIGURE 17-34 The VOR will be engaged with rotation of the head up to 40 degrees. Larger movements elicit a nystagmus, returning the eyes back to midline.

vestibular system, and their direction always is in the direction of the preceding rotation and opposite to the direction of post-rotatory nystagmus.

Nystagmus is induced by deflection of the cupula that occurs on angular acceleration and deceleration. In the clinical setting, one way nystagmus is elicited and evaluated is by rotating the subject seated in a swivel chair (or Barany chair). The clinician evaluates the duration and extent of nystagmus after the subject stops being rotated, or post-rotatory nystagmus. At the start of rotation, the inertia of the endolymph (see Figure 17-22) deflects the cupula in one direction, thereby stimulating the hair cells. This produces nystagmus in the direction of the rotation. After a period of rotation in the same direction, frictional forces cause the endolymph to begin moving, and eventually the endolymph will move at the same velocity as the head. At this point, the cupula will no longer be deflected, the hair cells return to their prerotation discharge levels, and the nystagmus ceases. When the rotation suddenly stops, inertia of the endolymph causes it to continue to move, with renewed deflection of the cupula, but this time in the opposite direction. **Post-rotatory nystagmus** will then be observed. Its direction (fast phase) will be opposite to the direction of the preceding rotation.

Thought Question

Nystagmus is a normal response to certain head movements, but it can also be indicative of pathological conditions. In preparation for understanding pathological manifestations of nystagmus, define nystagmus, identify several common daily situations in which nystagmus is appropriate, and indicate the pathways involved.

Nystagmus can be elicited in the horizontal canals using two different techniques: by rotating the subject, as described earlier, or by irrigating the external auditory meatus with warm or cold water or air, referred to as **caloric testing**. Caloric testing has the advantage of allowing each ear to be tested separately, but the disadvantage is imprecise control of the stimulus parameters (water or air temperature and stimulus duration). For caloric testing of the horizontal canal, the canal should be vertical, which is accomplished by having the patient tilt his or her head 60 degrees back from an upright position (Figure 17-35 ■). Irrigation of the external auditory canal with cold water sets up downwardly directed endolymphatic convection currents, while irrigation with warm water causes upwardly directed endolymphatic convection currents. In normal subjects, cold water irrigation elicits horizontal nystagmus to the opposite side after a latent period of about 20 seconds. Warm water irrigation induces nystagmus to the same side. This is the basis for the mnemonic "COWS"—cold opposite, warm same—referring to the direction of the fast phase of nystagmus. Nystagmus usually persists for 90 to 120 seconds.

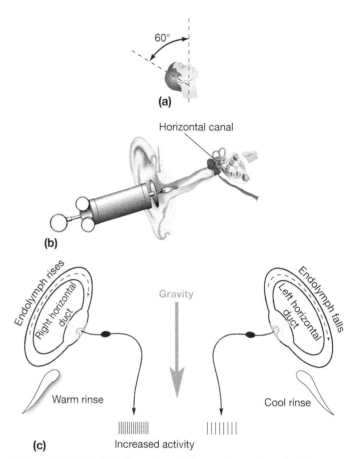

FIGURE 17-35 Caloric testing of the horizontal canal. (a) The head is tilted back 60 degrees. (b) The external auditory canal is irrigated with water. (c) Cold water irrigation causes the endolymph to fall on the same side, leads to decreased activity on the ipsilateral side, and elicits a nystagmus to the opposite side. Warm water irrigation caused the endolymph to rise and elicits a nystagmus to the same side.

Visual fixation may suppress nystagmus elicited by either rotation or caloric stimulation, the latter involving irrigation of the external auditory canal with cold or warm water. (Rotational suppression is dramatically illustrated with figure skaters and dancers.) To prevent visual fixation when testing a patient, his or her eyes should be kept closed or blindfolded during rotation. Alternatively, the patient may be fitted with Frenzel spectacles during caloric testing.

Thought Question

Compare the initial nystagmus observed in a healthy individual who is rotating with the post-rotatory nystagmus, and explain why the directions differ. Now relate these phenomena to the nystagmus that results when the external auditory canal is irrigated with hot or cold water.

Optokinetic Nystagmus

Given that the function of the VOR and labyrinthine (vestibular) nystagmus is to keep images from moving on the retina during head movement, it is not surprising that similar reflexive eye movements can be elicited by moving visual stimuli. A common example of such movements can be observed in the eyes of fellow train passengers as they watch the passing visual scene fly by the window. As regularly spaced telephone poles pass by, the passenger's eyes show a smooth pursuit phase as they track a specific pole toward the rear of the train, and then they snap back in a quick saccadic phase toward the front of the train to fixate on a new pole that is entering the visual field. This pattern of reflexive eye movements is called **optokinetic nystagmus (OKN)**. If the passenger were sitting on the left side of the train, this would be a right-beating horizontal nystagmus. In the clinical setting, horizontal OKN can be elicited by a rotating drum containing vertical stripes or by moving a ribbon with vertical stripes horizontally in front of the subject's eyes.

The smooth pursuit, or slow, phase of OKN is mediated by the ipsilateral parieto-occipital cortex that, via the vestibular nuclei and flocculonodular lobe of the cerebellum, project to the paramedian pontine reticular formation (PPRF), or lateral gaze center. In humans, unilateral lesions of the parietal region result in the slow pursuit phase of OKN being lost or diminished when the moving stimulus is rotated or shifted toward the side of the lesion. Thus, a lesion of the left parietal region results in an inability to track an object moving from right to left. In contrast, rotation of the drum to the side opposite the lesion elicits a normal response. The saccadic, or fast, phase of OKN is mediated by the frontal eye fields that project to the contralateral PPRF. Therefore, lesions involving the frontal cortex or anywhere in the saccadic pathways disrupt the fast phase of OKN. The presence of OKN can be used to determine whether an individual is blind. That is, monocular blindness can be excluded by testing each eye separately to elicit OKN.

Clinical Evaluation

A number of tests are used to assess vestibular function. Examples of commonly used tests include the following:

1. Observation of stance and gait in which the stance may be wide based and the subject may drift to the side of the lesion while walking.
2. Observation for spontaneous nystagmus that, if present, always signifies pathology.
3. Tests for **positional nystagmus**—that is, nystagmus that is present only with particular head positions.
4. Caloric tests of vestibular function in which there is an impairment or loss of thermally induced nystagmus on the involved side.
5. Rotational tests.
6. Tests of optokinetic nystagmus.
7. **Electronystagmography** detects the small voltage that exists between the cornea and retina. This voltage fluctuates with eye movement and is recorded by electrodes applied frontally and temporally. Electromyography has the advantage of permitting the recording of eye movements without being confounding by visual fixation.

Signs and Symptoms

Definitive signs and symptoms of vestibular dysfunction occur when there is an imbalance of activity occurring in the vestibular system of right and left sides. **Vertigo** is the cardinal symptom of irritative or destructive vestibular system lesions. The term *vertigo* is used to designate all subjective and objective illusions of motion or position. Vertigo can be elicited by caloric stimulation. The illusory movement of the environment is in the same direction as nystagmus. For example, cold-water irrigation of the right external auditory meatus produces a left-beating nystagmus, and the environment will appear to move to the left.

Caloric stimulation is used to test for unilateral or bilateral vestibular defects and elicits vertigo and nystagmus and other signs. Acutely, with eyes closed, the person will past-point (point to one side of a fixed visual target) in a direction opposite to the nystagmus. When standing with eyes closed, the individual will fall in a direction opposite to the nystagmus. Past-pointing and falling demonstrate semicircular canal influences on the spinal motor apparatus. Caloric stimulation with warm water mimics unilateral irritative labyrinthine disease because the threshold is increased, while cold-water irrigation mimics unilateral destructive disease because the threshold is inhibited.

Autonomic signs may accompany the vestibular signs and may be evoked, usually in lesser degree, by caloric stimulation. These include nausea, vomiting, pallor, perspiration, blood pressure drop, and tachycardia.

> **Thought Question**
>
> What autonomic signs are commonly associated with vestibular dysfunction, and why do they occur?

Vestibular Disease

Peripheral vestibular disease involves pathology of the labyrinth or vestibular nerve. Possible causes include trauma, BPV, neuritis, Meniere's disease, aminoglycoside (streptomycin, neomycin) toxicity, labyrinthitis, vestibular neuropathy, herpes zoster, and tumors. *Central* vestibular disease involves pathology of the vestibular nuclei, their secondary projections, or central sites of termination. Possible causes include infarcts, tumors, and viral infections.

Peripheral vestibular disease can be differentiated from central disease by a number of signs and symptoms. Peripheral disease tends to be abrupt in onset with symptoms of limited duration. These conditions may become recurrent. The transitory nature of symptoms is attributed to compensation in the function of the vestibular nuclei. Vertigo and nystagmus are common. In central disease, vertigo is commonly mild or may be absent. Accompanying brainstem signs, such as trigeminal or facial nerve dysfunction, are indicative of central disease. Failure of visual fixation to reduce the degree of nystagmus also is indicative of central disease.

Benign Positional Vertigo

Benign positional vertigo (BPV), also known as **benign paroxysmal positional vertigo (BPPV)**, is a common cause of episodic vertigo. BPV most commonly involves the posterior canal, but it can also involve the horizontal canal and, rarely, the anterior canal. This condition is characterized by transient episodes of vertigo lasting from 5 to 30 seconds caused by changes in head position, such as looking up, rolling over in bed, or bending over and straightening up. BPV is caused by otoconia and other cellular debris that have detached from the utricular macula and are displaced into the semicircular canal. Most commonly in BPV, the debris is free-floating (canalithesis), but otoliths can also attach to the cupula (eliciting the cupulolithesis form of BPV). During rapid changes of head position, the free-floating otoconia create convection waves on the endolymph that deflect the cupula of the affected semicircular canal.

Posterior canal BPV can be diagnosed by the **Dix-Hallpike maneuver** (Figure 17-36 ■). While seated in a long sitting posture upon the examination table, the person's head is held in the examiner's hands, turned 30 to 45 degrees to one side, and carried backward off of the end of the table into extension of about 25 to 30 degrees. After a latency of several seconds, the maneuver elicits a characteristic

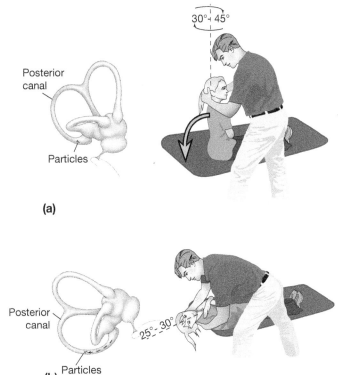

(a)

(b)

FIGURE 17-36 The Dix-Hallpike maneuver is used to detect posterior canal BPV. (a) The person begins in a long sit position with the head held by the examiner. The examiner rotates the head 30 to 45 degrees. (b) The examiner assists the person to lie down, carrying the head into 25 to 30 degrees of extension. This causes otoliths to move within the endolymph, thereby creating waves of the endolymph movement and bending of hair cells stereocilia in the involved canal, which induces vertigo and nystagmus.

vertigo accompanied by a vertical-torsional nystagmus typically lasting less than 15 seconds. This description pertains to canalithesis BPV of the posterior canal, but not the less common cupulolithesis BPV, wherein there is no latency.

It is important to note that the Dix-Hallpike test also detects the rare incidence of anterior canal involvement, with posterior versus anterior canal involvement determined by direction of nystagmus. In addition, another variant of BPV can occur in the horizontal canal, causing horizontal nystagmus. This condition is identified and treated using different positions than for BPV of the posterior canal. Therapy is designed to reposition the displaced otoconia from the canal back into the utricle via a sequence of head movements specific to the canal that is affected.

Thought Question

Contrast the movements that would produce vertigo in posterior versus horizontal canal BPV.

Vestibular Neuritis

Vestibular neuritis is a unilateral vestibular disorder that manifests as a sudden partial labyrinthine failure on one side. This disorder occurs because of inflammation of the vestibular nerve. It is important to recognize that this disorder involves only the vestibular nerve (not the labyrinth) and does not involve the auditory nerve.

On examination, the individual has a diminished or absent response to caloric stimulation of the horizontal semicircular canal on one side. There are profound disturbances of motion and body perception as well as a false sense of rotation. The individual may experience nausea and vomiting. Symptoms result in an abnormal weight shift toward the side of the lesion. The continuous severe vertigo and other symptoms diminish and disappear within a matter of several days. The specific cause of vestibular neuritis is unknown, but it may be the result of a viral infection affecting the vestibular nerve after it exits the labyrinth.

Vestibular neuritis illustrates an important aspect of the vestibular system—namely, its exquisite ability for adaptation through central changes. If the central nervous system is otherwise intact, and if the individual remains active (stimulating vestibular neurons to fire), adaptation can occur within days to weeks. The clinician helps the individual to resume activities that activate the vestibular system. If the person does not resume activities that require the vestibular system to fire, the functioning visual somatosensory system will compensate to some degree; he or she may still be dizzy and often is less mobile and less functional than previously. Forcing the vestibular system to work allows for a recalibration, based on the remaining pathways.

Meniere's Disease

Meniere's disease is a syndrome in which both auditory and vestibular functions are disturbed. Symptoms are episodic and vary considerably in frequency and severity, lasting several minutes to as much as 24 hours and recurring several times weekly for sometimes months on end. There may be remissions that last more than a year or two or even longer. Attacks of vertigo are abrupt and may be so severe the individual cannot stand, walk, or drive. The hallmark symptoms include sensorineural hearing loss, tinnitus, aural fullness, nausea, and vomiting that lasts up to 24 hours. Nystagmus also is present. The presence of both auditory and vestibular dysfunction is explained by the continuity of the cochlear duct and membranous vestibular labyrinth via the ductus reuniens. Inadequate drainage of endolymph through the endolymphatic duct and sac leads to distention of the endolymphatic system (endolymphatic hydrops) that causes the delicate cochlear hair cells to degenerate and ruptures the membranous labyrinth. Rupturing of the membranous labyrinth causes a disruption of vestibular receptors and liberates potassium-containing endolymph into the perilymph. This influx hyperpolarizes vestibular afferents.

Thought Question

Which signs and symptoms occur with disorders such as Meniere's disease and vestibular neuritis that are unlikely to occur with central disorders of the vestibular system?

Other Causes of Vertigo and Nystagmus

Cerebellar lesions may produce vertigo and nystagmus directly. Furthermore, the proximity of the cerebellum to the brainstem means that cerebellar lesions may affect the vestibular nuclei directly by pressure or secondarily by vascular disorders. Involvement of the upper cervical dorsal roots or the muscles and ligaments they innervate may produce signs of vestibular dysfunction (cervicogenic vertigo). Irritation of upper cervical dorsal roots may evoke nystagmus, vertigo, and disequilibrium. However, drug intoxication is the most frequent cause of induced nystagmus. Alcohol, barbiturates (as well as other sedative-hypnotic drugs), and phenytoin are typical offenders.

Summary

This chapter began with a discussion of the general structural features of the inner ear and its receptors that are common to both the cochlear and vestibular divisions of cranial nerve VIII. Despite the fact that both divisions receive information from hair cell mechanoreceptors, the receptors are embedded in dramatically different peripheral environments that account for the fact that hair cells of the auditory system respond to sound, while those of the vestibular division respond to gravitational forces and head movement. Sensory transduction is accomplished by a bending of the hair cell's stereocilia.

Airborne sound waves are gathered by the external ear and transferred to the fluid-filled inner ear via the middle ear, whose structures provide an impedance match between vibrations in air and those in perilymph. Hair cells of the organ of Corti are arrayed in a single inner row and multiple outer rows with more than four times as many receptors in the latter. Despite this numerical difference, auditory sensations are mediated by the relatively few inner hair cells, with the outer hair cells serving as an amplifier of inner hair cell transduction. Beyond the level of the cochlear nuclei, where primary auditory afferents synapse, the auditory system projections are bilateral—although with a more robust representation from the contralateral side. This means that damage to central auditory pathways

results in a diminution of hearing in both ears, although the deficit is greater in the contralateral ear.

The second major section of this chapter focused on the vestibular system. Hair cells belonging to the vestibular system reside in environments equipping them to respond either to static gravitational forces and linear acceleration (utricle and saccule) or to angular acceleration (semicircular canals). Essential to understanding the transduction process is the concept of inertia, applicable to both the otoliths and endolymph of the peripheral vestibular organs. The central vestibular system is unique because not only is it the most fundamental sensory system in the brain, it also is a vital UMN system. It is a bilaterally acting system with both sensory and motor capacities, but its operations are conducted largely out of the realm of consciousness, except under pathological or unusual stimulatory conditions. It also is the most integrative sensory system in the neuraxis because perceptions of posture, movement, and equilibrium, as well as their regulation, depend not only on vestibular input, but on visual and somatosensory as well.

For both audition and the vestibular system, we discussed important reflexes and their pathways. We then considered evaluation of conditions associated with disorders of the systems.

Applications

1. Practice clinical evaluation of hearing by administering the Rinne and Weber tests. You will need tuning forks for this activity. Identify what each test determines.

2. Kaitlin was a high school freshman who had bacterial meningitis that was treated with IV gentamicin. She went back to school but experienced difficulty.

She complained of headaches, dizziness and imbalance, and fatigue that increased in severity as the day progressed. She now walked up and down stairs by holding onto the handrail. She was also having difficulty hearing in crowded noisy places, such as the cafeteria or mall.

a. What neuroanatomical structures are affected by bacterial meningitis?

b. The administration of gentamicin is related to Kaitlin's symptoms. Identify the neuroanatomical structures affected by gentamicin. Explain how a lesion of these neuroanatomical structures relates to her symptoms.

c. Given what you know, what is the prognosis for these structures to heal?

d. Do you think Kaitlin can benefit from physical therapy? Explain your answer.

References

Auditory System

Baloh, R.W. Superior semicircular canal dehiscence syndrome. *Neurology* 62:684–685, 2004.

Hudspeth, A. J. Ch. 30 Hearing. In: Kandel, E. R., Schwartz, J. H., and Jessell, T. M., eds. *Principles of Neural Science*, 4th ed. McGraw-Hill, New York, 2000.

Hudspeth, A. J. Ch. 31 Sensory transduction in the ear. In: Kandel, E. R., Schwartz, J. H., and Jessell, T. M., eds. *Principles of Neural Science*, 4th ed. McGraw-Hill, New York, 2000.

Vestibular System

Agrup, C., Gleeson, M., and Rudge, P. The inner ear and the neurologist. *J Neurol Neurosurg Psychiatry* 78:114–122, 2007.

Angelaki, D. E. The physiology of the peripheral vestibular system: The birth of a field. *J Nueophysiol* 93:3032–3033, 2005.

Baloh, R. W., Yee, R. D., Kimm, J., and Honrubia, V. Vestobulo-ocular reflex in patients with lesions involving the vestibulocerebellum. *Exp Neurol* 72:141–152, 1981.

Bense, S., Bartenstein, P., Lochmann, M., et al. Metabolic changes in vestibular and visual cortices in acute vestibular neuritis. *Ann Neurol* 56:624–630, 2004.

Brandt, T., Dieterich, M., and Danek, A. Vestbular cortex lesions affect the perception of verticality. *Ann Neurol* 35:403–412, 1994.

Brandt, T., Bartenstein, P., Janck, A., and Dieterich, M. Reciprocal inhibitory visual-vestibular interaction. Visual motion stimulation deactivates the parieto-insular vestibular cortex. *Brain* 121:1749–1758, 1998.

Brandt, T., Schautzer, F., Hamilton, A., et al. Vestibular loss causes hippocampal atrophy and impaired spatial memory in humans. *Brain* 128:2732–2741, 2005.

Dieterich, M., Bartenstein, P., Spiegel, S., et al. Thalamic infarctions cause side-specific suppression of vestibular cortex activations. *Brain* 128:2052–2067, 2005.

Dieterich, M., Bense, S., Lutz, S., et al. Dominance for vestibular cortical function in the non-dominant hemisphere. *Cereb Cortex* 13:994–1007, 2003.

Furman, J. M., and Hain, T. C. "Do try this at home." Self-treatment of BPPV. *Neurology* 63:8–9, 2004.

Goldberg, M. E., and Hudspeth, A. J. Ch. 40 The vestibular system. In: Kandel, E. R., Schwartz, J. H., and Jessell, T. M., eds. *Principles of Neural Science*, 4th ed. McGraw-Hill, New York, 2000.

Imai, T., Ito, M., Takeda, N., et al. Natural course of the remission of vertigo in patients with benign paroxysmal positional vertigo. *Neurology* 64:920–921, 2005.

Jones, G. M. Ch. 41 Posture. In: Kandel, E. R., Schwartz, J. H., and Jessell, T. M., eds. *Principles of Neural Science*, 4th ed. McGraw-Hill, New York, 2000.

Nolte, J. *The Human Brain: An Introduction to Its Functional Anatomy*. Mosby Elsevier, Philadelphia, 2009.

Zhou, W., Tang, B. F., Newlands, S, D., and King, W. M. Responses of monkey vestibular-only neurons to translation and angular rotation. *J Neurophysiol* 96:2915–2930, 2006.

PEARSON **myhealthprofessionskit**

Use this address to access the Companion Website created for this textbook. Simply select "Physical Therapy" from the choice of disciplines. Find this book and log in using your username and password to access self-assessment questions, a glossary, and more.

18

Visual System

LEARNING OUTCOMES

This chapter prepares the reader to:

1. Recall the meaning of the following terms related to the transduction and transmission of light: rods, cones, optic disk, and rhodopsin.

2. Compare and contrast the role of rods and cones in transduction of light and the mechanism by which this occurs.

3. Differentiate the role of the scotopic and photopic systems and identify the type of receptor used in each system.

4. Discuss the functional consequences of normal aging of the eye and macular degeneration and relate the symptoms to the specific physiologic changes.

5. Discuss the role of each of the following in the transmission, perception, and interpretation of light: the optic nerve, optic tract, optic chiasm, lateral geniculate body, optic radiation, and Brodmann's areas 17, 18, and 19.

6. Describe how input from the left and right eyes is organized within the optic nerve, optic tract, and lateral geniculate body.

7. Analyze why lesions in the visual system, beyond the optic nerve, result in a visual field loss as opposed to loss of vision of an eye.

8. Explain hemianopsia in terms of the pathways involved and the visual field(s) affected and differentiate bitemporal from homonymous hemianopsia.

9. Contrast the projections from the superior colliculi that travel caudally to the spinal cord with those that travel rostrally to the thalamus, both in terms of anatomy and function.

10. Compare the visual loss associated with a lesion in Meyer's loop with the loss associated with a lesion in the optic radiation.

11. Contrast the functions of the on-center and off-center ganglion cells in the retina.

12. Compare the function of orientation columns, ocular dominance columns, and blobs.

13. Explain the clinical significance of each of the following: papilledema, scotoma, macular degeneration, hemianopsia, and cortical blindness.

14. Compare the pathways affected in bitemporal hemianopsia, homonymous hemianopsia, and heteronymous hemianopsia and describe the consequences of each.

15. Identify the specific lesions that lead to prosopagnosia and visual anosognosia.

16. Contrast the role of blobs, interblobs, and cortical columns in extraction of information about visual patterns, location of objects, and stereopsis.

17. Analyze the functional relevance of the projection of information from M- and P-ganglion cells of the retina to the magnocellular and parvocellular layers of the LGB to specific cortical regions.

18. Contrast the cortical and subcortical areas associated with the pupillary, fixation, and accommodation–convergence reaction reflexes.

19. Contrast the functional consequences of damage from the periphery to the midbrain to the visual cortices.

ACRONYMS

AMD Age-related macular degeneration
cGMP Cyclic GMP
CNS Central nervous system
CSF Cerebrospinal fluid
ICP Intracranial pressure
LGB Lateral geniculate body
MGB Medial geniculate body
MS Multiple sclerosis
RPE Retinal pigment epithelial cells
VOR Vestibulo-ocular reflex

Introduction

Vision is by far our dominant sense: about 70 percent of the receptors of the entire body are retinal photoreceptors; the massive optic nerves represent about one-third of all afferent fibers carrying information to the CNS. The physical stimulus for vision is light, the band of electromagnetic radiation with wavelengths between 400 and 700 nm. However, this represents only about 1/70 of the entire electromagnetic spectrum, so there is much that humans are incapable of seeing. The visual system is remarkable for the enormous range of light intensity over which it operates: the most intense light that can be viewed without damage to the eyes is 10^{13} times more intense than the dimmest visible light. This is possible because of adaptation, which is the capacity of the neural structures of the retina to adjust their operating levels to match ambient illumination.

The function of the visual system is to generate visual perceptions out of visual inputs. That is, what arrives at the retina is a two-dimensional pattern of light and dark, and the visual system converts this rather meager input into a three-dimensional visual world filled with recognizable objects performing familiar functions. Visual perception is used both to interpret the external environment and as one of the three critical components to postural control.

The visual system consists of interconnected neuronal networks at the retina, thalamus, and visual cortex by which attributes of the external world that emit or are illuminated by light waves are processed and apprehended. A unified visual image results from hierarchical neural processing occurring simultaneously in multiple distinct, but parallel, visual pathways. Because the retina is an outgrowth of the embryonic prosencephalon, it is part of the CNS. Accordingly, considerable information processing occurs within retinal neurons themselves.

Damage to the visual system can occur anywhere along this neural network, with very different consequences, depending on the location of the injury. When damage results in blindness, the person does not experience blackness, but simply nothing. Large regions of the retina can be damaged and go unnoticed. It may only be by clinical testing, or by accidents such as bumping into unseen objects, that an individual is made aware of the absence of sight.

This chapter follows the organization of previous chapters on sensory systems. Thus, the first section considers the sensory end organs in the retina: the rods and cones. The second major section presents projections of the visual system. Here, we trace the system's synaptology as it projects to the cerebral cortex via the geniculocalcarine tract as well as its projections to subcortical structures. The third and final section summarizes some of the mechanisms by which visual information is segregated and processed for purposes of function. In studying this section, it is important to recognize that a number of details are known regarding the manner in which visual information is processed to develop a functional appreciation of the visual world. However, much is yet to be learned before we will fully understand how the eye and brain work together to allow for the rich perceptions available to us. This section ends with a discussion of clinical connections, including assessment, visual field defects that result from damage to different parts of the system, and disorders of the visual system. The visual system, like the vestibular system, is among the most plastic of all sensory systems in the brain. Its mature functional characteristics determined by early visual experience that must occur during a certain critical period in development. Visual system plasticity is discussed in greater detail in Chapter 25.

Clinical Preview

In your clinical practice, you treat many older adults who have a variety of visual disorders. Some of these common disorders affect the visual system at the level of the sensory end organ (e.g., the retina, lens). Among the conditions that these older adults have are the following: macular degeneration, loss of visual acuity, and presbyopia. As you read through the first section, consider the following:

- What is the cause of these conditions?
- What is the likelihood that each condition will improve or worsen?
- How might these conditions affect postural control and other aspects of function?

SENSORY END ORGANS AND PRIMARY AFFERENTS

The Retina

Cell Types and Connections

The fact that the retina is part of the CNS is reflected in its complexly organized, multilayered arrangement of specialized cell types distributed in 10 histologically distinct layers. Seven major classes of cells reside in discrete layers of the retina (Figure 18-1 ■). **Rods** and **cones**, populating the deepest layer known as the photoreceptor layer, are the actual photoreceptors. Rods and cones synapse with bipolar cells. **Bipolar cells**, whose cell bodies are distributed in an intermediate layer known as the inner nuclear layer, are information-integrating neurons that, in turn, synapse with ganglion cells. **Ganglion cells**

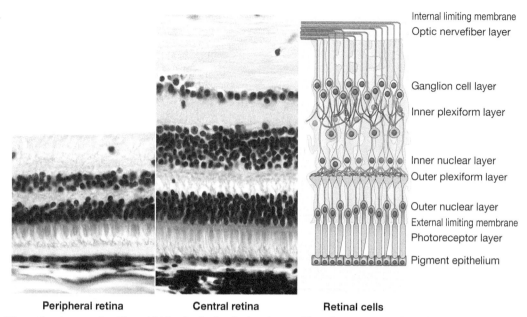

Internal limiting membrane
Optic nervefiber layer
Ganglion cell layer
Inner plexiform layer
Inner nuclear layer
Outer plexiform layer
Outer nuclear layer
External limiting membrane
Photoreceptor layer
Pigment epithelium

Peripheral retina   **Central retina**   **Retinal cells**

FIGURE 18-1 The retina is organized into 10 histologically distinct layers. The photoreceptor layer is comprised of rods and cones.

Source: Image copyright 2008 by David G. King, used with permission.

reside in the most superficial cell layer of the retina (closest to the lens) known as the ganglion cell layer. Ganglion cells are information-integrating neurons and have axons that exit the eyeball as the **optic nerve**; these are the output neurons of the retina. In addition to bipolar cells, the inner nuclear layer contains two other types of interneurons called **horizontal** and **amacrine cells**. The cell bodies of horizontal cells reside near the outer edge of the layer, while those of amacrine cells are found near the inner edge. Photoreceptors thus synapse not only with bipolar cells, but also with horizontal cells, and bipolar cells synapse not only with ganglion cells, but also with amacrine cells.

The rods and cones are at the back of the retina, adjacent to a light-absorbing, pigmented epithelium that prevents light reflection from the back of the retina. Light must pass through the other retinal layers, which are transparent, to reach the rods and cones. The rods and cones give the retina dual functions: the **scotopic**, or rod, system works at low levels of illumination (is very sensitive to light), is insensitive to color, and has limited resolution; the **photopic**, or cone, system works at high levels of illumination, is responsible for color vision, and handles sharp vision (visual acuity). Each eye has 80 to 110 million rods and 4 to 5 million cones.

Rods and cones are positioned in the posterior portion of the eyeball, where light can be focused on them. The distribution of rods and cones varies across the retina. Cones are concentrated in the center of the retina directly behind the lens, in line with the optical axis of the eye. They are densest in the **macula lutea** (L., yellow spot). The **fovea centralis** (L., small pit), within the macula, is a small, depressed region containing only cones (199,000 to 300,000 per square millimeter) and has been referred to as the "valley of keenest vision" (Figure 18-2 ■). This depression is formed because bipolar and ganglion retinal cells are displaced laterally, leaving only cone photoreceptors in the center. There is a capillary-free zone in the center of the fovea such that light passes unobstructed to the cones. Rods, and some cones, are distributed in the remainder of the retina, called the peripheral retina.

Both rods and cones have four major functional regions (Figure 18-3 ■). From the outer surface of the retina toward its interior, these regions are an outer segment, an inner segment, a nucleus, and a synaptic terminal that makes contact with the receptor's target cells within the retina. In the case of rods, the synaptic terminal is called a **spherule**, whereas in cones, the terminal is called a **pedicle**. Both spherules and the larger pedicles contain invaginations into which processes of bipolar and horizontal cells penetrate. Rod spherules contain only one invagination, whereas cone pedicles have multiple (12 to 25) invaginations.

A specific type of synapse occurs within these invaginations and is termed a triad. Triad synapses reflect the complexity of information processing that occurs within the retina. Each triad consists of the dendrite of a single

Thought Question

Based on the anatomy of the retina, what would be the consequences of degeneration of the macula?

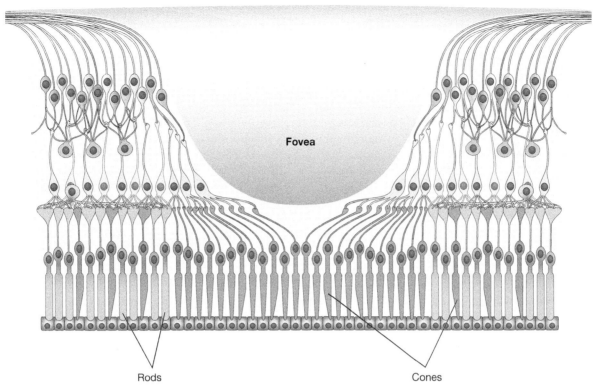

Fovea

Rods

Cones

FIGURE 18-2 The photoreceptor layer in the peripheral retina has a high density of rods. The photoreceptor layer in the central retina has a high density of cones. The fovea is a small, depressed region centrally located in the retina, which contains only cones. As illustrated here, vision is most acute in the foveal region.

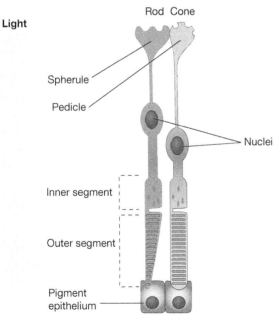

Light

Rod Cone

Spherule

Pedicle

Nuclei

Inner segment

Outer segment

Pigment
epithelium

FIGURE 18-3 Rods and cones have four major functional regions: an outer segment, inner segment, a nucleus, and a synaptic terminal. The synaptic terminal of a rod is called a spherule, while the synaptic terminal of a cone is called a pedicle.

bipolar cell flanked on either side by a process originating in two different horizontal cells. Triads are not the only types of synapses that occur between bipolar and photoreceptor cells.

Thought Question

Which cells and synapses are important for conveying light through the retina, and which are important in modulating the activity of neurons that convey visual information?

Synapses in the retina occur in vertical and horizontal arrays. The vertical array is from photoreceptor to bipolar cells to ganglion cells, and this three-step pathway carries the neural signal through the retina. The horizontal array is represented by the synapses established by horizontal and amacrine cells. Horizontal cells and amacrine cells are interneurons that mediate lateral interactions in the retina that modify the signal traversing the retina and integrate retinal function. Horizontal cells mediate lateral interactions between receptor cells and bipolar neurons. Amacrine cells mediate lateral interactions between bipolar and ganglion neurons.

Given the differential distribution of rods and cones in the central versus peripheral parts of the retina, it is to be expected that the synaptic connections between the photoreceptors and bipolar cells vary in different parts of the retina. The dendrites of a single-rod, bipolar cell form triad synapses with 15 to 20 different rods in the central retina but with up to 80 rods in the peripheral retina. In the central retina, each cone is innervated by only one invaginating bipolar cell, called an invaginating midget bipolar cell.

However, in the peripheral retina, several different cone pedicles are contacted by one midget bipolar cell.

Sensory Transduction in Rods and Cones

The process of transduction from light waves to electrochemical signals used by neurons occurs in the rods and cones. The photoreceptor *outer segment* is specialized for phototransduction. The outer segment of both rods and cones is filled with hundreds (600 to 1,000 per rod) of membranous sacs, called **disks**, arranged like a stack of dimes in a bank wrapper. The disks develop as invaginations of the plasma membrane. Those in rods pinch off from the membrane and are entirely intracellular, or free floating, whereas in cones, the disks do not pinch off so that their interiors remain continuous with the extracellular space. The outer segment membranes of rods and cones are filled with visual pigment protein. All rods contain the same protein, called **rhodopsin**. But three different types of cones exist, each with a unique type of visual pigment that preferentially captures photons from different components of the light spectrum and does not bear a universally accepted specific name. Thus, they often are referred to simply as *cone pigments*.

The inner segment contains abundant mitochondria in addition to other organelles such as endoplasmic reticulum and Golgi complexes. The mitochondria fuel the process of sensory transduction, as well as supply the energy required for the synthesis of visual pigment that occurs in the inner segment. Visual pigment is synthesized continuously, transported to the outer segment, and incorporated into disk membranes. Disks are continuously renewed. Old disks at the tips of the photoreceptors are removed by the phagocytotic activity of pigment epithelial cells.

The first step in transduction is the bleaching of visual pigment. Bleaching is caused by the photopigment's absorption of packets of light energy called *photons*. Different photopigments absorb photons of different wavelengths.

Because rods all contain rhodopsin, the visual pigment undergoes the same configurational change no matter what the wavelength of the stimulating light captured by a rod. Thus, rods are incapable of responding differently to different wavelengths and, therefore, cannot signal color.

Rods signal the event of photon capture and are capable of distinguishing brightness differences.

As noted, the three different types of cones each contain a unique visual pigment. One pigment is sensitive primarily to short wavelengths and contributes mainly to the perception of blue. A second pigment is sensitive to wavelengths in the middle range and contributes largely to the perception of green. A third pigment is sensitive to longer wavelengths and contributes strongly to the perception of red. Color is determined by the particular combination of different levels of excitation in each cone type and is virtually unlimited in tonal possibilities. The final perceived color of an object is determined in relation to the background against which the object is viewed.

> **Thought Question**
>
> People are able to see in dim and bright light and to differentiate many colors from each other. How does the structure of the visual system confer these abilities?

The events of transduction are similar in rods and cones and involve a G-protein-coupled, second-messenger system. Recall from Chapter 4 that in G-protein-coupled receptors, the binding of the neurotransmitter to the receptor activates G-proteins in the membrane, which in turn stimulates effector enzymes. The effector enzymes alter the intracellular concentration of cytoplasmic, second-messenger molecules that change the conductance of membrane ion channels, thus altering membrane potential. The unique aspect of transduction in photoreceptors is that photon capture by visual pigment leads to a membrane *hyperpolarization* rather than depolarization. In the dark, receptors are maintained in a depolarized state and the transmitter is continuously released from vesicles at the photoreceptor's basal surface. However, when stimulated by light, the membrane is hyperpolarized, and the amount of transmitter released from the receptor decreases. This response is graded, meaning that the more photons that are captured, the greater is the hyperpolarization of the photoreceptors, which in turn means that the decrease in release of neurotransmitter is greater.

Neurophysiology Box 18-1: Transduction in Photoreceptors

The depolarized state of photoreceptors in the dark is caused by a steady influx of Na^+ through channels in the outer segment membrane that are gated by an intracellular second messenger called *cyclic guanosine monophosphate*, or *cGMP*, that is continuously produced in the photoreceptor. High levels of cGMP in the dark keep the Na^+ channels open (Figure 18-4 ■).

When a photon of light is absorbed by a visual pigment, its protein component (called an *opsin*) rapidly changes its configuration. The altered opsin then activates an intracellular G-protein called *transducin*. The activated transducin, in turn, activates a *phosphodiesterase*, an enzyme that hydrolyzes cGMP. The breakdown of cGMP decreases its intracellular levels, causing the Na^+ channels to close and the outer segment membrane to hyperpolarize. The result is a decrease in the release of neurotransmitter from the photoreceptor. This process occurs at an incredibly fast speed, with the conformational changes occurring within picoseconds.

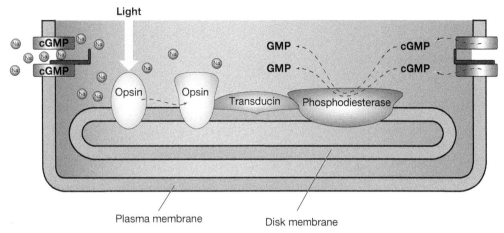

FIGURE 18-4 Sequence of events from the effect of light on configuration of opsin to activation of phosphodiesterase, which breaks down cGMP. The result is hyperpolarization of the outer segment membrane and decrease of neurotransmitter.

Ganglion Cells

The ganglion cell layer is much thinner than the layers containing photoreceptors and bipolar neurons. These neurons reside within the retina, and their axons form the optic nerve (discussed later). There are only about 1 million ganglion cells in comparison to about 100 million rods and 4 to 5 million cones. Retinal processing thus involves massive convergence onto ganglion cells. Significantly, the degree of convergence is not uniform across the retina. Regions specialized for high acuity (cones in the fovea centralis) have little convergence. In contrast, regions specialized for high sensitivity (rods in the peripheral retina) have a great deal of convergence.

Two types of ganglion cells are found in the retina: large cells called **type M** and small cells called **type P**. This classification is based on size. Additionally the cell's axon terminates in different layers of the lateral geniculate body. The small type P ganglion cells are the most common and have small dendritic fields and correspondingly small receptive fields. In this regard, the receptive field of ganglion neurons in the retina refers to that portion of the retina that alters its firing rate in response to a particular stimulus. They distinguish between the signals received from the three different types of cone photoreceptors and, therefore, signal information about color. Type P ganglion cells project to the **parvocellular layers of the lateral geniculate body (LGB)** of the thalamus (layers 3 through 6) (Figure 18-5 ■). The large type M ganglion cells have large dendritic fields and large receptive fields; they do not distinguish between the signals arriving from the three different types of cone cells but simply add them. Therefore, they are not concerned with color. These neurons provide information concerning patterns, are very sensitive to small contrasts in illumination, and are able to follow rapid changes in the stimulus. They appear to be involved with the analysis of the gross features of a stimulus and its movement. M ganglion cells project to the **magnocellular layers of the LGB** (layers 1 and 2). The M (magnocellular) and P (parvocellular) terminology is important because it is used to distinguish those components of the visual system that mediate different aspects of visual

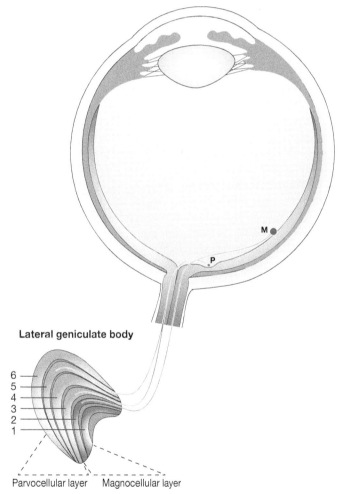

FIGURE 18-5 Type M and type P ganglion cells project from the retina to specific layers of the lateral geniculate body (LGB). Type M ganglion cells project to the magnocellular layers of the LGB (layers 1 and 2) and are concerned with patterns and contrasts. Type P ganglion cells project to the parvocellular layers of the LGB (layers 3 through 6) and are concerned with color transmission. Shown here are projections from the ipsilateral eye, which terminate in layers 2, 3, and 5. Layers 1, 4, and 6 receive input from the contralateral eye, not shown here.

perception. As will be discussed in detail later, the distinction between M and P ganglion cells is of critical importance because of their roles in separate parallel pathways that convey very different information to the visual cortex.

> ### Thought Question
>
> What is the difference between the type P and type M cells of the retina, and what is the functional relevance of this difference?

Three classes of interneurons reside between the photoreceptors and ganglion cells: bipolar, horizontal, and amacrine cells. These interneurons combine signals from multiple photoreceptors such that each ganglion cell monitors an area of the retina consisting of a circumscribed group of neighboring photoreceptors. This group makes up the receptive field for that ganglion cell. Thus, the electrical responses occurring in ganglion cells depend critically on the precise spatial and temporal patterns of light falling on the retina. It should be noted that only ganglion cells fire action potentials. All other cells in the retina respond to stimulation with graded changes in their membrane potentials.

The same *population* of ganglion cells signals the entire range of light intensities from scotopic threshold to bright sunlight and color. The most direct route for information flow across the retina is from a photoreceptor to bipolar cell to ganglion cell. At each of these synaptic relays, responses are modified by the lateral interactions of horizontal and amacrine interneurons. At photopic levels of illumination, this direct route originates in cone photoreceptors, but at scotopic levels of illumination (e.g., starlight, mediated by rods only), the neural signal originates in rod photoreceptors that reach a special population of bipolar cells dedicated just to rod function. Rod bipolar axons are large and unbranched and rarely synapse directly with ganglion cells, but instead synapse with amacrine cell processes that then signal ganglion cells. At levels of illumination mediated by both rods and cones (e.g., moonlight), receptor currents flow directly from rod terminals into the synaptic terminals of cones via the opening of modulated gap junctions. Thus, rod and cone photoreceptors share some of the same retinal circuitry, and one set of ganglion cells is able to carry information from either rod or cone pathways.

Optic Disk and the Blind Spot

The optic papilla, or optic disk, is a circular, elevated region where ganglion cell axons gather to leave the eye as the stout optic nerve. It is devoid of rods and cones and represents the **blind spot** in the visual field. Figure 18-6 ■ can be used to demonstrate your right eye's blind spot to yourself.

> ### Thought Question
>
> What is the physiological basis for the blind spot?

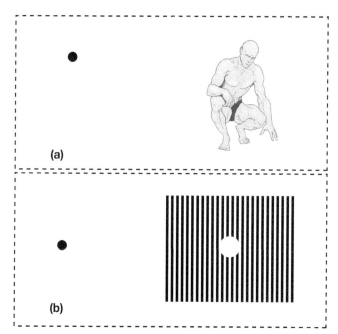

FIGURE 18-6 Demonstration of the blind spot in the visual field. (a) With your left eye closed, hold this image at arm's length. Focus on the spot to the left side of the figure. Slowly move the image toward you. At some point, the man's head will disappear. (b) With your left eye closed, hold this image at arm's length. Focus on the spot at the left side of the figure. Slowly move the image toward you. At some point, when the hole in the striped pattern falls on your blind spot, your brain will see the stripes fill in where none exist.

Blood Supply

The neural retina receives its blood supply from two sources. The outer retinal layers receive nutrients by diffusion from the choroidal capillary bed. Inner retinal layers are nourished by the **central retinal artery**, a branch of the **ophthalmic artery** (the latter being the first branch given off by the internal carotid artery). The central retinal artery runs forward in the optic nerve and enters the retina through the optic disc.

CLINICAL CONNECTIONS
Aging in the Eye

A number of age-related changes occur in the eye, not all of which adversely affect visual function in ways that can be documented clinically. One change that does affect vision is **presbyopia**, which is a loss of the power of accommodation. In presbyopia, the lens becomes progressively harder and less elastic with advancing age. Thus, this condition results in impairment of the ability to focus on near objects due to a compromise of accommodation. While a variety of factors may play a role, an established one involves the lens. There is a loss of elasticity in the lens capsule, and the fibers of the lens become more resistant to deformity with advancing age. Thus, the increase in the curvature of the lens required for near vision when the ciliary muscle contracts is insufficient to maintain focus.

A second condition, **age-related macular degeneration (AMD)**, increases in prevalence after the sixth decade of life and involves a degenerative process occurring at the retina-choroid interface in the area of the macula. AMD is the leading cause of legal blindness among elderly Caucasians in the Western world, but it is comparatively rare in other races. Advanced AMD affects more than 1.75 million individuals in the United States. Because of the demographic trend toward increased numbers of elderly in the population, the number of persons with advanced AMD in the United States is expected to approach 3 million by 2020. This is a bilateral disease, although its manifestations may be asymmetric. The average age of visual loss in the first eye is 65 years, with both eyes being involved at the age of 70. Peripheral vision is unaffected such that the person can still lead an independent life, especially if provided with appropriate low-vision aids and training.

> **Thought Question**
>
> A major problem among older individuals is that of macular degeneration. What might be the functional consequence of this disorder?

Two types of AMD are recognized: dry, or nonexudative, and wet, or exudative (also called neovascular). Dry AMD is the most common type. It typically causes a gradual mild to moderate impairment of vision over several months or years. Slow and progressive atrophy of the retinal pigment epithelium (RPE) and photoreceptors predominates. Wet AMD is more severe. Its effects on vision may be devastating, with a loss of all central vision in a matter of days. Two features characterize wet AMD: detachment of the RPE and subretinal neovascularization. Neovascular membranes grow out from the choriocapillaris. The stimulus for this proliferation apparently is the release of vascular endothelial growth factor as a response to local cellular hypoxia due to the changes in Bruch's membrane (which is the innermost layer of the choroid). The vessels grow through defects in Bruch's membrane to invade the subpigment epithelial space and then the subretinal space. Like neovascular tissue elsewhere, Bruch's membranes leak and bleed, resulting in subretinal exudates and fibrosis as the extravasated blood organizes. Invasion of the subpigment epithelial space causes hemorrhagic detachment of the RPE. Within a week or two, the leaky vessels enter the subretinal space, and extravasated blood leads to detachment of the neurosensory retina.

No surgical or any other definitive treatment for AMD exists. Those treatment options that are available are limited, invasive, and expensive. FDA-approved medications currently involve injections of agents designed to arrest the abnormal growth of neovascular membranes into the vitreous chamber of the eyeball. Some clinicians believe that dietary supplementation with antioxidants and minerals slows progression of mild AMD.

> **Thought Question**
>
> Both normal and pathological processes can alter visual capabilities. Consider how visual deficits may be addressed in rehabilitation.

Implications for Rehabilitation

Loss of visual acuity, presbyopia, and macular degeneration can have profound implications for the ability of an individual to function. As discussed in Chapter 17, the visual system is one of three key contributors to postural control. Thus, people with diminished visual acuity may need to rely more heavily on the other two systems: proprioceptive and vestibular. However, often the capacity of all three systems gradually diminish as a person ages. Hence, relatively small losses of capacity in each system can have a cumulative impact on postural control that are way beyond the contributions of any one system alone.

When working with an individual who falls—and who has a history of postural instability—it is important to test for visual acuity to determine the extent to which impairments in this system contribute to the problem and to assist the person to compensate appropriately for losses. As an example, the clinician can guide a person to use simple strategies, such as turning on a bedside light when getting up at night, which can be instrumental in preventing falls and potential fractures. Furthermore, enhancement of visual ability can help to compensate for impairments of the proprioceptive and vestibular systems.

PROJECTIONS
Overview of Terminology

To understand projections of the visual system, it is first helpful to understand some of the relevant terminology and concepts. First, to understand how visual images are perceived by the nervous system, it is important to differentiate between the receptive fields of the retina and the visual fields. The **receptive field** of the retina refers to that portion of the retina that alters its firing rate in response to a particular stimulus. In contrast, the **visual field** is defined as that portion of space that can be viewed by the retina when the eye is fixated straight ahead. These images are projected in a reverse and inverted relationship onto the retina. For example, the temporal visual field is projected to the nasal retinal field. The superior visual field is projected to the inferior retinal field. Understanding this relationship is paramount to understanding visual field deficits and is further discussed in the next section.

Next, in order to describe the visual fields, each retina (and macula) is conceptually divided into a temporal and nasal half (hemiretina) by a vertical line running through the fovea centralis (Figure 18-7 ■). Each hemiretina is also divided into upper and lower quadrants by a horizontal line passing through the fovea.

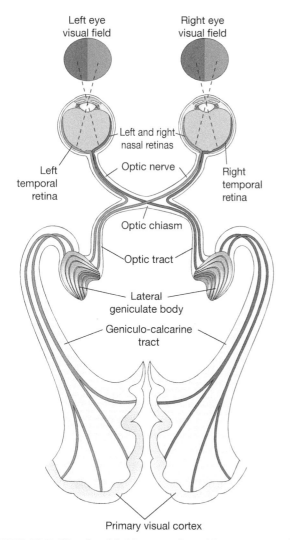

FIGURE 18-7 The visual fields are projected in a reverse and inverted relationship onto the retina. Projections from the retina form the optic nerve. There is a partial decussation at the optic chiasm; the projections from the nasal retinas decussate, while the projections for the temporal retinas remain ipsilateral. After the optic chiasm, these mixed fibers from the optic tract project to the lateral geniculate bodies of the thalamus. From there, third-order neurons project to the visual cortex.

Thought Question

What is the origin of the image processed by the right superior visual portion of the retina? What about images seen in the right superior visual field of each eye? Shortly, you will learn about visual field defects. As you proceed through the content, consider how a visual field defect relates to the visual field of each eye.

The third important concept is that the projection of visual information from the retina to the primary visual cortex (Brodmann's area 17) involves a significant remixing of retinal fibers from the two eyes. Because of its clinical importance in interpreting the location of damage within the projection from each eye, we shall discuss this

remixing before discussing the second- and third-order neurons of the cortical projection pathway. The visual field of each eye is divided into left and right halves, and each half is divided into superior and inferior quadrants. Figure 18-7 depicts the left and right visual fields of each eye and their projections onto the retina. Note that posterior to the optic chiasm, each optic tract contains information from the contralateral half of the visual field and that this laterality is preserved all the way to the cerebral cortex. Thus, the primary visual cortex in one hemisphere contains the representation of the contralateral half of the visual field.

Visual defects are always named according to the visual field loss and not according to the area of the retina that is damaged. Recall, the visual field is the area of physical space visible to an eye. The lens of each eye reverses and inverts all images in the visual field such that the retinal image is reversed and inverted. Thus, damage to temporal areas of the retina cause nasal visual field losses, and damage to nasal areas of the retina cause temporal visual field losses. Similarly, damage to inferior areas of the retina cause superior visual field losses, and damage to superior areas of the retina cause inferior visual field losses. With these important concepts in mind, it is now possible to trace visual information from the periphery to the visual cortex.

Thought Question

Based on the anatomical organization of the visual system, explain why visual deficits resulting from damage after the optic nerve must be named by the field that is affected and not with respect to a specific eye.

Primary Afferents

Our consideration of sensory systems up to this point has always included a set of primary afferent neurons whose peripheral processes belong to the PNS. However, the visual system has no primary afferent neurons in this sense because the retina is part of the CNS. This is due to the fact that the retina is an outgrowth of the embryonic prosencephalon. Nevertheless, it is conceptually useful to organize our thinking around a chain of neurons that link receptors with the cerebral cortex. In so doing, this would make the rods and cones independent transduction entities that synapse with bipolar neurons. This would then make retinal bipolar neurons analogous to primary afferent neurons of other sensory systems and retinal ganglion neurons analogous to second-order neurons. We shall follow this scheme throughout our discussion.

To understand the projection of a visual stimulus to the visual cortex, it is helpful to understand the convention used in naming the components of the system. Important components of the system include the retina and optic nerve, as well as the optic chiasm, optic tract, and optic radiation, all of which are depicted in Figure 18-7. The right and left optic nerves travel to the **optic chiasm**, where a partial decussation occurs. These fibers then form the left and right **optic tracts**. The optic tracts continue to the left and right LGB of the thalamus. Fibers then leave the LGB and project ipsilaterally to the visual cortex; these projections are called the **optic radiation**.

Second-Order Neurons

OPTIC NERVE, CHIASM, AND TRACT Each optic nerve containing the second-order axons of ganglion cells is composed of about 1 million fibers. The optic nerve is mis-named as being a cranial nerve, but in fact, it is a *tract* of the CNS; nonetheless, we will follow convention and refer to this collection of axons as the optic nerve. This means that axons of the nerve are myelinated by oligodendrocytes, not by Schwann cells as is the case for axons of the PNS. It also means that the membranes investing the optic nerves are similar to those of the CNS. The dural sheath of the nerve is continuous with the sclera of the eyeball. The nerve is surrounded by arachnoid and pia and is bathed by cere-bral spinal fluid (CSF) in the subarachnoid space. Elevated CSF pressure is thus transmitted to the subarachnoid space around the optic nerve. Increased pressure around the op-tic nerve can result in compression and compromise of ve-nous blood flow. The resulting edema is characteristic of papilledema (discussed in Clinical Connections).

The optic nerve, chiasm, and tract are all made up of the axons of retinal ganglion cells, but the nerve and tract of the *same side* have different axonal compositions due to the crossing of some fibers in the optic chiasm (see Figure 18-7).

Each optic nerve consists of axons that all originate in the ipsilateral eye. In contrast, each optic tract consists of axons that had originated from both eyes. Axons from the *nasal half* of each retina cross in the optic chiasm to enter the contralateral optic tract. Axons from the *temporal half* of each retina run through the lateral portion of the chiasm without crossing and enter the ipsilateral optic tract.

Each optic tract is composed of axons arising from the temporal retina of the ipsilateral eye and the nasal retina of the contralateral eye. This mixing results in each optic tract carrying information from the contralateral half of the visual field. Visual information projecting centrally in second-order neurons of the optic tract destined to reach the primary visual cortex in the occipital lobe synapses on neurons of the lateral geniculate body.

Third-Order Neurons

Most axons of the optic tract synapse on third-order neu-rons of the lateral geniculate body (LGB) of the thalamus. The lateral geniculate bodies are crescent-shaped struc-tures situated on the posterior and ventral aspect of the thalamus, lateral to the medial geniculate body (MGB) (see Figure 2-10). Cells of the LGB are arranged in six distinct layers, numbered, ventral to dorsal, from 1 to 6. Layers 1 and 2 contain comparatively large neurons and are referred to as the **magnocellular layers**, while the cells in layers 3

through 6 are small and are referred to as the **parvocelluar layers**. The magnocellular and parvocellular layers receive input from the M and P retinal ganglion cells respectively, as noted earlier. Furthermore, axons of the magnocellular and parvocellular neurons project to distinct cortical tar-gets and process different aspects of the visual message. So, there exists a magnocelluar visual system, or channel, and a parvocellular system, or channel. These channels are func-tionally and anatomically distinct; they operate in parallel from the retina to the primary visual cortex (see Processing of Functional Information). Optic tract axons terminate in a precise **retinotopic** pattern, with the fovea (which have the greatest density of retinal ganglion cells) occupying about half the neural mass of each LGB. Each LGB con-tains a map of the contralateral half of the visual field. That is, the projection from each eye contains information from the same portion of the image of the object being viewed (Figure 18-8 ■). However, the corresponding images are not fused because each layer of the LGB receives input from only one eye. Layers 1, 4, and 6 receive input from the contralateral eye, while layers 2, 3, and 5 receive input from the ipsilateral eye.

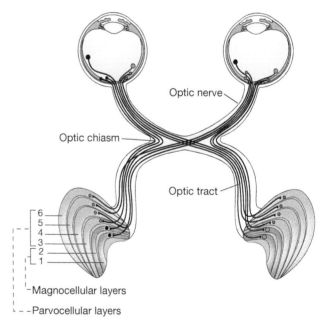

FIGURE 18-8 Three important points are illustrated here. (1) The optic tracts from the left retinal field (right half of visual field) of each eye project to the left LGB, illustrated in red, while the optic tracts from the right retinal field (left half of visual field) of each eye project to the right LGB, illustrated in blue. (2) The projections from the M and P retinal ganglia cells end in different layers in the LGB. The M cells end in the magnocel-lular layers (layers 1 and 2) of the LGB, while the P cells end in the parvocellular layers (layers 3 through 6). This is illustrated on the left, but occurs in each LGB. (3) The layers of the LGB receive inputs from both eyes, with layers 1, 4, and 6 receiving inputs from the contralateral eye, while layers 2, 3, and 5 receive input from the ipsilateral eye. This is illustrated on the right, although it, too, occurs bilaterally.

Third-order axons from the LGB form the optic radiation, or **geniculocalcarine tract**, whose axons terminate in a number of areas in the occipital lobe. This projection forms the last link in the geniculostriate (geniculocalcarine) system. Most axons end in the **primary visual (striate) cortex**, or **Brodmann's area 17**. The optic radiation maintains the retinotopic organization characterizing previous components of the system. After emerging from the LGB, most axons enter the so-called retrolenticular part of the posterior limb of the internal capsule. This portion of the internal capsule extends caudally behind the lentiform nucleus. Not all axons of the optic radiation follow the same trajectory toward the occipital cortex (Figure 18-9 ■). The most dorsal axons project almost directly backward toward the occipital lobe. However, the most ventral of the fibers first sweep anteriorly and downward into the temporal lobe and over and around the anterior limit of the inferior horn of the lateral ventricle, before looping backward toward the striate cortex. These fibers form **Meyer's loop**. Meyer's loop axons carry information from superior visual quadrants (inferior retinal quadrants) so that temporal lobe damage can produce

a specific visual field defect (see Visual Field Defects). Axons of the radiation then turn posteriorly in the region adjacent to the lateral wall of the inferior and posterior horns of the lateral ventricle. Finally, the axons swing medially to terminate in Brodmann's area 17.

Thought Question

From which visual field(s) of the retina do axons arise that make up the optic radiation? What about the axons that make up Meyer's loop? How would symptoms differ for lesions in these two regions?

The primary visual cortex is located almost entirely on the medial surface of the occipital lobe. The visual pathway ends retinotopically in the cortex above and below the **calcarine sulcus** (Figure 18-10 ■). Axons carrying information from the macula terminate most posteriorly, in the caudal one-third of the striate cortex on both sides of the calcarine sulcus. The macular representation

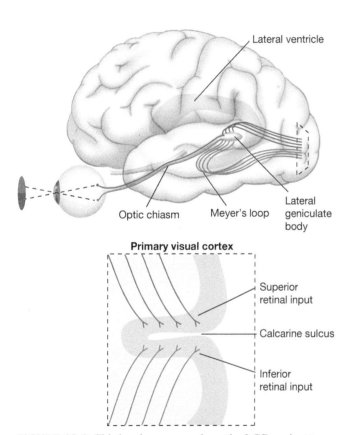

FIGURE 18-9 Third-order neurons from the LGB project to the primary visual cortex. The ventral fibers sweep anteriorly and downward and then progress posteriorly to the primary visual cortex. These projections form Meyer's loop. Meyer's loop carries information from the inferior retinal quadrants (i.e., the superior visual fields) and terminate *below* the calcarine sulcus. Axons carrying information from the superior retinal fields (i.e., the inferior visual fields) terminate *above* the calcarine sulcus.

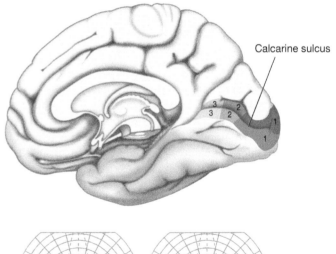

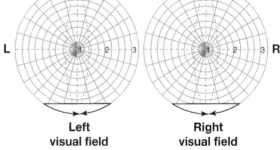

FIGURE 18-10 Three points are illustrated here. (1) The superior visual field (pink) terminates below the calcarine sulcus, while information from the inferior visual fields (purple) terminates above the calcarine sulcus. (2) Information from the macular representation of the central visual field (labeled 1) terminates in the caudal one-third of the visual cortex and occupies a disproportionately large area of the visual cortex. The most lateral portion of the visual field (labeled 3) terminates in the more rostral parts of the visual cortex.

occupies a disproportionately large area of the striate cortex, reflecting the fact that the macula is the part of the retina in which receptors are most densely packed and where visual acuity is sharpest. Axons carrying information from the paracentral and peripheral portions of the retina terminate in progressively more rostral parts of the calcarine area. Axons representing lower quadrants of the visual field end in the cortex above the calcarine sulcus, while axons representing upper quadrants of the visual field end in the cortex below the calcarine sulcus (see Figure 18-9).

Some axons of the optic radiation end in the **visual association cortex**, or **Brodmann's areas 18 and 19**. Brodmann's area 18 (the parastriate area) surrounds area 17. Area 19 (the peristriate area) surrounds and is larger than area 18. Areas 18 and 19 are horseshoe shaped and extend from the medial onto the lateral surface of the occipital lobe; together, they occupy virtually all of the lobe's lateral convexity (see Figure 7-5).

Thought Question

You are working in a rehabilitation unit with a woman who has a relatively small lesion affecting Meyer's loop. Would you expect her to have hemiplegia? What about language deficits? Why or why not?

Other Projections of Second-Order Optic Tract Axons

Axons of second-order optic tract neurons (ganglion cells) synapse in three subcortical structures besides the lateral geniculate body of the thalamus: the suprachiasmatic nucleus of the hypothalamus, the superior colliculus of the midbrain, and the pretectal area of the midbrain (Figure 18-11 ■).

Hypothalamic

A contingent of optic tract axons terminates in the **suprachiasmatic nucleus** of the hypothalamus. These fibers comprise the **direct retinohypothalamic projection**. They function in entraining circadian rhythms to the day–night cycle.

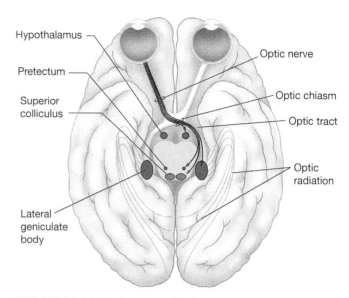

FIGURE 18-11 Optic tract projections to the suprachiasmatic nucleus of the hypothalamus, pretectal area, superior colliculi, and LGB.

Midbrain

A substantial number of optic tract axons bypass the LGB and terminate in two midbrain structures: the **superior colliculus** in rostral midbrain (most of the axons), and the **pretectal area** that is rostral to the superior colliculus at the junction of the midbrain and diencephalon.

Optic tract axons that bypass the LGB enter the **brachium of the superior colliculus** within which the axons are conveyed to the superior colliculus and pretectal area. Recall that the superior colliculi are two flattened eminences forming the rostral half of the tectum of the midbrain. Note that the brachium of the superior colliculus is *afferent* to the superior colliculus itself and is not part of the major pathway from receptor to cerebral cortex. This contrasts with the brachium of the inferior colliculus that is *efferent* from the inferior colliculus and is part of the major pathway from receptor to auditory cortex.

The major inputs to the superior colliculus are visual: one arising from the retina (from a distinct subpopulation of ganglion cells) and the other from the striate cortex. There are nonvisual input to the superior colliculus, including

---

Neurophysiology Box 18-2: Photoreception and Circadian Rhythms

Two classes of photoreceptors were described earlier. A third class, found in the mammalian retina, has been described. These photoreceptors are actually ganglion cells. They have been linked to a variety of physiological responses, including modulation of melatonin release, regulation of pupil size, and synchronization of circadian rhythms. These retinal ganglion cells are the main source of retinal input to the suprachiasmatic nucleus of the hypothalamus.

somatosensory (mostly via collaterals from somatosensory projections ascending to the thalamus) and auditory (via projections from the inferior colliculus). Efferent connections of the superior colliculus include projections to the cervical spinal cord via the **tectospinal tract**, to the brainstem reticular formation, and to the thalamus (discussed later).

The superior colliculus is concerned with detecting the direction of movement of objects in the visual field to facilitate visual orientation—that is, searching and tracking. A major function of the superior colliculus is orienting the eyes, head, and body toward visual and acoustic stimuli in the environment. This is sometimes referred to as the *visual grasp reflex*. Turning of the eyes and head occurs in an integrated movement sequence: the eyes move first, and the head starts to turn 20 to 40 msec later. Turning of the head elicits compensatory eye movements that are mediated by the vestibular system to maintain visual fixation (see Chapter 17). The pathways by which the superior colliculus produces head and body movements include the tectospinal tract and a tectoreticulospinal route.

Output from the superior colliculus has access to the cerebral cortex via the thalamus. The superior colliculus projects to the **lateral posterior nucleus** and the **pulvinar** of the thalamus. The lateral posterior nucleus projects to Brodmann's areas 5 and 7 of the parietal lobe. The pulvinar projects to areas 18 and 19 of the visual association cortex. Area 7 contains neurons related specifically to visual stimuli and eye movements. Experiments with monkeys have shown that some neurons discharge maximally when the animal simultaneously fixes its eyes on a target of interest and reaches for it. The projections from the superior colliculus to area 19 of the cerebral cortex could explain a puzzling visual capacity that sometimes remains in humans following selective lesions of the striate cortex. Such patients have no conscious awareness of visual stimuli in the blind portions of their visual fields, yet they may be able to accurately point to the stimulus. This capacity has been referred to as **blind sight** or **cortical blindness**.

PROCESSING OF FUNCTIONAL INFORMATION

The visual system has a tremendous variety of functional capabilities. After all, we can differentiate color and intensity. We are constantly perceiving, interpreting, and comparing shapes, depth, and movement. Often, a person can infer texture simply by observing an object. Neurophysiologists have developed a rudimentary understanding of a few of the physiological bases by which animals process and interpret the vast array of visual information that comes into the central nervous system in order to make meaning of the richly variable world in which we live. However, not enough is known yet to fully explain the processes that occur as we navigate our environment. In this section, we describe some of what has been learned, recognizing that the vast majority of these processes are yet to be explained.

Neurons of the Geniculocalcarine System

One of the ways by which the function of the visual system has been assessed is by determining the receptive field properties of neurons in the visual system. As noted earlier, the receptive field of a single neuron in any part of the visual system is the area of the retina in which light stimulation causes either excitation of the neuron or inhibition of the cell's resting discharge. The receptive fields of retinal ganglion cells, cells of the lateral geniculate body, and neurons of the visual cortices all have been thoroughly analyzed. Such analyses have shown that the visual system is hierarchically organized. That is, the properties characterizing the receptive fields at a given synaptic locus are determined by the properties of neurons at previous way stations that converge onto the next-higher-order cell. This analysis also has revealed that the visual cortices are organized into vertical units called **functional (cortical) columns**, introduced in Chapter 7. Three overlapping but independent systems of columns have been shown to exist in the visual cortex. Namely, these are **orientation columns**, **ocular dominance columns**, and **blobs**. Each is discussed in this section. The system of columns, and their interactions, allows for rapid and simultaneous parallel processing of our complex visual world. Understanding the specificity of the information that an independent cortical column processes helps to explain selective deficits. This columnar organization is a general feature of cortical organization for the entire neocortex.

Retinal Ganglion Cells

The responses of individual retinal ganglion cells are determined by shining small spots of light on the retina. Each ganglion cell responds to stimulation of a small circular patch of the retina. This restricted region of the retina defines the cell's receptive field and corresponds to a small region of the retina's visual field. Retinal ganglion cells discharge spontaneously. Their receptive fields possess a center–surround structure and fall into two major classes, both of which respond best to light contrast.

 On-center ganglion cells respond best when the central portion of its receptive field is illuminated by a spot of light and the light is restricted to this central region (Figure 18-12 ■). Illumination of the surrounding area of the receptive field reduces the response if a spot of light is used and eliminates the response if the entire surrounding ring is illuminated. Illumination of the entire receptive field causes a weak response because center and surround illumination oppose one another's effects (i.e., there is a lack of contrast). Conversely, **off-center** ganglion cells increase their discharge when the surround is illuminated and decrease their spontaneous discharge when the center of their receptive field is illuminated.

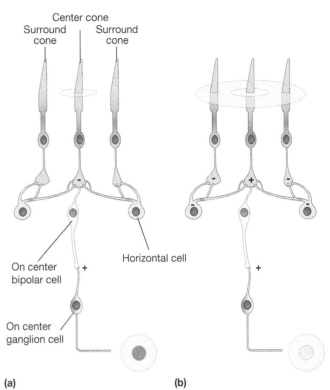

FIGURE 18-12 The mechanism that subserves visual contrast. (a) The central cone cells in the receptive field are illuminated, while the surround cones are not. This excites the on-center bipolar cell and ganglion cell, resulting in a sharp contrast between the center and the surround. Sharp contrast can occur only when illumination is focused on the central portion. (b) The surround is illuminated, resulting in a lack of contrast because the center and surround illuminations oppose one another's effects, resulting in a weaker response and less contrast.

> **Thought Question**
>
> In preparation for understanding how the nervous system identifies edges of objects—and, therefore, defines objects—explain the difference between on-center and off-center ganglion cells.

Neurons of the Lateral Geniculate Body

The function of the LGB remains unknown, although the response characteristics of its neurons have been analyzed. LGB neurons have response characteristics similar to those of retinal ganglion cells. Each cell responds to stimulation of a circumscribed region of the retina. Each neuron has either an "on" or "off" center with an opposing surround. Neurons in different layers of the LGB are driven from receptive fields in only one eye. Recall that at the level of the LGB, magnocellular and parvocellular systems are anatomically segregated, both in terms of origin of inputs (from M and P cells, respectively) and in terms of the eventual destination of fibers. Only 10 to 20 percent of the synaptic input to neurons in the LGB originate from the retina, with the majority of synaptic input originating in the brainstem reticular formation and the visual cortex. Because the latter are feedback connections, they may control the flow of information from the retina to the cortex.

Neurons of the Primary Visual Cortex

Cells in each layer of the primary visual cortex receive a unique combination of inputs and, in turn, project to a unique combination of neuronal targets. The primary visual, or striate, cortex is unique in that layer IV is subdivided into three distinct sublayers labeled IVa, IVb, and IVc; layer IVc is itself further subdivided into two tiers. Most LGB axons terminate in layer IVc, but the magnocellular (M) and parvocellular (P) neurons differentially terminate in the two tiers. Moreover, a second group of LGB parvocellular neurons terminates in layers II and III on patches of cortical neurons called blobs—peg-shaped columns spanning layers II and III (Figure 18-13 ■). (The functional importance of blobs is discussed later.) Thus, there are three systems of visual input: one magnocellular and two parvocellular channels, each with a unique function but operating in parallel.

Recall that the most effective stimuli for influencing retinal ganglion and LGB neurons are small spots of light. This also is true for the neurons in layer IV of the primary visual cortex and for the blobs in layers II and III. However, none of the other cells in the primary visual cortex have circular receptive fields. Rather, they respond best to lines and bars so that these cells have transformed concentric receptive fields into linear fields. This is accomplished by the connections among the cortical cells in different layers (see Figure 18-13).

The connections of cells in layer IV with cells in the layers above and below are arranged vertically in a unit called a **functional column**. Not all of these columns uniformly span all six layers of the striate cortex. Each functional column contains several types of cells: cells of layer

IVc that receive axons from the LGB, simple cells located in layers above and below layer IV that receive a converging input from neurons of layer IVc, and complex cells located in layers above and below layer IV that receive a converging input from simple cells. The function of simple and complex cells is presented in a later section.

Three overlapping and independent systems of columns occur in the visual cortex: orientation columns, the blobs, and the larger ocular dominance columns. Orientation columns are narrow (30 to 100 μm wide), vertical arrays of cells in which the cells all have the same receptive field axis of orientation (see Figure 18-13). That is, the simple and complex cells in the column may respond best to a bar of light, but only when it has a specific axis of orientation (say, vertical). In each adjacent column, there is an orderly shift in the axis of orientation of about 10 degrees. The orderly shifts in the axis of orientation in moving from one column to the next are regularly interrupted by blobs.

Ocular dominance columns, about twice as large as the orientation columns, are independent, alternating columns in which cell responses show a preference for either the left or right eye (see Figure 18-13). Cells in layer IV of the column are monocular because they receive projections only from the layers of the LGB concerned with one eye. (Layer IV cells are segregated into a series of alternating stripes, with one set related to the left eye and the other to the right eye.) However, cells in the column located in layers above and below layer IV respond binocularly, but with a definite dominance by one eye. This is because they receive most of their input from their own layer IV cells; but in addition, they receive some input from an adjacent ocular dominance column concerned with the other eye. Ocular dominance columns begin the process of fusion of images from corresponding points on the two hemiretinas into one image. Such fusion is essential to binocular vision and depth perception (**stereopsis**).

The blob is a peg-shaped column spanning layers II and III that receives input directly from the LGB (see Figure 18-13). (The term *blob* is derived from its appearance upon histological staining with cytochrome oxidase.) Intervening between the blobs are regions referred to as the **interblob regions**. Again, as with the M and P systems, the blob and interblob systems are important because they mediate different aspects of vision. The blobs are concerned with color vision, while the interblob system is concerned especially with form vision.

In addition to the vertical functional columns, the primary visual cortex is organized into six horizontal layers, as noted earlier. By virtue of its afferent and efferent connections and its particular cell type, each layer performs a unique task. Extensive horizontally arrayed connections exist that link cells within a layer with one another and, by this means, connect adjacent functional columns possessing the same response properties.

The vertical columns and horizontal layers together provide for a complex mechanism by which visual stimuli are processed and interpreted. Many of the details are yet to be understood.

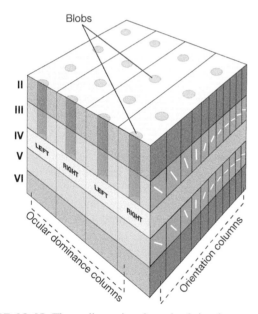

FIGURE 18-13 Three-dimensional patch of visual cortex. This figure illustrates three important mechanisms by which information received by the retina is parceled out for processing, allowing the brain to organize and interpret complex visual stimuli. (1) Ocular dominance columns alternate with cells in the columns, showing a preference for either the right or left eye. Furthermore, layer 4 of the ocular dominance columns are monocular (either right or left), but the layers above and below this layer respond binocularly, but with a definite dominance. (2) Orientation columns allow for parceling out information from visual stimuli, based on the axis of orientation. (3) Blobs are peg-shaped columns that span layers II and III only and are concerned with color vision. Recall that the interblob system (not shown) is especially concerned with form vision.

Thought Question

What is the functional importance of the ocular dominance column and the orientation column in the primary visual cortex? What is the functional difference between these two columns? And where do the stimuli originate for these two types of columns?

Extraction of the Visual Pattern by Cells of the Visual Cortex

Extraction of information about a visual pattern depends importantly on the way in which information, conveyed into the nervous system by lower-order neurons in the visual cortex, converges on higher-order neurons in the cortex. The convergence pattern of neurons in the visual system is determined by examining the receptive field properties of neurons at progressively higher levels of the system. For example, as described earlier, within the retina and LGB, individual neurons have a center–surround structure in their response to small spots of light, thus contributing to the appreciation of luminance contrasts. However, neurons of the striate cortex do not respond to small spots of light but rather, respond to light/dark bars or edges. Furthermore, the response of individual cells depends on the orientation of the bar. Some cells respond to bars that are presented vertically, others to those presented horizontally, and still others to every angle in between. Some cells respond to the length of the bar that is presented and some to the direction in which the bar of light is moved.

Each portion of the retina activated by a point in the visual world is analyzed by a specific set of cortical neurons in the primary visual cortex. In order to perform the analysis, the set must receive information about ocular dominance, stimulus orientation, movement, and color of the point in the visual world. This set of cortical neurons is called a **cortical**

module and consists of a 2×2 mm section of primary visual cortex (Figure 18-14 ■). Each module contains a complete set of orientation columns representing 360 degrees, a set of right and left dominance columns, and 16 blobs for the analysis of color. Adjacent modules are linked by horizontal connections. Thus, analysis of a complete complex shape in the visual world depends on the simultaneous activity in an array of modules in the primary visual cortex.

Another important difference between neurons of the striate cortex and those of the retina and LGB relates to the origin of inputs. Individual neurons in the striate cortex receive inputs that derived from both eyes, whereas those of the retina and LGB respond either to inputs from one eye or the other. The arrangement of bilateral inputs into neurons of the striate cortex appears to be related to the capacity for binocular vision, although the mechanisms by which binocular vision occurs are not fully understood.

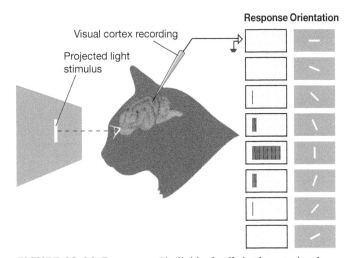

FIGURE 18-14 Response of individual cells in the cat visual cortex to the *orientation* of stimuli. As illustrated here, these particular cells respond most strongly to a vertical orientation.

Neurophysiology Box 18-3: Visual Development and Deprivation

Despite the fact that much in the circuitry of the developing visual system is genetically determined, the mature visual system is also very much a product of its early experience. Children with visual deprivation resulting from pathologies such as corneal scarring or congenital cataract often have poor vision even after the ocular condition has been corrected, and children with congenital strabismus often develop poor vision in one eye. These topics are discussed in greater detail in Chapter 25, which deals with plasticity in the human brain.

Animal experiments have shown that specific (but not all) organizational features of the striate cortex depend on the visual experience that occurs during a specific **critical** **period** in development. If vision of one eye is occluded during the critical period, cells in the striate cortex respond only to the *unoccluded eye*. Furthermore, for the eye that remains open (unoccluded), the ocular dominance columns are larger than normal. There is a loss of vision in the eye that is occluded, the severity of which depends on when the eye is closed during the critical period and for how long. The changes are partially reversible if the eye is reopened during the critical period, but not if it is reopened later. If occlusion occurs after the critical period, these changes do not occur, demonstrating that the phenomenon is one of development during periods and not due to disuse atrophy.

Higher Visual Processing

Thought Question

Here is a question to stretch your mind. What mechanisms can you think of that might allow the nervous system to differentiate the texture, size, and shape of an object versus the color versus its motion?

The processing of visual information at the level of the occipital cortex takes place in the primary visual cortex, also referred to as the *striate cortex* (Brodmann's area 17) and the visual association cortex, also referred to as the *extrastriate cortex* (Brodmann's areas 18 and 19). However, the processing of visual information is not limited to the striate and extrastriate areas of the occipital lobe. Rather, projections from the primary visual cortex diverge within the occipital lobe into two major pathways with different nonoccipital sites of termination (Figure 18-15 ■). A *dorsal pathway* terminates within the parieto-occipital cortex, while a *ventral pathway* ends in the occipitotemporal cortex.

Numerous channels of information are processed in parallel in the cortex—the best understood of which are three parallel channels for analyzing motion, form, and color. The first of these channels is involved in processing information about motion and spatial relationships (spatial vision or location of an object within the visual field). This information is conveyed by inputs that arise from M cells in the retina and are directed to the magnocellular layer of the LGB. From there, this information is conveyed to the visual association cortex (area 18) and then to the dorsolateral parietotemporal cortex for high-order visual processing.

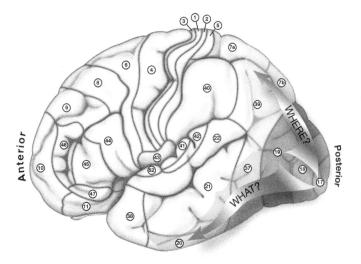

FIGURE 18-15 The dorsal pathway relays information from the primary visual cortex to the parieto-occipital cortex about *where* an object is located in space. The ventral pathway relays information about *what* an object is from the primary visual cortex to the occipitotemporal cortex.

The second channel is involved in processing of information related to form (i.e., with the intrinsic qualities of an object in terms of size, texture, and shape). Specifically, information about form is conveyed via retinal P cells to the parvocellular layers of the LGB and from there to area 17, the primary visual cortex. This information then is directed to the inferior occipitotemporal cortex for interpretation of form.

Thought Question

M and P cells of the retina end up in different areas of the visual cortex where they have very different functional roles. What is the pathway by which each of these retinal cells arrives at the cortex, and what is the role of each in terms of higher visual processing?

Finally, information about color likewise originates in the retinal P cells but is conveyed to both the parvocellular and intralaminar layers of the LGB and eventually to the inferior occipitotemporal cortex. A small population of cells in the inferotemporal cortex has been shown to be selectively responsive to complex stimuli, such as a hand or face. The latter represent the so-called grandmother cells postulated to exist in the 1960s, now also referred to as face cells. Some of the face cells respond best to frontal views, while others respond best to profiles. Distortions of the face cause the cell to stop responding. Such face cells have attracted considerable interest because of the clinical syndrome in humans called prosopagnosia (Gr., *prosopon*, face, + *a-*, negative, + *gnosis*, knowledge) (discussed later).

To summarize, the dorsal pathways (projections to the parieto-occipital association cortex) are necessary to determine *where* in the visual field an event occurred and do so by analyzing motion and spatial relationships between objects and between the body and the visual stimuli. The ventral pathways (projections to the occipitotemporal association cortex) are important in determining *what* the object in the visual field is and do so by analyzing form and color. These pathways are important in identification of colors, faces, letters, and other visual stimuli. As will be seen later, the consequences of CNS damage with respect to vision are quite different depending on whether a lesion occurs in the parieto-occipital or occipitotemporal area.

Visual Reflexes

Thought Question

What do you recall from Chapter 14 about visual reflexes?

Pupillary Size

Constriction of the pupil occurs with excitation of the parasympathetic innervation of the smooth muscle fibers of the sphincter muscle of the iris. *Dilatation* of the pupil occurs with excitation of the sympathetic innervation of the smooth muscle fibers of the radial (dilator) muscle of the iris. Pupillary size is determined by the balance of parasympathetic and sympathetic innervation of smooth muscle of the iris.

Dilatation occurs reflexively on shading the eye and is a feature of painful stimulation as well as emotional state and attitude. For example, the pupils of hungry people dilate significantly when they are shown a plate of food, whereas those of persons who have recently eaten a meal do not. Such dilatation is due primarily to inhibition of the parasympathetic innervation of the sphincter muscle. Under normal circumstances, dilatation of the pupil is due to a varying tonic influence of the parasympathetic innervation. It is likely that *maximal* dilatation of the pupil requires both parasympathetic inhibition and sympathetic excitation. The pathway for pupillary dilatation is incompletely known but appears to include a projection from the frontal cortex to the hypothalamus, a projection from the hypothalamus to the intermediolateral (sympathetic) cell column of upper thoracic segments of the spinal cord, preganglionic fibers from the intermediolateral cell column to the superior cervical ganglion, and postganglionic fibers to the dilator muscle of the iris. **Horner's syndrome** is caused by a lesion to the central or peripheral sympathetic pathways to the eye and was discussed in Chapter 12.

Thought Question

Describe how Horner's syndrome will alter normal pupillary responses.

Fixation Reflex

The fixation reflex functions to maintain the position of the eyes so that the image of the object of interest is kept on the fovea of both eyes. The reflex pathway is incompletely known. Its afferent limb involves the normal visual projection to cortical visual areas. Its efferent limb consists of cortical projections to the superior colliculus; the pretectal region; and, finally, to lower motor neurons of the oculomotor, trochlear, and abducens nuclei. Attention and interest directed toward specific objects in the visual field are required to elicit the reflex. When fixation occurs during head and body movement, this cortical fixation reflex is supported by vestibulo-ocular reflexes (see Chapter 17).

The Accommodation–Convergence Reaction (Near Reflex)

The accommodation–convergence reaction occurs when the gaze is shifted from a distant object to a near one and involves the following: an increase in the refractive power (curvature) of the lens, accomplished by contraction of the ciliary muscle; convergence of the two eyes, accomplished by simultaneous contractions of both medial recti muscles; and pupillary constriction. The increase in the curvature of

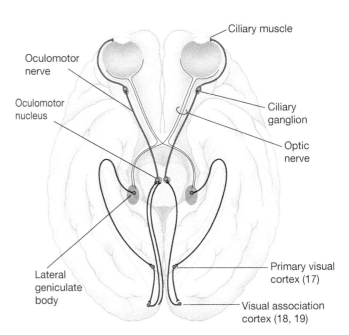

FIGURE 18-16 The accommodation reflex includes visual information projected to the visual cortex and then to the superior colliculus (illustrated in green), pretectal area, and then via interneurons to the oculomotor nucleus. The connections to the motor neuron and nerve are also illustrated in green.

the lens is due to its inherent viscoelastic properties: contraction of the ciliary muscle causes the ciliary ring to narrow; narrowing of the ciliary ring reduces the outward pull on the lens by the ring of filaments (of the suspensory ligament) that attach to the margins of the lens, which allows the lens to thicken.

The accommodation reflex differs from the simpler pupillary light reflex. The pathway includes the normal visual projection from the eye to the cerebral cortex, a projection back from cortical area 19 to the superior colliculus and pretectal region, and interneuronal connections to the oculomotor complex that stimulate motor neurons innervating the medial rectus muscles and preganglionic motor neurons of the Edinger-Westphal nucleus (Figure 18-16 ■).

CLINICAL CONNECTIONS
Role of Vision in Postural Control

Functionally, vision serves an essential role in interpreting objects within the environment and in intrapersonal space as well as for navigation through the environment. Visual

Thought Question

In order to maintain postural control during movement, it is necessary to have some level of stability during movement. One of the key contributors is that of stabilizing the visual information during movement of the head and body. Explain how this is accomplished.

inputs also provide one of the three critical components for postural control, along with inputs from the vestibular and proprioceptive systems. When individuals have deficits in the proprioceptive or vestibular systems, they may rely on visual information to substitute for these modalities. However, especially as people age, they often experience presbyopia, begin to lose visual acuity, and may have a number of other visual deficits, thereby limiting their ability to compensate for losses in the vestibular and proprioceptive systems. In combination, even relatively mild impairments in each system can result in increasing frequency of falls.

Further compounding problems with postural control when visual deficits occur with lesions of the brainstem, these defects may result in an inability for visual fixation as well as deficits of the **vestibulo-ocular reflex (VOR)**. As discussed in Chapter 17, these deficits have profound ramifications for postural control.

Finally, with cortical damage, individuals can have severe deficits of higher-order processing. These deficits may not interfere with the postural control mechanisms per se; nevertheless, they may have profound implications for falls and injuries. For example, some individuals can have visual field deficits, compounded by loss of awareness of one side of space. These individuals are at risk for trips, slips, and other injuries. Cortical deficits are discussed further in Chapter 24.

As such, assessment of the visual system from peripheral to central control is necessary to interpret the cause, location, and extent of visual deficits. With the resulting information, the rehabilitation professional can also identify strategies to improve postural control and overall function. Depending on the nature of the injury, intervention may rely on compensatory strategies, strategies to improve postural control through improved use of the VOR, or some combination thereof.

> **Thought Question**
>
> Given what you now know, which specific reflexes act together from the visual, vestibular, and proprioceptive systems to control posture in space? Now identify as many pathways as possible that might mediate the action of these reflexes. Finally, what examples can you think of in which a person performs a task that requires overriding one or more of these reflexes?

Assessment

For purposes of rehabilitation, the visual system is assessed from a variety of perspectives. These assessments are important in localizing damage to the system, in determining implications for postural control and movement, and in designing intervention strategies.

First, it is important to know whether an individual has sufficient acuity to function. The ocular examination includes the following components: measurement of visual acuity; ophthalmoscopic inspection of the refractive media and the optic fundi (posterior inner part of the eyeball), particularly the macular region and optic disc; and plotting of the visual fields. Retinal inspection is an important part of the neurological evaluation because the retina is part of the CNS, and its neurons, glia, and vasculature are subject to many of the diseases that affect other parts of the CNS (e.g., multiple sclerosis).

Typically, acuity is assessed using the Snellen eye chart and notation of 20/X, where 20/20 refers to normal acuity. In addition, visual capability is assessed along the neuroanatomic pathway from the reflexive responses to the peripheral stimulus (light) to visual fields to perception. The visual system is routinely assessed during neurological examinations and in emergency settings to determine integrity of the brainstem.

Also important is identification of scotomas. A **scotoma** is a visual field defect manifested as a circumscribed region of visual loss surrounded by normal vision. Scotomas are named according to their position or shape. Infarcts, hemorrhages, or infections of the retina can cause a monocular scotoma.

Pupillary Light Reflex (and the Swinging Flashlight Test)

> **Thought Question**
>
> The Edinger-Westphal nucleus is important in mediating pupillary size and reactivity. In preparation for understanding the following tests of the visual system, review the pathways associated with the Edinger-Westphal nucleus (Chapter 12).

The testing of pupillary size and reactivity yields important, often vital, clinical information. The term **anisocoria** denotes pupillary inequality. Light shown on the retina of one eye causes both pupils to constrict to a similar degree. The response in the eye stimulated is called the **direct pupillary light reflex**, while the response in the opposite, nonstimulated eye is called the **consensual pupillary light reflex**.

To understand this test, it is important to recall that the pathway for the pupillary light reflex consists of three parts (Figure 18-17 ■): (1) an afferent limb that consists of axons of retinal ganglion cells that pass via the optic nerve, optic tract, and brachium of the superior colliculus to the pretectal area of rostral midbrain; (2) interneurons of the pretectal area that terminate bilaterally in the **Edinger-Westphal nuclei** of the oculomotor complex; and (3) an efferent limb that consists of a two-neuron link to the sphincter muscle of the iris—*preganglionic* parasympathetic fibers from the Edinger-Westphal nuclei that course with fibers of the oculomotor nerve to synapse on cells of the ciliary ganglion and *postganglionic* fibers from the ciliary ganglion that terminate in the sphincter muscle.

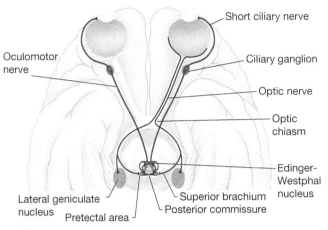

(a)

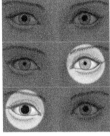

Right optic nerve damage
(b)

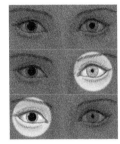

Right oculomotor nerve damage
(c)

FIGURE 18-17 The pupillary light reflex, in contrast to the accommodation reflex, does not involve the cortex. (a) Afferent projections from retinal ganglion cells end in the pretectal area of the midbrain, interneurons from the pretectal area terminate bilaterally in the Edinger-Westphal nucleus, and the parasympathetic efferent limb from the Edinger-Westphal nucleus projects to the ciliary ganglion and then to the pupillary sphincter muscle. When all pathways are intact, pupillary responses to a light stimulus in one eye would be symmetrical in both eyes. (b) Afferent limb damage—when the right optic nerve is damaged, light shone in the right eye will not produce either a direct or a consensual pupillary response (bottom panel). When light is shone in the left eye, a direct and consensual response is observed (middle panel). (c) Efferent limb damage—when the right oculomotor nerve is damaged, light shone in the right eye will not produce a direct pupillary response but will result in a consensual response (bottom panel). Light shone in the left eye will produce a direct but not a consensual response (middle panel).

Both pupils constrict when light is shone in just one eye because the retinopretectal afferents and the pretecto-Edinger-Westphal fibers are both crossed and uncrossed. Retinopretectal afferents partially cross in the optic chiasm. Pretecto-Edinger-Westphal neurons partially cross in the **posterior commissure**.

With complete interruption of the optic nerve on one side, illumination of the affected (blind) eye is not followed by constriction in either eye, while illumination of the non-affected eye elicits both the direct and consensual reflex. With complete interruption of the oculomotor nerve or ciliary ganglion on one side, illumination of the affected eye

Thought Question

As you have learned, the pupillary light reflex has three components (afferent, interneuron, and efferent). When testing the pupillary light reflex, how would you expect the findings to differ, depending on which component of the reflex is damaged?

does not elicit a direct reflex but does elicit a consensual reflex, while illumination of the healthy eye elicits a direct reflex but not a consensual reflex.

The **swinging flashlight test** is a procedure designed to test the *afferent limb* of the pupillary light reflex. With the patient looking into the distance, the clinician swings a light rhythmically from eye to eye, taking care to illuminate each pupil for two or three seconds. If both afferent pathways are normal, there will be equal pupillary constriction in both eyes when the light is directed to either eye. The response is symmetrical, but there is actually little or no change in pupil size because one eye will not recover from its consensual response before it is subjected to the direct light beam. However, when the afferent pathway from one eye is affected, the response is asymmetrical and is characterized by larger pupils when the light is directed into the affected eye than when it is direct into the unaffected eye (see Figure 18-17).

Visual Fields

Recall that the visual field is the field of view of the external world seen by one or both eyes without movement of the head and is defined in relation to a line through the fovea. Visual fields can be plotted at the bedside in alert, cooperative patients or determined more accurately with the use of a perimeter or tangent screen. Visual field deficits may involve half of the visual field (i.e., temporal or nasal half), referred to as **hemianopsia**, or may involve just the upper or lower quadrant, referred to as **quadrantanopsia**.

With one eye of the patient covered and the open eye looking straight ahead at a fixation point, visual fields are tested by moving a small object (pencil, white disc mounted on a stick, finger, etc.) from the periphery, where it cannot be seen centrally, until it can be seen "out of the corner" of the patient's eye. This is repeated from multiple different directions of approach, enabling the examiner to chart the visual field. Each eye can see nearly 90 degrees from the vertical visual axis in a temporal direction, but the field is less extensive in other directions because of the prominent obstructions imposed, in particular, by the nose but also by the eyebrows and cheeks. The visual field seen by the right eye is nearly the same as that seen by the left eye. More specifically, the nasal part of the field for one eye is the same as that for the temporal field seen by the other eye, with the exception of the far temporal periphery, called the **temporal crescent**. The temporal crescent is imaged on the nasal retina of one eye but not on the temporal retina of the other eye because of the obstruction by the nose.

The simplest procedure for testing visual fields is the so-called confrontation test. In this test, the examiner confronts (i.e., faces) the patient being tested. In one popular variant, the examiner and patient cover opposite eyes so that the uncovered eyes have mutually congruent visual fields. The patient is instructed to fix his or her gaze on the opened eye of the examiner and to inform the examiner when he or she first sees a target move into the field of vision. The target is brought slowly from the outside toward the center of the visual field. Because the patient's and examiner's peripheral visual fields are congruent, the presence of a visual field defect is verified when the object is visible in the examiner's field but there is no response from the patient. The four fields of vision—the upper, lower, nasal, and temporal quadrants—are tested separately for each eye. Visual impairments due to lesions of the central pathways generally affect only a part of the visual fields, so that plotting the visual fields provides information on lesion site.

Disorders of the Visual System

A number of conditions of the central nervous system can affect vision. Among the most prominent are stroke, traumatic brain injury, neonatal disorders, and multiple sclerosis. The relationship of damage from stroke to symptoms is discussed in detail in Chapter 24. In this chapter, some of the key visual disturbances are discussed.

Amaurosis Fugax

The term **amaurosis fugax** refers to a transient ischemic event affecting the retina. This transient event results from an occlusion in the central retinal artery or a branch from that artery. This condition is discussed further in Chapter 24.

Optic Neuritis

Optic neuritis is an inflammatory demyelinating disorder often related to multiple sclerosis (MS). Typically, this condition begins with eye pain, especially with movement, and monocular visual problems. The visual impairment typically includes visual loss in the center of the field (referred to as a central scotoma), decreased visual acuity, and impaired color vision. Optic neuritis can occur as an acute event or can progress slowly. Recovery is common and typically occurs within six to eight weeks, although it may take several months. While most people with optic neuritis eventually are diagnosed with MS, about 30 percent of individuals have a process limited just to the optic nerve.

Results of Elevated Intercranial Pressure

The term **papilledema** refers to optic disc swelling associated with and caused by elevated intracranial pressure (ICP) (discussed in Chapter 25). Even when papilledema is severe, the visual field defect may consist of nothing more than an enlargement of the blind spot. Papilledema is detected by observation with an ophthalmoscope. The optic disc appears edematous and engorged.

Visual Field Defects

Lesions located in different parts of the visual pathway from the retina to primary visual cortex result in characteristic visual field defects (Figure 18-18 ■). **Prechiasmal lesions of the retina** or optic nerve are manifested by either scotomas or by contractions of the visual field that involve just one eye (a monocular field defect). A monocular field defect is due to a prechiasmal lesion.

Because retinal ganglion cell axons converge toward the optic disc, damage near the center of the retina (fovea centralis) results in a larger field defect than does the same extent of damage in the periphery of the retina. Damage to the fovea causes a loss of central vision and results in considerable visual handicap because of the loss of visual acuity.

Damage to one optic nerve results in a monocular visual field defect; if complete, the patient complains of blindness in that eye (see Figure 18-18). This defect is accompanied by an afferent pupillary light reflex defect and atrophy of the affected optic nerve fibers that eventually is manifest as pallor in the optic disc.

The optic chiasm brings visual system fibers from the two eyes together. Damage to the chiasm, therefore, may result in field defects in both eyes. If the medial aspect of the optic chiasm is compromised, decussating axons from each nasal *retinal* hemifield are damaged. This results in a loss of the temporal visual fields in both eyes, a **bitemporal hemianopsia** (see Figure 18-18). This may also be referred to as a **heteronymous hemianopsia** because the field losses are nonoverlapping. The most common cause of damage to the central region of the chiasm is a result of pressure from a tumor of the pituitary gland, and the visual field defect is often the first clinical sign.

Damage to the lateral aspect of the chiasm compromises the non-crossing fibers from the temporal retinal field of the ipsilateral eye. This causes a loss of the ipsilateral nasal visual field, a **nasal hemianopsia**. This may result from a saccular aneurysm at a bifurcation of the internal carotid artery that lies adjacent to the chiasm. The aneurysm on one side may displace the chiasm against the opposite internal carotid artery, resulting in involvement of both lateral sides of the chiasm. Such bilateral involvement would produce a **binasal visual field defect**.

In the postchiasmal visual pathways, the nasal fibers of the contralateral eye join the temporal fibers of the ipsilateral eye. A defect that affects the nasal field of one eye and the temporal field of the other eye is described as *homonymous* because it involves deficits for similar regions

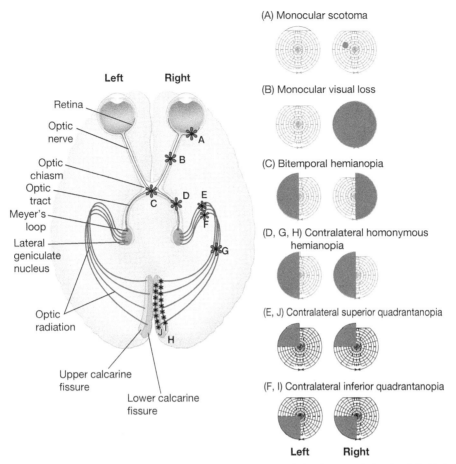

FIGURE 18-18 Lesions in the pathway from the retina to the visual cortex result in characteristic visual field defects. The nature of the defect is used clinically to localize the lesion as described in the text.

of the visual field for both eyes. A number of other terms are applied to lesions involving the postchiasmal visual pathways. The field deficits resulting from single lesions in the postchiasmal pathways are *contralateral* to the side of the lesion because the right postchiasmal pathways (optic tracts, LGBs, geniculocalcarine tracts, or optic radiations) carry information from the left side of the visual field from both eyes, and vice versa. Thus, the visual field loss is on the side of the visual field contralateral to the lesion. This laterality also applies to lesions of the primary visual cortex involving a single occipital lobe. Additionally, homonymous field deficits may be congruent or incongruent. If the defects in the homonymous field have the same shape they are said to be *congruent*, whereas if the shapes of the two defects are dissimilar, they are *incongruent*.

The optic tract is relatively small in cross section. Therefore, a unilateral lesion often damages all of its fibers, causing a contralateral homonymous field defect that affects the entire half of the field (Figure 18-18d). There is an afferent pupillary light reflex deficit, and optic nerve atrophy manifested as optic disc pallor eventually results.

A lesion involving the LGB also results in a contralateral homonymous hemianopsia, as well as atrophy of the optic nerve. However, there is no accompanying pupillary light reflex deficit because the anatomically distinct

ganglion axons that project to the pretectal nucleus and form the afferent component of this reflex are undamaged.

Because the optic radiations do not contain axons of retinal ganglion cells, their damage does not cause optic nerve atrophy but does result in a contralateral homonymous hemianopsia. However, because geniculocalcarine axons are spread out over a wide area, damage to the optic radiations often affects only a single quadrant rather than the entire hemifield. A lesion in the anterior part of the temporal lobe, for example, involves the axons of Meyer's loop that carry information from inferior *retinal* quadrants. The resultant contralateral homonymous field defects involve the upper quadrants. The defect sometimes is referred to as the "pie-in-the-sky" defect and goes by the cumbersome name of **contralateral homonymous superior quadrantanopsia** (see Figure 18-18). Lesions involving the parietal lobe may interrupt geniculocalcarine axons carrying information from superior retinal quadrants, resulting in contralateral homonymous inferior field defects.

A characteristic feature of the contralateral homonymous field defects resulting from damage to the primary visual cortex is congruency. The extent of congruency depends on how closely fibers from corresponding points in each retina and carrying the identical visual field information are positioned to each other at the lesion site. The primary visual cortex is the first place where single neurons receive input from both eyes; therefore, there is an exact point-to-point representation of the visual field. Consequently, damage to the primary visual cortex results in complete congruency. Lesions involving the upper bank of the calcarine fissure result in a contralateral homonymous inferior quadrantanopsia, while lesions to the lower bank cause a contralateral homonymous superior quadrantanopsia (see Figure 18-18). Damage involving the entire primary visual cortex results in a contralateral homonymous hemianopsia, while smaller lesions cause homonymous scotomas in the appropriate portion of the contralateral visual field.

Vascular lesions of the occipital lobe may produce a contralateral homonymous hemianopsia in which the central few degrees of the field are spared, a circumstance called **macular sparing**. Because of its dense sensory innervation, the fovea has a very large representation in the primary visual cortex. Additionally, the central visual field is represented in the occipital pole that receives a variable degree of collateral circulation from the middle cerebral artery in addition to its main supply from the posterior cerebral artery. A vascular occlusion of the posterior cerebral artery may result in a contralateral visual field loss that does not involve central vision in individuals in whom this collateral circulation is robust.

Some people with homonymous hemianopsia may still be capable of experiencing some visual sensations in the blind fields. Colored targets may be detected, while achromatic ones cannot. People lacking pattern discrimination in the hemianopic field may still be able to accurately reach and look at a moving light in the blind field (see the earlier discussion of projections from the superior colliculus, lateral posterior, and pulvinar nuclei).

Thought Question

What is the difference in cause and consequence of homonymous hemianopsia, cortical blindness, and anosognosia?

Deficits Associated with Higher Cortical Processing

The capacity to recognize visually presented objects depends not only on the integrity of the primary visual cortex (Brodmann's area 17), but also on areas 18 and 19 and the angular gyrus of the dominant hemisphere. People with **visual agnosia**, unlike those who are blind, are able to perceive, but they cannot understand the meaning of what they see. Basic visual perception is intact, in that these individuals may be able to describe accurately the size, shape, and color of an object such that they are unable to identify the object unless they are able to palpate, taste, smell, or hear it.

Bilateral lesions of area 17 of the occipital lobes may result in **cortical blindness** if the lesions are complete. This condition can occur as a result of bilateral posterior cerebral artery occlusion. The extent of loss of sight is equivalent to that following complete lesions of the optic nerves.

The pupillary light reflexes can still be elicited because the visual cortex is not part of the reflex pathway, but reflexive closing of the eyelids to bright light or threat is lost. The eyes can still move through a full range, but the person is not able to interpret anything in the visual realm. When the lesion is incomplete, the individual may have varying degrees of visual perception.

One cause of cortical blindness is embolic or thrombotic occlusion of the posterior cerebral arteries. Because the posterior cerebral arteries also supply the medial temporal lobe and thalamus, other symptoms may accompany the blindness. This condition may also result from anoxic damage, as with prenatal and perinatal injury, traumatic brain injury, or a failed suicide attempt.

When the lesions extend beyond area 17 to include visual association cortices, the obviously blind person may either be indifferent to the blindness or may deny being blind altogether. In the latter case, these individuals act as though they can see. This curious disorder is known as **Anton's syndrome**, or **visual anosognosia**.

DAMAGE TO THE PARIETO-OCCIPITAL CORTEX To understand visual disturbances associated with the parieto-occipital cortex, it is important to recall that this area is associated with identifying *where* an event occurred. Lesions in this area, especially those in the nondominant hemisphere, can result in impairments of construction and other deficits of visual–spatial processing. People with these lesions may have difficulty with such seemingly simple and routine tasks as dressing. For example, they may put clothes on backward, try to put an arm in the leg of a pair of pants, and related errors. Balint's syndrome is specifically associated with damage to this region and consists of the following: simultagnosia, optic ataxia, and ocular apraxia. **Simultagnosia** refers to a condition in which the individual can perceive only a small region of the visual field at a time. These individuals have particular difficulty scanning a complex visual field or identifying moving objects. Rather than seeing the entire field, they tend to describe only small random parts. **Optic ataxia** refers to impaired ability in reaching for or pointing to an object. The difficulty occurs because of difficulty localizing the object as opposed to ataxia of the extremity per se. Once the location is reached, the individual can repeat the motion, even with eyes closed, without ataxia. **Occular apraxia** refers to difficulty directing gaze toward objects in the peripheral vision by using saccades.

DAMAGE TO THE OCCIPITOTEMPORAL CORTEX The occipitotemporal cortex is the area of the cortex that processes the *what*, or the form, of objects. One of the most distressing disorders associated with lesions in this region is referred to as **prosopagnosia**, in which the individual is unable to recognize people by looking at them. The person with this disorder can recognize people by clothes, voice, or other attributes but not by face—even when the person is well known (e.g., a husband or daughter).

Other phenomena associated with lesions in this area include **micropsia**, in which objects appear unusually small, and **metamorphosia**, in which objects have a distorted shape or size. This is sometimes referred to as "Alice in Wonderland" syndrome and has been reported to occur with migraine, vascular lesions, and tumors of this area. In cerebral diplopia or polyopia, such people see two or more images of a single object.

Thought Question

Damage to the occipitotemporal cortex leads to very different symptoms than does damage to the parito-occipital cortex. This distinction will be of great importance when designing rehabilitation approaches for people who sustain CVAs to these regions. What is the difference in the expected symptoms?

To fully appreciate this distinction, this is a good time to synthesize how information from the retina is used to determine what an object is (form) and where it is (location).

Multiple Sclerosis

For many people, one of the first signs of multiple sclerosis (MS) is visual disturbances. About 25 percent of patients have, as the initial manifestation, an episode of optic neuritis, resulting in visual loss. Typically, this loss evolves quickly (over a period of days) and in most cases improves significantly or completely. Other visual disturbances can occur with MS, including a scotoma, involving the macular area and blind spot, visual field defects (sometimes a homonymous hemianopsia), and disturbances of the VOR in cases of brainstem lesions. The wide variety of visual deficits associated with MS reflect the fact that lesions associated with MS can occur anywhere within the CNS, without a consistent pattern from one patient to the next. Recall that the optic nerve is not a true cranial nerve. It is a CNS structure and, therefore, subject to demyelination in a central disorder such as MS.

Migraine

The prodromal phase of classic **migraine** (affecting about 1 percent of the population) frequently involves the visual cortex. A visual aura occurs in about one-third of migraine sufferers and consists of unformed flashes of white or colored light or scattered scotomata, either across the visual fields or in the periphery. About 10 percent of migraine sufferers experience a scintillating scotoma that continues to enlarge over 20 to 30 minutes, then disappears. Dazzling, zigzag lines surround the scotoma and give rise to the name *fortification spectrum* because they were fancifully likened to the battlements of a fortification. Although people may attribute the visual aura to only one eye, in actuality it is nearly always bilateral because it originates from the occipital cortex.

Summary

The visual system is one of the most plastic systems in the human brain, in that its adult function is significantly shaped by early visual experience. The structural and functional organization of the system is known in elaborate detail, beginning with the cells and their synaptology in the retina and extending to its robust cortical representation, wherein cells are organized into several different types of functional columns for analysis of input from the LGB. The organization of cells within these columns is deterministically hierarchical in that the response properties of a given neuron are defined by the projections it receives from its presynaptic neurons. Important subcortical projections are established by retinal ganglion cells. These subserve a variety of functions. For example, those projections to the superior colliculus provide an alternate route of access of visual information to visual association areas of the cortex via association nuclei of the thalamus. Unfortunately, the function of this projection is not understood. Those projections to the hypothalamus are involved in maintenance of circadian rhythms such as the sleep–wakefulness cycle. Those projections to the pretectal area mediate the pupillary light reflex.

The visual system can be affected by a variety of conditions affecting the central nervous system. Testing of the visual system is often key to localizing that damage and, in addition, can be of central importance to interpreting the implications of reduced or altered vision for postural control, perception, and interpretation of the world around us.

Applications

1. Jennifer was a 27-year-old graduate student who sought assistance for frontal and temporal headaches, which she had been experiencing for six weeks. She described difficulty seeing objects on the left, as well as numbness and clumsiness of her left hand. Provide an explanation for each of the following findings from her neurological examination.

    a. Bilateral papilledema.
    b. Left homonymous hemianopsia that was incomplete: the lower visual field was more extensively involved.
    c. Left lower facial weakness.
    d. Moderate weakness of left arm.
    e. Slight increase in reflexes at left bicep and brachioradialis tendons.

f. Sensory disturbances of the left hand:
   i. Diminished appreciation of touch and of sense of position and movement of the fingers.
   ii. Comparison of sizes and shapes and recognition of substances and textures by feel was lost.
   iii. Two-point discrimination was also defective.
   iv. Diminished discriminative response to pain was observed.
g. Where do you think her lesion is located?

2. A 38-year-old woman had experienced double vision for two weeks. She also noticed her left eyelid began drooping during the previous week. On further questioning, she stated she has not had a menstrual period for a full year and had mild bifrontal head pain intermittingly for six months. Examination revealed the following:

- Left eye deviated down and to the left.
- Left palpebral fissure was 3 mm narrower than right.
- Left pupil measured 5 mm in diameter, right 2 mm.
- Left pupil reacted sluggishly when light was directed into either eye.
- Right eye reacted to light directed into either eye.

- Visual acuity was 20/20 bilaterally.
- Confrontational visual field testing: unable to see fingers in the superior temporal field of either eye.
- Able to accurately detect mild fragrances with either nostril.
- Sensation to light touch and pinprick in all three divisions of CN V was normal.
- Motor, sensory, tendon reflexes, coordination, and gait examination were also normal.

a. What is the technical term for double vision? What are possible causes? Diagram the visual effects.
b. Identify the cranial nerve(s) affected in this case.
c. Identify where in the visual pathway a lesion can occur to produce such visual field loss.
d. She has two symptoms seemingly unrelated to the visual system that helped her neurologist to localize the lesion.
   i. Why is the head pain relevant to her condition? What does it suggest regarding the underlying type of lesion?
   ii. What does the symptom of amenorrhea suggest as to the location of the lesion?
e. Locate the area of the lesion.

References

Barton, J. J. S., Hefter, R., Chang, B., Schomer, D., and Drislane, F. The field defects of anterior lobectomy: A quantitative reassessment of Meyer's loop. *Brain* 128:2123–2133, 2005.

Berson, D. M. Phototransduction in ganglion-cell photoreceptors. *Eur J Phyiol* 454:849–855, 2007.

Kandel, E. R., and Wurtz, R. H. Ch. 2.5 Constructing the visual image. In: Kandel, E. R., Schwartz, J. H., and Jessell, T. M., eds. *Principles of Neural Science*, 4th ed. McGraw-Hill, New York, 2000.

Lennie, P. Ch. 29. Color vision. In: Kandel, E. R., Schwartz, J. H., and Jessell, T. M., eds. *Principles of Neural Science*, 4th ed. McGraw-Hill, New York, 2000.

Nolte, J. *The Human Brain: An Introduction to Its Functional Anatomy*, 6th ed. Mosby Elsevier, Philadelphia, 2009.

Remington, L. A. *Clinical Anatomy of the Visual System*, 2nd ed. Elsevier, St. Louis, 2005.

Schneider, K. A., and Kastner, S. Visual responses of the human superior colliculus: A high-resolution functional magnetic resonance imaging study. *J Neurophysiol* 94:2491–2503, 2005.

Tessier-Lavigne, M. Ch. 26. Visual processing by the retina. In: Kandel, E. R., Schwartz, J. H., and Jessell, T. M., eds. *Principles of Neural Science*, 4th ed. McGraw-Hill, New York, 2000.

Wurtz, R. H., and Kandel, E. R. Ch. 27. Central visual pathways. In: Kandel, E. R., Schwartz, J. H., and Jessell, T. M., eds. *Principles of Neural Science*, 4th ed. McGraw-Hill, New York, 2000.

Wurtz, R. H., and Kandel, E. R. Ch. 28. Perception of motion, depth, and form. In: Kandel, E. R., Schwartz, J. H., and Jessell, T. M., eds. *Principles of Neural Science*, 4th ed. McGraw-Hill, New York, 2000.

PEARSON
myhealthprofessionskit™

Use this address to access the Companion Website created for this textbook. Simply select "Physical Therapy" from the choice of disciplines. Find this book and log in using your username and password to access self-assessment questions, a glossary, and more.

Cerebellum and Basal Ganglia

LEARNING OUTCOMES

This chapter prepares the reader to:

1. Recall the meaning of the following terms related to cerebellar dysfunction: intention tremor, dysmetria, decomposition of movement, dysdiadochokinesia, ataxia, and nystagmus.

2. Analyze the cellular architecture of the cerebellum.

3. Differentiate the archicerebellum and neocerebellum based on the origin of inputs, destination of outputs, and the functional importance of each.

4. Relate the following major cerebellar tracts to the peduncle through which they travel, the phylogenetic portion of the cerebellum in which they reside, and the information that they carry: DSCT, CCT, VSCT, RSCT, trigeminocerebellar projection, interpositorubral projection, and the dentothalamic fibers.

5. Discuss the overall importance of cerebellar functions with respect to control of purposeful movement.

6. Compare the destination and role of projections from the vermis with those of the anterior lobe of the paleocerebellum.

7. Relate cerebellar syndromes to the role of the related structures of the cerebellum.

8. Describe signs that typically occur with lesions to the neocerebellum and contrast them with signs associated with lesions of the archicerebellum.

9. Explain what is meant by *disinhibition* as it relates to circuits of the basal ganglia and describe the sequence of events and outcomes involved in this process.

10. Contrast the direct and indirect pathways through the basal ganglia.

11. Recall the meaning of the following terms related to basal ganglia dysfunction: tremor, rigidity, bradykinesia, and postural instability.

12. Discuss the epidemiological factors related to Parkinson's disease (PD).

13. Explain the consequences of loss of dopamine-producing cells in the midbrain in relation to the function of the basal ganglia (BG) and the signs and symptoms of PD.

14. Compare three types of pharmacologic therapies for PD in terms of site of action and consequences: dopamine replacement, dopamine agonist, and inhibitors of dopamine metabolism.

15. Relate the basic components of the physical examination for people with PD to the underlying condition.

16. Contrast the role of pharmacological, surgical, and physical interventions in the management of individuals who have PD.

17. Contrast the location of damage associated with Huntington's disease (HD) to that associated with PD and contrast the neurotransmitters affected; relate these differences to the resulting symptoms.

18. Describe the basic components of the physical examination and interventions for people with HD.

ACRONYMS

BG Basal ganglia

CBL Cerebellum

CCT Cuneocerebellar tract

COMT Catechol-O-methyltransferase

DN Dentate nucleus

DA Dopamine

DBS Deep brain stimulation

DSCT Dorsal spinocerebellar tract

EPSP Excitatory postsynaptic potential

GABA Gamma-amino butyric acid

GDNF Glial cell line–derived neurotrophic factor

GPe Globus pallidus, external segment

GPi Globus pallidus, internal segment

HD Huntington's disease

L-Dopa Levadopa

LMN Lower motor neuron

MAO Monoamine oxidase

PD Parkinson's disease

RF Reticular formation

RSCT Rostral spinocerebellar tract

SN Substantia nigra

SNpc Substantia nigra pars compacta

SNpr Substantia nigra pars reticulata

STN Subthalamic nucleus

VSCT Ventral spinocerebellar tract

VTA Ventral tegmental area

Introduction

The gross anatomy and blood supply of the cerebellum were presented in Chapter 6 and those of the basal ganglia in Chapter 7. This chapter revisits both of these important structures, but primarily from the perspective of their role in movement and because both the cerebellum and basal ganglia are important and common targets of neurological disease. Their involvement gives rise to distinctive constellations of neurologic signs and symptoms, depending importantly on the location of the pathology in a particular structure.

The first major section of this chapter deals with the cerebellum. We begin with a discussion of the circuitry within the cerebellum itself, which is uniform throughout the entire structure. Despite this uniformity, the cerebellum may be subdivided into three regions that subserve different functions: the archicerebellum, the paleocerebellum, and the neocerebellum. The functional specificity of each region derives from the uniqueness of its input and output connections—that is, the circuitry through the cerebellum. These connections are defined for each of the three regions. Next, the role of the cerebellum is discussed with respect to motor learning. This section ends with clinical connections, including examples of the syndromes seen in humans following lesions that affect each of the three regions as well as implications for physical rehabilitation.

The second major section of this chapter concerns the basal ganglia. As in the first section, we begin with a discussion of the circuitry of the basal ganglia. This time, however, we do not consider the intrinsic circuitry within the basal ganglia but, rather, focus on the circuitry through the basal ganglia. This circuit comprises a loop that begins in the cerebral cortex, projects to the striatum where it synapses, then synapses in the *internal* segment of the globus pallidus–substantia nigra pars reticulata, and returns to the motor cortices via the thalamus. This is called the direct circuit, and its function is to facilitate movement. A second circuit is routed through the *external* segment of the globus pallidus and subthalamic nucleus before it reaches the internal segment of the globus pallidus–substantia nigra pars reticulata. This is called the indirect circuit, and its function is to suppress movement. The remainder of this section is clinical. Two diseases of particular importance to the rehabilitation specialist affect specific components of the circuitry through the basal ganglia. The first, Parkinson's disease, is by far the most frequent, and it is considered in depth—both its pathophysiology and treatment—including pharmacological, surgical, and physical rehabilitation. Huntington's disease (chorea) is the second of the diseases discussed. Significantly, major components of the symptomatology of these diseases can be explained by changes in the function of the direct and indirect pathways through the basal ganglia. Implications for physical rehabilitation are considered. The final portion of this section discusses a clinical disorder that follows damage to the subthalamic nucleus: hemiballismus.

CEREBELLUM

Clinical Preview ·················

In your rehabilitation practice, you work with individuals who have a wide range of cerebellar disorders. Mrs. Karch is one such individual. She sustained a gunshot wound with damage restricted to the left side of her neocerebellum. Mr. Ogelthorpe has long-standing alcoholism with substantial degeneration of the paleocerebellum. And Laney is a 3-year-old child who was recently diagnosed with a medulloblastoma, located along the nodulus of her cerebellum. As you read through this section, consider the following:

- What constellation of symptoms, based on region of the cerebellum involved, would be expected for each of these individuals?

- How do the symptoms relate to the physiological role of these three areas of the cerebellum?

- What clinical examinations could you perform with each of these three individuals?

Thought Question

In preparation for understanding the content of this chapter, review content in Chapter 6 related to the cells that make up the cerebellum, the overall structure of the cerebellum, the nuclei, the peduncles, and the different nomenclatures used to define portions of this important structure.

As intensively studied as the structure and function of the cerebellum has been ever since the early 20th century, there still is a lack of consensus as to the nature of the fundamental cerebellar operation and how it is accomplished. There is, however, an abundance of information on its histological features and synaptology, its extensively known neuronal physiology, its well-established input and output connectivity patterns, and the documented characteristic clinical signs that result from its damage. Additionally, one of the more formidable problems in understanding the functions of the human cerebellum is that the cerebella of nonhuman primates and mammals, such as the cat (the subjects of experimental research), differ from that of the human.

Many theories have been advanced as to the specialized functions of different regions of the cerebellum. Most are just that—theories. Perhaps the prime example of this is the voluminous literature relating to the discharge of single neurons in the cerebella of monkeys trained to perform isolated movements of single joints. Correlations between discharge patterns and movement parameters were weak at best and sometimes nonexistent, as well as being inconsistent across studies. One reason is that the cerebellum is not concerned with single joint movements, but with multijoint movements. The cerebellar regulation of compound multijoint movement has, in fact, been inferred from clinical observation by neurologists such as Sir Gordon Holmes, who was among the first (1917) to carefully document the deficits following cerebellar damage. Holmes believed that defective multijoint movement was the result of cumulative errors in the regulation. Among the errors that he described with respect to compound movements are delay of initiation and abnormalities in the rate, range, and contraction force of the constituent, single-joint movements of which the compound movement was composed. Current thinking is that the cerebellum has an important comparator function, allowing for comparison of the intended movement with the actual movement as a means of detecting movement errors and then providing for ongoing corrections as the movement evolves.

The arrangement of cerebellar neurons is so regular that a description of the microcircuitry in one cerebellar area is uniformly descriptive of that in all other portions of the cerebellum. The extraordinary constancy of this microcircuitry has driven the search for a corresponding unitary functional principle that forms the basis for all cerebellar operations. Yet, despite its elegantly simple structure and transparent neuronal circuitry, a coherent model of cerebellar function remains elusive. In fact, despite the considerable uniformity of cytoarchitectural structure across the cerebellum, the functions of different regions of the cerebellum are widely different. The differences are conveyed by the origin of inputs and destination of outputs from the cerebellum. Thus, we shall look at the input–output relations of different cerebellar regions in attempting to define function. But first, the microcircuitry of the cerebellum will be defined.

Circuitry of the Cerebellum

Recall from Chapter 6 that the cerebellar cortex has a uniform and simple three-layered structure. Thus, unlike the cerebral cortex (described in Chapter 7), the cerebellum shows no cytoarchitectural subdivisions. As described later, two of the three layers of the cerebellum are each comprised of different cell types. The third layer is comprised mostly of dendrites and axons from cells originating in the other layers, with a much lower density of neurons. An appreciation of the three layers of the cerebellar cortex is of importance in understanding its functional role.

Layers

Most superficial is the **molecular layer**, which has a low cell (neuron) density. This layer primarily contains the dendritic arborizations of cells that reside in the deeper layers—numerous thin axons that run parallel to the long axis of the folia. In addition, this layer contains two types of inhibitory interneurons: stellate cells in its outer portion and basket cells in its inner portion. The extensive dendritic tree of each Purkinje cell, whose flask-shaped cell bodies form the single-cell-thick, middle Purkinje cell layer, extends into the molecular layer. The unique feature of Purkinje cell dendrites is that they are flattened into a single plane oriented perpendicular to the long axis of the folium in which the dendritic tree is situated.

The **Purkinje layer**, or middle layer, contains the cell bodies of the Purkinje cells (which are neurons, but typically identified as *cells*). The Purkinje cells are inhibitory to the neurons on which they synapse, primarily neurons of the deep cerebellar nuclei. They release the transmitter gamma-amino butyric acid (GABA).

Finally, the innermost cortical layer, or **granular layer**, is comprised of tightly packed granule cells (neurons) that are excitatory, releasing glutamate onto the Purkinje cells. Granule cells send their axons into the molecular layer, where each bifurcates to form a fine unmyelinated parallel fiber that extends about 5 mm along the long axis of a folium. Each parallel fiber passes through and synapses on the dendritic tree of as many as 500 Purkinje cells. The granular layer also contains the cell bodies of inhibitory interneurons called Golgi neurons (Figure 19-1 ■).

Thought Question

In earlier discussions about the spinal cord, we related damage and expected symptoms to the specific area of the cord and the levels of the spinal column that were affected. The relationships are more complicated with respect to lesions of the cerebellum. As you proceed through this section, identify major differences between the spinal cord and cerebellum that make it difficult to draw functional relationships between symptoms and site of lesion for the cerebellum.

Thought Question

Which of the three layers of the cerebellum contain neurons that release inhibitory neurotransmitters and which contain neurons that release excitatory neurotransmitters? What is the overall action of the output of the cerebellum—excitatory or inhibitory?

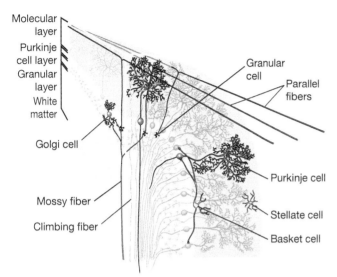

FIGURE 19-1 Three layers of the cerebellum and the cells (neurons) that comprise them.

Peduncles, Inputs, and Outputs

Three peduncles connect the cerebellum with the remainder of the CNS, as described in Chapter 6. The **inferior cerebellar peduncle** (also called the restiform body) connects the cerebellum with the spinal cord. The **middle cerebellar peduncle** (also called the brachium pontis) has massive connections with the pons. These two peduncles primarily carry inputs to the cerebellum. In contrast, the **superior cerebellar peduncle** (also called the brachium conjuctivum), mainly carries outputs from the cerebellum.

Input to the cerebellum, as indicated in Chapter 6, is primarily via two main fiber systems: mossy fibers and climbing fibers. The most direct route to Purkinje cells is via climbing fibers, all of which originate in the contralateral inferior olivary nucleus. Named for the morphology of their terminations on Purkinje cells, each climbing fiber climbs the dendrites of a single Purkinje cell like ivy winding around a trellis. The climbing fiber–Purkinje cell synapse is excitatory and is one of the most powerful in the nervous system. A single climbing fiber action potential elicits a huge excitatory postsynaptic potential (EPSP) that produces a short high frequency burst of Purkinje cell action potentials.

Mossy fibers are most numerous and also project to Purkinje cells, but not directly. They originate from a variety of sources, including the vestibular nuclei, spinal cord, and cerebral cortex. Those from the cerebral cortex reach the cerebellum via the pontocerebellar projection system. These fibers travel in the middle cerebellar peduncle, one of the most massive pathways in the brain. Mossy fibers terminate on the dendrites of granule cells whose axons, in turn, synapse on the spines of Purkinje cell dendrites via parallel fibers. Mossy fibers are also excitatory to the neurons on which they synapse.

Output from the cerebellum is only via the Purkinje cells. These neurons either project directly to the vestibular

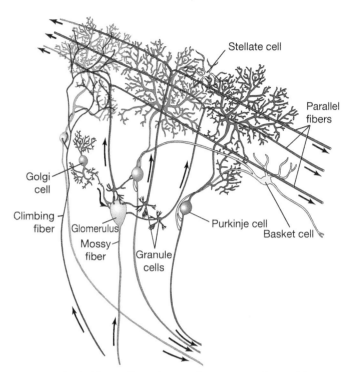

FIGURE 19-2 Mossy fibers have *indirect* connections with Purkinje cells, whereas climbing fibers have *direct* connections with the Purkinje cells. Mossy and climbing fibers are input fibers to the cerebellum, whereas axons of Purkinje cells are the output fibers.

nuclei or synapse in deep cerebellar nuclei, which in turn project to destinations outside the cerebellum. Because they are inhibitory, the net effect of Purkinje cell output is inhibitory.

Outputs from the cerebellum are modulated as follows: Both mossy and climbing fibers send collaterals to neurons of the deep cerebellar nuclei before continuing on to end on neurons of the cerebellar cortex (Figure 19-2 ■). These projections excite neurons of the deep cerebellar nuclei and provide a background excitatory drive on neurons of the deep nuclei. This represents the main excitatory loop through the cerebellum. This excitatory loop is then modulated by an inhibitory side loop that passes through neurons of the cerebellar cortex and is mediated by Purkinje neurons. Purkinje neurons are driven by the same excitatory inputs as the main excitatory loop, as well as by inhibitory interneurons of the cortex. The latter include basket cells and stellate cells that synapse, respectively, on the cell body and dendrites of Purkinje cells. Golgi cell interneurons receive excitatory inputs from granule cell parallel fibers (in the molecular layer). They then provide feedback inhibition onto the granule cell dendrites in the granule layer. The inhibitory action of Purkinje neurons has been depicted as *sculpting* (shaping) the background excitatory output from the deep nuclei. Increasing the discharge of Purkinje cells via their excitatory drives decreases output from the deep cerebellar nuclei, whereas decreasing the discharge of Purkinje cells via their inhibitory cortical drives increases deep nuclear output through disinhibition.

Which cerebellar loops are excitatory and which are inhibitory? Which neurotransmitters are responsible for these two types of neuronal influences?

Cerebellar Input–Output Connections in Relation to Function

As discussed in Chapter 6, the cerebellum is divisible into three regions based on four different criteria:

1. Its gross anatomy as determined by its two major fissures (flocculonodular lobe, anterior lobe, and posterior lobe).
2. The phylogeny of its gross anatomy (archicerebellum, paleocerebellum, and neocerebellum).
3. The source of afferent fibers projecting to different regions of the cerebellar cortex (vestibulocerebellum, spinocerebellum, and pontocerebellum).
4. The pattern of projections from the cerebellar cortex to its underlying deep nuclei (medial zone, intermediate zone, and lateral zone).

Thus, a number of different nomenclatures have been developed to describe the components of the cerebellum. Despite all of the nomenclature, none of the options precisely correlates structure with function in a manner that can be used to explain all clinical conditions. However, archicerebellum, paleocerebellum, and neocerebellum are often used interchangeably with vestibulocerebellum, spinocerebellum, and pontocerebellum, respectively. No naturally occurring lesions exist that fit any of these terms in isolation. For example, cerebellar lesions may involve more than one phylogenetic region; inputs from different sources may go to more than one cerebellar lobe. In some instances, we use phylogentic terminology, whereas in others it is more appropriate to use functional terminology. The relationship between phylogenetic and functional terminology is summarized in Table 19-1 ■.

Thinking ahead and based on your knowledge of neuroanatomy to date, what do you suppose might be the role of each of the following inputs to the cerebellum: vestibular, spinal, and cortical?

Phylogenetic terminology is used, despite the limitations just described, to name two clearly defined syndromes of particular importance in rehabilitation. The first is the **archicerebellar syndrome**, resulting from damage to the flocculonodular lobe and deep parts of the vermis. Note that the archicerebellum is sometimes referred to as the vestibulocerebellum, and as such we often see vestibular-like symptoms with the archicerebellar syndromes. The second is the **neocerebellar syndrome**, resulting from damage to the largest part of the cerebellum, the lateral hemispheres of the anterior and posterior lobes We shall use this phylogenetic terminology because not only is it the most accurate anatomically in terms of correlating clinical deficits with anatomy, but it provides a framework for understanding the cognitive functions of the cerebellum presented in Chapter 21. By default, then, we are left with a **paleocerebellar syndrome**. Recall the paleocerebellum is comprised of the intermediate zone and most of the vermis. Because the paleocerebellum consists of components residing in both the anterior and posterior lobes and includes both midline and paravermal cortex (see Figure 6-17) the lesion would have to extend from the superior to inferior surface of the cerebellum and be confined to vermal and paravermal cortex, an exceedingly unlikely occurrence. Thus, a clearly defined paleocerebellar syndrome does not appear to occur in humans. What we call the paleocerebellar syndrome involves just the component of the paleocerebellum residing in the anterior lobe

Archicerebellar Connections and Function

Connections to the flocculonodular lobe and fastigial nucleus from the vestibular nuclei (Figure 19-3 ■), along with projections from the retina, are central to the role of the cerebellum in influencing and maintaining equilibrium (stance and gait). Vestibular afferents project to the archicerebellum from two sources: fibers from the ipsilateral vestibular division of CN VIII that project directly to the archicerebellum without synapsing in the brainstem (primary fibers) and axons that originate from cell bodies within ipsilateral vestibular nuclei (secondary fibers). Vestibular afferents convey information from the labyrinths concerning the position of the head in space (static information) and changes in head position (dynamic information). Such information reflexively influences the distribution of tone in the limb, trunk, neck, and extraocular musculature. These reflexively induced muscular adjustments are in a direction

Table 19-1 Terminology Used to Discuss the Cerebellum

PHYLOGENY	LOBES	LONGITUDINAL ZONES	FUNCTIONAL REGIONS
Archicerebellum	Flocculonodular	Vermis	Vestibulocerebellum
Paleocerebellum	Anterior	Intermediate	Spinocerebellum
Neocerebellum	Posterior	Lateral	Pontocerebellum

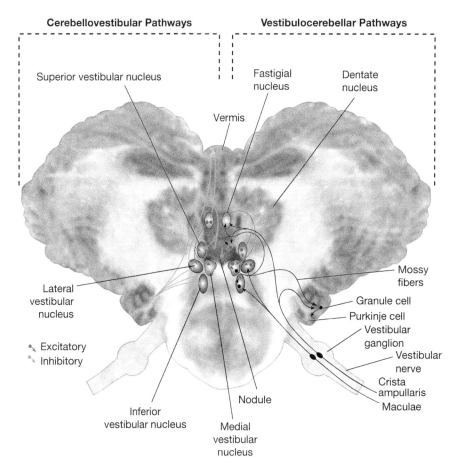

Cerebellovestibular Pathways

Vestibulocerebellar Pathways

Superior vestibular nucleus

Fastigial nucleus

Dentate nucleus

Vermis

Mossy fibers

Granule cell

Lateral vestibular nucleus

Purkinje cell

Vestibular ganglion

Excitatory

Vestibular nerve

Inhibitory

Crista ampullaris

Maculae

Nodule

Inferior vestibular nucleus

Medial vestibular nucleus

FIGURE 19-3 Connections of the archicerebellum. Vestibular afferent project directly and indirectly by way of the fastigial nuclei to the archicerebellum.

that opposes the disturbing force; therefore, they act to maintain a normal upright posture and horizontal head position (refer to Chapter 17).

In addition to vestibular information, the flocculonodular lobe receives information from the retina via an indirect route that involves climbing fibers from the inferior olivary nucleus. Purkinje cells of the flocculus have been shown to respond selectively to the direction in which a visual stimulus moves across the retina. This information is important in regulating the vestibulo-ocular reflex (see Chapter 17).

Archicerebellar efferents leave the cerebellum (see Figure 19-3) and project to two brainstem structures: the vestibular nuclei and reticular formation. Influences on the vestibular nuclei are mediated by direct as well as indirect cerebellar projections. The direct projection consists of Purkinje cell axons that end directly on vestibular nuclear neurons. The indirect projection consists of Purkinje cell axons that end on neurons of the fastigial nucleus whose axons, in turn, terminate on vestibular neurons. The vestibular nuclei receive incoming labyrinthine information and, after intranuclear processing, distribute it to segmental motor neurons via descending vestibulospinal tracts and to extraocular motor neurons via ascending medial longitudinal fasciculus fibers (MLF). However, portions of the vestibular nuclear complex serve also as a major cerebellar

output station so that ascending and descending projection systems emanating from the vestibular nuclei carry both labyrinthine and cerebellar information.

Thought Question

What important roles did you learn about previously for the MLF?

The outputs from the archicerebellum (along with other regions), their main motor function, and the upper motor neuron pathway influenced by these connections are summarized in Table 19-2 ■.

Archicerebellar influences on the reticular formation (RF) are conveyed to the spinal cord via descending reticulospinal tracts and to brainstem extraocular motor nuclei via ascending fibers of the RF. Neurons of the RF receive abundant secondary projections from the vestibular nuclei; thus, they are importantly modulated by labyrinthine information. To sum up, the muscular adjustments that maintain equilibrium and regulate position of the eyes are managed by the vestibular nuclei and RF—both of which receive and process labyrinthine information, both of which send their

Table 19-2 Regions of the Motor Cerebellum

REGION	MAIN FUNCTION	UPPER MOTOR NEURON PATHWAY INFLUENCED
Flocculonodular lobe	Equilibrium and vestibulo-ocular reflexes	Medial longitudinal fasciculus, vestibulospinal and reticulospinal tracts
Vermis of anterior and posterior lobes	Movement coordination of proximal limb and axial muscles	Anterior corticospinal, reticulospinal, vestibulospinal, and tectospinal tracts
Intermediate zone of hemisphere	Movement coordination of distal limbs	Lateral corticospinal and rubrospinal tracts
Lateral zone of hemisphere	Motor planning	Lateral corticospinal tract

output to segmental and extraocular motoneurons, and both of which are strongly influenced by the cerebellum.

Removal of the flocculonodular lobe in monkeys results in a syndrome of disequilibrium, characterized by falling, oscillations of the head and trunk, and a gait characterized by staggering and a wide base of support. That these are deficits in the vestibular control of posture and movement is clear from the fact that voluntary and postural reflex movements are not impaired if the trunk is supported against gravity, a maneuver that reduces vestibular contributions to movement. Isolated lesions of the fastigial nucleus in monkeys prevent the animal from sitting, standing, and walking, with frequent falls to the side of the lesion. Much of the body musculature is involved, but only for stance and gait. Given the efferent connections of the flocculonodular lobe, it is clear that an archicerebellar lesion would have two interrelated effects. Because the vestibular nuclei are under continual cerebellar control, the lesion would disrupt the processing of labyrinthine information in the nuclei as well as alter the motor output from them. An analogous effect would be exerted on the brainstem reticular formation.

Animal experimentation has revealed two additional functions for the flocculonodular lobe. First, ablation of the nodulus (and uvula) confers an apparent immunity to motion sickness upon an animal, thus implicating the nodulus in the genesis of motion sickness. The nodulus is the vermal portion of the flocculonodular lobe. The uvula is the vermal portion of the cerebellar tonsils (see Figure 6-12). Secondly, removal of the vestibulocerebellum reduces the plasticity of the vestibulo-ocular reflex.

Paleocerebellar Connections and Function

Based on the input–output connections of the paleocerebellum, it is likely that one of its fundamental roles is its comparator function, by which intended movement is compared with the movement as it is executed, with appropriate adjustments made to the ongoing movement. Information about the intended movement (referred to as an **efference copy**) also is sent to the cerebellum. As initial phases of a movement are executed, patterns of peripheral receptor discharge change, and the cerebellum receives a

description of the portion of the movement actually effected (e.g., limb position, velocity, muscle contractile forces, agonist–antagonist relations). Such input enables the cerebellum to assess whether the next portion of the cerebral motor command is appropriate to the efference copy and to the prevailing limb status upon which it is to be superimposed. If the comparison does not match, it is thought cerebellar output modifies the command. The cerebellum thus constantly updates movement as it is evolving through a modification of command signals directed to the LMNs. As such, this automatic comparator-based mechanism does not operate as a follow-up corrective system, but rather occurs simultaneously with the movement.

Unlike the archicerebellum, the functions of the paleocerebellum, as defined anatomically in Chapter 6, are not definitively apparent, yet, somewhat paradoxically, a voluminous animal literature exists on its input–output connections, as will become evident later. Various authors have considered the paleocerebellum to be the part of the cerebellum most concerned with the regulation of muscle tone and with the coordination of postural activities (e.g., standing) and gait. All authors agree that its regulatory sphere embraces the musculature of the whole body. Our discussion will focus largely on the anterior lobe component of the paleocerebellum because this is the component that has the most clinical applicability.

As described in Chapters 17 and 18, regulation of postural activities such as standing (the maintenance of an upright stance) depends on three sensory modalities: proprioception, vision, and vestibular. All three of these modalities are heavily represented in the vermis throughout the whole of the corpus cerebelli. The stretch reflexes mediated by muscle spindles represent the raw material of standing, and in a sense, their regulation is more fundamental to standing than equilibrium. Equilibrium is one aspect of this control in which vestibular input is important. But, in addition, proprioception and vision are important factors. Proprioception is important because interruption of its input either in the dorsal roots (as in tabes dorsalis) or in the dorsal columns of the spinal cord results in **sensory ataxia**, wherein standing without swaying is difficult,

Thought Question

This is a good time to synthesize important information related to postural control. Lesions involving the archicerebellum result in very different symptoms from lesions involving the paleocerebellum. How do the symptoms associated with these two types of lesions compare, and what are the important differences in the connections of these two regions that explain the difference in symptoms?

particularly with the eyes closed (Romberg sign), and gait is uncoordinated. The role of vision in standing is readily apparent when we stand on a single foot and compare the amount of body sway with the eyes closed and with them open.

Cells of origin of the spinocerebellar systems possess a more complex organization than originally assumed. Some cells process proprioceptive and exteroceptive information separately; others respond to both types of input. Furthermore, significant integrative activity may occur in these cells—some, for example, integrate information from descending supraspinal pathways with various combinations of input from the periphery. Finally, a given peripheral input may concurrently activate neurons belonging to several spinocerebellar projections.

Given this segregation of somatosensory input by body part, it is to be expected that the *spinocerebellum* contains somatotopic sensory maps. Indeed, the entire body is mapped in two different areas of the cerebellar cortex, although the mapping is not nearly as precise as that in the primary sensorimotor cortex. One map is located mainly in the anterior lobe, whereas the other lies in the posterior lobe. In each map, the head is located nearest the primary fissure (Figure 19-4 ■) such that the two maps are inverted relative to one another. In the anterior lobe representation, the neck and trunk are immediately adjacent to the midline, and the arms and lower extremities are represented in the paravermal cortex (i.e., in the intermediate zone). Furthermore, as we noted in Chapter

6, each of the deep cerebellar nuclei contains a complete output map of the entire body.

FIVE TRACTS OF THE PALEOCEREBELLUM Five main afferent tracts are associated with the paleocerebellum that are of importance in the control of movement. This afferent input to the cerebellum is presumably used in the comparator function of the cerebellum, providing information about what actually occurred during ongoing movement. As will be discussed later, efferent inputs to the cerebellum arise from the motor cortex and can provide information about the intended movement. The comparator function suggests that these two sources of information are compared; ongoing adjustments then are made as necessary. Thus, considering the comparator function of the cerebellum, it is appropriate that somatosensory inputs reach the cerebellum broadly from the lower and upper extremities; torso; and head, neck, and face.

The five ascending projections convey afferent information from the spinal cord and brainstem to the paleocerebellum, terminating chiefly in the anterior lobe. Two of these tracts are related to the lower limbs and lower trunk (the dorsal and ventral spinocerebellar tracts); two to the upper limbs, upper trunk, and neck (the cuneocerebellar and rostral spinocerebellar tracts); and one to the head and intraoral structures (the trigeminocerebellar projection).

The **dorsal spinocerebellar tract (DSCT)** originates from neurons of the **nucleus dorsalis**, or **Clarke's column**, located medially at the base of the dorsal horn in spinal cord segments T1 to L2 or L3 (see Figure 5-4). Axons of Clarke's column cells course laterally into the ipsilateral lateral funiculus and take up a position in the dorsolateral periphery of the funiculus, where they turn rostrally and ascend as the DSCT (Figure 19-5 ■). The DSCT is not present caudal to L3 because the nucleus dorsalis does not exist below this level. However, afferents derived from segments caudal to L3 are represented in the DSCT. Such afferents reach the nucleus dorsalis by ascending in the fasciculus gracilis. The DSCT enters the cerebellum via the inferior cerebellar peduncle. It terminates ipsilaterally in both anterior and posterior lobe components of the spinocerebellum, but primarily in the intermediate zone of the anterior lobe. Fibers end only in those cerebellar regions containing the representations of the lower limbs.

The DSCT conveys information from muscle spindles (primary and secondary endings), Golgi tendon organs, joint receptors, pressure receptors, and cutaneous receptors from the lower extremities and lower trunk. Based on responses to peripheral receptors, the DSCT has been divided into proprioceptive and exteroceptive subdivisions,

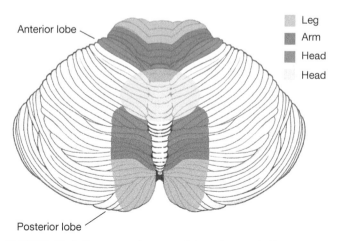

Anterior lobe

Leg
Arm
Head
Head

Posterior lobe

FIGURE 19-4 Somatotopic maps of the spinocerebellum.

Thought Question

Compare and contrast the somatosensory information conveyed by the DSCT and the CCT.

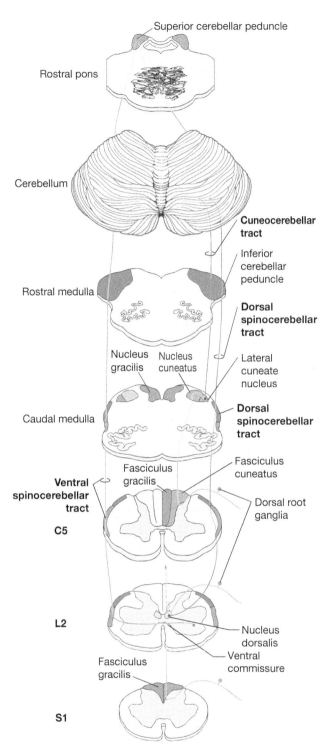

FIGURE 19-5 Three of the five afferent cerebellar tracts are depicted: the DSCT, VSCT, and CCT.

and the tract is capable of conducting modality-specific and space-specific information to the cerebellum. This projection is usually referred as conveying *unconscious proprioception* because it does not go to the cerebral cortex.

The **cuneocerebellar tract (CCT)** is for the upper extremities, neck, and upper trunk what the DSCT is for the lower extremities and lower trunk in that the two possess similar organizational features. The cells of origin of the

CCT are located in both the **lateral (external) cuneate nucleus** and the **main cuneate nucleus (nucleus cuneatus)** of the medulla (see Figure 19-5). Branches of dorsal root fibers from cervical and upper thoracic nerves pass over the posterior horns, turn rostrally, and ascend in the fasciculus cuneatus. Upon reaching the caudal medulla, they synapse on neurons of the lateral cuneate nucleus whose axons then enter the adjacent ipsilateral inferior cerebellar peduncle within which they project to cerebellar cortex. CCT axons end in those spinocerebellar regions related to the representations of the upper extremities. Like the DSCT, the CCT conveys proprioceptive and exteroceptive functional subdivisions (unconscious proprioception). Most axons of the proprioceptive subdivision are derived from the lateral cuneate nucleus and respond most effectively to group Ia muscle spindle input, although some respond to activation of Golgi tendon organs. Axons of the exteroceptive subdivision originate primarily from cells of the main cuneate nucleus and respond to cutaneous stimuli.

The **ventral spinocerebellar tract (VSCT)**, like the DSCT, is related to the lower trunk and lower extremities. Fibers of the VSCT arise from a scattered cell column located primarily in the dorsolateral portion of the ventral horn (see Figure 19-5). These cells are distributed over lumbar and sacral spinal cord segments. Axons of the cells cross to the opposite side of the cord and take up a position at the periphery of the lateral funiculus, ventral to the DSCT. Unlike the DSCT, the VSCT does not enter the cerebellum via the inferior cerebellar peduncle; rather, it ascends through the medulla and most of the pons. At upper pontine levels, the tract enters the cerebellum by coursing along the dorsal surface of the superior cerebellar peduncle. After decussating again, the fibers terminate in the regions of lower extremity representation in the anterior lobe and paramedian lobule.

One of the major differences between the DSCT and VSCT has been revealed by recording the activity of DSCT and VSCT neurons during locomotion. Both types of neurons are phasically active during locomotion. However, after sectioning the dorsal roots, DSCT neurons no longer show phasic activity, while VSCT neurons continue to discharge in phase with the step cycle. This shows that VSCT neurons, unlike DSCT neurons, did not receive excitatory drive from peripheral receptors, but rather from spinal cord interneurons and descending motor tracts. All of the major descending pathways are capable of powerfully influencing the cells of origin of the VSCT. Thus, the two tracts are forwarding fundamentally different types of information to the cerebellum: the DSCT (and CCT) signals the cerebellum about the movement being executed via unconscious proprioception (i.e., the actual movements), whereas the VSCT informs it about the motor commands being transmitted to motor neurons (i.e., the intended movements).

The upper extremity equivalent of the VSCT is the **rostral spinocerebellar tract (RSCT)**. Its cells of origin are distributed over cervical segments but have not been identified with certainty. RSCT fibers ascend uncrossed,

Thought Question

What are the fundamental differences in the anatomical structures and functional roles of the DSCT and CCT compared with the VSCT and RSCT?

with some entering the cerebellum by way of the superior cerebellar peduncle and others by way of the inferior cerebellar peduncle. Unlike the CCT, the RSCT terminates in both upper and lower extremity representations of the anterior lobe. Neurons of the RSCT respond to group Ib afferents and flexor reflex afferents. These four tracts (DSCT, CCT, VSCT, and RSCT) project ipsilaterally to the cerebellum. They do so either by remaining ipsilateral or by crossing twice. This helps explain why motor deficits after unilateral cerebellar lesions are ipsilateral to the lesion.

Projections from the face and intraoral structures to the cerebellum have been investigated less intensively than those from the spinal cord, particularly with respect to function. However, the mesencephalic nucleus, main sensory nucleus, and spinal trigeminal nucleus (with the exception of the subnucleus caudalis) all contribute to the **trigeminocerebellar projection**. Some fibers enter the cerebellum via the superior cerebellar peduncle, others via the inferior cerebellar peduncle (e.g., those from spinal trigeminal nucleus). Trigeminocerebellar afferents terminate ipsilaterally in the posterior lobe areas containing the face representation.

Visual (and auditory) input likewise projects to the paleocerebellum. This projection overlies that of somatosensation of the head and provides the visual component in the maintenance of the body's orientation in space and upright stance.

Efferent projections from the paleocerebellum are fundamentally different for its vermal and intermediate zones (see Table 19-2). Projections from the vermis are similar to those outlined previously for the vestibulocerebellum: vermal cortex influences the vestibular nuclei either directly or by way of the fastigial nucleus. Vermal Purkinje cells exert an especially pronounced direct inhibitory effect on cells of the lateral vestibular nucleus (Deiter's nucleus). It is noteworthy that this is the only example of Purkinje cells projecting out of the cerebellum and is the only inhibitory output of the cerebellum; all other Purkinje cells project to cerebellar deep nuclei, which are the primary efferent output of the cerebellum and have excitatory effects on postsynaptic targets. This cerebellar influence is then conveyed to segmental levels via the lateral vestibulospinal tract. The lateral vestibulospinal tract exerts an excitatory action on spinal cord motoneurons supplying extensor muscles. Axons from the fastigial nucleus also project to the contralateral ventrolateral nucleus of the thalamus. Thalamocortical axons then terminate on neurons of the primary motor cortex that regulate the axial and proximal limb musculature. Thus, the primary influence of the medial cerebellum is on the ventromedial component of the descending motor system important for the regulation of posture during voluntary movement.

Projections from Purkinje cells of the anterior lobe intermediate zone go to the nucleus interpositus. Some axons from the nucleus interpositus project, via the superior cerebellar peduncle, to the large cell (magnocellular) component of the red nucleus of the midbrain. Such axons form the **interpositorubral projection**. However, the size of the magnocellular RN in humans is very small, meaning that the size of the rubrospinal tract that arises from its cells is correspondingly small. The significance of the rubrospinal tract to normal motor behavior in humans is unknown but is likely to have comparatively little significance given its small size. Most axons from the interposed nucleus bypass the RN and continue rostrally to synapse in the ventrolateral nucleus of the thalamus whose axons, in turn, terminate in the primary motor cortex concerned with the control of the limb muscles. Ablation of the interpositorubral projection in monkeys results in a marked tremor of 3 to 5 Hz during reaching movements, but not during sitting, standing, or walking.

Neocerebellar Connections and Function

Connections of the neocerebellum indicate that it plays an important role in the governance of voluntary movement, a concept strongly supported by clinical as well as experimental data. This applies particularly to the synthesis of signals that relate to the planning of movement. However, it is not the only cerebellar component contributing importantly to voluntary movement; the paleocerebellum does as well.

Thought Question

Differentiate the archi- and neocerebellum based on the input and output functions and the functional importance of each.

Unlike the paleocerebellum, the neocerebellum does not receive input from peripheral receptors. Afferent projections to the neocerebellum originate in motor and association cortices located in the cerebral cortex (see Chapter 7). The association cortex then projects to the cerebellum via the pons (Figure 19-6 ■). Axons of cerebrocortical neurons descend in the internal capsule and cerebral peduncle to pontine levels, where they synapse on cells of the pontine nuclei. Within the cerebral peduncle, **frontopontine fibers** are located within the approximate medial third of each side. Fibers from parietal, occipital, and temporal cortices to the pons are located laterally within the cerebral peduncles. Mossy fiber axons from pontine nuclei cells of each side enter the contralateral middle cerebellar peduncle and terminate on dentate nucleus (DN) cells and granule cells of the lateral zone cortex. The complete pathway is usually referred to as the *corticopontocerebellar projection*, but note that such a term could apply to fibers from any cerebrocortical area to any cerebellar area. Understanding the relationship of the cortical projections to the cerebellum is helpful in understanding the localization of lesions. Recall that damage to the cerebellum

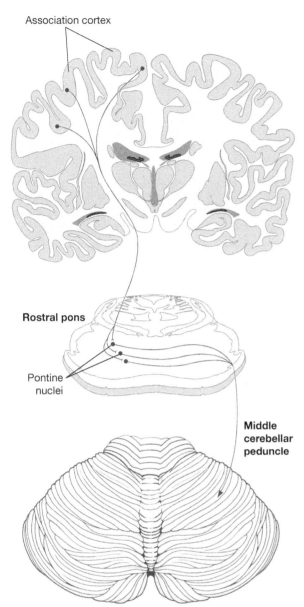

peduncle sweep ventromedially into the brainstem tegmentum prior to decussating at the level of the inferior colliculus. The crossed fibers continue their ascent, passing through and surrounding the red nucleus. DN axons terminate in two main structures: the contralateral red nucleus and the contralateral ventrolateral nuclear complex of the thalamus. Ablation of the DN in monkeys causes deficits in reaching—resulting in the overshoot of a target as well as incoordination of compound finger movements, wherein the monkey relies on an increased use of single-digit movements as opposed to pinching movements in picking up pieces of food.

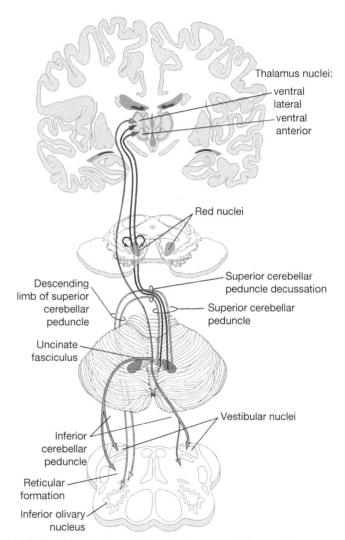

FIGURE 19-6 Afferent projections to the neocerebellum (frontopontine fibers) originate in the motor and association areas of the cortex. These fibers synapse in nuclei in the pons whose neurons decussate and enter the cerebellum by way of the middle cerebellar peduncle. This pathway in its entirety is also referred to as the corticopontocerebellar projection.

globally, or to the ascending cerebellar tracts specifically, will result in motor deficits on the ipsilateral side. However, damage to the cortical projections to the pons would result in contralateral motor deficits.

Purkinje cells of the neocerebellum project onto neurons of the DN. Dentate efferents exit the cerebellum via the ipsilateral superior cerebellar peduncle (Figure 19-7 ■). Fibers from the interposed nuclei also run in this peduncle. The superior cerebellar peduncle courses rostrally into the upper pons, where it forms the dorsolateral wall of the fourth ventricle. At the junction of pons and midbrain, fibers of the superior cerebellar

FIGURE 19-7 Efferents from the deep cerebellar nuclei. Projections from the dentate nuclei exit the cerebellum via the ipsilateral superior cerebellar peduncle, decussate, and then terminate in two main structures: the contralateral red nucleus and the contralateral thalamus. Some projections from the interposed nuclei also decussate and travel to the red nucleus and the VA/VL of the thalamus. Other projections ascend, decussate, and then descend to the contralateral inferior olivary nucleus. Projections from the fastigial nucleus are bilateral, traveling by way of the inferior cerebellar peduncle to the vestibular nuclei and inferior olivary nucleus and reticular formation.

The **dentatothalamic fibers** can be identified immediately dorsolateral to the red nucleus. Dentate efferents terminate in a number of thalamic zones collectively known as the *ventral lateral complex*, a component of which is the nucleus ventralis lateralis (VL). Axons of these thalamic cells ascend in the internal capsule and synapse on neurons of the primary and premotor cortices (Brodmann's areas 4 and 6). In total, this pathway comprises the dentatothalamocortical projection. It is important to note that the cerebellum represents the major driving force on VL neurons and, thus, on cells of the primary and premotor cortices whose neurons influence LMNs via the lateral corticospinal tract.

Damage to the superior cerebellar peduncle and dentate nucleus give rise to the most severe and enduring cerebellar symptoms. Damage to the superior cerebellar peduncle may follow occlusion of the superior cerebellar artery and result in the incoordination of voluntary movement on the side ipsilateral to the lesion. Such a lesion would interrupt fibers from the dentate and interposed nuclei emanating from virtually the whole of the ipsilateral cerebellar hemisphere.

A variety of clinical signs are recognized in the neocerebellar syndrome (discussed later), but one of the more prominent deficits occurs in the timing of agonist and antagonist muscle contractions. Disorders in the timing of voluntary movement have been amply documented in people with neocerebellar pathology. Studies of people in which the cerebellar hemispheres have been surgically removed indicate that the lateral zone contributes importantly to organizing the reciprocal behavior of motoneurons supplying agonist and antagonist muscles. Functional ablation (cooling) of the DN in monkeys performing self-paced, alternating arm movements prolongs movement duration by delaying the termination of agonist muscle activity and, hence, the initiation of antagonist muscle contraction used to perform a return movement. If the movement is triggered by a visual *go* signal, DN cooling results in a delay in the onset of cortical motor cell discharge and increased reaction time. Such experiments indicate that the signals passed from DN to motor cortex contain information relating to the generation and timing of voluntary muscle contraction.

Dentate efferents to the red nucleus synapse in the parvocellular portion of that nucleus. The parvocellular potion is by far the largest part of the red nucleus. The parvocellular red nucleus projects to the whole of the inferior olivary nuclear complex in the medulla whose axons, in turn, project back as climbing fibers to the entirety of the contralateral cerebellum, where they terminate on Purkinje neurons. The function of the DN–parvocellular

RN–inferior olivary nucleus–cerebellar cortex–DN feedback loop is uncertain, but it is generally considered to be involved in motor learning.

Table 19-3 ■ summarizes the major input pathways to the cerebellum; Table 19-4 ■ summarizes the main output pathways from the motor cerebellum.

Motor Learning and the Cerebellum

The cerebellum is involved with motor learning. One of the first observations showing this in humans relates to the vestibulo-ocular reflex (VOR) that was discussed in Chapter 17. As anyone who wears corrective lenses can attest, when a new lens prescription is first worn that significantly magnifies or reduces the retinal image, objects in the environment seem to move when the head moves. This is because automatic stabilization of the retinal image has been compromised. (There may be visual blurring during head movement, as well as a compromise in the visual control of posture.) Such stabilization of the retinal image is automatically maintained by the VOR. The VOR normally has a gain of one, meaning that each degree of head movement elicits a compensating degree of eye movement. Time is required for an adaptive change in the gain of the VOR to occur in order to recover automatic image stabilization.

An even more dramatic example of the plasticity of the VOR has been documented in animals as well as humans. When a subject is fitted with reversing prisms such that head movement in one direction causes apparent movement in the opposite direction, an unaltered gain of one in the VOR would exaggerate retinal instability of the image and be counterproductive. However, if the reversing prisms are worn continuously as the subject moves about in the environment, the gain of the VOR eventually reverses direction so that eye movement is in the same direction as head movement. When the prisms are then removed, the gain of the reflex slowly reverts to one such that the eyes again move in the direction opposite the head displacement.

Table 19-3 Major Cerebellar Input Pathways

INPUT PATHWAY	MAIN ORIGIN(S) OF INPUT	CELLS PROJECTING TO CEREBELLUM	MIDLINE CROSSING	PEDUNCLE OF ENTRY
Spinocerebellar pathways	Lower extremity proprioceptors	Nucleus dorsalis (Clarke's nucleus)	None	Inferior
Dorsal spinocerebellar tract	Movement-related interneurons, intended movement signals for lower extremeity	Spinal border cells (T12–L5)	Once in cord, again in cerebellum	Superior
Ventral spinocerebellar tract	Upper extremity and neck proprioceptors	External cuneate nucleus	None	Inferior
Cuneocerebellar tract	Unknown	Cells of dorsal horn of lower cervical segments	None in spinal cord	Superior and inferior
Rostral spinocerebellar tract				
Trigeminocerebellar	Proprioceptors and exteroceptors of head	Spinal trigeminal nucleus (subnucleus interpolaris)	None	Inferior
Vestibulocerebellar	Labyrinth	Direct from vestibular ganglion and indirect via vestibular nuclei	None	Inferior
Olivocerebellar (climbing fibers)	Cerebral cortex, red nucleus, brainstem, and spinal cord	Inferior olivary nucleus	In medulla	Inferior
Pontocerebellar	Cerebral cortex	Pontine nuclei	In pons	Middle
Tectocerebellar	Auditory and visual impulses	Inferior and superior colliculi	Unknown	Superior

If the flocculus of the archicerebellum is removed in experimental animals, or a particular part of the inferior olivary nucleus is ablated, these adaptive changes in the VOR do not occur, demonstrating that the cerebellum is involved in motor learning. People with lesions involving the archicerebellum have an almost total inability to modulate the VOR with vision.

The cerebellum also is involved in the learning of voluntary movement. Take, as an example, the learning of eye–hand coordination in throwing of a dart. An individual who is proficient in dart throwing must learn to alter the trajectory of the dart if fitted with wedge prisms. The prisms bend the optic path to the right, and the eyes have

Table 19-4 Main Output Pathways of the Motor Cerebellum

REGION	OUTPUT NUCLEI	PEDUNCLE	OUTPUT TARGET INFLUENCED
Flocculonodular lobe	Fastigial nuclei, vestibular nuclei	Inferior	Medial longitudinal fasciculus, reticular formation, vestibular nuclei
Vermis of anterior and posterior lobes	Fastigial nuclei	Superior	Ventrolateral nucleus of thalamus (VL), tectum, reticular formation, vestibular nuclei
Intermediate zone of hemisphere	Interposed nucleus	Superior	VL, red nucleus (magnocellular)
Lateral zone of hemisphere	Dentate nucleus	Superior	VL, red nucleus (parvocellular)

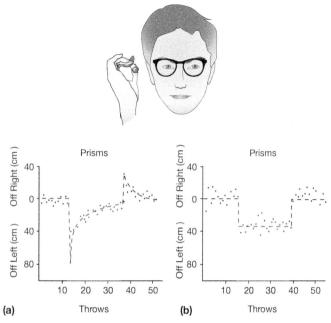

FIGURE 19-8 The cerebellum, prism glasses, and the VOR. (a) A representation of successive throws that illustrates motor learning by an individual with an intact cerebellum. Initially, after being fitted with prisms that bend the optic path to the right, the direction of the throw is off center to the left. Over a number of trials, the cerebellum learns to compensate, and the throws become more accurate. When the prisms are removed, the throws initially are offset to the right due to the previous learning, but the cerebellum quickly recalibrates. (b) A representation of successive throws that illustrates lack of motor learning in an individual with cerebellar dysfunction. While wearing the prisms, the throws are always offset to the left; when the prisms are removed, the throws return to the baseline accuracy.

to look to the left to see the target (Figure 19-8 ■). The direction of throw is in the direction of gaze because the eyes fixate the target and serve as the reference aim for the arm in throwing. When the prisms initially are placed on the subject, her arm throws are wide to the left of the target. But the coordination between eye position and the synergy of the gaze–arm throw is a voluntary motor skill developed and maintained with practice. Thus, with practice, the calibration between gaze and arm throw direction gradually recalibrates such that each successive throw is closer to the target; finally, throws are on-target. When the glasses are then removed, the eyes are now on target but the dart throws are now wide to the right because the gaze–arm throw calibration previously learned while wearing the prisms persists for the initial throws. But with continued throws, the gaze–arm throw trajectory recalibrates back to its original setting and throws again are on-target. People with degenerative disease of the inferior olivary nucleus are unable to recalibrate the gaze–arm throw trajectory such that throws are wide to the left for as long as the prism glasses are worn. After removal of the prisms, the darts land where they did before their introduction.

CLINICAL CONNECTIONS

Dysfunction resulting from cerebellar damage tends to follow certain general rules. First is that the severity of cerebellar deficits may not reflect the magnitude of cerebellar damage. This can be due to a variety of factors. Cerebellar disturbances resulting from non-progressive pathological changes tend to diminish with time, sometimes resulting in a remarkable degree of compensation. Similarly, disturbances due to slowly progressive involvement of the cerebellum may produce only slight symptoms, even when the damage is quite extensive. The age at which damage is sustained has been thought to be an important variable. Owing to the greater plasticity in an immature brain, damage sustained at a young age is better compensated than similar damage occurring later in life. While this may be true generally, in the case of cerebellar damage, recovery of function and age of insult are not necessarily linearly related: the site of the lesion is critical for motor compensation, and lesions involving the deep cerebellar nuclei may not be fully compensated at any developmental age.

Second, it is often difficult to determine the location of a focal cerebellar lesion on the basis of the patient's symptoms, which usually occur as a constellation of related disturbances due to the involvement of more than one of the functionally different cerebellar subdivisions. In large part, this results from the fact that there is little room for expansion in the infratentorial part of the cranial vault. A space-occupying lesion such as a tumor in the posterior fossa is thus likely to cause symptoms from mechanical pressure on surrounding cerebellar structures, or, indeed, even on the medulla and pons of the brainstem. For this reason, the symptoms produced in experimental animals by discrete lesions in particular anatomical or functional zones bear only an imprecise relationship to the symptoms of many of the cerebellar diseases in humans. Third, owing to their large size, the cerebellar hemispheres are likely to become involved, even with lesions that may begin in the vermis. Fourth, unilateral lesions produce ipsilateral deficits. Fifth, even total removal of the cerebellum does not abolish movement. Thus, it appears that the consequences of cerebellar lesions occur because intact neural structures continue to function but no longer have the modulatory and controlling influence of the cerebellum.

Only two of the three syndromes identified in animal experimentation have been very well defined in humans: the archicerebellar and neocerebellar syndromes.

Thought Question

Thinking ahead, what are the fundamental differences of the neocerebellum as compared to the paleocerebellum and archicerebellum with respect to their inputs and outputs and how does this information relate to cerebellar syndromes?

Syndromes

Archicerebellar Syndrome

The most common lesion involving the archicerebellum of humans is a **medulloblastoma**, a highly malignant tumor occurring predominantly in children 4 to 8 years of age. This rapidly growing embryonic tumor arises in the nodulus and neuroepithelial roof of the fourth ventricle, often filling the ventricle. Although its origin has not been established with certainty, the tumor is believed to be derived from undifferentiated embryonic cells in the nodulus or inferior medullary velum. A typical clinical picture is that of a listless child who vomits frequently and complains of morning headaches, often leading to an initial diagnosis of gastrointestinal disease. The vomiting and headaches, along with **papilledema**, are general symptoms associated with elevated intracranial pressure. The elevated intracranial pressure results from the location of this tumor along the course of exit of CSF from the fourth ventricle (obstructive hydrocephalus is produced, see Chapter 25). In fact, elevated intracranial pressure is the most serious problem accompanying cerebellar medulloblastomas because the tumor can compress the brainstem, interfering with such vital functions as respiration. These signs and symptoms are soon followed by development of true cerebellar deficits: an unsteady, stumbling gait with frequent falling. In the archicerebellar syndrome, it is vestibular control of the limbs and trunk against gravity that is compromised. Movements are normal when the child is lying in bed.

> **Thought Question**
>
> What is papilledema, and why does it result from increased intracranial pressure associated with cerebellar lesions?

Vestibulo-ocular control also is compromised in people who have lesions of the vestibulocerebellum. It is uncertain whether all such symptoms are due to the cerebellar involvement or to associated damage of the underlying vestibular nuclei or their projections. Positional nystagmus has been described as an early sign in medulloblastoma. Resting gaze may be deviated from the midline, away from the side of the lesion. Another oculomotor disturbance is a loss of the adjustability (or gain) of the vestibulo-ocular reflex. The cerebellum is involved in compensating for retinal slip during head turning accomplished by fine-tuning the gain of the VOR.

In addition to pure cerebellar signs, some syndromes result in complex symptoms of the brainstem and cerebellum combined. For example, occlusion of the posterior inferior cerebellar artery, a major branch of the vertebral artery, affects the inferior cerebellar peduncle, which (among other projections) carries vestibular fibers to the cerebellum. This gives rise to archicerebellar symptoms in conjunction with other signs characterizing Wallenberg's syndrome (see Chapter 15).

Paleocerebellar Syndrome

A paleocerebellar syndrome can be produced in experimental animals, although this syndrome has not been unequivocally delineated in humans, as noted earlier. Involvement of the anterior lobe component of the paleocerebellum, however, results from chronic alcoholism, wherein degeneration of the anterior parts of the anterior lobe cortex occurs. Such people demonstrate a capacity to stand and walk against gravity, unlike people with vestibulocerebellar involvement. However, the person with anterior lobe damage cannot properly control his or her muscles in either standing or walking. The lower extremities are spread wide apart (wide-based stance) in a voluntary attempt to maintain postural stability. Steps are hesitant and small, and he or she staggers to both sides. Attempts at voluntary movement (heel-to-shin, heel-to-knee tests) reveal marked incoordination of the lower extremities, even when the individual is lying in bed. The anterior lobe syndrome is thus shown to be a deficit in the control of muscles generally, not just in their use in opposing gravity. The upper extremities may display mild clinical signs that correlate with a general lack of degeneration in the cerebellar upper extremity representations in the more posterior anterior lobe.

Neocerebellar Syndrome

A neocerebellar syndrome is the most commonly encountered type of cerebellar disease in humans. Many causes have been identified, including cardiovascular pathology; metastatic tumors, in particular, bronchiogenic; primary gliomas, such as astrocytomas; multiple sclerosis; and degenerative diseases, the majority of which are hereditary. The syndrome is due to involvement of the hemispheres, and if the damage is unilateral, the symptoms appear on the side of the lesion.

A variety of clinical signs are associated with the neocerebellar syndrome. **Intention tremor** is characteristic, meaning that the tremor is present during actions. **Hypotonia** refers to a decrease in the normal resistance offered by muscle in response to palpation or passive movement of a limb. It is more apparent with acute than with chronic cerebellar lesions. However, some neurologists maintain that hypotonia is not typically seen. Hypotonia, when present, may be demonstrated in a number of ways. The hypotonia results in part from depressed stretch reflexes so that the knee jerk reflex becomes pendular. With a **pendular knee-jerk reflex**, the lower extremity swings back and forth four or five times, as contrasted with only one or two that occur normally. Another method of testing for hypotonia is to tap the wrists of the outstretched arms: the involved arm will be displaced through a wider range than normal due to a lack of postural fixation of the arm at the shoulder. **Asthenia** (weakness or a loss of muscular power) may also be seen occasionally.

The cerebellum is importantly concerned with coordination of complex movements that involve antagonistic muscle groups acting over two or more joints. Its action enables such movements to take place with smoothness and precision. It is not unexpected, therefore, that the primary motor manifestations of neocerebellar disease are seen in voluntary, goal-directed movement. Several generic terms have been used to describe these deficits: **asynergia**, defined as a lack of cooperation between muscles that normally act in unison, and **ataxia**, defined as an inability to coordinate the muscles in the execution of voluntary movement. Ataxic deficits are due to disturbances in the rate, range, force, and direction of movement. There also is slowness in the initiation of voluntary movement, and once initiated, movements may be slower or faster than intended. Excessive range of motion may be observed, and the force applied may be too much or too little.

> **Thought Question**
>
> You are working in rehabilitation with an individual who had a gunshot wound to the back of his head, with damage restricted to the cerebellum. What symptoms would you expect if the damage was solely to the neocerebellum?

Cerebellar Dysarthria

Cerebellar lesions often give rise to a motor speech disorder in which the deficits resemble those in the limbs except they are manifest in the orofacial, laryngeal, and respiratory musculature. This is referred to as **ataxic dysarthria** or **cerebellar dysarthia**. Uniform agreement on the localization of cerebellar lesions that produce ataxic dysarthria does not exist. Some maintain that vermal and paravermal regions of the anterior and/or posterior lobes are the regions primarily concerned with speech. Others believe that midline (vermal), intermediate (paravermal), and lateral (hemispheral) pathology can all result in speech deficits. Still others consider that ataxic dysarthria is a manifestation primarily of hemispheral damage and is thus a component of the neocerebellar syndrome. Whatever the case, certain features characterize ataxic dysarthria.

People with cerebellar pathology may have defects that occur in the synergic patterns of contraction, both within a given muscle group as well as across different groups. Thus, the normal coordination existing among the muscles of articulation, phonation (laryngeal), and respiration may be compromised such that, for example, excessive expiratory force is exerted against laryngeal muscles that themselves are too forcefully contracted, or the expiratory contractile force needed for phonation is not properly timed with respect to contractions of the laryngeal or articulatory muscles. Agonist–antagonist contraction timing relations within a given articulator may be disrupted such that an articulatory contact cannot be terminated at the proper time by contraction of the antagonist muscle. Thus, the tongue may remain in contact with the teeth or hard palate, or the lips may remain together too long. Because of deficits in the rate, force, and timing of speech muscle contraction patterns, speech may be too slow or monotonous and syllables uttered with too little or too much force, the latter being referred to as

explosive speech. Or, words may be broken up into their constituent syllables with an unnatural separation, resulting in **scanning speech**. Some people with ataxic dysarthria will repeat given syllables or phonemes to the point where they seem to be **stuttering**. However, unlike the person who truly stutters, the person with ataxic dysarthria does not lock on or repeat a specific consonant or sound (phoneme) that occurs in a consistent position within words.

Physical Rehabilitation

Examination Strategies

A variety of tests of voluntary movement are routinely used to assess coordination. Some of these relate to coordination of limbs; others relate to coordination of posture and gait. Descriptions of several follow.

Several tests are used to assess limb coordination. In the *finger-to-nose test*, the patient is instructed to touch his own nose with his own index finger with his eyes closed. The test is begun from a position of full extension and varying degrees of abduction of the upper extremity. In the *nose-finger-nose test*, the patient places the tip of his index finger on his own nose, reaches to a position of full extension to touch the examiner's finger, then returns to touch the tip of his own nose (Figure 19-9 ■).

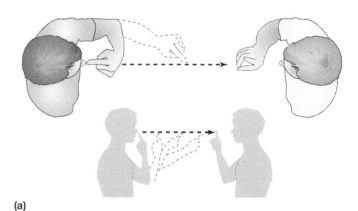

(a)

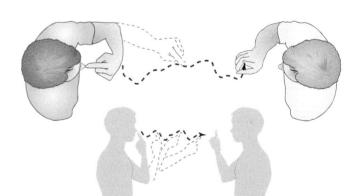

(b)

FIGURE 19-9 Finger-to-nose test. (a) The accuracy of performance of an individual with an intact cerebellum. (b) The dysmetria of an individual with cerebellar dysfunction. The trajectory is wavy instead of straight (dysmetria) and is offset from the nose.

The examiner moves his own finger to different positions during the test. A variation of this test is for the examiner to hold a finger in one position, have the patient close his or her eyes, and then perform the test with the eyes closed, alternately touching the examiner's finger and his or her nose. In the *alternate heel-to-knee, heel-to-toe test*, the patient is asked, while in a supine position, to touch the knee and big toe alternately with the heel of the opposite extremity. In the *heel-on-shin test*, the patient, while in a supine position, is asked to slide the heel of one foot up and down the shin of the opposite lower extremity.

In such tests of voluntary movement, the movement may stop before the target is attained, or the limb may actually overshoot the target. The latter is referred to as **dysmetria** (also, *hypermetria* and *past-pointing*). The target is then approached by a series of side-to-side movements of the finger, which, if they assume a rhythmic quality, are referred to as **intention tremor**. Tremors are seen best when the responding extremity is in a position of full extension. The basis of the tremor is uncertain. Some believe the tremor is due to the patient's voluntary attempts to correct the overshoot, while others believe the tremor is due to a defect in the cerebellum's utilization of proprioceptive information and, therefore, is not voluntary. Most believe that the dentate nucleus must be implicated for intention tremor to occur. In compound movements such as bringing finger to nose or heel to knee, the movement may be broken down into its constituent parts rather than being performed in a smooth and precise manner. Different components of the movement may be executed at the wrong time. This is referred to as **decomposition of movement**. For example, in reaching toward an object, the patient may first flex the shoulder, then extend the elbow, and then extend the wrist, although normally all three movements would occur together as one smooth movement. This sign is a reflection of the fact that the cerebellum is involved in the control of compound multijoint movements as opposed to single-joint movements. Thus, the deficit in compound movement is a cardinal neocerebellar deficit and does not result simply from the sum of individual single joint movement deficits.

Deficits in the rate, range, force, and direction of movement may become especially apparent in tests that require alternate motion. One such test is the *knee pat* (pronation-supination) in which the patient, while in the sitting position, is instructed to pat his or her knee alternately with the palm and dorsum of the hand. Irregularities of rhythm result in a decrease in alternate motion rate, and the patient may not consistently hit the same spot on the knee. This deficit is given the impressive name of **dysdiadochokinesis**. Another test of alternate motion is the successive touching of each finger to the thumb.

Several tests are used to assess the function of the cerebellum in control of eye movements, postural control,

and gait. With respect to eye movements, ataxia may occur with overall poor coordination. Ocular dysmetria may be apparent, saccades may be slowed, and nystagmus may occur. (These tests were described in Chapter 17.)

Postural control and gait can be assessed by testing standing balance and observing gait. A common clinical assessment is the Romberg test, wherein the patient stands with feet together, arms at his or her side, and is observed for sway and loss of balance. In the sharpened Romberg, the patient is asked to close his or her eyes for one minute, eliminating visual information and strategies from the balancing task. The gait of an individual with cerebellar dysfunction may be staggering, and the base of support is typically wider than would normally be expected.

Thought Question

For each of the following symptoms associated with lesions of the archicerebellum, what specific connections are most likely implicated: staggering gait, nausea and vomiting, positional nystagmus, and loss or gain of the VOR?

Intervention Strategies

Physical interventions for people with cerebellar disorders are complicated by the very nature of the disorder—namely, dysfunction in the comparator function during evolving movement. It is clear that the role of the cerebellum relates not to individual joints or movements of segments, but rather to the fundamental organization of movements. As a consequence, when damage occurs, it is not possible to simply remediate individual movements; indeed, remediation may be difficult or impossible, given the fundamental central nervous system flaw in motor control.

Deficits of motor control associated with cerebellar damage are further compounded by impaired motor plasticity often associated with the damage. Impaired motor plasticity can further compromise the individual's ability to learn new tasks. For this reason, much of the intervention strategy relies on compensatory approaches, such as having the patient slow down and providing support, especially of the trunk. Additionally, it is important that people with cerebellar damage preserve whatever cerebellar function still is available. Hence, it is important to educate them to make appropriate changes such as discontinuing the use of alcohol.

In general, the prognosis for restoration of normal function is very poor. However, the role of the rehabilitation professional is to assist these individuals to learn how best to compensate for the damage in order to maximize functionality and quality of life.

It is noteworthy that people can live with significant loss of cerebellum if they are born with this condition. For these individuals, the deficit is apparent only when the system is highly stressed.

BASAL GANGLIA

You work in a clinic that evaluates people with a wide range of movement disorders. Mr. Archibald was diagnosed with Parkinson's disease about six years ago. At this time, he has substantial difficulty with balance and has fallen frequently in the past month. It takes him much longer to complete basic daily activities such as dressing and bathing. Furthermore, he doesn't like to be seen in public because his right hand is constantly shaking due to tremor. Mrs. Kramer was genetically screened recently and knows that she has the gene for Huntington's disease. She is beginning to exhibit subtle clumsiness. As you read through this section, consider the following:

- What is the normal function of the basal ganglia with respect to control of movement?
- How does Parkinson's disease affect specific circuitry of the basal ganglia, and what is the role of the midbrain in this disease process?
- How is the circuitry differentially affected in Parkinson's disease and Huntington disease?
- What are the similarities and differences in symptoms, causes, and treatment of Parkinson's disease compared with Huntington's disease?

Recall from Chapter 7 that a number of distinct, but parallel, operating circuits run through specific parts of the basal ganglia, each with a relationship with a specific part of the cerebral cortex. Thus, each circuit is a loop that originates in a distinct part of the cerebral cortex, projects to a distinct region of the basal ganglia (BG), then returns via the thalamus to the area of cerebral cortex from which it originated (see Figure 7-10). Our concern in this chapter is primarily with the motor loop that begins and ends in the motor and somatosensory cortices. However, it is to be understood that a naturally occurring disease process, such as that occurring in Parkinson's disease (PD) and Huntington's disease (HD), does not affect more than one loop through the basal ganglia. Thus, the symptoms in disorders such as PD and HD do not confine themselves just to the motor system, but affect also cognitive processes and emotional status.

Thought Question

In preparation for learning more about the basal ganglia, it is important to review content presented in Chapter 7. Specifically, recall the names and locations of the nuclei associated with this structure. Identify the nuclei in cross section, noting the relationship of the nuclei of the basal ganglia to the nuclei of the thalamus. Also, note the location of the internal capsule to these structures. Are there two basal ganglia (one on each side), or is there a single structure referred to as the basal ganglia?

Anatomy and Function of Circuits through the Basal Ganglia

To understand the circuitry and function of the basal ganglia, it is necessary to understand several key points. These relate to the role of disinhibition in permitting movement, the direct and indirect pathways of the basal ganglia, and the multiple channels (hence, functions) of the basal ganglia.

The Concept of Disinhibition

The basal ganglia stimulate movement through a process of *disinhibition of the thalamus*. To understand this concept, it is helpful to begin with connections between the thalamus and motor cortex and work backward to the basal ganglia. Specifically, the thalamocortical connections (from the VA/VL nuclei of the thalamus to the motor and premotor cortices) use the neurotransmitter glutamate (which is excitatory to the motor cortices), thus depolarizing cortical upper motor neurons and facilitating movement. However, motor nuclei of the thalamus (VA/VL) are tonically inhibited by the output nuclei of the basal ganglia. In other words, there is a persistent inhibition of the output. Therefore, in order for the thalamus to excite the motor cortices, it is necessary to *phasically disinhibit the motor nuclei of the thalamus* (VA/VL).

To understand how phasic (or transient) disinhibition of the VA/VL of the thalamus is accomplished, we now start from the cerebral cortex and work our way through the basal ganglia to get to the thalamus. Specifically, massive projections from the cerebral cortex provide the main input to the basal ganglia. Most of these cortical inputs to the basal ganglia are directed to the striatum and use glutamate as the neurotransmitter. Recall that glutamate is excitatory; hence, inputs from cerebral cortex to striatum excite the striatum. Note that a second input to the striatum is from the substantia nigra pars compacta of the midbrain and releases dopamine in the striatum via the dopaminergic nigrostriatal pathway. This contribution is key to understanding Parkinson's disease, as discussed later.

About 90 percent of striatal neurons project to other nuclei of the basal ganglia. All of these striatal projection neurons use GABA as their neurotransmitter (along with different neuropeptides). Recall that GABA is inhibitory; hence, these striatal projections are inhibitory to their postsynaptic targets. Striatal neurons fire at a low rate and tend to be phasically active under the influence of excitatory drive from the cerebral cortex. Some of these striatal projection neurons project directly to two basal ganglia output nuclei. These are the globus pallidus *internal* segment (GPi) and the substantia nigra pars reticulata (SNpr). The projection of the GABAergic striatal neurons onto the GPi/SNpr result in inhibition of the output from these nuclei. Thus, these phasic projections onto the GPi/SNpr effectively inhibit the inhibition of the VA/VL of the thalamus. This phenomenon is called **disinhibition** (Figure 19-10 ■).

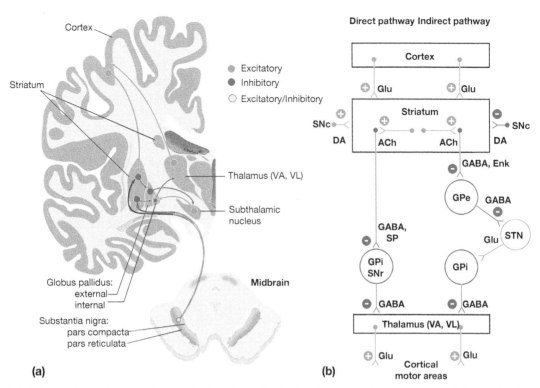

FIGURE 19-10 (a) The nuclei and connections of the basal ganglia depicted in coronal cross sections of the forebrain and midbrain. Note that the substantia nigra, a component of the basal ganglia, is located in the midbrain. Excitatory (+) connections are depicted in red, inhibitory (−) in green. (b) Schematic of the direct and indirect pathways of the basal ganglia.

To summarize, facilitation of movement through these loops begins with projections from the cerebral cortex that are excitatory to the striatum. The striatum then sends inhibitory projections to the GPi/SNpr. The GPi/SNpr (also referred to as the output nuclei of the basal ganglia) is phasically inhibited, thus phasically disinhibiting the motor thalamus (VA/VL). The net effect is that the phasic disinhibition allows the motor thalamus to phasically excite the motor cortex and thereby facilitates generation of voluntary movement.

> **Thought Question**
>
> What specific sequence of actions is required to facilitate purposeful movement? What is the role of *disinhibition* in this sequence?

Direct and Indirect Pathways

The striatum influences the tonic activity of GPi/SNpr output neurons via two different pathways, referred to as the direct pathway and indirect pathway (Figure 19-11 ■). These two pathways are separate, parallel circuits that originate in the striatum and converge onto the basal ganglia output nuclei (GPi, SNpr) with opposite effects on these basal ganglia output nuclei, thereby having opposite effects on the motor thalamus. Hence, these two pathways have opposite effects on the motor cortex and, therefore, opposite effects on the initiation of voluntary movement.

The pathway from the striatum to GPi/SNpr is referred to as the **direct pathway** because of the direct synaptic actions of the striatum to the GPi/SNpr output nuclei. Intermingled with these striatal neurons of the direct pathway is a separate population of GABAergic striatal neurons that do not project to the GPi/SNpr, but instead project to the *external* segment globus pallidus (GPe), referred to as the **indirect pathway**. These two pathways from striatum to globus pallidus have opposite effects on the thalamus and, therefore, the cortex.

Specifically, this indirect pathway also begins with cortical projections to the striatum. However, striatal neurons of the indirect pathway give rise to an inhibitory projection to the GPe, whose neurons have an inhibitory (GABAergic) projection to neurons of the **subthalamic nucleus (STN);** the STN has an excitatory glutamatergic projection to GPi/SNpr output neurons. Corticostriate excitation of this indirect pathway has a net effect on GPi/SNpr output neurons that is the opposite of that mediated by the direct pathway. This occurs as follows: Striatal projections to GPe neurons release GABA and thus inhibit GPe neurons. The GPe projection onto neurons of the STN also releases GABA and thus inhibits STN neurons. Because GPe neurons inhibit neurons of the STN, a reduction in GPe activity removes inhibition from STN neurons whose activity thus increases (the STN is disinhibited when striatal neurons of the indirect pathway are phasically activated). (Any time two distinct GABAergic projections are in tandem, neurons in the final target are disinhibited

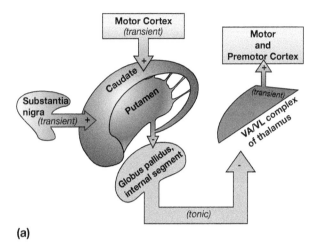

(a)

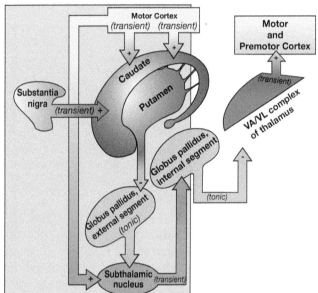

FIGURE 19-11 Tonic and transient (phasic) connections of the basal ganglia. (a) Direct pathway. (b) Indirect pathway.

when the first set of GABAergic neurons are active.) STN neurons project to the GPi/SNpr output neurons and excite them by releasing glutamate. The increased activity of the inhibitory GPi/SNpr (GABAergic) output neurons further inhibits thalamic neurons. The activity of thalamic neurons decreases phasically, which lessens the excitatory drive on upper motor neurons of the premotor and supplementary motor cortices. Thus, activation of the indirect pathway suppresses the initiation of voluntary movement.

Thought Question

Diagram the events illustrating the following statement with respect to facilitation of movement: When striatal neurons of the direct pathway are phasically active, the net effect is a facilitation of movement, whereas when striatal neurons of the indirect pathway are phasically active, the net effect is less facilitation of movement.

To summarize, activation of striatal neurons of the direct pathway facilitates initiation of movement by inhibiting basal ganglia output nuclei, which in turn disinhibits the motor thalamus. The resulting increased excitatory drive from the motor thalamus to the motor cortex ultimately leads to increased activity of cortical UMN, which facilitates initiation of movement. In contrast, activation of striatal neurons of the indirect pathway leads to increased firing rate of the basal ganglia output nuclei, which increases the inhibition of the motor thalamus and ultimately decreases excitation of the motor cortex, thereby failing to facilitate movement.

Finally, it should be noted that this *firing rate* model of basal ganglia function is overly simplistic in that it converts synaptic networks of the basal ganglia to simple plus and minus signs. Nevertheless, this conceptual model effectively explains many (though not all) of the clinical signs associated with basal ganglia pathology, as discussed later in this chapter.

One additional interconnection among nuclei of the basal ganglia is of clinical relevance in Parkinson's disease and should be considered here. This is the dopaminergic projection from the pars compacta of the substantia nigra (SNpc) to the striatum that is involved in Parkinson's disease. Dopamine exerts both excitatory and inhibitory influences on striatal neurons, but these opposing effects are exerted on separate sets of neurons. Excitatory effects are exerted on striatal neurons that are part of a pathway that facilitates movement, whereas inhibitory effects are exerted on striatal neurons that are part of a pathway that suppresses movement. A loss of dopamine such as occurs in Parkinson's disease (see Clinical Connections) would remove excitation from the pathway that facilitates movement (i.e., the direct pathway) and increase the excitation (via disinhibition) of the pathway that suppresses movement (i.e., the indirect pathway). The result would be a decrease in movement.

It is important to recognize that dopamine has many complex pre- and postneuromodulatory synaptic actions in the striatum and that these actions work through different types of dopamine receptors. The *net effect* of dopamine is excitation of striatal neurons of the direct pathway via D1 receptors and inhibition of striatal neurons of the indirect pathway via D2 receptors.

Thought Question

Dopamine is a single neurotransmitter. Yet, in some situations it can have excitatory influences, and in other situations it can have inhibitory influences. Given that it is a single neurotransmitter, what could account for its ability to have opposite effects? Note, you may need to revisit Chapter 4.

Parallel Channels

Well-defined loops or channels of information processing are associated with the basal ganglia. The first is the **motor channel** (described earlier), associated with disorders of movement seen in Parkinson's disease (PD) and Huntington's disease (HD). Inputs are mainly to the putamen and outputs are from the GPi and SNpc. The **oculomotor channel** is important in the regulation of eye movements. Inputs are from the body of the caudate nucleus, while the cortical destination is the frontal eye fields and the supplementary eye fields. The **prefrontal channel** appears to be important in cognition. Inputs are from the head of the caudate, and the destination is to the prefrontal cortex. Finally, the **limbic channel** is associated with regulation of emotions and motivational drives. Inputs are from a wide number of structures, including the limbic cortex, hippocampus, and amygdala with projections to the nucleus accumbens and ventral striatum. Outputs are from the ventral pallidum to the medial dorsal and ventral anterior nucleus of the thalamus and to the limbic cortex. Given these five channels, with their widespread connections, it is not surprising that disorders such as PD and HD have wide-ranging consequences (see Clinical Connections). Of these channels, the motor channel is best understood.

> ### Thought Question
>
> The basal ganglia is involved with processing of a number of different kinds of information in addition to motor information. What are they?

CLINICAL CONNECTIONS
Parkinson's Disease

PD is classified as a degenerative disease that is progressive. It is the second most common neurodegenerative disease of the brain, following Alzheimer's disease. For years, PD has been considered the prototypical basal ganglia disease, although the pathophysiology is not confined just to these subcortical nuclei. The most conspicuous symptoms of PD are caused by the death of neurons, primarily in the **substantia nigra pars compacta (SNpc)** of the midbrain (see Chapter 7). The number of SNpc dopaminergic neurons that die increases over time so that the signs and symptoms of PD steadily worsen. It appears that PD results from accelerated neuron death of these midbrain dopaminergic neurons, for reasons that are not understood in most cases.

Approximately 1 million Americans are diagnosed with PD, with more than 50,000 new people diagnosed each year. The mean age at onset is in the early to middle 60s, with young onset PD occurring in 5 to 10 percent of cases. People with young-onset PD typically are diagnosed between the ages of 21 and 40. Chronic cocaine abuse, which acts to deplete the brain of its dopamine content, may hasten the appearance of PD symptoms by 20 years. The disease has been observed in all socioeconomic classes, ethnic groups, and countries in which it has been investigated. There is no known treatment that halts the continued

death of substantia nigra neurons. For some people with PD, the symptoms remain mild, but, in most individuals, the disease progresses to the point of severe disability. More than 60 percent of people with PD are disabled within 5 years of disease onset and 80 percent after 10 years.

In a description of the disease that later would bear his name, James Parkinson stated in 1817 that it is characterized by "involuntary tremulous motion, with lessened muscular power, in parts not in action and even when supported; with a propensity to bend the trunk forward, and to pass from a walking to a running pace, *the senses and the intellect being uninjured*" (italics added). The italicized portion of this statement began a controversy that has been resolved only fairly recently.

Today, the cardinal signs of PD are described as tremor, rigidity, bradykinesia, and postural instability. The first three signs are typically apparent early in the disease, whereas postural instability typically becomes apparent later.

Tremor is the first sign in 70 percent of people with PD. Tremor occurs when the limb is at rest and is worse with anxiety, with contralateral motor activity, and during ambulation. Hence, tremor associated with PD is referred to as a *resting tremor*. Tremor usually presents asymmetrically with a frequency of 4 to 6 Hz, classically resembling pill rolling, and is predominant at rest. Note that the resting tremor of PD differs markedly from the intention tremor of cerebellar disorders because the former occurs at rest, whereas the tremor associated with cerebellar disorders only occurs with action. However, people with PD do experience tremor during activity later in the disease process.

> ### Thought Question
>
> How does tremor associated with PD differ from tremor associated with cerebellar disorders?

Bradykinesia, or slowness of movement, is the most characteristic feature of PD, as well as the most disabling of the symptoms of early PD. Initially, it is seen as difficulty with handwriting and reduced arm swing during gait, but it can also be observed with finger or foot tapping, alternating movements of the hands, and fist opening and closing. Three terms are used to describe problems with speed of movement: (1) *bradykinesia* refers to both reduced amplitude and speed of movement, (2) *hypokinesia* refers to a paucity of movement, and (3) *akinesia* refers to difficulty initiating movement. Initially, bradykinesia manifests itself clinically in overall slowing of movement, as well as lack of facial expression (referred to as *masked facies*). As the disease progresses, the individual may have difficulty initiating movement or may experience motor blocks (referred to as *freezing*).

Rigidity, characterized by increased resistance to slow passive movement, is identified during passive movement of extremities, torso, or neck. *Lead pipe rigidity* refers to a slow and sustained contraction; *cogwheel rigidity* has tremor superimposed and manifests as a catching and releasing throughout the range. Rigidity can increase with contralateral motor activity or mental task performance. This is apparent in response to reinforcing maneuvers, such as having the person make a strong fist with one hand while rigidity is tested on the contralateral extremity.

Postural instability develops gradually, resulting in poor balance and leading to an increased risk for falls. Postural instability results from impaired postural reflexes that would normally produce motor responses necessary for recovery of balance when perturbations occur.

In combination, the impairments associated with PD lead to gait disorders (slow shuffling gait with a tendency for retropulsion and propulsion). The patient's gait may become *festinating* (L., *festinare*, to hasten). Festinations are short steps that can occur while the patient is moving either forward or backward, and the steps become progressively more rapid as if the patient were chasing his or her own center of gravity to avoid falling.

As the disease continues to progress, associated movements are lost, leading to *en bloc* movements in which the torso moves as a single unit without dissociation of the thorax from the pelvis. Episodes of freezing become problematic as the disease progresses, and there is a loss of ability to perform two tasks simultaneously. Voice projection becomes problematic, making it difficult to hear and understand the patient. Handwriting becomes small, referred to as micrographia. A large proportion of patients eventually experience *dyskinesias*, or wearing off and on–off difficulties associated with pharmacological managements.

Although typically thought of as a motor system disorder, PD is now recognized to be considerably more complex, with most patients experiencing disabling nonmotor impairments. Included are cognitive decline (observed in as many as 80 percent of patients, see Chapter 20), dementia (between 40 and 80 percent), daytime sleepiness (79 percent), hallucinations (50 percent), and depression (up to 50 percent). Autonomic disorders are common, including urinary incontinence (41 percent) and symptomatic postural hypotension (35 percent). Finally, sensory disturbances have been identified with PD, including pain as well as burning, tingling, and numbness in the affected limb. These symptoms affect approximately 40 percent of people with the disorder. Pain has been identified in up to 80 percent

of these individuals. And fatigue is reported for about 50 percent of patients. Clearly the nonmotor symptoms of PD are pervasive. They can be as disabling (and sometimes more so) as the motor symptoms. Some of these symptoms could relate to pathophysiology of one or more of the channels of the BG, whereas others might relate to degeneration of other projections that do not involve the BG.

Etiology

In most cases, no known cause of degeneration of dopaminergic neurons resulting in PD can be identified, although there are a few known environmental and genetic causes. It is likely that PD results from the combination of a number of factors, including age, genetic susceptibility, and environmental factors.

With regard to genetics, a number of monogenic forms of parkinsonism have been identified that result in classic features of PD. These include mutations in the SNCA gene with forms identified associated with the LRRK2, Parkin, and PINK1 genes. However, simple Mendelian inheritance explains only a small fraction of the cases of PD. Only about 5 to 10 percent of people with PD have a familial pattern of inheritance. These genetic forms are more likely to be the cause of parkinsonism in the people who have their onset of symptoms at a younger age.

Since the 1980s, the main hypothesis of the etiology of PD has been the environmental theory. Epidemiological studies have identified risk factors, the most common of which include rural living, exposure to well water, pesticides, herbicides, and wood pulp mills. The theory is based largely on the occurrence of irreversible signs of PD and selective destruction of cells in the SNpc in people who took a chemical they mistakenly thought was synthetic heroin. The chemical has been identified as MPTP (1-methyl-4-phenyl-1,2,3,6-tetrahydropyridine). After intravenous injection of MPTP, these people developed acute and severe PD. Could PD result from exposure to an unknown MPTP-like compound? PD is more frequent in industrialized countries and agrarian areas in which toxins are commonly used. Despite an extensive search, no such poison has been found. The fact that PD occurs all over the world and has been described in one fashion or another for thousands of years suggests that there is not just a single toxin that causes the disease.

Disorders 19-1: Hoehn and Yahr Stages of Parkinson's Disease

Stages of PD were identified by two neurologists, Margaret Hoehn and Melvin Yahr, to characterize symptoms and function. A commonly used modification of the classification is as follows:

Stage 1:   Unilateral symptoms.
Stage 1.5: Unilateral symptoms with some axial involvement.

Stage 2:   Bilateral symptoms without impaired balance.
Stage 2.5: Mild bilateral symptoms; recovery on pull test.
Stage 3:   Mild/moderate bilateral symptoms; some postural instability; can live independently.
Stage 4:   Severe disability; can walk independently.
Stage 5:   Depends on a wheelchair for mobility; bedridden unless assisted.

Environmental toxins may not be the only factors contributing to the development of PD. If all cases of PD have a similar pathological mechanism, then an environmental toxin capable of triggering this mechanism must have been present since at least 1817 when the James Parkinson first described the disease. Manmade chemicals similar to MPTP are thus not likely to be the only toxins. A variety of factors probably contribute to the development of PD. Such factors could include a combination of genetic or constitutional predisposition, dietary factors, environment, and aging. This combination could vary among people.

Whatever the precipitating cause of the neurodegeneration associated with PD, evidence is mounting to suggest that a signal-mediated apoptotic process occurs. **Apoptosis** (see Chapter 3) refers to a form of cell death that occurs with little inflammation, but with chromatin clumping and fragmentation of DNA. Factors that have been implicated in this process include mitochondrial dysfunction (associated with PD), perhaps precipitated by the free radicals formed during oxidative metabolism of dopamine.

Thought Question

PD is thought of as a disorder of the BG, yet it is well known that the cell loss occurs in the brainstem. What two nuclei of the midbrain are particularly affected, and how does that cell loss affect the function of the BG?

The Brain Disorder in PD: Pathophysiology

Although PD is considered a disorder of the BG, the actual cell death begins in the brainstem. The most consistent change in the brains of people with PD is the death and resulting loss of neurons in the **substantia nigra (SN)**, comprised of black, pigmented, dopaminergic-producing cells (Figure 19-12 ■). Although the pathology may not begin in the SN, the most conspicuous loss of neurons occurs in the SNpc, whose neurons synthesize and release the

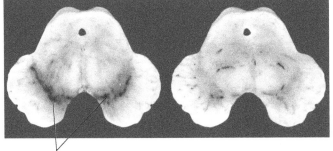

Normal substantia nigra   PD substantia nigra

Pigment cells

FIGURE 19-12 Substantia nigra of the midbrain. In the normal condition, the substantia nigra pars compacta is seen as a black pigmented area. In the midbrain of people with PD, there is a loss of the black pigmented cells in substantia nigra pars compacta and, therefore, a loss of dopamine (DA) production.

transmitter dopamine. A significant loss of cells also occurs in other pigmented nuclei, including the **ventral tegmental area (VTA)** located in the midline adjacent to the substantia nigra, whose neurons also synthesize and release the transmitter dopamine; the **locus coeruleus** of the pons, whose neurons synthesize and release the transmitter norepinephrine; and the **dorsal motor nucleus of the vagus** of the medulla, whose neurons also synthesize and release the transmitter norepinephrine.

The disease-related loss of neurons in PD occurs against a background of cellular degeneration and loss that is part of the process of normal brain aging. The process of aging may increase the brain's vulnerability to PD. In people who are neurologically normal, the number of neurons in the SNpc drops by about 50 percent between the ages of 20 and 60. Overt signs of PD appear when the cell loss reaches 75 to 80 percent of the neurons in the SNpc, so the disease has a fairly distinct threshold. During the process of this cell loss, still-surviving DA neurons increase their metabolic activity, but eventually it is not enough to compensate for the continuing loss of DA neurons.

The axons of the midbrain dopamine (DA) neurons project to many brain structures in addition to the striatum. DA is released onto the neurons of these structures. When neurons of the SNpc die, these structures are deprived of a normal amount of the transmitter DA and then do not function properly. Within the striatum, the putamen is the most severely involved with a DA loss of about 95 percent. This loss occurs in early in PD. The caudate nucleus suffers a DA loss later in the disease, and the loss may amount to more than 80 percent.

Although typically thought of as a disorder of the BG, the consequences of PD are much more widespread, including cognitive and emotional consequences associated with other parts of the CNS outside the BG. For completeness, other features are discussed here. Midbrain DA neurons also project into the cerebral cortex (mesocortical projection) and into subcortical structures of the limbic system (mesolimbic projection) (Figure 19-13 ■). The **mesocortical projection** sends its axons to parts of the frontal and temporal lobes. In the frontal lobe, dopaminergic projections terminate on neurons of the medial frontal lobe, including the anterior cingulate cortex, as well as on neurons of the dorsolateral prefrontal cortex. In the temporal lobe, dopaminergic projections terminate on neurons of anteromedial cortical regions, including the entorhinal cortex. The **mesolimbic projection** projects to the hippocampus, nucleus accumbens (ventral striatum), amygdala, and septal area. The cognitive consequences of Parkinson's disease are discussed in Chapter 21.

Particular attention has been paid to the loss of dopamine projections from the VTA to the association cortex of the frontal lobe because of the similarity between certain symptoms of PD and those following restricted damage to parts of the frontal lobe following a stroke or head trauma. Dopamine losses of about 60 percent have been found in the frontal association cortex of people with PD. Thus, some of the symptoms of PD are caused by a loss of the transmitter

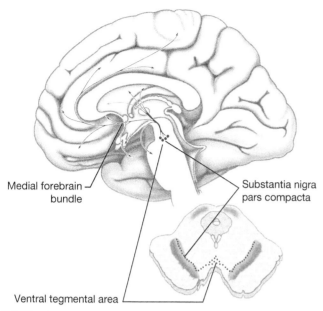

Medial forebrain bundle

Substantia nigra pars compacta

Ventral tegmental area

FIGURE 19-13 Dopaminergic neurons of the midbrain project to the basal ganglia, cerebral cortex, and subcortical areas. There are mesocortical projections to the frontal and temporal lobes and mesolimbic projections to subcortical areas.

DA in the striatum and some by a loss of DA in the frontal association cortex (as will be discussed in Chapter 21).

In the striatum, dopamine normally excites the direct pathway and inhibits the indirect pathway. These opposite effects are due to the presence of different dopamine receptors on the neurons of origin of the direct and indirect pathways from the striatum. The direct pathway whose neurons of origin contain excitatory D1 dopamine receptors terminate on neurons of the internal segment of the globus pallidus. In contrast, the neurons of origin of the indirect pathway contain inhibitory D2 dopamine receptors whose axons terminate on neurons of the external segment of the globus pallidus. Thus, the loss of dopamine in the putamen results in decreased activity in the direct pathway that facilitates movement and increased activity in the indirect pathway that suppresses movement (sew Figures 19-10 and 19-11). Collectively, these synergistic changes result in increased activity in GPi/SNpr output neurons so that inhibition of thalamic neurons is increased. Thus, the excitatory thalamocortical drive on cortical motor neurons is reduced, resulting in the hypokinetic signs of Parkinson's disease (akinesia, bradykinesia).

There is no known curative treatment for PD that stops the neuronal degeneration of DA-releasing cells in the SNpc and VTA. Symptomatic treatment can be medical or surgical. In addition, physical intervention has been shown to improve functional ability and may possibly be implicated in slowing down disease progression.

Pharmacological Management

Therapeutic drugs include dopamine replacement (e.g., levodopa), dopamine agonists (e.g., bromocriptine, pramipexole, ropinirole), inhibitors of dopamine metabolism

(e.g., COMT inhibitors such as entacapone and MAO-B inhibitors such as selegiline), and anticholinergic agents (e.g., trihexyphenidyl). The best combination of drugs and their dosages vary from patient to patient and are based on the constellation of symptoms. Doses are determined largely by trial and error. Patients who benefit most from drug treatment are those with a relatively mild form of the disease. In patients with more severe disease, symptomatic relief is only partial. These patients eventually reach a level of incapacity that is not significantly responsive to any medication.

> ### Thought Question
>
> As you read through the next sections, compare the role and site of action of each of the following drug therapies used in treating PD: dopamine replacement therapy, dopamine receptor agonist therapies, and inhibitors of dopamine metabolism. Give examples of each type of therapy.

LEVODOPA (L-DOPA) The vast majority of patients are treated medically, through the administration anti-parkinsonian drugs, in particular, levodopa (L-Dopa). More than 30 years following its introduction, L-Dopa therapy remains the most effective treatment for the symptomatic relief of PD signs and symptoms. A variety of adjunctive medical therapies are used to enhance the effectiveness of L-Dopa. However, a continuing unresolved problem has been to develop a mode of drug delivery that stimulates striatal neurons at pharmacological levels in a sustained manner, particularly in advanced disease, and can be used easily by patients and/or caregivers.

Treating PD with levodopa (L-Dopa, Larodopa, Dopar) is categorized as *replacement therapy*. Levodopa is a chemical compound from which the neurotransmitter dopamine (DA) is formed during the natural synthesis of DA that occurs inside neurons of the SNpc and VTA. Levodopa is taken orally, crosses the blood–brain barrier, and enters the extracellular fluid surrounding neurons within the brain. Levodopa is then taken inside of SNpc and VTA neurons and converted into DA by an enzyme, L-Dopa decarboxylase. Note that DA cannot cross the blood–brain barrier; thus, if this conversion occurs outside of the brain, levodopa has no therapeutic effect on PD.

A critical number of SNpc neurons and their support cells must remain alive in order for dopamine replacement therapy to work. The administration of large amounts of levodopa then causes the still-surviving SNpc neurons to release more than their usual amount of DA, thus making up for (i.e., replacing) the DA lost due to the death of some SNpc neurons. Levodopa therapy does not cure PD, so the death of SNpc (and VTA) neurons continues. This means that levodopa therapy is eventually bound to fail because, ultimately, there will not be enough surviving neurons to compensate for those that have died.

One of the problems with levodopa replacement therapy is the large dose that must be administered in order for a sufficient dose to cross the blood–brain barrier before it is converted to DA. One strategy to reduce the amount of levodopa required is to prevent its breakdown by L-Dopa decarboxylase before it crosses the blood–brain barrier. This is accomplished by administering L-Dopa with another drug—either carbidopa or benserazide. These drugs block the levodopa-to-DA conversion in the gut (i.e., outside of the brain). More levodopa is thus available to enter the brain, which lowers the amount of levodopa that has to be taken by the patient by four- to fivefold. The dose of levodopa or the carbidopa and levodopa combination is different for different patients.

Levodopa therapy usually is started when the disease begins to interfere with the activities of daily living. The rationale for postponing therapy this long is that drug-induced adverse side effects (e.g., dyskinesias) and response fluctuations (i.e., wearing off, on–off) relate to treatment duration, although there is still controversy regarding whether these complications are due to treatment duration or disease duration. There is some evidence that earlier initiation of appropriate therapy may delay functional disability. The longer the person is on levodopa therapy, the more likely the patient is to suffer response fluctuations and adverse side effects. There also was a concern that levodopa itself may be injurious to neurons, but recent evidence suggests that this is not the case. However, some clinicians believe that levodopa therapy should be initiated at the time of diagnosis, rather than waiting until functionally significant disability develops. Levodopa is taken orally either in divided doses two to four times a day or as controlled-release tablets two or more times a day. The rationale behind the use of extended-release tablets is to create a smooth, sustained release of the drug into the blood—with the thought that fluctuations in dopamine levels may contribute more to motor complications than does the total dose.

While levodopa is the single, most effective agent in the treatment of PD, not all of the symptoms of PD respond to the drug to the same degree. Akinesia, bradykinesia, and rigidity respond best. Tremor is variably affected. Postural stability is, for the most part, unresponsive to levodopa. Mental changes, autonomic nervous system dysfunction (excessive sweating, constipation), and sensory changes are not affected and may even be made worse.

In most people, the response to levodopa is reasonably stable for the first several years of treatment, but thereafter additional adverse side effects and motor fluctuations develop in about 80 percent of patients and increase in severity the longer the duration of treatment. The most common adverse side effect of levodopa is that it causes various types of abnormal involuntary movements (**dyskinesias**). The dyskinesias may be so severe as to interfere with speech (when they involve the facial, tongue, and lip musculature), swallowing, respiration, and balance. The severity of dyskinesia may force a reduction in the dose of levodopa. In many patients, some degree of dyskinesia must be accepted as the price to pay for the reduction of PD symptoms. Dyskinesias can be as uncomfortable and disabling as the rigidity and akinesia of PD, but many individuals would rather be dyskinetic than immobile, and many people appear not to notice their dyskinesia.

Psychiatric side effects may be seen after taking levodopa—typically, after three or more years of treatment and more frequently in elderly patients and patients with dementia. They often limit the amount of levodopa that can be taken and seriously reduce the effectiveness of therapy. Common initial symptoms include vivid dreams, disturbed sleep patterns, and visual illusions. Occasionally, a psychosis resembling schizophrenia may occur. Visual hallucinations are common. These consist of formed objects such as people or animals and are generally non-threatening. In many people, the best that can be expected is a compromise between some visual hallucinations and a less than optimal control of the movement disorders.

Motor (response) fluctuations include end-of-dose deterioration and on–off episodes. Early in the course of PD, the period during which levodopa is effective may be longer than the lifetime of the drug in blood plasma. This suggests that the nigrostriatal DA system has the capacity to store and release DA. As SNpc neurons continue to die, this "buffering capacity" of the nigrostriatal system is lost. The patient's motor state then may fluctuate dramatically with each dose of levodopa because the brain has an increasing dependence on the oral administration of levodopa, in which there are changing blood plasma concentrations of the drug.

End-of-dose deterioration, or the wearing-off phenomenon, consists of a progressively shortening period of time during which levodopa is effective, with a rapid return of rigidity and akinesia at the end of the dosing interval. Increasing the dose and frequency of administration can help end-of-dose deterioration, but this may cause the appearance of dyskinesia.

The **on–off phenomenon** occurs in the later stages of PD. Individuals with this problem fluctuate rapidly between being *off*, having no beneficial effects from the levodopa, and being *on*, but with severe dyskinesia. This is very disabling because the individual never knows when he or she will become severely immobilized. This loss of movement may last from a few minutes to several hours and occurs unexpectedly over and over again.

DOPAMINE RECEPTOR AGONISTS Dopamine receptor agonists stimulate DA receptors in the striatum directly and have several potential advantages over the use of levodopa. First, enzymatic conversion of these drugs is not required for them to be effective. Therefore, they do not depend on the presence of surviving nigrostriatal neurons for their effectiveness. This may make them useful in the treatment of the late stages of PD. Second, dopamine agonists may be more selective in their actions. The use of levodopa (after its conversion to DA) activates DA receptors of all subtypes throughout the entire brain. Dopamine receptor agonists, on the other hand, are selective to varying degrees for different subtypes of DA receptors. Third, many DA receptor agonists are effective for a period of time substantially longer than levodopa. Fourth, dopamine agonists are associated with lower rates of developing dyskinesias and motor fluctuations, especially when administered in low doses. Finally, some data suggest that levodopa actually contributes to the death of DA neurons from the formation of free radicals and putative toxicity from the metabolism of DA by SNpc neurons (although other findings contradict this). In any event, DA receptor agonists avoid this potential problem.

Dopamine receptor agonists can be used to stimulate dopamine receptors directly or to stimulate the release of dopamine centrally. For example, bromocriptine (Parlodel) stimulates dopamine receptors directly, while amantadine stimulates the release of dopamine centrally. Recently, several additional dopamine agonists have been tested and are now used, including pramipexole, ropinerole, and rotigotine. The actions these drugs have on PD symptoms are similar to those of levodopa. Adverse side effects also are similar, but DA receptor agonists cause dyskinesia less

often than levodopa. Their duration of action after a single dose is usually longer than that of levodopa so that motor fluctuations are reduced.

All of the dopamine agonists have to be started at very low doses; the dosage is then built up over several months due to psychological side effects. These agents are more likely to induce hallucinations and psychosis than levodopa. Another major problem with these agents is a potential to induce compulsive behaviors, such as gambling, and these problems need to be monitored. The available dopamine agonists also can cause leg edema.

DOPAMINE METABOLISM INHIBITORS Once the dopamine is released into the synaptic cleft (in the CNS) it is vulnerable to metabolism (breakdown) by two enzymes: **catechol-O-methyltransferase (COMT)** and **monoamine oxidase (MAO)** (Figure 19-14 ■). Both COMT and MAO are widely distributed throughout the body, including the brain. The highest concentrations of each are in the liver

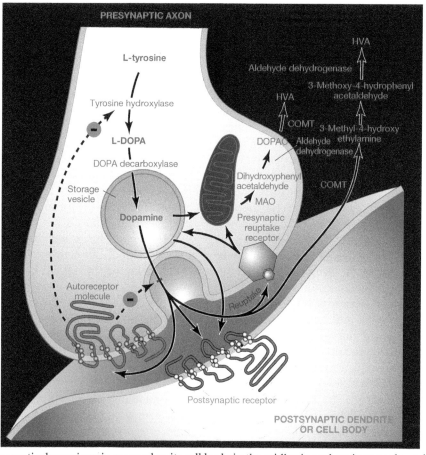

FIGURE 19-14 The presynaptic dopaminergic neuron has its cell body in the midbrain and projects to the striatum. Within the presynaptic terminal, the amino acid tyrosine is converted by L-Dopa by tyrosine hydroxylase, which in turn is converted to dopamine by Dopa decarboxylase. Dopamine is released as a neurotransmitter into the synaptic cleft, where it binds to postsynaptic receptors. Two mechanisms serve to control the amount of dopamine in the synapse and adjacent extracellular space: (1) a negative feedback loop mediated by the autoreceptor on the presynaptic membrane that modifies release and biosynthesis of dopamine and (2) re-uptake of dopamine by presynaptic receptors. These two mechanisms serve to modulate the dopamine synaptic and extracellular concentration on an ongoing basis. In addition, some of the dopamine is converted to metabolites by COMT to 3-methyl-4-hydroxy ethylamine and some is converted by MAO to dihydroxyphenyl acetaldehyde. COMT and MAO inhibitors (not shown) prevent these conversions, thereby preventing the reduction of available dopamine.

and kidney. There are distinct differences in the cytological locations of the two enzymes. MAO is associated chiefly with the outer membrane of mitochondria, including those within the terminals of adrenergic fibers, whereas COMT is located largely in the cytoplasm, but little is found in adrenergic neurons. Inhibitors of these two enzymes can reduce the overall requirements for levodopa.

Two COMT inhibitors are currently used as adjuncts to levodopa: tolcapone inhibits peripheral and, to a lesser extent central, COMT, whereas entacapone inhibits COMT only in the periphery. Tolcapone is more effective clinically, but it is associated with liver toxicity and is therefore reserved for people who do not respond adequately to entacapone.

MAO inhibitors block the oxidation of dopamine and, because of the presence of MAO in the terminals of dopaminergic neurons, increase dopamine levels in the synapse with striatal neurons. Two commonly used MAO inhibitors are selegiline and rasagiline. Both can be used as monotherapy in early PD and as adjuncts to levodopa in advanced PD. Some neurologists initiate the treatment of all newly diagnosed individuals with selegiline or rasagiline. There was great hope that MAO inhibitors would prove to have a neuroprotective effect, but this has not been convincingly demonstrated. The basis for the belief that the drug is neuroprotective was that selegiline protects monkeys from MPTP-induced symptoms of PD and prevents the MPTP-induced degeneration of cells of the SNpc. Because selegiline is an antioxidant, it would prevent the generation of free radicals that result from the breakdown of dopamine. Rasagiline is an irreversible inhibitor of MAO-B and is more selective and potent than selegiline. Unlike selegiline, rasagiline does not generate amphetamine or methamphetamine metabolites that can cause side effects such as insomnia.

ANTICHOLINERGIC AGENTS Anticholinergic agents related to the drug atropine have long been used in the treatment of PD, and, in fact, were used before levodopa was discovered. They have little or no corrective effect on rigidity and bradykinesia, the most disabling aspects of PD, but they can be effective in treatment of tremor. Therefore, they are used in the treatment of early PD, before symptoms have become severe, or for patients in whom tremor is the predominant symptom. They can be used alone in patients who cannot tolerate levodopa or in conjunction with levodopa. The optimum dosage level is achieved when there is the greatest relief from tremor with adverse side effects that the patient can tolerate. Anticholinergic drugs cannot be withdrawn suddenly because the patient is likely to become completely immobilized and incapacitated from a severe and sudden increase in rigidity and tremor.

Anticholinergic agents block muscarinic acetylcholine (ACh) receptors and thus prevent the action of ACh. This action occurs on neurons in the striatum. The actions of the two transmitters, DA and ACh, are normally in balance in the striatum. The purpose of anticholinergic agents is to counterbalance the predominance of ACh activity that is caused by the loss of striatal DA. Several anticholinergic drugs are used, including trihexyphenidyl (Artane), benztropine mesylate (Cogentin), and diphenhydramine hydrochloride (Benedryl).

The adverse effects of these drugs are a result of their anticholinergic properties and include dry mouth, which may be of benefit in cases where there is a drooling of saliva; blurring of vision through dilation of the pupil and loss of accommodation; and constipation and (sometimes) urinary retention. Most troublesome side effects, and the reason these are rarely used, include sedation, mental confusion, mental slowing, impairment of memory, and hallucinations.

AMANTADINE Amantadine, an antiviral agent that is used in the prevention and treatment of influenza A, has an anti-parkinsonian effect. Amantadine has only a modest effect on the symptoms of PD. Therefore, it is used in early PD, before the symptoms have become severe. It may also be used as an adjunct to levodopa in patients experiencing involuntary movements with relatively small doses of levodopa. The mechanism of action of amantadine is not known clearly. It is thought to act by releasing DA from striatal neurons or to block the inactivation of DA (by reuptake). Amantadine also has anticholinergic properties.

The side effects of amantadine are similar to those of levodopa, but considerably milder. Possible side effects include nausea and vomiting, dizziness, lethargy, sleep disturbance (nightmares), confusion, and hallucination. Edema of the lower extremities may be troublesome to some patients.

NEUROTROPHIC FACTORS Because neurotrophic factors regulate the survival of neurons in the developing nervous system, it has been hoped that they could be exploited in the treatment of neurodegenerative diseases such as PD. One such factor is glial cell line–derived neurotrophic factor (GDNF). However, direct infusion of GDNF into the putamen of PD patients has not been shown to result in significant improvement in the clinical manifestations of the disease. Indeed, it is not fully understood what endogenous GDNF does in the adult human brain.

Surgical Interventions

The surgical treatment of PD has had an interesting history. Surgery is not a new treatment for PD. In the early 1950s, it was discovered that destroying the globus pallidus (a procedure known as a *pallidotomy*) relieved the tremor and rigidity of PD. Deep within the interior of the brain, the globus pallidus (GP) is located through the use of a procedure called *stereotaxy* in which the locations of deep brain structures are defined by a set of three-dimensional coordinates referenced to a standard point. Lesioning of the GP is performed by stereotactic neurosurgery. As noted earlier, because neurons of the striatum function abnormally due to the loss of DA, neurons of the GP also function abnormally. Suppressing the abnormal neural activity in the GP by lesioning it reduces tremor and rigidity but has little effect on the other symptoms of PD. The pallidotomy could only be done on one side of the brain—on the GP opposite the side of the patient's most severe symptoms—because bilateral ablation resulted in loss of swallowing ability. Also, the procedure was limited because parkinsonian symptoms would often re-occur and side effects were common because brain structures adjacent to the GP also could be inadvertently destroyed.

By the 1960s, pallidotomy was largely replaced by another stereotactic surgical procedure that was directed to the ventrolateral thalamus. The procedure is called a *ventrolateral thalamotomy*. The rationale for this procedure was the same as that for lesioning the GP, except that the ventrolateral nucleus of the thalamus is further downstream in the circuit from the striatum. Ventrolateral thalamotomy relieves contralateral tremor in up to 90 percent of patients. There is a decrease in rigidity, but akinesia and bradykinesia are unaffected.

With the introduction of L-Dopa therapy in the 1960s, stereotaxic neurosurgery was largely abandoned. However, the occurrence of L-Dopa-induced motor fluctuations and dyskinesia in patients on long-term medication led to the revitalization of neurosurgical approaches using more sophisticated modern neurophysiological and brain-imaging technologies to guide the stereotaxic placement of the lesion. The internal segment of the globus pallidus (GPi) and the subthalamic nucleus (STN) are currently the favored targets of modern stereotaxic neurosurgery. In both procedures, patients are maintained postoperatively on L-Dopa medication, although the doses can be substantially reduced.

MODERN PALLIDOTOMY AND SUBTHALAMOTOMY The renewed interest in pallidotomy as a treatment for PD has been encouraged by reports in the popular media of the dramatic benefits experienced by PD patients who underwent pallidotomy using newly developed surgical techniques, including single-cell microelectrode recording to delineate regions with the aberrant discharges. These newer techniques enable the neurosurgeon to more accurately locate the GPi and to place a lesion in just a particular part of the nucleus (the posteroventral GPi). All of the cardinal symptoms of PD (tremor, rigidity, and bradykinesia) show improvement following modern pallidotomy, and the procedure also reduces L-Dopa-induced dyskinesias. The most impressive improvement is the reduction of levodopa-induced dyskinesia. Following the procedure it is usually possible to reduce the levodopa dosage. With unilateral pallidotomy, the motor benefits are predominantly on the side of the body contralateral to the lesion. Still, the procedure can cause unwanted side effects due to inadvertent damage to brain structures adjacent to the GPi. Bilateral pallidotomies are not performed because, although the motor benefits are greater, the risk of unwanted side effects also is greater. There is a high incidence of cognitive impairment, dysarthria, and swallowing problems with bilateral pallidotomy.

As with all stereotaxic neurosurgery, the procedure is permanent, so it would not be possible to use future medical or surgical procedures if they are found to be superior to pallidotomy. At the current time, there is insufficient information about the optimal target site in the GP, about exactly which patients are the best candidates for surgery, and about the long-term risks and benefits of the procedure to recommend the widespread application of pallidotomy in routine clinical practice.

Because overactivity of the subthalamic nucleus is one of the hallmarks of the parkinsonian brain, it has also been looked at with interest as a possible site of surgical intervention. In contrast to pallidotomy, unilateral or bilateral subthalamotomies do not result in severe complications, while providing long-lasting significant amelioration of all of the cardinal features of PD, as well as significantly reducing L-Dopa-induced dyskinesias. However, clinical outcomes vary from patient to patient, and some do manifest motor problems and dysarthria that may or may not resolve over time.

DEEP BRAIN STIMULATION Deep brain stimulation (DBS) is an alternative to destructive surgery. The basis for this procedure came from studies on monkeys that were made parkinsonian by the injection of the neurotoxin MPTP. In these animals, lesions and electrical stimulation of the subthalamic nucleus (STN) reduced tremor, rigidity, and akinesia. As noted earlier, the STN receives information from the striatum indirectly via the external segment of the GP. Because of the abnormality in the activity of striatal neurons caused by the DA deficiency, the STN also functions abnormally, overactivity of the subthalamic nucleus being a hallmark of PD (i.e., the nucleus is disinhibited).

Thought Question

What are the similarities and differences between surgical ablation and deep brain stimulation in treatment of PD?

DBS of the STN is the most significant and effective therapeutic advance in the symptomatic treatment of PD since the introduction of L-Dopa in the 1960s. In this procedure, electrodes are implanted stereotactically in the STN of both sides. The nuclei are stimulated bilaterally with pulse generators implanted in the patient. Bilateral DBS can be safely performed and produces motor benefits significantly greater than those occurring after unilateral stereotaxic neurosurgery. Akinesia, tremor, and rigidity improve significantly as do daily living activities.

A major advantage of DBS is that the procedure is reversible should superior medical or surgical therapies be developed in the future. People with PD receiving DBS, like those undergoing neurosurgery, continue to receive L-Dopa therapy but at significantly reduced dosages. DBS thus reduces L-Dopa-induced dyskinesias, eliminating them altogether in some people. The procedure is not without its adverse side effects, however.

Cognitive impairment (e.g., working memory) and mood disturbances (e.g., depression, emotional lability) as well as speech difficulties, postural instability (equilibrium), and gait disorders, may develop.

Because similar therapeutic outcomes are achieved with both DBS and lesions in the STN, it was believed that the high-frequency electrical stimulation inactivates the STN. But whether this actually is the mechanism of the efficacy of DBS is unclear. DBS has a long-term (measured at least to five years) therapeutic effect on the cardinal features of PD and reduces L-Dopa-induced dyskinesias.

Recently, stimulation sites other than the STN have been targeted for DBS and may produce even more favorable symptomatic relief. For example, the zona incerta, a structure contiguous to the STN, may be a better target for DBS, as may the GPi. Recent findings from a large, randomized, controlled intervention study suggest little difference between DBS at the STN compared with the GPi. And most recently investigators have begun to examine benefits of stimulation of the pedunculopontine tegmental nuclei in an attempt to address the impairments of postural instability and gait that are not well remediated with other stimulation targets.

FETAL NIGRAL TRANSPLANTATION Another experimental surgical procedure that does not require making a lesion in the basal ganglia circuitry is the transplantation of substantia nigra cells from aborted fetuses into the striatum of people with PD, a procedure referred to as *neurorestorative* whose objective is to restore the anatomicophysiological organization of the nigrostriatal system. The first transplantation trials were begun in 1987; since then, hundreds of people have received transplants into the neostriatum of human mesencephalic fetal tissue.

Neurons from the midbrain that will develop into DA-releasing neurons are extracted from aborted fetuses. These cells are then stereotactically transplanted (injected either as a cell suspension or solid tissue graft) into the caudate nucleus and/or putamen—in most people on the side of the brain contralateral to the most severe symptoms. The transplanted fetal nigral cells have been shown to survive with axon growth into the striatum and little evidence of immunological rejection of the grafts. With grafting in only one side of the brain, a graft-derived functional improvement would be counteracted by continuing degeneration of the intrinsic DA system, especially on the nonoperated side, due to the ongoing disease process.

However, even with bilateral fetal nigral transplantation, little, if any, benefit is detectable after 24 months, even though positron emission tomography (PET) scanning shows survival and function of the transplanted dopaminergic neurons. While many scientific, safety, logistical, financial, legislative, regulatory, religious, and ethical concerns exist about using aborted human fetal tissue for grafting in the treatment of advanced Parkinson's disease, to some extent they have become moot with the publication of studies in 2001 and 2003. A number of the younger people who received transplants developed severe (in some cases, incapacitating) dyskinesias to the point where one patient was no longer able to feed himself. One of the researchers in the study stated that the dyskinetic patients "...chew constantly, their fingers go up and down, their wrists flex and distend." Patients writhe and twist, jerk their heads, fling their arms about. "It was tragic, catastrophic...It's a real nightmare. And we can't selectively turn it off." Note that these involuntary movements, termed *runaway dyskinesias*, are due to the transplantation and are independent of continuing L-Dopa medication. A moment's reflection indicates why the procedure is tenuous at best. Transplanting fetal cells into a fully developed adult nervous system and expecting them to replicate the normal anatomical and functional organizational pattern created during development is questionable. After all, the factors that guide axonal outgrowth and synaptogenesis during development are no longer present in the adult nervous system. Even though the transplanted cells survive to synthesize and release dopamine, feedback-controlled neuronal inputs that normally modulate that release are not present.

Serious ethical concerns also surround the use of placebo controls in the surgery used to implant fetal grafts in order to validate the efficacy of the transplant itself. The sham surgery in control PD patients uses an invasive procedure that insults the integrity of the body and exposes the patient to a substantial risk with no potential benefit. Bioethicists, as well as many neurosurgeons, consider the use of placebo controls in transplant surgery to be inherently unethical.

Physical Rehabilitation

EXAMINATION STRATEGIES The examination strategy for people who have PD includes assessment of the cardinal signs (tremor, rigidity, bradykinesia, and postural instability). Tremor is typically described in terms of each of the

Neuropathology Box 19-1: Rigidity Differs from Spasticity

Rigidity associated with PD differs from spasticity associated with UMN damage (see Chapter 9). Rigidity is not velocity dependent, nor is it responsive to peripheral somatosensory stimuli. Furthermore, rigidity can be reduced, at least temporarily, through behavioral strategies such as relaxation, whereas spasticity cannot.

affected extremities, as well as the effect on the neck and trunk. Rigidity is measured as resistance to passive movement of the extremities or neck, both with and without reinforcement maneuvers. Bradykinesia can be assessed by having the patient repeat maneuvers of the upper and lower extremity as fast as possible and comparing the patient's performance to that of a healthy individual. For the upper extremity, examples include making a fist and then opening and closing the hand as quickly as possible or moving the arm back and forth from forearm supination to pronation as fast as possible. For the lower extremity, the seated person can raise the knee and tap the heel on the ground repeatedly. To measure postural instability, the examiner typically pulls the patient backward from the pelvis or shoulders and determines his or her ability to correct for the displacement; this test is part of determining the Hoehn and Yahr stage of disease. Other issues of importance include response to medication; history of falls (including when, where and why); and nonmotor signs such as sleep disturbance, fatigue, and pain.

> **Thought Question**
>
> What difference would you expect to find in a test of supination and pronation for a person with PD compared with a person with cerebellar dysfunction? What is the physiological basis for the difference?

Two rating scales are available to quantify the impairments and functional limitations associated with PD. The first is the Unified Parkinson's Disease Rating Scale (UPDRS), which is the gold standard used by neurologists and researchers. The second is the PROFILE PD, which is specifically designed for rehabilitation specialists. These two scales provide quantitative data for the major signs and symptoms associated with the disorder.

INTERVENTION STRATEGIES In recent years, evidence has clearly demonstrated that physical intervention can greatly improve function of individuals who have PD. There are two different, and complementary, approaches to intervention. The first approach is based on the abnormalities of motor processing associated with the disorder. For example, people with PD often have difficulty initiating movement volitionally because of the consequences of loss of dopamine, interfering with the ability to disinhibit the thalamus in order to facilitate movement. However, it is often possible to facilitate movement through auditory, visual, and tactile stimuli, bypassing the thalamic projections to the motor cortex. Relaxation approaches have been shown to be beneficial because of the connections between the limbic system and movement. These issues are discussed further in Chapter 20.

The second approach is directed at sequelae of PD that are not neurologically based. There is considerable evidence that intervention strategies for people with PD

should also be directed toward remediating the musculoskeletal and cardiovascular sequelae that accompany the disease because of loss of activity.

Of particular interest, recent evidence from animal studies suggests that high-intensity exercise (either aerobic exercise or exercise that is highly skill dependent) may actually protect against the degeneration associated with PD. This is discussed further in Chapter 26.

> **Thought Question**
>
> What pathways would be involved in the use of auditory and visual stimulation to overcome difficulty that people with PD have initiating and sustaining movement?

Huntington's Disease (Chorea)

Huntington's disease (HD) owes its name to the American physician George Huntington, who first described the disease in a published report in 1872. HD is an inherited, progressive, neurodegenerative disease characterized by a triad of manifestations: motor changes, including choreoathetosis, abnormal muscle stretch reflexes, and impaired, rapid, alternating movements; cognitive decline leading to frank dementia; and a variety of psychiatric disorders, including depression, anxiety, irritability, and apathy. While this triad of symptoms characterizes HD, in clinical practice, a diagnosis of HD is typically made only when the motor signs become prominent. This practice has established the motor deficits as the classical feature of HD, although the disturbances in motor function may not be the first or the most distressing feature of the disease—either to the person or family of the afflicted individual. Rather, the cognitive and neuropsychiatric disorders may dominate the clinical picture. These topics are discussed in Chapter 21. This chapter focuses on the motor deficits characterizing HD.

HD affects all races; males and females inherit the disease with equal frequency. About 30,000 people in the United States are affected by HD, with an additional 150,000 at risk of developing the disorder. The typical age of onset is in the fourth and fifth decades of life. HD, notable for killing the folk singer Woody Guthrie in 1967, is relentlessly progressive; most people with the disorder deteriorate to a vegetative state within 10 to 15 years and die, on average, within 15 to 20 years of onset of symptoms, generally as a result of infectious complications of immobility. A juvenile form of HD progresses more rapidly, typically leading to death within 7 to 10 years after disease onset.

> **Thought Question**
>
> HD, like PD, affects the basal ganglia. However, the nuclei affected differ markedly. What is the difference? Relate the nuclei affected to the symptoms of HD and contrast these symptoms with those of PD.

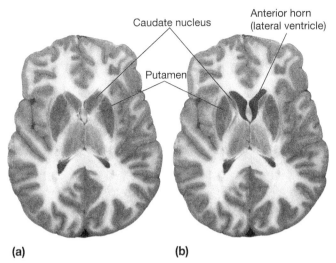

Caudate nucleus

Anterior horn
(lateral ventricle)

Putamen

(a) **(b)**

FIGURE 19-15 Horizontal sections of cortex illustrating (a) normal size of caudate nucleus in people without HD and (b) atrophy of the head of the caudate nucleus and enlargement of the anterior horn of the lateral ventricle as manifested in people with Huntington's disease (HD).

The characteristic neuropathologic feature of HD is bilateral gross atrophy of the head of the caudate nucleus (CN) and anterior putamen (Figure 19-15 ■). The atrophy of the head of the CN alters the configuration of the anterior horns of the lateral ventricle such that the bulge normally produced by the head of the CN is absent on CT or MRI scans. MRI scans reveal that striatal atrophy begins long before the onset of diagnosable motor symptoms. Although it is uncertain when striatal atrophy begins, the volume of the head of the CN is only one-half of normal and that of the putamen one-third to one-half of normal at the time of diagnosis of HD, and volumes are significantly reduced in gene-carrying preclinical individuals. The neurodegeneration in the striatum is accompanied by a decrease in striatal metabolism, also discernable prior to symptom onset in gene carriers. After the manifestation of HD symptoms, the striatal hypometabolism progresses and is associated with a decrease in cortical metabolism. The cortical hypometabolism is attributed to the dysfunctions induced in the cortico-striato-thalamo-cortical loops by the striatal atrophy.

In the early stages of HD, spontaneous movement abnormalities are slight and give the impression of fidgetiness and clumsiness. With progression of the disease, the involuntary jerking and writhing movements (chorea) become more pronounced and affect, in particular, muscles of the face, tongue, and upper extremities. The extraocular muscles also are involved in most people, resulting in a loss of smooth pursuit in eye tracking. Ultimately, however, all of the body musculature may be involved. Eventually, voluntary movements are initiated and executed more slowly than normal. The coordination of voluntary movement becomes more difficult as the disease progresses, eventually becoming impossible. Muscle tone typically is decreased until late in the disease.

The loss of striatal neurons in early stages of HD when motor dysfunction is the most prominent aspect of the disease involves GABAergic neurons that project to the external segment of globus pallidus (GPe) that are components of the indirect pathway (see Figure 19-11). This loss reduces inhibition of GPe neurons whose activity thus increases. This increases inhibition of STN neurons via the GABAergic projection from GPe to STN. The STN is thus functionally inactivated. The result is that output from the basal ganglia (via GPi/SNpr GABAergic neurons) is decreased because of the loss of excitation from the STN. This change in BG output in HD is the opposite of that occurring in PD, where the STN is disinhibited, resulting in increased BG output. Correspondingly, the motor deficits in HD and PD are opposites of one another, with hypotonia and dyskinesia characterizing HD and hypertonia and akinesia characterizing PD.

Glutamate is the excitatory transmitter released by axons of the massive cortical input to the striatum. GABAergic output neurons from the striatum are excited by glutamate via NMDA glutamate receptors. Overexposure to glutamate due either to excessive release of the transmitter or to a failure in the re-uptake mechanism by glial cells in the striatum causes excitotoxic cell death of the medium-sized spiny GABAergic output neurons of the neostriatum. Thus, glutamate may be the proximate causative neurotoxin in the striatum in HD.

Excitotoxicity leads to oxidative stress and cell death by apoptosis. The Bcl-2 family of anti-apoptotic molecules normally opposes changes in mitochondrial function that are caused by oxidative stress. However, glutamate excitotoxicity diminishes Bcl-2 activity, allowing cytochrome c to be liberated from mitochondria. Once in the cytoplasm, cytochrome c activates caspase-3, obligating the cell to die by apoptosis.

Thought Question

Which neurotransmitters are implicated in HD? What is their site of action and how do they compare with neurotransmitter imbalances associated with PD?

The Genetic Abnormality in HD

HD is an autosomal-dominant disorder caused by an expanded number of cysteine, arginine, glycine (CAG) repeats in the Huntington gene on chromosome 4. Identification of the HD gene in 1993 permitted the development of a test for detection of the defective gene in motor asymptomatic individuals. HD survives because the average age of onset is in the mid-30s, at which time most carriers of the defective gene have had children. However, because there is no cure for the disease, predicting a progressive, incapacitating, and fatal neuropsychiatric disease in, at the time, healthy persons raises serious ethical problems.

Medical Management

The dopamine antagonist haloperidol currently is the most effective drug in the symptomatic treatment of the movement disorder in HD. The mechanism of haloperidol's therapeutic effect is unclear. This drug is administered only when the chorea is functionally disabling because medication with neuroleptic agents can cause **Tardive dyskinesia**. Tardive dyskinesia is characterized by repetitive, purposeless, and involuntary movements of the facial, oral, and lingual regions.

Spurred by fetal transplantation in Parkinson's disease, attempts have been made to treat people with Huntington's disease using fetal cell implants of striatal neurons. To date, these have been unsuccessful. The numbers of people so treated are far too few to permit any statistical validity because the incidence of HD is so low compared with PD. While pathological studies of fetal cell transplantation in PD have demonstrated that fetal cells integrate into striatal synaptic circuitry and release DA in the intended areas (with non-therapeutic, disastrous consequences), there is little evidence to date that transplanted cells integrate into striatal synaptic circuitry in people with HD.

Deep brain stimulation and ablation of the internal segment of the globus pallidus also have been used to treat HD.

Physical Rehabilitation

EXAMINATION STRATEGIES Examination of an individual with HD will vary depending upon the stage of the disease. A standardized tool, the United Huntington Disease Rating Scale (UHDRS), may be used to examine cognitive and motor function. Determination of an individual's abilities to perform activities of daily living (ADLs), assessment of muscle strength and tone, and observation of gait and extraneous movements will inform the clinician of the impact of the disease on the motor system. Furthermore, observation and assessment of the person's mental state and psychological status will reveal the cognitive and psychiatric deficits associated with this progressive neurological disorder.

INTERVENTION STRATEGIES It is reported that individuals affected with HD are underserved in rehabilitation. This may be due in part to the complexity of the disease, in that it is progressive and involves cognitive and psychiatric decline. Additionally, because the disease is an autosomal dominant disorder, parents and children of the patient may also be affected by the disorder. Hence, the typical caregivers may not be available to assist the patient. Furthermore, it is important to consider whether there are psychological ramifications for the offspring of a person diagnosed with HD.

The motor complications are addressed by interventions to increase trunk stability and control and to improve postural control. Similar to people with PD, relaxation may help to decrease extraneous movements, and auditory stimulation may help to organize and improve gait patterns. It is important for the rehabilitation clinician to understand the extent of cognitive and psychiatric involvement. The clinician may need to simplify instructions to ensure comprehension, especially in later stages of the disease when cognitive function becomes compromised. Furthermore, the patient may be prone to experiencing depression, anxiety, irritability, and apathy—all of which have an impact on response to intervention.

Thought Question

Compare and contrast the examination strategies used for assessing a person with PD and one with HD.

Hemiballismus

Hemiballismus is a severe and dramatic form of dyskinesia. The involuntary movements of hemiballismus consist of wild, unpatterned flinging movements of an entire extremity. The uncontrollable movements may occur intermittently several times a minute or may be nearly continuous. As with Parkinson's disease, hemiballismus has a well-defined pathologic substrate. The disorder is caused by a discrete lesion of the subthalamic nucleus, most commonly resulting from a vascular disorder in a penetrating branch of the posterior cerebral artery. The abnormal movements occur on the side of the body contralateral to the lesion. A primary difference between hemiballism and PD and HD is that the former has an acute (usually vascular) onset, whereas PD and HD are progressive disorders of the basal ganglia.

In contrast to Parkinson's disease, in which there is overactivity in the indirect pathway from the striatum to GPi/SNpr, in hemiballism there is underactivity in the indirect pathway. The subthalamic lesion eliminates an excitatory drive on GPi/SNpr neurons whose inhibitory output to the thalamus is thereby reduced. The thalamus is disinhibited by the subthalamic nuclear lesion. It is not clear precisely how the increased excitatory drive from the thalamus on cortical motor neurons acts to produce the involuntary movements.

It is helpful to put signs and symptoms associated with disorders of the cerebellum and basal ganglia into a broader context. Table 19-5 ■ summarizes the clinical signs resulting from lesions to different components of the motor system.

Table 19-5 Clinical Signs of Lesions to Different Components of the Motor System

LESION LOCATION	VOLUNTARY STRENGTH	ATROPHY	STRETCH REFLEXES	TONE	INVOLUNTARY MOVEMENTS[A]
Muscle (myopathy)	Weak (paresis)	Potentially severe	Hypoactive	Hypotonic	No
Neuromuscular junction	Weak with continued exertion	Minimal	Depends on when elicited	Depends on when tested	No
LMN	Weak (paresis, paralysis)	Potentially severe (neurogenic atrophy)	Absent or hypoactive	Hypnotic (flaccid)	No[b]
UMN	Weak (paresis or paralysis)	Mild (disuse atrophy)	Hyperactive (spastic)[c]	Hypertonic	No
Cerebellar circuitry	Normal	No	Hypoactive	Hypotonic	No
Basal ganglia	Normal	No	Normal (?)	Variable, dependent on specific disorder[d]	Yes (dyskinesias)[d]

[a] By definition, involuntary movements occur spontaneously against the person's will. To be distinguished from abnormal movement that is initiated voluntarily (e.g., ataxia, intention tremor).

[b] Fasciculations are not considered movements.

[c] After a massive UMN lesion resulting in spinal shock, reflexes are absent with hypotonia during the period of spinal shock.

[d] The dyskinesias include athetosis, chorea, ballismus, and resting tremor. Dystonia also may be seen.

Summary

Our consideration of the cerebellum began with a discussion of the five types of neurons residing in the three layers of the cerebellar cortex and their geometric and synaptic relationships. Four of these neurons are inhibitory and include stellate, basket, Golgi, and Purkinje neurons. Only one is excitatory, the granule cell. The main excitatory loop through the cerebellum includes the excitatory climbing and mossy fibers synapsing on neurons of the deep cerebellar nuclei, providing them with a background excitatory drive. This drive is modulated by an inhibitory side loop through the cerebellar cortex, in which Purkine cells synapse on neurons of the deep nuclei to either decrease or increase the latter's discharge.

The afferent and efferent connections established by the archicerebellum, paleocerebellum, and neocerebellum were presented. Those of the archicerebellum underlie the cerebellar control of equilibrium and the vestibulo-ocular reflex. The afferents focus on connections from the vestibular nuclei, while the efferents focus on projections via the fastigial nucleus to the vestibular nuclei and reticular formation, which then relay descending information to spinal cord and ascending information to extraocular lower motor neurons. Damage to

the archicerebellum in humans causes an unsteady and stumbling gait, with frequent falling and deficits in vestibulo-ocular control. Afferents to the paleocerebellum originate in the spinal cord and brainstem and carry proprioceptive and exteroceptive information from the extremities, trunk, and face. The efferent projections from the paleocerebellum are to the lateral vestibular nucleus via the fastigial nucleus and to the red nucleus and ventrolateral nucleus of the thalamus via the nucleus interpositus. The role of the paleocerebellum in human motor control is not clearly defined. Chronic alcoholism may cause a degeneration of cortical neurons in the lower extremity representation of the anterior lobe, resulting in marked loss of control of the lower extremities in standing, walking, and other voluntary movements. Afferent projections to the neocerebellum do not originate from peripheral receptors, but rather are derived from motor and association cortex of the cerebral cortices that relay first in the pontine nuclei. Neocerebellar efferent projections are to the red nucleus and ventrolateral nucleus of the thalamus via the dentate nucleus. Damage to the neocerebellum in humans, in addition to hypotonia and a pendular knee jerk, causes a wide array of deficits in voluntary movement: ataxia, dysmetria, intention tremor, decomposition of movement, dysdiadochokinesis, and ataxic dysarthria. Finally, the role of the cerebellum in motor learning in humans was addressed. This has been demonstrated by studying the effects of reversing prisms on the vestibulo-ocular reflex, as well as the effects of wedge prisms on the trajectory of dart throws. Both the reflex and voluntary movement compensations occasioned by fitting a subject with prisms are impaired by damage to the cerebellum or its input.

Our consideration of the basal ganglia focused on the anatomy and function of the motor loop through the basal ganglia. The motor loop begins in the motor and association cortices and synapses in the striatum (putamen), and striatal neurons that project to the internal segment of the globus pallidus/substantia nigra par reticulata (GPi/SNpr) whose output is to the thalamus. The loop is completed by the thalamocortical projection back to the motor and sensory cortices. However, there are two pathways by which the striatum can influence the output nuclei GPi/SNpr of the basal ganglia: (1) a direct pathway that projects directly to the GPi/SNpr and (2) an indirect pathway that synapses first in the external segment of the globus pallidus, in turn projects to the subthalamic nucleus (STN), and then projects to the GPi/SNpr. We discussed how the direct pathway facilitates movement and the indirect pathway suppresses movement. Parkinson's disease results in decreased activity in the direct pathway and increased activity in the indirect pathway, thereby accounting for the hypokinetic signs of the disease (akinesia, bradykinesia). This is because of the existence of a projection from the pars compacta of the substantia nigra (SNpc) to the neurons of origin of the direct and indirect pathways. Normally, dopamine excites (via D1 receptors) the direct pathway and inhibits (via D2 receptors) the indirect pathway, thereby facilitating movement. But the loss of dopamine due to a degeneration of cells in the SNpc results in less activity in the direct pathway and more activity in the indirect pathway, thus accounting for the hypokinetic signs of PD.

Huntington's disease, having a cause and pathophysiology different than that of PD, results in a decreased output from the GPi/SNpr because the indirect pathway is inactivated, leaving the direct pathway unopposed in the early stages of the disease. Because the indirect pathway is affected in opposite ways in PD and HD, the signs are correspondingly the opposite: HD is characterized by excess motor activity (dyskinesia).

The symptoms and treatments in PD and HD were addressed. PD is treated with a wide array of drugs and with surgical approaches such as deep brain stimulation (DBS). HD, a genetic disease, is not effectively treated with medication, surgery, or DBS, at least thus far, although such treatments are being explored.

Hemiballismus, the most severe of the dyskinesias, typically results from a stroke that damages the subthalamic nucleus. The indirect pathway is affected in the same way as in HD, thus resulting in excess motor activity.

Applications

1. Mrs. Patel is a 70-year-old retired music teacher. She has a history of hypertension, atrial fibrillation, and migraines. One morning she awoke with a severe headache. Upon getting out of bed, she fell to the right and required help from her husband to get up. She then had an episode of nausea and vomiting. They went to the emergency department. Significant findings from her neurological examination included unsteadiness with standing and walking, dysmetria with finger-to-nose testing and heel-to-knee testing on the right, intention tremor on the right, and dysdiochokinesia on the right.

   a. Given this information, what is the most likely location of the lesion?
   b. Given her medical history and an abrupt onset, what is the most likely diagnosis?

2. Mr. Bartlett is a 65-year-old retired miner. He reports to his family physician with complaints of trembling in his left hand, minor difficulties in walking, and several episodes of coughing/choking while eating. His wife reports that he is spending more time just sitting around the house. She feels like he is becoming more quiet and withdrawn, and he seems to have some problems remembering things. Mr. Bartlett states he feels like he is having trouble getting out of his recliner and wonders if he should get a different kind of chair. Findings from the neurological examination include:

   - Cranial nerves are intact; however, his face is relatively expressionless throughout the exam.
   - Questions are answered in short phrases with staccato-like delivery.
   - Gross motor screen reveals good general strength throughout all limbs.
   - Resistance to passive movements is apparent during active movements of his left upper extremity.
   - Difficulty with balance testing is present.
   - Gait is shuffling with decreased arm swing.

   a. Does Mr. Bartlett's work history raise any questions that require exploration? If yes, what are they?
   b. If the cranial nerves are intact, what could account for his lack of facial expression and difficulty swallowing?
   c. What do you think is Mr. Bartlett's diagnosis? Explain your answer.

References

Cerebellum

Allen, G., and Tsukahara, N. Cerebrocerebellar communication systems. *Physiol Rev* 54:957–1006, 1974.

Barinaga, M. The cerebellum: Movement coordinator or much more? *Science* 272:482–483, 1996.

Dum, R. P., and Strick, P. L. An unfolded map of the cerebellar dentate nucleus and its projections to the cerebral cortex. *J Neurophysiol* 89:634–639, 2003.

Holmes, G. The symptoms of acute cerebellar injuries due to gunshot injuries. *Brain* 40:461–535, 1917.

Holmes, G. Clinical symptoms of cerebellar disease and their interpretation. The Croonian lectures II. *Lancet*:1177–1182, 1922.

Holmes, G. The cerebellum of man. The Hughlings Jackson memorial lecture. *Brain* 62:1–30, 1939.

Jansen, J., and Brodal, A. *Aspects of Cerebellar Anatomy.* Johan Grundt Tanum Vorlagm, Oslo, 1954.

Konczak, J., Schoch, B., Dimitrova, A., Gizewski, E., and Timmann, D. Functional recovery of children and adolescents after cerebellar tumour resection. *Brain* 128:1428–1441, 2005.

Larsell, O. Morphogenesis and evolution of the cerebellum. *Arch Neurol Psychiat* 31:580–607, 1934.

Larsell, O., and Jansen. J. *The Comparative Anatomy and Histology of the Cerebellum: The Human Cerebellum, Cerebellar Connections, and Cerebellar Cortex.* University of Minnesota Press, Minneapolis, 1972.

Middleton, F. A., and Strick, P. L. Basal ganglia and cerebellar loops: Motor and cognitive circuits. *Brain Res Rev* 31:236, 2000.

Nitschke, M. F., Kleinschmidt, A., Wessel, K., and Frahm, J. Somatotopic motor representation in the human anterior cerebellum. A high resolution functional MRI study. *Brain* 119:1023–1029, 1996.

Perlmutter, J. S., and Thach, W. T. Writer's cramp: Questions of causation. *Neurology* 69:331–332, 2007.

Richter, S., Schoch, B., Kaiser, O., et al. Children and adolescents with chronic cerebellar lesions show no clinically relevant signs of aphasia or neglect. *J Neurophysiol* 94:4108–4120, 2005.

Thach, W. T., Goodwin, H. P., and Keating, J. G. The cerebellum and the adaptive coordination of movement. *Ann Rev Neurosci* 15:403–442, 1992.

Basal Ganglia

Alexander, G. E., DeLong, M. R., and Strick, P. L. Parallel organization of functionally segregated circuits linking basal ganglia and cortex. *Annu Rev Neurosci* 9:357, 1986.

Alvarez, L., Macias, R., Lopez, G., et al. Bilateral subthalamotomy in Parkinson disease: Initial and long-term response. *Brain* 128:570–583, 2005.

Aosaki, T., Graybiel, A. M., Kimura, M. Effect of nigrostriatal dopamine system on acquired neural responses in the striatum of behaving monkeys. *Science* 265:412–415, 1994.

Asanuma, K., Tang, C., Ma, Y., et al. Network modulation in the treatment of Parkinson disease. *Brain* 129:2667–2678, 2006.

Aylward, E. H., Sparks, B. F., Field, K. M., et al. Onset and rate of striatal atrophy in preclinical Huntington disease. *Neurology* 63:66–72, 2004.

Baron, M. S., Vitek, J. L., Bakay, R. A. E., et al. Treatment of advanced Parkinson disease by posterior GPi pallidotomy: 1-year results of a pilot study. *Ann Neurol* 40:355–366, 1996.

Burn, D. J. Sex and Parkinson disease: A world of difference? *J Neurol Neurosurg Psychiatry* 78:787, 2007.

Damier, P, Kastner, A., Agid, Y., and Hirsch, E. C. Does monoamine oxidase type B play a role in dopaminergic nerve cell death in Parkinson disease? *Neurology* 46:1262–1269, 1996.

Davis, G. C., Williams, A. C., Markey, S. P., et al. Chronic parkinsonism secondary to intravenous injection of meperidine analogues. *Psychiatry Research* 1:249–254, 1979.

de la Fuente-Fernandez, R., Ruth, T. J., Sossi, V., et al. Expectation and dopamine release: Mechanism of the placebo effect in Parkinson disease. *Science* 293:1164–1166, 2001.

DeLong, M. R., and Wichmann, T. Circuits and circuit disorders of the basal ganglia. *Arch Neurol* 64:20–24, 2007.

Esselink, R. A. J., de Bie, R. M. A., de Hann, R. J., et al. Unilateral pallidotomy versus bilateral subthalamic nucleus stimulation in PD. A randomized trial. *Neurology* 62:201–207, 2004.

Fazzini, E., Dogali, M., Sterio, D., et al. Stereotaxic pallidotomy for Parkinson disease: A long-term follow-up of unilateral pallidotomy. *Neurology* 48:1273–1277, 1997.

Follett K. A, Weaver F. M., Stern M., et al. Pallidal versus subthalamic deep-brain stimulation for Parkinson's disease. *N Eng J Med* 362:2077–2091, 2010

Frank, S., and Biglan, K. Long-term fetal cell transplant in Huntington disease. *Neurol* 68:2055–2056, 2007.

Goetz C. G., Tilley B. C., Shaftman S. R., et al. Movement Disorder Society-sponsored revision of the Unified Parkinson's Disease Rating Scale (MDS-UPDRS): Scale presentation and clinimetric testing results. *Mov Disord.* 23:2129–2170, 2008.

Goldman, P. S., and Nauta, W. J. H. An intricately patterned prefrontocaudate projection in the rhesus monkey. *J Comp Neurol* 171:369, 1977.

Grafton, S. T., Waters, C., Sutton, J., Lew, M. F., and Couldwell, W. Pallidotomy increases activity of motor association cortex in Parkinson disease: A positron emission tomographic study. *Ann Neurol* 37:776–783, 1995.

Gerfen, C. R. The neostriatal mosaic: Multiple levels of compartmental organization in the basal ganglia. *Annu Rev Neurosci* 15:285–320, 1992.

Goetz, C. G. New lessons from old drugs Amantadine and Parkinson disease. *Neurology* 50:1211–1212, 1998.

Graybiel, A. M., Aosaki, T. Flaherty, A. W., and Kimura, M. The basal ganglia and adaptive motor control. *Science* 265:1826–1831, 1994.

Hamani, C., et al. The subthalamic nucleus in the context of movement disorders. *Brain* 127:4, 2004.

Hershey, T., and Mink, J. W. Using functional neuroimaging to study the brain's response to deep brain stimulation. *Neurology* 66:1142–1143, 2006.

Hershey, T., Revilla, F.J ., Wernle, A., et al. Stimulation of STN impairs aspects of cognitive control in PD. *Neurology* 62:1110–1114, 2004.

Holthoff-Detto, V. A., Kessler, J., Herholz, K., et al. Functional effects of striatal dysfunction in Parkinson disease. *Arch Neurol* 54:145–150, 1997.

Hornykiewicz, O. Metabolism of brain dopamine in human parkinsonism: Neurochemical and clinical aspects. In: Costa, E., Cote, L. J., and Yahr, M. D., eds. *Biochemistry and Paramacology of the Basal Ganglia*, Raven Press, New York, 1966.

The Huntington's Disease Collaborative Research Group. A novel gene containing a trinucleotide repeat that is expanded and unstable in Huntington's disease chromosomes. *Cell* 72:971–983, 1993.

Joynt, R. J., and Gash, D. M. Neural transplants: Are we ready? *Ann Neurol* 22:455, 1987.

Koller, W. C., and Tse, W. Unmet medical needs in Parkinson disease. *Neurology* 62(Suppl 1):S1–S8, 2004.

Kolota, G. Parkinson research is set back by failure of fetal cell implants. *The Brain in the News* 8(5):1–2, 2001.

Kotzbauer, P. T., and Holtzman, D. M. Expectations and challenges of the therapeutic use of neuroprophic factors. *Ann Neurol* 59:444–447, 2006.

Krack, P., Batir, A., Van Blercom, N., et al. Five-year follow-up of bilateral stimulation of the subthalamic nucleus in advanced Parkinson disease. *N Eng J Med* 349:1925–1934, 2003.

Landau, W. M. Mucking around with Peter Pan. *Ann Neurol* 24:464, 1988.

Landau, W. M. Clinical neuromythology VII—Artifical intelligence: The brain transplant cure for parkinsonism. *Neurology* 40:733–740, 1990.

Lang, A. E. The progression of Parkinson disease: A hypothesis. *Neurology* 68:948–952, 2007.

Lang, A. E. and Obeso, J. A. Time to move beyond nigrostriatal dopamine deficiency in Parkinson disease. *Ann Neurol* 55:761–765, 2004.

Limousin, P., Pollak, P., Benazzouz, A., et al. Effect on parkinsonian signs and symptoms of bilateral subthalamic nucleus stimulation. *The Lancet,* 345:9195, 1995.

Lindvall, O., Sawle, G., Widner, H., et al. Evidence of long-term survival and function of dopaminergic grafts in progressive Parkinson disease. *Ann Neurol* 35: 172–180, 1994.

Marsden, C. D., and Obeso, J. A. The functions of the basal ganglia and the paradox of stereotaxic surgery in Parkinson disease. *Brain* 117:877, 1994.

Nauta, W. J. H., and Domesick, V. B. Crossroads of limbic and striatal circuitry: Hypothalamo-nigral connections. In: Livingston, K. E., and Hornykiewicz, O., eds. *Limbic Mechanisms: The Continuing Evolution of the Limbic System Concept.* Plenum Press, New York, 1978.

Nolte, J. *The Human Brain: An Introduction to Its Functional Anatomy.* Mosby Elsevier, Philadelphia, 2009.

Olanow, C. W. GPi pallidotomy—Have we made a dent in Parkinson disease? *Ann Neurol* 40:341–343, 1996.

Olanow, C. W., Kordower, J. H., and Freeman, T. B. Fetal nigral transplantation as a therapy for Parkinson disease. *Trends Neurosci,* 19102–109, 1996.

Olanow, C. W., Stern, M. B. and, Sethi, K. The scientific and clinical basis of the treatment of Parkinson disease. *Neurology* 72(Suppl 4):S1–S136, 2009.

Pahapill, P. A., and Lozano, A. M. The pedunculopontine nucleus and Parkinson disease. *Brain* 123:1767–1783, 2000.

Palhagen, S., Heinonen, E., Hagglund, J., et al. Selegiline slows the progression of the symptoms of Parkinson disease. *Neurology* 66:1200–1206, 2006.

Parent, A., and Hazrati, L.-N. Functional anatomy of the basal ganglia. I. The cortico-basal ganglia-thalamo-cortical loop. II. The place of subthalamic nucleus and external pallidum in basal ganglia circuitry. *Brain Res Rev* 20:91,128, 1995.

Patel, N. K., Heywood, P., O'Sullivan, K., et al. Unilateral subthalamotomy in the treatment of Parkinson disease. *Brain* 126:1136–1145, 2003.

Peppard, R. F., Martin, W. R. W., Carr, G. D., et al. Cerebral glucose metabolism in Parkinson disease with and without dementia. *Arch Neurol.* 49:1262–1268, 1992.

Petersen, A., Mani, K., and Brundin, P. Recent advances on the pathogenesis of Huntington's disease. *Exp Neurol* 157:1–18, 1999.

Plaha, P., Ben-Shlomo, Y., Patel, N. K., and Gill, S. S. Stimulation of the caudal zona incerta is superior to stimulation of the subthalamic nucleus in improving contralateral parkinsonism. *Brain* 129:1732–1747, 2006.

Pujol, J., Junque, C., Vendrell, P., et al. Reduction of the substantia nigra width and motor decline in aging and Parkinson disease. *Arch Neurol.* 49:1119–1122, 1992.

Rajput, A. H. Environmental causation of Parkinson disease. *Arch Neurol* 50:651–652, 1993.

Rascol, O. Assessing the risk of a necessary harm. Placebo surgery in Parkinson disease. *Neurology* 65:982–983, 2005.

Redgrave P., Rodriguez M., Smith Y., et al. Goal-directed and habitual control in the basal ganglia; implications for Parkinson's disease. www.Nature/reviews/neuro, 11:760–772, 2010.

Ridding, M. C., Inzelberg, R., and Rothwell, J. C. Changes in excitability of motor cortical circuitry in patients with Parkinson disease. *Ann Neurol* 37:181–188, 1995.

Rinne, J. O., Roytta, M., Paljarvi, L., et al. Selegiline (deprenyl) treatment and death of nigral neurons in Parkinson disease. *Neurology* 41:859–861, 1991.

Sawle, G. V., Playford, E. D., Burn, D. J., et al. Separating Parkinson disease from normality. *Arch Neurol* 51:237–243, 1994.

Schapira, A. H. V. Treatment options in the modern management of Parkinson disease. *Arch Neurol* 64:1083–1088, 2007.

Schapira, A. H. V., and Obeso, J. Timing of treatment initiation in Parkinson disease: A need for reapprasial? *Ann Neurol* 59:559–562, 2006.

Schenkman M. Current concepts in rehabilitation of individuals with Parkinson disease. Home Study Course. American Physical Therapy Association, 2010.

Schenkman, M., McFann, K., Barón, A. E. "PROFILE PD": **Pr**ofile **O**f **F**unction and **I**mpairment **L**evel **E**xperience with **PD**. Clinimetric properties of a rating scale for physical therapist practice. *JNPT* 34:182–192, 2010.

Schupbach, W. M. M., Maltete, D., Houeto, J. L., et al. Neurosurgery at an earlier stage of Parkinson disease: A randomized controlled trial. *Neurology* 68:267–271, 2007.

Shannon, K. M. Dopamine: So "last century." *Neurology* 69:329–330, 2007.

Tanner, C. M., Ottman, R., Goldman, S. M., et al. Parkinson disease in twins. *JAMA* 281:341–346, 1999.

Whittier, J. R. Ballism and the subthalamic nucles (nucleus hypothalamicus; corpus Luysi): Review of the literature and study of thirty cases. *Arch Neurol Psychiatry* 58:672, 1947.

Wichmann, T., and Delong, M. R. Deep brain stimulation for neurologic and neuropsychiatric disorders. *Neuron* 52(1):197–204, 2006.

Wirdefeldt, K., Gatz, M., Schalling, M., and Pedersen, N. L. No evidence of heritability of Parkinson disease in Swedish twins. *Neurology* 63:305–311, 2004.

Voluntary Movement

LEARNING OUTCOMES

This chapter prepares the reader to:

① Recall the location of the following areas of the frontal cortex that are involved in the control of movement: primary motor cortex (M1); premotor cortex, including the supplementary motor area (SMA); and the lateral premotor cortex.

② Compare the roles of each area of the frontal cortex involved in control of movement.

③ Discuss the location of the posterior parietal cortex and its role in the control of movement.

④ Identify components of the limbic system that are involved in control of movement and explain the functional relevance of these connections.

⑤ Explain the meaning and importance of haptic sensing and the relationship to the perceptual action system.

⑥ Constrast the cortical and brainstem areas involved in orientation for voluntary movements of reach, grasp, and gait.

⑦ Describe various disorders of gait and relate each disorder to the neuroanatomic location involved.

⑧ Differentiate ideational, ideomotor, kinetic, and oral apraxia and the neuroanatomic locations involved in each.

⑨ Analyze the areas of the CNS that are involved in learning and executing goal-directed purposeful movement and contrast the roles of the different areas.

ACRONYMS

CM Corticomotoneuronal

CMA Cingulate motor area

CPG Central pattern generator

DLPFC Dorsolateral prefrontal cortex

M1 Primary motor area

M2 Supplementary motor area

M3 Anterior cingulate motor area

M4 Posterior cingulate motor area

PAS Perceptual action system

PPC Posterior parietal cortex

rCBF Regional cerebral blood flow

SC Superior colliculus

SMA Supplementary motor area

Introduction

Everyday, voluntary movement typically is initiated because of an underlying motivation prompting us to take a particular action. In this respect, voluntary movement is unique and differs fundamentally from reflex action. Reflexive movements are automatically triggered by an environmental stimulus, and the muscles that contract and the joints that move are predetermined by the nature and characteristics of the stimulus. In contrast, although a given voluntary movement can be triggered by an environmental stimulus (e.g., swinging the bat at an approaching baseball), most everyday, voluntary movement is generated internally in the absence of any proximate external stimulus that dictates a specific action. Also, unlike reflexes, the precision and efficiency of voluntary movement improves markedly with practice and experience, whereas a reflexive action may be performed faultlessly the first time it is executed.

The sequence of neural processes that leads from thought to movement and the areas of the brain involved remain incompletely understood despite years of research. What seems clear, however, is that to perceive, to think about, and to act effectively upon the environment, the brain must possess an internal representation of the world that is built up over years of experience as the developing human interacts with his or her environment.

The anatomical substrate for voluntary movement was first discussed in Chapters 8, 10, and 11. There we introduced the concepts of systems of upper and lower motor neurons. In Chapter 11, we indicated that the pyramidal system is the major descending UMN system that mediates voluntary movement. The important roles of the cerebellum and basal ganglia in mediating voluntary movement were presented in Chapter 19. In this chapter, the topic of voluntary movement is addressed again, but this time from a broader perspective. In this chapter, the term *voluntary movement* is applied to those movements that are goal-directed and preplanned by the individual. Such movements are distinct from the simplistic voluntary movements studied experimentally, where exact parameters of the movement must be specified. In the performance of thusly defined voluntary movement, the brain may exploit hard-wired reflex connections as well as automatic motor subroutines that, for example, regulate posture. All of the cortical motor areas contributing to the performance of such movement are discussed and, as we shall see, they do not all reside in the agranular cortex of the frontal lobe but also include parts of the parietal lobes and limbic system. We discuss the concurrent roles voluntary movement and sensation play in determining our perceptual experience of the environment and the regulation of independent finger movement, as well as reaching and grasping. The recently introduced concept that the superior colliculus represents a UMN system contributing to these functions is discussed. We discuss the clinical disorder apraxia that follows cerebral damage. Apraxia is a high-level motor disorder in which the individual loses the capacity to execute highly complex and previously learned motor skills and gestures despite having no weakness, ataxia, or other motor deficit. Finally, we then bring together roles that might be played in the execution of voluntary movement by *all* of the functional systems presented in earlier chapters in a hypothetic scheme wherein a baseball pitcher learns how to throw strikes.

Clinical Preview

Marion Walsh, Nadya Pavlovna, and Arnold Schwartz all were admitted to the rehabilitation unit for rehabilitation following a stroke. These three individuals have lesions in different parts of the nervous system. Ms. Walsh's lesion is in the frontal lobe, Ms. Pavlovna's lesion affected the posterior parietal cortex, and Mr. Schwartz has involvement of the limbic system. Each of these individuals has deficits in control of movement. As you read through this section, consider the following:

- What functions do the frontal lobes play with regard to movement, and which specific areas of the frontal lobe relate to each function?

- The parietal cortex is generally associated with the sensory system, and the limbic system is associated with emotion; yet these areas also have specific roles with regard to voluntary movement. What are those roles?

THE CEREBRAL CORTEX AND VOLUNTARY MOVEMENT

Cortical Areas Subserving Voluntary Movement

To this point, a number of tracts associated with the motor system (Chapters 8, 13, 14, and 15) and cortical areas have been presented that are associated with the control of movement. However, the control of purposeful movement requires a complex integration of information not only from the motor system, but also from other systems, including the somatosensory, vestibular, visual, and limbic systems to name a few. Some of the most important cortical areas are presented here.

The term *motor area* is most often applied only to those cortical areas residing in the frontal lobe. However, the parietal and cingulate gyrus of the limbic system are also intimately involved in the generation of voluntary movements. Note that we are beginning our discussion of the cortical control of voluntary movement in a conventional way in that we start with the motor cortices of the frontal lobe and then progress through the parietal lobe and limbic system. In the actual generation of some types of voluntary movement, the sequence is initiated in the limbic system, progresses into the parietal lobe, and is executed from the frontal lobe.

The frontal lobe contains three motor areas: the primary motor cortex (M1), the supplementary motor cortex (M2), and the lateral premotor cortex. These areas also are differentiated as follows: the premotor area has been defined as Brodmann's area 6, including the supplementary motor area and the lateral premotor cortex. The parietal lobe includes the postcentral gyrus (Brodmann's areas 3, 1, and 2), the posterior parietal cortex (Brodmann's areas 5 and 7). And the limbic system contains two motor areas: the anterior cingulate (M3) and the posterior cingulate (M4) motor areas. These three major areas of the cortex are importantly involved in the generation and guidance of voluntary movement.

Frontal Cortex

The focus of this chapter is on the role of the cerebral cortex in voluntary movement. The large frontal lobes contain four general functional areas of importance: the primary motor, the premotor and supplementary areas, Broca's area, and the prefrontal cortex. The frontal lobes play a particularly important role in motor planning and programming for motor control. *Motor control* refers to the ability to regulate or direct the mechanisms essential to movement, with *planning* referring to the preliminary organization prior to the movement and *programming* referring to specifications that allow for the movement to progress.

PRIMARY MOTOR CORTEX (M1) The **primary motor cortex (M1)**, Brodmann's area 4, is located in the precentral gyrus, the largest component of which is buried in the anterior wall of the central sulcus and cannot be seen from the surface. The sequential, but distorted, somatotopic representation of body parts depicted in the motor homunculus has been noted previously, wherein the leg and foot are represented on the medial hemispheral surface and the trunk, arm, hand, digits, and face in progressively more ventral zones on the lateral surface (see Figure 7-7). The motor homunculus thus implies that spatially separate cortical zones control the movements of different body parts with, for example, each digit of the hand having a separate cortical territory with adjacent muscle groups represented in adjacent cortical areas. In actuality, however, this orderly somatotopic representation greatly oversimplifies the manner in which muscles are represented in M1. For one thing, the same muscle is represented multiple times in M1. For example, corticomotoneuronal (CM) neurons that control a particular digit are not grouped together in a somatotopically segregated population in the hand control area of M1 but are distributed throughout the area. Thus, the

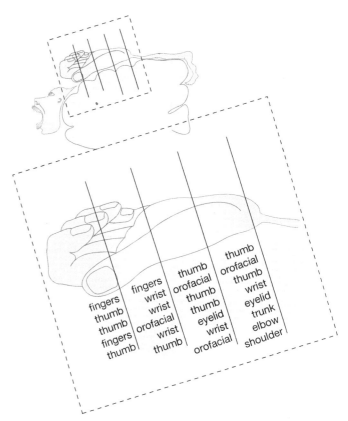

FIGURE 20-1 The individual corticomotoneuronal projections are distributed throughout the area of M1 so that they can ultimately control muscles from more than one body segment.

somatotopic organization of M1 is a *fractured somatotopy*. Furthermore, CM neurons that control independent finger movements have axons that diverge to terminate on LMNs innervating several muscles (Figure 20-1 ■) so that many cortical neurons influence more than one finger muscle.

Electrical stimulation of the surface of M1 in conscious patients undergoing neurosurgery evokes discrete isolated movements of the limbs on the contralateral side of the body. Usually, such movements involve the functional muscle groups concerned with a specific movement, but individual muscles also may be contracted separately. The evoked movements are never skilled movements comparable to those of complex acquired movements. No soley ipsilateral body movements are elicited, but bilateral movements of the upper face, jaw, tongue, pharynx, and larynx are elicited.

> **Thought Question**
>
> What evidence suggests that M1 is involved in the control of movement?

No general consensus exists regarding the nature of the motor representation that is expressed in the discharge of M1 neurons despite many years of research. It may be that M1 functions at a low level in the cortical hierarchy near the final motor output to muscles in that its neurons encode the *kinetic* features of a movement—such as the muscle forces required to rotate the joints (torques) to produce the desired movement. Alternatively, it may be that M1 functions at a higher level in the control hierarchy further removed from the motor periphery in that its neurons encode the *kinematic* features of a desired movement—such as the direction, speed, and spatial path of, for example, hand displacement. Kinematic features comprise the observable spatiotemporal form of a movement. Lastly, it is possible that M1 may encode both muscle forces and trajectory during performance of a task.

PREMOTOR CORTEX The term *premotor cortex* applies to all of Brodmann's area 6, occupying both the lateral and medial hemispheral surfaces. The term *premotor* derives from the fact that area 6 lies rostral to area 4, the primary motor cortex. The premotor cortex contains several distinct motor areas that can be differentiated from one another in terms of their afferent and efferent connections, as well as function. Described here are the connections and roles of the SMA and lateral premotor cortex.

The **supplementary motor area, SMA (M2),** was the first of the premotor areas to be recognized as a functionally distinct area of the premotor cortex. M2 occupies Brodmann's area 6 of the superior frontal gyrus on the medial surface of the hemisphere, immediately rostral to the leg representation in area 4 (Figure 20-2 ■). It contains a complete representation of the body, with the face, arm, and leg being represented in rostrocaudal sequence.

Surface electrical stimulation of the SMA (in conscious patients undergoing neurosurgery) elicits movement, but more intense current is required than with stimulation of M1, and the movements are more complex. Responses may consist of the turning of the trunk to the opposite side (orienting movement) or the assuming and holding of a contralateral limb posture as opposed to the quick, phasic movements that are elicited with stimulation of area 4. The movements are synergistic (e.g., involving an entire limb) and consist of tonic contractions of the postural type that are often maintained for many seconds after the stimulation ceases. Many of the movements elicited from stimulating M2 are bilateral. The movements involving the proximal muscles are mediated by direct projections from the SMA to the spinal cord. Some SMA projections make monosynaptic connections with alpha LMNs.

Regional increases in cortical neuronal activity are accompanied by local increases in blood flow to the area. Regional cerebral blood flow (rCBF) can be determined by injecting a radioactive isotope of xenon gas dissolved in saline into a subject while performing a motor task and then measuring the radioactivity over different parts of the cortex with arrays of detectors placed over the scalp. When this is done with a subject performing the simple, repetitive, motor task of flexing the finger against a spring-loaded cylinder, rCBF increases in the hand area of the

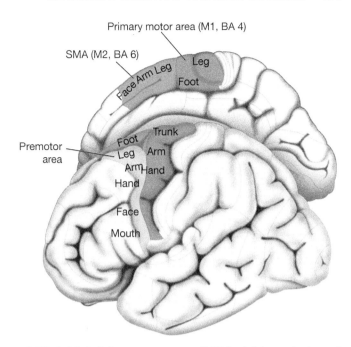

FIGURE 20-2 Primary motor area (M1) is visible on the lateral surface of the cerebral hemisphere with a small portion, representing the foot and leg, visible on the medial surface. Motor area 2 (M2), also referred to as the supplementary motor area (SMA), is located on the medial surface of the hemisphere, rostral to the M1. Note that a small portion of M2 is visible on the lateral surface. The SMA contains a complete homunculus, which is organized from rostral to caudal. This contrasts with the homunculus of M1, which is organized from ventral to dorsal.

primary motor and somatic sensory cortices of the contralateral hemisphere (Figure 20-3 ■). (The increase in activity in the postcentral gyrus is due to the increased somatosensory input generated by the repetitive finger flexion.) When a subject performs a more complex movement, such as sequentially touching each finger of the left hand to the left thumb, rCBF again increases in the hand area of the right sensorimotor cortex, but the rCBF increases expand to include the SMA bilaterally. Most interesting, however, is that when the subject simply mentally rehearses the complex sequence of finger movements, rCBF increases only in the area of the SMA bilaterally. This suggests that the SMA is a supramotor region involved in the planning of movement, specifically with the internal generation of complex movement sequences. In addition to planning self-initiated complex sequences of movement, the SMA is involved in coordinating bimanual movements, as well as the postural adjustments that precede voluntary movement. It may also be involved in the generation and control of visually guided, simple reaching movements.

People with damage to the SMA have difficulties with bimanual coordination. They experience great difficulty, for example, making a fist with one hand while simultaneously turning their other hand palm up. Rather, they perform the same movement with both hands or execute the movements sequentially as opposed to simultaneously.

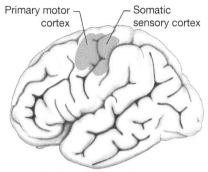

(a) Finger flexion performance

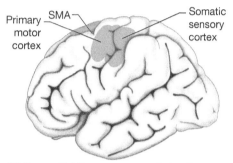

(b) Sequential finger movements (performance)

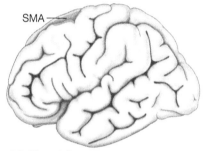

(c) Mental finger movement rehearsal

FIGURE 20-3 Studies utilizing regional cerebral blood flow (rCBF) have identified the areas of cortical involvement for (a) performance of a simple (single movement) task, (b) performance of a more complex task (involving sequential movements), and (c) mental rehearsal of a finger task without movement.

Thought Question

What cortical areas comprise MI, SMA, and area 6? Compare the role of each of these areas in control of movement. What evidence supports the identification of these regions and their roles?

Area 6 on the lateral hemispheral surface, the **lateral premotor cortex**, is divisible into at least two areas (see Figure 20-2). The first area, area 6a alpha, occupies most of the precentral gyrus and, like area 4, contains a complete and ordered representation of body parts. Electrical stimulation of area 6a alpha results in movements similar to those elicited from area 4, but the current intensities required are higher. Such movements are mediated by

corticospinal fibers originating from the pyramidal neurons of area 6a alpha. The second subdivision of area 6 is area 6a beta. It occupies the caudal part of the superior frontal gyrus immediately rostral to area 6a alpha. Electrical stimulation of area 6a beta evokes more general movement patterns consisting of rotation of the eyes, head, and trunk to the opposite side. Synergic patterns of flexion or extension of the contralateral limbs also may be elicited.

Thought Question

How do the effects of stimulation of 6a alpha and 6a beta differ?

A variety of functions have been advanced for the lateral premotor cortex. It is, for example, responsible for the initial phases of orienting the body and arm toward a desired target and controlling the proximal movements that project the arms to the target (reaching). The latter would be consistent with the fact that corticospinal projections from parts of the lateral premotor cortex terminate primarily on LMNs innervating proximal limb muscles.

Parietal Cortex

The parietal lobe, located posterior to the central sulcus and superior to the lateral sulcus, is primarily considered in terms of its somatosensory functions. However, other functions also reside in the parietal lobe, including processing and integration of visual and auditory stimuli. Here, we discuss the integrated role of the parietal lobes in relationship to movement.

Within the parietal lobe, the **posterior parietal cortex (PPC)** is of particular importance in control of voluntary movement. The PPC comprises Brodmann's areas 5 and 7 of the superior parietal lobule (see Figure 7-5). The PPC is involved in regulating movement, in particular of the extremities. Goal-directed movements such as reaching for and grasping an object require elaborate sensory analyses and guidance. First, the environment in which the movement transpires must be accurately represented such that the performer knows the spatial relationships among potential obstacles and the location of the sought-after object. Second, the orientation of the body toward the object must be known, as well as the position of the limbs relative to the object, in order to accurately determine which limb is to be the effector as well as the muscles that can best be used in the movement. Third, the physical properties of the object itself such as its shape and size also must be known. Both areas 5 and 7 receive somatosensory (tactile and proprioceptive) and visual information. Within these areas, particular subareas process primarily visual information; others process predominantly somatosensory information; still others integrate somatosensory and visual information. Recall from Chapter 18 that the dorsal pathway of visual information projects to the parieto-occipital association cortex and is used in determining where an event occurred. Given the elaborate somatosensory input to the superior parietal lobule, it is not surprising to find that the PPC, like the frontal motor cortices, contains a multiplicity of face, arm, and leg representations.

Each of the different *frontal and limbic* motor areas (M1, M2, lateral, premotor, and cingulate motor area) receives afferents predominantly from one subarea of the PPC. The input from the motor areas forms a **parieto-frontal circuit**. Functionally, these inputs are of critical importance to movement because they allow for initiation of movement in response to the decision to move or in response to somatosensory, auditory, or visual stimuli. A number of such circuits exist, each of which specifies the particular array of sensory information that is to be used to specify the critical features of the movement required to attain the movement's desired goal. These sensory representations are transformed into muscle control signals in the motor cortex—that is, these specialized circuits, which work in parallel, transform sensory information into action. The relationship of sensory and motor circuitry is elaborated later when we discuss haptic sensing.

Limbic Areas

The limbic system is involved in mediating emotion and memory and drive-related behavior, each of which is of importance in the decision to move. Recall that the limbic system is a functionally defined area comprised of parts of the frontal, parietal, and temporal lobes.

The **cingulate motor areas (CMAs)** are located in the base (fundus) and banks of the cingulate sulcus on the medial surface of each hemisphere and are subdivided into rostral and caudal areas (Figure 20-4 ■). The rostral cingulate motor area (CMAr, M3) is located in Brodmann's

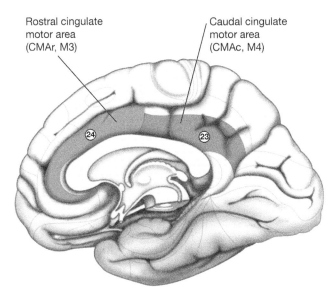

FIGURE 20-4 The cingulate motor areas of the limbic system are located in the cingulate gyrus.

area 24, while the caudal cingulate motor area (CMAc, M4) resides in area 23. M3 and M4 both contain complete body representations with face, arm, and leg representations organized in rostral to caudal topography. Each CMA is reciprocally connected to the primary (M1) and supplementary motor (M2) cortices.

Projections from each CMA to the spinal cord are topographically organized so that those originating in the arm representations terminate in the contralateral cervical enlargement, while those from the leg representations end in the contralateral lumbosacral enlargement. (Projections originating in the face representations synapse in the facial nucleus, as noted in Chapter 14.) Cingulospinal projections from the arm representations in both CMAs have a mode of termination in the spinal cord similar to that of the pyramidal system. That is, most cingulospinal projections terminate in the intermediate zone of the spinal gray and, therefore, influence LMNs indirectly via interneurons. A smaller contingent of cingulospinal projections terminate directly (i.e., monosynaptically) on LMNs in the dorsolateral portion of Rexed's lamina IX, which innervates the distal flexor muscles.

Thought Question

What is the functional implication of the anatomical link between the limbic system and the motor system?

The cortical connections of the CMAs (in addition to those with motor areas) are key to understanding their function. Both areas receive widespread connections from the prefrontal cortex, the amygdala, and cortex of the limbic system (i.e., non-motor areas of the cingulate gyrus). Such inputs provide the CMAs with information about motivational state and the internal status of the subject as well as cognitive information about the environment, including its suitability for the successful attainment of the particular motor act. Thus, when the subject is appropriately motivated to act, the CMAs select voluntary movements designed to fulfill the goal of the performance (i.e., with a reward value) when environmental conditions permit attainable execution of the act.

Connections of the Cortical Motor Areas

Cortical Connections

The primary motor cortex receives direct projections from a number of sources (Figure 20-5 ■). The projections from the primary somatosensory cortex (Brodmann areas 3, 1, and 2) are via short association fibers and are somatotopically organized so that, for example, the hand area of primary somatosensory cortex projects to the hand area of M1. As a result of these direct connections, neurons in M1

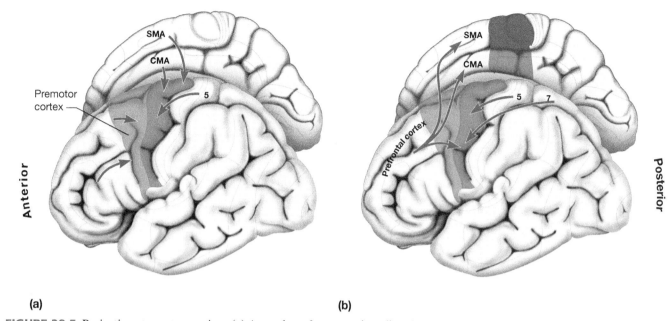

(a)   **(b)**

FIGURE 20-5 Projections to motor cortices. (a) A number of areas project directly to the primary motor area, M1, including the following: primary somatosensory cortex (areas 3, 1, 2); all of the premotor cortices and area 5 of the posterior parietal cortex (PPC); and the cingulate motor area (CMA) and supplementary motor area (SMA). (b) A number of areas project directly to the premotor cortex, including the following: somatosensory association cortices, areas 5 and 7, and the dorsolateral prefrontal cortex (DLPFC). Additionally, the DLPFC projects to the CMA and SMA.

have peripheral somatosensory receptive fields. Neurons in M1, for example, receive muscle spindle input from the muscles whose movements they influence. All of the premotor cortices project to M1, as does area 5 of the PPC. Additionally, M1 receives projections from the cingulate motor area (CMA) and supplementary motor area (SMA).

The premotor cortex has abundant connections as well, including those from somatosensory association cortices (Brodmann's areas 5 and 7) and area 46 of the prefrontal cortex, called the **dorsolateral prefrontal cortex (DLPFC)**. Finally, the DLPFC connects to the SMA and CMA. Both of these areas then connect to M1 as described earlier. The DLPFC is involved in short-term memory for action-related sensory information, preparatory motor set, and the inhibition of motor responses to distracting stimuli (see haptic sensing).

Subcortical Connections

> **Thought Question**
>
> To this point in the chapter, we have been focusing on the cortical areas associated with movement. What important roles can you think of for the cerebellum, basal ganglia, and brainstem areas with respect to movement?

In Chapters 6 and 19, connections to the motor area were introduced, including connections between the cerebellum, the basal ganglia, and the thalamus. Here, we revisit their roles in context of voluntary movement.

M1 and the premotor cortices are reciprocally connected to two subcortical structures, the cerebellum and basal ganglia. Projections between these structures are from two distinct cortical-subcortical circuits: a cortico-basal ganglia-thalamo-cortical circuit and a cortico-cerebello-thalamo-cortical circuit. Each of these cortical and subcortical loops functions as an integrated circuit. As shown in Figure 20-6 ■, these cortical-subcortical loops synapse in different portions of the ventrolateral thalamus that, in turn, project to distinct cortical territories. The internal segment of the globus pallidus synapses in the

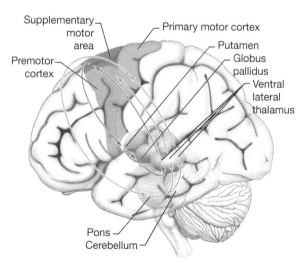

FIGURE 20-6 Cortical and subcortical loops. The primary motor cortex and the premotor cortex are reciprocally connected with the cerebellum and basal ganglia.

ventrolateral nucleus that, in turn, projects to the SMA. Output from the cerebellum synapses in two areas of the ventrolateral thalamus, one of which projects to the premotor cortex while the second projects to M1. These two loops are differentially deployed depending (1) on the type of voluntary movement being executed and (2) on the extent to which the motor skill has been learned.

THE CONTROL OF VOLUNTARY MOVEMENT

Clinical Preview ·················

You are working in a rehabilitation center where you treat many people who have had strokes resulting in impaired control of voluntary movements. Some people have particular difficulty with upper extremity reaching and/or with hand control, while others have difficulty performing functional movements, but only on request, a condition referred to as apraxia. As you read through the following sections, consider how the nervous system controls these different functions. In particular, consider the following:

- How do the sensory and motor systems work together for exploration by the hand, referred to as *haptic sensing*?

- How does neuroanatomic control of reaching activities differ from neuroanatomic control of haptic sensing?

- How does apraxia differ in its consequences on the control of movement from paresis, and what is the neuroanatomic basis for conditions of apraxia?

The neurological control of purposeful voluntary movement is difficult to study because true purposeful movements are those complex movements that are executed in everyday life activities. They lie beyond the scope of current experimental techniques. However, some of the components and neuroanatomic correlates can be inferred from investigations on simplified voluntary movement whose parameters can be controlled experimentally. In this section, we begin with an examination of the integration of perception and action in functional tasks. This interaction is of essential importance in many aspects of purposeful movement and, in particular, in the use of the hand. Next, we consider the relatively simplified upper extremity tasks of reaching and grasping. This information is followed by a summary of the role of the superior colliculus in mediating voluntary movement, especially as it relates to head/trunk orientation during movement. Then, we address a more complex movement, that of gait. We next address the complex processes that occur in planning of movement (before movement even is initiated). And, finally, we end the section with examples illustrating some of the important clinical consequences of disorders of voluntary movement.

Perceptual Action System and Haptic Sensing

To understand purposeful movement, we first consider the role of perception. The term **perceptual action system (PAS)** emphasizes that purposeful movement does not occur in isolation from the sensory perceptual experience of the environment, but rather that the two systems work in concert as movement evolves. This concept is illustrated using the example of the hand. We typically do not think of the critical role that the hand plays in perception; in most day-to-day activities, we attend to its purposeful motor performance, and the associated visual input dominates perceptual awareness. However, the sensory feedback derived from the exploratory manipulation itself is even more important than visual feedback in guiding the evolving exploratory movements.

The term **haptic sensing** refers to exploration by the hand. Haptic is derived from the Greek word *haptikos*, meaning "able to lay hold of." Thus, haptic sensing is the derivation of information about an object's intrinsic properties, such as its size, shape, and texture, by means of exploratory finger movements performed during manipulation of the object by the hand. In haptic sensing, the hand itself not only has a motor role, but also an exploratory role for conscious sensory perception and cognition—that is, object identification. For example, in identifying the shape of sculptured objects without the use of vision, people typically (1) curve their fingers around its face, using all of the fingers and fitting them into the cavities—this is done repetitively as the orientation of the object is changed (i.e., precision grasping and releasing); (2) move their fingers in a way that is exploratory, in that the movements do not become stereotyped or occur in a fixed sequence that is obviously repeated; (3) repetitively oppose the thumb and other digits, but with different fingers used in the repetitions—the object may be rubbed with one or more fingers, or sometimes a single finger may be used to trace the curvature of the object.

Thought Question

Contrast the roles of receptors for touch, proprioception, and pain with respect to haptic sensing. How is each sensory modality used?

We especially depend on haptic perception when we work in the dark or without vision, such as when retrieving a particular denomination of coin or particular key from a purse or pocket. Haptic sensing by object manipulation depends on two processes. First, it requires the integration of different modalities of sensory signals. Second, it requires the integration of this disparate sensory information with the motor commands that themselves are responsible for the temporal modulation of the sensory signals. The sensory modalities involved are cutaneous and proprioceptive. The most important cutaneous information is derived from the volar surfaces of the fingertips and activation of both slowly and rapidly adapting mechanoreceptors (see Chapter 9). The most important proprioceptive information is derived from muscle spindles in the finger muscles. As noted in Chapter 9, muscle spindles underlie the discrimination of joint angles. The discrimination of finger joint angles, in turn, determines the perception of hand posture or shape, thereby providing information about the three-dimensional geometry of the object. It is the *integration* of cutaneous and proprioceptive information that generates the haptic feedback underlying object identification. That the identification does not rely on cutaneous feedback alone is evident from the fact that while a given object can be correctly identified across subjects (or repeatedly by a given subject), the pattern of cutaneous pressures varies at any given time, as well as over time, as different fingers touch the object in various combinations as the hand manipulates it. Rather, the identification depends on the concurrent influx and integration of information from the skin and from proprioceptors conveying information about hand posture. Eliminating either cutaneous or proprioceptive feedback impairs object identification, but eliminating both prevents correct identification. Thus, haptic feedback generates information about solid objects in three dimensions.

Thought Question

What do the connections between the motor cortical area M1 and the DLPFC imply about short-term memory and movement? What might be the implications for motor learning and movement rehabilitation following damage from strokes and traumatic brain injury?

Haptic processing is sequential and so depends on the integration of information that evolves over time. In other words, object identification depends on the totality of skin–joint input generated during an entire sequence of hand movements. Thus, the sensory input generated during an early stage of the movement sequence is no longer present during later stages so that the temporal gap between mutually contingent sensations must be bridged. This means that the information generated during earlier stages must be stored in what is called **working memory**. Working memory is information storage that is temporary and enables a particular task to be accomplished. In this case, sensory information is stored for later retrieval when the movement sequence is complete and the totality of the information can be integrated. Storing this

information in working memory is the function of the dorsolateral prefrontal cortex (DLPFC). DLPFC is reciprocally connected to all of the premotor areas of the frontal lobe, as well as to the PPC, and so is in a position to oversee haptic sensing.

Thought Question

We have focused on the PAS with respect to haptic sensing. But perception is also critical to any type of movement. What do you suppose might be the motor and functional consequences of sensory loss of the upper extremity without motor loss or with minimal motor loss? What types of lesions might result in this type of loss?

Independent Finger Movements in Other Functions

Now let us consider the complexity of the motor side of the control of movement by examining the control of individual finger movements. Typing or playing a musical instrument depends on the capacity to move the fingers rapidly and independently in precise and complex temporal sequences involving accurate, individuated finger placements. Such learned motor skills are executed by the complex interplay of some 27 intrinsic and extrinsic hand muscles. However, the digits are not anatomically independent, being biomechanically coupled to one another by common tendons, although the thumb has greater biomechanical independence compared with the other digits. Thus, moving single digits independently in complex sequences such as occur in playing a keyboard musical instrument requires a precise pattern of activation and inhibition of many muscles acting on multiple fingers. Movements of an individual finger are controlled by neurons in the hand area of the primary motor cortex via direct corticomotoneuronal (CM) projection.

One of the seemingly puzzling features of this privileged monosynaptic input to LMNs innervating the extrinsic hand muscles is the extent to which their axons diverge to innervate multiple LMN nuclei (see Figure 20-1), as well as to innervate many LMNs in a given nucleus that supply a specific muscle. This innervation pattern would seem to pose a special problem for the three multitendon extrinsic finger muscles located in the forearm that control flexion and extension of the fingers. Each of these muscles gives rise to four parallel tendons that insert into the four digits. In the face of the divergence in the direct CM projection, how are these muscles controlled to give rise to individual finger movements? The answer is that the direct CM projections are not uniformly distributed across the LMNs innervating these multitendon muscles. Rather, they tend to be segregated to supply subsets of LMNs innervating individual fingers (i.e., the muscles regulate individual tendons).

Grasping

The hand is so important to normal human behavior that the major function of the shoulder and arm is to place the hand in a position where it can perform its specific function. Thus, many of the voluntary hand movements performed by humans in their everyday lives are divisible into several components, beginning with a reaching phase and ending with grasping and manipulation phases. Reaching and grasping in stylized patterns has been extensively investigated and has greatly helped us to understand mechanisms subserving the control of movement. However, it is important to recognize that the movements studied are, indeed, highly stylized—and, hence, somewhat limited in application to everyday movements.

The act of seizing or grasping an object can be expressed in fundamentally different types of grips that depend on different motor control circuits. A **precision grip** is used in grasping the bow of a violin or a pen, for example. In the precision grip, forces are directed between the thumb and finger. A **power grip** is used in tasks such as holding a hammer to strike a nail. In the power grip, the fingers and thumb direct forces toward the palm to transmit a force to an object (Figure 20-7 ■). The precision grip requires independent movement of the fingers and is mediated by the primary motor cortex. M1 is virtually unique among the motor areas of the cerebral cortex in controlling independent finger movements. Individual CM

neurons in the primary motor cortex discharge during such precision grips. However, during contraction of the same muscles in a power grip—such as occurs when holding a hammer or climbing a rope, where all of the fingers are flexed in unison around the object with counterpressure from the thumb—the same CM neuron does not discharge. The power grip does not require independent movements of the fingers and so can be mediated by non-CM neurons. Such neurons may originate either within or outside of M1. Furthermore, they may terminate either in the brainstem or synapse indirectly on LMNs, thereby mediating synergistic contraction of more muscles. Still other control circuits may mediate utilization of the hand to form a fist in an outburst of anger.

Thought Question

What cortical areas are important for grip and for shaping the hand? Are they similar or different? What is the evidence for their contributions?

Neuroanatomical Areas Controlling Grasping

Reaching for and grasping an object requires that the object is accurately located in three-dimensional space surrounding the body and that the location of the object is transformed for appropriate arm movement toward the object. In addition, the intrinsic properties of the object (size and shape) must be perceived and transformed into an appropriate posturing of finger movements in order to grasp it. Grasping involves a straightening and progressive opening of the fingers until an appropriate aperture is attained. This is followed by a closure of the grip until it matches the size and shape of the object. Both of these visuomotor transformations are mediated by the anterior intraparietal area of the PPC and ventral part of the lateral premotor cortex. The anterior intraparietal area is located in the anterior lateral bank of the intraparietal sulcus and is activated during normal precision grasping. People with damage to the PPC involving the cortex lining the anterior part of the intraparietal sulcus exhibit impaired preshaping of the hand during goal-directed grasping.

Orienting Movements of the Eyes, Head, and Neck

Thought Question

Before proceeding, it will be helpful to refresh your memory about the anatomy of control of eye movements related to visual and vestibular brainstem pathways. Diagram these pathways, and add in the pathways between the superior colliculus and the cortex.

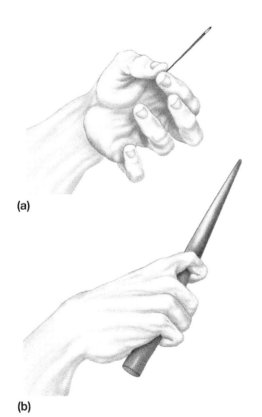

(a)

(b)

FIGURE 20-7 Types of grip. (a) Precision grip is mediated by corticomotoneuronal (CM) projections. (b) Power grip is mediated by non-CM projections.

In Chapters 11 and 18, automatic eye movements referred to as saccades were introduced. We now consider the anatomy and function of these movements as they relate to goal-directed purposeful movement. Furthermore, a number of other automatic movements involving the head and neck are also critical during purposeful movement. Movements of the eyes, head, and neck are discussed in relation to purposeful movement.

The role of the superior colliculus (SC) is of particular functional relevance in relation to the oculomotor system: it participates in the generation of saccadic eye movements and is a command center for gaze shift in that it controls the coordinated movement of the eyes and head. Recall that in Chapter 17, it was noted that the **tectospinal tract** originates from neurons of the superior colliculus (SC), comprising a component of the ventromedial descending UMN system. **Saccades** are ballistic, step-like, voluntary, conjugate eye movements that are used to capture a visual image on the fovea of the retina (i.e., to change the point of foveal fixation). These voluntary eye movements occur in all directions and are used for reading and other forms of visual scanning, such as looking at pictures or scenes. They also are used in more automatic functions such as looking over at objects that first appear in peripheral vision. The motor programs (sometimes called central pattern generators) for saccades reside in the reticular formation of the midbrain and pons and are controlled by corticobulbar fibers descending from the cerebral cortex in a manner analogous to the cortical control of other voluntary movements (Figure 20-8 ■). The motor system controlling saccades is organized in a manner similar to the organization of the system controlling other voluntary movement. Thus,

there is a primary motor cortex, and there are connections of the primary motor cortex with other cortical motor areas residing in the same or different lobes. Additionally, the basal ganglia and cerebellum interact with the cerebral cortex in the production of saccades.

The primary motor cortex for saccades is the **frontal eye field** located in the posterior portion of the middle frontal gyrus (part of Brodmann's area 8). Electrical stimulation of the frontal eye field evokes horizontal conjugate deviation of the eyes to the contralateral side.

These movements are mediated by descending projections to the paramedian pontine reticular formation containing a central pattern generator for horizontal saccades. Some of the projections are direct; some projections relay in the SC, which in turn projects to the pontine reticular formation. Two other cortical areas elicit saccades when stimulated. One is located in the supplementary motor area on the medial hemispheral surface and is termed the **supplementary eye field**. The second area is in the parietal lobe and is termed the **parietal eye field**. Both of these fields project directly to the brainstem as well as projecting to the frontal eye field, thus paralleling the organization of outputs from the cortical motor areas controlling voluntary movement of the limbs. The functional roles of the supplementary and parietal eye fields have not been clarified.

A lesion involving the frontal eye field in one hemisphere results in an inability to look voluntarily to the contralateral side (vertical eye movements are not impaired). Interestingly, this deficit generally recovers in a matter of days. However, when both the frontal eye field and SC are damaged, a long-lasting loss of ability to generate saccades results.

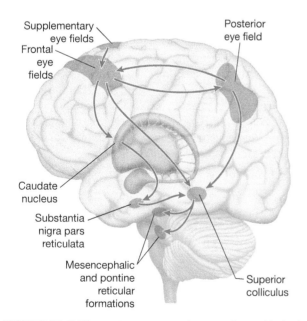

FIGURE 20-8 The motor programs for saccades reside in the reticular formation and are controlled by corticobulbar fibers that originate in the frontal eye field, supplementary eye field, and posterior eye fields. The basal ganglia and cerebellum also participate in control of saccadic eye movements.

Thought Question

The superior colliculus appears to play a number of different roles in the control of movement. What are they?

In addition to controlling saccades, it now appears that neurons of the SC play a considerably broader role in voluntary movement. The SC plays a role in the execution of voluntary orienting movements—not only for gaze, but also for the head and arm. The parts of the SC involved in the voluntary control of neck and arm movements are its deeper layers from which the tectospinal and other tectofugal projections arise. In addition to gaze-related neurons, these deeper layers of the SC contain a separate and independent population of neurons related only to head movement, irrespective of whether the head movement leads to a gaze shift. Direct projections from the SC descend in the tectospinal tract to terminate on LMNs of the spinal cord that control neck muscles. Electrical stimulation of the SC is capable of eliciting activity in neck muscles and head movement without any accompanying gaze shift. But the role of the SC in voluntary movement seems even more encompassing than the control of head movement and gaze. The activity of SC neurons is also related to arm movement, in particular to the activity of shoulder muscles in reaching tasks. Additionally, the SC may play a role in grasping and hand conformation.

> **Thought Question**
>
> From a functional perspective, what would be the consequence of loss of saccadic movements of the eyes?

Gait

Gait is a voluntarily deployed movement, and all of its components can be adjusted voluntarily to fit prevailing environmental circumstances (e.g., the nature of the terrain on which the person walks, the predictability of surface variations such as firmness and height). However, it is a unique type of voluntary movement because an important aspect of gait is instinctual and not learned. It inevitably appears as part of the human motor repertoire under natural conditions. The basic movement pattern of stepping is present at birth in that it can be elicited by contacting the sole of a neonate's foot with a flat surface and shifting the center of gravity, first laterally onto one foot, permitting the opposite foot to be raised, then forward, allowing the body to move onto the advancing foot. This stepping pattern indicates the presence of operational, hard-wired spinal cord circuitry responsive to peripheral input that is modulated by descending input from the vestibular system, a system that is functional at birth. Central pattern generators (CPGs), introduced in Chapter 11, are important in this regard.

What the infant does learn during the first year of life is to maintain balance in relation to gravity during the continuously unstable equilibrium that characterizes walking. That is, during walking, the center of gravity shifts from side to side and forward as the infant's weight is borne first on one foot and then on the other. It is a maturation of the systems that maintain successful balance control that enable the infant to learn to control locomotion voluntarily, that is, to deploy walking toward the attainment of a goal. This depends on information from a number of systems, including the vestibular, visual, and proprioceptive systems. Initially, under conscious regulation and with continued practice (and numerous falls), balance control does become automatic like other voluntary movement.

Additionally, other aspects of gait are also learned. The cadence of gait and the lightness or heaviness of tread vary from person to person such that an individual may be identified by the sound of his or her footsteps. Likewise, the carriage of the body and swing of the arms may impart a highly individualistic style to a person's gait.

Higher Cortical Processing and Control of Movement

All goal-directed voluntary movement is learned, as discussed earlier. Some such movements have been mastered through long practice (the slow learning phase) and have become habitual (the retention phase). Others still demand continuous attention and thought as the initial conceptualization of the movement's final purpose is attained only by continuously modifying individual components of the motor sequence until the goal is achieved. Diverse areas of the cerebral cortex are involved in such goal-directed voluntary movement. Activity in these areas reflects the highest level of motor planning and programming. The posterior parietal lobe is important because skilled movements involve dynamic transformations in space and spatial representations reside in the posterior parietal cortex.

The neural substrate for organizing movements resides primarily in the dominant left hemisphere and involves the sequential activation of specific cortical areas (Figure 20-9 ■). When a person is requested to perform a gesture with the right hand, information is first projected to the primary auditory cortex and then to Wernicke's area, where the command is decoded. Information is then sent to the posterior parietal cortex (e.g., the supramarginal gyrus, superior parietal lobule), where the command (intent of the movement) is integrated with information concerning the sensory context in which the movement will occur and the status of the body parts that will make the movement. This information is forwarded to the premotor cortex (area 6) over the **superior longitudinal fasciculus**. The superior longitudinal

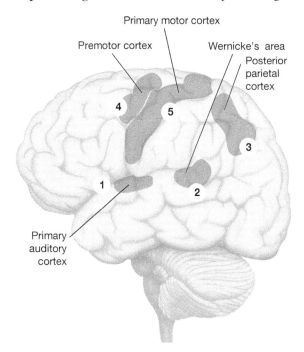

FIGURE 20-9 The neural substrate for a movement on command of the right hand resides in the left (dominant) cerebral hemisphere and involves activation of the highlighted areas. The numbers indicate the sequential order of their activation.

fasciculus (also known as the arcuate fasciculus) is a long association bundle of fibers. Within the premotor cortex, these sensory representations are transformed into a motor code (program) that specifies the essential features of the gesture required to achieve its intended goal. The motor program is forwarded to the left primary motor cortex that mediates execution of the gesture with the right hand. If the gesture is to be executed with the left (usually nondominant) hand, the motor program generated in the left premotor cortex is transmitted to the right premotor cortex over fibers in the trunk of the corpus callosum. Short association fibers link the right premotor cortex with the right primary motor cortex that then mediates execution of the gesture with the left hand. If the person is imitating a gesture performed by the examiner, the posterior parietal cortex is reached over visual system projections originating in the primary visual cortex, rather than by language system projections from Wernicke's area (which is involved in the interpretation of spoken language).

Thought Question

Control of movement involves more than the execution of the motion. First, there must be planning, then programming of the movement. In addition, motor memory is essential. Considering everything discussed in this chapter, what cortical areas are involved with each of these functions?

CLINICAL CONNECTIONS
Disorders of Gait

Gait is a function of integration of a wide range of neurological processes, including such diverse cortical areas as the motor cortex, parietal cortex, cerebellum, basal ganglia, brainstem, and spinal cord. Therefore, abnormalities of gait can occur as a result of dysfunction in almost any part of the nervous system. The consequences of dysfunction in these various areas are quite different, depending on which combination of systems are involved (e.g., motor, somatosensory, vestibular, and visual). Indeed, the specific abnormalities of gait often are so distinctive that the experienced clinician can sometimes make a determination of the person's underlying disorder simply by observing gait. Some of the typical abnormal gait patterns are presented in Table 20-1 ■. Still, definitive localization of a lesion causing a gait disorder—particularly when the disorder is mild—can only be made in the context of a full neurological examination.

Thought Question

Consider the disorder of sensory ataxic gait. Why might people with sensory loss have ataxia? How might a rehabilitation professional teach the individual with this disorder to compensate for this type of gait problem?

Table 20-1 Localization and Features of Gait Disorders

NAME	ALTERNATIVE NAMES	GAIT CHARACTERISTICS	LOCALIZATION OF LESION SITE	INTERPRETATION OF THE DEFICIT
Cerebellar gait	Ataxic gait	Wide-based, erratic shifting of weight, irregular cadence, unsteady, staggering, falling toward the side of greater pathology.	Midline and paravermal cerebellum.	Unable to modulate by correcting the ongoing movement.
Sensory ataxic gait	Tabetic gait	Wide-based, brusque, high-stepping movement of the legs and flapping (stamping) of the feet, irregular cadence; ataxia markedly exaggerated when walking in the dark.	Somatosensory nerve fibers subserving kinesthesia, posterior columns, medial lemniscus.	Unable to sense where the lower extremities are in space because of proprioceptive loss.
Spastic gait	Plegic gait, Hemiplegic gait	Stiff-legged, circumduction, slow cadence, scuffing sound as the foot scrapes the floor; stiff, flexed arm with decreased swing.	Unilateral or bilateral damage to the cortical motor system or the corticospinal tracts. (Note that this is one type of gait disorder associated with stroke and, furthermore, that there are a number of possible causes of abnormal gait that might appear to fit this description, not all of which relate to the motor system specifically.)	Unable to fractionate movements.

Table 20-1 **(Continued)**

NAME	ALTERNATIVE NAMES	GAIT CHARACTERISTICS	LOCALIZATION OF LESION SITE	INTERPRETATION OF THE DEFICIT
Parkinsonian gait	Festinating gait	Forward-leaning, narrow-based, slow cadence, short, shuffling steps until festination; difficulty with gait initiation; decreased or absent arm swing, turning en bloc.	Substantia nigra.	Forward leaning posture due to altered musculoskeletal alignment secondary to bradykinesia and rigidity; slowness of movement and inability to initiate due to bradykinesia, akinesia.
Dyskinetic gait	Dystonic and choreoathetotic gaits	Continuous intrusion of involuntary movements during walking in which there may be unilateral or bilateral writhing (athetoid), dance-like (choreic), or flinging (ballistic) movements of the arms and legs; abnormal torsion of the trunk (flexion, lordosis, scoliosis) and flexion of one or both legs at the hip assert themselves during walking.	Striatum, subthalamic nucleus, or other components of the basal ganglia.	Inappropriate extraneous movements initiated due to spontaneous release, resulting from inappropriate disinhibition.
Vertiginous gait	Toppling gait	Wide-based, slow, short steps, with tottering and falling.	Semicircular canals, vestibular nerve, vestibular nuclei.	Ineffective sense of equilibrium due to incongruence of somatosensory, visual, and vestibular inputs.
Frontal gait	Apraxia of gait	Wide-based, slow, shuffling, short-steps; one or both feet appear to be stuck to the ground as the body moves forward (torso and legs not in phase); difficulty starting and stopping.	Frontal lobes and/or their subcortical white matter.	Ineffective motor planning associated with frontal damage.

Apraxia

Damage to the dominant posterior parietal cortex results in an inability to recognize a complex movement when it occurs in another person, as well as an inability to generate such movements when asked to do so. As we noted earlier, the transformation of such a representation into action demands the participation of the frontal lobe—specifically, the premotor and prefrontal cortices. Damage to the frontal lobe, therefore, can result in an inability to generate a movement when asked to do so but may not disrupt the capacity to perceive such actions when occurring in another person. Impairments in these functions are reflected in a clinical disorder called *apraxia*. Tests

for apraxia involve having patients produce goal-directed motor acts. Note that a set of conditions, referred to as *constructional apraxia* and *dressing apraxia*, occur with damage to the nondominant posterior parietal cortex.

The term **apraxia** defines a unique category of movement disorder in which the person is unable to carry out—on request and/or by imitation—a skilled, learned movement. Apraxia is not due to paresis, ataxia, sensory changes, or deficiencies of understanding resulting from a language disturbance (such as can occur in Wernicke's aphasia) or to impaired intellectual capacity (such as with confusion or dementia). The key to revealing an apraxic deficit is the mode of eliciting the motor act or gesture from the patient.

The gesture is always elicited in the artificial context of the examination room and can be done in a variety of ways: by giving the patient a verbal command or request to perform the act, by presenting the patient with an object or tool and asking him or her to pretend to use it, or by requesting the patient to imitate an action or gesture performed by the examiner. Actually handing the patient a familiar object or tool and asking him or her to use it should also be done, but this mode of eliciting a gesture simulates a natural context and may not reveal all types of apraxic deficits.

Apraxic deficits are subdivided into specific types that represent disturbances at different points in the sequence of neural events leading to the performance of a skilled voluntary motor act: ideational (or conceptual), ideomotor, and kinetic. The planning of complex activities involves conceptualizing their final purpose, as well as the appropriate order of the individual components of the motor sequence that will achieve the goal of the act. The failure to conceive a performance strategy results in ideational apraxia. Ideomotor apraxia results when there is a dissociation between an intact conceptualization of the act and its translation into a motor program. Kinetic apraxia occurs when the motor program itself is defective.

The clinical pattern of, for example, an ideomotor apraxic deficit depends on where in this praxis system the causative lesion is located. The following account assumes that a verbal request has been made by the clinician to perform a movement and, therefore, the left hemisphere is involved exclusively or initially. A lesion situated in the posterior parietal cortex or in the superior longitudinal fasciculus would result in an apraxia involving both right and left upper extremities. A similar pattern would result from a lesion involving the left premotor cortex, but because such damage is also likely to extend to the adjacent primary motor cortex, the clinical picture would be of an apraxia of the left (nondominant) hand and a right-sided paresis that masks an attendant apraxia. A lesion involving the fibers of the corpus callosum would result in a left-sided apraxia with no involvement of movements on the right side. A similar clinical picture should result from damage to the right premotor cortex, but in actuality, associated damage to the contiguous right primary motor cortex results in a left-sided paresis that masks the apraxia.

Ideational Apraxia

In **ideational apraxia,** there is a loss of knowledge about objects and tools in terms of the actions and functions they serve. In addition, there is an inability to organize single actions into a sequence so as to achieve an intended purpose. These deficits are present, even though the person is able to recognize and name the articles he or she attempts to manipulate. Thus, ideational apraxia presents as an inability to perform multiple-step tasks (e.g., preparing a letter to mail, lighting a candle) and to associate single tools and objects with their corresponding action (e.g., an inability to select a hammer to drive a nail, using a toothbrush to comb the hair, or correctly pantomime a movement that is markedly

different from the one requested by the examiner). People with ideational apraxia are impaired in everyday life, as well as in the clinical setting, because they do not use tools or objects properly, they choose an incorrect tool or object to perform a desired activity, or they perform a complex sequential activity in an improper order. Thus, there is no voluntary–automatic dissociation. No single anatomical site has been identified that, when damaged, causes ideational apraxia, although the cortex of the left parieto-temporo-occipital junction is believed to play an important role. Ideational apraxia is commonly seen in people with dementia and especially in people with Alzheimer's disease.

Ideomotor Apraxia

Ideomotor apraxia is a disorder of goal-directed movement wherein the goal of the action usually can be recognized. The person knows what he or she wants to do but is unable to translate the idea of the action into an appropriate motor program. Ideomotor apraxia primarily reflects a disturbance in the timing and spatial organization of gestural movements. Temporal errors manifest themselves as either an increased or decreased rate of production of a pantomime or an improper sequencing of a complex movement that requires multiple positionings, such as striking a match before taking out a cigarette. Spatial errors include abnormal movement amplitude; for example, when asked to pantomime teeth brushing, a patient uses his or her own finger to represent the toothbrush and leaves no space between the finger and mouth to represent the imagined toothbrush.

One of the most striking features of ideomotor apraxia is a voluntary–automatic dissociation. This means that the movement deficit shows up in the clinical setting, where movements are required out of their natural context, but not in the person's everyday spontaneous behavior. Even in the clinical setting, task performance may normalize when the patient is given an actual tool or object to use. Thus, ideomotor apraxia results in little or no interference with everyday function such that the person may not even be aware of having a movement disorder. Lesions causing ideomotor apraxia typically involve the left hemisphere and are centered in the supramarginal gyrus and superior parietal lobule. Such lesions may involve the cerebral cortex as well as the underlying white matter that would interrupt the superior longitudinal fasciculus connecting the PPC with the premotor area and produce bilateral limb apraxia.

Kinetic Apraxia

Kinetic apraxia manifests itself as a loss of hand and finger dexterity that cannot be accounted for by paresis, ataxia, or sensory loss. Manipulatory finger movements are clumsy and coarse, and all movements are affected—whether they involve the use of tools and instruments (e.g., hammer, scissors, hairbrush, toothbrush), gestures (e.g., waving goodbye, saluting), or are meaningless (e.g., touch your nose, wiggle your fingers). Moreover, the apraxic deficit is consistent in that it is manifest both in everyday activities as well in the clinical setting so that for this form of apraxia, the mode by which a movement is elicited makes no difference in contrast to the situation in ideomotor apraxia. That is, there is no dissociation between voluntary movement requested by an examiner out of its natural context and automatic (habitual) movement elicited by internal motivations and natural settings. Lesions that result in limb kinetic apraxia involve frontal lobe damage that is centered in the premotor cortex, but associated involvement of the parietal cortex may occur.

> **Thought Question**
>
> What differentiates ideational, ideomotor, and kinetic apraxia functionally and anatomically?

Oral Apraxia (Facial-Oral Apraxia)

Oral apraxia may be the most common form of apraxia and may be associated with apraxia of the limbs. In oral apraxia, people are unable to execute facial movements on command, such as pantomiming blowing out a match or candle, blowing a kiss, whistling, puffing out the cheeks, or clearing the throat. Performance may improve when the person is asked to imitate the examiner or is presented with an actual object. Oral praxis may be subserved by a neural substrate different from that mediating limb praxis, although both primarily involve the left hemisphere. For one thing, oral apraxia more often results from damage to the premotor cortex anterior to the mouth area of the primary motor cortex than from damage to the parietal lobe. Given that this anterior area is contiguous with Broca's area, oral apraxia often is associated with Broca's aphasia.

Apraxia and Aphasia

Apraxia and aphasia often co-exist, owing to the anatomical proximity of the distributed neural networks subserving praxis and language in the left, dominant hemisphere. Thus, a Wernicke's aphasia frequently accompanies ideomotor and ideational apraxias resulting from damage to the PPC. The comprehension deficit characterizing Wernicke's aphasia makes it difficult to demonstrate an associated apraxia because spoken or written requests to perform an act will not be understood. The clinician must find a way to persuade the patient to imitate his or her movement. Conduction aphasia also may accompany limb apraxia due to damage to fibers of the superior longitudinal fasciculus, but in conduction aphasia, comprehension is intact so that testing for apraxia can still be carried out effectively.

HYPOTHETICAL SCHEME FOR THE LEARNING AND EXECUTION OF GOAL-DIRECTED PURPOSEFUL MOVEMENT

Rehabilitation therapists play critical roles in assisting individuals to regain and refine control of movement. For this reason, it is essential to understand the control of normal movement in preparation for considering restoration of movement following orthopedic injuries (e.g., tear of the medial meniscus, ankle sprains) and neurological disorders such as brain injury and stroke.

To this end, we present a hypothetical scheme illustrating how various regions of the CNS work together in the generation of movement. Our purpose is to explore the integrated and parallel operations of different cortical and subcortical structures as they interact to generate and guide purposeful motor acts. This information then assists the clinician to predict what aspects of motor control might be affected with different types of injury. As will be seen, this section illustrates the complexity of processes that subserve movement as well as the many cortical and subcortical areas that are involved. Damage in many different areas of the CNS can potentially lead to abnormalities of control of movement. The specific nature of the abnormality depends on the site of damage. Likewise, the site of damage may dictate the approach to intervention.

Motivation, the Decision to Act, and Learning

For purposeful movements, the individual must be motivated to act. As noted in Chapter 8, voluntary movements are unique in terms of their motivational aspects. Such motivation is generated in limbic areas of the cerebral cortex (portions of the prefrontal cortex and limbic system as well as in specific components of the basal ganglia). That these structures are, in fact, involved with motivation comes from humans with a variety of clinical conditions. For example, lack of initiative, spontaneity, and a general diminution of motor activity are characteristic features of particular focal damage to the prefrontal cortex (discussed in Chapter 21). Two diseases involving the basal ganglia—Parkinson's disease and Huntington's disease—are characterized in part by an apparent rupture between motivation and movement (discussed in Chapter 22). In these clinical conditions, the person is not paralyzed, apraxic, or confused, yet the person cannot carry out necessary daily activities. With motivating stimulation, these people can perform motorically. What is impaired is the ability to initiate spontaneously a desired or automatic motor task.

Once the decision is made to act, a complex sequence of events occurs before and during the execution of the movement. As an example, consider a pitcher learning how to throw strikes. We first consider what is going to be automatic (already learned) in the process of throwing a pitch and does not have to be learned de novo. This concerns the postural adjustments that occur in preparation for the throw, during the throw, and after the throw. Clearly, the pitching movement would be highly destabilizing in the absence of compensating postural adjustments. The pitcher raises the leg contralateral to the throwing arm, rocks back on the supporting leg, and thrusts the body forward. This dramatically changes the pitcher's center of gravity. Simultaneously, the throwing arm moves forward in a great arc; the pitcher's body continues to move forward until the throw is completed. The pitcher lands on the initially flexed leg and raises the initially extended supporting leg. The body's entire center of gravity has shifted markedly from the start to the end of the throw. The compensatory postural adjustments are mediated by static and dynamic vestibulocollic and vestibulospinal reflexes. Our pitcher is also aware of the nature of the surface that will support his body as the throw is executed. The hardness of the support surface would be signaled by somatosensory input, its slope by vestibular and visual input. These inputs condition the automatic postural adjustments that will maintain body stability during these dramatic shifts in its gravitational axis occasioned by the dynamics of the pitching motion.

Initially, the pitcher must position his body appropriately toward the plate. This depends on his having a three-dimensional mental construct of his own body—that is, a coordinated mental image of the relationship of the parts of his body to one another and knowledge of the portion of space occupied by his body. Such a body schema depends on the posterior parietal cortex (PPC), where an integration of proprioceptive, visual, and vestibular input occurs. Additionally, the lateral premotor cortex, perhaps via a parieto-frontal circuit from the PPC, seems to be involved at least in the initial phases of orienting the body and arm toward a selected (desired) target.

Now let us turn to the learning of the pitching throw. The process of learning a voluntary movement with continued practice is divisible into several more or less distinct phases. There is, first, an early, short-term, fast learning phase in which performance improves rapidly, even within a single training session. This is followed by a long-term, slow learning phase in which performance gains are incremental and are observable across multiple training sessions or weeks of practice. Once the motor skill has been overlearned with extended practice, further performance gains do not occur. The motor skill has now entered the retention phase, in that the skill becomes resistant to the passage of time such that it can be readily retrieved and performed with reasonable accuracy despite a long intervening period without practice. To illustrate these concepts, our focus will be on the pitcher's throwing arm, not the other effectors participating in the pitch (e.g., the legs).

Given appropriate motivation, the novice pitcher must determine the goal of the throw, which may include the selection of the appropriate effector, the right or left arm. In this case, the target of the throw is the catcher's mitt. The goal is visually derived. The eyes fixate the target and serve as the reference aim for the arm in throwing such that the direction of the arm throw is in the direction of gaze. This was discussed in Chapter 19. With an awareness of the environment in which the pitch is to unfold, the brain plans a strategy for the intended movement, the first component of which is reaching for and grasping the ball resting in his own mitt. As discussed earlier, this involves

the posterior parietal cortex and a parieto-frontal circuit projecting into the lateral premotor area.

Planning

The throw itself must then be planned. Which shoulder and arm muscles will contract as prime movers and which as supporters and in what sequence? Which muscles will be inhibited? How long and with what force will the muscles contract? What is the direction and speed of the movement? In other words, both the kinetic and kinematic features of the movement are selected. From the regional cerebral blood flow studies referred to earlier, we can infer that at least M1 is involved in this process, although other cortical areas and structures may be involved as well. EEG studies reveal that wide areas of the cerebral cortex become active approximately 0.8 second before the onset of a voluntary movement. These areas include not only M2, but also the lateral premotor cortex. These potentials have been referred to variously as *readiness potentials, motor potentials,* or the *contingent negative variation*. Presumably, this early cortical activity reflects an initial planning of movement occurring in motor association cortices.

Recall that the supplementary motor cortex (M2), the lateral premotor cortex, and the primary motor cortex (M1) represent the origins of two massive loops projecting to the basal ganglia and cerebellum and then back again to cerebral motor cortices via the thalamus (see Chapter 19). Activity ongoing in the motor cortices is projected to the basal ganglia—specifically, the putamen—and cerebellum—specifically, to the lateral cerebellum via the corticopontocerebellar pathway. What can be said from animal studies is that neurons in the putamen and internal segment of the globus pallidus (the principal output nucleus of the basal ganglia) begin to change their discharge rates before the onset of a stimulus-triggered voluntary movement. Likewise, neurons in the dentate nucleus of the cerebellum (representing the output nucleus of the lateral hemispheres) also change their discharge rates before the onset of a voluntary movement. These changes in neuronal firing rates have been interpreted to suggest that both the basal ganglia (its motor circuit) and cerebellum are involved in the planning of voluntary movement. What could they be contributing to the motor plan? And if they do contribute anything at all to the impending movement, the dramatically different internal neuronal organizations of the putamen and cerebellum means the contribution each structure makes is unique.

Consider first the putamen. The signal sent back to the motor cortices prior to movement onset may not be related at all to the execution of the throwing movement per se. Rather, the signal may be predictive of the potential reward value of the throw. In this way, the putamen contributes to the sensorimotor leaning process, wherein our thrower labors to become a skilled pitcher. If so, this would imply that the responses of putaminal neurons should change as the behavioral sensorimotor task is being learned. This is not known in humans, although it is the case in animals. What is clear, though, is that we cannot simply discuss motivation and reward early on and then ignore them as the motor task is being learned and refined. They must be ongoing phenomena. Thus, it is significant that dopamine neurons of the SNpc project strongly to the putamen. They fire in response to primary rewards. After an animal has learned a conditioned response, it responds to reward-related stimuli.

In the case of the discharge of cerebellar dentate nucleus neurons prior to movement onset, there is no evidence to suggest that this relates to the specific contraction patterns in the muscles selected by the motor cortices to execute the movement. For one thing, the lateral cerebellum contains no sensory information from proprioceptive or tactile receptors (or indeed any information from peripheral receptors at all) about the current status of muscles and joints. But the signal could relate to the multijoint coordination required for the arm throw to be accurately directed toward its target.

Thus, both the putamen and cerebellum appear to contribute to the formulation of the motor plan being generated in the cerebral cortex. But they do so in dramatically different capacities.

Execution

At some point, the plan has been sufficiently specified to be sent to the primary motor cortex for execution. Although, as noted earlier, it is not clear exactly what features of the movement are encoded in the discharge of UMNs of M1, their discharge does initiate and guide the execution of the movement. This is accomplished via three synaptic organizations: (1) by their direct effect on LMNs via the corticomotoneuronal projection (CM) projection, (2) by their indirect effect on LMNs via spinal cord interneurons, and (3) by their effect on UMN systems originating in the brainstem that, in turn, project to LMNs. This effect may include the recruitment into the evolving movement pattern of hard-wired spinal cord reflex connections.

As an individual movement unfolds during the short-term, fast learning phase, it is being consciously monitored by the sensorimotor cerebral cortex. But how would the sensorimotor cortex determine whether the movement was on or off target? Visual information is one obvious cue as, for example, when the ball sails five feet above the catcher's mitt. There is also somatosensory feedback resulting from the person's own movement. This is called reafferent information, or simply reafference, to distinguish it from sensory input from external causes, called afference. Still, how would sensorimotor cortices know whether reafference accurately reflected what the motor program intended to accomplish (i.e., the ball landing squarely in the center of the stationary catcher's mitt)? Clearly, the monitoring cortices must have a referent against which they can compare reafferent information. Thus, the idea of an **efference copy**, or **corollary discharge**, was invoked. Corollary discharge is a postulated neural message (a copy) sent out by the motor command centers that initiate voluntary movement. The message is a corollary of the command and is sent to monitoring areas. The efference copy is thought to be a specific central expectation of input that predicts the altered sensory input expected to result from actual execution of the movement. The actual sensory return (the reafference) is then matched with the predicted return. Obviously, based on past experience in throwing balls, the brain is able to predict what a likely sensory return will be when the ball is actually thrown. This efference copy is approximate for initial throws but is refined as successive throws more closely approach the target.

An efference copy of intended movement is also sent to the cerebellum, as discussed in Chapter 19. During the long-term, slow phase of the learning process, the movement becomes progressively more automatic as the brain relies less on conscious monitoring by the cerebral cortex and more on unconscious monitoring by the cerebellum. The cerebellum receives an exquisitely detailed report on the ongoing status of all muscles and joints of the body. This is compared to the efference copy. Motor cortex discharge conveyed to the cerebellum via the cerebropontocerebellar pathway is continuous as the movement is evolving. As initial phases of the movement are executed, patterns of peripheral receptor discharge change, and the cerebellum receives a description of the portion of the movement actually affected (e.g., limb position, velocity, muscle contractile forces, agonist–antagonist relations). Such input enables the cerebellum to assess whether the next portion of the cerebral motor command is appropriate to the efference copy and to the prevailing limb status upon which it is to be superimposed. If the comparison does not match, it is thought cerebellar output modifies the command. The cerebellum thus constantly updates movement as it is evolving through a modification of command signals before they impinge on LMNs. As such, this automatic, comparator-based mechanism operates as an "online" and "follow-up" corrective system. A compromise of cerebellar function by disease may well force the motor system entirely into a follow-up mode of correcting movement through the action of the cerebral cortex. A slowing and deterioration of motor performance would then result.

Automatization

Eventually, during the end of the long-term phase of motor learning, performance becomes asymptotic, and further gains do not occur even with repeated throws. The motor skill has become automatic in the sense that the thrower does not need to pay conscious attention to somatosensory feedback. In the case of pitching a baseball, the movement is said to be ballistic: that is, its execution is too fast to be monitored by somatosensory feedback. Still, the skilled basketball player may know immediately when she has launched a brick, and the professional pianist may know when an incorrect key has been struck even before hearing it.

Significantly, automatization of the motor skill is characterized by plastic changes in the deployment of cortical and subcortical components of the motor system. These changes persist through the retention phase of the motor skill. Brain-imaging studies in humans using functional magnetic resonance imaging and positron emission tomography have revealed that during the early learning phase of acquiring a motor sequencing skill, the cerebral motor cortices (the primary motor cortex, premotor cortex, SMA, and anterior CMA) as well as prefrontal and parietal cortices, the striatum, and the cerebellum are all actively deployed during the movement. However, with extended practice and automatization of the sequencing skill, the motor system relies less on activity of the cerebellum and more on activity in the striatum. In addition to activity levels, the physical size of the representations of the hand increase both in the contralateral primary motor and primary somatosensory cortices after extended practice of the skill (discussed in Chapter 26).

Lastly, continuing dynamic exchanges occur between all of the cortical motor areas and their subcortical partners. These processes are ongoing and parallel.

Now, on to learn how to throw curves, sliders, and flutter balls.

Summary

This chapter sought to broaden our perspective and understanding of voluntary movement: the goal-directed movements subserved by the whole of the neuraxis and all functional systems of the brain and spinal cord. Six areas of the cerebral cortex are involved in mediating voluntary movement: the primary motor cortex, the supplementary motor area, the lateral premotor cortex, rostral and caudal cingulate motor areas, and the posterior parietal cortex. All are reciprocally interconnected in various patterns. Additionally, M1 and the premotor cortices are reciprocally interconnected with the cerebellum and basal ganglia. Various motor acts were described in terms of their neural substrates. These included haptic sensing, independent finger movements, and reaching and grasping. Contrary to previous thinking that considered the superior colliculus as a system involved only in gaze, this structure now is thought to have an additional role as a UMN system in the regulation of arm and neck movement independent of gaze control (i.e., in reaching and grasping). Gait—a complex interaction of postural control, stepping routines, and adaptively modulated, hard-wired spinal cord circuitry—was then addressed in the context of voluntary movement. Next, we considered apraxia, the inability of a person to perform skilled movements and gestures upon request or by imitation. Such movements were previously within the person's voluntary movement repertoire but are lost following lesions involving the cerebrum. People with apraxia have no other motor deficits. Four different types of apraxia were discussed: ideational, ideomotor, kinetic, and oral, which may be the most common form. The relationship between aphasia and apraxia was considered because the two disorders often co-exist. Finally, a hypothetical scheme was developed showing how the various functional systems of the neuraxis might be sequentially deployed as a baseball pitcher throws a ball, then refines his skill as he learns how to throw strikes. Certainly, this scheme is not the last word in the control of voluntary movement. With this information as a background, we can begin to explore the different ways in which movement is affected in individuals who have damage from strokes and traumatic brain injury.

Applications

1. People with Parkinson's disease are often seen in rehabilitation for difficulty with gait. One rehabilitation technique that may be used to is rhythmic auditory stimulation (RAS), which refers to the skilled use of audible rhythm (a steady beat) to elicit movement.

    a. What pathways are used to initiate movement in response to RAS and which are bypassed?

    b. Explain why this technique may be helpful for people with PD.

    c. Visual stimuli (such as lines on the floor) also can be used to assist people with Parkinson's disease to take larger steps. Explain how this phenomenon relates to the use of RAS.

2. Ms. Balenscu has had a stroke that left her with some peculiar symptoms. During her neurological examination, the physician asked her to demonstrate through pantomime some specific movements: brush her teeth, light a match, and comb her hair. Ms. Balenscu stated she understood the directions. However, her actions included her finger on her teeth, repeatedly shaking her hand, and placing both hands on her head in response to the commands. Her husband was present and reported that she is able to brush her teeth, light her own cigarette, and comb her hair at home without such difficulty.

    a. What is the name of this deficit?

    b. Where do you hypothesize her lesion is located?

References

Bates, J. F., and Goldman-Rakic, P. S. Prefrontal connections of medial motor areas in the rhesus monkey. *J Comp Neurol* 336:21--228, 1993.

Binkofski, F., Dohle, C., Posse, S., Stephan, K. M., Hefter, H., Seitz, R. J., and Freund, H. J. Human anterior intraparietal area subserves prehension. A combined lesion and functional MRI activation study. *Neurology* 50:1253–1259, 1998.

Beurze, S. M., de Lange, F. P., Toni, I., and Medendorp, W. P. Integration of target and effector information in the human brain during reach planning. *J Neurophysiol* 97:188–199, 2007.

Doyon, J, Penhune, V., and Ungerleider, L. G. Distinct contributions of the cortico-striatal and cortico-cerebellar systems to motor skill learning. *Neuropsychologia* 41:252–262, 2003.

Floyer-Lea, A., and Matthews, P. M. Distinguishable brain activation networks for short- and long-term motor skill learning. *J Neurophysiol* 94:512–518, 2005.

Gibson, J. J. *The Senses Considered as Perceptual Systems.* Houghton Mifflin, Boston, 1966.

Goodwin, A. W., and Wheat, H. E. Sensory signals in neural populations underlying tactile perception and manipulation. *Annu Rev Neurosci* 27:53–77, 2004.

Henriques, D. Y. P., and Soechting, J. F. Approaches to the study of haptic sensing. *J Neurophysiol* 93: 3036–3043, 2005.

Karni, A., Meyer, G., Jezzard, P., Adams, M. M., Turner, R., and Ungerlieder, L. G. Functional MRI evidence for adult motor cortex plasticity during motor skill learning. *Nature* 377:155–158, 1995.

Lederman, S. J., and Klatzky, R. L. Haptic identification of common objects: effects of constraining the manual exploration process. *Perception Psychophys* 66:618–628, 2004.

Leiguarda, R. C., and Marsden, C. D. Limb apraxias—Higher-order disorders of sensorimotor integration. *Brain* 123:860–879, 2000.

McIsaac, T. L., and Fuglevand, A. J. Motor-unit synchrony within and across compartments of the human flexor digitorum superficialis. *J Neurophysiol* 97:550–556, 2007.

Morecraft, R. J., and Van Hoesen, G. W. Cingulate input to the primary and supplementary motor cortices in the rhesus monkey: Evidence for somatotopy in areas 24c and 23c. *J Comp Neurol* 322:471–489, 1992.

Morecraft, R. J., Louie, J. L., Schroeder, C. M., and Avramov, K. Segregated parallel inputs to the brachial spinal cord from the cingulate motor cortex in the monkey. *Neuroreport* 8:3933–3938, 1997.

Nolte, J. *The Human Brain: An Introduction to Its Functional Anatomy.* Mosby Elsevier, Philadelphia, 2009.

Picard, N., and Strick, P. L. Activation of the supplementary motor area (SMA) during performance of visually guided movements. *Cerebral Cortex* 13:977–986, 2003.

Rizzolatti, G., Luppino, G., and Matelli, M. The organization of the cortical motor system: New concepts. *Electroenceph Clin Neurophysiol* 106:283–296, 1998.

Roland, P. E., Larsen, B., Lassen, N. A., and Skinhof, E. Supplementary motor area and other cortical areas in organization of voluntary movements in man. *J. Neurophysiol* 43:118–136, 1980.

Schieber, M. H., and Hibbard, L.,S. How somatotopic is the motor cortex hand area? *Science* 261:489–492, 1993.

Shima, K., and Tanji, J. Role for cingulate motor area cells in voluntary movement selection based on reward. *Science* 282:1335–1338, 1998.

Stuphorn, V. New functions for an old structure: Superior colliculus and head-only movements. *J Neurophysiol* 98:1847–1848, 2007.

Walton, M. G., Bechara, B., and Gandhi, N. J. Role of the primate superior colliculus in the control of head movements. *J Neurophysiol* 98:2022–2037, 2007.

Zadikoff, C., and Lang, A. E. Apraxia in movement disorders. *Brain* 128:1480–1497, 2005.

PART VI

Special Functional Systems of the CNS: Cognitive Systems

One of the attributes that sets humans apart from other primates is the ability to think, remember, reason, and then formulate these constructs into a complicated language, both orally and in writing. These attributes are essential ingredients in the human ability to express emotion in poetry, prose, paintings, and sculpture. This attribute also underlies the human ability to create skyscrapers and airplanes from elemental materials, not to mention computers and iPads. And, sadly, this is the attribute that allows humans to turn technological advances toward increasingly sophisticated destructive uses associated with wars and terrorism. To date, neuroscientists have only begun to scratch the surface in characterizing the neurophysiological basis for emotions, memories, and cognition. Additionally, scientists are only recently beginning to understand the neurophysiology underlying morality, ethical behavior, and spirituality, with increasing evidence for the relationship of disease to these attributes. Understanding of these latter relationships is only now emerging, and the neurophysiological bases have not yet been sufficiently developed to include this content in the current chapters. However, we can anticipate advances in this area over the coming years.

Generally, it is through diseases or other malfunctions of the nervous system that neuroscientists commonly elucidate those aspects of neurophysiology and neuroanatomy that provide the basis for higher cortical processing. For this reason, each chapter of Part VI begins with foundational information, followed by a discussion of some of the clinical conditions that help elucidate the role of the nervous system.

Chapter 21, the first chapter in Part VI, addresses cognition at both the cortical and subcortical levels. The first major section of this chapter begins with a discussion of concepts related to spatial and facial recognition. These constructs are subserved by the posterior cortical association areas. Next we present constructs related to

executive function, which is related to the capacity to generate behaviors that are appropriate to the circumstances in which they unfold. Executive function manifests itself in the context of such functions as contingency planning, self-monitoring, and modifying behavior in the face of changing circumstances. Executive function is subserved by the anterior association cortex. In the second major section of this chapter, we turn our attention to the subcortical areas and explore the emerging roles of the basal ganglia and cerebellum as they relate to cognition and motivation, drawing on clinical conditions, including Parkinson's disease, obsessive-compulsive disorder, and Tourette's syndrome.

Chapter 22 addresses emotion, memory, and language. This chapter begins with a discussion of emotion and memory, utilizing the condition of epilepsy to illustrate the relationship between these two constructs. The stories of two individuals who sustained significant neurological damage for different reasons are then used to illustrate the role of different nervous system structures in emotion and memory. The second major section of this chapter focuses on language, drawing liberally from individuals who sustained strokes to differentiate the portions of the nervous system that play roles in understanding versus producing spoken or written language.

We end Part VI with Chapter 23, which focuses on normal aging and Alzheimer's disease (AD), because both have implications for cognition, language, emotion, and memory. The first major section of this chapter focuses on processes that change as an individual ages. This sets the stage for understanding the differences in brain changes associated with Alzheimer's disease, which is the topic of the second major section of this chapter. Here, we begin with the types of AD and risk factors followed by a discussion of brain changes that occur with this disorder. We end this chapter with the clinical consequences of AD and implications for the rehabilitation professional.

Cognition: Cortical and Subcortical Contributions

LEARNING OUTCOMES

This chapter prepares the reader to:

1. Contrast unimodal and multimodal association cortices and explain the functional implications of their anatomical location.

2. Relate cognitive function to Brodmann's areas associated with the following: primary motor, premotor, primary somatosensory, somatosensory association areas, and executive functions.

3. Differentiate the anterior association cortex and the limbic association cortex with respect to location and function.

4. Identify the structures that comprise each of the following: anterior association cortex, posterior association cortex, and limbic association cortex.

5. Discuss the following with respect to interpretation of visual and somatosensory information: simultaneous agnosia, unilateral hemispatial neglect, and prosopagnosia.

6. Define the following terms related to higher cortical functions of the frontal cortex: contingency planning and executive function.

7. Define the following term related to denial of disease: anosognosia (or asomatognosia).

8. Discuss lesions related to executive functions of the frontal cortex with respect to location of the lesion and the possible difficulties that people might experience.

9. Explain the role of the following tests in identifying disorders of cognition related to the association cortices: block design, drawing of a clock face or house, Tower of Hanoi test, Tower of London test, Stroop test, and Wisconsin Card Sorting Test (WCST).

10. Analyze the role of the cerebellum in cognition.

11. Discuss the location and role of three parallel loops connecting the association cortices, limbic system, and the basal ganglia.

12. Compare and contrast cognitive dysfunction associated with the following disorders of the basal ganglia, including the neuroanatomic substrates involved and the functional consequences: Huntington's disease, Parkinson's disease, obsessive-compulsive disorder, and Tourette's syndrome.

ACRONYMS

ACC Anterior cingulate cortex

ADHD Attention deficit/hyperactivity disorder

DLPFC Dorsolateral prefrontal cortex

DM Dorsomedial nucleus of the thalamus

DA Dopamine

fMRI Functional magnetic resonance imaging

GPi Globus pallidus internal segment

HD Huntington's disease

OCD Obsessive-compulsive disorder

PD Parkinson's disease

PET Positron emission tomography

SNpc Substantia nigra pars compacta

SNpr Substantia nigra pars reticulata

TBI Traumatic brain injury

TS Tourette's syndrome

VTA Ventral tegmental area

WCST Wisconsin Card Sorting Test

Introduction

The term *cognition* is broad in scope and refers to the mental processes by which the brain manipulates information that is generated internally or externally (i.e., by emotional and sensory inputs). In its broadest context, cognition refers to information-processing abilities related to perception, learning, remembering, analyzing, judging, and solving problems. Thus, the familiar construct of mental ability as measured by intelligence quotient (IQ) tests only taps into a very small aspect of cognitive function. Indeed, by the broader definition, animals possess cognitive capacities in that they sense, perceive, recognize, demonstrate emotion, and exhibit other memory-dependent actions. However, humans are unique from other mammals in the far greater richness of their cognitive capacities. The depth and variety of these capacities allow the creation of sophisticated generalizations from collated memories of individual events. They enable us to generate subtle analogies through insight, foresight, intuition, and imagination. They endow man with the capacity to speak, to write, and to render art.

The idea that complex cognitive abilities are localized to specific areas of the brain was first confirmed by clinical neurologists in the late 1800s. Without exception, these cognitive capacities (such as language, judgment, foresight, planning, and memory) depend on activity in the association cortices of the cerebral hemispheres. The most sophisticated of these cognitive capacities—namely, manifestations of the creative process—remain largely out of the reach of modern neuroscience, although inroads may be possible through the use of imaging technology (assuming it is possible to develop behavioral tasks that actually tap true creativity).

Within the past several decades, neuroscientists have come to increasingly recognize that while cognitive capacities do, in fact, depend on association cortex, subcortical structures and the cerebellum also participate in cognition. As we shall see in this chapter, subcortical structures do this through their massive and reciprocal relationships (circuits) with association cortices. Subcortical structures, such as the caudate nucleus of the basal ganglia and part of the dentate nucleus and lateral hemisphere of the cerebellum, maintain

reciprocal relationships with association cortices. The inputs and outputs of these circuits are distinct from those of other parts of the cerebellum and basal ganglia, which connect with primary motor and sensory cortical areas. Thus, for example, the thalamic nuclei through which these cognitive subcortical structures relay to reach the association cortex are different than those relaying motor or sensory information to the cerebral cortex. An interesting clinical observation is that the behavioral deficits resulting from, for example, a lesion affecting the caudate nucleus may qualitatively parallel the deficits resulting from damage to the cortical area to which the caudate nucleus projects. This, of course, does not mean that the neural mechanisms causing the deficits in the caudate and cerebral cortex are the same, only that their end result affects a similar constellation of behaviors.

This chapter begins our exploration into cognitive function. We first define the cortical contributions to cognition. Here, we specifically address issues associated with perception, judgment, foresight, and planning. In the second major section, we turn to subcortical contributions to cognition, focusing on the basal ganglia and cerebellum. In this section, we draw primarily from two conditions of the basal ganglia: Parkinson's disease and Huntington's disease. We also discuss the cognitive consequences of obsessive-compulsive disorder and Tourette's syndrome, which further illustrate clinical consequences of subcortical nuclei as they relate to cognition.

The distinction is not always clearly delineated between cognition and other aspects of higher cortical processing related to emotion and memory. The boundaries are somewhat blurred, both in terms of cortical processing and the behavioral manifestations of that processing. For example, emotional self-control and adaptive responses to changing conditions are critical to intelligent behavior and are juxtaposed with emotions. As a consequence, some topics that are introduced in this chapter (e.g., motivation and emotion as relates to cognition) are developed in greater depth in Chapter 22, which specifically focuses on emotion, memory, and language.

CORTICAL CONTRIBUTIONS TO COGNITION

Clinical Preview

You are working in a rehabilitation center that specializes in rehabilitation of people who have had a traumatic brain injury. Many of these individuals have significant problems with cognition. Often, these deficits are even more disabling than are their motor and sensory deficits. Examples of cognitive deficits that you encounter in your

patients on a daily basis include the following: impulsivity and difficulty inhibiting inappropriate responses such as emotional outbursts; difficulty planning and organizing their day, adjusting to unexpected circumstances, and solving unanticipated problems; and difficulty with facial recognition, path finding, and other aspects of spatial perceptual discrimination.

As you read through this section, consider the following:

- What are the anatomical regions that subserve these functions?
- What clinical tests are available to assess these deficits?

Role of the Association Areas of the Cerebral Cortex

A fundamental role of the association cortex is that of cognitive processing. Two types of association cortex have been defined: unimodal and multimodal (polymodal). The **unimodal association cortex** surrounds each of the primary sensory areas of the cerebral cortex (Figure 21-1 ■). It is concerned with the elaboration of messages sent from the primary receiving areas related to the particular sensory modality. For example, in the case of somatosensory cortices, information transmitted via the medial lemniscus to the thalamus to the primary somatosensory cortex is forwarded in modality-segregated channels (i.e., unimodal). The convergence and integration of this information to yield more complex perceptions such as stereognosis occurs in the unimodal somatosensory association cortex. In the case of the visual system, the unimodal visual association cortex integrates information about form, color, and motion that arrives in the brain in separate pathways.

The **multimodal association cortex** receives information from several unimodal association cortices and thus functions in integration of information from different modalities (cross-modal). For example, the multimodal association cortex of the posterior parietal lobe is concerned with awareness of one's body and the extrapersonal space in which it moves. Such awareness depends on an integration of vestibular, visual, and proprioceptive inputs. Our concern in this chapter is with the multimodal association cortex.

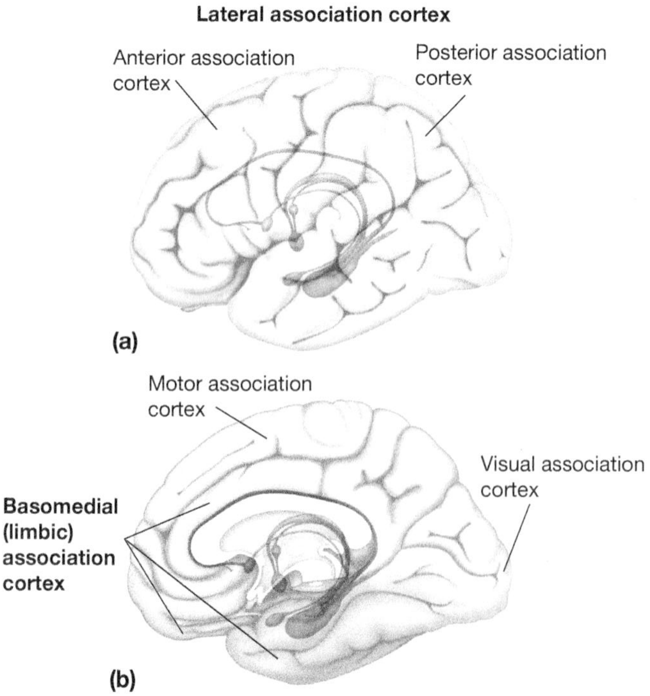

Thought Question

Distinguish unimodal from multimodal association cortices in terms of their anatomical location and their functional roles.

Multimodal association cortices are divisible into two main groups: lateral and basomedial (also called limbic) association cortices. The **lateral association cortex** resides primarily on the lateral convexity of each hemisphere, in the frontal lobe rostral to Brodmann's area 6 and in the parietal, temporal, and occipital lobes that border the unimodal association cortices of the auditory, visual, and somatosensory systems. Because of their anatomical positions, the areas of the lateral association cortex are further differentiated into two areas referred to as the **anterior association cortex** and the **posterior association cortex** (see Figure 21-1). The **basomedial association (limbic) cortex** consists of a less well-defined set of cortical areas that include the orbital surface of the frontal cortex, as well as the medial frontal lobe, the medial temporal lobe, and the cingulate gyrus. The cingulate gyrus and medial temporal lobe (parahippocampal gyrus) comprise important components of the traditionally defined limbic system. Note that the frontal lobe contains the dorsolateral association cortex as well as a large portion of limbic association cortex.

Three features distinguish the lateral and basomedial association cortices from other areas of the neocortex. First, this association cortex is multimodal (i.e., multisensory) in contrast to both the primary sensory and unimodal sensory association cortices that border each of the primary areas. The polysensory nature of these association cortices results from the fact that they receive information from other areas of the neocortex. Projections beginning in each of the primary sensory cortices (i.e., somatosensory, auditory, and visual) progress through a series of orderly cortical synapses. They terminate, first, in the unimodal association cortices bordering each of the primary sensory receiving areas. Each unimodal cortex directs its output to the posterior multimodal association cortex (Figure 21-2 ■). The posterior multimodal association cortex, in turn, projects to other sectors of multimodal association cortices. Thus, it projects to the anterior association cortex as well as to the inferotemporal cortex. Furthermore, both the anterior and posterior multimodal association cortices share common, overlapping projections to and from the inferotemporal cortex and entire limbic multimodal association cortex. There are also common projections to subcortical structures such as the striatum. At each neocortical synaptic way station, information processing occurs so that the association cortices have a repeatedly preprocessed multisensory internal representation of the environment. Such representations enable association cortices to generate behaviors appropriate to ongoing external events. The limbic association cortex,

FIGURE 21-1 Lateral and basomedial (limbic) association cortices. (a) The lateral association cortex is differentiated into the anterior and posterior association cortices. (b) The basomedial or limbic cortex is less well defined but includes the orbital surface of the frontal lobe, the temporal lobe, and the cingulate gyrus. Note that the basomedial limbic cortex surrounds other (unlabeled) structures of the limbic system.

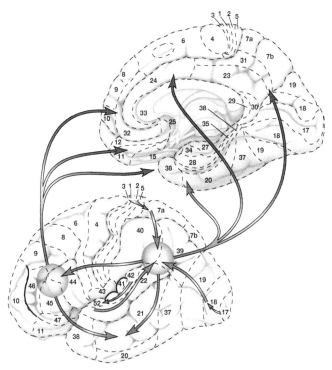

FIGURE 21-2 Each primary sensory cortex (Brodmann's 3, 1, 2; 17; and 41, 42) projects to the adjacent unimodal association cortex. Each unimodal cortex projects to the posterior multimodal association cortex. Both the posterior and anterior association cortices (represented as spheres) project to other association cortices, with overlapping projections to the inferior temporal cortex. Areas 3, 1, and 2: primary somatosensory cortex; area 17: primary visual cortex; and areas 41 and 42: primary auditory cortex.

in addition, receives input representing the internal state of the organism, enabling it to generate motivated behaviors imbued with affect as well as behaviors in response to proximate external events (also imbued with affect).

A second unique feature of the multimodal association cortex is that it receives input from distinct nuclei of the thalamus. The lateral association cortex receives its input from the two largest nuclei of the thalamus. Specifically, the anterior association cortex receives its thalamic input from the dorsomedial (DM) nucleus, the second largest nucleus in the human thalamus (Figure 21-3 ■), while the posterior association cortex receives its input from the pulvinar (P), the largest of the human thalamic nuclei. The cingulate and parahippocampal gyri of limbic association cortex receive their input primarily from the anterior nucleus of the thalamus.

Thought Question

Now is a good time to synthesize information learned in this chapter and in previous chapters related to the unimodal and multimodal association cortices. To this end, make a list of the areas that you have learned about, their anatomical location (including Brodmann's areas, if known), and their functional importance. Which of these areas are unimodal and which are multimodal?

It should be noted that the DM nucleus is structurally and functionally heterogeneous. It has at least three cytologically distinct sectors that project to different regions of association cortex. Its largest sector (the parvocellular portion) has a massive projection to virtually the entire frontal cortex rostral to areas 6 and 32, including the dorsolateral prefrontal cortex. A smaller (magnocellular) portion projects to the limbic association cortex of the frontal lobe.

Thought Question

Distinguish between the lateral and basomedial association cortices in terms of their location and hypothesize their functional differences.

In addition to receiving input from a sector of the DM nucleus, the limbic association cortex receives a projection from the anterior nucleus of the thalamus. Projections of the DM and anterior nuclei partially overlap.

The third unique feature of the multimodal association cortex is that the cortices in the two cerebral hemispheres do not have equivalent functions. One hemisphere is dominant for a particular function, while the corresponding area in the opposite hemisphere has a different function. Specifically, the so-called dominant hemisphere (left hemisphere in most people) is of particular importance in language, whereas the so-called nondominant hemisphere (right hemisphere) is of particular importance in interpreting spatial relationships. This contrasts with other neocortical areas such as the primary motor and sensory cortices, where the two hemispheres are functionally equivalent but are related to lateralized structures of the body. This concept of cerebral dominance was first developed in conjunction with the representation of language, wherein only one hemisphere (the left in the vast majority of people) is dominant but now is known to embrace other functions as well, as discussed later with respect to spatial cognition.

Thought Question

Contrast the thalamic inputs to the anterior, posterior, and limbic association areas. For each thalamic nucleus that you have identified, review what you know regarding inputs and outputs to this nucleus generally. (You may need to review content in Chapters 6 and 7.) How does this information assist you to understand the role of the different thalamic inputs to their related association functions?

Multimodal association cortices are just as important in the processing of motor information as they are in the processing of sensory information. The motor association areas (referred to as the **motor association cortex**) are located in Brodmann's area 6 and lie anterior to the primary motor cortex. The motor association cortex differs fundamentally from

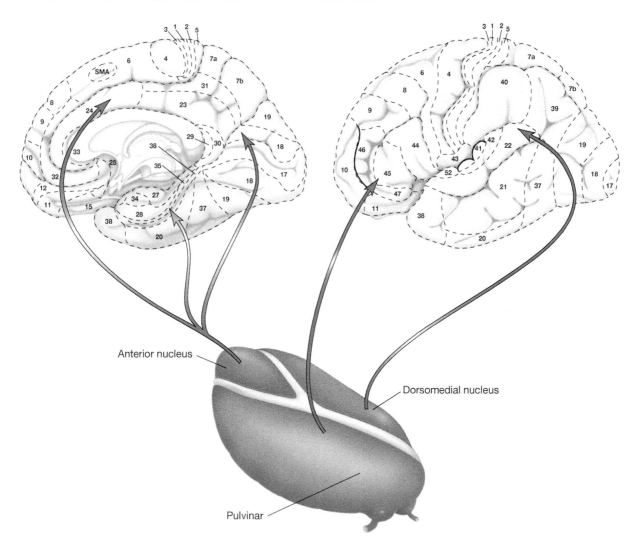

FIGURE 21-3 Thalamic inputs to the multimodal association cortices. The anterior association cortex receives input from the dorsomedial nucleus, the posterior association cortex receives input from the pulvinar nucleus, and the basomedial (limbic) association cortex receives input primarily from the anterior thalamic nucleus.

the sensory association cortex. First, as we saw in Chapter 20, the motor association cortex receives sensory information from the multimodal association cortex in the parietal lobe, reflecting the fact that the planning of movement depends on the sensory environment in which it unfolds. Second, the relationship between the primary and motor association cortices is reversed: information flows *from* motor association cortex *to* the primary motor cortex.

The orbitomedial prefrontal cortex and the dorsolateral cortex are reciprocally interconnected, as would be expected. However, their other dominant reciprocal cortico-cortical connections are different. The dorsolateral prefrontal cortex connections are with somatosensory, auditory, and visual association cortices, whereas the orbitomedial prefrontal cortex connections are dominated by relations with the olfactory, gustatory, and visceral association cortices. Likewise, the dominant reciprocal relations with subcortical structures are different. Orbitofrontal connections are dominated by reciprocal connections with the amygdala, hippocampus, and hypothalamus, while such

reciprocal connections with these structures do not occur in the case of the dorsolateral prefrontal cortex. Moreover, even in those situations where both prefrontal cortices are related to the same subcortical structures (e.g., the basal ganglia or particular thalamic nuclei), the projections are with different sectors of these structures, as was noted earlier for the DM nucleus. A variety of other connectivity pattern differences are known to exist.

Lateral Association Cortex: Posterior Association Areas

Concepts related to the posterior association area were introduced in Chapter 18 in the context of disorders of the visual system. Here, we synthesize these concepts in the context of general cognitive roles of the posterior association cortex.

SPATIAL COGNITION Spatial cognition is a global concept that applies to a surprisingly wide variety of behaviors, some of which may seem, at first glance, to be unrelated to one another. Accordingly, a deficit in spatial cognition can express itself in a wide variety of specific behaviors that can occur in isolation or in variable combinations. Such deficits may include:

1. Inability to localize objects in space so that there are deficits in reaching and pointing to visual targets.
2. Deficits in learning or remembering routes so that an individual is unable to trace a route from one place to another.
3. Inability to relate (synthesize) spatially separated objects or events such that the individual is unable to describe the action portrayed in a picture, although he or she can describe the individual items making up the picture (the deficit is called **simultaneous agnosia**).
4. Difficulty with visuoconstructive ability such that, for example, the individual may be unable to reproduce a three-dimensional block design.
5. Inability to spell the beginning of words or to coherently read a long passage, skipping whole lines and beginning reading in the middle of another line. (Tasks such as reading, counting, and spelling depend on an accurate spatiotemporal perception of a stimulus sequence.)
6. Deficits of spatial cognition extending to imagery and memory, such that a person may be unable to recall the arrangement of furniture in a room or the layout of rooms in his or her house.

The most prominent clinically demonstrable example of these deficits is **unilateral hemispatial neglect**, defined as a failure of directed attention to the body (personal space) and extrapersonal space on the side contralateral to the lesion. People with this disorder behave as if one side of the body and extrapersonal space had ceased to exist and live in only half of the world. For example, the individual may shave only one side of the face, may apply lipstick to one side, or may eat the food only on the right side of the plate. Individuals with unilateral hemispatial neglect may bump into objects located on the neglected side (e.g., door jambs, furniture).

Lesions most consistently responsible for unilateral neglect are localized in the right hemisphere and are centered in the inferior parietal lobule and the parieto-occipito-temporal junction. Thus, the most common neglect is left-sided. Significant numbers of people with right hemisphere damage (e.g., from stroke, traumatic brain injury, tumor) manifest symptoms of left-sided neglect. Of interest, the presence of a neglect syndrome in right hemisphere strokes is more predictive of functional disability and poor outcome than is the motoric severity of the stroke per se. Here, it is important to recall that the right cerebral hemisphere is dominant for spatial cognition, although the unilateral dominance is not as clear-cut as that for language.

FACIAL RECOGNITION **Prosopagnosia** was introduced in Chapter 18 as a hallmark of lesions involving the temporal lobe association cortex. In this most fascinating of the agnosias, the person is unable to identify familiar faces (either in person or by picture), perhaps even that of his or her own spouse, and is unable to learn to recognize new faces. This disorder has been brought to general awareness by the neurologist, Oliver Sacks, in his stories compiled in *The Man Who Mistook His Wife for a Hat*.

The person with prosopagnosia may still be able to identify a known person, but does so on the basis of other cues such as a mustache, glasses, or the sound of the voice. The basis of the disorder is unclear, but some neurologists have speculated that the person's accurate perception of a face cannot be matched to the memory of that face. Acquired prosopagnosia has been said to follow unilateral occipitotemporal lesions, bilateral occipitotemporal lesions, bilateral occipital lesions, and anterior temporal lesions. Prosopagnosia is a disorder of sufficient rarity that attributing it to a lesion involving a particular region of association cortex with a given laterality is of uncertain validity.

Lateral Association Cortex: Anterior Association Areas

The frontal lobe comprises the neural substrate of complex cognitive processes such as planning capacity, foresight, insight, empathy, altruism, abstract reasoning, self-awareness, and the governance of emotion. Thus, this lobe does not have a clearly identified single purpose. This is understandable considering that the definition of the frontal lobe is an anatomical one (as noted in Chapter 2), that it represents nearly half of the entire cerebral cortex, and that it is composed of subregions that are anatomically and functionally heterogeneous.

The motor functions of the frontal lobe (agranular cortex) were defined as early as 1870. In that year, the great neurologist Hughlings Jackson postulated the presence of a somatotopically organized motor cortex in the brain based on his study of the spread of muscular contractions during a type of epileptic seizure that now bears his name. That this brain area included the precentral gyrus of the frontal lobe was independently, experimentally confirmed by electrical stimulation of the frontal lobe in animals, also in 1870, and in humans as early as 1874. However, a unified concept of the function of the more extensive areas of the frontal lobe rostral to the agranular motor cortex (areas 4 and 6)—the so-called granular prefrontal cortex—has not emerged to this day, despite a vast literature and endless speculation on its function. Nevertheless, individuals with specific clinical conditions related to frontal lobe function have shed considerable light on the matter.

Indications that the prefrontal association cortex was divisible into at least two major subareas was propsed by Kleist as early as 1934, when two different clinical syndromes were first described following prefrontal damage. The dorsolateral convexity was postulated to be concerned mostly with intellectual functions. The **dorsolateral prefrontal cortex (DLPFC)** consists of Brodmann's areas 8, 9, 10, 11, 44, 45, 46, and 47 (see Figure 7-5). In contrast, the orbital and medial surfaces of the prefrontal cortex were postulated to be concerned with emotional and visceral activities. The orbital surface consists of Brodmann's areas 10, 11, 12, 13, and 14, while the medial surface consists of Brodmann's areas 8, 9, 10, 11, and the anterior part of 12.

> **Thought Question**
>
> How do motor and cognitive processes of the frontal lobe differ in terms of their general location, Brodmann's areas involved, and functional importance?

These neuroanatomical differences are reflected in the fact that two distinct clinical syndromes have been definitively documented since 1934 as a consequence of frontal lobe damage. One syndrome follows lesions of the dorsolateral prefrontal convexity and consists of affective flatness and reduced cognitive and motor activity. The second syndrome results from lesions affecting the orbitofrontal cortex and consists of behavioral disinhibition, loosened social controls and judgment, and wide oscillations of affect. Neither of these two classical syndromes is associated with primary deficits in movement, sensation, language, long-term memory, or intelligence. This fact is consistent with the idea that the prefrontal cortex functions in an executive as opposed to operational (essential, obligatory) capacity in the regulation of neural activity.

EXECUTIVE FUNCTION (CONTINGENCY PLANNING)
Contingency (context-dependent) planning refers to the capacity to generate behaviors that are appropriate to the circumstances in which they unfold. It thus applies both to social and nonsocial contexts. The anterior association cortex (dorsolateral) is involved in mediating behaviors that are fundamentally nonsocial in nature. Here, contingency planning manifests itself as the capacity to alter goal-directed behavior when the conditions in which the behavior is occurring change. This adaptability ensures that the original conception will still be attained. A variety of higher-order cognitive processes, referred to collectively as **executive functions**, are involved. These processes apply to both intellectual and social contexts. Executive functions refers to the higher cognitive ability to generate behaviors that are appropriate to the circumstances in which they unfold. These functions include the following:

1. The generation of multiple strategies to attain a specific goal or solve a specific problem.
2. Choosing, sequencing, and initiating subroutines that collectively achieve the goal.
3. Self-monitoring the adequacy of the sequence of actions.

4. Modifying behavior when conditions change.
5. Inhibiting incorrect responses in the face of distraction.

Socially appropriate behavior is unique in that it demands a proactive regulatory influence that considers the potential consequences of a behavior on the feelings and reactions of others with whom the person is interacting (i.e., it demands foresight and insight). This is a function of the limbic association cortex rather than the anterior association cortex and is considered in Chapter 22.

> **Thought Question**
>
> What is *executive function*, and how does this important aspect of anterior association cortex relate to the concept of *contingency planning*? Thinking ahead, and utilizing prior knowledge, what types of injuries or diseases do you think might possibly cause disorders of executive function?

Basomedial (Limbic) Association Cortex

One of the best-understood portions of the basomedial (limbic) association cortex is the **anterior cingulate cortex** (ACC). The cingulate cortex received its name because it forms a collar, or *cingulum*, around the corpus callosum. When it was first described by Broca, the focus of understanding about the cingulate cortex was related to its role in emotion. It is now recognized that the ACC has involvement not only with emotional processing, but also with performance evaluation and optimization.

Overall functions of the ACC related to performance evaluation and optimization include focused problem-solving, error recognition, a role in anticipation of movement, and adaptive responses to changing conditions. This area of the cortex is of particular importance in focusing on difficult problems, as well as monitoring performance in response to rewards and adjusting behavior accordingly. Functions of the ACC related to emotion include production of intense fear or pleasure, as well as emotional self-control, social insight, and maturity. Experiments have demonstrated that activity of the ACC was greater in subjects who had a higher level of social awareness (based on objective tests). Developmental and cognitive alterations such as attention deficit disorders and obsessive-compulsive behaviors have been correlated with structural and metabolic changes in this region.

The cellular basis for some of these phenomena is beginning to be decoded. For example, the multimodal association cortex of the ACC in the human has highly developed and dense contributions of neurons called spindle cells. These cells are involved in reward and reward-associated behaviors and are especially sensitive to dopamine availability. Therefore, alteration of available dopamine in some common disorders not only affects motor function (as discussed in Chapter 19), but can have cognitive consequences as well.

CLINICAL CONNECTIONS

Alexander Luria was among the first to describe problems associated with frontal lobe pathology, in general, and executive function, specifically. His clinical observations, along with others such as Kleist, set the stage for more recent work related to motor and executive function. These types of deficits are well recognized in individuals who have sustained traumatic brain injury (TBI).

The functions of human association cortices are best revealed by understanding their dysfunctions following localized damage to the cerebral hemispheres coupled with careful postmortem examination of the brain. Modern neuroimaging technologies are making an increasingly important contribution to the study of cognitive function. It must be appreciated that such techniques still suffer from limited resolution. They also face a more daunting problem in terms of accurately defining what constitutes a resting mental state against which task-dependent changes in brain activity can be assessed. Difficulties also exist with developing behavioral tasks that unequivocally isolate the cognitive function of interest from contaminating cognitive or motoric-related brain activity. Some have urged that functional neuroimaging be used very cautiously as a sole technique in establishing a neuroanatomy of cognition.

The rehabilitation clinician may work with individuals who have difficulty resulting from damage to the association cortices. These individuals may have variation of clinical consequences due to different pathological conditions. Consider, for example, a person who has had a stroke restricted to the middle cerebral artery or a person with a tumor in the frontal lobe compared with a person who has had traumatic brain injury (TBI). The individual with a stroke or a tumor will have a fairly restricted location of injury, whereas the person with trauma to the brain usually has multifocal and diffuse pathological consequences. TBI results from an insult to the brain caused by external forces. For example, a TBI may occur from a motor vehicle accident, fall, violent act, or a sports injury and often results in damage to various areas that may or may not be contiguous. Of importance, TBI often leaves the individual with changes in perceptual abilities and executive functions. Therefore, it is important not only to assess the integrity of the sensory system, motor system, and reflexes, but also to investigate the individual's abilities with cognition. Consequences of stroke and TBI are discussed in greater detail in Chapters 24 and 25. In the following sections, we present some of the tests of cognition as they relate to the functions of the posterior and anterior association cortical areas. These standardized tests are used to diagnose specific types of cognitive dysfunction and the relevant cortical areas. The rehabilitation professional draws on findings from these tests to interpret examination findings, specifically related to the individuals' function, and to design appropriate interventions. Much is left to be learned about the correlation between performance on many of these neuropsychological tests and functional implications in relation to the individual's daily activities.

Thought Question

By now, you should be developing an appreciation of the broader context of *cognitive* functions of the brain, beyond those related to intelligence as measured by IQ. This is a good time to synthesize some of the key issues. List examples of cognitive deficits associated with vision, emotion, and higher-level decision making. For each example, name the deficit and then think about ways that you might test for the deficit. Now read on to learn of some of the standardized tests that are used in diagnosing these deficits.

Tests of the Posterior Association Area

A variety of simple tests have been devised to assess the functions of the posterior association area. A number of these tests are used to elicit the presence of neglect. One of the most traditional is to have the person draw a clock face from memory. The person with neglect may do one of several things: leave out the numbers on the left, transpose all of the numbers to the right side of the clock face, or place both hands of the clock on the right side when requested to indicate 9:20 (Figure 21-4 ▪). Other tests used to elicit different aspects of spatial cognition include drawing a map, copying a three-dimensional figure such as a cube or other complex figure, and reconstructing a three-dimensional block design or a puzzle. Benson's Three-Dimensional Constructional Praxis Test is one such example.

When a lesion in the posterior parietal area of the right hemisphere extends into the primary sensory and motor cortices, a dense left-sided hemiplegia may result. Despite the paralysis, the person may act as if nothing were the matter. When asked to raise the paralyzed left arm, the person may do nothing but still claim it has been raised. Here, there is a cognitive negation of the disorder; in extreme cases, the person even may deny ownership of the paralyzed and insensate limb, claiming it to be that of the person in the next bed or of a cadaver, perhaps even a snake. This denial (unawareness) of disease is called **anosognosia** or **asomatognosia**.

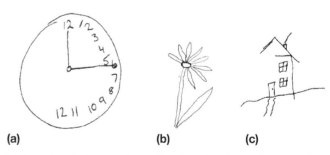

FIGURE 21-4 Illustrations of typical drawings when people with unilateral neglect are asked to draw a clock, a flower, and a house. Note that the left side is consistently omitted from each figure.

Thought Question

Neglect is quite different from somatosensory loss and is one of the most difficult disorders to remediate with physical rehabilitation. Draw on your understanding of the meaning of *neglect* and the role of the association cortex to explain why this is the case.

Tests of the Anterior Association Area

A number of tests of the anterior association area provide insight into the way executive functions manifest themselves in behavior. For example, the Wisconsin Card Sorting Test (WCST) is a problem-solving task that measures the ability of a person to identify (i.e., to form hypotheses about) the relevant category for sorting a pack of cards according to a set of stimulus cards that vary in three dimensions: in symbol form, color, and number (Figure 21-5 ■). The relevant sorting category switches across trials without advance instruction to the person being tested so that performance depends on flexible thinking (the ability to shift set) and the capacity to inhibit previously correct responses. In this test, the individual is given a pack of 64 cards on which are printed one to four symbols (a star, square, circle or cross) in different colors (red, green, yellow, or blue). Each card is different. The task is to place the cards one at a time under four stimulus cards (one red cross, two green stars, three yellow crosses, and four blue circles) according to a principle that the individual must determine from the pattern of the examiner's responses to the subject's placement of the cards. The individual simply begins placing cards and the examiner tells him or her whether each placement is correct or incorrect. The examiner begins the test with color as the basis for sorting, shifts to form, then to number, returns again to color, and so on. When, for example, the principle is color, the correct placement of a <u>red</u> card is under one <u>red</u> cross, regardless of the card's number or form, and the examiner responds accordingly. After 10 consecutive correct placements, the examiner shifts the principle to form (e.g., the <u>cross</u>), indicating the shift only by the change in his pattern of right and wrong responses. The test continues until

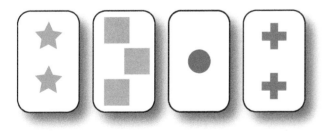

FIGURE 21-5 Example of cards used in the Wisconsin Card Sorting Test. The examiner asks the individual to identify the pattern of cards according to color, symbol design, or number of symbols.

the individual has made six runs of 10 correct placements. People with frontal lobe damage achieve fewer sorting categories, indicating an impaired ability to form concepts.

The Stroop test measures the ease with which a subject can shift his or her perceptual set to conform to changing external demands and suppress a habitual response in favor of a novel one. In this test, words naming colors are printed in a color that is different from the name (e.g., the word *blue* might be printed in the color red). The person being tested might first be asked to either indicate the color or the word. The test thus assesses cognitive flexibility. The most demanding part of the Stroop test is the subtest in which the subject must name the color in which a word is written while suppressing the distracting tendency to read the word itself. In other words, after years of reading experience, the person must overcome the inclination to read the word and focus instead on the color of the ink in which it is written. When people without neurological problems are asked to name the color of the ink (blue, green, red, yellow) rather than read the word itself, the speed at which they complete the task decreases significantly. This normal decrease in color-naming speed is called the "color–word interference effect" or "Stroop interference." In people with frontal lobe lesions, this difference is even greater.

Several tower tasks measure planning and foresight. The person must perform a mental rehearsal of the act he or she is about to undertake by breaking down the goal into subgoals that then must be executed in an appropriate order. In the Tower of Hanoi test (see Figure 21-5), the person must transfer a series of colored rings of different sizes from the first to the third peg such that the transferred rings are in the same order as they were at the start. The rule governing acceptable moves is that no ring can be placed on top of a smaller one. In the Tower of London test, the person must rearrange three colored balls from an initial configuration so as to match a presented goal configuration with as few moves as possible. Over the course of the test, different goal configurations are presented that vary in difficulty according to the minimal number of moves required to attain a given configuration.

People with frontal lobe lesions involving the anterior (dorsolateral frontal) association cortex have difficulty with tests of executive function and spatial perception such as those just described.

In addition to formal testing, observation provides insight into difficulties with frontal lobe function. People with anterior association cortex lesions exhibit a lack of initiative and spontaneous initiation of activity; they do not seek novelty. These impairments combine to give the appearance of apathy and loss of interest in interpersonal exchange. Significantly, such people are not paralyzed, apraxic, or confused; and they do not have sensory deficits or impairments in perception, long-term memory, or general intelligence. The impairment in initiating and sustaining mental activity results in an inability to maintain a coherent reasoning process, leading to easy distraction by irrelevant stimuli and perseveration. This affective flatness (referred to as *flattened affect*), coupled with reduced motor and cognitive activity, typifies certain frontal lobe syndromes. In contrast to people with lesions involving the anterior association cortex, individuals with orbitofrontal lesions (i.e., lesions of the frontal limbic association cortex) may show very little impairment on these neuropsychological tests.

Tests of the Basomedial (Limbic) Association Cortex

Several tests are thought to specifically tap into the function of the basomedial association cortex. One such test is the Counting Stroop test (a variant of the test described earlier). This test is thought to activate the dorsal part of the ACC. In contrast, the emotional Stroop test (in which emotionally charged words are used) is thought to activate the ventral part of the ACC. Additionally, the Spot the Change 5 test is a test of visual working memory.

Thought Question

Here is something to consider. What do you think might be the clinical value and limitations of the tests of cognition just discussed?

CONTRIBUTIONS OF BASAL GANGLIA AND CEREBELLUM TO COGNITION

Clinical Preview ·················

You are working in a movement disorders clinic to which individuals come for examination who are experiencing extraneous movements and/or cognitive deficits resulting from a variety of diagnoses. Included are people with Parkinson's disease, Huntington's disease, Tourette's syndrome, and obsessive-compulsive disorder. As you read through this section, consider the following:

- In what ways are the cognitive symptoms similar and in what ways are they different for people with these four disorders?

- What cortical and subcortical areas are involved in each condition?

- At what ages are these disorders most likely to occur?

- What types of pharmacological and physical intervention strategies are available for each condition?

In the previous section of this chapter, we discussed association areas in relation to cognition. In this section, we will see that both subcortical and cerebellar structures have projections to these same association areas. And furthermore, these structures are intimately involved with cognition.

Cognitive Functions of the Basal Ganglia

Historically, the basal ganglia were long thought of in terms of their motor function. However, the concept that the basal ganglia have functions other than the regulation of motor behavior has recently been established. Neuroanatomical data, as noted in Chapter 7, indicate that parallel yet structurally and functionally segregated pathways run through the basal ganglia and that each is related to an area of the cerebral cortex that mediates a distinct function. Modern imaging technology has allowed clinicians and cognitive neuroscientists to demonstrate nonmotor areas and structures of the brain that malfunction in disease states known to involve pathology of the basal ganglia. Thus, beginning in the 1980s, concepts of basal ganglia function have undergone a dramatic revision.

A whole host of cognitive functions have been attributed to the circuitry in which the caudate nucleus of the basal ganglia is central, leading to a greatly expanded understanding of the clinical manifestations of basal ganglia disease. Diseases once thought to be mainly motor in nature, such as Parkinson's disease and Huntington's disease, now are recognized to have important consequences for cognition and emotion. In some individuals, the initial presenting signs are cognitive and emotional in nature; in other individuals, signs related to cognition and emotion appear later in the course of the disease, after motor-presenting signs. In either event, the cognitive and emotional consequences of these disorders may be even more debilitating than the motor consequences. Furthermore, disorders that were considered behavioral or social disorders are now recognized as disorders affecting the basal ganglia and other subcortical structures and may include alterations in motor function. For example, obsessive-compulsive behavior, previously believed to be psychogenic, is now viewed as a result of alterations in the metabolism of caudate nucleus neurons (as well as the anterior cingulate gyrus). Abnormal caudate metabolism also may contribute to a form of so-called subcortical dementia.

This change in thinking about basal ganglia function is particularly well illustrated in the case of Huntington's disease (chorea). Historically, Huntington's disease (HD) was considered to be essentially motoric in nature, and it is typically discussed in the context of the motor system when basal ganglia disorders are considered. Yet, the motor impairment (chorea) in the disorder seems secondary in importance to the emotional and cognitive (dementia) alterations that characterize HD.

Complex Basal Ganglia Loops

Several parallel loops were introduced in Chapter 19 that connect the basal ganglia with other cortical areas are of importance for sensorimotor, association, and limbic function.

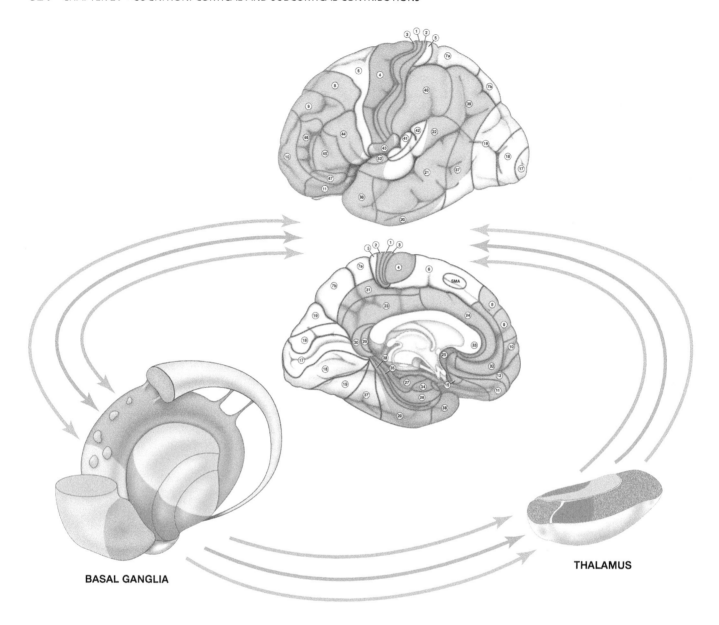

BASAL GANGLIA

THALAMUS

FIGURE 21-6 Three parallel loops interconnect the basal ganglia and functionally associated cortical areas. These loops link cortical areas through the basal ganglia to the thalamus and back to the same cortical area.

Each such loop begins in a different cortical area, synapses in a different part of the basal ganglia, relays in distinct parts of the globus pallidus internal segment (GPi)/substantia nigra reticulata (SNpr), and synapses on neurons in distinct parts of given thalamic nuclei before projecting back to its site of cortical origin (Figure 21-6 ■). The loops involving association and limbic cortices are referred to as complex loops. Three specific complex loops originating and terminating in the frontal lobe have been identified: a dorsolateral prefrontal circuit, a limbic circuit, and a lateral orbitofrontal circuit.

Of the three parallel loops, the *dorsolateral prefrontal circuit* has been easiest to identify with specific clinical findings (discussed later) with specific clinical significance in cognition. The dorsolateral prefrontal circuit originates in the dorsolateral prefrontal cortex (DLPFC; Brodmann's areas 9 and 10) and projects to the head of the caudate nucleus. From

the head of the caudate nucleus, direct and indirect projections synapse in distinct regions of the GPi/SNpr whose neurons project to the dorsomedial nucleus of the thalamus from which thalamocortical projections return to the DLPFC.

Thought Question

Contrast the role of the loop involved in the DLPFC from that involved in the limbic circuit in terms of connections and functional importance.

The *limbic circuit* arises from the cingulate gyrus and medial and orbital frontal cortex, as well as from the parahippocampal gyrus (see Figure 21-6). It projects to the ventral striatum (nucleus accumbens) that also receives substantial direct projections from the hippocampus and amygdala, the latter structures considered to be the *head ganglia* of the limbic system. The ventral striatum projects to the ventral pallidum whose efferents terminate in a unique sector of the dorsomedial nucleus of the thalamus. From the DM nucleus, projections are sent back to cerebral cortex of the limbic system. This circuit has an important side loop that is involved in movement. The ventral striatum projects to dopamine (DA) neurons in the substantia nigra pars compacta (SNpc). DA neurons, in turn, project back to the nonmotor caudate nucleus, the motor putamen, and the ventral striatum. This side loop appears to provide a link between the limbic system (motivation) and the putamen of the motor system (movement).

The last loop, the *lateral orbitofrontal circuit*, seems to combine elements of both association and limbic loops. The functional significance of the lateral orbitofrontal circuit is unclear in terms of contributing something unique to cognitive function. Functional neuroimaging is in its infancy in adding to the understanding of the cognitive contributions of lateral orbitofrontal and limbic association cortices.

Two ideas are important in understanding cognitive alterations in diseases that affect the basal ganglia. First, although each loop synapses on a distinct sets of neurons, it is unlikely that that these loops are selectively damaged by diseases that affect the basal ganglia. This means that people with basal ganglia disorders may typically have both motor and cognitive dysfunction. In Parkinson's disease (PD), for example, the degeneration in the SNpc and ventral tegmental area (VTA) dramatically affect the DA content in the putamen, caudate nucleus, and ventral striatum. Similarly, the massive degeneration that occurs in the striatum of people with HD would be expected to affect multiple nonmotor circuits. Also, the hypermetabolism of neurons in the head of the caudate nucleus that characterizes obsessive-compulsive disorder is unlikely to confine itself to the neurons of a specific circuit. Thus, the cognitive deficits that are observed in naturally occurring disease processes that affect the basal ganglia should, to some extent, be shared across different disease states.

Second, damage to the *caudate nucleus* results in clinical signs and symptoms that are related to those that occur after damage to the area of the cerebral cortex to which the caudate nucleus is related. This was dramatically illustrated in the case of a 25-year-old woman who sustained bilateral damage to the head of the caudate nuclei of undetermined cause. Her symptoms, described by Richfield and colleagues, bear an uncanny similarity to those following damage to the *prefrontal cortex* (see Chapter 22). This woman had been a high school honor student. She worked full-time, lived independently, and was about to be married. Over a period of a month, she experienced daily headaches with occasional nausea and vomiting. Subsequently, her personality changed dramatically, with episodes of vulgarity, impulsivity, violent outbursts, and indifference. She had hypersomnia, increased appetite, and hypersexuality. These changes manifested in altered affect, motivation, cognition, and ability to care for

herself. She engaged in minor criminal behaviors, including shoplifting and exposing herself. This woman married, but she was divorced shortly thereafter. She was hospitalized twice for psychiatric care without benefit.

Cognitive Functions of the Cerebellum

That the cerebellum is importantly involved in cognitive and affective functions is an increasingly accepted idea. The idea of a role for the cerebellum in mental functions is supported by anatomical, clinical, and neuroimaging data. From an anatomical perspective, a large part of the dentate nucleus, the ventrolateral, is definitively present only in humans and is called the *neodentate*. This part contrasts with the phylogenetically older part of the dentate nucleus, the dorsomedial part, in terms of its morphology, histology, histochemistry, and pattern of anatomical connections.

> **Thought Question**
>
> Which parts of the cerebellum are present only in humans? What unique functions do these neuroanatomic substrates serve?

The dorsomedial part of the dentate nucleus, present in subhuman primates, is the motor domain of the nucleus concerned with generation of movement and its regulation. It contains a somatotopic map of the body and face and projects in a topographically organized manner to the primary and premotor cortices. In contrast, the ventrolateral neodentate represents the nonmotor domain of the nucleus and is concerned with mental skills. Unlike the motor domain, the nonmotor domain contains small neurons and large and pronounced infoldings of the nucleus, and its output neurons project to association and limbic system cortices in the frontal, parietal, and temporal lobes.

The anatomical relationships between the cerebral cortex and cerebellum are organizationally similar to those between the cerebral cortex and basal ganglia, the latter also being involved in both motor and cognitive functions. First, there are multiple, closed-loop circuits between the cerebral cortex and ventrolateral dentate in that the multiple cortical areas that are the targets of its output project back to the cerebellum. Second, these circuits are anatomically segregated from one another in that the neurons projecting to a given cortical area are clustered together and do not overlap with dentate neurons projecting to a different cortical area.

The closed-loop circuits linking the cerebral cortex with the cerebellum consist of a massive input limb from the cerebral cortex to the pons and from the pons to the cerebellum (corticopontine and pontocerebellar pathways terminating as mossy fibers in the cerebellum) and an output limb from the cerebellar deep nuclei to the thalamus and from the thalamus to the cerebral

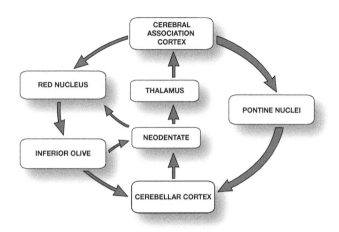

FIGURE 21-7 Closed-loop circuits link the cerebellum with the cerebral cortex. One loop is comprised of a massive projection via the pontine nuclei to the cerebellar cortex, then back to the cerebral cortex. The other loop is comprised of projections via the red nucleus and inferior olive to the cerebellar cortex and then via the neodentate nucleus back to the red nucleus.

cortex (cerebellothalamic and thalamocortical projections) (Figure 21-7 ■). Robust and highly organized projections to the pons arise not only from sensorimotor cortices, but also from association and limbic cortices. The prefrontal cortex and posterior parietal and superior temporal cortices, as well as parahippocampal and cingulate cortices, all project to the pons.

A second, also newly evolved, route has been identified by which cerebral association cortices can reach the cerebellum via the red nucleus, whose axons, in turn, provide the inferior olivary nucleus with its single-most massive input. Axons of the inferior olivary nucleus then project as climbing fibers to terminate in the cerebellum (on Purkinje cells as well as neurons of the deep nuclei) (see Figure 21-7). The inferior olivary nucleus is connected to the neodentate nucleus whose axons, in turn, project back to the red nucleus. This neural loop may participate in language function (as well as motor learning, noted earlier) in that the red nucleus receives a projection from Broca's language area in the prefrontal cortex and, perhaps as well, from Wernicke's language area in the posterior parietal and superior temporal lobes.

Involvement of the cerebellum in nonmotor functions also draws support from a clinical perspective. Stereotaxically placed neurosurgical lesions in the ventrolateral dentate of humans fail to result in classical motor signs of cerebellar damage such as ataxia and tremor. Instead, a cognitive affective syndrome occurs following cerebellar damage. This syndrome is characterized by deficits in executive function (e.g., planning and foresight, set-shifting, abstract reasoning, working memory), visual spatial capacities (e.g., drawing or copying geometric figures), and language production (e.g., mild anomia, dysprosodia, agrammatism). In addition, deficits in affect occur—for example, there may be a flattening of affect, disinhibited and inappropriate behavior may

occur, or there may be an alternation between these two states. These deficits combine to result in a general lowering of intellectual function. The mechanism by which the cerebellum affects these behaviors is not known. Furthermore, it is not possible to differentiate the contribution of the damaged cerebellum to these cognitive and emotional deficits from that of the cerebrocortical association and limbic areas to which the cerebellum projects, which become hypoperfused as a consequence of losing their cerebellar input (see later discussion of diaschisis).

The behavioral manifestations characterizing the cognitive affective syndrome of cerebellar injuries are transient. The syndrome is most pronounced following bilateral and acute cerebellar lesions involving the posterior lobe. Damage to the anterior lobe results in only minor alterations in executive and visual–spatial functions, while damage to the midline vermis results in the most dramatic alterations in affect (i.e., the vermis is the *limbic* cerebellum).

The existence of the cognitive affective syndrome is entirely consistent with neuroimaging data obtained in healthy people. Positron emission tomography (PET) and functional magnetic resonance imaging (fMRI) have revealed that activation of the cerebellum occurs during a wide variety of cognitive tasks. Cerebellar activation occurs in tests of language function, working memory, explicit memory retrieval, mental imagery, cognitive planning, and other nonmotor tests.

Finally, the cerebellum apparently contributes to the cognitive (as well as motor) deficits that occur in children who were born prematurely. From 25 to 50 percent of schoolage children who have survived a premature birth demonstrate cognitive impairments, learning disabilities, and academic challenges. Acute focal disturbances in a given structure of the brain may result in anatomical and functional deficits in a structure distant from the site of injury when the two structures are connected by fiber tracts. This phenomenon is called **diaschisis**. The robust excitatory reciprocal connections between the cerebellum and cerebral cortex mean that a lesion restricted to either structure may result in diaschisis of the other. Injury to the pathways connecting the cerebral cortex to the cerebellum on one side results in crossed cerebellar diaschisis manifested by hypometabolism, cell loss, and atrophy of the contralateral cerebellar hemisphere. A reduction in cerebellar gray matter and myelinated white matter volumes can be detected by MRI in prematurely born neonates as young as 10 weeks of age who have sustained cerebral parenchymal injury. Conversely, cerebellar injury sustained as a complication of premature birth causes crossed cerebellocerebral diaschisis in which there is a contralateral decrease in cerebral volume that can be detected by MRI as early 10 weeks postnatally. Thus, the long-term behavioral and cognitive impairments among children who have survived an extremely preterm birth and sustained either primary cerebellar injury or cerebral parenchyma injury can be explained, in part, by the role of the cerebellum in cognition and its reciprocal anatomical relations with cerebrocortical association areas.

Neuropathology Box 21-1: Autism Spectrum Disorders and Cognition

Autism spectrum disorders refers to a wide range of disorders, all of which have autism at their core. These disorders range from Asperger's syndrome, in which individuals are somewhat limited socially and emotionally, to those with profound autism. The defining characteristics of autism spectrum disorders are qualitative impairments related to cognitive function, especially as relates to social communication and interactions, verbal and nonverbal communication, and stereotypical behaviors. A high percentage of individuals with autism also demonstrate cognitive delays. In addition, increasing evidence suggests that this may also be associated with motor deficits. Thus, this disorder affects emotion and language,

cognition (especially social cognition), and potentially motor control.

Imaging approaches—including MRI, diffusion tensor imaging, and regional cerebral blood flow—have demonstrated wide-ranging effects on the brain in people with autism spectrum disorders. Areas of the brain that have been implicated include the corpus callosum and parts of the brainstem, amygdala, hippocampus, and cerebellum. Also implicated are the caudate nucleus, inferior parietal lobules, middle temporal gyrus, and precentral gyrus. Given this wide range of structures with apparent abnormalities, it is not surprising that autism spectrum disorders have been associated with a wide range of impairments.

CLINICAL CONNECTIONS

Cognitive symptoms associated with several disorders are helpful to understanding the roles of subcortical structures as relates to cognitive function. Two conditions that are particularly useful to understanding the role of the basal ganglia in cognition are Parkinson's disease and Huntington's disease. These two conditions are particularly useful in that they illustrate the intertwining of cortical and subcortical structures and motor and cognitive domains. It is important to recognize that these are complex disorders, and only some of the associated impairments are related to cognitive functions. Some of the other important symptoms associated with PD and HD were presented in detail in Chapter 19.

First, we address cognitive deficits, followed by deficits of motivation in relationship to movement. We then address two additional disorders—obsessive-compulsive disorder (OCD) and Tourette's syndrome (TS)—that add to an understanding of cognitive roles of subcortical structures.

Cognitive Deficits Associated with Basal Ganglia Disorders

Parkinson's disease and Huntington's disease provide particularly useful insight into cognition, as well as social and emotional dysfunction, in conditions that are typically considered motor disorders. Both of these disorders are associated with clearly described motor deficits of the basal ganglia. Yet, here we see that they also are characterized by important cognitive, social, and emotional deficits.

Parkinson's Disease

Cognitive deficits may occur even in the early stages of PD and before some of the motor manifestations. In order to understand such deficits, it is necessary to be aware

of the fact that dopaminergic targets other than the striatum are affected by the midbrain cell loss in the SNpc and VTA, although generally not to the same extent. Levels of dopamine and its metabolites are reduced in allocortical structures like the hippocampus and in neocortical structures such as the entorhinal, cingulate, and frontal association cortices. Particular attention has been paid to the dorsolateral prefrontal association cortex, initially because of the similarity between certain symptoms of advanced Parkinson's disease and those observed following restricted dorsolateral prefrontal lesions resulting, for example, from strokes. Unknown at the time of this initial interest was the fact that the dorsolateral prefrontal cortex is a recipient of the dopaminergic mesocortical projection from the VTA as well as being a target of some pars compacta efferents. Moreover, the dorsolateral prefrontal convexity represents the end-stage processor of the dorsolateral prefrontal nonmotor loop through the basal ganglia. Thus, not only would this frontal association cortex receive an abnormal outflow from the basal ganglia (via the dorsomedial thalamic nucleus) due to the dopamine deficiency in the caudate nucleus, but the cortical processing of that defective outflow would itself be abnormal owing to the cortical dopamine deficiency. Dopamine depletions of 60 percent have been found in the frontal association cortex of people with PD before they begin levodopa replacement therapy.

In many clinical situations, cognitive deficits are not clinically evident, especially early in the disease, but can be revealed with specific neuropsychological testing. Indeed, the application of comprehensive neuropsychologic test batteries with people who have PD has gone far to characterize the cognitive manifestations of this disease. An important, but unresolved, question concerns the nature of the pathology underlying the cognitive changes. There does appear to be a dissociation between cognitive and motor performance in that people with PD who perform less well than controls

Neuropathology Box 21-2: Attention Deficit/ Hyperactivity Disorders

Attention deficit/hyperactivity disorder (ADHD) is the most common neurobehavioral disorder presenting in children. A percentage of children who have had problems in childhood will continue to have problems in adulthood, where it is manifested by significant social psychopathology, school and occupational failure, and emotional difficulties.

In children, ADHD is characterized by difficulty paying attention, distractibility, impulsivity, and hyperactivity that are inappropriate for the developmental stage of the child. There may also be symptoms of low frustration tolerance, frequent shifting of activities, difficulty with organization, and excessive daydreaming. Adults with ADHD may have manifestations of impulsivity with intrusiveness, impatience, fidgetiness, and restlessness. These individuals are at risk of developing co-existing psychopathology, including anxiety, mood disorders, oppositional disorders, and conduct disorders. Behaviors such as smoking, drug, and alcohol abuse are common in adults who have ADHD.

The understanding of the neuropathology causing ADHD and the pharmacology of treatments is evolving as advances are made in neuroimaging. Some of the regions with abnormalities associated with ADHD include the splenium of the corpus callosum, cingulate gyrus, caudate nucleus, cerebellum, striatum, and frontal and temporal cortices. With regard to cortical areas that have been implicated in ADHD, the dorsal frontostriatal system appears to be associated with emotional impulsivity, the left orbital/medial frontal cortex and striatum with interference inhibition, and

the left lateral inferior/dorsolateral prefrontal cortex with attention allocation. Taken together, it has been proposed that the core symptoms of ADHD might derive from dysregulated modulation of cortical plasticity in the developing brain, resulting in altered patterns of corticocortical connectivity.

At this time, there is a belief that two neurotransmitter systems may be altered in a person who has ADHD: the dopaminergic and the noradrenergic. There is a decrease of dopamine control over background firing rates of cortical and subcortical areas involved in reward and motivation. Furthermore, the neuropathology of the syndrome has been correlated with genetic studies to the D2 and D4 receptor subtypes. The noradrenergic systems modify impulsivity and attention. These systems are involved in monitoring new stimulus features and detecting changing or new stimuli.

Treatment of people with attention deficits includes pharmacologic interventions as well as nonpharmacologic and behavior modifying approaches. Examples of the latter for school-aged children include specialized educational planning for individualized education environments, with input from guidance counselors and school psychologists, as well as frequent checks with family and teachers. Typical educational structures include predicable routines, learning aids, resource room time, and checked homework. Assistance to parents is useful to optimize home behavior. Strategies can be continued as these individuals enter college, at which time the student can utilize the institution's study programs. Focused therapy using cognitive-behavioral features can be used with people of all ages.

---

on tests of cognitive function are not necessarily the ones with the most severe motor deficits. This has led to the suggestion that two groups of people with PD may exist: one with a relatively pure deficiency of dopamine in the motor putamen and another with an additional dopamine deficit in the caudate nucleus. Positron emission tomography (PET) scan data in people with early PD who do not have dementia indicate that a dopamine deficiency can appear in the putamen while the caudate still shows normal dopamine levels. But this does not necessarily mean that, when cognitive deficits do appear, they are the result of incorporation of the caudate nucleus into the dopamine deficiency. This is because of the potential dopamine loss in the frontal cortex. Thus, the two groups of individuals could be separable on the basis of both having deficiencies of striatal dopamine but with the cognitively compromised group having an additional deficit in cortical dopamine.

Agreement is not uniform on the nature of mental status changes in PD. This is, in part, due to inconsistencies across studies in experimental design and methodology, as well as across patient populations. There is, nonetheless, an emerging consensus that the mental status changes present

themselves as a constellation of specific deficits, not as a global dementia or generalized disruption of cognitive function. However, dementia is a complication of PD, and the risk of developing dementia increases with disease progression.

The cognitive deficits observed in people with PD manifest themselves only on particular types of tasks: specifically, on tasks in which successful performance depends on the individual's ability to internally (subjectively) formulate a performance strategy based on cues derived from the context in which the task is being carried out. Perhaps the best-known test requiring the individual to organize, or reorganize, behavior according to the shifting requirements of a task is the Wisconsin Card Sorting Test. This is a task in which feedback-related information is used to modify performance.

A number of studies have shown that people with PD achieve significantly fewer card-sorting categories in the WCST than matched normal controls. Several additional deficits have been observed. For example, people with PD may require significantly more trials to complete the first correct category. This deficit has been suggested to reflect an inability to initiate concepts because feedback information cannot be used effectively to initiate a change in performance. Further, people with PD may verbalize correct responses even though failing to execute them, stating, for example, "it must be color" while continuing to respond in a random pattern.

It is of more than passing interest that qualitatively similar performance deficits in the WCST also are observed in people who have sustained selective lesions of the prefrontal cortex. In people with more extensive removals of the frontal lobes (e.g., lobectomies for the relief of intractable epilepsy), there is a marked tendency to perseverate incorrect responses in addition to the inability to sort cards into categories. Such perseverative thinking can also be demonstrated in people with PD when appropriate scoring procedures are applied to the WCST. Indeed, the WCST is regarded as a test of prefrontal cortex cognitive function: administration of the test to normal subjects selectively increases prefrontal cortex regional cerebral blood flow. These and a number of other similarities in the neuropsychologic profiles seen following prefrontal lesions and those observed in people with PD indicate that dysfunction of the prefrontal cortex underlies at least some of the cognitive symptomatology of that disorder.

Such a hypothesis is entirely consistent with the pathway anatomy of the dorsolateral, prefrontal, nonmotor circuit through the basal ganglia. Thus, the consequence of loss of dopamine-containing neurons in the VTA and SNpc places functions dependent on the prefrontal cortex in double jeopardy: the dopamine deficiency in the caudate nucleus disrupts its neural processing, thereby depriving the prefrontal cortex of normal input via the thalamic DM nucleus. In addition, the midbrain dopaminergic cell loss deprives the prefrontal cortex of its direct, extrinsic supply of dopamine.

Another clinical manifestation of basal ganglia involvement in cognitive function is observed in some people with PD who are treated with dopaminergic medication. Such behaviors are linked by being reward based and repetitive in nature. These individuals may exhibit behaviors that include pathological gambling, hypersexuality, compulsive shopping or eating, compulsive medication use, and hobbyism. It is not clear whether such behaviors are the result of dopaminergic medications interacting with an underlying individual vulnerability or whether they are manifestations of the primary pathology in PD.

Huntington's Disease

Huntington's disease is another disorder of the basal ganglia that helps to illustrate the subcortical contributions to cognitive function. The long-standing clinical practice of basing the diagnosis of HD on motor symptoms has obscured the relationship between the actual onset of each of the triad of behavioral manifestations of the disease. Until recently, the first manifestations of HD—that is, prior to the development of frank motor disorders—remained unclear. Today, it is certain that many people present with psychotic manifestations prior to a clinical diagnosis of HD. Such people are classified as being in the *preclinical* period but are, in fact, manifesting symptoms of HD. Approximately half the people with HD have changes in their character as initial symptoms. They also display depression, anxiety, irritability, and apathy. Depression also has been identified as the first symptom in as many as half of people with HD. People with HD may begin to find fault with everything, complain constantly, and nag family members. They may develop suspicious behaviors, irritability, and impulsivity. Other manifestations, related to poor self-control, include outbursts of temper, alcoholism, sexual promiscuity, and periods of despondency. Such symptoms are essential aspects of the disease because they arise out of structural changes in the brain involving frontal-striatal complex loops. These symptoms are not reactive in nature. They do not occur, for example, as a result of an individual's knowledge of being at risk because of genetic testing or from the burden of growing up in a family with affected members. This gradual decline in intellectual function—without aphasia, agnosia, apraxia, or memory loss—has been characterized as **subcortical dementia**.

Initially, the cognitive deficits observed in HD were attributed to the degeneration of cerebrocortical neurons once thought to be a characteristic neuropathologic feature of the disease. However, there is no significant loss of cortical neurons even in people with moderately advanced cases of HD, although a moderate degree of gross atrophy of the cerebral cortex is observed in most autopsied brains of people with the disease.

The loss of striatal neurons in HD is preceded by a biochemical lesion in the striatum in that PET scans show that glucose metabolism is characteristically decreased before the neuronal loss can be detected. PET scans also show that glucose metabolism is reduced in the frontal cortex in people with HD. This depression of prefrontal neuronal function occurs secondary to the loss of striatal neurons and involves *all* of the complex loops through the basal ganglia. Destruction of the head of the caudate nucleus in HD anatomically disconnects the cortex and striatum. Deprived of normal facilitating information from the caudate nucleus that determines appropriate action, the frontal lobe cortex is unable to properly regulate emotional behavior or personality attributes or perform its executive functions. Executive functions, discussed earlier, refer to goal-directed skills that permit the efficient use of intelligence in organizing, decision making, planning, impulse control, awareness of social skills, and ordering of priorities. It should be noted that people with HD also have gross degeneration and changes of the anterior cingulate cortex (ACC). Hence, cognitive consequences of this disorder are not solely predicated on changes to the basal ganglia.

Thought Question

With regard to Huntington's disease, which cortical loops explain motor dysfunction and which explain cognitive dysfunction?

Cognition, Motivation, and Planning of Movement

We have just examined the cognitive consequences of two motor disorders of the basal ganglia. Here, we turn to another aspect of cognitive dysfunction of the basal ganglia—namely, the effects of cognitive processing on motor expression. To understand this relationship, it is important to recall that, as noted earlier in this chapter, multimodal association cortices associated with cognition relate to motor as well as intellectual aspects of cognition. That is, cognition is not just intellectual but also has implications for higher-level processing as relates to movement. In this context, cognition of the subcortex plays a role in motivation and planning of motor activities. Not only are there cortical association areas of importance, but also subcortical areas.

Thought Question

This is a good time to synthesize clinical with neuroanatomical information. What are two possible reasons people with disorders of the basal ganglia might have cognitive dysfunction?

With regard to the neuroanatomical basis of motivation and related motor activities, dopamine-producing neurons of the SNpc and VTA are in an anatomical position to provide a link between the limbic system and movement. This link involves the side loop of the limbic circuit through the basal ganglia mentioned earlier. Dopaminergic neurons of the SNpc receive their cortical input preferentially from neurons of the cerebral cortex whose input, in turn, is from the hippocampus and amygdala. Dopaminergic neurons, in turn, project to the motor portion of the basal ganglia (putamen). The loss of DA neurons in PD results in an interruption of this limbic-to-motor link. In PD, there is no paralysis or paresis such that, with appropriate stimulation, these individuals are capable of rapid, effective movement. Thus, the link between motivation and movement is interrupted, causing a disinclination to move and akinesia.

Similarly, in HD there is a disconnect between motivation and motor activity. In a study of people with early stage HD, it has been observed that the inability to plan and organize motor activities is more troubling to the individual than the chorea associated with the disease. Although people with HD rarely initiate independent activity—and are happy to sit, doing nothing—they can participate in activities that are planned out for them and are supervised. In other words, these individuals lack the motivation to plan on their own a goal-oriented (unified) pattern of motor actions. This problem with motivation may explain why people with basal ganglia disorders have such a difficult time embracing exercise programs even when they understand the importance.

Two conditions that were long considered psychiatric disorders are particularly helpful in illustrating the motivational aspects of movement: obsessive-compulsive disorder (OCD) and Tourette's syndrome (TS).

Obsessive-Compulsive Disorder

Obsessive-compulsive disorder (OCD) is a relatively common neuropsychiatric disorder estimated to affect 1 to 3 percent of the general population. This is an anxiety disorder, characterized by intrusive thoughts (obsessions) and compulsions. Between one-third and one-half of all people with this disorder first experience symptoms in childhood or adolescence. People with OCD typically have normal general intelligence (full-scale IQ) and language abilities. In fact, people who are mildly affected with OCD may seem so regular that even close friends and relatives may be unaware of their stressful secret lives.

Obsessions are repetitive, repellant ideas or impulses that are experienced as intrusive, senseless, and unreasonable. Many obsessions concern violence, doubt, or contamination by germs or dirt. Examples of obsessions include a mother who is horrified by the repetitive thought of stabbing her newborn child, or a boy who is agonized by the recurrent thought that he will be contaminated if he comes into contact with dirt. **Compulsions** are repetitive, purposeful behaviors that result from obsessions in an attempt to assuage them or behaviors that must rigidly follow specific rules. They, too, are experienced by the individual as irrational and unnecessary. The most common compulsions are checking, counting, and washing. The mother who experiences the thought of exacting violence on her newborn by stabbing him acts to prevent the stabbing by repeatedly checking that all of the kitchen knives are securely locked away. Likewise, the boy with obsessions of contamination may repetitively wash his hands to alleviate his distress about contact with dirt.

A range of obsessions and compulsions may be present in any given person with one, two, or even all of the common manifestations being present. Insight into the irrationality of the obsessions and compulsions and the struggle to resist them are what distinguish obsessions from delusions. The symptoms of OCD are time-consuming and may eventually interfere with normal social, school, or occupational functions.

A number of neuropsychological deficits can occur in people with OCD. Visuospatial deficits and impairment of nonverbal memory are relatively common. Most interesting in terms of helping to define the sites of neuropathology are impairments of executive function. Any given complex behavior demands a number of ongoing evaluations, as well as an oversight of memory of similar past experiences. The sensory inflow emanating from the behavior and the context in which it is occurring must be considered. The affective (agreeable or disagreeable) feeling generated by the situation must be determined and its significance evaluated. Executive function depends on the capacity to use this information as the situation evolves, and behavioral strategies must shift to maintain successful performance. People with OCD have difficulty changing strategies (set-shifting) when the rules for successful performance of a task change. Such behavioral deficits suggest alterations in the function of the fronto-striatal circuitry.

The first indication that OCD is associated with dysfunction in specific brain circuitry occurred after pandemics of the early 1900s, when the observation was made that people with PD from Von Economo's encephalitis developed OCD symptoms when lesions of the striatum were present. Eventually, it was noted that people with neurological conditions that exhibit obsessive and compulsive symptoms typically have disorders involving the basal ganglia or inferior frontal cortex. Functional brain imaging (PET scanning and glucose metabolism) shows that the orbitofrontal cortex, cingulate cortex, and head of the caudate nucleus are hyperactive (hypermetabolic) in people with OCD. There is a normalization of activity in this corticostriatal circuit following successful treatment of symptoms with drugs or behavior therapy. Thus, it is likely that the limbic circuit through the basal ganglia is involved in the pathogenesis of OCD. This functional alteration in the limbic circuit is paralleled by structural alterations in the orbitofrontal and cingulate cortices and ventral striatum.

Pharmacotherapy and behavioral therapy are currently the most utlized options in the treatment of OCD. Behavior therapy consists of systematic desensitization, wherein the person is exposed to a graded series of representations of the object, such as a feared contaminant, and is finally exposed to the object itself. Neurosurgery, with deep brain stimulation of the subthalamic nucleus, although confirming involvement of the limbic circuit, is a procedure of last resort used, if at all, only in the most severe situations in which the person is totally disabled.

Tourette's Syndrome

Tourette's syndrome (TS), first described in 1885, was considered to be a psychological disorder until the 1960s. Thus, psychotherapy was the accepted mode of treatment. Today, TS is unequivocally regarded as an organic brain disorder involving, in particular, complex circuits through the basal ganglia and the neurotransmitter dopamine (DA). TS occurs in all cultures and races in which it has been sought and is estimated to affect 1 percent of children. TS is three to four times more common in males than females.

The etiology of TS is unclear. Although a familial cause has been established, the exact genetic basis has not. It is likely that multiple genes are involved that interact with potential environmental factors (such as gender) to influence the phenotypic expression of TS.

Motor and phonic (noise-producing, often called vocal) tics are the cardinal features of TS. It should be recognized at the outset that the distinction between motor and phonic tics is artificial in that phonic tics are motor tics, just ones that result in sound. Nonetheless, both forms of tic must be present, although not necessarily concurrently, for a diagnosis of TS. The tics manifest themselves in a variety of forms and change frequently. Except for the occurrence of tics, the standard neurological examination is typically normal.

Both motor and phonic tics may be simple or complex. Simple motor tics are fast, darting, meaningless muscular events, while complex motor tics involve several muscle groups, are more sustained, and may appear more purposeful or to be contextually inappropriate and exaggerated fragments of ordinary motor behaviors. Examples of simple and complex motor tics are listed in Table 21-1 ■. Phonic tics may also be simple or complex. Simple phonic tics are meaningless, explosive sounds or noises, whereas complex phonic tics consist of linguistically meaningful utterances, phrases, and even statements. Table 21-1 also lists examples of simple and complex phonic tics.

Coprolalia, the explosive utterance of foul or obscene words or phrases, is a dramatic complex phonic tic and often is exploited in media portrayals of TS. However, coprolalia occurs in less than one-third of patients and is not necessary to diagnosis. Likewise, *copropraxia*, an obscene motor tic, is uncommon.

A number of useful diagnostic features occur in association with tics. First is the capacity to voluntarily suppress the tics. Although this capacity varies from one individual to the next, some can control their symptoms for an hour or two or even longer, depending on the circumstances. Suppression complicates diagnosis when it occurs in the doctor's office. However, voluntary suppression comes at the expense of increasing anxiety, tension, and discomfort resulting from the unfulfilled urge to tic. The latter is related to a second useful diagnostic feature, namely, the feeling of relief and tension reduction experienced when the patient tics. Third, tic symptoms are fluid in that they change in anatomic location, variety, and intensity on a daily, weekly or monthly basis, particularly in younger people.

In most individuals with this disorder, anxiety, stress, and excitement exacerbate symptoms. In contrast, relaxation—in particular, intense mental concentration on a particular activity—alleviates or even eliminates symptoms altogether. Thus, tasks requiring full attention and full focus wherein the person is not self-conscious—such as acting, participating in a sport, or performing surgery—may be performed symptom-free. In the majority of people with TS, the symptoms are mild to moderate and may not be sufficiently debilitating to everyday life activities to warrant medical intervention. Only a minority of people is severely affected.

While tics are the hallmark of TS diagnosis, the disorder is often associated with one or more typical co-morbid conditions. In general, when co-morbid conditions are present, they are more debilitating than the tics themselves. Furthermore, they are independent diagnostic categories and follow their own natural progression so that it is common to see the tics improve over time, whereas the symptoms, caused by a particular co-morbid condition, worsen.

It is noteworthy that more than half of people diagnosed with TS have symptoms of attention deficit/hyperactivity disorder (ADHD). In addition, OCD and learning disorders can also co-occur. Notably, though, intelligence is normally distributed across the population of children with TS.

Table 21-1 Examples of Simple and Complex Tics

	SIMPLE	COMPLEX
Motor tics	Eye blinking	Touching
	Nose twitching	Holding facial expressions
	Lip pouting	Sustained staring
	Eye rolling	Picking at the nose
	Facial grimacing	Finger drumming
	Shoulder shrugs	Kissing
	Abdominal tensing	Hopping
	Head and extremity jerks	Clapping
	Kicks	Gyrating
	Finger movements	Bending
	Tooth clicking	Touching the ground
	Jaw snaps	"Dystonic" postures
		Echopraxia (imitation of someone else's movements)
		Copropraxia (sudden, vulgar, sexual, or obscene gestures like giving the finger)
Phonic tics	Gasps	Single words or phrases
	Chirps	Echolalia (repeating the last heard sound, word, or phrase of another)
	Barks	Palilalia (repeating one's own sounds or words)
	Squeaks	Coprolalia (expression of a socially unacceptable word or phrase, such as an obscenity, or ethnic, racial, gender, or religious slur)
	Grunts	
	Snorts	
	Clicks	
	Growls	
	Throat clearing	
	Coughs	
	Sniffing	

The onset of TS is usually between the ages of 5 and 7. Most children (one-half to two-thirds) with TS experience a dramatic decline in the severity of symptoms during adolescence. In some individuals, symptoms remit completely by early adulthood. Therapy for people with TS potentially involves psychological counseling, psychotherapy, and/or medical intervention, depending on the array and severity of unique features in a given person. The majority of individuals have symptoms that are mild to moderate, as noted earlier. In such people, it is essential to evaluate whether medication should be administered at all, given the side-effect burden (occasionally disastrous) associated with commonly used drugs.

No drug entirely eliminates tics. The mainstay treatment of tics has been the use of potent dopamine postsynaptic receptor blockers that inactivate DA (D$_2$) receptors. These drugs include haloperidol and pimozide. The fact that DA receptor blockers are the most effective treatment is strong, although circumstantial, evidence that the transmitter DA plays an essential role in TS. However, side effects of these drugs include parkinsonism, dystonia, dyskinesia, and akathisia (a feeling of inner restlessness) in the short term, and, in the long term, with tardive dyskinesia, a disastrous outcome that sometimes outlasts, even permanently, the termination of medication.

What OCD, ADHD, and TS Tell Us about the Brain

The neuropathology and pathogenesis of TS have not been adequately defined. Most attention has been directed at the complex loops that feed through the caudate nucleus, whose dysfunction result in the symptoms of TS. However, abnormalities of the midbrain, the source of dopaminergic innervation of the forebrain, may well be the precipitating neuropathology. What seems reasonable is the idea that the neuropathology underlying TS, ADHD, and OCD are related. For one thing, the behaviors characterizing each of these disorders share a common phenomenological thread. All may be linked by the inability of the brain to properly filter, and thus inhibit, influences that normally shape socially appropriate (and thus successful) behavioral sequences. Clearly, the capacity to shift or switch behavior adaptively in the face of changing environmental circumstances is vital to success (physical and social), and sometimes even for survival.

In people with TS alone, the volume of the caudate nucleus is reduced across all age groups, and this is one of the most consistent neuroimaging findings in people with TS. In fact, the extent of reduction in caudate nucleus in children with TS predicts the severity of tic (and OCD) symptoms in early adulthood. As the spatial extent of basal ganglia pathology increases, people with TS with co-morbid conditions are incorporated into the clinical profile. People with TS and co-morbid OCD have, in addition to the reduced caudate nucleus volume, smaller volumes of the putamen and globus pallidus. Dysfunction in the putamen and globus pallidus would disrupt additional neuroregulatory loops through the basal ganglia, further compromising operation of the filter (i.e., inhibition). Finally, people with TS and co-morbid ADHD, in addition to having reduced caudate nucleus volumes, exhibit larger volumes in the cortical regions to which the caudate nucleus interacts via its complex loops.

Summary

We began this chapter with a consideration of cortical cognition. We first discussed association areas of the neocortex, noting that two types exist—unimodal and multimodal. The unimodal cortex is concerned with elaborating perceptions for a specific modality (somatosensory, visual, or auditory), while the multimodal association cortex integrates input from multiple sensory modalities and mediates such complex cognitive functions as spatial cognition involving both personal and extrapersonal space. The lateral association cortex (including both posterior and anterior areas) and the basomedial or limbic multimodal association cortex were defined and discussed in terms of their unique anatomy and functions. Spatial cognition is a function of the posterior association cortex, lesions of which result in unilateral hemispatial neglect wherein the contralateral half of the body and extrapersonal space are no longer recognized. Anterior association cortex of the frontal lobe is involved in executive function, which is the capacity to alter goal-directed behavior to ensure that the goal is still attained when the conditions in which the behavior unfolds change. A number of neuropsychological tests specifically sample executive function. These include the Wisconsin Card Sorting Test, the Stroop test, and the Tower of Hanoi and Tower of London tests. Performance on these tests deteriorates in people with a lesion of the anterior association cortex.

The second major section of this chapter dealt with the basal ganglia and cerebellum in cognitive function. Participation of these structures in cognition results from their interconnection with specific multimodal association cortices. We began this section with the cognitive functions of the cerebellum. Among the cognitive disorders seen with damage to the cerebellum is the cognitive affective syndrome that is characterized by deficits in executive function, language production, and affect. We concluded this section by discussing clinical consequences of disorders affecting the basal ganglia as it relates to cognitive dysfunction. Here, we considered two disorders that are traditionally thought of as mainly motor in nature (i.e., PD and HD) and two disorders that are traditionally thought of as psychiatric in nature (i.e., OCD and TS).

Applications

1. A 63-year-old woman with a past medical history of diabetes, hypertension, and osteoporosis went to bed early one evening with a severe headache. The next morning when she got out of bed, she fell to the floor. Her husband helped her up and noticed something was wrong: she wasn't moving her left arm or leg. She denied anything was wrong and was reluctant to go to the emergency department (ED); however, he insisted. At the ED, it was determined that she had sustained a stroke. Upon examination, it was found she was unable to discriminate touch on the left extremities, but could do so on the right. She was not spontaneously moving her left extremities, nor did she move them upon command. She was spontaneously using her right extremities and demonstrated good strength when asked to hold against resistance. She seemed to be unaware of the left side of her body and to that side of the environment. She was admitted for acute care and subsequently to a rehabilitation facility.
   a. Given her somatosensory and motor losses, and the presence of neglect, identify the cortical regions most likely affected by the stroke.
   b. How does the presence of neglect affect prognosis for an individual with stroke?

c. Once she was in the rehabilitation facility, what tests could be used to confirm that she had a left hemispatial neglect?

d. This individual seemed unaware of her deficits and even denied them when diagnosed by the neuropsychologist in the rehabilitation facility. What term would you use to describe her denial of deficits?

2. The basal ganglia are of great importance in control of movement. However, these structures likewise have important roles in cognitive and affective functions. Consider what you have learned about people with PD.

a. Identify motor and nonmotor symptoms that manifest in individuals with PD.

b. Create a list of tests and measures used to identify each of these symptoms.

References

Cortical Cognition

Allman, J. M., Hakeem, A., Erwin, J. M., Nimchinsky, E., and Hoff, P. The anterior cingulate cortex. The evolution of an interface between emotion and cognition. *Ann NY Acad Sci* 935(1):107–117, 2001.

American Psychiatric Association. Practice guideline for the treatment of patients with obsessive-compulsive disorder. *Am J Psychiatry* 164(suppl):1, 2007.

Baxter, D. M., and Warrington, E.K. Neglect dysgraphia. *J Neurol Neurosurg Psychiatry* 46:1073–1078, 1983.

Bird, C. M., et al. The impact of extensive medial frontal lobe damage on "Theory of Mind" and cognition. *Brain* 127:914–928, 2004.

Bisiach, E., and Luzzatti, C. Unilateral neglect of representational space. *Cortex* 14:129–133, 1978.

Buxbaum, L. J., Ferraro, M. K., Veramonti, T., et al. Hemispatial neglect. Subtypes, neuroanatomy, and disability. *Neurology* 62:749–756, 2004.

Feinberg, T. E., Haber, L. D., and Leeds, N. E. Verbal asomatoagnosia. *Neurology* 40:1391–1394, 1990.

Fulton, J. F. *Functional Localization in the Frontal Lobes and Cerebellum*. Oxford University Press, London, 1949.

Groenewegen, H. J., and Uylings, H. B. M. The prefrontal cortex and the integration of sensory, limbic, and autonomic information. In: Uylings, H. B .M., et al., eds. *Progress in Brain Research*, Vol. 126. Elsevier, Amsterdam, 2000.

Hobbs N. Z., Pedrick A. V., Say M. J., et al. The structural involvement of the cingulate cortex in premanifest and early Huntington's disease. *Mov Disord* 26: 1684–1690, 2011.

Karnath, H.-O., and Dieterich, M. Spatial neglect — A vestibular disorder? *Brain* 129:293–305, 2006.

Kolb, B., and Whishaw, I. Q. *Fundamentals of Human Neuropsychology*, 4th ed. W. H. Freeman, New York, 1995.

Mallet, L., Polosan, M., Jaafari, N., et al. Subthalamic nucleus stimulation in severe obsessive-compulsive disorder. *N Engl J Med* 359:2121, 2008.

Mesulam, M.-M. Ch. 2. The human frontal lobes: Transcending the default mode through contingent encoding. In: Stuss, D. T., and Knight, R.T., eds. *Principles of Frontal Lobe Function*, Oxford University Press, New York, 2002.

Sacks, O. *The Man Who Mistook His Wife for a Hat and Other Clinical Tales*. Harper & Row, New York, 1985.

Saper, C. B., Iversen, S., and Frackowiak, R. Ch. 19. Integration of sensory and motor function. In: Kandel, E., Schwartz, J. H., and Jessell, T.M., eds. *Principles of Neural Science*, 4th ed. McGraw-Hill, New York, 2000.

Basal Ganglia

Alexander, G. E., DeLong, M. R., and Strick, P. L. Parallel organization of functionally segregated circuits linking basal ganglia and cortex. *Ann Rev Neurosci* 9: 357–381, 1986.

Anderson, K. E., and Savage, C. R. Cognitive and neurobiological findings in obsessive-compulsive disorder. *Psychiatr Clin N Am* 27:37–47, 2004.

Banaschewski, T., Woerner, W., and Rothenberger, A. Premonitory sensory phenomena and suppressibility of tics in Tourette syndrome: Developmental aspects in children and adolescents. *Dev Med Child Neurol* 45:700, 2003.

Baxter, L. R., Schwartz, J. M., Bergman, K. S., et al. Caudate glucose metabolic rate changes with both drug and behavior therapy for OCD. *Arch Gen Psychiatry* 49:681–689, 1992.

Bloch, M. H., Leckman, J. F., Zhu, H., and Peterson, B. S. Caudate volumes in childhood predict symptom severity in adults with Tourette syndrome. *Neurology* 65:1253–1258, 2005.

Brownell, G. L., Budinger, T. F., Lauterbur, P. C., and McGeer, P. L. Positron tomography and nuclear magnetic resonance imaging. *Science* 215: 619–626, 1982.

Caine, E. D., Hunt, R. D., Weingartner, H., and Ebert, M. H. Huntington's dementia. Clinical and neuropsychologic features. *Arch. Gen. Psychiatry* 35:377–384, 1978.

Cavedini, P., Riboldi, G., D'Annucci, A., et al. Decision-making heterogeneity in obsessive-compulsive disorder: Ventromedial prefrontal cortex function predict different treatment outsomes. *Neuropsychologia* 40:205–211, 2001.

Coffey, B. J., Biederman, J., Geller, D. A., et al. The course of Tourette's disorder: A literature review. *Harvard Rev Psychiatry*, 8:192, 2000.

DeLong, M. R., and Wichmann, T. Circuits and circuit disorders of the basal ganglia. *Arch Neurol* 64:20–24, 2007.

DiFiglia, M. Excitotoxic injury of the neostriatum: A model for Huntington's disease. *Trends Neurosci* 13: 286–289, 1990.

Freeman, R. D., Fast, D. K., Burd, L., et al. An international perspective on Tourette syndrome: Selected findings from 3,500 individuals in 22 countries. *Dev Med Child Neurol*, 7:436, 2000.

Garraux, G., et al. Increased midbrain gray matter in Tourette's syndrome. *Ann Neurol* 59:381–385, 2006.

Goetz, C. G., and Klawans, H. L. Gilles de la Tourette on Tourette syndrome. In: Friedhoff, A. J., and Chase, T. N., eds. *Gilles de la Tourette Syndrome*. Raven Press, New York, 1982.

Heaton, R. K. *Wisconsin Card Sorting Test Manual.* Psychology Assessment Resources, Odessa, FL, 1981.

Jenike, M. A. Neurosurgical treatment of obsessive-compulsive disorder. *Br J Psychiatry* 35:79–90, 1998.

Knowlton, B. J., Mangels, J. A., and Squire, L. R. A neostriatal habit learning system in humans. *Science* 273:1399–1401, 1996.

Lehericy, S., et al. Diffusion tensor fiber tracking shows distinct corticostriatal circuits in humans. *Ann Neurol* 55:522–529, 2004.

Lezak, M. D. *Neuropsychological Assessment*, 3rd ed. Oxford University Press, New York, 1976.

MacLean, P. D. *The Triune Brain in Evolution.* Plenum Press, New York, 1990.

Marsh, R., Alexander, G. M., Packard, M. G., ct al. Habit learning in Tourette syndrome. *Arch Gen Psychiatry* 61:1259–1268, 2004.

Marshall, J., White, K., Weaver, M., et al. Specific psychiatric manifestations among preclinical Huntington disease mutation carriers. *Arch Neurol* 64:116–121, 2007.

Mataix-Cols, D., Wooderson, S., Lawrence, N., et al. Distinct neural correlates of washing, checking, and hoarding symptom dimensions in obsessive-compulsive disorder. *Arch Gen Psychiatry* 61: 564–576, 2004.

Middleton, F. A., and Strick, P.L. Anatomical evidence for cerebellar and basal ganglia involvement in higher cognitive function. *Science* 266:458–461, 1994.

Mink, J. W. Neurobiology of basal ganglia circuits in Tourette syndrome: Faulty inhibition of unwanted motor patterns? *Adv Neurol*, 85:113, 2001.

Muslimovic, D., Post, B., Speelman, J. D., and Schmand, B. Cognitive profile of patients with newly diagnosed Parkinson disease. *Neurology* 65:1239–1245, 2005.

Nolte, J. *The Human Brain: An Introduction to Its Functional Anatomy*. Mosby Elsevier, Philadelphia, 2009.

Pappert, E. J., Goetz, C. G., Louis, E. D., et al. Objective assessments of longitudinal outcome in Gilles de al Tourette's syndrome. *Neurology*, 61:936, 2003.

Pauls, D. L. An update on the genetics of Gilles de la Tourette syndrome. *J Psychosom Res* 55:7, 2003.

Peterson, B. S., Thomas, P., Kane, M. J., et al. Basal ganglia volumes in patients with Gilles de la Tourette syndrome. *Arch Gen Psychiatry* 60:415–424, 2003.

Pujol, J., Soriano-Mas, C., Alonso, P., et al. Mapping structural brain alterations in obsessive-compulsive disorder. *Arch Gen Psychiatry* 61:720–730, 2004.

Rauch, S. L., and Baxter, L. R., Jr. Neuroimaging in obsessive-compulsive disorder and related disorders. In: Jenicke, M., Baer, L., and Minichiello, W.E., eds. *Obsessive-Compulsive Disorder: Practical Management*, 3rd ed. Mosby, St. Louis, 1998.

Richfield, E. K., Twyman, R., and Berent, S. Neurological syndrome following bilateral damage to the head of the caudate nuclei. *Ann Neurol* 22:768, 1987.

Ropper, A. H., and Brown, R. H. Ch. 39. Degenerative diseases of the nervous system. In: *Adams and Victor's Principles of Neurology*, 8th ed. McGraw-Hill, New York, 2005.

Rosenblatt, A. Understanding the psychiatric prodrome of Huntington disease. *J Neurol Neurosurg Psychiatry* 78:913, 2007.

Sandor, P. Pharmacological management of tics in patients with TS. *J Psychosom Res*, 55:41, 2003.

Shohamy, D., et al. Cortico-striatal contributions to feedback-based learning: Converging data from neuroimaging and neuropsychology. *Brain* 127:851–859, 2004.

Singer, H. S. Tourette's syndrome: From behavior to biology. *Lancet Neurol* 4:149, 2005.

Swerdlow, N. R., and Young, A. B. Neuropathology in Tourette syndrome: An update. *Adv Neurol* 85:151, 2001.

Temel, Y., and Visser-Vandewalle, V. Surgery in Tourette syndrome. *Mov Disord* 19:3–14, 2004.

Volkow, N. D., Wang, G. J., Kollins, S. H., et al. Evaluating dopamine reward pathway in ADHD. *JAMA* 302:1084–1091, 2009.

Voon, V., and Fox, S. H. Medication-related impulse control and repetitive behaviors in Parkinson disease. *Arch Neurol* 64:1089–1096, 2007.

Cerebellum

Allen, G., Buxton, R. B., Wong, E. C., and Courchesne, E. Attentional activation of the cerebellum independent of motor involvement. *Science* 275:1940–1943, 1997.

Barinaga, M. The cerebellum: Movement coordinator or much more? *Science* 272:482–483, 1996.

Desmond, J. E., Chen, A., and Shieh, P. Cerebellar transcranial magnetic stimulation impairs verbal working memory. *Ann Neurol* 58:553–560, 2005.

Dum, R. P., and Strick, P. L. An unfolded map of the cerebellar dentate nucleus and its projections to the cerebral cortex. *J Neurophysiol* 89:634–639, 2003.

Kim, S.-G., Ugurbil, K., and Strick, P.L. Activation of a cerebellar output nucleus during cognitive processing. *Science* 265:949–951, 1994.

Konczak, J., Schoch, B., Dimitrova, A., Gizewski, E., and Timmann, D. Functional recovery of children and adolescents after cerebellar tumour resection. *Brain* 128:1428–1441, 2005.

Leiner, H., Leiner, A. L., and Dow, R. S. Cognitive and language functions of the human cerebellum. *Trend Neurosci* 16:444–447, 1993.

Limperopoulos, C., Soul, J.S., Haidar, H., et al. Impaired trophic interactions between the cerebellum and cerebrum among preterm infants. *Pediatrics* 116: 844–850, 2005.

Nolte, J. *The Human Brain: An Introduction to Its Functional Anatomy*. Mosby Elsevier, Philadelphia, 2009.

Ravizza, S. M., et al. Cerebellar damage produces selective deficits in verbal working memory. *Brain* 129:306–320, 2006.

Richter, S., Schoch, B., Kaiser, O., et al. Children and adolescents with chronic cerebellar lesions show no clinically relevant signs of aphasia or neglect. *J Neurophysiol* 94:4108–4120, 2005.

Schmahmann, J. D., and Sherman, J. C. The cerebellar cognitive affective syndrome. *Brain* 121:561–579, 1998.

Timmann, D., Drepper, J., Maschke, M., et al. Motor deficits cannot explain impaired cognitive associative learning in cerebellar patients. *Neuropsychologia* 40:788–800, 2002.

PEARSON
myhealthprofessionskit™

Use this address to access the Companion Website created for this textbook. Simply select "Physical Therapy" from the choice of disciplines. Find this book and log in using your username and password to access self-assessment questions, a glossary, and more.

Emotion, Memory, and Language

LEARNING OUTCOMES

This chapter prepares the reader to:

1 Define the terms *emotion* and *memory*.

2 With respect to memory, explain the role of the following: memory trace or engram; declarative, procedural, and semantic memory; prospective memory; and anterograde and retrograde memory.

3 Discuss the steps that take place from the acquisition of memory to storage and relate the steps to neuroanatomical structures.

4 Relate amnesia to areas of neuroanatomic injury or disease.

5 Discuss what has been learned about the neurological basis of memory and emotion from people who have epilepsy.

6 With respect to memory, discuss core components of the limbic system and their functional importance.

7 Identify major inputs and outputs of the limbic system and discuss their relationship to emotion and memory.

8 Compare and contrast the following language deficits: Broca's aphasia, Wernicke's aphasia, global aphasia, conduction aphasia, and transcortical aphasia.

9 Differentiate propositional (symbolic) from emotional language and discuss the neuroanatomic correlates of each.

10 Differentiate the functional roles of different neuroanatomic regions associated with language from reception to speech.

ACRONYMS

ACA Anterior cerebral artery

LTM Long-term memory

MCA Middle cerebral artery

PCA Posterior cerebral artery

PNS Peripheral nervous system

STM Short-term memory

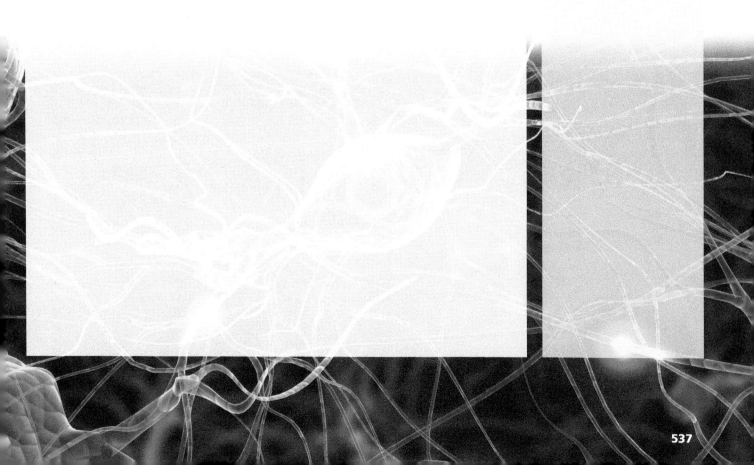

Introduction

This chapter presents three of the cognitive functions that attain their most complete elaboration in humans: emotion, memory, and language. Emotion and memory are mediated in large part by components of the limbic system. In contrast, language is mediated by cortical areas that include the frontal and temporal cortices and connections between the two. Emotion, memory, and language are inextricably linked to other constructs of cognition such as attention, executive function, and decision making. Thus, the content in this chapter complements and builds on information presented in Chapter 21, recognizing that there is no clear distinction between these interrelated functions.

The first major section of this chapter discusses emotion and memory, beginning with emotion. Emotion is the most fundamental and significant attribute of human cognition. It has a major substrate in the highest level of the brain, the frontal cortex. Not only does it color our everyday activities, but it is the fundamental mechanism used to guide behavior in a social milieu. While we may tend to think of emotion as dictating socially pathologic behavior, it is a far more pervasive navigational guidepost that is used in directing virtually all

behavior. Next, we address memory—which is a multifaceted function. Some memory mechanisms operate on a short-term time scale, others on a long-term (even permanent) scale; some function to encode explicit facts and events, others to record skills and habits. Moreover, there is not a single, unitary system in the brain that mediates these different aspects of memory. Memory and emotion are intimately related. Our most durable and vivid memories are those associated with the strongest emotions.

The second major section of this chapter discusses language, a uniquely human behavior in terms of its richness, that provides a vehicle for the expression of emotion and memory. Indeed, there appears to be a specific neural substrate for the expression of emotion and for our capacity to recognize emotion in the language of others. Language *is* memory and emotion in action. Language is truly remarkable: simple words act as symbols for everything in our world; simple marks on paper are able to transmit a rich cultural heritage across generations. No wonder language disorders resulting from brain damage can be so devastating. What could be worse than losing the capacity to communicate?

EMOTION AND MEMORY: THE LIMBIC SYSTEM

Clinical Preview

You are working in a rehabilitation center that specializes in rehabilitation of people who have had a traumatic brain injury. In Chapter 21, you learned about some of the cognitive issues these individuals face. Many of these individuals also have significant problems with emotion and memory. Examples of the deficits encountered on a daily basis include the following: emotional outbursts, inappropriate behaviors (e.g., sexual innuendos), and loss of short-term memory but ability to remember experiences from the past.

As you read through this section, consider the following:

- How are deficits of emotion and memory related?
- What are the anatomical regions that subserve these functions?

Contemporary neuroscience views emotion as playing an indispensable role in our mental lives in two vital and expansive functional realms: in guiding complex behavior in social contexts and in the formation of easily accessible memories of self-involved experience. Thus, rather than

considering emotion as an interfering, chaotic state of mentation, it emerges as a most fundamental and significant attribute of human nature.

Attempting to understand the genesis of human emotion in terms of brain structure and function continues to vex neuroscientists. The search for a single, more or less discrete system that mediates emotion is prompted by the fact that despite the great range of emotional states, such states normally have three elements in common: (1) a set of associated physiologic (largely autonomic) responses, (2) characteristic forms of expressive behavior, and (3) distinct subjective feelings. (Consider experiences of test anxiety or nervousness the first time you speak publically.) On the other hand, the rich variety of possible emotional states has prompted some to question the utility of attempting to define a single neural system that mediates emotion.

Thought Question

Which specific structures of the limbic system were discussed in Chapter 21 in context of cognition, and what was the role of each? As you proceed, consider how those structures, and others discussed in this chapter, relate to emotion and memory.

In 1937, James Papez suggested that a specific brain circuitry subserves emotional experiences, much as the occipital cortex is specific to vision. This circuit includes the

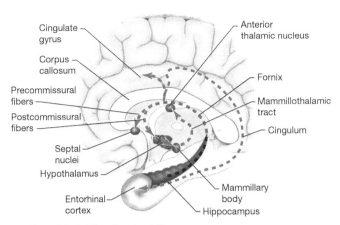

FIGURE 22-1 The circuit of Papez.

hypothalamus (and specifically the mammillary bodies), the anterior nucleus of the dorsal thalamus, the cingulate cortex, the hippocampus, and the fornix (Figure 22-1 ■). As will be seen, many of these structures are still considered of importance both in emotion and memory.

Our approach to understanding emotions is to draw from the role of the limbic system in the context of a prominent clinical disorder, **psychomotor epilepsy**. This disorder results in excessive neuronal discharge often confined just to neurons in structures comprising the limbic system. As we will see, such excessive discharge unequivocally reveals that the limbic system is, in fact, involved in the mediation of emotion and memory.

Emotion

> ### Thought Question
>
> Can a person's emotional experience be characterized objectively by another?

Emotion is, first and foremost, a *subjective* experience imbued with a *physical quality* that is either agreeable (pleasant) or disagreeable (unpleasant). In addition to this good–bad valence, emotional reactions vary along a second dimension, namely, that of intensity, or state of arousal. Emotions are entirely private mental phenomena, known only to ourselves, because only we as individuals have access to the interoceptive signals elicited by environmental (exteroceptive) events or by thought. ("The thought of it makes me ill.") The existence of emotion in another person must be *inferred* on the basis of the behavior displayed by the person in a given social context. Thus, in contrast to other forms of mental activity, emotion is invested with a unique and pervasive *social aspect*. That such inferences are typically successful is attested to by the fact that we can discuss emotion and say or hear *I feel angry, sad,* or *overjoyed* and be

reasonably certain that mutual understanding exists of what is being experienced.

As a consequence, attempts to define a set of basic, universal emotions often focus on the public display of emotion. One of the more prominent manifestations of emotion occurs in facial expression. Significantly, the capacity to recognize emotional state solely in terms of facial expression is consistent across literate cultures and the set of basic emotions so defined consists of six: anger, fear, disgust, happiness, sadness, and surprise (Figure 22-2 ■). However, facial expression is not the only behavioral manifestation of emotion. Sadness, for example, can be expressed in the form of dejected behavior; fear can result in protective behavior, anger in aggressive behavior, and happiness in affectionate and joyful behavior. Additionally, emotion is distinguished from other forms of mental activity by virtue of the fact that it alters the status of the body through activation of the autonomic nervous system. The pounding heart, the parched mouth, the sweating, the shaking legs that accompany fear are all well-known manifestations of emotion.

From a broader perspective, American psychologist William James eloquently described the vital and all-pervasive role emotion plays in human experience, noting that it is through emotion that one attributes meaning to experiences; indeed, it is through emotion that experiences are deemed as favorable or unfavorable in nature. He goes on to suggest that without emotion, nothing would have significance, character, expression, or perspective.

Memory

Memory is defined as "the mental registration, retention, and recall of *past* (emphasis added) experience, knowledge, ideas, sensations, and thoughts" (*Taber's Cyclopedic Medical*

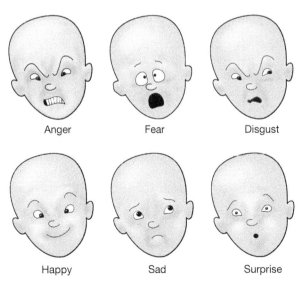

FIGURE 22-2 Examples of facial expressions for six basic emotions that are found consistently across cultures.

Dictionary, 16th ed.). While memory has this retrospective, one-sided link with time, it importantly defines both our *present* and *future* reality and behavior. Although we do not know what will come to pass, how we face future events is determined by memory. This is because memory quickly and effectively orients and drives us toward behavior that is projected into the future. So there is a *memory of the future*, called **prospective memory**. Prospective memory is the capacity to remember what we should or must do in order to successfully negotiate a future event based on past experience, knowledge, ideas, sensations, or thoughts. For example, a wide receiver in a football game knows how many steps he must take, and the direction, in order to catch a football that has not yet been thrown. As another example, we may know how we must react to negotiate a particular social situation when it actually is encountered. Past, present, and future all are woven into a single fabric. We do not isolate the present and future as intervals torn from the fabric of the past. Memory defines who we are in the here-and-now.

Thought Question

Describe the process involved in translating an experience or observation to a memory.

The term *memory* embraces two related processes. The first process is the *acquisition of a memory*, and this involves the learning of a novel skill, items(s) of information, or pattern of behavior. The second process occurs at some later time and is called *retrieval of the memory*. Retrieval involves the recall of the information or the re-expression of the skill or behavior. These two processes are linked by a change in the brain called the **memory trace** or **engram**. However, no one knows exactly what the change is, and its localization in the brain appears to vary depending on the nature of the specific memory. The engram stores the learned information in such a form that it can be retrieved in response to appropriate cues. When an individual sustains a blow to the head resulting in unconsciousness, the victim may not remember events associated with the accident itself, although events occurring earlier in time (e.g., minutes before an automobile accident) can be remembered. This is referred to as **retrograde amnesia**. The presence of retrograde amnesia suggests that a change occurs in the brain at the moment of formation of a memory. That is, because of the blow, the memory is never captured in a neurological change. The term **anterograde amnesia**, in contrast, refers to a loss of ability to create new memories, following an event that led to amnesia.

Acquisition of a memory (the learning process) involves three stages. The first is short-lived, lasting only seconds to minutes, and represents a period during which the learned event can be remembered; it is called **short-term memory (STM)**. The event is then forgotten unless it is consolidated by the intermediate process whereby STM is transferred to long-term memory; this stage is called **memory consolidation**. The duration of the consolidation phase is uncertain. It may be a matter of hours, days, or years, depending on the specific memory; in any case, it involves the hippocampus. The third and final stage is called **long-term memory (LTM)** in which the event can be recalled over a period of days or years, even a lifetime. STM and LTM are mediated by different neural mechanisms and different areas of the brain.

Many items are placed in STM (e.g., telephone numbers, names, dishes on a breakfast menu, ingredients for a recipe, arrangement of furniture in a house), but not all are consolidated into LTM. This is functionally advantageous for a number of reasons. First, the functional utility of recalling most items present in STM over a longer time period is limited. Second, it is likely that the capacity of the normal brain to store and retrieve information from LTM is finite. Perhaps most important, however, is the fact that to consolidate every phenomena or item in STM into LTM would be behaviorally incapacitating. This was most dramatically demonstrated by A. R. Luria in his classic book, *The Mind of the Mnemonist* (1968). For nearly three decades, Luria studied a single individual who possessed an apparently unlimited capacity not only to consolidate every item that entered STM into LTM, but to retain all items indefinitely. Yet, despite his unlimited capacity for remembering details, he was not able to generalize from those memories. If every event is remembered, sophisticated generalizations, metaphors, abstractions, concepts, inferences, and other elements of normal mentation would be impossible because they depend on forgetting parts of the individual events that contribute to them. The mnemonist, for example, could not draw inferences from those details regarding the importance of changes to that content. On meeting someone whose appearance had changed because of a haircut, the mnemonist might ask, "Have we met?" rather than saying, "You've cut your hair!" This contrasts with the response of most people who can recognize an acquaintance despite age-related changes in appearance, changes in dress, hairstyle, presence or absence of a mustache or beard, and the like.

Recently, scientists have studied individuals with seemingly limitless memory (hyperthymesia). An increased ability to recall autobiographical information may be related to an enhanced ability to store information or a decreased ability to suppress retrieval of stored information. In these recent studies, the hippocampus appears to be functioning appropriately, while the prefrontal cortex has been postulated to be involved in this phenomenon.

To understand utilization of memory for functional purposes, one more term is helpful: **working memory**, the ability to hold information in mind that is needed to complete complex tasks or sequential actions, including reasoning and learning. Working memory involves holding a particular concept briefly in awareness while a mental operation (e.g., arithmetic) is performed. Thus, working memory refers to the small amount of information we can keep in mind at one time. It has been described as *running commentary*. Working memory may be transferred into long-term memory or may be lost once its purpose is fulfilled.

Thought Question

Identify the types of memory that might be most important to the rehabilitation specialist when teaching a person a new skill, and discuss the role of each.

Although we tend to think of memory as a unitary function, LTM is divisible into two major forms that depend on different sets of brain structures (Figure 22-3 ■). **Declarative (or explicit) memory** is the memory for facts and events that occurred at a unique time or place and can be consciously recalled (i.e., declared). Declarative memory can be further subdivided into **episodic memory**, which relates to autobiographical information, and **semantic memory**, which relates to nonautobiographical information. **Procedural (or implicit) memory** refers to memories of procedures and skills acquired through repeated practice but that are not accessible to conscious recollection. Riding a bicycle and playing a musical instrument are examples of procedural memory retrievals.

The process of memory storage itself may be robust and enduring. This is suggested by electrical stimulation of the cerebral cortex in conscious patients in whom exceptionally detailed and vivid memories of past events are elicited in the emotional context in which they originally were experienced. However, these memories are not necessarily available to conscious recall, which has also been revealed in pathological states, in which forgotten memories are recalled, again in vivid and emotional detail. What this tells us is that normal memory is not a literal replaying of past events, but is a reconstitution, in both content and form, from incomplete parts that are affected by the internal and external cues that elicit the memory. Indeed, we may not be able to recall particular events when the internal and external environment is markedly different from the conditions prevailing during memory acquisition. Thus, memory is an *emergent phenomenon*—that is, an entity unpredictable from the actual events that were entered into LTM. For example, several people who witness the same robbery may all report the event differently.

The most reductionistic level of memory analysis concerns the molecular and cellular events occurring within and between neurons that underlie all plastic responses of the brain to experience (refer to Chapter 4). But some believe it would be an act of faith to think that such analysis would be capable of revealing the nature of such a durable feature of the human brain as memory. That is, the capacity of the brain to distinguish between a memory from childhood and one of a friend's face does not depend on the existence of particular molecules or molecular events, changes in the efficiency of a particular transmitter, or alterations in the efficiency of synaptic transmission. On the contrary, it depends on circuits in the brain and where they are located. Analyzing the cell biology of memory has been likened to analyzing the design of the laser pickup on a DVD player. Although knowing the design is important to understanding how a DVD player works, it would tell you nothing about the story on a particular disc. For that, you have to hit the play button.

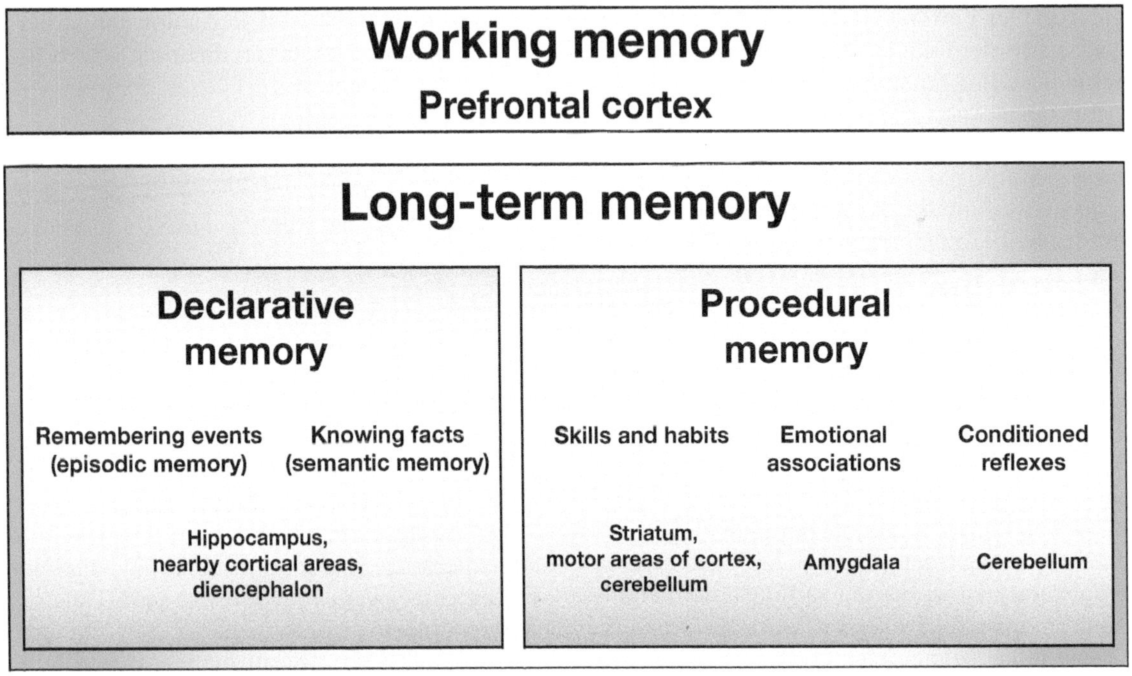

Working memory
Prefrontal cortex

Long-term memory

Declarative memory	**Procedural memory**
Remembering events (episodic memory) Knowing facts (semantic memory)	Skills and habits Emotional associations Conditioned reflexes
Hippocampus, nearby cortical areas, diencephalon	Striatum, motor areas of cortex, cerebellum Amygdala Cerebellum

FIGURE 22-3 Aspects of memory and the associated structures.

Emotion and Memory Are Related

One important commonality shared by emotion and memory is that excesses as well as deficiencies of each can compromise behavior. Beyond this, we all know that emotionally tinged events occupy a special place in our memories. Thus, for example, a movie that aroused emotion is much more readily retrieved from memory than those that were nonarousing. It is the visceral component of emotion that serves as a vital cue for the retrieval of specific events from memory because it sets them apart as being distinct from the ordinary catalogue of everyday events.

Autonomic arousal occurs whenever there is a conflict or discrepancy between a situation that is unfolding in the real world and the expectations we bring to the situation. When our expectations of the world fail, the resulting autonomic arousal directs and focuses our attention on potentially important aspects of the environment to ensure that every detail of sensory input is processed such that the right action can be taken.

Lessons from Psychomotor Epilepsy

The limbic system represents a critical link in the neural processes mediating emotion and memory as is evident from **psychomotor epilepsy**. Psychomotor epilepsy also may be referred to as temporal lobe epilepsy, limbic system epilepsy, and complex partial seizure.

Epilepsy, a disorder found in both adults and children, may be defined as the repeated occurrence of sudden, excessive, and synchronous discharges in large groups of neurons resulting in an almost instantaneous disruption of consciousness, disturbance of sensation, convulsive movements, impairment of mental function, or some combination of these behavioral signs (referred to as *seizures*). The word *epilepsy* is derived from a Greek word meaning *to seize upon*. Because of their sudden nature, seizures are called *ictal events*, from the Latin *ictus*, meaning *to strike*. Currently, epilepsy is differentiated into three forms: simple, complex, and generalized. *Simple epilepsy*, by definition, does not have an alteration of consciousness. *Complex epilepsy* has an alteration of consciousness, and *generalized epilepsy* has a loss of consciousness.

An epileptic discharge is capable of originating in only certain structures of the brain—most notably the cerebral cortex and amygdala. However, the ensuing abnormal discharge of neurons may involve cells in any structure of the CNS. The latter circumstance accounts for the wide variety of clinical manifestations of a seizure, which reflect the functions of the brain regions involved in the abnormal discharge. The symptoms of a seizure may be broadly categorized as positive or negative. **Positive signs** are an exaggeration of normal function, such as the jerking of a limb (convulsions) or seeing flashing lights. **Negative signs**, on the other hand, reflect the loss of particular functions, such as loss of the capacity to form new memories of activity ongoing during the seizure.

Simple seizures can include motor, sensory, and/or psychological manifestations. The nature of the manifestations depends on the specific areas of the nervous system that are involved. Motor manifestations include movements associated with the motor strip of the homunculus, aversive movements associated with the premotor cortex, and postural signs associated with the premotor cortex. A classic clinical example of a focal motor seizure is often referred to as the Jacksonian March, named after neurologist Hughlings Jackson who first described the condition. The seizure consists of an orderly progression or "march" of movements, reflective of the organization of the motor homunculus. The lesion associated with the Jacksonian seizure is distinctly located in the motor strip of the cortex contralateral to the side where the movements begin. Sensory manifestations can be visual (occipital and temporal), somatosensory (parietal), or auditory (temporal). Psychological manifestations occur in response to discharges within the temporal lobe or limbic system.

One of the unique aspects of the limbic system is that its structures collectively share a low threshold for epileptic discharge such that the seizure activity can remain confined to the limbic system and not trespass on other parts of the brain (although the seizure discharge may secondarily spread to other structures). Psychomotor epilepsy is a form of partial seizure in which consciousness is altered but not necessarily lost. Thus, there is no complete loss of control of thought and action, but rather a period of altered behavior and altered consciousness for which the person may be amnesic.

The full-blown psychomotor seizure consists of a number of phases. The seizure initially announces itself to the individual in an *aura*, a sometimes complex, psychic experience that may manifest itself in one or more of a wide variety of vivid forms: as an illusion, hallucination, dyscognitive state, or as an emotional (affective) experience.

Most common are *illusions*, or distortions of ongoing experience (perception), that have an immediate environmental event that causes them. Thus, in the visual sphere, objects or persons in the environment may seem smaller and more distant or nearer and larger. Similar distortions may occur with auditory sensations. Pain, coldness, warmth, burning, pressure, or tingling in a body part may be experienced. Patterns of illusions that distort time are referred to as dyscognitive states. These illusions usually assume one of two forms. Either there is a disturbing feeling of excessive familiarity with ongoing events as though all of this had been experienced at another time (*déjà vu*) or, conversely, a feeling of strangeness, discomfort, or unreality (*jamais vu*). Déjà vu has been correlated with activity of the entorhinal cortex of the medial temporal lobe.

Purely emotional experiences may also occur with illusions. Experiencing some kind of fear is perhaps the most common aural symptom. The person may feel anxious (the unpleasant feeling that accompanies anticipation of the future) or profoundly lonely. In contrast, happiness or sexual excitement may also be experienced

Hallucinations are perceptions that occur without a proximate stimulus to cause them. Typically, these are visual or auditory and are composed of formed (or unformed) images, sounds, or voices. Or they may be vestibular in nature such that the person feels like he or she is falling, dizzy, or floating. Less often, the hallucination is olfactory or gustatory in nature, and, when these occur, the odor or taste is usually disagreeable (e.g., like "burning rubber" or "spoiled tuna in a dirty outhouse"). People may experience visceral feelings in the "pit of the stomach" when experiencing a hallucination (e.g., nausea) that are commonly associated with intense feelings of fear.

What these aural experiences reveal is that components of the limbic system are multisensory—that is, olfactory, gustatory, gastrointestinal, visual, auditory, vestibular, and somatosensory input all reach the limbic system immediately (illusions), or information from them is stored in the system (hallucinations). In addition, such symptoms show that components of the limbic system are capable of attaching emotional significance to sensory stimuli and internally generated perceptions (thought).

Such psychic experiences may comprise the entire psychomotor seizure. When they do not, the seizure progresses into its second phase, a period of altered consciousness such as unresponsiveness, or dreamy state, during which the motor components of the seizure occur.

During psychomotor seizures, the individual may also have motoric behaviors. For example, in what are called *spontaneous automatisms*, there may be smacking of the lips, chewing, sucking, or swallowing movements that seem to echo the hunger or thirst experienced during the aura. Such automatisms may include also aimless fumbling with articles of clothing or walking about in a daze. Yet, the individual is out of contact with reality; if given a command or asked a specific question, he or she may not respond at all or may respond incoherently or in a confused manner. Other automatisms are elicited by environmental stimuli and are called *reactive automatisms*.

Perhaps the most remarkable reactive automatism ever recorded (in 1888) was that by the famous neurologist Hughlings Jackson, the founder of neurology as a science. It involved a young doctor (Doctor Z) suffering from psychomotor epilepsy as a consequence of a small lesion in the medial temporal lobe in the region of the uncus. During one of his seizures, the doctor examined a person, made a correct diagnosis, and wrote an appropriate prescription, but had no recollection of it after the seizure terminated. An *uncinate seizure* includes the following: déjà vu, olfactory hallucination, and a sense of fear. This anterograde amnesia indicates that components of the limbic system are involved in the formation of new memories, but are not involved in the storage of old memories, because complex habitual acts that draw on stored memory may be performed faultlessly during the seizure. People may continue to perform acts in progress at the time of the seizure, such as washing dishes. Complex automatisms, however, more generally involve behavior that is inappropriate to the circumstances—for example, undressing in public. This observation suggests that components of the limbic system are also involved in successful (appropriate) social behavior.

Limbic System

The array of structures and pathways identified with the limbic system is inconsistent across authors largely because no single criterion has been established by which to include or exclude given structures from membership in the system. However, certain structures comprise what are considered *core* structures because most authors include them as limbic system constituents: the cingulate and parahippocampal gyri, the hippocampus, the amygdala, the

Neuropathology Box 22-1: Arousal, Attention, and Emotion

In an interesting experiment, novice volunteers were strapped to a bungee cord and allowed to free-fall for 150 feet. While free-falling, they were tested on their ability to read numbers from the screen of a small computer strapped to their wrists. During the high-adrenaline rush of the free-fall, they could read numbers at a significantly higher rate than does a normal person. Thus, because there was higher arousal, they could read more numbers. Additionally, it is important to recognize that the emotional content could have a personal point of view. Whether the free-fall experience was considered exhilarating or dreadful (good or bad) depends on the expectations the jumper brought to the event.

septal nuclei, and the hypothalamus. Additionally, contemporary evidence reveals that the orbitomedial prefrontal association cortex is an integral component of the limbic system; indeed, it appears to be its integrating and orchestrating entity.

The cingulate and parahippocampal gyri occupy the medial hemispheral surface and form a readily visible (but incomplete) ring around the diencephalon and rostral brainstem. These two structures comprise the major anatomical components of the limbic system as noted in Chapter 2. The hippocampus consists of two interrelated gyri (the dentate gyrus and the hippocampus proper) that have been folded into the inferior horn of the lateral ventricle and are housed by the overlying parahippocampal gyrus (see Figure 2-19). The interrelationship of the dentate gyrus and hippocampus proper is such that (in cross section) they form two interlocking Cs (Figure 22-4 ■). The amygdala (a subcortical nucleus on each side) is a collection of more or less distinct nuclei situated beneath the uncus of the parahippocampal gyrus at the anterior end of the hippocampus and inferior horn of the lateral ventricle (see Figure 6-7). Although the term *amygdala* means *almond*, the structure is more the size and shape of a walnut. The septal nuclei are located next to the anterior end of the hypothalamus immediately adjacent to the midline and septum pellucidum. The location of the hypothalamus was presented in Chapter 6 and that of the orbitomedial (basomedial) prefrontal association cortex in Chapter 21.

The anatomical connections among these limbic system structures are complex, and to detail them here is beyond the scope of this book. But we shall mention several general principles in this connectivity pattern. First, these structures are all interrelated to one another with reciprocal connections that are either direct or indirect via synaptic relays in other structures such as the thalamus. Second, the strength of these interrelationships varies across different sets of structures. Both trends befit a system mediating functions that, while being different, are intimately related to one another—namely, emotion and memory.

Connections among Limbic System Structures

We begin our exploration into connections with the limbic system by defining output and input ends of the limbic system. We then specify the direct reciprocal connections between them. Finally, we indicate other connections that must exist in order for the limbic system to accomplish its functions.

> **Thought Question**
>
> What is the medial forebrain bundle? With what structures is it connected? And why is this an important component of the limbic system?

The output end of the limbic system is a functional and anatomical continuum represented by the septum and hypothalamus (Figure 22-5 ■). Through its connections with brainstem autonomic and somatic structures (largely through the **medial forebrain bundle**), the output end mediates the behavioral expression of emotional states. In such mediation, we should not forget the functions of the secretory hypothalamus. The behavioral expression of emotion includes manifestations such as changes in respiration, heart rate, flushing, pallor, sweating, dry mouth, facial expression, postures, gestures, fluidity of motor activity, and so on. Major direct access to this output end derives from three structures: the hippocampal formation (comprised of the hippocampus, the dentate gyrus, and a region of cerebral cortex, the subiculum), the amygdala, and the orbitomedial prefrontal association neocortex (see Figure 22-5). In turn, both the hippocampal formation and amygdala are reciprocally and massively connected to the orbitomedial prefrontal cortex. Thus, two major subsystems derive from the orbitomedial prefrontal cortex: hypothalamic and hippocampal-amygdaloid. This places the orbitomedial prefrontal association cortex in a position to orchestrate the general activities of the limbic system. So what, then, must the input end itself receive to enable it to fulfill its functions?

Memories and emotions are both multimodal phenomena. That is, memories can be elicited by any mode of interoceptive or exteroceptive stimulus, just as any interoceptive or exteroceptive stimulus can be invested with emotional significance. A prerequisite to these functions is that the *input end* of the limbic system must receive highly processed sensory reports of ongoing experience from every sensory modality: olfactory, gustatory, visceral, somatosensory, visual, and auditory. And this they do. The orbitomedial prefrontal cortex receives input from association cortices mediating auditory,

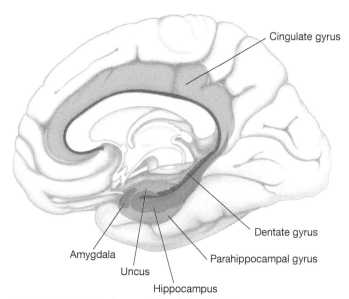

Cingulate gyrus

Dentate gyrus

Parahippocampal gyrus

Amygdala

Uncus

Hippocampus

FIGURE 22-4 The interrelationship of the dentate gyrus and hippocampus proper are such that they form two interlocking Cs.

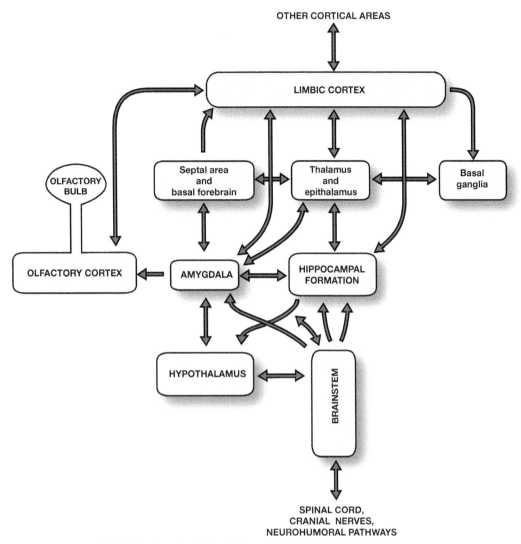

FIGURE 22-5 Overview of the limbic circuitry depicting the input and output projections.

visual, and somatosensory input as well as from the hypo-thalamus mediating interoceptive input. Likewise, neurons of both the amygdala and hippocampus are responsive to interoceptive as well as exteroceptive sensory inputs, again being highly processed by cortical association areas before impinging on neurons of these structures.

AMYGDALA *Specific* involvement of the amygdala in emo-tion was cleverly highlighted in an experiment conducted by J. L. Downer in 1961. Downer selectively removed the amygdala on one side in a monkey who, in addition, had the optic chiasm sectioned, as well as all of the commis-sural fibers linking structures of one cerebral hemisphere with their fellows in the opposite hemisphere. The result-ing animal possessed a single amygdala that had access to visual information *only* from the eye on the same side as the *intact* amygdala (Figure 22-6 ■). With both of its eyes open, this animal exhibited a monkey-typical aggressive response at the sight of a person: it would grimace, bare its teeth, and jump around in its cage. Closing the eye on the side of the amygdalectomy did not result in any observ-able behavioral change. However, opening this eye and

closing the opposite eye (the eye with input to the intact amygdala) resulted in a dramatic change in behavior. The animal showed no signs of aggression or fear at the sight of human observers and would approach the front of the cage and take raisins from the experimenter's hand. Thus, in the absence of the amygdala, the monkey was unable to inter-pret the emotional significance of a visual stimulus (i.e., an approaching human representing a potential threat) in the same way as does an animal with an intact amygdala. This placidity occurred only in response to visual stimulation: if the animal's arm was touched or prodded, a momentary aggressive response would result. Thus, somatosensory in-put still had access to the remaining intact amygdala.

Thought Question

Experiments creating the Kluver-Bucy syndrome in monkeys have been important to our understanding of the role of the limbic system. Has this syndrome been identified in hu-mans? What is known and what is not known in this regard?

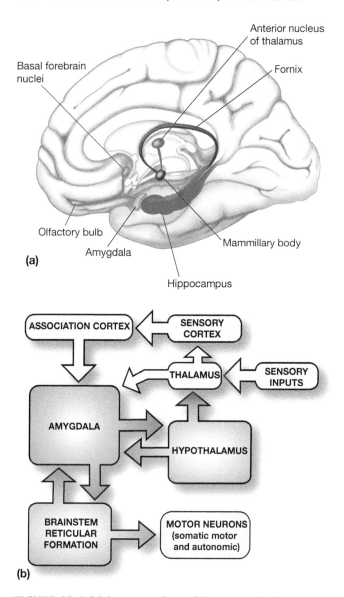

(a)

(b)

FIGURE 22-6 Major connections of the amygdala. (a) Location of the amygdala within the limbic circuitry. (b) Schematic of connections of the amygdala.

That medial temporal lobe structures, including the amygdala, are involved in emotional behavior was first demonstrated in a series of investigations carried out by Kluver and Bucy in the late 1930s. In these studies, large portions of the temporal lobes were removed bilaterally in adult rhesus monkeys, resulting in a constellation of deficits that came to be known as the **Kluver-Bucy syndrome**. Not only did such lesions destroy the amygdala, they also destroyed the hippocampal formation, inferotemporal cortex, anterior parts of the parahippocampal gyrus, and the uncus. Normally aggressive and intractable monkeys because placid, tame, and friendly. They showed an absence of emotional response, displaying neither fear nor anger to normally emotionally arousing stimuli, such as threats or social gestures from other animals. The monkeys were unusually hyperattentive and responsive to the environment; they were constantly active

and compulsively mouthed everything in reach, including such objects as nails, dirt, or a hissing snake. Male animals became markedly hypersexual, exhibiting a monumental increase in sexual activity as well as a diversity of sexual manifestations (e.g., mounting a garbage can). From these observations, it seems clear that the monkeys lost the ability to recognize the meaning of objects visually—for example, they were unable to distinguish edible from inedible objects. In other words, the animals displayed a type of **visual agnosia**. Although scientists have looked for this constellation of behavioral changes of Kluver-Bucy syndrome in people, it has not been described. The primary manifestation of the syndrome in humans is the compulsive oral tendency.

The amygdala receives a vast array of convergent sensory information from all exteroceptive and interoceptive sensory cortices. Thus, converging on neurons of the amygdala are inputs from visual, auditory, and somatosensory systems arising from the neocortex of unimodal association areas as well as from the polymodal association neocortex in the inferotemporal (direct) and dorsolateral (indirect) prefrontal cortices. In addition, limbic association cortices, in receipt of interoceptive input, project strongly to the amygdala. Given the projections of the amygdala to the hypothalamus and brainstem autonomic centers, these connections provide a route whereby exteroceptive and interoceptive stimuli can *activate* emotions and their behavioral expression. But the amygdala does not just activate emotional expression—it *modulates* its intensity. The amygdala can augment or suppress the effectiveness of the hypothalamus on emotional expression. All autonomic responses that can be elicited by stimulation of the hypothalamus also can be elicited by stimulation of the amygdala, but their duration is more natural in character, and the influence can be either facilitatory or inhibitory.

Essential to the understanding of amygdalar function is the presence of reciprocal projections from the amygdala back to unimodal, polymodal, and limbic association cortices. These connections allow the amygdala to modulate sensory input *according to* affective state. That is, the amygdala is in a position to participate in the way the brain attends to its present environment.

An anecdote related by Nauta and Feirtag (1986) effectively illustrates the point. When a hungry child enters a restaurant, he or she sees only what the diners have on their plates. But on leaving, the child observes that the diners also have faces. There is a broader social context to this anecdote. As the hungry child enters the restaurant, sees and smells the wonderful aromas wafting from the food, what prevents him or her from grabbing it off a diner's plate and gobbling it down, or crying in frustration? So yet another pivotal, socially integrative, cerebral element exists in this process of emotionality—namely, an entity that governs emotion according to social propriety and comportment, and this entity is the orbitofrontal cortex.

Selective bilateral damage to the amygdala in humans is rare. However, in people who have sustained such damage as, for example, with experimental lesions of the amygdala to relieve intractable epilepsy, social cognition is compromised. The recognition of facial expressions of, in particular, fear and anger are impaired. Further, such impairment extends to the recognition of emotion as revealed in another person's pattern of vocal expression (prosody, discussed later). The recognition of vocal expressions of fear and anger are the most severely compromised. Both lesion and functional neuroimaging indicate that the amygdala plays a significant role in monitoring the direction of eye gaze essential to determining the emotional state of other people based on their appearance. All of this indicates that the amygdala plays a pivotal role in the perception of the emotional status of others with whom we are interacting in a social environment. Amygdalar damage also occurs in disorders such as Alzheimer's disease, schizophrenia, and the autism spectrum of disorders that are characterized by deficits in emotional expression as they relate to interaction with others.

DORSOLATERAL AND ORBITOMEDIAL CORTICES OF THE PREFRONTAL CORTEX As noted in Chapter 21, the distinction between a dorsolateral and orbitomedial (limbic) part of the prefrontal cortex is based not only in differences in the patterns of cortico-cortical and cortico-subcortical connections, but also in the two classical syndromes resulting from localized prefrontal damage. Several additional features of the connectivity pattern of orbitomedial prefrontal cortex are worth noting because they inform us about function. The projections between the hypothalamus and orbitomedial prefrontal cortex are reciprocal, as noted earlier (see Figure 22-4). What this indicates is that the orbitomedial prefrontal cortex is not only in a position to receive reports from the hypothalamus about the status of the autonomic (visceral and endocrine) periphery, but that it can influence its *own* hypothalamic input. The same operational principle is true for the reciprocal connections between the amygdala and orbitomedial prefrontal cortex, as well as those between the orbitomedial prefrontal cortex and hippocampus. One additional reciprocal relationship of the orbitomedial prefrontal cortex is significant. The nature of cerebrocortical functioning depends on inputs from cholinergic nuclei in the basal forebrain and from monoaminergic input from nuclei in the brainstem. Thus, the orbitomedial prefrontal cortex is able to regulate not only its own levels of cholinergic and monoaminergic neurotransmission, but also the input of other cortical areas as well as subcortical structures such as the hypothalamus receive. What all this means is that the connections of the orbitomedial prefrontal cortex indicate that it represents the *highest control system* not only of autonomic function, but also of mnemonic function as they relate, in particular, to social-emotional behavior.

People with deficits in **executive function** experience problems with real-life situations that require the organization of goal-oriented behavior in open situations where there

are relatively few constraints. In contrast to individuals with dorsolateral prefrontal damage, people with orbitomedial prefrontal damage may perform well on neuropsychological tests conducted in an office setting. However, they may act with a complete lack of judgment and restraint in the relatively unstructured setting of everyday life.

Everyday life is filled with events that may or may not fulfill our expectations and with people whose behavior does or does not fulfill our predictions. Effective adaptive organization of behavior in everyday life depends on numerous factors, one of which is the capacity to shift perspective. This entails the ability to project ourselves into the future so as to predict the potential consequences of contemplated behavior (foresight) as well as the capacity to enter someone else's shoes to understand what other people might believe and feel in response to our actions (insight or empathy). This is the *public forum* of social cognition, where we as individuals are interacting with other behaving entities. It depends (1) on the accurate perception of the emotional states of others and (2) on the capacity to reason about these mental states. In other words, the perceptions must be manipulated in such a way that they permit us to attribute to others an independent mental state helping us to interpret and predict their behavior. The perceptual aspect of this public forum is mediated by the amygdala. The reasoning aspect depends on the reciprocal relationships of the orbitomedial prefrontal cortex with the amygdala and hippocampal formation. Such relationships would enable the orbitomedial prefrontal cortex to bring online public social-emotional and memory processes such that they may participate in developing the cognitions mediating complex socio-emotional, contingency-dependent situations.

But there also is a *private element* in social cognition that is the subjective agreeable–disagreeable (physical) valence of emotion. Social cognition (reasoning) is continuously being updated as it is evolving. Thus, the reciprocal relationship between the orbitomedial prefrontal cortex and hypothalamus may enable the neocortex to send to the hypothalamus neural codes representing cognitions related to prospective social actions. What is sent back from the hypothalamus is a neural signal that enters into the evolving cognition indicating that the prospective action elicits an interoceptive feeling of agreeableness or disagreeableness: in other words, the anticipatory visceral response, the "gut feeling" enters into cognition. In 1971, Nauta proposed that these anticipatory visceral responses serve as "navigational markers" in guiding complex behavioral programs. That such interactions occur is expressed in statements such as "The thought of it makes me sick." Damage to the orbitomedial prefrontal cortex would disconnect decision making from the constraining influence of the anticipatory visceral response. This would short-circuit adaptive long-term planning in favor of an immediate egocentric gratification of selfish desires. Given this, it is little wonder that people who have sustained orbitomedial prefrontal damage lack empathy and engage in thoughtless acts, being unconcerned about the outcome of events involving themselves and others. Interestingly, it appears that not only may there be laterality differences in the hemisphere mediating socio-emotional behavior, but that this laterality may be gender dependent.

Beyond the dilemma of the individual, a societal interest in the orbitomedial prefrontal cortex looms large. Paul MacLean (1990), coiner of the term *limbic system*, asks questions about altruism, dependent on both foresight and insight (empathy): what is it about humans that impels us to build hospitals and conduct medical research concerning people who are not yet sick, or even born, and to build libraries so that those yet unborn may learn about their rich cultural heritage?

HIPPOCAMPAL FORMATION The hippocampal formation includes the following structures: hippocampus proper, the dentate gyrus, and a region of cerebral cortex, the subiculum, interposed between the hippocampus proper and cortex of the parahippocampal gyrus. The hippocampus proper is also referred to *Ammon's horn* (*cornu ammonis*, which derives from Ammon, an Egyptian deity whose symbol was a ram with curved horns) because of the way the hippocampi, from a superior position, curve outward and downward into the temporal lobes (see Figure 2-18). The dentate gyrus is so named because of its toothed appearance, caused in part by a series of arteries that penetrate the dentate gyrus from the adjacent subarachnoid space. As noted in Chapter 2, in transverse section, the hippocampus proper and dentate gyrus assume the form of two interlocking Cs (see Figure 22-4).

The hippocampal formation is part of the medial wall of the temporal lobe and may be considered a submerged gyrus of the cerebral cortex. The position of the hippocampal formation is usually described in relation to the ventricular system, where it makes up the medial wall and floor of the inferior horn of the lateral ventricle. Largest at the temporal extremity of the inferior horn, the hippocampal formation tapers progressively as it arches posteriorly, superiorly, and medially to end at about the level of the splenium of the corpus callosum, a distance of about 5 cm.

The subcortical connections of the hippocampal formation are dominated by reciprocal projections to the output end of the limbic system—namely, the septal area and hypothalamus (see Figure 22-5). The hippocampal formation is also reciprocally connected with a large expanse of the neocortical surface, including association areas of the frontal, parietal, temporal, and occipital lobes. Particularly noteworthy are the reciprocal connections between the hippocampal formation and orbitomedial prefrontal cortex.

Thought Question

The orbitomedial prefrontal cortex is intimately connected to the limbic system. What do you already know about this structure? How is it related to the limbic system, and what are the specific input and output connections related to this structure?

CLINICAL CONNECTIONS

Two individuals who had significant damage to relevant structures—Phinneas Gage and H.M.—contributed to our understanding of functional consequences of neuroanatomic damage as it relates to memory and emotion. Their stories, and the resulting conditions, are illustrative and are described next.

Thought Question

Through an exceptionally unfortunate work-related event, Phinneas Gage sustained an injury related to the executive functions of the cortex. What are executive functions? What aspects of Phinneas Gage's symptoms are related to these functions? And what does this suggest about the location of damage that he sustained?

Phinneas Gage: Emotional Consequences of Damage to the Orbitomedial Prefrontal Cortex

Perhaps the first documented insight into the function of the frontal lobes in emotional experience and behavior was by J. M. Harlow in 1848. Harlow was a physician who attended a patient by the name of Phinneas Gage who had sustained, then survived for more than 12 years, extensive frontal lobe damage. Indeed, it has been claimed that contemporary research on frontal lobe function began at 4:30 p.m. on September 13, 1848. On that late summer day in Cavendish, Vermont, a work crew was blasting rock to clear the way for extending track on the Rutland & Burlington Railroad. Gage, the foreman of the crew, was responsible for filling holes drilled in the rock with blasting powder, a fuse, and sand. The force of the explosion was increased significantly by tightly packing the powder into the hole. The iron was blunt at the end used to tamp the powder but tapered to a point 1/4 inch in diameter at the opposite end. While Gage was tamping the blasting powder, his attention was diverted by his men and the iron struck rock, causing a spark that ignited the powder. The explosion propelled the iron obliquely upward. It passed completely through Gage's head and high into the air, falling to the ground some 30 or so feet behind him, smeared with blood and brain.

Incredibly, Gage remained conscious and was able to describe the accident to his men and then to the physician an hour or so later. He remained lucid for approximately a day following the accident. The tamping iron had penetrated Gage's head below the left cheek, torn through the base of the cranium and the overlying prefrontal cortex of the left frontal lobe, and exited his head though the top of the frontal bone anterior to the coronal suture (Figure 22-7 ■). So massive was the damage that Harlow could pass the index finger of his right hand through the opening in the frontal bone in the direction of the wound in the cheek until, unobstructed by brain tissue, it met his left index finger inserted through the cheek wound.

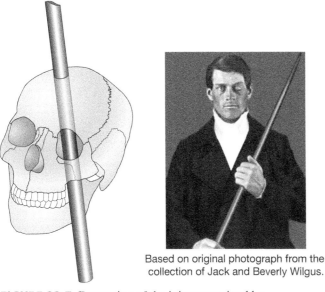

Based on original photograph from the collection of Jack and Beverly Wilgus.

FIGURE 22-7 Recreation of the injury sustained by Phinneus Gage.

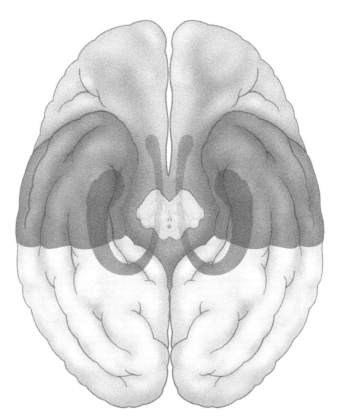

FIGURE 22-8 Depiction of the bilateral removal of H.M.'s medial temporal lobes, including the anterior portions of the hippocampus and the amygdala, resulting in a loss of short-term memory.

Gage subsequently developed a marked brain infection and lapsed into a stupor and delirium that lasted approximately a month. But he then improved rapidly such that by the 56th day following the accident, Gage was walking the streets of the town, again interacting with his friends and others. The most remarkable aspect of this case is its sheer improbability. Indeed, the case was met with great skepticism by the medical community such that, for example, one highly regarded surgeon referred to it as a "Yankee invention."

In the physical sense, Gage had recovered. He no longer had pain in his head. However, mentally, he was substantially changed. Prior to the injury, he had been balanced—a shrewd, smart business man, who was energetic and focused. After the injury, he was no longer able to work as a foreman because his mental status changed so profoundly. He became irreverent, profane, impatient, and obstinate. Indeed, so changed was he that his friends said he was "no longer Gage."

The case of Phineas Gage illustrates the importance of the prefrontal areas as they relate to social cognition. Here, a previously well-adjusted member of society became socially inappropriate following severe damage to the frontal lobe. Important parallels to the changes observed in Gage are discussed in Chapter 25 for individuals who sustain traumatic brain injuries affecting the prefrontal cortex.

H.M.: Excision of the Hippocampal Formation and Implications for Memory

Since the 1950s, it has been traditional to associate the hippocampal formation with memory. This association resulted from the now classical case of H.M. who, in 1953 at the age of 27, had an operation in which an 8-cm length of the medial temporal lobe was excised bilaterally, including the anterior two-thirds of the hippocampus, the amygdala,

and the overlying cortex (Figure 22-8 ■). The operation was performed by the neurosurgeon Dr. William Scoville, with the goal of relieving H.M. of the severe intractable epilepsy he had suffered from since the age of 16. Dr. Scoville noted that this frankly experimental operation was considered justifiable because H.M. was totally incapacitated by the severity and frequency of his seizures, which had proven refractory to a medical approach. H.M.'s ensuing loss of recent memory was unexpected, profound, and permanent. (The literature refers to this person as H.M. After his death in 2008, his name, Henry Molaison, was released.)

H.M. was intensively studied by Scoville and Milner, who described his profound loss of ability to form new memories, even years after the surgery. After the excision, H.M. lived each day as an entirely new experience, remembering nothing of the day-to-day events of his life. For example, he was unable to recognize staff members who worked with him on a daily basis, was unable to find his way to the bathroom, and could not remember what he had for lunch, even a half hour after eating. He never learned the address of the home to which his family moved subsequent to the surgery, nor could he reliably find his way home. At the same time, he appeared relatively normal in other respects. He was able to reason and understand. His personality was essentially unchanged, and remarkably, his early memories were unaffected.

Comprehensive neuropsychological testing of H.M. established the important principle that the ability to acquire new memories is a distinct brain function, separable from perceptual and cognitive capacities and from personality attributes as well. Moreover, the memory deficit was categorically selective for only certain types of memory recall.

H.M.'s IQ was above average and his long-term memory was intact, so he could recollect past events that were formed before the surgery. H.M.'s short-term memory also was quite normal so that as long as he was not distracted, he could communicate ongoing experiences, understandings, and details. Likewise, *procedural memory* was intact. For example, H.M. could learn the new task of drawing by looking at his hand in a mirror, but subsequently he had no memory of ever having practiced the mirror-drawing task. However, the capacity to acquire new information about facts and events and enter them into long-term memory was lost. What H.M. lost was the capacity to *consolidate* memory, and this resulted in *anterograde amnesia*, sometimes called *hippocampal amnesia*. H.M.'s case illustrates the important ideas that the neural substrates for procedural and declarative memory are different and that the substrates involved in consolidation (disrupted in anterograde memory) are different than those used to consciously recall memory (disrupted in retrograde amnesia).

Thought Question

The hippocampus was removed bilaterally from H.M. Why was this surgery performed, what were the consequences, and what was learned about nervous system processing as a result? Would this surgery likely be performed today? Why or why not?

In H.M.'s case, the surgical procedure destroyed the anterior two-thirds of the hippocampus bilaterally, as well as the amygdala and adjacent cortex. As a consequence, the relative contributions of these various structures to memory could not be assessed unequivocally. However, a role for the hippocampus itself was established in cases with selective hippocampal damage in 1986 and again in 1990. Experimentation with monkeys has established that in addition to the hippocampus, the cortex adjacent to the amygdala (but not the amygdala itself), as well as the entorhinal and parahippocampal cortices, are important components of the memory system.

Thought Question

It should be evident that the limbic system includes a number of structures that link to other parts of the nervous system. To more fully appreciate the limbic system, it is important to recall the other connections of the various structures identified with the limbic system. To synthesize this information, make a table of the major structures associated with the limbic system, as well as their input and output connections as identified in other chapters of this text.

LANGUAGE

Clinical Preview

When working in the intensive care unit, acute care rehabilitation, subacute rehabilitation, and home care settings, you are likely to encounter individuals who have a variety of difficulties related to communicating through spoken language, despite the fact that they have the motor ability that is needed for speech. As you read through this section, consider the following:

- What are different ways in which we communicate through language?
- Which cortical areas subserve these functions?
- What are the different types of language deficits that occur with cortical damage?
- What tests can be used to identify these deficits?
- Given the location of the deficits, what motor, somatosensory, or perceptual deficits would potentially co-occur?
- What would be the emotional and social impact of deficits of language?

We now turn our attention to language, a cognitive function of great intricacy that develops naturally as a component of our biological endowment, unique to humans. In this section, we seek to identify the neural substrates for language processing that account for the observed clinical patterns of language breakdown as manifested in the aphasias.

Overview

Language is not a unitary entity. **Propositional (or symbolic) language** is unique to humans in terms of its natural appearance, development, and robustness. While it is true that great apes possess a certain language capacity in that they can be taught rudimentary and fragmentary elements of propositional language, this is not their normal inheritance. By contrast, **emotional language**, wherein communication between members of a species via vocalization and behavioral displays, is present in all animals and undergoes increasing differentiation in the animal kingdom, as documented by Charles Darwin. Such emotional language (expressing responses to immediate environmental circumstances) does not depend exclusively on structures of the cerebral hemisphere as does propositional language.

Although there is a long history of debate in the literature of philosophy and psychology as to whether language and thought should be considered as synonymous functions, there are important distinctions between

Thought Question

Differentiate the following: (1) propositional from emotional language and (2) thought, language, and speech. Why are these different elements of language of importance to the rehabilitation specialist?

them. Language and thought are constant companions in that language plays a central role in the internalization and subsequent expression of symbolic terms for thought. However, to state that language is inextricable from thinking is to narrowly define thought. For one thing, to believe that the preverbal infant lacks thought hardly seems reasonable, just as we cannot offhandedly discard the concept that mental phenomena guide the development of language. For another, it is not clear that destruction of cortical language areas impairs thinking, only that it may compromise the *exchange* of thought between people. Language seems to be for the purpose of communicating thought, but is not essential for thought itself. Additionally, areas of the brain that participate in language function have been localized, whereas complex mental phenomena such as imagination and creativity have not.

Likewise, the relationship between language and consciousness is not easily resolved, in part because definitions of consciousness are so variable. If we define *consciousness* as the state of being aware of our own thoughts and actions, then we do use language to structure the experiences that appear in consciousness. (In this context, it is important to note that consciousness refers to a state of awareness of self beyond the basic level of consciousness conveyed by the reticular activating system of the brainstem.) But this does not mean that all thought depends on language or that all of the behaviors humans generate are consciously mediated. Actions that are performed without our being aware of their origin—that is, without our consciousness being

engaged—can later be given a credible rationale. This occurs when our language system witnesses the behavior. It then attributes cause to the action in terms of our consciously held, language-based attitudes and beliefs, even though the language system itself may be unaware of why the action occurred.

A distinction between language and speech is more readily drawn. Deficits in language function are always a reflection of cerebral injury, the most dramatic deficits being a reflection of damage to the dominant (usually left) cerebral hemisphere. Although a derangement of speech may also result from cerebral injury, this is not the most usual cause. Speech deficits follow damage not only to the cerebellum and brainstem, but also to the PNS as well as to the muscles of speech articulation themselves (see dysarthria discussion). Moreover, the term *speech* refers more to the mechanistic aspects of verbal expression involving articulation. The term *language*, on the other hand, refers to the use of conventionalized verbal symbols ordered sequentially according to accepted rules of grammar and by which ideas and feelings are communicated from one person to another.

Thought Question

Differences among consciousness, language, and speech are of more than passing philosophical interest. Consider a person who is unable to communicate because of a brain tumor or stroke that affected the language centers. Can you assume this person has no thought? How might you begin to establish the degree to which this person understands and the means to communicate with the individual?

With respect to speech, a number of characteristics are of importance to rehabilitation practice. **Prosody** is a term used to describe the melodious aspect of speech, wherein stress (inflection), pitch (tone), timbre, and

Neurophysiology Box 22-2: Critical Periods in the Development of Language

Language development has periods of sensitivity during which it is necessary to develop specific skills related to language. For example, pitch and prosody are acquired by age 3. Grammar structures are developed by age 12. If a child is exposed to a language (second language) after age 3, the child will not be able to become a native speaker. If not exposed to the second language by age 12, the child will not achieve a full vocabulary or contextual grammar. Furthermore, language of non-native speakers of English is less proficient with respect to lexical and syntactic ability if the individual moves to a place where English is the main language after a child is about 7 or 8 years old. Furthermore, there are examples of children raised under conditions of essential total deprivation as relates to language (e.g., until age 13). Such children never develop speech skills. These observations suggest that the language system, like the visual system (see Chapter 18), has critical periods of development.

rhythm are used to convey meaning. The term was introduced by Monrad-Krohn in 1947. It is divisible into different types. *Emotional prosody*, as the term connotes, imparts emotion to speech, including attitudinal elements. Emotional prosody includes such paralinguistic expressions as sighs and grunts, as well as stress and rhythm patterns that convey an opinion about the topic or person being addressed. (How many different expressions of the sentence "He is funny" can be used to convey an attitude about the person?) *Linguistic prosody*, on the other hand, is used syntactically or grammatically (discussed later).

The term **aphasia** is used with respect to abnormalities of speech and/or language due to disease or injury and is defined as a disturbance in the use of language due to cerebral injury, and not due to sensory or motor disturbances or to generalized mental deterioration. The key criterion in this definition is one of linguistic impairment: in aphasic disorders of speech production, the verbal output must be linguistically compromised, whereas the muscles of articulation may be used normally in nonlinguistic activities. Likewise, in aphasic disorders of comprehension, spoken or written language may not be understood, but hearing and vision may be normal when tested nonverbally.

Neural Substrates of Language

Limbic Substrate

Components of the limbic system are involved in the production of language. They seem to represent a starter, or facilitating, mechanism essential to the initiation of speech in that their damage results in varying degrees and duration of mutism. This facilitating system is bilateral, without hemispheric dominance, and extends from the periaqueductal gray of the midbrain through the reticular thalamus to the anterior cingulate gyrus and supplementary motor area of the frontal lobe. The syndrome referred to as **apathetic akinetic mutism** follows damage to the periaqueductal gray matter in the rostral midbrain. Individuals with this syndrome appear awake in that they can track visually, have intact motor and sensory systems, but do not respond to commands. Damage to the anterior cingulate gyrus and adjacent supplementary motor cortex may cause spontaneous speech to be lost entirely (although recovery of spontaneous speech may occur with time). Given involvement of the limbic system in motivation, impairment of this starter mechanism may explain the loss or reduction of spontaneous speech (i.e., mutism) in certain types of aphasia. Additionally, in the neocortical damage that results in nonfluent aphasia, there may be a selective preservation of emotionally charged, vulgar, and profane speech, along with a temporary improvement in speech, when such people are under emotional stress. These phenomena indicate that the limbic substrate remains functional in the presence of neocortical damage.

Neocortical Substrate

PROPOSITIONAL LANGUAGE Unlike the limbic substrate, which is bilateral, the neocortical substrate for propositional language resides predominantly in the association cortex of only one cerebral hemisphere. In the great majority of people, language representation is lateralized to the left hemisphere, which is referred to as the **dominant hemisphere**. This is true regardless of whether a person is right- or left-handed. However, left-handed people are more likely than right-handed people to have language represented in the right hemisphere, or in both hemispheres. Still, only some 15 percent of left-handers have right hemisphere language dominance, while about 15 percent have bilateral language representation.

Because the neocortical language areas border the lateral (Sylvian) fissure, if there is an anatomical basis for the lateralization of language, it should be found in the region of the lateral fissure. Indeed, in some 70 percent of brains, the upper surface of the superior temporal gyrus posterior to the primary auditory cortex—a region called the **planum temporale**—is significantly larger in the left than in the right hemisphere. Because the planum temporale forms the lower bank of the posterior part of the lateral fissure, the lateral fissure extends further posteriorly in the left hemisphere (Figure 22-9 ■). Given that these hemispheric differences are present in utero, language dominance must fundamentally be genetically determined.

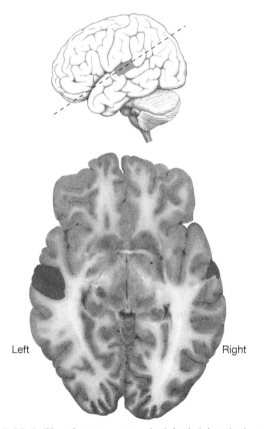

FIGURE 22-9 The planum temporal of the left hemisphere, which houses the primary auditory cortex, extends further posteriorly than it does in the right hemisphere.

Significantly, language development itself seems to be intrinsic to the human brain. The growth and maturation of language are guided by our genetic endowment because all children, regardless of culture, acquire language within a few years without explicit instruction in grammar.

As noted earlier, language areas of the neocortex are clustered around the Sylvian (lateral) fissure and, therefore, these areas are collectively called the **perisylvian language zone** (Figure 22-10 ■). Included in the zone are the classically recognized language areas: an anteriorly located **Broca's area**, encompassing the posterior third of the inferior frontal gyrus and corresponding to Brodmann's areas 44 and 45, and a posteriorly situated **Wernicke's area**, encompassing the posterior part of the superior temporal gyrus

corresponding to the posterior part of Brodmann's area 22. We should note that Broca's area is immediately anterior to the inferior portion of the primary motor cortex subserving upper motor neuron innervation of the lips, tongue, soft palate, pharynx, and larynx and that these two neocortical areas are interconnected by short association fibers.

It now is accepted that neocortical lesions causing aphasia also involve cortex surrounding these classically defined areas, so it is more accurate to speak of an anteriorly positioned **Broca's territory** and a posteriorly located **Wernicke's territory**. Broca's territory includes not only Brodmann's areas 44 and 45, but also the posterior parts of the middle frontal gyrus, the inferior precentral gyrus (Brodmann's area 43, ventral to the

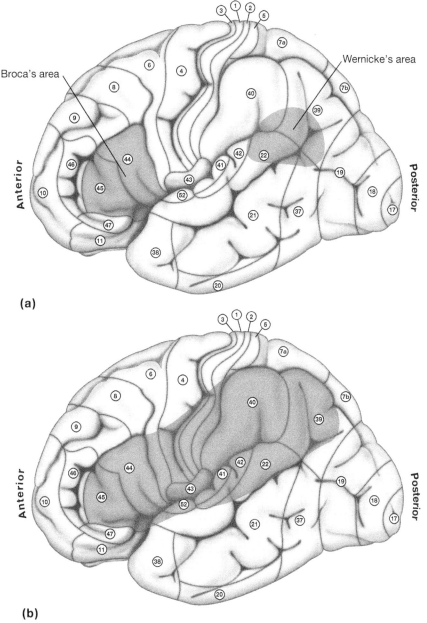

(a)

(b)

FIGURE 22-10 Language areas of the neocortex. (a) Broca's and Wernicke's areas. (b) The perisylvian language zone includes both Broca's and Wernicke's areas.

primary motor area), and the anterior insula. Similarly, Wernicke's territory includes not only the posterior part of the superior temporal gyrus (area 22), but also the posterior part of the middle temporal gyrus, the opercular portions of the inferior parietal lobule (the angular and supramarginal gyri, Brodmann's areas 39 and 40, respectively), and the posterior insular gyri. Neuroimaging has revealed additional areas of the temporal lobe to be involved in language. Interestingly, the perisylvian language zone in females is proportionately larger than in males, and this may account for the sexual dimorphism in verbal ability.

> **Thought Question**
>
> When carrying on a conversation with another individual, where is the auditory information associated with speech received and interpreted? Where are the processes associated with responding verbally processed, and how does information get from the former site to the latter?

These areas are interconnected by a rich network of long association fibers. Most prominent are fibers belonging to the **superior longitudinal fasciculus (arcuate fasciculus)** (see Figure 2-24) that directly interconnect Wernicke's and Broca's territories. They pass around the posterior end of the Sylvian fissure, with some traversing subcortical white matter dorsal to the insula and some traversing the extreme capsule in the subcortical white matter of the insula. Broca's and Wernicke's territories also are interconnected indirectly by projections that have an intervening synapse in the inferior parietal lobule. These indirect projections thus have a posterior segment projecting from Wernicke's territory to the angular and supramarginal gyri and an anterior segment projecting from the inferior parietal lobule to Broca's territory.

EMOTIONAL LANGUAGE While the right (nondominant) hemisphere plays a minimal role in propositional language, it does play a vital role in the expression of emotion in spoken language, as well as the capacity to detect emotion in the speech of others. The right hemisphere system for generating emotional prosody in one's speech and for comprehending emotional prosody in the speech of others is organized in a manner similar to the organization of the system mediating propositional language in the dominant hemisphere. That is, the area in the right hemisphere analogous to Broca's territory is involved in the production of emotional prosody, while the area in the right hemisphere analogous to Wernicke's territory is involved in comprehending emotional prosody. Emotional prosody is obviously a capacity exercised in a social context, so it is worth noting that right hemisphere damage can affect other aspects of social intercourse—for example, the capacity to assess social situations properly and the nonverbal recognition and expression of emotion by facial expression.

CLINICAL CONNECTIONS

Aphasia is one of the frequent impairments of higher mental function resulting from stroke and head injury. Many schemes and test batteries of varying complexity have been developed to classify the different types of aphasia. We should note that formal tests involving score-based diagnosis, including the Western Aphasia Battery, give only the appearance of objectivity for several reasons: (1) score assignments are defined by criteria developed by the author of the test, and, (2) actual scoring is based on a clinician's judgment. Fortunately, as will be discussed later, thoughtful clinical examination usually enables a clinician to accurately determine the type of aphasia being manifest by a patient.

Two broad categories of aphasia are recognized and summarized in Figure 22-11 ■: (1) those resulting from damage to the perisylvian language areas, and referred to here as *primary aphasias*, and (2) those resulting not from lesions of the perisylvian language areas themselves, but from lesions of the surrounding multimodal association cortex. Such lesions result in the perisylvian language areas being isolated (separated) from the adjacent association

Syndromes	Aphasia Type	Fluency	Repetition	Comprehension
Primary Aphasic	Broca's 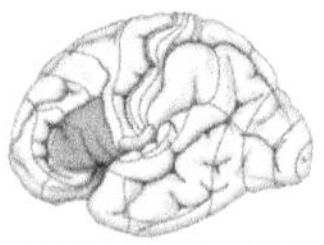	-	-	±
Primary Aphasic	Wernicke's 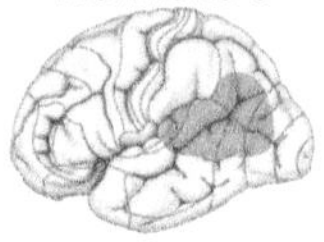	±	-	-
Primary Aphasic	Global 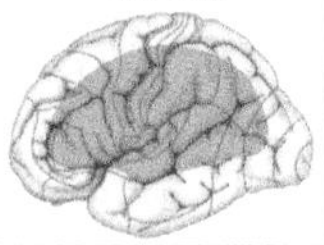	-	-	-
Aphasic Dis-connection	Transcortical motor 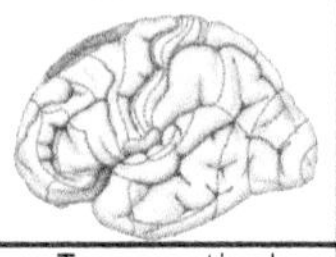	-	±	±
Aphasic Dis-connection	Transcortical sensory 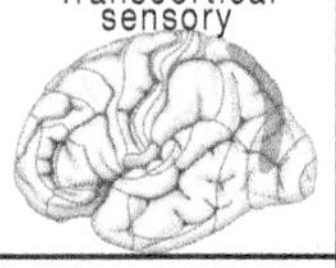	±	±	-
Aphasic Dis-connection	Conduction 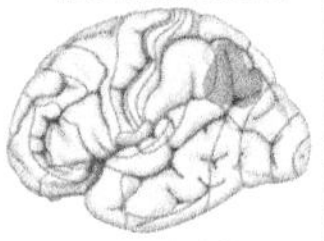	±	-	±

FIGURE 22-11 Language deficits. Location of the lesions and their consequences for fluency, repetition, and comprehension. "+" indicates that the language function is intact; "−" indicates that the language function is impaired; "+/−" indicates that the language function may or may not be impaired.

cortex. The aphasias that are produced by such isolation are referred to here as *aphasic disconnection syndromes*.

Primary Aphasias and Causative Lesions

Broca's Aphasia

Broca's aphasia—also called *motor, expressive, anterior,* or *nonfluent aphasia*—derives its name from the initial observation in 1861 by neurologist Paul Broca that a specific type of aphasia resulted from damage to the posterior part of the inferior frontal gyrus that primarily affected language expression and largely spared language comprehension. This area was subsequently identified by Brodmann as areas 44 and 45—areas that are now collectively known as Broca's area. This localization by Broca was based on postmortem examination of the brain of a single patient called "Tan," so named by other patients in Broca's clinic because he was unable say anything but the nonsense word *tan* and an occasional curse word. Only the surface of Tan's brain was examined, and for some unknown reason, Broca dismissed more extensive surface lesions from consideration; there was no sectioning of Tan's brain. It is now known that the lesion causing the complete syndrome that traditionally characterizes Broca's aphasia is much larger than originally described in this single patient. The causative lesion involves not only the inferior frontal gyrus, but also the subjacent white matter and even the head of the caudate nucleus and putamen, the anterior insula, and frontoparietal operculum, and adjacent cerebrum. Thus, Broca's aphasia does not equate with a lesion in Broca's area.

The impact of Broca's aphasia cannot be underestimated. There is a before and after in the life of a person who has Broca's aphasia, separated sometimes only by an instant in time, an explosive brain bleed, or a blow to the head. It is the "after" that the individual, family members, therapists, and others must deal with. When people with Broca's aphasia have their language function taken from them, they are aware of their inability and struggle to communicate. The language deficit makes it difficult for them to be a part of the social fabric and can thus lead to psychological and social impairments.

Wernicke's Aphasia

Wernicke's aphasia derives its name from the neurologist who originally described the syndrome in 1874, Carl Wernicke. It is also called *sensory, receptive, posterior,* or *fluent aphasia*. Wernicke's aphasia is characterized predominantly by a deficit in language comprehension with relatively fluent, but error-filled, language production. Lesions responsible for Wernicke's aphasia include not only the classically defined Wernicke's area (the posterior part of area 22 on the superior temporal gyrus), but the additional neocortical regions comprising Wernicke's territory specified earlier. Long-lasting Wernicke's aphasias are related to lesions involving both the supramarginal and angular gyri. Thus, similar to the situation with Broca's aphasia, Wernicke's aphasia does not equate with a lesion confined to Wernicke's area. In contrast to the person with Broca's aphasia, people with Wernicke's aphasia are not so acutely aware of their deficit. (They think

that the words they speak make sense.) For these individuals, the psychological difficulty lies in not understanding why those around them cannot communicate with them.

Thought Question

What symptoms (aside from language symptoms) might you anticipate when working with a person who has Wernicke's aphasia? Explain these symptoms in terms of the regions of the nervous system most likely to be affected in conjunction with damage resulting in Wernicke's aphasia.

Global Aphasia

Global aphasia is caused by a lesion that destroys nearly all of the perisylvian language zone. The lesion includes Broca's territory anteriorly and Wernicke's territory posteriorly, as well the neocortex between them. All aspects of language are severely impaired. Language fluency is virtually nonexistent, with the person being able to say, at most, a few words. Likewise, language comprehension is severely impaired, although a few words may be understood. Not only is a person unable to express him- or herself, but he or she is not able to comprehend spoken language. For the clinician, people who are globally aphasic may be the most difficult of all to work with in rehabilitation. Despite the extreme impact of their injuries on speech and language, it is important to note that even people who are globally aphasic learn, over time, to communicate with their loved ones, presumably drawing heavily on emotional language rather than symbolic language.

Thought Question

When working in rehabilitation with a person who is globally aphasic, which aspects of thought, language, and speech are likely to be the best avenues for communication?

Aphasic Disconnection Syndromes and Causative Lesions

Conduction Aphasia

Conduction aphasia represents the classic disconnection syndrome, wherein both Broca's and Wernicke's territories are intact and functional but the connection between them is damaged (i.e., fibers of the superior longitudinal fasciculus have been destroyed). Wernicke himself actually predicted the clinical symptoms that should follow such a lesion. Language comprehension is relatively spared (as in a Broca's aphasia with an intact Wernicke's area) and the person's language production is fluent but filled with errors (as in a Wernicke's aphasia with an intact Broca's area). The cardinal feature of conduction aphasia is a gross deficit in the ability of the person to repeat words, phrases, or sentences spoken by the examiner. For some unknown reason, the deficit in repetition is sometimes greatest for small grammatical words such as *the*, *if*, and *is*.

The gross deficit in repetition was predicted from the following model for language processing. Sounds of incoming speech that reach the auditory cortex must be transferred to Wernicke's territory, where they are processed into meaningful words. In order to repeat the words, word-based signals must be forwarded from Wernicke's territory to Broca's territory over the superior longitudinal fasciculus. Within Broca's territory, the word-based signal is transformed into a code specifying the muscular movements required for speaking the word. This motor program is then forwarded to the primary motor cortex that actually generates contraction of the muscles of the lips, tongue, larynx, and respiration that vocalize the word. When fibers of the superior longitudinal fasciculus are destroyed, information is not forwarded directly from Wernicke's territory to Broca's territory, so the word cannot be repeated.

The syndrome of **conduction aphasia** was originally attributed to damage involving the long association fibers of the superior longitudinal fasciculus that directly link Wernicke's territory with Broca's territory. People with conduction aphasia actually comprise a heterogeneous group ranging from Broca-like to Wernicke-like. And, while the cerebral injury causing conduction aphasia involves the superior longitudinal (arcuate) fasciculus, damage to this structure alone is insufficient to produce the syndrome. In addition, portions of the inferior parietal lobule (the supramarginal gyrus, in particular), the insula, and the indirect connections between Wernicke's and Broca's territories (see Figure 22-11) may also be involved in the different variants of conduction aphasia.

> **Thought Question**
>
> What aspects of language do you anticipate would be functional for a person with conduction aphasia? When working with such a person in a rehabilitation setting, what types of communication do you anticipate would be effective, and which would not? How does this compare with a person who has Broca's aphasia? What about a person who has Wernicke's aphasia?

Transcortical Aphasias

The signs seen in the transcortical aphasias were first described by Lichtheim in 1885, although he did not name these aphasias "transcortical." Transcortical aphasias are either Broca-like or Wernicke-like except that repetition is spared. The most common cause of transcortical aphasia is infarction of the **watershed area**, representing the border zone of multimodal neocortex lying within the peripheral territories of the major cerebral arteries (see Chapter 7). Such infarcts spare Broca's area, Wernicke's area, and the interconnections between them (Figure 22-12 ■).

A person with impaired fluency (reduced spontaneous speech) and intact language comprehension (such as

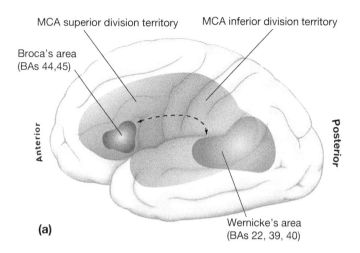

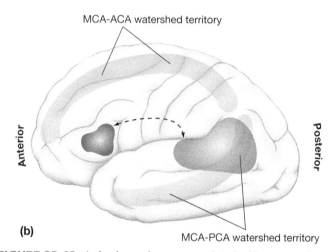

FIGURE 22-12 Aphasia syndromes correlated with vascular lesions. (a) Common infarcts of the middle cerebral artery, resulting in transcortical aphasia. (b) Infarct at the border between the middle cerebral artery and posterior cerebral artery (referred to as the watershed territory) resulting in transcortical aphasia.

in a person with Broca's aphasia) but with intact repetition has a **transcortical motor aphasia**. A frequent cause is a lesion involving the frontal lobe watershed area between the anterior cerebral artery and middle cerebral artery (ACA and MCA, respectively) in the dominant hemisphere. Wernicke's and Broca's territories are both intact, as is the connection between them, thereby enabling repetition of spoken words. But the corticocortical connections essential for Broca's territory to function normally in the formulation of language are destroyed.

A person with intact fluency and impaired language comprehension (such as in a Wernicke's aphasic) but with spared repetition has a **transcortical sensory aphasia**. A common cause is infarction of the watershed area in the posterior parietal and occipital lobes. This involves the peripheral territories of the ACA-MCA in the parietal lobe and the PCA-MCA in the occipital lobe. Such a lesion would destroy corticocortical connections between the parietal and occipital lobe multimodal association cortex required for Wernicke's territory to function normally.

Thought Question

What are the similarities and what are the differences between conduction aphasias and transcortical aphasias?

Clinical Evaluation

By focusing just on the spontaneous speech of people with aphasia, it is possible for a clinician to accurately diagnose the aphasia subtype in the great majority of these individuals. Table 22-1 ■ summarizes the characteristic features of spontaneous speech evaluated in determining aphasia subtype. Significantly, Carl Wernicke himself emphasized in 1874 the importance of evaluating the spontaneous speech of the person with aphasia, noting that the main distinction between people with Broca's and Wernicke's aphasia was to be found in the speech of the patient. Deficits in reading and writing parallel in form and severity those seen in the oral communication of aphasic patients.

In evaluating the spontaneous speech of an individual, one of the most significant discriminating factors is the prosody of speech. Our concern here is with so-called linguistic prosody as opposed to emotional prosody. Linguistic prosody includes such speech-production elements as raising the voice at the end of a statement to indicate a question; placing stress on certain syllables of a word to clarify its grammatical class, for example, *con'-vict* is a noun, whereas *con-vict'* is a verb; or pauses and stresses to define syntactical relations, for example, *The man* [pause] *and woman dressed in black* [pause] *came to visit* tells us that it was only the woman who was dressed in black. Other factors in the production of speech that are important include the rate of speaking, wherein less than 50 words per minute is considered nonfluent and 150 words per minute or more as fluent, and the effort required to speak, wherein the person has difficulty initiating speech, sometimes grimacing, puffing, grunting, or pounding the hand to start speaking. Word choice also is assessed. What types of words does the individual use? Are they substantive words conveying the essence of the communication (e.g., nouns and action verbs), or are they predominantly relational (e.g., adverbs and adjectives) obscuring the essence of the communication?

Is paraphasic speech present? **Paraphasia** is a process of substitution and assumes three forms. *Literal paraphasia* is where one phoneme is substituted for another, for example, instead of "the house is white" the person says "the house is whil." *Verbal paraphasia* is where one word is substituted for another, for example, instead of "the house is white," the person says "the house is whale." *Neologistic paraphasia* is where a nonword (a new or made-up word) is substituted for a real word, for example, instead of "the house is white," the person says "the house is gleft."

Certain language deficits are found in virtually all types of aphasia, suggesting that they follow damage anywhere in the perisylvian language zone. Most important is a *word-retrieval deficit*. A person with a word-retrieval deficit cannot find a word he or she wants to use to express a thought or respond to a question or find the meaning of a word he or she hears or sees. Thus, there is a reduction in available vocabulary that is most evident on the expressive side, but it is seen also in the receptive side. This word-retrieval deficit has been called *anomic aphasia* (also *nominal or amnesic aphasia*) or just *anomia*. The word-retrieval deficit is considered to be the basic deficit in all aphasias.

When the brain damage that gives rise to this word-retrieval deficit is anteriorly placed, involving the region of Broca's territory, then a *primary verbal dyspraxia* occurs in addition to the anomia, resulting in defective word production. This combination of deficits defines the essence of a Broca's aphasia. Verbal dyspraxia affects the initiation of speech movements as well as the selection, organization, and blending of phonemes. The actual initiation of verbal expression depends on the integrity of Broca's territory and its relation to the primary motor area, and when Broca's territory has been damaged, the initiation of speech appears effortful or laborious. Indeed, the person may physically struggle to start speaking. The selection of phonemes may be inexact as is their production, and the organization of phonemes into syllables and syllables into words may be incorrect. The normal harmonious blending of phonemes may be inexact because articulatory transitions are improperly executed. In mild cases, speech may seem sloppy (drunk-like).

The rate of speaking is low such that the Broca's aphasic is nonfluent. But by using a few highly informative substantive words, or even a single word, the person may be able

Table 22-1 Spontaneous Speech in Broca's and Wernicke's Aphasia

SPEECH CHARACTERISTIC	BROCA'S APHASIA	WERNICKE'S APHASIA
Related terms	Motor, expressive, anterior, or nonfluent aphasia	Sensory, receptive, posterior, or fluent aphasia
Rate	Low (<50 wpm)	High (>150 wpm)
Prosody (linguistic)	Abnormal	Normal
Effort (initiation of speech)	Marked	Minimal
Word choice	Substantive (i.e., nouns, action verbs)	Relational (i.e., adjectives, adverbs)
Paraphasia	Present and literal	Frequent, verbal, and neologistic

Table 22-2 Differential Features of the Main Types of Aphasia

CATEGORY OF APHASIA	TYPE OF APHASIA	SPONTANEOUS SPEECH	AUDITORY COMPREHENSION	CAPACITY FOR REPETITION	TYPICAL LESION LOCATION*
Primary Aphasias	Broca's	Nonfluent Effortful Prosody impaired Paraphasia, literal Word-choice, substantive	Largely preserved for single words and grammatically simple sentences	Impaired	Posterior part of the inferior frontal gyrus Subjacent white matter, head of the caudate nucleus and putamen
	Wernicke's	Fluent Well articulated Prosody normal Paraphasia, verbal, and neologistic Word-choice, relational	Impaired	Impaired	Posterior part of the superior temporal gyrus, supramarginal and angular gyri
Aphasic Disconnection Syndromes	Global	Nonfluent	Impaired	Impaired	Superior longitudinal fasciculus, Broca's and Wernicke's areas
	Conduction	Fluent	Intact or largely Preserved	Impaired	Superior longitudinal fasciculus and portions of the inferior parietal lobule
	Transcortical motor	Nonfluent	Intact or largely preserved	Intact or largely preserved	Frontal lobe watershed area
	Transcortical sensory	Fluent	Impaired	Intact or largely preserved	Posterior and occipital lobe watershed area

*Typically involves deep structures as well.

to communicate his entire idea. This is called *telegraphic* or *agrammatic speech*. Paraphasic errors are confined mainly to literal paraphasia. Prosody is defective so that, for example, inflectional endings are omitted and speech is, or tends to be, monotone. Comprehension is largely intact, at least for single words and grammatically straightforward sentences. However, the preservation of comprehension is a dual-edged sword because it means that the person is aware of his or her defective speech. This can lead to great frustration ("I can't talk, I can't talk") and even profound depression. Repetition is impaired and writing shows the same deficiencies as are manifest in spontaneous speech.

When the damage causing anomia is posteriorly situated in the perisylvian language zone, a markedly different syndrome results. The auditory perception of

Thought Question

Given the location of the lesion associated with a Broca's aphasia, what other motor symptoms affecting extremities, torso, and/or speech might co-occur?

language plummets, which is most dramatically reflected in the spontaneous speech of the person. The anomia coupled with this auditory imperception defines the essence of a Wernicke's aphasia. The expressive abnormalities in Wernicke's aphasia are thought to be due to the release of an intact Broca's territory from the normal auditory controlling influence that Wernicke's territory exerts over Broca's territory (possibly as a result of speech disinhibition). Because language production is such a highly overlearned capacity, the idea is that Broca's territory is able to execute its basic functions autonomously.

In the person with Wernicke's aphasia, the rate of speaking is normal or high such that the speech is characterized as being fluent. The execution of speech is intact. Yet, the content of the output is low in terms of its informational load. The Wernicke's aphasic uses many relational (filler) words as opposed to substantive words, known as *empty speech* or *word salad*. Paraphasic errors are abundant; particularly striking may be neologistic paraphasia, wherein the picture of a pen may be stated to be a "tiz," replete with the person providing a correct spelling of *tiz*. Prosody is normal. This normality has been depicted in the following way:

if you knew only what a language sounds like (and didn't know its vocabulary, grammar, and syntax), the speech of a Wernicke's aphasic would sound normal. Comprehension of both spoken and written language is impaired such that, for example, questions asked or instructions given by the examiner will not be understood. The comprehension deficit, however, means that the person is unaware of his or her own jumbled, often bizarre, speech and therefore does not experience the frustration of the person with Broca's aphasia. Repetition is impaired, sometimes to the point where even single words and nonsense syllables cannot be repeated. The person's writing reveals the same types of deficits as are observed in his speech. Table 22-2 ■ summarizes the differential features of the main types of aphasia.

Summary

This chapter began with a discussion of emotion and memory. With respect to emotion, we differentiated physical from social aspects. In the context of memory, we discussed the process of consolidation, wherein events stored in short-term memory are transferred to long-term memory. We next considered the various types of information that are stored in memory and differentiated declarative from procedural functions. Within this chapter, we also considered the relationship between these two important human experiences of emotion and memory and used epilepsy as an excellent example of how these two fundamental properties are interrelated. In particular, by understanding the positive and negative symptoms that occur in people with epilepsy, the neural processes were illustrated for mediating emotion and memory. The structures and

pathways of the limbic system were identified and related to both emotion and memory. Next, we turned to two classic case examples, one of Phinneas Gage and the other of H.M., which illustrate the functional roles of two specific cortices: the orbitomedial prefrontal cortex and the hippocampal formation, respectively.

The second major section focused on language. We examined the difference between emotional and linguistic prosody and identified the neuroanatomical locations that are responsible for generating each of these important elements of communication in language. Then, we described the class of deficits of language known as aphasia, identified the main types of aphasia, and linked each to the underlying neuroanatomical substrates. Finally, we ended this section with examples of the clinical expression and evaluation of various forms of aphasia.

Applications

1. When people have psychomotor seizures, they may experience both positive symptoms and negative symptoms.

   a. Define positive symptoms, and generate a list of positive symptoms as they relate to seizure activity.
   b. Define negative symptoms, and generate a list of negative symptoms as they relate to seizure activity.
   c. Explain how these symptoms are related to the location of the seizure activity.
   d. We met other examples of positive and negative symptoms associated with neurological damage in earlier chapters. Provide examples of both positive and negative signs not associated with seizures.

2. Alphonso Gonzales had a large infarct of the left middle cerebral artery (MCA) that left him with global aphasia.

   a. What is global aphasia?
   b. Thinking broadly about his future ability to communicate, what is his prognosis for various aspects of communication? In other words, what avenues of communication will be available to him, and how might he relearn communication skills, given the losses associated with global aphasia?
   c. Knowing the location and size of his stroke, what deficits, other than language impairments, do you predict he may have?

References

Emotion and Memory

Aggleton, J. P. The contribution of the amygdala to normal and abnormal emotional states. *Trend in Neurosci* 16:328–333, 1993.

Aron, A., et al. Reward, motivation, and emotion systems associated with early-stage intense romantic love. *J Neurophysiol* 94:327–337, 2005.

Bartolomei, F., et al. Cortical stimulation study of the role of rhinal cortex in déjà vu and reminiscence of memories. *Neurology* 63:858–864, 2004.

Brain Work. The Neuroscience Newsletter 16(1):11, 2006.

Coricelli, C., et al. Regret and its avoidance: A neuroimaging study of choice behavior. *Nature Neurosci* 8:1255–1262, 2005.

Devinsky, O., Morrell, M. J., and Vogt, B. A. Contributions of anterior cingulate cortex to behavior. *Brain* 118:279–306, 1995.

Dostoevsky, F. *The Idiot.*

Downer, J. L. deC. Changes in visual gnostic functions and emotional behavior following unilateral temporal pole damage in the "split-brain" monkey. *Nature* 191:50–51, 1961.

Harlow, J. M. Recovery after severe injury to the head. *Mass Med Soc Publ* 2:329–347, 1868.

Knowlton, B. J., Mangels, J. A., and Squire, L. R. A neostriatal habit learning system in humans. *Science* 273:1399–1401, 1996.

MacLean, P. D. *The Triune Brain in Evolution.* Plenum Press, New York, 1990.

Mesulam, M.-M. The human frontal lobes: Transcending the default mode through contingent encoding. In: Stuss, D. T., and Knight, R.T., eds. *Principles of Frontal Lobe Function.* Oxford University Press, New York, 2002.

Nauta, W. J. H. The problem of the frontal lobe: A reinterpretation. *J. Psychiatry Res* 8:167–187, 1971.

Nauta, W. J. H., and Feirtag, M. Ch. 9 Affect and motivation: The limbic system. In: *Fundamental Neuroanatomy.* W. H. Freeman, New York, 1986.

Nicotra, A., et al. Emotional and autonomic consequences of spinal cord injury explored using functional brain imaging. *Brain* 129:718–728, 2006.

Nolte, J. *The Human Brain: An Introduction to Its Functional Anatomy.* Mosby Elsevier, Philadelphia, 2009.

Penfield, W., and Rasmussen, T. *The Cerebral Cortex of Man.* Macmillan, New York, 1950.

Purves, D., Augustine, G. J., Fitzpatrick, D., et al., eds. *Neuroscience*, 2nd ed. Sinauer Associates, Sunderland, MA, 2001.

Raine, A., et al. Reduced prefrontal gray matter volume and reduced autonomic activity in antisocial personality disorder. *Arch Gen Psychiat* 57:119–127, 2000.

Rempel-Clower, N. L., Zola, S. M., Squire, L. R., and Amaral, D. G. Three cases of enduring memory impairment after bilateral damage limited to the hippocampal formation. *J Neurosci* 16:5233–5255, 1996.

Schacter, D. L., Addis, D. R., and Buckner, R. L. Remembering the past to imagine the future: The prospective brain. *Nature Rev Neurosci* 8 (9):657–661, 2007.

Scott, S. K., et al. Impaired auditory recognition of fear and anger following bilateral amygdala lesions. *Nature* 385:254–257, 1997.

Scoville, W. B., and Milner, B. Loss of recent memory after bilateral hippocampal lesions. *J Neurol Neurosurg Psychiat* 20:11–21, 1957.

Shaw, P., et al. The impact of early and late damage to the human amygdala on "theory of mind" reasoning. *Brain* 127:1535–1548, 2004.

Squire, L. R., Stark, C. E. L., and Clark, R. E. The medial temporal lobe. *Ann Rev Neurosci* 27:279–306, 2004.

Squire, L. R. and Zola-Morgan, S. The medial temporal lobe memory system. *Science* 253: 1380–1385, 1991.

Tranel, D., et al. Does gender play a role in functional asymmetry of ventromedial prefrontal cortex? *Brain* 128:2872–2881, 2005.

Language

Benowitz, L. I., Finkelstein, S., Levine, D. N., and Moya, K. Ch. 19. The role of the right cerebral hemisphere in evaluating configurations. In: Trevarthen, C., ed. *Brain Circuits and Functions of the Mind: Essays in Honor of Roger W. Sperry.* Cambridge University Press, Cambridge, UK, 1990.

Benson, D. F. Fluency in aphasia: Correlation with radioactive scan localization. *Cortex* 3:373–394, 1967.

Blonder, L. X, Bowers, D., and Heilman, K. M. The role of the right hemisphere in emotional communication. *Brain* 114:1115–1127, 1991.

Canter, G., Trost, J., and Burns, M. Contrasting patterns of speech in apraxia of speech and phonemic paraphasia. *Brain Lang*, 24:204–222, 1985.

Catani, M., Jones, D. K., and Ffytche, D. H. Perisylvian language networks of the human brain. *Ann Neurol* 57:8–16, 2005.

Chomsky. N. *On Nature and Language*. Cambridge University Press, Cambridge, UK, 2002.

Compston, A. On aphasia. By L. Lichtheim, MD, Professor of medicine in the University of Berne. *Brain*, 129:1347–1350, 2006.

Dorsaint-Pierre, R, Penhune, V. B., Watkins, K. E., et al. Asymmetries of the planum temporale and Heschl's gyrus: Relationship to language lateralization. *Brain* 129:1164–1176, 2006.

Freedman, M., Alexander, M. P., and Naeser, M. A. Anatomic basis of transcortical motor aphasia. *Neurology* 34:409–417, 1984.

Harasty, J., Double, K. L., Halliday, G. M., et al. Language-associated cortical regions are proportionately larger in the female brain. *Arch Neurol* 54:171–176, 1997.

Hillis, A. E., Work, M., Barker, P. B., et al. Re-examining the brain regions crucial for orchestrating speech articulation. *Brain* 127:1479–1487, 2004.

Josse, G., and Tzourio-Mazoyer, N. Hemispheric specialization for language. *Brain Res Rev* 44:1–12, 2004.

Kertsz, A., and McCabe, P. Recovery patterns and prognosis in aphasia. *Brain* 100:1–18, 1977.

Monrad-Krohn, G. H. Dysprosody or altered melody of language. *Brain* 70:405–415, 1947.

Paus, T., Zijdenbos, A., Worsley, K., et al. Structural maturation of neural pathways in children and adolescents: In vivo study. *Science* 283:1908–1911, 1999.

Price, C. J. The anatomy of language: Contributions from functional imaging. *J Anat* 197:335–359, 2000.

Robinson, B. W. Limbic influences on human speech. *Ann NY Acad Sci*, 280:761–771, 1976.

Ross, E. D. The aprosodias. In: Feinberg, T. E., and Farah, M. J., eds. *Behavioral Neurology and Neuropsychology*. McGraw-Hill, New York, 1997.

Sommer, I. E. C., Aleman, A., Bouma, A., and Kahn, R. S. Do women really have more bilateral la. *Brain* 127:1845–1852, 2004.

Segarra, J. M. Cerebral vascular disease and behavior. *Arch Neurol* 22:408–418, 1970.

Urban, P. P., Rolke, R., Wicht, S. et al. Left-hemispheric dominance for articulation: A prospective study in acute ischaemic dysarthria at different localizations. *Brain* 129:767–777, 2006.

Normal and Abnormal Aging of the Central Nervous System

Introduction

An appreciation of the nervous system changes that occur with normal aging is of critical importance to the rehabilitation specialist, in that many of the people who seek rehabilitation are young-old (ages 65 to 74) or even among the old-old (ages 75 to 84). Many such individuals seek assistance with medical or orthopedic conditions that do not directly affect the nervous system. Yet, age-related changes to the nervous system can potentially influence treatment choices. In addressing normal and abnormal aging, it is important to distinguish between life span and life expectancy. *Life span* is the average age at which an individual would die were he or she able to avoid disease and accidents. This age is set by some unknown genetically programmed biological clock, although it is not certain precisely when this death clock is set to run down. *Life expectancy*, on the other hand, is a statistical figure. It is the number of years a person may expect to live in the face of disease, injury, and accidents. Medical science has dramatically lengthened life expectancy, but not life span. Almost invariably, though, life expectancy falls short of life span due to the progressively increasing susceptibility to disabling fatal diseases as we grow older. Indeed, some believe the changes that occur in old age represent the cumulative effects of injury and disease. Two other terms are of importance in this regard: *senescence* refers to the state of being old or the process of growing old; *senile* relates to exhibiting characteristics of aging, especially in relation to cognitive loss (memory).

Medical advances as well as increased attention to factors promoting personal health have extended life expectancy in the United States from 47 years at the beginning of 1900 to its present 71 years for men and 78 years for women. In 1950, people 65 and over comprised only 7.7 percent of the population. Today, the number stands at 12 percent, and by 2020 it will have reached 17.3 percent. Fastest growing of all is the group of people 85 and older. The first major section of this chapter addresses changes that occur with aging. Included are changes to the cell volume, as well as changes to cellular structures (e.g., dendrites, membranes) and to blood flow. Clinical correlations then are discussed as they relate to posture, balance, and gait.

As the longevity of the population has increased, so too has the incidence of age-related brain pathology. Alzheimer's disease (AD), for example, has emerged as a major health risk among those over 65 years of age. Because of the devastating emotional burden on the family members of those with AD, and the staggering financial burden on society of caring for these individuals, the need to understand the process of brain aging is a matter of utmost importance. Thus, the second major section of this chapter addresses nervous system changes associated with AD, contrasting these changes with those associated with normal aging. This section ends with a discussion of clinical ramifications of AD.

NORMAL AGING

Clinical Preview

You are working in a clinic that specializes in treatment of people with deficits of postural control. Among those you work with are Mr. Garfield, who has macular degeneration; Mrs. Zheng, who has diabetes; and Mrs. Greenfield, who has general cognitive changes, although she does not have frank Alzheimer's disease.

Recall that in Chapters 9, 17, and 18, you learned about the proprioceptive, vestibular, and visual systems and how these systems work together in postural control and stability. In Chapter 20, you also learned that the motor system plays a critical role in postural stability because it is the effector system through which these responses are generated.

As you read through this section of the text, it is timely to integrate previously learned information with information about aging. Consider the following:

- How does aging affect these various systems?
- How do changes in these various systems affect postural control and stability?

across individuals. This is reflected, for example, in the fact that standardized tests such as the Wechsler Adult Intelligence Scale are age adjusted to compensate for this anticipated decline. Thus, at age 75, it is possible to obtain an IQ of 100 while answering only half as many items correctly as at age 21. That this decline is the behavioral manifestation of an aging brain seems beyond dispute. During the past several decades, a large volume of literature has accumulated on the gross and cellular morphologic changes that occur in the aging CNS, as well as the changes that occur in cellular function, system physiology, and behavior. Given the organizational complexity, as well as the number of neurons and their mechanisms of communication, it seems reasonable to assume that cellular aging in the brain would possess unique features that distinguish it from the general process of cellular aging involving the entire organism.

Thought Question

Compare performance on the Wechsler Adult Intelligence Scale for 21-year-olds with that of 75-year-olds, and explain why the difference occurs. Also explain why this scale provides a reasonable solution to characterizing intelligence of people of different ages.

Cognitive decline is considered a universal feature in people living to old age, even though the age of onset varies

It has been pointed out that the relationship between mental deterioration and brain pathology rests on correlations that, though statistically significant, are far from perfect. Not infrequently, studies will cite cases from individuals who manifested severe mental impairment during life but did not display the anticipated brain pathology on postmortem examination, or, conversely, individuals possessing ostensibly normal premorbid mental function that exhibited marked morphologic changes. While potential reasons for this lack of correspondence are numerous, as will become evident later, it is abundantly clear that wide individual variation characterizes not just the structural changes associated with aging, but other age-related brain alterations as well.

It seems a commonplace observation that those who age successfully are individuals who have maintained active mental and physical lives. True enough that the brain is not a muscle, but when it comes to the effects of inactivity, the brain may turn out to be very much like a muscle. If so, then it is entirely possible that some, perhaps even much, of what we interpret today as behavioral expressions of an aging brain turn out instead to be expressions of disuse atrophy.

Thought Question

Here is a philosophical question to ponder. Although it is generally agreed that people living to old age have *cognitive decline*, how does one weigh the impact of experience, judgment, and wisdom against the impact of slowed working memory when determining whether or not cognitive decline has occurred? Is cognition declining or changing?

Brain Changes

Normal aging of the brain involves gradual, progressive changes in the morphology, the physiology, and the biochemistry of the CNS. A variety of hypotheses have been advanced to explain this complex process. Among these are genetically programmed cell death, hormonal imbalance, the cross-linking of macromolecules, enzyme deterioration, autoimmune reaction, oxidative damage to cellular constituents, and somatic mutation.

Furthermore, when interpreting the literature on brain aging, it is important to keep in mind a number of factors. First, it is unlikely that a specific, singular pattern of brain aging will emerge owing to the diverse influences heredity, diet, lifestyle, and other environmental factors exert on the nervous system. Second, it is important to understand that brain aging is a nonuniform, regionally variable phenomenon. Within the cerebrum, for example, a given cortical area may experience a marked neuronal loss, while an immediately adjacent area remains normal. Third, just as in development, the temporal profile of age-related structural and functional changes varies in different parts of the brain. Some neuronal populations begin to change as early as the first decade of life, while others do so only in the seventh decade.

Cerebrocortical Changes

NEOCORTEX: FALLOUT VERSUS SHRINKAGE The brain undergoes a number of morphologic changes as a function of age. It is well known, for example, that whole brain weight decreases by about 18 percent (with the predominant decline occurring after 55) and that the width of the cortical mantle narrows by some 10 to 15 percent. It was commonly believed that the hallmark of the aging neocortex is a profound loss of neurons. Neocortical neuronal depopulation has been claimed to amount to 0.8 percent per year and to begin in early maturity. This would mean that over a 60-year span of adulthood, 50 percent of cortical neurons would be lost. However, it now appears that a number of methodological flaws in some of the early studies gave rise to this pessimistic view, most important of which was the small numbers of brains analyzed. Wide individual variations are now known to characterize cortical cell populations in people of similar age. Consequently, large numbers of brains must be studied if true, age-related changes are to be distinguished from normal variability.

Thought Question

What might be the implication of changes in brain size based on cell shrinkage versus fallout?

Recent data derived from suitably sized samples (more than 50) indicate that the major age-related neocortical modification is not cellular fallout (loss of cell) but rather a shrinkage of large-sized neurons. Frontal, temporal, and parietal lobes of people over 70 years of age all show diminished numbers of large neurons, with the parietal lobe being the least affected. In both the frontal and temporal lobes, this loss is counterbalanced by increased numbers of small neurons such that no age-related decrease in neuron density occurs. The implication here is that shrinkage causes some large neurons to shift into the small-neuron class. Although some cellular loss does occur, the loss amounts to only 10 to 15 percent. This is hardly the profound, high-rate loss suggested by earlier reports. It is important to note that, at least in this regard, the process of normal aging distinguishes itself from Alzheimer's disease in which extensive neocortical neuron depletion does occur. This indicates that Alzheimer's disease is not simply an accelerated process of normal aging.

DENDRITIC MODIFICATIONS A second age-related neocortical modification involves degenerative changes in both the basilar and apical dendrites of pyramidal neurons (see Chapter 7). The sequence of these degenerative changes

---

Thought Question

Review the role of horizontally oriented dendrites that was presented in Chapter 7. How does this role relate to the functional implications of loss of these dendrites?

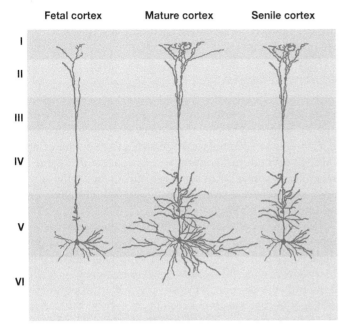

Fetal cortex   Mature cortex   Senile cortex

I
II
III
IV
V
VI

FIGURE 23-1 Neurons in the mature cerebral cortex, as compared with the fetal cerebral cortex, have an extensive system of dendritic branching and bundling, most pronounced in the basilar shafts of pyramidal neurons. In the senile cerebral cortex, the dendrites again begin to decrease in mass.

occurs in reverse order to their perinatal development. A major difference between the fetal and mature cortex is the appearance in the latter of an extensive system of dendritic branching and bundling most pronounced in the basilar shafts of pyramidal neurons in layers 3 and 5 (Figure 23-1 ▪). This strongly interlacing system is oriented horizontally, that is, approximately parallel to the brain surface. Senile neocortex reverses this developmental sequence in that there is a marked loss of this horizontal dendritic mass compared with that seen in a mature cortex.

The most frequently cited functional correlate of these dendritic systems is that they provide a massive postsynaptic receptive surface for the enormously dense presynaptic input characteristic of mature neocortex. But further significance has been attached to these interlacing dendritic bundles—namely, that they store or code central programs for cortical output. In this context, it is important that horizontally oriented dendrites establish preferential synaptic relationships with intracortically originating fibers.

Thought Question

What explanation might account for the dendritic proliferation that occurs during early aging in certain cortical areas that is followed by dendritic regression in the "oldest old"? In what brain regions or areas is this observed?

Several functional consequences have been hypothesized for the loss of these horizontally running plexuses in senescence. First, this loss would disrupt intracortical

processing—and thus cortical efficiency—thought to be responsible for the more subtle, modulatory aspects of cortically generated behaviors. A second hypothesized consequence would be a progressive reduction in the size of the reservoir containing the central programs for cortical output, thereby reducing the flexibility and eventually the repertoire of cortically mediated functions. This may manifest itself in the declining motor strength, the reduced motor dexterity and agility, and the declining cognitive capacities observed in senility.

It is commonly assumed that the cardinal changes in the brains of elderly people are degenerative in nature (i.e., loss of cells in given structures and concomitant reduced concentrations of particular neurotransmitters). This is not entirely the case, however. Certain of the structural manifestations of aging are, in fact, proliferative in character, but this seems to be true only over a restricted (and as yet undefined) time period. In neurons of the parahippocampal gyrus the process of normal aging (from 51 to 79 years of age) is associated with a proliferation of dendrites. Such proliferation is thought to be a compensatory response elicited in surviving cells by the loss of neighboring neurons. An increase in the receptive surface of still-viable neurons would accommodate the additional synaptic input formerly residing on the dendritic surface of defunct cells. The brains of deceased people with Alzheimer's disease do not show the age-related increase in dendritic extent in neurons of the parahippocampal gyrus. It is uncertain whether dendritic regression is an actual feature of the disease or simply represents a failure of the compensatory proliferation response to occur.

Dendritic proliferation does not occur in all parts of the normally aging brain. It is not observed in neurons of the neocortex. Furthermore, in very old age (between 73 and 90 years), dendritic proliferation may be followed by regression, as, for example, occurs in neurons of the dentate gyrus.

Neurotransmitter Changes

Normal aging involves decreases in the concentrations of a number of transmitters. Such declines affect particular, identifiable systems earlier than others so that some detectable order should be manifest in the behavioral changes associated with the aging process. Alterations in brain transmitter levels may be caused by a disturbance at any step in the transmitter's metabolism. Thus, changes in the enzymes required for synthesis or degradation, disruption of storage, transport, release, or re-uptake mechanisms or factors that alter transmitter–receptor binding may be singly or multiply causal.

Thought Question

Relate decreases in the following neurotransmitters to their known roles, and hypothesize regarding the possible functional consequences: dopamine, norepinephrine, serotonin, and acetylcholine. Note that you may need to review information presented in Chapter 4.

Changes in the amount of a neurotransmitter normally elicit an adaptive regulatory response in the number of postsynaptic receptors such that a deficiency of transmitter availability at the synapse causes postsynaptic receptors to proliferate. During aging, neurons gradually may lose their capacity to respond to transmitter reductions in this manner. This would compromise the ability of the brain to maintain its homeostatic balance, especially under stress. Such loss of neuronal plasticity has been proposed as one of the causal mechanisms of brain aging.

Three monoamines (dopamine, norepinephrine, and serotonin) undergo age-related concentration declines, although at different ages, in conjunction with the documented cellular losses occurring in each system. Thus, for example, the 50 percent reduction in cell number seen in the substantia nigra between 20 and 60 years of age manifests itself in significantly reduced dopamine concentrations in neurologically normal-aged individuals. The intracellular enzymes responsible for catecholamine synthesis exhibit parallel declines: tyrosine hydroxylase and L-dopa decarboxylase decrease most rapidly during the first three decades of life and thereafter exhibit a steady but less precipitous decline. Between the ages of 10 and 60 years, tyrosine hydroxylase activity in the striatum of neurologically normal individuals drops by 70 percent.

The other two monoamines, norepinephrine and serotonin, also undergo significant concentration reductions during aging. The drop in these two biogenic amines may underlie the increased incidence of depression in elderly individuals, one of the most serious psychiatric problems associated with aging. Although heterogeneous in symptomatology and etiology, depression is often divided into *endogenous* (internally elicited) and *reactive* (externally evoked) forms. Most depression in elderly individuals is of the endogenous variety, whereas that in the young more typically is reactive. While it currently seems unlikely that endogenous depression is due solely to a simple deficiency of norepinephrine, serotonin, or both, as originally postulated by the "biogenic amine hypothesis," it is clear that noradrenergic and serotonergic neurons are implicated in the pathogenesis of depression, as well as in the response to therapeutic agents.

Just as surviving, intact neurons mount a structural response to the loss of neighboring cells, so also do they respond biochemically. In neurologically normal-aged individuals (74 years), the metabolites of the monoaminergic transmitters are not reduced, and in fact, the ratio between the metabolites and the amine increases. This suggests an increased speed of transmitter turnover in surviving neurons and has been interpreted as a plastic (adaptive) response to the cellular loss. Interestingly, dopamine and serotonin concentrations are reduced in the brains of people with Alzheimer's disease, but a concomitant reduction is also seen in their metabolites, indicating that surviving neurons are neurochemically deficient. Changes in neurotransmitter systems in senescence and Alzheimer's disease are not confined to biogenic amines but embrace a number of neuropeptides as well. At present, the peptidergic alterations cannot be interpreted in functional terms, so they will not be discussed.

Neuronal Changes

LIPOFUSCIN Lipofuscin (age pigment) is a membrane-bound organelle containing waste products the cell is unable to degrade or eject. The fate of postmitotic neurons, therefore, is to accumulate lipofuscin as a function of age. This age-related intraneuronal accumulation of lipofuscin is a reliable biomarker of brain age and, in fact, is the single most consistent age-related morphological alteration thus far detected in brain.

Lipofuscin consists primarily of the by-products of intracellular membrane destruction such as occurs with lysosomal degradation of mitochondria. Although inert, it is not clear that this age pigment is entirely benign. Congestion of the cell with pigment may interfere with the degradative efficiency of the lysosomal system, thereby slowing down organelle membrane turnover and/or endocytotic and exocytotic mechanisms. Thus, while lipofuscin itself may not be causal to brain aging, it may be a by-product of cellular reactions that do play a role in this phenomenon.

There are two important observations about the accumulation of lipofuscin: (1) it displays a predilection for certain sets of neurons, and (2) the rate of accumulation with age varies across these sets. The accumulation is most marked in neurons belonging to the motor system: the inferior olivary nucleus, the dentate nucleus, the globus pallidus, and lower motor neurons of the spinal cord and brainstem. Neurons of the inferior olivary complex and dentate nucleus accumulate lipofuscin within the first decade of life such that by the sixth decade, lipofuscin fills most of the soma. Neurons of the globus pallidus do not contain significant amounts of pigment until the seventh or eighth decade of life. Neurons of the cerebral cortex also accumulate increasing amounts of lipofuscin with advancing age.

LIPIDS AND MEMBRANE FLUIDITY Both the content and composition of whole brain lipid change continuously throughout life. Total lipid content in the brain increases most rapidly up to about 2 years of age but continues a less steep rise up to a peak at 30 to 40 years of age. The period of most rapid increase reflects the marked structural differentiation of the nervous system occurring during this time span as, for example, myelinization of the large corticospinal tract. This neural system contributes importantly to the control of voluntary movement and completes its myelinization during the second year of life. From a peak at 30 to 40 years, total whole brain lipid declines at a steady rate after the age of 50 years. The lipid classes, including cholesterol, showing the greatest losses between 40 and 70 years of age are those enriched in myelin. The finding is consistent with the significant reduction in myelin content seen in the aged brain.

Chemical synaptic transmission depends on a host of membrane-mediated events as outlined in Chapter 4. Thus, the biochemical and biophysical properties of the participating membranes are of crucial importance to proper synaptic transmission. A number of these properties change with aging.

The function of the integral and other membrane-associated proteins depends on the fluidity of their lipid microenvironment. Changes in lipid fluidity affect the lateral mobility of the proteins and, hence, their capacity to interact within the lipid bilayer and with peripheral proteins (see Figures 3-1 and 4-28). Shifting of a protein vertically across the membrane could alter the extent of its surface exposure, thereby changing its accessibility to intra- and extracellular chemical constituents. Important determinants of membrane lipid fluidity are the extent of saturation of the fatty acid side chains and the amount of cholesterol. One notable change in the membranes of brain tissue during aging is a marked increase in the ratio of cholesterol to phospholipids and a consequent decrease in membrane fluidity.

Increases in membrane viscosity with age can be expected to affect some, but not all, of the various receptor types residing in neuronal membrane. An increase in membrane rigidity may squeeze a receptor vertically across the membrane, compromising its function either by altering its surface exposure or actually causing it to be shed from the membrane.

NEURITIC PLAQUES AND NEUROFIBRILLARY TANGLES
Neuritic (senile) plaques develop in the parenchyma of the brain and are not strictly intraneuronal although they do involve degenerating axonal and dendritic processes. **Neuritic plaques** are discrete, spherical lesions averaging about 30 µm in diameter (Figure 23-2 ■). They are characterized by three major components: a central core of beta-amyloid protein (hence, the name *cored* plaque) surrounded by neurites (axonal and dendritic processes) in varying stages of degeneration with an outer margin composed of reactive glial cells (astrocytes and microglia). Neurofibrillary tangles, on the other hand, are entirely intraneuronal and lead to the death of neurons. The

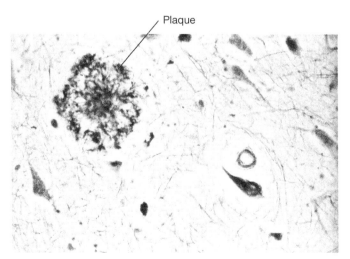

FIGURE 23-2 Neuritic plaques are discrete, spherical lesions averaging about 30 µm in diameter that develop in the parenchyma of the brain.

development and morphology of neurofibrillary tangles are described later.

In the brains of nondemented people, there is an increasing tendency for neuritic plaques to appear with advancing age. Plaques appear first in the hippocampus and parahippocampal gyrus but later become more widespread. While neuritic plaques are almost universally present in the brains of people in their late 80s, mentally intact elderly people have relatively fewer than do those with Alzheimer's disease. In contrast to neuritic plaques, very few neurofibrillary tangles are found in the brains of mentally intact elderly individuals. Those that do occur are located mainly in the hippocampus and parahippocampal gyrus. This paucity of neurofibrillary tangles in the nondemented elderly stands in marked contrast to their abundant and diffuse distribution in the brain's of people with Alzheimer's disease.

> **Thought Question**
>
> Differentiate neuritic plaques from neurofibrillary tangles in terms of their structure, location within the nervous system, and functional implications.

Blood Flow

Blood flow to the brain of neurologically normal people, which amounts to 750 to 1,000 ml/min, declines by some 23 percent between the ages of 33 and 61. However, the brain compensates for this decrease by extracting a larger proportion of the oxygen carried by the blood. The factors responsible for the flow decline are unclear, but the small neurons controlling dilation and contraction of brain arterioles that tend to disappear with normal aging have been implicated.

Behavioral Changes

MOTOR AND SENSORY CHANGES Brain changes with aging would be of little consequence if it were not for their impact on the individual as a whole. Some changes have consequences for morbidity and mortality such as, for example, the changes in vision (Chapter 17) and changes in blood vessels that lead to stroke. Acuity diminishes for senses of taste and smell, which can diminish a person's interest in and enjoyment of eating food, with potential consequences for weight loss among older adults. Other neurological system changes have consequences for safety and contribute to diminished postural control and potential falls of older adults. Specifically, both sensory and motor processing gradually slows down, affecting purposeful movement through changes in somatosensory processing and movement reaction time.

With respect to the somatosensory system, documented age-related changes include diverse declines in the morphology and physiology of a number of cutaneous and mechanoreceptors and large sensory structures, including preferential loss of large myelinated sensory fibers. Age-related decline is also apparent in sensory nerve conduction velocities and sensory nerve action potentials in humans. Of importance, sensory fibers appear to be affected at a younger age than are motor fibers. A reduction of neurotrophins within the skin and neurotrophin receptors of primary sensory neurons has been implicated in the distal sensory impairments that are associated with aging. (Neurotrophins are polypeptides that are essential in the development and survival of neurons both in the CNS and PNS.)

These age-related changes result in somatosensory changes, including declines in vibratory sense and discriminative touch. Declines in distal lower extremity proprioception and vibration occur among older individuals, resulting in a decline in joint position sense. Changes in position sense appear to affect the distal joints (ankle, knee) more than the proximal joints (hip). Of importance, animal studies suggest that denervation and mechanoreceptor loss actually precede joint degeneration and might possibly be among the causative factors contributing to knee osteoarthritis. Vibrotactile sensitivity, associated with Pacinian corpuscles and related pathways, declines as do touch thresholds and perception of discriminative touch associated with decreases in Meissner's corpuscles.

Similar age-related changes are apparent in the motor system, including a gradual decline in nerve conduction velocities as well as loss of muscle mass. With regard to nerve conduction velocities, there is a decremental reduction by decade between 20 and 90 years, with a 10-msec difference between the youngest and oldest decades. Reaction times are also delayed among older individuals. For example, young adults can perform a driving test in which they respond to a change from a green to red light by moving the foot from the accelerator to the brake with a reaction time within 150 to 250 msec (well within the 500-msec cutoff used by most motor vehicle departments). Older adults between ages of 70 and 85, in contrast, have a reaction time of 350 to 1,200 msec. This slowing with aging appears to be centrally mediated for the most part, although loss of myelin on peripheral nerves has been reported and would be expected to contribute to a slowing of conduction velocities. These deficits in motor conduction are compounded by losses of muscle itself. It has been estimated that 50 percent of the decline in muscle mass is accounted for by an age-related fallout or loss of motor neurons themselves and, in particular, axonal loss.

Changes to the sensory and motor systems can have significant functional consequences. Older adults demonstrate a decreased ability to integrate postural adjustments necessary for anticipatory and reactive responses. These deficits are, in part, related to changes that occur peripherally in the sensory and motor systems.

CIRCADIAN RHYTHMS Homeostasis—the maintenance of a constant internal milieu—has long been a cardinal tenet of physiology. However, it now is evident that the functional integrity of all living organisms depends as well on the maintenance of a number of interdependent body rhythms. These oscillating physiological behavioral responses are called **circadian rhythms** (L., *circa*, about, + *dies*, a day) because they are entrained to the day–night cycle. Circadian rhythms are intrinsic—that is, they are generated, run, and coordinated by the brain. They are also autogenous in that the rhythms continue under conditions of constant dark, although these periods may vary somewhat from 24 hours. It has been hypothesized, though not proved, that the functional deterioration characterizing aging is, in part, the consequence of loss of coordination among the many interdependent rhythms. Whatever the validity of this hypothesis, documented changes in a variety of circadian rhythms do occur in the elderly, along with a degeneration of cells in that portion of the brain participating in regulating such oscillations.

The sleep–wake cycle is one of the more obvious light-entrained endogenous rhythms of the body. The major ontogenetic changes in the sleep pattern, at least thus far documented, involve rapid eye movement (REM) and stage 4 non-REM sleep. The latter, the stage of deepest non-REM sleep that is highly responsive to the amount of prior wakefulness, declines exponentially from childhood to middle age and may be absent after 60 years of age. REM sleep declines from 50 percent of total sleep time at birth to 25 percent of total sleep time at approximately 10 years of age. It then remains steady to the seventh or eighth decade of life, after which further declines occur. Additionally, elderly people experience more frequent awakenings during the night and take more daytime naps. They appear, then, to return to the biphasic sleep pattern of the infant.

Circadian variations have been documented for a variety of transmitters (serotonin, dopamine, norepinephrine, and acetylcholine) and neuropeptides in various brain structures as well as in cerebrospinal fluid. Daily fluctuations also occur in receptor numbers and/or affinity for some neurotransmitters and neuropeptides in the maturing brain.

It is believed that the amplitude of a circadian oscillation directly reflects the stability of the rhythm. Thus, decreases in the amplitudes of body temperature and endocrine (e.g., aldosterone, renin, testosterone, growth hormone, thyroid-stimulating hormone, and estradiol) rhythms in old age possibly represent alterations in circadian timekeeping. Lastly, elderly people seem to exhibit a greater incidence of dissociation among the normally intricately synchronized circadian rhythms.

A specific group of neurons within the hypothalamus, the **suprachiasmatic nucleus (SCN)**, represents one of the two primary circadian clocks. Light stimulus, which entrains activity of the SCN to the day–night cycle, reaches a specific luminance-sensitive subpopulation of SCN cells via a direct projection from the retina, the **retinohypothalamic projection** introduced in Chapter 18. Light, of course, simply entrains SCN function to the 24-hour period because even in the absence of this afferent, input neurons of the SCN display a clear circadian rhythmicity in metabolic and electrophysiologic activity. Total lesions of the SCN in animals result in a loss of circadian rhythms for sleep–waking, drinking and locomotor activity, body temperature, and adrenal corticosterone and in the number of benzodiazepine and adrenergic receptors. Conversely, stimulation of the SCN produces phase shifts in circadian behaviors. That the SCN is not the sole circadian clock is indicated by the preservation of some rhythms following SCN lesions. However, the SCN is thought to orchestrate the activity of this as-yet-anatomically-unknown oscillator during normal light–dark cycles.

The neural substrate underlying circadian rhythm changes in old age and, even more dramatically, in senile dementia of the Alzheimer's type. Immunocytochemical studies on the human hypothalamus have shown a 45 percent reduction in the number of SCN cells in the elderly (80 and older) and a 73 percent reduction in people with Alzheimer's disease. This neuronal degeneration is likely antedated by a functional compromise of these same neurons, thus accounting for the observation that changed circadian rhythms occur at an earlier age than the observed cell loss. With the SCN cellular fallout, remaining neurons seem to clump closer together, producing a decrease in overall SCN volume. These changes help to explain the difficulties that older people experience with sleep, a problem that can interfere with their ability to participate fully in rehabilitation.

> **Thought Question**
>
> It is not yet clear to what extent changes in the brain are programmed and inevitable and to what extent they reflect *disuse atrophy*. What might be the implications of these two possibilities in terms of rehabilitation strategies and expectations? If changes are *programmed*, what would account for the wide range of findings among older adults of similar ages?

CLINICAL CONNECTIONS
Effect of Aging on Posture, Gait, and Falling

In individuals free of neurologic disease, a number of neurologic signs of aging are observed consistently. The most conspicuous manifestations of the aging process are changes in posture and gait. Such changes are exploited by actors who portray elderly people with stooped posture, and short, shuffling steps. Changes in stance and gait are universal features of aging. Almost imperceptibly, a tendency to stoop develops, the steps shorten, and walking slows. Walking becomes more cautious, and elderly indvdiuals use handrails to prevent a misstep in negotiating stairs or a ramp. The common gait changes seen in elderly individuals have been associated in part with the normal cellular loss (caused by the occurrence of neurofibrillary tangles) in the substantia nigra and resultant loss of the neurotransmitter dopamine. This also is true in the case of the stooped posture.

Also common among older individuals are deficits of balance, with falls representing a major health problem.

Indeed, a fall often is the precipitating event of the cascade of medical complications that end in the death of an elderly person. Due to a compromise in postural control mechanisms, older people may be unable to make rapid postural adjustments during routine activities such as walking, descending stairs, changing position, or putting on pants while standing (which requires standing alternately on one leg). Related changes known to occur among older individuals include depression of tendon reflexes at the ankles in comparison with those at the knees (indeed people over 80 years of age may lose Achilles reflexes altogether) and a loss of alpha lower motor neurons in the ventral horn with altered motor signs, including reduced speed and amount of motor activity, increased reaction time, and reduced muscular power especially in the lower extremities.

With regard to sensory processing related to posture and gait, somatosensory changes occur, including elevated thresholds for the perception of cutaneous stimuli and impairment or loss of vibratory sensibility in the toes and ankles. Vision is one of the most important senses used in maintaining balance. Neuro-ophthalmologic signs of concern include progressively decreasing pupillary size, resulting in decreased responsiveness to light; impairment of accommodation (presbyopia), resulting in farsightedness (hyperopia); impaired convergence; restricted range of upward conjugate gaze; impaired visual pursuit; decreased dark adaptation; and increased sensitivity to glare (see Chapter 18).

These motor and somatosensory changes can have a profound impact on stability (and falls). Specifically, as discussed in Chapters 9, 17, 18 and 20, the balance response mechanisms rely on inputs from the vestibular, visual, and proprioceptive systems for inputs and on muscle strength and postural alignment for the output systems.

Although we have focused on sensory and motor processing associated with posture, postural control, and gait, it should be noted that sensory and motor changes also affect upper extremity function, including, for example, impairment of fine motor coordination (e.g., deteriorating handwriting) with arm and hand movements that are more clumsy. Similarly, changes in hearing can occur. For example, high-frequency sensorineural hearing loss (presbycusis) occurs due to a loss of hair cells in the organ of Corti with an accompanying reduction in speech discrimination. And finally, there may be a reduction of the sense of smell and, to a lesser degree, the sense of taste.

Effect of Aging on Cognition and Memory

As discussed previously, cognitive and structural changes are associated with normal aging. Some of these changes are measurable by performance on standardized tests; some result in observable changes of the neocortex, dendrites, and neurotransmitters. In aging individuals, the development of neurotic plaques is first apparent in the areas related to memory: the hippocampus and parahippocampal gyrus. It stands to reason then that memory will be affected by normal aging. It has been observed that normally aging individuals may have prolonged cognitive processing speeds and decreases in working and short-term memory. Additionally, there may be losses in spatial processing and problem solving as well decreases in executive functioning. Much variability exists among older individuals. While these changes may be of concern for some individuals, they should not be confused with pathological aging of AD, in which the changes are more pronounced and of substantially greater functional consequence.

Known risk factors for cognitive aging include low level of education and having a history of head injury with loss of consciousness. Additionally, there are modifiable factors associated with cognitive decline such as hypertension, diabetes, and levels of physical, mental, and social activity. Much research is currently under way to understand what defines normal cognitive changes associated with aging and what interventions may prevent risk factors and cognitive decline. Further, several factors have been postulated that may protect against cognitive decline, such as vitamin E, statins, and omega-3 fatty acids. Additionally, lifestyle considerations such as social engagement and mental and physical activity may be important.

ABNORMAL AGING: ALZHEIMER'S DISEASE

Clinical Preview ················

Your 82-year-old grandmother was active and independent all of her life. Over the past four years, she has been experiencing increasing difficulty managing on her own. For example, she has difficulty recalling familiar recipes, has frequently left the stove on, misplaces her keys regularly, and most recently got lost on her way home from the grocery store. Just this week she was diagnosed with AD.
   As you read through this section, consider the following:

- How do her difficulties differ from those associated with normal aging?

- What kinds of structural and physiological changes do you anticipate that are different from those associated with normal aging?

- Given her age, and the prognosis for a person with AD, how would you expect this diagnosis to affect your grandmother?

The term **dementia** designates a symptom complex embracing intellectual, behavioral, and personality deterioration in an otherwise healthy adult that is severe enough to compromise occupational or social performance. It is the fourth leading cause of death in adults (following heart disease, cancer, and stroke). By far, the predominant cause of dementia is **Alzheimer's disease (AD)**, the most common degenerative disease of the brain. AD is becoming a major public health issue worldwide. The marked increase in life expectancy, largely through the cure of infectious diseases, has enabled many in the population to reach an age at which degenerative brain diseases such as AD become common. If treatments to prevent or delay the onset of AD are not developed, this demographic trend toward increased numbers of elderly persons in the population means that the number of people with AD is projected to grow in the United States from an estimated 5 million in 2008 to some 20 million by the year 2050. The tremendous annual monetary cost of AD, now estimated to be $150 billion, pales in comparison to the societal cost whereby family members and friends must cope with the suffering and stress engendered by watching a loved one deteriorate. Currently, there is no approved peripheral biochemical or imaging marker for AD. Consequently, at this time, a definitive diagnosis of AD can be made only by histologic confirmation obtained by performing either a cerebral biopsy or autopsy. Nonetheless, thorough analysis of the person's behaviors, coupled with careful mental-status examination, has allowed clinical identification of AD to attain a 90 percent accuracy rate.

Many of the clinical and pathologic features of AD overlap with those of normal aging. This is the underlying basis of the view that there is a transitional (evolutionary) relationship among normal aging, mild cognitive impairment, and AD. This view of a transitional relationship from normal aging fuels the unfortunate assumption that normal moments of forgetfulness in elderly people are harbingers of dementia. This should be a matter of concern for two reasons: it fosters unnecessary anxiety, and it is a false assumption.

While age is the single most important risk factor for Alzheimer's disease, it is important to emphasize that Alzheimer's disease is not a process of accelerated (exaggerated) brain aging. It is a degenerative disease of the brain. A substantial number of documented phenomena that occur in the neurons of those with Alzheimer's disease are simply not observed in age-matched normal controls. For example, during normal aging, the number of neurons in the hippocampal formation decreases little, if at all, whereas nearly 60 percent of neurons are lost in the hippocampus of people with AD. Other cellular changes that characterize Alzheimer's disease—for example, neuritic plaques and neurofibrillary tangles—may also be seen in the brains of normally aging people. Indeed, there is marked overlap between certain of the neuropathologic findings in the brains of normal aged people and people with AD. However, the extent of the changes and their topographical distribution are different in the two populations.

Clinically, the most common features of AD include an insidious onset, impairment of two or more areas of cognition and behavior, and progression leading to early death. The symptomatic course of this tragic illness extends over a period of 5 to 10 years, with a mean survival of 9 years from symptom onset, although the disease can last for as many as 20 years.

Thought Question

How is AD similar to normal aging and in what ways does it differ? Can AD be considered accelerated aging? Why or why not?

Types and Genetics of Alzheimer's Disease

Etiologically, two different types of AD exist. Both types are currently considered to be similar clinically and pathologically. Most cases of AD (90 to 95 percent) are sporadic (SAD), of late onset (after 65 years), and without any known genetic cause. In contrast, a minority of the people who have AD (about 5 to 10 percent) have genetic mutations, in which case the disorder is referred to as familial (FAD). Typically, this occurs before 65 years and is referred to early-onset AD.

Thought Question

What differentiates familial from sporadic AD?

Although all causes of SAD are not known, aging is the main risk factor for SAD in that the number of people with the disease doubles every five years after the age of 65. However, there must be additional factors besides aging to cause SAD because only 50 percent of people aged 85 years suffer from SAD. Environmental factors have been proposed to play a role. In addition, a susceptibility gene has been identified on chromosome 19 (the ApoE4 allele) that increases the risk of developing SAD.

FAD is caused by specific mutations in one of three genes: the amyloid precursor protein gene (APP) on chromosome 21, a presenilin 1 gene (PS1) on chromosome 14, and a presenilin 2 gene (PS2) on chromosome 1. All three genes act through a common, final pathway, resulting in an increase the production or deposition, or both, of amyloid beta protein, one form of which is cytotoxic to neurons. Considerable attention has been devoted to chromosome 21 because people with Down syndrome, who are born with three copies of chromosome 21 rather than the normal two, always develop the full range of brain lesions characteristic of AD, and in the same locations, by age 40 or 50. Indeed, individuals with Down syndrome overproduce amyloid beta protein from birth. Recently, beta amyloid levels, obtained from the cerebrospinal fluid, also have been used as a diagnostic marker for Alzheimer's disease.

Risk Factors

Age, family history, head injury, lack of education, and environmental factors are consistently considered to place a person at risk of developing AD. Age is the strongest risk factor, as noted earlier. A positive family history of AD increases the odds of developing the disease at any age by three- to fourfold. A history of head injury of sufficient severity to have led to hospitalization or a loss of consciousness results in a twofold increase in the risk of developing AD. Head injury has been speculated to increase the neuronal secretion of beta-amyloid protein and to cause the release from astrocytes of reparative proteins such as ApoE and others that speed the conversion of beta-amyloid to the compact, and potentially neurotoxic, amyloid that forms the core of the neuritic plaque.

Lack of education has an important correlation with the risk of an individual developing AD. The risk of developing AD doubles in individuals without education when compared to those with six to eight years or more years of education. The protective effect of education is assumed to be due to an increase in the brain's capacity to process, store, and generate information (a *brain reserve*) such that education buffers the onset of dementia. On the other hand, if those with a higher premorbid intelligence, or education, are at a biologically more advanced state of neurodegeneration by the time symptoms become apparent, then the disease may progress more rapidly. Factors such as lower levels of socioeconomic status, poor health care, and poor working and living conditions may co-exist with low levels of education. These may also be contributors to risk of AD.

Over the years, aluminum has received considerable attention as a potential cause of AD. However, evidence associating aluminum and AD is not definitive. A variety of other environmental toxins have also been studied as possible enhancers for contributing to the onset of AD, but, as yet, no specific agent has been identified.

Brain Changes in Alzheimer's Disease

Blood Flow

In neurologically normal persons between the ages of 33 and 61 years, blood flow to the brain declines by some 23 percent, and there is a compensatory increase in oxygen extraction from the blood. In AD, however, a further 30 percent decline in cerebral blood flow occurs. In addition, in contrast to the nondemented elderly, oxygen consumption is not increased and, in fact, declines by a similar 30 percent. A parallel decrease in glucose consumption is observed. Blood flow and chemical energy extraction from the blood continue to decrease as the clinical condition worsens. At one time, this impaired capacity of the brain to obtain chemical energy was thought to be a cause of AD, rather than a consequence of the disease's destruction of neurons.

General Markers of Brain Atrophy

Brain atrophy develops in people with AD as an inevitable consequence of the death of neurons, primary causes of which are the deposition of cytotoxic beta-amyloid protein and the development of neurofibrillary tangles. The rate of neuron loss accelerates as the disease progresses. This loss is responsible for the increased rate of cognitive decline accompanying disease progression.

Normal Brain

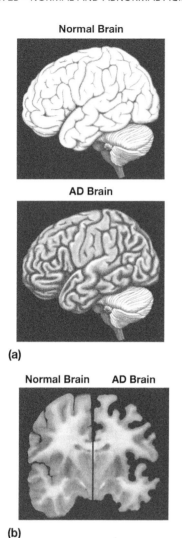

AD Brain

(a)

Normal Brain   AD Brain

(b)

FIGURE 23-3 The brain of people with Alzheimer's disease has diffuse atrophy as compared with older adults without AD.

Whole brain weight is decreased by 10 to 19 percent relative to age-matched normals. On gross visual inspection, the brain appears diffusely atrophied, although the atrophy may be more pronounced in one lobe than in another (Figure 23-3 ■). The most extensive atrophy may be observed in the gyri of association areas with relative sparing of primary motor, primary somatosensory, and primary visual cortices. Computerized tomography (CT scan) and magnetic resonance imaging (MRI) are useful diagnostic aids. Such measures show cerebral convolutions to be narrowed and sulci widened as well as atrophy of the hippocampal gyrus. The lateral and third ventricles are symmetrically enlarged to varying degrees—up to about twice normal size in advanced AD. Such indices of atrophy reveal group differences between the brains of persons with AD and those from age-matched normal controls. However, such changes in the brains of individual people with AD do not necessarily exceed those in many mentally intact older persons, so overlap between the two groups precludes the utilization of these measures in the diagnosis of individuals, especially early in the disease. The CT scan

and MRI are most useful in excluding subdural hematoma, multi-infarct dementia, brain tumor, and hydrocephalus as causes of the mental deterioration.

MEDIAL TEMPORAL LOBE STRUCTURES The pronounced memory deficit and emotional changes in AD call attention to potential pathology of temporal lobe structures. And, indeed, structures of the temporal lobe are nearly always the most severely involved, and the temporal lobe in general is affected to a greater extent than other lobes of the brain. Thus, some brain regions have higher vulnerability to AD pathology than others. A number of temporal lobe structures have proven vital to the memory process, in particular, the hippocampus. The volume of the hippocampal formation may be reduced by up to 60 percent in advanced AD. The distribution of hippocampal formation neuronal pathology effectively disconnects the hippocampus from the remainder of the brain: the entorhinal cortex-perforant pathway degeneration prevents other areas of the brain from sending information into the hippocampus, while other cell death prevents the hippocampus from sending its information back to other parts of the brain.

The volume of the amygdala in advanced AD may be reduced by 45 percent. Changes in the amygdala likely contribute to the changes in emotion seen in AD as well as to the inability of emotional content to influence memory retention.

The volume of the **nucleus basalis of Meynert** may be reduced by 69 percent in comparison to controls. This is significant because the cells of the nucleus basalis are cholinergic and supply the cerebral cortex with its major cholinergic input (Figure 23-4 ■). This would account for the drop, sometimes dramatic, in cortical acetylcholine

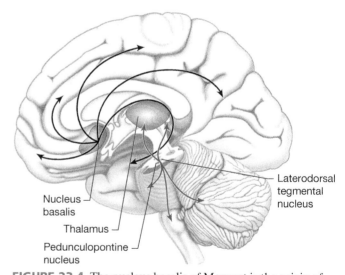

Laterodorsal tegmental nucleus

Nucleus basalis

Thalamus

Pedunculopontine nucleus

FIGURE 23-4 The nucleus basalis of Meynert is the origin of cholinergic projections to cortical areas and a decline of acetylcholine in the brain is the basis for symptomatic treatment of Alzheimer's disease with anticholinesterase drugs. Other cholinergic projections arise from the brainstem and include the pedunculopontine tegmental nuclei and the laterodorsal tegmental nuclei.

levels in AD. It also provides a neurochemical basis for the symptomatic treatment of AD with anticholinesterase drugs.

Microscopic Brain Changes

Several alterations visible in neuronal cells under the light microscope are diagnostic of AD. The brains of individuals with AD distinguish themselves from the brains of the nondemented elderly individuals not only in the extent of pathological alterations, but also in their topographic distribution, as well as in the nature of some of the alterations themselves. The three major, though not exclusive, pathologic signs of AD are the presence of senile plaques, the occurrence of neurofibrillary tangles within neurons, and the deposition of amyloid around and within cerebral blood vessels. These three pathologic changes are due to abnormalities in the metabolism of two distinctive proteins: **amyloid** and **tau**. Senile plaques involve the protein amyloid, while neurofibrillary tangles involve the protein tau. Recognition of the involvement of two different proteins in the pathology of AD is fundamental because they represent two distinct targets of potential therapy for AD.

The neurodegenerative process of AD begins long before the symptoms of clinical dementia are seen. AD-like neurofibrillary changes may begin 40 to 50 years before clear signs of cognitive impairment are apparent. Once the individual becomes symptomatic from AD, profound impairment and death become eminent, occurring within only 5 to 10 years.

SENILE PLAQUES AND NEUROFIBRILLARY TANGLES For years, neuritic (senile) plaques were considered the primary marker of AD. Recall from the section on normal aging that these plaques occur even in normally aging brains, but usually to a much lesser degree than in those with AD. The morphology of neuritic (senile) plaques was presented earlier. The distribution of plaques in the brains of people with AD is illustrated in Figure 23-5 ▇.

It is now recognized that the density of **neurofibrillary tangles (NFTs)**, as opposed to plaques, are best correlated with the severity of dementia. Neurofibrillary tangles are bundles of intracellular fibrous proteins that fill the cell bodies of neurons. They represent abnormal accumulations of proteins involved in the building of the neuron's cytoskeleton. Microtubules are the largest of the neuron's cytoskeletal fibers. They are made up of the protein tubulin (alpha and beta) that forms (polymerizes into) strands distributed about a hollow core (Figure 23-6 ▇). The assembly of alpha and beta tubulin into strands is regulated by a group of microtubule-associated proteins (MAPs), one of which is called tau. Tau protein promotes the assembly of microtubules and stabilizes their structure but a slight chemical change in tau (phosphorylation) diminishes this protein's ability to promote assembly. A lack of microtubules has dire consequences for a neuron. Recall from Chapter 3 that

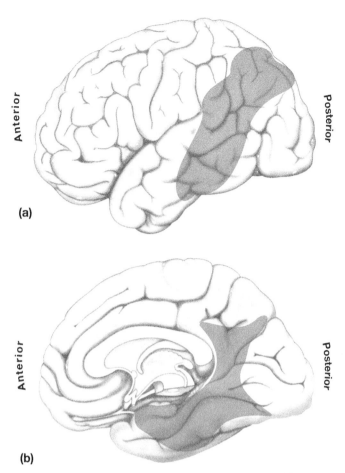

FIGURE 23-5 Areas with the highest density of neurtitic plaques in brains of people with Alzheimer's disease. The purple color represents the area with highest density.

microtubules are responsible for axoplasmic transport in that they form tracks along which motor proteins shuttle vesicles to and from the cell body.

In AD, the chemical change in tau results in a marked decrease in the assembly of tubulin into microtubules such that microtubules are only rarely seen in affected neurons. Instead, tau protein itself assembles into bundles of filaments that wrap around one another in pairs to form a helix (hence, the term *paired helical filaments*). This massive overdevelopment of pathological fibrillar protein interferes with the transport of substances from one part of the neuron to another, cutting off the transport of molecules and materials essential for survival of the neuron. Thus, affected neurons have been depicted as dying of strangulation.

CEREBROVASCULAR AMYLOID Cerebrovascular amyloid is a common pathologic alteration observed in the majority of brains of people with AD (found in more than 90 percent). Generally, the amyloid begins to aggregate in the middle, muscular layer of a blood vessel and then progresses into the outer vascular layers. Occasionally, the entire vessel wall may be overtaken by amyloid. This has been correlated with leukoencephalopathy or microvascular changes noted on MRI.

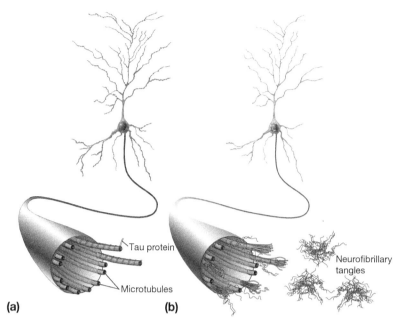

FIGURE 23-6 Neurofibrillary tangles and breakdown of tau proteins are characteristic of the brains of people with Alzheimer's disease. (a) Representative axon from a healthy individual with tau proteins that promote the assembly of microtubules, which stabilize the axon's structure. (b) Representative axon of a person with AD, illustrating the disintegration of the microtubules.

CLINICAL CONNECTIONS

Clinical Features

The clinical symptoms that characterize AD can be organized into five areas: memory, visual spatial function, personality changes, movement and reflex changes, and surviving capacities. The various symptoms may not manifest themselves in the same order in every person because the pattern of involvement of given brain areas may vary among people. The onset of symptoms usually is so insidious that neither the person nor family can accurately fix an exact date.

> **Thought Question**
>
> Can you relate deficits of memory and emotion associated with AD to specific neuroanatomic structures?

Memory

The major symptom of AD is the gradual, but progressive, development of forgetfulness. In the initial stages of the disease, appointments may be forgotten and possessions misplaced. Eventually, even the most familiar and rote aspects of learned behaviors are lost such as, for example, the capacity to properly use eating utensils. During the later stages, the recognition of family members—indeed, even self-recognition—may be lost. It is sometimes believed that recent memories are lost first, whereas those pertaining to remote events (long-term memory) are not affected until later in the illness, but not all clinicians agree with this. Thus, both recent and long-term memory may be impaired together. Interestingly,

healthy aging leaves intact the enhancing effects of emotion on memory (refer to Chapter 22), but in people with AD, the benefit bestowed on memory by emotional content is lost.

Language

The memory impairment spills over into the language sphere. The person's speech initially becomes halting due to an inability to retrieve a needed word. Names and common nouns are lost initially. Finally, the person fails to speak in full sentences. Writing is similarly affected. As the disease progresses, comprehension suffers a similar fate such that eventually nothing that is either written or said is understood. At this point, the deterioration of language and verbal skills has progressed to a frank clinical aphasia. Arithmetic skills suffer a similar progressive deterioration. Ideomotor apraxia—the inability to carry out on request or by imitation a complex voluntary movement (see Chapter 20)—may be demonstrated, but whether this is due to the comprehension deficit, the memory deficit, or both, is uncertain.

Visuospatial Function

Visuospatial deficits appear at some point in the disorder. Difficulties with dressing, an inability to distinguish right from left or to interpret a road map, turning in the wrong direction, or becoming lost in once familiar surroundings are but some of the manifestations of this loss of spatial orientation. With the worsening of visuospatial orientation, even the simplest of geometric forms or patterns cannot be copied or duplicated in block constructions (see Chapter 21).

Personality Changes

A prominent feature in the development of AD is the occurrence of personality changes. Outward emotional reactions coarsen and the person becomes more egocentric.

Social graces deteriorate as he or she becomes insensitive to the needs and wishes of others and ignores personal hygiene. Social avoidance, fearfulness, agitation, paranoia, and irritability are common, but the opposites of these conditions may also develop—namely, inertness and placidity. Verbal and even physical aggression toward family members may develop, in particular, as the dementia progresses and the person senses an increased loss of control over his or her life. Not infrequently, a poorly organized paranoid delusional state develops. People with AD become suspicious and may spy on family members. They may be convinced that their possessions are being stolen and thus hide them. Hallucinations occasionally accompany the paranoia. Such behavioral changes are the major cause of institutionalization.

Movement and Reflex Changes

A number of movement and reflex alterations appear during the course of the disease. Unsteady, short steps characterize a gait disorder that usually appears later in the illness. Parkinsonian symptoms of tremor, rigidity, and akinesia may be added to the disturbance in locomotion. Ultimately, though, the person loses the capacity to either stand or walk and, bedridden, sinks into a state of relative mutism and akinesia. Appetite, sometimes initially increased, is eventually lost, and he or she becomes emaciated. A number of pathological reflexes, such as the sucking or grasping reflex (supposedly signs of frontal lobe dysfunction), are released and can be readily elicited, especially late in the disease. Finally, and possibly as a result of inattention and immobility, the person may experience frequent aspiration, ultimately leading to infections such as aspiration pneumonia.

Surviving Capacities

Throughout the period of mental deterioration, other neural functions survive relatively unaltered. Thus, visual acuity and visual fields remain relatively intact, as do corticospinal and corticosensory functions. If hemiplegia or visual problems do develop, then either the AD has been complicated by a stroke, tumor, or subdural hematoma or the diagnosis of AD is itself incorrect.

Treatment

Pharmacological Management

Several decades ago, people with AD were treated with metabolic enhancers and vasodilators, even though AD is not a disease either of cerebral metabolism or cerebral blood flow. Although changes in metabolism and cerebral blood flow do, indeed, occur, they are now recognized as consequences rather than causes of the disorder. Discovery of the deficit in the transmitter acetylcholine (ACh) provided the first basis for development of a rational management protocol.

Cerebral ACh levels can be enhanced via three pharmacologic strategies: drugs can be administered that augment synthesis or release, act directly on the postsynaptic receptor, or prevent inactivation of ACh by blocking the degradative enzyme acetylcholinesterase (AChE). Replacement therapy, the strategy of choice in Parkinson's disease that increases transmitter synthesis and release (in this case DA), proved disappointing: administration of choline and lecithin, the precursors of ACh, does not produce improvement either in memory or psychological performance.

Four acetylcholinesterase inhibitors that are approved by the Food and Drug Administration (FDA) include donepezil, rivastigmine, galantamine, and tacrine. Of these, tacrine has very limited clinical use because the drug is toxic to the liver (hepatotoxicity), causes a number of unfavorable side effects, and requires four-times-a-day dosing. None of the acetylcholinesterase inhibitors treat the underlying neurodegenerative process that continues unabated. Consequently, if their administration is stopped, the person's cognitive functions will return to the level expected if the drug had never been administered. Furthermore, the benefits themselves are only modest. Once the maximum dosage is reached, cognitive functions do not continue to improve, and the net effect of the drug is to only to delay the person's cognitive and social decline. Cognitive deterioration continues, even though he or she stays on the medications.

Current research on therapeutic approaches to treating AD is focusing on targeting the proteins whose abnormal metabolism causes the brain pathology. Virtually all of the research that has progressed to clinical trials has been devoted to amyloid because of the "amyloid cascade hypothesis," which suggests that amyloid plays a central role in the pathogenesis of AD. The accumulation of beta-amyloid in the brain initiates a cascade of events that leads to neuronal dysfunction, neurodegeneration, and dementia. None of these efforts has been successful, including development of a vaccine that stopped the development of senile plaques but did not affect dementia. It may be that attacking the abnormal metabolism of the protein tau is a more appropriate target, but this is not currently known.

Antipsychotic agents such as chlorpromazine are sometimes given to calm a behaviorally unmanageable individual and make life more bearable for family members. Whatever current treatment is adopted as a therapy for AD, educating the family and planning for the still-inevitable decline of behavior and cognition are vital.

Physical and Psychosocial Interventions

AD is a disease that affects not just the person in question, but also profoundly affects the family and caregivers. In fact, from the perspective of the rehabilitation professional, perhaps some of the most important aspects of AD relate to the psychosocial consequences of the disorder.

People with AD undergo progressive losses of memory and language and concomitantly experience profound changes in personality, with a progressive loss of ability to care for self. Although these individuals also have altered postural control, gait, and functional movements, such deficits are often of lesser importance than are the cognitive and emotional difficulties.

Given the profound implications of AD for the individual and the family, the rehabilitation professional works with both. For example, the rehabilitation professional may work with people who have AD to improve balance, gait, and safety. Equally importantly, the clinician may work with family members and caregivers who live with and care for that individual, providing guidance, encouraging respite, and assisting in developing long-term strategies to cope with the progression through the disorder. Rehabilitation professionals can support family members through education about the disorder, assist them in their grief related to the loss of the loved one's former personality and self, help evaluate the home or living facilities for safety, and assist them to adjust their expectations and roles as their loved one changes.

Summary

This chapter summarized some of the important changes that occur in the nervous system with typical aging and contrasts these changes to those that occur with the disorder of Alzheimer's disease. This information is important to the rehabilitation professional for two reasons. First, many of the individuals who come to a rehabilitation professional for assistance with a specific disorder or injury are in their fifth, sixth, or later decades of life. These individuals have likely experienced changes in the nervous system associated with aging that should be taken into consideration when designing rehabilitation strategies. Second, the incidence and prevalence of AD is widespread and will only increase as the population ages.

This chapter began by defining and contrasting important terms, including aging, life span, life expectancy, and senility. We then examined the changes that occur in the brain, including cerebrocortical, neurotransmitter, and neuronal changes. Included was a discussion of specific structures (e.g., dendrites), specific neurotransmitter changes, and changes to structural components of neurons (e.g., lipids, plaques). We concluded the section with a summary of some of the important sensory and motor consequences that result from these structural changes.

Alzheimer's disease (AD) was the focus of the second topic of this chapter. Included was a discussion of risk factors and genetics, as well as a discussion of the brain changes in AD that differentiate this disorder from normal aging. We then turned our attention to the consequences of AD for memory, language, and perception. Finally, we summarized some of the major implications for rehabilitation of people who have AD.

Applications

1. Antonio Yglesias is 67 years old. He is and has been rather active and healthy his whole life, essentially experiencing normal aging. Recently, he has had some trouble with balance and gait. When he takes a walk each morning, he is concerned that he might stumble or fall. Additionally, he reports it is taking longer to complete his typical walking route.
   a. What nervous system components could be implicated in his difficulty with balance and gait? Consider all of the contributors from peripheral to cortical, including sensory, motor, and cognitive systems.
   b. Comment on how each of these components could be affected by normal aging.

2. Alec Keeney is 77 years old and was diagnosed with AD three years ago. Alec has trouble with word finding, misplaces important items, and frequently asks his wife the same questions throughout the day. He has recently started having emotional outbursts, sometimes yelling or crying without any apparent precipitating event. His posture is stooped forward, and he has frequent losses of balance when walking outside with his wife. He has fallen twice in their home.
   a. Identify areas of the cortex that could be implicated in each of these findings.
   b. How does Alec's prognosis compare to that of Antonio?

References

A randomized, placebo-controlled, clinical trial of high-dose supplementation with vitamins C and E, beta carotene, and zinc for age-related macular degeneration and vision loss: AREDS report no. 8. *Arch Ophthalmol* 119(10):1417–1436, 2001.

AD2000 Collaborative Group. Long-term donepezil treatment in 565 patients with Alzheimer's disease (AD2000): Randomized double-blind trial. *Lancet* 363:2105, 2004.

Anstey, K. J., and Low, L. F. Normal cognitive changes in aging. *Australian Fam Phys* 33(10):783–787, 2004.

Bennett, D. A., and Holtzman, D. H. Immunization therapy for Alzheimer disease? *Neurology* 64:10–12, 2005.

Bennett, D. A., Schneider, J. A., Arvanitakis, Z., et al. Neuropathology of older persons without cognitive impairment from two community-based studies. *Neurology* 66:1837–1844, 2006.

Black, S. E., Doody, R., Li, H., et al. Donepezil preserves cognition and global function in patients with severe Alzheimer disease. *Neurology* 69:459–469, 2007.

Braak, H., and Braak, E. Staging of Alzheimer's disease-related neurofibrillary changes. *Neurobiol Aging* 16:271–278, 1995.

Buckner, R. L., Snyder, A. Z., Shannon, B. J., et al. Molecular, structural, and functional characterization of Alzheimer's disease: Evidence for a relationship between default activity, amyloid, and memory. *J Neurosci* 25:7709–7717, 2005.

Friedman, D. S., O'Colmain, B. J., Munoz, B., et al. Prevalence of age-related macular degeneration in the United States. *Arch Ophthalmol* 122(4): 564–572, 2004.

Galasko, D. R., Gould, R. L., Abramson, I. S., and Salmon, D. P. Measuring cognitive change in a cohort of patients with Alzheimer's disease. *Stat Med* 19: 1421–1432, 2000.

Hardy, J. Alzheimer disease: Genetic evidence points to a single pathogenesis. *Ann Neurol* 54:143, 2003.

Hardy, J., and Selkoe, D. J. The amyloid hypothesis of Alzheimer disease: Progress and problems on the road to therapeutics. *Science* 247:353, 2001.

Hart, Jr., W. M. *Adler's Physiology of the Eye, Clinical Application*, 9th ed. Mosby Year Book, St Louis, 1992.

Mayeux, R. Dissecting the relative influences of genes and the environment in Alzheimer's disease. *Ann Neurol* 55:156–158, 2004.

Perry, R. J., and Hodges, J. R. Attention and executive deficits in Alzheimer's disease. *Brain* 122:383, 1999.

Remington, L. A. *Clinical Anatomy of the Visual System*, 2nd ed. Elsevier, St Louis, 2005.

Ropper, A. H., and Brown, R. H. Ch. 39. Degenerative diseases of the nervous system. In: *Adams and Victor's Principles of Neurology*, 8th ed. McGraw-Hill, New York, 2005.

Scarmeas, N., Albert, M., Brandt, J., et al. Motor signs predict poor outcomes in Alzheimer disease. *Neurology* 64:1696–1703, 2005.

Scheibel, M., Lindsay, R. D., Tomiyasu, U., and Scheibel, A. B. Progressive dendritic changes in aging human cortex. *Exp Neurol* 47:392, 1975.

Schneider, J. A., Li, J., Li, Y., et al. Substantia nigra tangles are related to gait impairment in older persons. *Ann Neurol* 59:166–178, 2006.

Selkoe, D. J. The origins of Alzheimer disease: A is for amyloid. *JAMA* 283:1615–1617, 2000.

Selkoe, D. J. Alzheimer's disease: Genes, proteins, and therapy. *Physiol Rev* 81:741–766, 2001.

Spalton, D, J., Hitchings, R. A., and Humter, P. A. *Atlas of Clinical Ophthalmology*. Lippincott, Philadelphia, 1984.

Tiraboschi, P., Hansen, L. A., Thal, L. J., and Corey-Bloom, J. The importance of neuritic plaques and tangles to the development and evolution of AD. *Neurology* 62:1984–1989, 2004.

Welsh, E. M., ed. *Frontiers in Alzheimer's Disease Research*. Nova Science, New York, 2006.

Wilson, R. S., Li, Y., Aggarwal, N. T., et al. Education and the course of cognitive decline in Alzheimer disease. *Neurology* 63:1198–1202, 2004.

PART VII

Injury, Disease, and Recovery of Nervous System Functions

The final part of this text provides a link between the content of neuroscience and clinical practice by the rehabilitation professional. The role of the rehabilitation professional is to assist individuals to improve function to the greatest extent possible, given the underlying conditions. Best practice relies on an understanding of the nervous system changes, both physiological and anatomical, and their implications for function. Thus, a major goal of this part of the text is to illustrate how an understanding of neuroscience is applied by the rehabilitation professional as he or she assists individuals with injuries of the nervous system. Furthermore, it is often through a thorough appreciation of the impact of diseases and disorders on function that one is well positioned to integrate and synthesize an understanding of the neurophysiology and neuroanatomy of the nervous system. The second major goal of Part VII, then, is to provide just such opportunities for solidifying understanding of neurophysiology and neuroanatomy of the cortical and subcortical structures. For these two reasons, it is fitting to end this text with clinical conditions of particular importance with respect to rehabilitation.

It should be noted that this part of the text lays the groundwork for application to examination, evaluation, and intervention strategies for people with neurological injury and disease. This part of the text is not intended to provide detailed discussions related to rehabilitation, which comprise its own area of study—that of rehabilitation science. Nor is it our intention to provide an in-depth discussion of neuropathology of neurological conditions, which likewise comprises a distinct topic and is beyond the scope of this text.

Chapter 24 focuses on stroke. The first major section provides a physiological basis for understanding ischemic stroke. The second major section of the chapter provides a detailed discussion of the specific consequences associated with syndromes of the middle, anterior, and posterior cerebral arteries; the internal carotid artery; and the lacunar infarct. This section ends with implications for rehabilitation. The third major section of the chapter presents the physiology of hemorrhagic stroke, differentiating this type of stroke from ischemic stroke. The final major section presents several important hemorrhagic stroke syndromes, again ending with implications for rehabilitation.

The topic of Chapter 25 is the brain's environment and brain injury. The first three major sections of this chapter focus on the meninges, cerebrospinal fluid, and the blood–brain barrier, respectively. Disorders specific to each of these brain structures are presented (e.g., meningioma, meningitis, and hydrocephalus). This content provides the basis for understanding traumatic brain injury, which is the topic of the fourth major section of this chapter. Included in this section are causes and mechanisms of traumatic brain injury, a discussion of concussion versus coma, and implications for rehabilitation.

Brain plasticity is the topic of the final chapter in this text, Chapter 26. It is a fitting end to this text because brain plasticity is at the frontier of investigations of importance for rehabilitation. This chapter begins with an overview of brain plasticity, drawing on information presented in Chapter 4 about plasticity at the level of cells but expanding it substantially to encompass plasticity of neural networks and behavioral implications. Here, we also discuss the difference between neural recovery and neural compensation. The second major section focuses on plasticity of cortical structures, first presenting some of the classic experiments related to development of vision, followed by experiments related to cortical maps for hand function. The topic of the third major section focuses on emerging evidence related to plasticity following brain damage in humans. The final major section of this chapter focuses on exercise and brain plasticity. In this section, we draw from both animal models of stroke and experiments in people who have sustained strokes and other types of brain damage. This area of investigation is just beginning to blossom; over the next decades, it has the potential to radically alter approaches to physical as well as cognitive intervention.

Cortical Strokes

LEARNING OUTCOMES

This chapter prepares the reader to:

1. Define the following terms: ischemia, necrosis, infarct, thrombus, and embolus.

2. Differentiate ischemic strokes, hemorrhagic strokes, and transient ischemic attacks (TIAs).

3. Discuss the relationship between cardiac disease and ischemic stroke.

4. Discuss the relationship between atherosclerotic disease and thrombotic stroke.

5. Explain why a disruption of blood flow for as little as five to six minutes leads to cell infarct and necrosis.

6. Compare and contrast the process and consequences of thrombotic and embolic strokes, including time course and prognosis.

7. Discuss the specific attributes of the circle of Willis that help to protect the nervous system from the effects of occlusion of specific blood vessels.

8. Compare white to red thromboses and describe the process by which one is converted to the other.

9. Compare and contrast the impairments anticipated with occlusion of the following major blood supplies: anterior, middle, and posterior cerebral arteries.

10. Predict the extent of damage and anticipated impairments, depending on whether a stroke occurs in distal versus proximal territories and whether it is in the right or left hemisphere.

11. Hypothesize regarding the location of a lesion associated with an ischemic stroke, based on the resulting constellation of impairments.

12. Interpret prognosis for functional recovery based on lesion size and the constellation of impairments.

13. Discuss implications of different lesions for the rehabilitation professional's strategy for examination and intervention.

14. Contrast the causes, time course, and consequences of hemorrhagic stroke to that for ischemic stroke.

15. Contrast three common causes of hemorrhage with respect to the anatomical basis, symptoms, and prognosis: primary intracerebral hemorrhage, aneurysm, and arteriovenous (AV) malformation.

16. Provide a rationale for strategies used in rehabilitation to focus the examination of people who have sustained a stroke.

ACRONYMS

ACA Anterior cerebral artery

AF Atrial fibrillation

AVM Arteriovenous malformation

CT Computerized tomography

CTA Computerized tomography angiogram

CVA Cerebrovascular accident

CSF Cerebrospinal fluid

FES Functional electrical stimulation

HDL High-density lipoprotein

LDL Low-density lipoprotein

MCA Middle cerebral artery

MRA Magnetic resonance angiography

MRI Magnetic resonance imaging

PCA Posterior cerebral artery

TIA Transient ischemic attack

tPA Tissue plasminogen activator

UMN Upper motor neuron

Introduction

Cerebrovascular disease is a generic term referring to any disease that affects the blood vessels of the brain. The general term for these problems is *stroke*. Cerebrovascular disease can cause symptoms that may be brief and transient or cause long-term deficits that often result in extraordinary personal upheavals with lifelong consequences. Strokes rank first as a cause of chronic and permanent functional disability in the United States. Stroke also represents the third leading cause of death, after heart disease and cancer, in the adult population in the United States. Because stroke is so common, an appreciation of the causes and consequences of stroke is central to rehabilitation practice.

Strokes can occur in the cerebrum, brainstem, cerebellum, or spinal cord. This chapter focuses only on cortical strokes; strokes in other major structures (e.g., spinal cord, brainstem) were addressed in other chapters.

Most cerebrovascular disease falls into one of two categories: either ischemic or hemorrhagic. **Ischemic strokes** are due to inadequate blood flow resulting in tissue death. Ischemic stroke accounts for about 80 percent of all strokes. The term *ischemia* means to keep back blood. Ischemic strokes occur when cells of the nervous system are perfused with too little blood. **Hemorrhagic strokes** occur when there is a hemorrhage (or bleeding) into the nervous system tissues and potentially into ventricles. These two types of stroke are different in terms of risk factors, causes, time course, and consequences. Hence, they are discussed separately. It should be noted that despite all the newer technology and better clinical awareness, no obvious cause can be identified in fully one-third of ischemic strokes. In these cases, the classification of cryptogenic stroke is used.

The defining feature of a stroke is the time course over which clinical deficits unfold. Most typically, the functional disability develops rapidly. Almost a third of patients sustain strokes while they are asleep; they are unaware that anything is wrong until they wake up. When they awaken, they may have problems with facial movement, weakness of one side of the body, difficulty with balance and walking, or difficulty with speech and language. If the event occurs while a person is awake, the neurologic deficit is usually abrupt and reaches its worst state almost at once. Some people have a *stroke in evolution*, which is characterized by stepwise progression of deficit. Each step is characterized by the appearance of a new deficit or set of deficits. People who sustain a stroke then experience stabilization or even an improvement of their deficits. When people have a complete resolution of the deficit within minutes after the onset of the event, it is referred to as a **transient ischemic attack (TIA)**.

In most cases, once a person sustains a stroke, the deficits will stabilize, with improvements occurring over a matter of minutes or within a day or even over months. This stabilization distinguishes stroke from progressive neurological disorders such as tumors, Parkinson's disease, or Alzheimer's disease in which there is a steady or stepwise deterioration of function. In sum, the hallmark of a stroke is its rapid onset compared with other diseases of the brain. This timeframe may apply to all types of stroke syndromes: its onset and the development of deficits, the attainment of stabilization, and the resolution, if any, of the deficits.

Through an appreciation of the risk factors for stroke, clinicians can assist individuals to develop appropriate preventive strategies. The impact of these preventive strategies can be seen in the dramatic change in the severity of strokes over the past 20 years and the dropping incidence of stroke in younger individuals. Furthermore, an understanding of the consequences of stroke and knowledge of the expected findings (based on location of lesions) assist the clinician to develop the most appropriate intervention strategies for specific patients.

This chapter is organized into four major sections. The first section presents an overview of the physiology and consequences of ischemic stroke. This is followed by the second section, which introduces the relationship of the lesion site of ischemic strokes to likely impairments and the implications for rehabilitation. In the third and fourth sections of the chapter, we turn to hemorrhagic strokes, presenting the physiology and consequences of hemorrhages (third section) and ending with the consequences of hemorrhages and implications for rehabilitation (fourth section).

Neuropathology Box 24-1: Immediate Action following Stroke: FAST

The American Heart Association and the American Academy of Neurology have tried to educate patients and families about the symptoms of stroke. They have developed the FAST mnemonic to do so, referring to abrupt loss of function in the **face**, **arms**, and **speech** and the **time** (need) for immediate action.

If a patient gets to a hospital that can manage acute ischemic stroke within four and a half hours, it may be possible to minimize the damage from the stroke. After that, too much time has elapsed, and a window of opportunity for treatment has closed. Unfortunately, the vast majority of people who suffer a permanent stroke do not seek or access treatment until it is too late to limit the extent of brain damage. Therefore, the most important aspect of stroke management today is early recognition of the symptoms so that the patient can get medical attention as soon as possible. The expression for treatment success is "time is tissue."

ISCHEMIC STROKE

Clinical Preview ·················

Mrs. Vandemere was admitted to the acute care hospital where you work following a stroke. She had some loss of movement on her left side on admission, but over the first day of her admission, the symptoms worsened. From the medical record, you learn that her stroke was thrombotic in nature. Mrs. Nguyen was admitted on the same day. Earlier that day, she experienced almost total loss of movement on her left side and loss of ability to talk. Yet within a half hour, her symptoms had resolved. And Mr. Carlson was admitted two days later with moderate loss of movement on the right side as well as some language deficit. Three days later, his symptoms were similar to the day of admission. As you read through this chapter, consider the following:

- What type of stroke would likely evolve over the first few days, which would resolve quickly, and which would be fairly stable?

- What was the likely reason for Mrs. Nguyen's hospitalization, given that her symptoms had resolved?

- Drawing on information that you learned in Chapters 7, 21 and 22, also consider why it is important to know the side on which the stroke occurred.

Risk Factors

Often times, effective treatment of people who have had a stroke is not possible soon enough after a stroke to prevent brain damage; hence, it is important to identify who is at risk and modify that person's lifestyle to reduce as many risk factors as possible. Unfortunately, one of the factors that correlates with increased stroke incidence is simply age which is non-modifiable. The passage of time allows chronic risk factors to exert a progressively increasing effect. However, other risk factors can be modified with appropriate treatment.

Thought Question

The rehabilitation professional can play an important role in educating people regarding healthy living, designed to prevent strokes. What specific factors should the rehabilitation professional be aware of when working with any person who might be at risk?

Of potentially modifiable risk factors, cardiac disease is the largest risk factor for stroke because emboli can break off abnormal cardiac tissue and lodge in the cerebrovascular system, therefore obstructing blood flow. *Atrial fibrillation (AF)* is a common cardiac condition often resulting in emboli associated with ischemic stroke. Other cardiac conditions have the potential of producing emboli

as well: myocardial infarction, endocarditis, mitral valve prolapse, and other heart conditions. One increasingly apparent cause of embolic stroke is a "paradoxical embolus," in which the blood clot is formed on the venous side of the circulation, breaks off, and passes through a *patent foramen ovale* in the heart and enters the cerebrovascular systems.

Hypertension is another major risk factor for ischemic stroke. For one thing, hypertension is associated with atherosclerotic (plaque) formation in the larger arteries. This is correlated with injury to the intima, the promotion of platelet aggregation, and the formation of the plaque. This process can be associated with the vessels becoming occluded or with creation of embolic material.

Blood lipids are associated with increased risk of ischemic stroke in various ways. People with high levels of cholesterol and low-density lipoprotein have a higher risk of stroke. These lipids can actually make up part of the plaque and stimulate the pathological chain reactions that form the arterial disease. However not all lipids are bad. High-density lipoprotein (HDL) picks up cholesterol from tissue cells and transports it to the liver for disposal. Therefore, HDLs help prevent atherosclerosis (i.e., they are antiatherogenic). The ratio of the HDL to LDL (low-density lipoprotein) or HDL to cholesterol is a good biological marker for risk to heart attacks or stroke.

Diabetes mellitus is a risk factor because the disease accelerates the rate of atherosclerosis. People who have diabetes are also at risk for pathological changes in the smaller vessels of the brain that can become occluded and cause specific types of strokes that are not due to atherosclerosis.

Other risk factors associated with stroke include obesity, smoking (cigarettes in particular), and excessive alcohol consumption. Some oral contraceptives increase the risk of stroke, especially in women who have migraine and who also smoke cigarettes. Increasingly, risks of abuse of other substances are of concern, including cocaine, amphetamines, and even over-the-counter medications that include sympathomimetics (e.g., ephedrine) and mimic the effects of the sympathetic nervous system.

Physiology of Ischemic Stroke

In Chapter 2, it was noted that neurons do not store significant amounts of either of their essential nutrients, oxygen or glucose, to fuel their high metabolic rate, and therefore, neurons are very vulnerable to reduced blood flow. Additionally, without adequate blood flow, the brain loses its ability to wash out the metabolic products of brain metabolism, and toxic metabolic products accumulate. Typically, a complete loss of blood flow can be tolerated only for a maximum of five or six minutes before there is death of not only the neurons, but also the supporting glial cells and the cells of the circulation. This results in infarction and necrosis. However, some people tolerate occlusive disease with few, if any, symptoms. This means that the relationship between vessel occlusion and clinical deficits sometimes is unpredictable. In other words, no one-to-one relationship exists between arterial occlusion at a specific site and the state of the brain tissue supplied by the occluded vessel.

Ischemic strokes result from lack of oxygen due to mechanical obstruction of one or more arteries that prevents adequate blood supply to the vessels and brain tissue distal to the site of blockage. Whether or not ischemia results in cell death in that location depends on several factors, including the completeness and duration of occlusion and collateral circulation. When ischemia is severe enough that neurons and other cells in brain tissue are deprived of blood, they soon die. This is called **ischemic necrosis**. The term *necrosis* comes from the Latin *necros*, meaning "to make dead." The local area of necrotic brain tissue is referred to as an **infarct**.

Infarcts may occur as a result of thrombosis or embolism. A **thrombus** or **atheroma** is a clot from cells normally circulating in the blood. Attached to the vessel wall, a thrombus may completely or incompletely occlude the lumen of a vessel. The term **thrombosis** refers to the formation or presence of a thrombus. An **embolus** is a plug composed of a detached fragment of a thrombus. Emboli can also be composed of other substances, such as pure cholesterol or even fat that travels in the arterial circulation and eventually gets stuck in an artery whose lumen is too small to allow further passage of the material. The term **embolism** refers to this process.

Thought Question

This is a good time to begin to tabulate ways in which emboli and thromboses are similar and ways in which they differ. As you continue through this chapter, you can continue to add to the list.

Infarcts due to ischemia, whether from thrombosis or embolism, often have a pale appearance (called **pale infarcts**) because there are no red blood cells in the area of the infarct. This type of stroke generally affects the older population. If the infarct has also injured the blood vessels, and the blood vessel walls break, blood can leak into the infarction, and a **red** or **hemorrhagic infarction** develops.

In summary, while causes of focal cerebral ischemia vary widely, the end result in brain tissue is the same—namely, lack of an adequate blood supply. Occlusive cerebrovascular disorders resulting in ischemia are caused primarily by atherosclerosis of blood vessels or embolization, both leading to occlusion of an artery. In rare instances, ischemic infarction can be caused by inflammation, trauma to a vessel (dissection of the artery), or coagulation disorders.

Stroke-Modifying Factors

The actual effect of arterial occlusion on brain tissue depends on a number of factors specific to each person. As a result, the clinical deficits present in a patient cannot always be accurately predicted, even when the vessel that has been occluded is known. Much of this unpredictability stems from individual differences in vascular architecture.

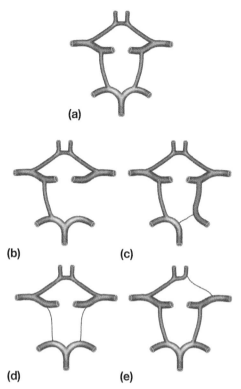

(a)

(b)   (c)

(d)   (e)

FIGURE 24-1 Anomalies in the circle of Willis. (a) Typical circle of Willis. (b) Incomplete circle (posterior communicating artery is missing). (c) One posterior cerebral artery arising from an internal carotid artery. (d) Abnormally small posterior communicating arteries. (e) Both anterior cerebral arteries are perfused primarily by one internal carotid artery.

Other factors are systemic in nature and relate to the individual's overall body and brain metabolism.

First, the structure of the **circle of Willis** may vary considerably in different people (Figure 24-1 ■). Recall from Chapter 2 that the circle of Willis is the ring of arteries at the base of the brain where the internal carotid and vertebrobasilar systems form anastomotic links. In only 50 percent of people is the circle fully intact with all of its pieces of significant size to provide collateral blood supply if one of the vessels to the brain has become occluded. In the ideal situation, the structure of the circle of Willis allows effective collateral circulation when there is occlusion of one of the arteries in the neck. This would permit the intracranial arteries on the occluded side to be filled from the opposite, unoccluded arteries, thereby preventing or reducing the severity of brain infarction. It should be noted that the posterior communicating arteries are too small in almost all human brains to subserve this function.

A second issue is the variability in end-to-end meningeal anastomoses between branches of the three major cerebral arteries discussed in Chapter 7 (see Figure 7-18). These may vary considerably in extent and robustness across individuals. Third, anastomoses between the internal and external carotid arteries occur to a variable degree in different individuals. One region in which such anastomoses occur is around the orbit of the eye, with blood passing from the external carotid

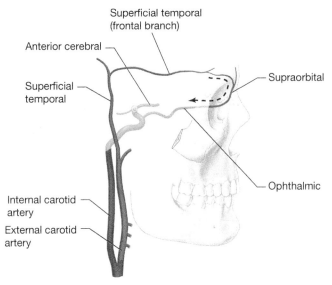

Superficial temporal
(frontal branch)

Anterior cerebral

Superficial
temporal

Supraorbital

Ophthalmic

Internal carotid
artery

External carotid
artery

FIGURE 24-2 Anastomoses between the internal and external carotid arteries around the orbit of the eye, via the ophthalmic artery.

into the internal carotid artery via the **ophthalmic artery** (Figure 24-2 ■). Such anastomoses may serve to lessen ischemic damage when the internal carotid artery is occluded.

Fourth, the speed of occlusion may affect the ischemic outcome. When an occlusion develops slowly, more time is allowed for collateral circulation to open up. When the occlusion develops rapidly, if the functioning collateral channels are not sufficient and even if they increase with time, this usually occurs far too late to reduce the original risk of ischemia and infarction.

Finally, general systemic and metabolic factors may affect the degree of ischemia resulting from occlusion of a vessel. Blood pressure is one such factor. Thus, a narrowed vessel may still deliver sufficient blood when blood pressure is 190/100 but fail to do so when blood pressure falls to 120/70. Such a drop in blood pressure may occur on sudden standing after a long period of recumbence, such as occurs during sleep. These drops in blood pressure can occur in an individual who is being treated with medication designed to lower blood pressure or if the person has underlying neurologic or systemic disorders that affect the ability of the person to maintain adequate blood pressure. Concurrent metabolic conditions can add to the risk of stroke. A fall in the level of sodium in blood serum, development of a fever, changes in the level of oxygen in the blood (as in people

with pulmonary disease), and lowered blood glucose levels (as in people with diabetes who use insulin incorrectly) may all result in the appearance of focal neurologic symptoms.

To understand the role of glucose, it is important to recognize that in the normal brain, glucose is metabolized to carbon dioxide and water. If the metabolism is inefficient, then the aerobic metabolism converts to anaerobic metabolism, and lactic and pyruvic acids accumulate. These acids change the pH of the brain tissue and further damage neurons. When the circulation is not adequate to wash out these acids, there is increased damage to the neurons and the blood vessels in the area of reduced blood flow.

Thrombosis

Hardening of the arteries, or **atherogenesis**, is the formation of an **atheroma**, also referred to as **plaque** or **stenosis**, in the larger- and medium-sized vessels of the body. The process is referred to as **atherotic disease** and is the same for the cerebral circulation as it is in the coronary arteries, or aorta, or the arteries to the legs. It begins because of a combination of factors, including the anatomy and biology of the blood vessels, the hemodynamics of the vessels, and coagulation factors. Atherotic disease may begin in childhood with the formation of fatty streaks in the intima and increases with age (Figure 24-3 ■).

Histologically, the fatty streak is a focal thickening of the intima with invasion of smooth muscle cells followed by infiltration of the cells with lipids such that the vessel wall becomes less pliable. The deposition of cholesterol and other lipids start a chain reaction. Inflammatory cells migrate into the streak; apoptosis occurs; and the fatty streak turns into a fibrous plaque, an atherosclerotic plaque, or an atheroma. As the plaque matures, revascularization occurs, and the center becomes more necrotic and filled with a lipid core that can be calcified. In the meantime, the external elastic membrane compensates by allowing both dilation and constriction of the vessel. Eventually, the constriction starts to obstruct the lumen, resulting in stenosis.

The hemodynamics of the vessel adds insult to the injury. The most common location for neurovascular atherogenesis is at the bifurcation of arteries (Figure 24-4 ■). The common carotid bifurcation in the neck is by far the most common location of neurovascular pathology. The turbulence physically irritates the intima, and it tends to wash away any protection the chemistry of the intima has to prevent clot formation. As the stenosis continues, it causes worsening of the turbulence.

Neuropathology Box 24-2: Diabetes and Stroke

A person with diabetes who has a hypoglycemic reaction can present with focal neurological symptoms that mimic a stroke. In fact, one of the first tests an emergency medical team will carry out on a person suspected of having a stroke is to check the blood sugar—and correct it if necessary. On the other hand, if the person's blood sugar is too high, as also can occur in diabetes, then possible recovery from the event is impaired, resulting in greater disability.

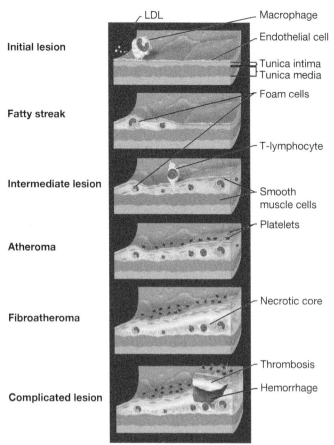

Initial lesion

Fatty streak

Intermediate lesion

Atheroma

Fibroatheroma

Complicated lesion

LDL — Macrophage
— Endothelial cell
— Tunica intima
— Tunica media
— Foam cells
— T-lymphocyte
— Smooth muscle cells
— Platelets
— Necrotic core
— Thrombosis
— Hemorrhage

FIGURE 24-3 Temporal development of atherosclerotic lesions. The initial lesion and fatty streak can begin from the first decade of life. The intermediate lesion and the atheroma can develop from the third decade. The fibroatheroma and complicated lesions can begin in the fourth decade. These early stages often are clinically silent, with symptoms becoming overt in the fourth decade or later. LDL: Low density lipoprotein.

Often, it is possible to hear the turbulence by using a stethoscope and listening to the noise, referred to as a bruit. The turbulence also ruffles up the platelets. When the platelets become traumatized, coagulation factors are activated and a thrombus forms. Initially, the thrombus forms a **white plaque** made up mainly of platelets. This eventually adds to the activation of other coagulation factors, and fibrin is formed. The white plaque now adds to the stenosis in the atheroma; the plaque is now atherothrombotic.

Thought Question

Atherosclerosis and thrombosis are intimately related. Discuss common locations for occurrence, and explain the consequences.

The developed atherothrombosis can cause neurovascular problems in three ways: by decreasing blood flow, by fragmenting and breaking off the thrombus or even part of the plaque (an embolus), or by hemorrhaging into the

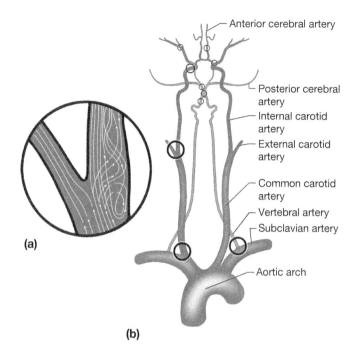

(a)

(b)

— Anterior cerebral artery
— Posterior cerebral artery
— Internal carotid artery
— External carotid artery
— Common carotid artery
— Vertebral artery
— Subclavian artery
— Aortic arch

FIGURE 24-4 (a) Distortions in the laminar pattern of blood flow occur at points where the blood vessels bifurcate or branch. The swirling motion of blood flow favors the development of atherosclerosis at these sites. (b) Major sites of atherosclerosis involving the blood vessels that supply the brain are indicated by the black circles.

weakened center of the thrombus, thereby causing complete occlusion of the artery (Figure 24-5 ■). When hemorrhage into the thrombus occurs, it is referred to as a **red plaque**.

Generally a slow reduction of the lumen of the carotid artery does not cause symptoms. However, once the blockage becomes greater than 70 percent of the remaining lumen, the individual may have transient ischemic symptoms (TIA). This can occur when there also is a compromise of

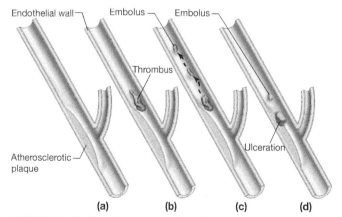

Endothelial wall — Embolus — Embolus —
Thrombus
Atherosclerotic plaque
Ulceration

(a)   (b)   (c)   (d)

FIGURE 24-5 Complications associated with atherosclerosis. (a) Plaque encroaching on the lumen of an artery, leading to stagnation of blood flow distal to the plaque. (b) Formation of a thrombus on the plaque. (c) Fragments of the thrombus breaking off from the main mass to form emboli. (d) Ulceration of the vessel wall, allowing material of the atherosclerotic plaque to embolize.

cardiac output, a failure of the collateral circulation due to other stenotic disease, or even congenital variations of the circle of Willis. Once a person has transient symptoms due to stenosis, definitive treatment with surgery is indicated (i.e., an endartectomy or stent).

The most common problem of **atherothrombotic** pathology is the embolus. Sometimes, the embolus is simply crystals of cholesterol. When cholesterol emboli get into the retinal circulation, they can actually be seen on fundiscopic examination as bright, sparkling material in the arteries (Hollenhorst plaques) and cause transient monocular blindness (otherwise known as **amaurosis fugax**). More commonly, the embolus consists of a collection of the platelets and fibrin from the thrombus. Because this is pale in color, it is called a **white thrombus**. These are very soft and may break up, forming a white embolus, in which case the patient may then have a progression of symptoms that stagger over time, a stroke in evolution, or a TIA. More complicated thromboses may have red blood cells and even part of the atheroma in them (and can also include the necrotic debris, smooth muscle cells, and lipid junk). This is a **red thrombus**. These tend to be larger and tougher and do not break up as frequently. When they do break off, they form emboli referred to as **red emboli** that are more dangerous and tend to block the medium- sized intracranial arteries and cause abrupt and persistent deficits. An ulcer in an atheroma, detected with imaging, is a sign that an artery-to-artery embolization may have taken place, whether or not the person had any reportable symptoms. Such lesions may require an endartectomy or stent to prevent a more devastating stroke.

A complete occlusion by atheroma is rare in the carotid circulation. Often, the occlusion has occurred so slowly that the individual does not have any symptoms because collateral circulation has been able to be utilized to compensate for the gradual narrowing. With slow atheroma development, three of the four neurovascular vessels may close off and the person may have no symptoms because of the compensatory collateral circulation. When the person has a stroke due to occlusion of the common carotid artery, a hemorrhage into the artery wall usually occurs abruptly, without time for development of collateral backup.

In summary, the process of thrombosis combined with atherosclerosis produces stenosis that may lead to severe and even complete occlusion of the vessel. It is important to recognize that these changes and potential symptoms can occur in any arterial system, not just the carotid arteries. Pathology in the arch of the aorta, the vertebral arteries, or even in the intracranial larger vessels can result in all of the scenarios discussed in this section.

Thought Question

Thrombotic strokes can also lead to embolic strokes. Why and how would this occur?

Embolism

Cerebral embolism may result from a variety of disorders but is often a result of cardiovascular disease. Fully 75 percent of cardiac emboli lodge in the brain because the cerebrovascular vessels are the first to arise off the aorta. Emboli can also occur from atherosclerotic thrombus in the arch of the aorta, at the location where the cranial vessels branch off from the aorta, and as noted at the carotid bifurcation and siphons (see Figure 24-4). Following trauma resulting in fractures of major bones, fat may embolize to the brain or limbs. Some forms of cancers can also spread to the brain by embolization.

Thought Question

Atherosclerotic plaques often develop in specific locations. Where are these locations, and what is the common feature?

Thrombus in the heart commonly results from chronic atrial fibrillation due to atherosclerotic or rheumatic heart disease. The rapid and irregular contractions (fibrillation) of heart muscle result in the development of a clot in the left atrium because blood no longer flows smoothly through the heart. Sudden changes in cardiac rhythm, such as occurs when the fibrillating heart returns to a normal rhythm (as may occur with cardioversion), may also result in the breaking off of a fragment of thrombotic material that then enters the circulation as an embolus. A mural thrombus may also form on the damaged endocardium (inner lining of the heart) overlying an area of myocardial infarction.

Embolic material travels in the circulatory system until it reaches a vessel whose lumen is too small to permit further passage of the embolus (Figure 24-6 ■). Once lodged in a vessel, the embolus may remain and plug the lumen solidly. Often, however, the embolus breaks into smaller fragments that then enter smaller vessels, and sometimes the symptoms disappear entirely. This phenomenon can result in a staggering course of the deficits.

Thought Question

Strokes are frequently associated with cardiac disease. Now is a good time to begin tabulating all of the cardiac conditions that could result in stroke. What are the implications for the rehabilitation professional?

The infarct resulting from an embolic stroke may be pale, hemorrhagic, or mixed. Most embolic infarcts are pale because there are no blood cells in the brain tissue. However, the development of secondary hemorrhage into an area of pale embolic infarction may occur. This is due to the breaking up of the embolic material that had blocked the artery, a return of blood flow under full pressure, and an area of the artery that injured. As a result, when again perfused under a normal blood pressure, the weakened and ischemic arterial

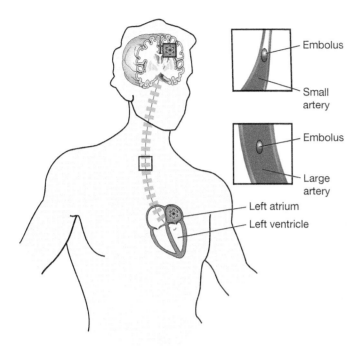

to 15 minutes, but rarely longer than 30 minutes. TIAs are a strong predictor of an impending major stroke with cerebral infarction. A stroke may follow one or more TIAs by hours, weeks, or months.

The symptoms associated with TIAs are similar to the symptoms of a completed stroke and, likewise, depend on the vessel involved. The only difference is the duration of the clinical difficulties. Hence, the transient symptoms vary and may include any of the following: (1) numbness, tingling, or weakness in the face, arm, or leg, especially on only one side of the body; (2) difficulty walking; (3) difficulty talking or understanding what others are saying; (4) confusion; (5) difficulty with vision in one or both eyes; and (6) dizziness and loss of coordination.

Thought Question

What key factor differentiates TIAs from embolic and thrombotic strokes? How are these events similar?

The clinical significance of a TIA is as an alert for the professional that the person should be referred to a physician who can then rigorously pursue the cause of the event and correct that cause. If a person has a single TIA, there is a 10 percent chance that that person will have another TIA within a week and a 2 percent risk that the person could complete an infarction within that week.

FIGURE 24-6 Cerebral embolism most commonly results from embolic material that originated in the heart. Cardiac disease, such as atrial fibrillation, sometimes leads to the development of a thrombus (clot) in the chambers of the heart. A fragment of the thrombus can break off to form an embolus. The embolus then travels in the arterial system until it reaches an artery in the brain whose diameter is too small for the embolus to travel any further. By blocking the artery, blood cannot reach brain tissue distal the embolus, resulting in infarction of the blood-starved tissue.

wall leaks, and blood escapes into the surrounding necrotic brain tissue. (See hemorrhagic strokes.)

Transient Ischemic Attacks

Sometimes, stenosis of a vessel may result only in episodes of transient signs and symptoms without actual tissue destruction. Most such transient ischemic attacks last from 2

CLINICAL CONNECTIONS
Time Course

By far, most strokes are completed within minutes of the precipitating event. However, as noted earlier, emboli can break up after the initial production of symptoms and cause a TIA or changing sequence of symptoms, referred to as a *stroke in evolution* (in progress). This is usually due

Neuropathology Box 24-3: Two Important Forms of TIA

Two important forms of TIA are transient monocular blindness and transient global amnesia. In **transient monocular blindness** (also called **amaurosis fugax**), the person reports a gradual loss of vision. The pattern of the visual loss can be just about anything, but it involves only one eye. Some people simply describe a blurring. Others describe a "curtain descending over their vision." Still others notice a visual loss traveling in from the lateral part of vision. On occasion, examination of the optic fundus during or soon after the transient monocular blindness can demonstrate embolic material in the retinal vessels. The embolic material may be aggregations of platelets or even cholesterol crystals.

With **transient global amnesia,** individuals have no loss of consciousness, and do not have any localizing neurologic deficits other than the inability to store and recall recent events; it is called an amnesia. They repeatedly ask, "Where am I?" and "How did I get there?" They can, however, tell you their name. And, in less than 24 hours, the amnesia has completely resolved. The unique feature of this diagnosis is that such individuals do not have any other cognitive loss. They can do calculations, can spell, can name, and are able to tell you the names of their grandchildren. These individuals, as well as people with transient monocular blindness, do not have any sensory or motor loss.

to tumbling of the clot into smaller and smaller arteries. However, once the embolus lodges in a vessel, the resulting deficits are completed within minutes. The stage of *completed stroke* refers to a sustained ischemic event resulting in neurologic deficits that can last for a day, weeks, or permanently. It should be noted that a person who has suffered one thrombotic stroke is at risk of having another stroke.

The onset of a thrombotic stroke may occur in several ways. Almost one-third of thrombotic strokes occur during sleep. The individual awakens unaware of any problem, may then fall because he or she is paralyzed, or look in the mirror and see facial weakness, or find that he or she cannot speak normally at the breakfast table.

The course of an atherothrombotic stroke cannot be predicted with confidence. This is particularly true early in the course of cerebral thrombosis. However, because time is of the essence when managing a stroke, a decision has to be made within 2 to 4.5 hours regarding appropriate emergency medical management. Emergency imaging is imperative to determine the nature (ischemic or hemorrhagic) and size of the stroke. If there is any hemorrhagic component, or if the size of the stroke is greater than one-third of a hemisphere, then thrombolytic management should not be used.

A number of factors related to time course help in differentiating embolic from atherothrombotic infarction. Most important is the suddenness with which an embolic stroke develops. The full-blown set of deficits evolves within several seconds or a minute with embolic occlusion. The event may be so sudden that the person stops speaking in midsentence with a total loss of speech. Second, a seizure with the onset of a stroke is usually a sign of an embolic as opposed to a thrombotic stroke. Third, embolic occlusions may occur during any time of the day and often occur during periods of activity. Finally, embolic occlusions often produce neurologic deficits, even severe deficits, which are only temporary. With disintegration of the embolic material blood flow is restored and signs and symptoms change. Also of importance, infarction resulting from embolic occlusion is more likely to become hemorrhagic than is infarction from atherothrombotic occlusion.

Anticoagulation

Thrombolytic management now includes intra-arterial administration of tissue plasminogen activator (tPA), as well as various techniques such as a combination of ultrasound with tPA or catherization and disruption of the occlusion to break up the clot. The time to treatment is important. The best results are when time of onset of the stroke to treatment is less than 1 hour. Current practice for intravenous tPA administration is to treat within 4.5 hours (and up to 6 hours) of the onset of the stroke. Unfortunately, almost a third of acute strokes occur while the person is asleep, and it is not possible to establish when the stroke took place.

Patient selection is important in decisions regarding how to treat a person with an acute ischemic stroke. First, the patient must be medically stable. Individuals who have uncontrollable hypertension are not usually appropriate for such interventions, nor are individuals with recent surgery. Patients who have had neurosurgical procedures are at high risk for treatment complications. If the infarct is seen on CT scan to involve greater than 33 percent of the distribution of the middle cerebral artery, the risk of complications of intracerebral hemorrhage increases from 5 to 6 percent to almost 40 percent.

Following the acute management of the stroke, treatment recommendations include the use of statins, antiplatelet agents (aspirin, aspirin + extended-release dipyridamole or clopidogel) and lifestyle changes. If the patient has atrial fibrillation, then anticoagulation with warfarin or dibigatran is suggested.

ISCHEMIC STROKE SYNDROMES

Clinical Preview

You met Mrs. Vandermere in the last section of this chapter. When reading her medical chart, you learn that she had a thrombotic stroke in the territory of the right middle cerebral artery, extending into the right parietal lobe. Furthermore on repeat MRI, performed a day later, it is noted that the stroke also involves the right temporo-parietal-occipital junction. Mr. Carlson's stroke, in contrast, was in his left middle cerebral artery, but the location of the lesion is much more anterior, barely extending into the parietal lobe. On examination, you find that both of these individuals have difficulty walking. As you read through this chapter, consider the following:

- Given what you have learned so far, what impairments would you expect to find in each case?

- How is the location of the lesion (i.e., blood vessel involved, where in the vessel, and which side) important in predicting likely impairments?

- To what extent can you predict the location of a lesion from the constellation of impairments that occur?

- How does this information assist the rehabilitation professional in making choices regarding examination and intervention strategies?

The pathology and clinical consequences of ischemic strokes can be categorized in terms of the size of the vessel involved. Vessel size is related to the location of the artery. Each of the three major intracranial cerebral arteries is divided into three portions: a stem, penetrating branches, and cortical branches. The tables provided in this section illustrate the clinical syndromes of the three major cerebral arteries and differentiating symptoms associated with the stem, penetrating, and cortical branches of that artery. The stem has the largest diameter of any portion of the artery. In the case of the anterior cerebral artery (ACA) and middle cerebral artery (MCA), the stem is that portion of the vessel from its origin at the circle of Willis to the point where its penetrating branches arise to nourish deep structures of the cerebrum. In the case of the posterior cerebral artery (PCA), the stem is that portion of the artery from its origin at the bifurcation of the basilar artery to the point where it gives rise to its penetrating branches, which nourish the midbrain and diencephalon. The cortical or circumferential portions are the more distal portions of the vessel, draping over the cortex or brainstem. Occlusion of the stem of an intracranial artery will result in ischemia in the territories nourished by both the penetrating and cortical branches of the artery and, therefore, would result in the widest possible array of deficits from occlusion anywhere in the distribution of that artery.

> ## Thought Question
>
> In preparation for understanding the impact of left versus right hemispheric strokes, review the content in Chapters 21 and 22, and make a table of the specific impairments that are expressed in only one hemisphere or the other. Also, identify the location of the lesion for each symptom.

The penetrating branches of each intracranial artery are the smallest branches of that artery and nourish discrete areas of the brain. They can be occluded without involvement of either the stem or cortical branches and, therefore, would result in the most restricted array of deficits from occlusion anywhere else in that artery. After each vessel has attained the surface of the cerebral cortex, artery diameter decreases progressively as the branches of the artery course over the hemisphere. The cortical branches divide repeatedly into the named cortical branches that finally terminate in the artery's peripheral area of supply (refer to Chapter 7).

In summary, it is evident that the more proximal the location of an occlusion in a major cerebral artery nourishing the cerebral cortex, the more widespread the area of cortical ischemia and the greater the array and severity of clinical deficits. As the location of an occlusion shifts distally, the deficits become more discrete. For example, in the case of the MCA, occlusion of its superior division to the pars triangularis (inferior frontal lobe or Brodmann's area 45) in the dominant hemisphere proximal to the point where superior division branches have arisen would result in a Broca's aphasia plus motor deficits. In contrast, a more distal occlusion involving only a single branch of the superior division could result just in a nonfluent pattern of aphasia in which repetition is spared or just in cortical sensory and motor deficits.

> ## Thought Question
>
> The location of a lesion within the vessel involved is of critical importance in determining the extent of damage that will occur. Compare and contrast damage and extent of impairments that would be associated with a lesion in the following three areas: within the stem of the vessel, at the distal end of the territory of the vessel, and restricted to the penetrating vessels that arise from the main vessel.

It is noteworthy that large vessel disorders result most often from atherosclerotic disease. In contrast, medium and small vessel involvement, or cortical branch syndromes, typically result from embolism. In addition, there is a unique disorder that is due to occlusion of small, penetrating arteries. This is referred to as the lacunar strokes, and the disorders are called **lacunar syndromes**. Most often, lacunar syndromes are correlated to the consequences of a combination of hypertension or diabetes and not to atherosclerosis of these small vessels.

The pathology and clinical consequences of ischemic strokes can also be categorized by the territory of the cerebrum supplied by a vessel. Strokes associated with the anterior cerebral artery affect the most anterior-medial portions on the cerebrum, those associated with the middle cerebral artery affect the middle-lateral portions of the cerebrum, and those associated with the posterior cerebral artery affect the most posterior portions of the cerebrum. Considering all of the territories together, strokes may result in an unbelievably wide array of impairments, ranging from complicated changes in personality to an inability to perceive sensations correctly or to move parts of the body. However, the specific impairments that will occur with any particular stroke, as noted, are vessel dependent. Thus, it is helpful to learn stroke syndromes, based on the vessels involved. This serves two purposes: (1) this approach assists the reader to solidify an understanding of the functional correlates of different regions of the cerebrum, and (2) the reader learns to link vascularity to distribution, resulting impairments, and prognoses. For this reason, each of the following sections is organized by vascular distribution. Within the vascular distribution, the information is further organized by considering lesions affecting the stem versus the more distal distributions.

> ## Thought Question
>
> This is a good time to synthesize information in order to prepare for learning about impairments associated with specific vascular lesions. Review the vascular supply of the cerebrum, Brodmann's areas, and specialized roles of different parts of the cerebrum (see Chapters 7, 21, and 23 to get started). Drawing from this foundational information, make lists of the impairments that might occur with strokes associated with the following vessels: ACA, MCA, and PCA. How many different symptoms can you relate to each vascular territory?

Neuropathology Box 24-4: Muscle Tone Revisited

It should be noted that strokes in several different vascular distributions can lead to changes in muscle tone, which was originally introduced in Chapter 8. Muscle tone is the resistance muscle displays to passive stretch (lengthening) of a muscle. Muscle tone is usually lost for a period of days or weeks following a stroke. This condition may be manifest as a dense hemiplegia, sometimes referred to as *flaccid paralysis*. Note that, strictly speaking, *flaccid paralysis* should be reserved for lower motor neuron disorder, while *dense hemiplegia* should be used in the case of upper

motor neuron damage (such as in cortical strokes). The hemiplegia may remain flaccid in some patients, where the arm dangles uselessly at the patient's side and the leg must be braced in order to support the patient's weight in standing. In many patients, muscle tone gradually increases; eventually, the increase may become marked, resulting in a condition referred to *spasticity with hemiparesis*. Recall from Chapter 11 that spasticity is one component of the upper motor neuron syndrome.

Middle Cerebral Artery

Ischemic events and infarcts are more common in the MCA than in either the ACA or PCA. In part, this is because the MCA nourishes a larger portion of the cerebrum than the other arteries. Additionally, the MCA is more of a continuation of the internal carotid than is the ACA, such that an embolus in the internal carotid will be much more likely to travel into the MCA than the ACA. The most common cause of occlusion of the stem of the MCA is embolism, with less than 10 percent of occlusions resulting from a thrombus. Likewise, embolism is the most common cause of occlusion of the cortical branches of the MCA. Depending on the size of an embolus, it may lodge in vessels of different diameter. In general, infarction in the cortical territory of the MCA causes symptoms that may include contralateral weakness of the upper motor neuron (UMN) type; sensory loss of the cortical type, cognitive problems, or homonymous hemianopsia; and depending on the hemisphere involved, either an aphasia or impaired spatial perception.

Thought Question

An occlusion of the left MCA can result in various types of aphasias. Where is the lesion that produces each? Based on presence of each type of aphasia, what impairments of the motor and/or sensory systems would you anticipate? Thinking ahead, why would the constellation of symptoms be of importance to the rehabilitation professional who is responsible for determining prognosis and plan of care for patients with these different injuries?

As a general rule, occlusion of the internal carotid artery most often produces ischemia of the cerebral cortex within the peripheral and central territories of supply of the MCA. When the artery's main stem is occluded, infarction occurs not only in the cerebral convexity, but in the deep structures of the cerebrum that are nourished by the

penetrating branches of the MCA. Deficits are most severe when the internal carotid is occluded at the stem (proximally) because both the penetrating and distal vessels then are affected.

Progressing distally over the convexity of the hemisphere, artery diameter decreases progressively as the peripheral territory of supply is approached and the area of nourished tissue decreases. Thus, deficits become fewer and less severe the more distal the location of an occlusion in the artery (this applies also to the ACA and PCA). Deficits associated with infarcts distal to the stem of the MCA are likely to affect the upper extremity to a greater extent than the lower extremity. The reason is apparent when reviewing the motor and sensory homunculi (Chapter 7). Cognitive deficits can occur with more distal infarction. Finally, occlusion of penetrating branches of the MCA affects deep structures. For example, the internal capsule may be affected in which all of the corticospinal tracts converge into a small bundle (see Lacunar Syndromes).

Recall from Chapters 21 and 22 that the consequences of lesions affecting the left and right hemisphere can be quite different. When the dominant hemisphere is involved in the infarct, aphasia may occur. The aphasia is most often an expressive (motor, Broca's) aphasia. However, there may be a sensory (receptive, Wernicke's) aphasia or a mixed (global) aphasia if both the anterior and posterior speech areas are involved. When the nondominant hemisphere is involved, rather than aphasia, there may be problems with prosody or unilateral visuospatial perceptual deficits.

Deficits seen with infarcts in the territories supplied by the stem, penetrating, and cortical branches of the MCA are summarized in Table 24-1 ■. The expected differences, based on laterality, also are differentiated.

Anterior Cerebral Artery

Occlusion of the ACA is much less common than occlusion of the larger MCA. Occlusion of the ACA is generally embolic; rarely will the lesion be due to atherosclerosis.

Table 24-1 Clinical Syndromes of the MCA

LOCATION	AFFECTED TERRITORY	DEFICITS
Cortical left	Superior division (1a)	Spasticity, hemiparesis, inability to isolate specific muscle groups, and cortical (discriminative) sensory deficits of the right face greater than the right arm greater than the leg. Nonfluent, Broca's or conduction aphasia. Dysarthria. Usually, transient deviation of the head and eyes to the left (left-gaze preference). Occlusions affecting individual distal branches of the superior division may result in just one of these symptoms.
	Inferior division (1b)	Fluent, or Wernicke's, aphasia and a right homonymous hemianopsia. Bilateral ideomotor apraxia. Occlusions affecting individual distal branches of the inferior division may result in just one of these symptoms.
Cortical right	Superior division (1a)	Spasticity, hemiparesis, inability to isolate specific muscle groups, and cortical (discriminative) sensory deficits in the left face and arm. Dysarthria. Usually, transient deviation of the head and eyes to the right (right-gaze preference). Occlusions affecting individual distal branches may result in just one of these symptoms.
	Inferior division (1b)	Left visuospatial neglect and other disorders of spatial perception (e.g., constructional apraxia). Left homonymous hemianopsia. When right hemisphere lesions involving the motor area of the frontal lobe extend into the parietal lobe, the patient may be unaware of, or indifferent to, the paralyzed arm (*anosoagnosia*). Defective recognition of the emotional content of speech.
	Penetrating (2)	Pure motor syndrome consisting of contralateral spasticity with hemiparesis in which there is equal involvement of the face, arm, and leg. Pure sensory syndrome and may affect only one limb.
	Stem (3)	Combination of the previous penetrating and cortical syndromes lateralized to the side of the main stem lesion. Generally, the motor and sensory deficits will be very severe. With left-sided main stem occlusion, the language deficit will be a global aphasia.

Occlusion of the stem of one ACA proximal to its connection with the anterior communicating artery is usually well tolerated and may cause no symptoms at all. This is because the ACA distal to the occlusion receives sufficient collateral circulation from the opposite ACA from the anterior communicating artery or numerous collaterals between the distal branches along the corpus callosum. In general, involvement of the cortical branches of one ACA causes UMN-type weakness and cortical-type sensory deficits primarily affecting the contralateral leg, as well as bowel and bladder function (Figure 24-7a ■). If the upper extremity is affected, the shoulder typically is more impaired than the hand (opposite to the consequences of MCA infarct). Maximal deficits are caused by bilateral infarctions when blood flow in both ACAs is arrested. This can occur when the person has a congenital anomaly of the circle of Willis and both ACAs arise from one ACA stem and the stem becomes occluded (Figure 24-7b). The resultant infarction would involve the medial frontal-parietal areas, including the orbital/mediobasal surfaces of both hemispheres.

In addition to a cortical sensory-motor syndrome involving both lower extremities from the bilateral paracentral lobule infarctions, a severe behavioral disturbance results from orbital/mediobasal prefrontal cortex infarctions. There are wide oscillations of affect with episodes of excitation and euphoria that may be superimposed on a background of abulia and apathy; behavioral disinhibition with outbursts of irritability; and loosened social control and judgment as manifested by erotic behavior, sexual exhibitionism, lewd remarks, and inappropriate jokes. There may also be a significant apraxia of the nondominant hand from damage to the corpus callosum, depriving the supplementary motor cortex and motor areas in the nondominant hemisphere of information from the dominant hemisphere. In this case, the person can imitate a gesture with the dominant hand but cannot do so with the nondominant hand. Deficits seen with infarction in the territories nourished by the stem, penetrating, and cortical branches of the ACA are summarized in Table 24-2 ■.

Table 24-2 Clinical Syndromes of the ACA

LOCATION	AFFECTED TERRITORY	DEFICITS
Cortical	Left	Spasticity with hemiparesis and cortical (discriminative) sensory deficits of the right leg. May include a frontal-type alien hand syndrome with reflexive grasping. Disorder of speech initiation.
	Right	Spasticity with hemiparesis and cortical (discriminative) sensory deficits of the left leg. May be frontal-type alien hand syndrome with reflexive grasping.
	Corpus callosum	Apraxia of the nondominant hand. May include a callosal-type alien hand syndrome.
Penetrating	Medial striate (Heubner)	With unilateral lesions, unpredictable combinations of dysarthria, abulia, agitation and hyperactivity, contralateral visuospatial neglect, and language difficulty. For bilateral lesions, see "Stem" entry.
Stem	Unilateral	Combination of the previous penetrating and cortical syndromes lateralized to the side of the stem lesion.
	Bilateral	Severe change in personality and affect in which there may be abulia (apathy), inattentiveness, forgetfulness, motor inertia, akinetic mutism, agitation, and psychosis. Urinary incontinence. Suck and grasp reflexes.

Thought Question

What is the likely basis for the apathy exhibited by some people after sustaining a stroke involving the ACA? Would you anticipate this deficit with lesions of the left ACA, right ACA, or both? Why?

Posterior Cerebral Artery

In general, unilateral occlusion of the PCA results in a contralateral homonymous hemianopsia that may be complete or incomplete. Examination of the visual field helps the clinician differentiate where the injury is. Injuries to the geniculocalcarine system closer to the lateral geniculate nucleus will result in a contralateral homonymous hemianopsia in which macular vision is likely to be lost. These symptoms indicate that the injury is deeper and more likely to involve the stem of the posterior cerebral artery, or even the middle cerebral artery deep vessels. If there is sparing of the macular vision (referred to as macular sparing), then the lesion is more likely to be in the distribution of the more distal vessels of the posterior cerebral artery involving the calcarine cortex. Even more distal artery involvement can result in quadrantic visual losses if the embolus lodges in the vessels supplying the superior or inferior calcarine cortex (see Chapter 18).

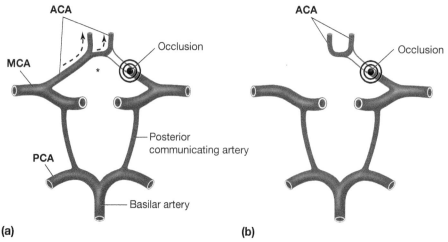

FIGURE 24-7 Ventral view of the circle of Willis. (a) When the left anterior cerebral artery is occluded as shown, the anterior cerebral artery distal to the occlusion may still receive adequate blood from the right anterior cerebral artery via the anterior communicating artery located above the asterisk. (b) When both anterior cerebral arteries arise from one ACA stem, occlusion of that stem results in an infarction involving both sides of the brain.

Table 24-3 **Clinical Syndromes of the PCA**

LOCATION	AFFECTED TERRITORY	DEFICITS
Cortical	Left	Right homonymous hemianopsia. Alexia without agraphia when the splenium of the corpus callosum also is involved.
	Right	Left homonymous hemianopsia.
	Bilateral	Billateral homonymous hemianopsia (blindness); Anton's syndrome (Chapter 18); Balint's syndrome's (Chapter 18); amnestic syndrome (transient global amnesia); retrograde and anterograde amnesia; prosopagnosia (Chapter 21).
Penetrating	Paramedian (Brainstem)	Weber's syndrome (Chapter 15); Benedikt's syndrome (Chapter 15).
	Thalamoperforate (Diencephalon)	Hemiballismus.
	Thalamoperforate (Diencephalon)	Thalamic syndrome (thalamic pain) (Chapter 16).
Stem		A mixture of the cortical and penetrating branch syndromes.

When a lesion in the PCA involves the dominant (usually left) hemisphere and includes the posterior corpus callosum (the splenium), **alexia** (inability to read) **without agraphia** (inability to write) results. Such people often have **anomia** (inability to name) for colors and various **visual agnosias**. Bilateral cortical lesions may occur as a result of a single embolic or thrombotic occlusion of the upper basilar artery, particularly if the posterior communicating arteries are especially small. Such lesions may result in bilateral homonymous hemianopsia (cortical blindness), but other visual field defects (scotomas) can occur depending on the size and location of the lesions. **Anton's** and **Balint's syndromes** (see Chapter 18) can also occur. When bilateral lesions involve the inferomedial temporal lobes, severe memory impairment can occur. These individuals may have relatively intact intelligence but may be unable to form new memories. They instead confabulate or make up responses. When the bilateral lesions involve both the inferomedial temporal and occipital lobes, a lack of facial recognition (**prosopagnosia**) may occur (see Chapter 21). Deficits seen with infarction in the territories supplied by the stem, penetrating, and cortical branches of the PCA are summarized in Table 24-3 ■. As indicated in that table, strokes in the PCA can affect the brainstem and subcortical structures.

Neuropathology Box 24-5: Bruits and the Internal Carotid Artery

The neurologic deficits resulting from atherothrombotic occlusion of the internal carotid artery are more variable than with occlusion of any other vessel. In some cases, occlusion of one internal carotid artery may not produce any deficits at all if the collateral supply from other vessels is adequate. In other cases, occlusion may result in a massive infarction of the anterior two-thirds of the entire cerebral hemisphere, which can lead to significant and permanent disability, or even death, in a few days. As noted earlier, favored locations for stenosis in this system are at the bifurcation of the common carotid artery into the external and internal carotid arteries and at the carotid siphon. The branches of the internal carotid artery in their order of occurrence are the ophthalmic artery, the posterior communicating artery, the anterior choroidal artery, the ACA, and the MCA (Figure 24-8 ■).

The presence of blockage in the common and internal carotid arteries can be evaluated directly in contrast to other cerebral arteries, where stenosis is determined either by the resulting clinical deficits or by diagnostic imaging procedures such as MRI or CT scanning. Direct evaluation is done by placing a stethoscope on certain sites in the neck and listening for sounds generated as a result of the turbulent flow of blood in the arteries. Turbulence is caused by a narrowing (stenosis) of the vessel lumen. The sound is called a bruit (Fr., noise). When bruit is heard at the angle of the jaw, the area of stenosis and turbulent flow is at the bifurcation of the common and internal carotid arteries (i.e., in the carotid sinus) (Figure 24-9 ■). When bruit is heard lower in the neck, just above the clavicle, the stenosis is in the common carotid or subclavian arteries. Stenoses that are not tight enough or those that are too tight may generate no bruit at all. An ominous sign is the loss of a previously heard bruit. This could imply the artery has been completely obstructed.

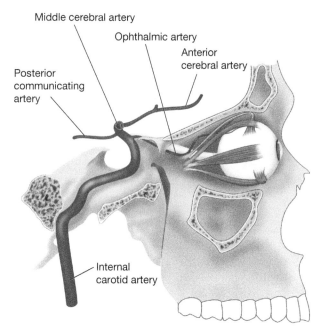

FIGURE 24-8 Branches of the right internal carotid artery.

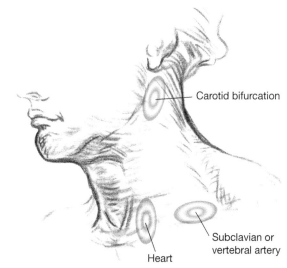

FIGURE 24-9 Diagram to show the localization of different cervical bruits. A bruit under the angle of the jaw results from stenosis at the carotid bifurcation. Bruits above the clavicle are caused by occlusions at the origin of either the subclavian or vertebral arteries.

Carotid Border-Zone Syndromes/ Watershed Infarcts

Carotid artery dysfunction can result in reduction of blood flow through the system as a whole. With an appreciation of middle and anterior syndromes, it is possible to understand the effects of this condition. Specifically, if there is blockage in the carotid artery, a drop in blood pressure further reduces blood flow. This results in hypoperfusion, especially to the distal areas where the most distal vessels of the MCA and ACA meet (Figure 24-10 ■). This is referred to as the watershed area. When hypoperfusion is sufficient to cause

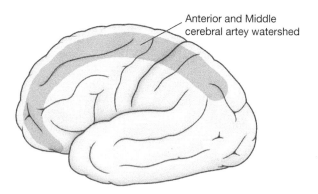

FIGURE 24-10 The watershed area on the lateral surface of the left hemisphere (shaded) formed by the middle and anterior cerebral arteries. The watershed area is in the peripheral territories of each artery and represents the zone of maximal ischemia, with stenosis of the internal carotid artery on that side. The peripheral territory of the posterior cerebral artery is not shown.

an infarct the consequence is referred to as the **watershed** or **carotid border-zone syndrome**. Note that the watershed infarcts can occur as a result of congestive heart failure and severe hypotension, in addition to atherosclerotic disease of the carotid vessels. Similarly, a watershed infarct can occur in the distribution at the border zone between the MCA and PCA.

The internal carotid artery usually is at least 70 percent occluded in order to produce the carotid border-zone syndrome. With this degree of stenosis, blood flow in the artery distal to the occlusion is decreased significantly but is not eliminated. In this situation, the peripheral territories of both the middle and anterior cerebral arteries represent the zone of maximal ischemia. This zone is called the watershed area.

Maximal ischemia occurs in the watershed area because it requires the greatest pressure for blood to reach the terminal ends of the two arteries, where the vessels have the smallest diameter. The area of maximal ischemia is also referred to as the border zone between the middle and anterior cerebral arteries—hence, the clinical name of carotid border-zone syndrome. The portion of the border zone representing the shoulder in the pre- and postcentral gyri is greater than the portion representing the hand. The border zone is also the most vulnerable cortical area in cases of transient ischemic attacks with stenosis of the internal carotid artery and cardiac output changes. If the lesion involves the dominant hemisphere, a pattern of aphasia can occur (transcortical motor aphasia, in which repetition is better than spontaneous speech). If the lesion involves the border zone between the middle cerebral artery and the posterior cerebral artery of the dominant hemisphere, a syndrome referred to as Gerstmann's syndrome may be clinically apparent.

Lacunar Syndromes

When an occlusion affects only the penetrating vessels (lacunes), sensory and/or motor deficits typically occur without cognitive deficits (Figure 24-11 ■). With penetrating vessel disease, the symptoms tend to affect the face, arm,

Neuropathology Box 24-6: Gerstmann's Syndrome

In 1940, Gerstmann described a syndrome consisting of acalculia, agraphia, finger agnosia, and right–left disorientation. He interpreted this constellation of symptoms to represent a disturbance of body schema arising from left parietal lobe disease. This syndrome, localizing a lesion to the posterior parietal region of the dominant hemisphere, was of importance in early recognition of laterality of the brain.

and leg equally. This is because the pathways are so tightly organized in the internal capsule. This contrasts markedly with the consequences of distal vessel occlusion of the MCA and ACA—in which case, it is possible for the face and arm to be more affected than the leg or vice versa. This is because the pathways are more diffusely organized within the cortex as illustrated by the homunculus (Chapter 8).

Thought Question

Which of the following types of impairments could potentially accompany lacunar strokes and which would not: motor, somatosensory, sensory perceptual, Broca's aphasia, emotional lability, graphaestheia, and ataxia?

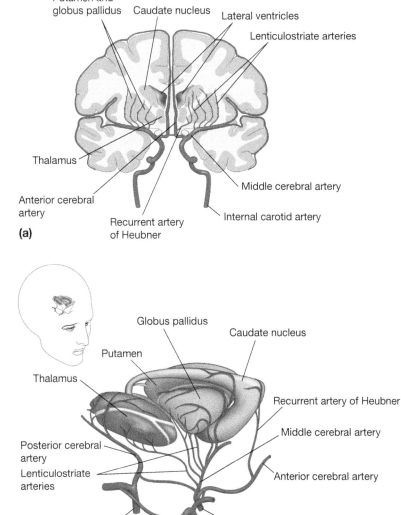

(a)

(b)

FIGURE 24-11 Deep-penetrating vessels. (a) Coronal section of the cortex illustrating the lenticulostriate arteries arising from the middle cerebral artery and the recurrent artery of Huebner arising from the anterior cerebral artery. (b) Illustration of the deep-penetrating vessels that arise from all of the major vessels to supply the basal ganglia and thalamus.

The lacunar stroke is pathologically unique in that it results from a different pathology than atherothrombotic disease and is due to small infarcts in the penetrating branches of the cerebral arteries. The term **lacune** is applied to the small cavity (*pit* or *lake*) that results in the process of healing when the dead brain cells are removed in the process. Lacunar pathology is correlated with chronic hypertension, diabetes, or a combination of these disorders. Lacunae can range from 3 to 15 mm in diameter. Whether they cause symptoms depends on their location. Lacunae occur most frequently in the caudate nucleus and putamen; in these locations, they are typically asymptomatic. In order of frequency, other locations susceptible to lacunar infarctions include the thalamus, basal pons, internal capsule, and deep white matter of the cerebral hemisphere. While there are many lacunar syndromes, the most common are pure motor hemiplegia, pure sensory stroke, dysarthria–clumsy hand syndrome, and ipsilateral ataxic hemiparesis, each of which is discussed.

When lacunae occur in the vascular territory of the **lenticulostriate arteries** (in the posterior limb of the internal capsule [anterior portion] or adjacent corona radiata), a **pure motor stroke**, resulting in pure motor hemiplegia, that involves the face (lower half), arm, hand, leg, and foot. This is referred to as *capsular hemiplegia*. Here, all descending corticofugal projections to the brainstem and spinal cord are tightly organized as they pass through the internal capsule. As a consequence, involvement of these body parts is of equal severity, which is in contrast to cortical branch (distal) syndromes, where there is a differential body part involvement as described earlier.

Lacunar involvement of the ventral pons (infarction in the territory of the penetrating branches of the basilar artery) may also result in a pure motor stroke, although not identical to that from lenticulostriate involvement. Lacunae involving the lateral thalamus (VPL/VPM) or, less often,

parietal white matter (corona radiata) cause a **pure sensory stroke**, resulting in a somatosensory loss to all primary modalities in the contralateral face, arm, and body extending to the midline. Lacunar involvement of the ventral pons may cause the **dysarthria–clumsy hand syndrome**, characterized by a clumsiness of the hand contralateral to the lesion site and dysarthria from intramedullary cranial nerve lesions. **Ipsilateral ataxic hemiparesis** may follow lacunar infarcts in ventral pons in the posterior limb of the internal capsule or parietal white matter (corona radiata). The ataxia is on the same side as the weakness. Table 24-4 ■ summarizes the most common lacunar syndromes.

It is not uncommon for a person with a lacunar infarction to develop more such infarctions. Multiple lacunar infarctions can produce the *lacunar state*. When multiple lacunar infarcts affect the posterior limb of the internal capsule *bilaterally*, **pseudobulbar palsy** may result. The usual history of a person who develops pseudobulbar palsy is that he or she suffered numerous lacunar infarcts involving corticobulbar fibers of the posterior limb of the internal capsule on one side of the brain at an earlier point in time that may have been asympotomatic. Because of the bilateral cortical innervation of some cranial nerve motor nuclei, infarcts involving corticobulbar fibers on just one side will not produce a permanent impairment in speech or swallowing. However, when both sides are involved, damage to the corticobulbar fibers in both the right and left internal capsules produces the syndrome referred to as pseudobulbar palsy. The symptoms characterizing pseudobulbar palsy are numerous. A major group of symptoms involve speech and include dysarthria (in which the person is unable to produce speech [articulate] normally) and dysphonia (in which the person is unable to properly make voiced sounds by vibration of the vocal cords). If the individual is asked to produce (phonate) a prolonged vowel, such as *ah*, there is more air than sound

Table 24-4 Common Lacunar Syndromes

SYNDROME	CLINICAL FINDINGS	SITE OF LESION (PREFERRED)	POSSIBLE VESSELS INVOLVED
Pure motor hemiplegia	Unilateral spasticity and weakness with equal involvement of face, arm, and leg	Posterior limb of internal capsule; ventral pons	Lenticulostriate penetrating branches of MCA; penetrating branches of basilar artery
Pure sensory stroke	Loss of all primary sensory modalities in contralateral face and body	VPL/VPM*	Thalamogeniculate penetrating branches of PCA
Dysarthria–clumsy hand	Deficit in speech articulation; clumsiness of contralateral hand	Ventral pons	Paramedian penetrating branches of basilar artery
Ataxic hemiparesis	Unilateral ataxia and weakness	Ventral pons	Penetrating branches of basilar artery

*VPL: ventral posterolateral nucleus of the thalamus; VPM: ventral posteromedial nucleus of the thalamus

in the vowel. A number of deficits occur related to eating. Dysphagia occurs in which the individual cannot swallow properly and cannot move his or her tongue. There is spasticity and paresis of the muscles of mastication so that the person cannot chew; this is accompanied by an exaggerated jaw-jerk reflex. The person cannot elevate the soft palate, so there is a nasal regurgitation of food.

In addition, there is spasticity and paresis of the entire face on both sides so that the individual cannot wrinkle the forehead, forcefully close the eyes, or elevate and retract the corners of the mouth in a voluntary smile. Movement of all these muscles may be preserved in spontaneous movements such as yawning, coughing, and clearing of the throat.

Also, spasmodic (pathologic) laughing and crying can occur. In pathologic laughing, the person is thrown into gales of laughter for no apparent reason or at the slightest provocation. Hilarious laughter may continue to the point of exhaustion. Pathologic crying occurs more often. This may be the reflexive response to something that may usually cause joy and laughter. The mention of possibly emotionally laden topics, even mentioning the family in conversation, may cause the individual to go into a bout of uncontrollable crying. These symptoms occur because the person loses inhibition from cortical structures over the brainstem centers involved in behaviors such as laughing and crying.

Finally, multiple lacunar infarctions can also cause a clinical picture referred to as pseudo-Parkinsonism. Additionally they can result in a pattern of dementia referred to as **subcortical dementia**.

Thought Question

In your rehabilitation practice, you notice that certain people with strokes are more likely to have emotional outbursts and difficulty initiating well-known movements than other patients with whom you work. What does this suggest to you about the blood supply that was likely affected? Thinking ahead, what does this suggest to you about prognosis and the appropriate rehabilitation strategies?

CLINICAL CONNECTIONS

Prognosis

If an individual survives a completed stroke, the long-term prognosis usually favors improvement. The extent of the infarct is important. At one extreme, recovery may begin and be virtually complete even within hours, or in a day or two in people with small infarcts. At the other extreme, people with severe deficits may not have meaningful improvement even after months of intense rehabilitation. The prognosis becomes poorer the longer the delay in the beginning of recovery. It is believed by many that, in general, whatever impairments remain after five or six months will be permanent, although their severity may decrease over time. On the other hand, some evidence suggests that improvement can

continue over extended periods, as long as 10 years. It should be noted that improvement should be considered both in terms of neurological improvement and functional improvement. There may be considerable potential for functional improvement, even in the case of lesions in which neurological changes have stabilized. The impact of high-intensity rehabilitation is currently under extensive investigation.

Medical Prognosis

When a patient is initially comatose or stuporous, it usually indicates that the infarction is large and there is considerable edema. Edema is the body's response to injury and occurs with all tissue injury, including injury to the brain. Brain edema in patients who have stroke reaches its maximum in three or four days, then slowly subsides. The degree of edema that develops and its location can markedly influence the short-term prognosis.

With regard to medical management, immediately poststroke, CT scans are necessary to indicate whether the stroke is ischemic or hemorrhagic. If the stroke is ischemic, thrombolytic therapy or anticoagulation can be used, with the goal of decreasing the extent of the lesion. If the stroke is hemorrhagic, those therapies are contraindicated. The CT also indicates the size of the infarct, which determines whether thrombolytic therapy can be used. An MRI can indicate which specific areas are infarcted and is particularly helpful in visualizing small embolic infarctions and lacunar infarctions. The MRI typically is administered a few days poststroke because it takes time for the full extent of the infarction to become apparent. Other diagnostic tests are used to determine what type of neurological insult has occurred (e.g., stroke, aneurysm, tumor) (see Box 24-7).

Functional Prognosis

The vessel that is occluded and the territories that undergo ischemic injury determine the functional effects of ischemic strokes. Hence, knowledge of location of a patient's lesion can greatly assist the rehabilitation specialist to develop a treatment plan based on prognosis. In some cases, the location of the insult is available from neurological reports; in other cases, the rehabilitation professional works backward from the patient's signs and symptoms to hypothesize the lesion location.

The location of the lesion and resulting impairments also provide the key pieces of information used in predicting the extent of functional recovery. With respect to location of lesion, disability from most to least severe is generally associated with the following: large strokes, the presence of edema or hemorrhage, strokes in more than one vascular territory, and strokes in a single vascular territory with greatest to least disability as follows: MCA, ACA, PCA, brainstem, cerebellar, and small vessels. In addition to knowing which vessel is involved, the rehabilitation specialist should know whether the involvement is in the distal or proximal territory of the vessel. Distal territory lesions of any of the three major vessels (MCA, ACA, and PCA) are smaller and have less severe consequences than

Neuropathology Box 24-7: Procedures Used in Diagnosis of Cortical Damage

- **Computed tomography (CT)** is used within 20 minutes of the time that the patient arrives at the hospital to determine whether there is a hemorrhage and the size of the infarct; with hemorrhage or large infarcts, tissue plasminogen activator (tPA) would be contraindicated.
- **Magnetic resonance imaging (MRI)** is used to define the specific tissue damage that cannot be picked up by the CT scan (e.g., small embolic infarcts and lacunes).
- **MRI diffusion-weighted studies** can be used within 30 minutes to an hour following the event to determine

whether a completed stroke has occurred or if the patient has experienced a TIA.
- **Contrast computerized tomography angiogram (CTA)** is particularly sensitive to thrombotic disease or embolic occlusion and is very sensitive in detecting aneurysms and AVMs and to image extracranial vasculature in the person who has a completed stroke.
- **Magnetic resonance arteriogram (MRA)** is useful to examine vascular structures (e.g., arterial venous malformations [AVMs] and aneurysms) and to image extracranial vasculature in the person who has a completed stroke.

do proximal territory lesions within the cortex in these vessels. With respect to impairments, the following are associated with greater functional deficits: older age, cognitive dysfunction, neglect, and ideomotor apraxia.

Finally, the location of the lesion provides insight regarding appropriate intervention strategies. If the MCA is occluded, the patient is likely to have both somatosensory and motor loss because of the areas of the cortex that are perfused by this artery. If the lesion primarily affects the parietal cortex, the primary involvement is somatosensory. Yet, this latter patient may have motor deficits stemming from the somatosensory loss. The intervention strategies for a patient with motor deficits related to both motor and somatosensory cortical involvement can differ substantially from the strategies used for the patient with somatosensory loss only leading to motor deficits. Imaging data can assist the clinician to determine whether loss of motor function results from involvement of the motor structures themselves (frontal cortex) or from motor and somatosensory structures (frontal and parietal cortex), or whether loss of motor function is a result of somatosensory loss alone (parietal cortex) without motor structure involvement. Similarly, damage to structures in the premotor cortex will have very different consequences than damage to structures in the prefrontal cortex, again with implications for rehabilitation.

The prognosis for neurological as well as functional recovery provides the rehabilitation professional with a starting point when making decisions about the type of strategy that will be used: remediation (or improvement of underlying deficits) versus compensation for those deficits. Often, in the acute and rehabilitation settings, the rehabilitation professional joins in making decisions regarding placement (home versus long-term care). Knowledge regarding the location and extent of the patient's lesion are of importance in assisting with these decisions. Furthermore, standardized measurement tools can be used to predict the likelihood of functional recovery following a stroke. The National Institute

of Health Stroke Scale (NIHSS) is highly recommended for this purpose (see Table 24-5, provided later).

Further complicating the prognosis for functional recovery from stroke is that many individuals have a number of co-morbid conditions. These co-morbid conditions (e.g., cardiac disease, diabetes, cognitive dysfunction) can greatly affect the overall prognosis for functional return.

Imaging and the Location of the Lesion

One of the skills needed by the rehabilitation professional is the ability to link cross-sectional representations of the cerebrum with their three-dimensional structure and to identify the structures that are located in the cross sections. This is analogous to linking cross sections of the brainstem with the three-dimensional structure, which was the topic of Chapter 15. The content of the cross section of the cerebrum depends on the plane from which the section was taken. Perhaps the most frequently used are those sections taken in the plane of CT scans or MRI scans. Figure 24-12 ■ provides just such representations. Furthermore, the distribution of the major arteries is highlighted within these representative cross sections.

Thought Question

Here is a task that will help synthesize all of the information you have learned about infarcts associated with the major vasculature of the brain. For infarcts of each of the main vessels: (1) make a list of key anatomical structures that are affected at each level represented in the cross sections of Figure 24-12, (2) differentiate cortical from subcortical structures, and (3) identify the likely constellation of symptoms associated with each infarct. Then consider what the distribution might look like if the infarct were in the distal vessel as opposed to the proximal vessels depicted here.

Examination

A detailed discussion of examination and intervention is beyond the scope of this text. However, some examples of the role that lesion location plays in this process are summarized in this section and the next.

Many people have difficulty with balance, postural control, and gait, following a stroke. Typically, these deficits are examined using a similar battery of tests and measures. A few representative measures, used widely in neurological physical therapy, are summarized in Table 24-5 ■. However, quantifying and describing these deficits is not sufficient for development of a targeted intervention strategy. In addition, it is necessary to understand the underlying causes of these deficits (e.g., somatosensory, motor). Hence, examination strategies are needed to identify the likely underlying impairments. For example, a person with a stroke in the ACA is most likely to have impairments of motor organization, could have apraxia and problems with motivation, but is not likely to have somatosensory loss. Thus, it is probable that the causes of deficits of balance, gait, and postural control are most directly related to the former impairments. In contrast, a person with a stroke in the MCA territory may have impairments of the motor system, somatosensory system, and potentially even the visual systems (from the penetrating vessels supplying the posterior limb of the internal capsule). Thus, loss or impairment of somatosensory awareness can contribute to the deficits of balance control and gait. And a person with a more posterior lesion from MCA (or a lesion of the PCA extending more anteriorly) is likely to have problems of association, resulting in neglect, spatial planning, prosopagnosia, and the like. Hence, the clinician should be particularly sensitive to testing for these impairments in that case. By knowing or hypothesizing the location of the lesion, the clinician can make judicious choices regarding the tests and measures that will be used in the examination process.

Second, the hemispheric location of the stroke should prompt the clinician to perform certain tests. For example, a patient with a right hemisphere lesion is more likely to have difficulties with construction and spatial perception, whereas a person with a comparable lesion in the left hemisphere is more likely to have difficulties with language and apraxia. Assessment of spatial perceptual ability would be indicated for people with a right MCA lesion, and assessment of language ability and praxis would be indicated for people with left MCA lesion.

In summary, by utilizing information about the size and location of a patient's lesion, the clinician can make informed decisions regarding appropriate examination strategies for specific patients. Additionally, this information provides the clinician with insight that assists in the interpretation of causes underlying deficits of balance, gait, and overall function.

Intervention

Knowledge regarding location of lesions associated with ischemic stroke can assist with decisions regarding the rehabilitation strategy. Prognosis, location of the damage, and extent of the damage all provide valuable information.

First is an estimation of the prognosis for the patient—both in terms of physiological recovery and in terms of functional recovery. It is important to recognize from the outset that these may be very different.

Table 24-5 Representative Examination Outcome Measures for Use with People Who Have Had Strokes

ASSESSMENT TOOL/OUTCOME MEASURE	APPLICATION/DESCRIPTION
Functional reach test (FR)	Single item test used to screen for balance and fall risk
Berg Balance Scale (BBS)	14-item test used to determine balance and fall risk
Dynamic Gait Index (DGI)	8-item test used to measure functional mobility in gait and fall risk
10-meter walk test	Used to measure gait speed over a 10-meter distance
6-minute walk test	Used to measure endurance/distance walked in 6 minutes
Fugl-Meyer Motor Performance and Sensory Assessment	A 50-item scale that investigates motor, somatosensory, and reflex function in people with hemiplegia; also available in a 12-item format
Stroke Impact Scale (SIS)	A self-report measure of 64 items in 8 domains to assess quality of life following stroke
The National Institutes of Health Stroke Scale (NIHSS)	11-item scale used to quantify stroke severity and predict recovery from stroke
Functional Independence Measure (FIM)	18-item scale used to quantify physical mobility, self-care, and cognitive abilities; primarily an inpatient tool

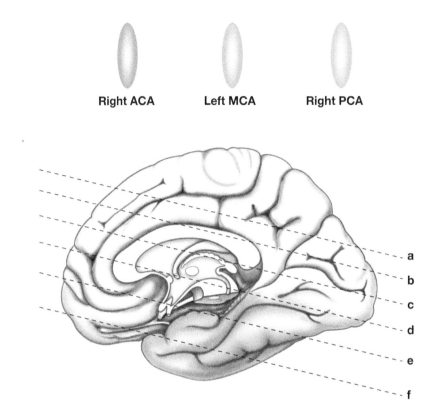

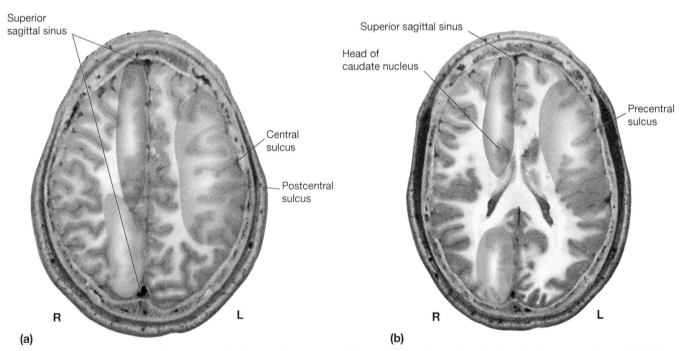

FIGURE 24-12 An example of infarcts to the three major vessels of the cerebrum, illustrating the broad affect spanning multiple levels. The distribution of lesions associated with proximal infarcts to the anterior, middle, and posterior cerebral arteries are depicted at six levels. The side of the vessel that was infarcted is indicated at the top of the figure. Note that the right side of the image represents the left side of the brain in a CT scan.

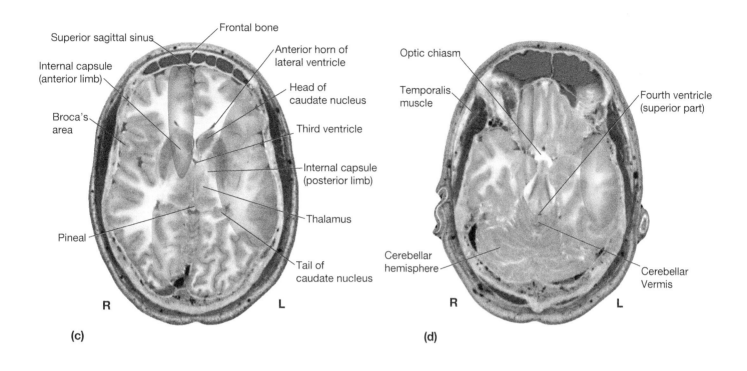

(c)

(d)

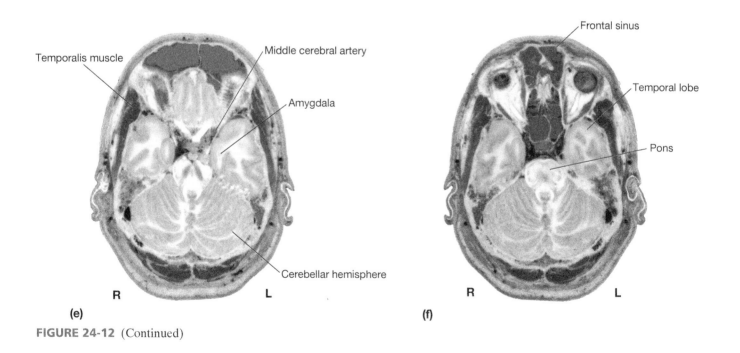

(e)

(f)

FIGURE 24-12 (Continued)

For example, a person may sustain permanent losses, including hemiplegia and global aphasia, and yet be able to compensate such that he or she has relatively limited functional loss. That is, some such persons are able to live independently. Both aspects of recovery should be thus considered separately.

Second, the rehabilitation professional is frequently part of the decision-making team that determines where a patient will go after discharge. For example, will a patient in an acute care setting be discharged to home, subacute rehabilitation, or a skilled nursing facility? Similarly, should a patient from a subacute facility be discharged home or to a skilled nursing facility? The rehabilitation specialist's contributions to these discussions can be greatly enhanced if he or she understands the underlying neuroanatomical damage and its implications for motor, sensory, and functional recovery.

Third, the clinician makes decisions about the approach to rehabilitation. Rehabilitation strategies almost always include a combination of *restorative strategies* designed to remediate underlying impairments and function, *compensatory strategies* designed to bypass underlying impairments and function that are not likely to improve, and *preventive strategies* designed to avoid future impairments and additional pathology that could further compromise the patient's ability to function. As examples, a person who has severe difficulty walking because of motor and somatosensory loss may need to compensate for these impairments by using a walker or wheelchair, whereas restorative strategies are appropriate for a person with more mild loss who may be able to overcome these deficits and return to independent walking without such assistive devices. For almost all patients, preventive strategies should be included to prevent skin breakdown, further injury and falls, loss of range of motion, altered postural alignment, deconditioning from changes in activity, and importantly, future stroke.

Fourth are the decisions related to the global focus of the intervention strategy. The overall purpose of rehabilitation is to improve a person's ability to function and participate in desired activities. To this end, it is increasingly clear that intervention strategies should focus on function (as opposed to overemphasizing underlying impairments). And indeed, a major focus of rehabilitation relates to restoration of function. However, decisions related to the approach to intervention should also take into account an understanding of the underlying impairments that interfere with function. In this regard, it is important to decide whether it is appropriate to improve an underlying impairment as a means of improving function. For example, it is likely that strategies to enhance sensory input will benefit the person who has somatosensory loss contributing to motor and functional loss if the person has some remaining somatosensation. On the other hand, somatosensory input will be of little value to the person who has a total loss of somatosensation. Similarly, an individual with a profound somatosensory loss who still has an ability to attend and compensate will benefit much more from sensory techniques that utilize other (intact) sensory systems than will an individual with a severe neglect (e.g., somatosensory or visual neglect). As another example, there is increasing evidence that people following a cerebrovascular accident (CVA) have specific muscle weakness that can be improved with rehabilitation. At the same time, the person needs to have sufficient motor control for this to be feasible. Knowledge of the location and extent of a lesion can assist the clinician to make educated decisions about which patients are likely to recover sufficient capacity in the sensory and motor systems such that it is appropriate to target specific underlying impairments in the intervention.

Fifth are the decisions related to specifics of the intervention strategy. Several specific strategies have received considerable experimental attention over the past two decades. Included are body weight–supported treadmill training and constraint-induced movement therapy. These strategies allow high-intensity practice of relevant functional tasks. In body weight–supported training, also called locomotor training, the person walks on a treadmill with some of the body weight supported by a harness. The clinician can vary the amount of body weight support provided to a particular patient depending on the degree of hemiparesis present in the lower extremity. In constraint-induced movement therapy, the person's uninvolved hand is gloved such that he or she is forced to use the involved hand for function. The clinician chooses relevant tasks and manipulates the difficulty of those tasks based on the constellation of impairments present. These strategies are further discussed in Chapter 26, which addresses brain plasticity.

Another strategy, functional electrical stimulation (FES), also deserves mention. FES is the use of neuromuscular electrostimulation in combination with functional tasks to improve recruitment of paretic or weak muscles. Common applications include hemiparetic wrist extensors with grasp and anterior tibialis during gait.

HEMORRHAGIC STROKE

Clinical Preview ················

Antonio Pescarelli was admitted to the ICU where you work. He had sustained a hemorrhagic stroke and now is in a stuporous state. You note on reading his medical chart that he is being treated with mannitol. As you read through this section, consider the following:

- Why is mannitol used to treat patients who have hemorrhagic strokes?

- Can you predict at the time that a patient is in the ICU what will be the functional outcome?

- To what extent can you predict the impairments that will result from a hemorrhage?

With hemorrhagic disorders, arteries rupture and blood floods from the broken vessel directly into intracranial structures, brain tissue, the ventricles of the brain, or the subarachnoid space. The main types of hemorrhagic strokes include primary intracerebral hemorrhage, rupture of aneurysms resulting from congenital factors or infection, rupture of arteriovenous malformations, trauma, and breakdown of small vessels that have been weakened by amyloid or bleeding into tumors, especially those that are metastatic. In primary intracerebral hemorrhage, there is a direct leakage of blood from an artery into brain tissue. Primary intracerebral hemorrhage is mainly associated with chronic hypertension and degenerative changes in cerebral arteries. **Subarachnoid hemorrhage** is bleeding into the subarachnoid space surrounding the brain and spinal cord, usually associated with the rupture of cerebral (also called saccular or berry) aneurysms. The rupture of an **arteriovenous malformation** also leads to brain hemorrhage. Trauma can result in **subdural hemorrhage**, wherein there is venous bleeding into the potential space beneath the dura mater covering the brain. Trauma can also induce **epidural hemorrhage**, which represents arterial bleeding from a torn meningeal artery with the blood accumulating outside the dura mater. These types of traumatic intracranial hemorrhage are discussed in Chapter 25. There is increasing recognition that intracerebral hemorrhage also can occur as a result of a rupture of very small vessels in the cortex that have been weakened by infiltration of the vessel walls by amyloid.

In addition to the causes of hemorrhage just discussed, recall that red infarcts occur in about 30 percent of people who have sustained an embolic stroke. Evidence of this hemorrhage is best seen on a CT scan or through MRI imaging. Rarely, blood may leak into the ventricular system and subarachnoid space; when this occurs, evidence of the hemorrhage appears in the cerebrospinal fluid (CSF) as red blood cells or a discoloration of CSF produced by products resulting from the breakdown of red blood cells (xanthochromia). The appearance of red blood cells in the CSF occurs only in a minority of cases of hemorrhagic infarct due to embolism.

Risk Factors

Hypertension is a risk factor for hemorrhagic stroke because the penetrating vessels are vulnerable to both thickening of the vessel in some places and thinning of the vessel wall in smaller penetrating vessels, deep in the brain. The thickening leads to a loss of lumen and, hence, to ischemic infarcts, while the thinning creates microaneurysms. Rupture of these microaneurysms leads to intracranial hemorrhage. Other risk factors include anticoagulation and/or an inherited coagulation deficit.

Physiology of Hemorrhagic Stroke

Intracranial hemorrhage has two major effects on brain tissue. The first is due to the fact that the volume of blood that has escaped from an artery takes up space within the cranial vault. Intracranial volume is taken up by three components: brain cells, the normal volume of blood, and cerebrospinal fluid. If the hemorrhage adds to the volume of blood inside the cranium, then it acts as a space-occupying mass. Because the cranium is a closed volume, any increase of volume from the hemorrhage will cause a mass effect and increase the intracranial pressure. If edema is present, this also adds to the increased intracranial pressure. This can result in a number of problems. For one thing, it may cause a rise in intracranial pressure. As far as the circulation is concerned, a sequence of events occurs because of the increased intracranial pressures. First, the intracranial pressure can exceed venous pressures. This impediment of venous drainage causes passive congestion and further leakage of blood into the intracranial space. On the arterial side, there is an initial increase of systemic blood pressure in a reflexive attempt to overcome the intracranial pressure. When this happens, the pulse rate goes down because of vagus reflexes from the carotid artery sensors. This is called the *Cushing effect*. However, if the intracranial pressure gets too high, blood simply cannot get into the cranium. These processes cause a cascade of further hemorrhages, infarctions, edema, and herniation, resulting in damage to the brain's tissues (neurons, axons, and glia)—even in locations distant from the location of the hemorrhage. The pathophysiology set off by a significant intracranial hemorrhage is a dynamic and constantly changing process.

The second major result of intracranial hemorrhage is caused by the escaped blood irritating structures adjacent to the hemorrhage. For some reason, this is most commonly associated with subarachnoid hemorrhage and is rarely seen with primary intracerebral hemorrhage or with bleeding from an arteriovenous malformation. A dreadful consequence of the pathology of subarachnoid hemorrhage is cerebral vasospasm. Initially, the spasm protects the brain, because it serves as a tourniquet on the vessel that has bled. But, if the blood diffuses through the subarachnoid space and gets trapped in other locations, other vessels can go into spasm. This may cause sufficient loss of blood flow to the territory of the vessel in spasm so that secondary infarctions result in brain tissue quite removed from the location of the original hemorrhage. Cerebral vasospasm may not occur until a few days after the original bleed and can persist for weeks, causing delayed clinical deterioration and delaying surgical interventions.

Thought Question

Hemorrhagic strokes, in contrast to most ischemic strokes, can affect tissues at a distance from the initial bleed. What are the various reasons that explain why this occurs, and what does this imply with respect to predicting the impairments that will result from these strokes?

Last, but not least, is that a blood vessel that has broken is very likely to break again. This risk of a rebleed is a major factor in deciding how to treat a person with intracranial hemorrhage. Hemorrhagic strokes involve specific anatomical structures that differ from those involved in ischemic strokes.

CLINICAL CONNECTIONS
Time Course and Prognosis

Most primary intracerebral hemorrhages begin during wakefulness and activity, in contrast to many ischemic strokes that begin during sleep. African Americans are affected more often than Caucasians. A common pattern is for the person to have a stroke in evolution. That is, initially the patient presents with a mild deficit like that of an ischemic lacunar infarction, but the symptoms progress—which is why it is imperative that imaging be done before any therapeutic intervention is initiated in any individual with a stroke. Anticoagulants or thrombolytic agents, which are appropriate for a person with an ischemic event, would be disastrous in a person with a hemorrhagic event. A person presenting with the mildest of symptoms, or even a TIA, may have an intracranial hemorrhage. The person with a primary intracerebral hemorrhage usually does not have a headache, in contrast to the person with a subarachnoid hemorrhage.

Nausea and vomiting at the onset of a hemorrhagic stroke occurs much more often than with ischemic strokes. Focal cerebral seizures occur in about 10 percent of people who have intracerebral hemorrhage. Drowsiness, confusion, loss of consciousness, and periodic increases in the depth and rate of respiration followed by respiratory decreases (*Cheyne-Stokes respiration*) also are more characteristic of hemorrhage than ischemia because the patient with a hemorrhage is more apt to have increased intracranial pressure.

About 30 to 35 percent of people with a primary intracerebral hemorrhage die due to the acute injury because of the hemorrhage-causing herniation as well as the cascade of other systemic problems (see Chapter 25). If the person does not have the catastrophic course described previously, the prognosis may be quite reasonable. Intracranial bleeding associated with hemorrhagic stroke does not necessarily cause anoxia of the tissue and, hence, may not destroy neuronal tissue. The extravasated blood can be removed from the brain tissue by the healing process if the person survives. This is in sharp contrast to ischemic strokes in which tissue death occurs within a few minutes. If the person survives, the neurologic deficits may slowly resolve over weeks or even months. As a consequence, with smaller hemorrhages, there may be a considerable recovery of function.

Thought Question

Patients with hemorrhagic strokes typically have a different time course of onset and often experience a number of symptoms that differentiate them from people with ischemic stroke. Identify as many of these differences as possible.

HEMORRHAGIC STROKE SYNDROMES
Primary Intracerebral Hemorrhage

Spontaneous (nontraumatic) hemorrhage is the third most common cause of stroke, following atherothrombosis and embolism. Our concern in this chapter is with intracerebral, or parenchymal, hemorrhages. About 90 percent of spontaneous intracerebral hemorrhages occur when a brain-penetrating artery is damaged and finally ruptures. There is a higher incidence of this problem in people who have had hypertension. Blood escapes from the ruptured vessel (extravasates) and forms a roughly circular or oval mass in the deep structures of the brain, basal ganglia, internal capsule, and thalamus. Recall that the penetrating vessels supply the "deep" structures of the brain. These are the same vessels that are involved in lacunar pathology. Therefore, these people can present with an apparent lacunar infarction, and imaging is necessary to make the distinction. In patients with hypertension, the occurrence of bleeding tends to parallel the intensity and duration of hypertension.

The extravasated mass of blood may displace and compress adjacent brain tissue. When large (several centimeters in diameter), the hemorrhage may displace midline brainstem structures thereby compromising vital centers leading to coma and death (Figure 24-13 ■). Large

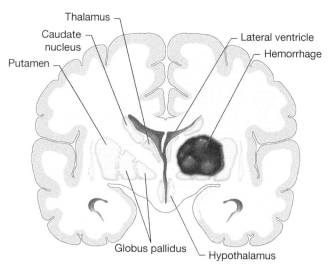

FIGURE 24-13 Frontal section of the brain. Intracerebral hemorrhage into the basal ganglia. Note that the extravasated blood forms a mass that displaces midline structures.

hemorrhages can break into the ventricular system, and also may be life-threatening.

Ruptured Intracranial Aneurysms

A ruptured intracranial aneurysm is the second most common hemorrhagic cause of stroke in the adult. The source of the bleeding is a ruptured **saccular**, or **berry**, **aneurysm**. Berry aneurysms are small, localized ball</br>oonings, or dilations, of a vessel wall, resulting from a defect in the elastic membrane of the vessel. The vast majority of saccular aneurysms (90 to 95 percent) occur in relation to the circle of Willis located at the base of the brain. Saccular aneurysms occur at points of bifurcation or branching of intracranial vessels (Figure 24-14 ■).

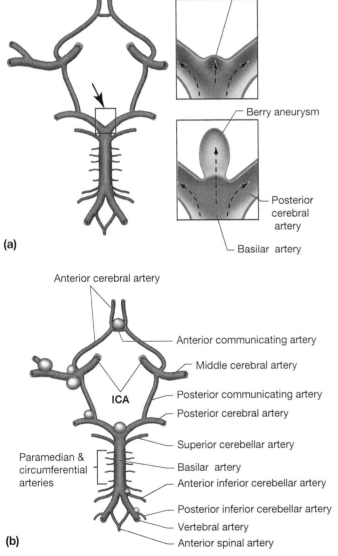

(a)

(b)

FIGURE 24-14 (a) Saccular (berry) aneurysms develop at weak points in the wall of an artery. Over time, especially in people with high blood pressure, the weak part of the vessel wall expands. (b) Common sites at which saccular aneurysms occur; typically they occur at branches in the vascular system. As depicted, the size of the aneurysm approximates the frequency at that site. About 90 percent of aneurysms occur on the anterior half of the circle of Willis. ICA: internal carotid artery.

Only some 10 percent occur in relation to the vertebrobasilar system. About 10 percent of individuals with an aneurysm will have more than one aneurysm.

An unruptured saccular aneurysm usually causes no focal signs or symptoms (Figure 24-15 ■). Notable rare exceptions to this are aneurysms that compress the optic nerves or chiasm; the hypothalamus; the pituitary gland; or the third, fourth, fifth, or sixth cranial nerves. Unruptured saccular aneurysms occur as an incidental finding in 2 percent of routine autopsies.

Rupture can occur at any age, but it is most common between the ages of 40 and 65 and in situations where the aneurysm is greater than 2 mm in size. In most cases, there are no warning symptoms of an impending rupture. Most ruptures occur during waking hours. Contrary to popular belief, the rupture is precipitated by straining, exercise, or sexual activity in less than one-third of patients.

Except as noted earlier, initial symptoms are related to rupture of the aneurysm when blood is forced into the subarachnoid space around the circle of Willis. The usual symptoms include sudden severe headache ("the worst headache ever") and neck pain and stiffness (nuchal rigidity).

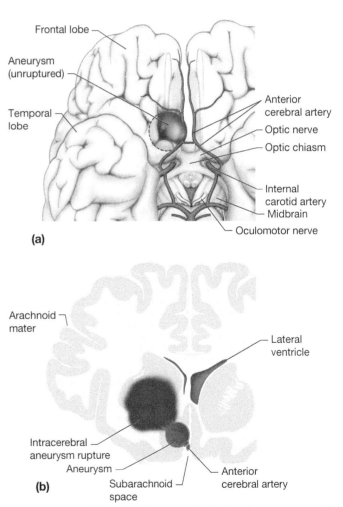

(a)

(b)

FIGURE 24-15 (a) Ventral view of the brain showing an unruptured aneurysm of the anterior cerebral artery. (b) Frontal section of the brain showing that the aneurysm has ruptured intracerebrally.

In addition, the person may experience loss or alteration of consciousness, as well as specific focal neurological deficits such as hemiparesis, aphasia, and visual deficits.

Blood from the ruptured aneurysm may also penetrate into the brain in about 30 to 40 percent of patients. The blood may also break into the ventricles, which is associated with a loss of consciousness and, ultimately, a poor prognosis.

If the blood stays confined to the local area around the circle of Willis, the patient may not have any signs or symptoms other than a headache. When the bleeding is associated with neurological localizing findings, however, the clinical course is more likely to result in permanent neurological problems. As mentioned earlier, the neurologic symptoms and tissue damage can be due to vasospasm. This may occur in areas of the brain far removed from the bleed and often causes an encephalopathy with alteration of awareness or loss of consciousness early during the course of the bleed. If the bleeding is severe enough so that it breaks into a ventricle or causes a global vasospasm and hypoperfusion, the patient can lapse into a coma. When there is a loss of consciousness at the time of the bleed, the patient has only a 10 percent chance of survival; if the patient survives, that person will then manifest significant persistent deficits.

Some patients have focal neurologic signs that do point to the location of the aneurysm (see Figure 7-1). Ptosis, diplopia, dilation of the pupil, and deviation of one eye laterally (divergent strabismus) may occur and are caused by involvement of the third cranial nerve. These signs indicate an aneurysm at the junction of the posterior communicating artery and the internal carotid artery or herniation of the brain (see Chapter 25). Monocular blindness suggests an aneurysm at the origin of the ophthalmic artery from the internal carotid artery. Transient paresis of one or both legs at the onset of the bleeding indicates an anterior communicating artery aneurysm that has interfered with blood supply in the territories of the ACAs. Hemiparesis or aphasia indicates an aneurysm at the bifurcation of the left middle cerebral artery that has bled into superior and inferior divisions. Deficits that occur after the first day may be due to vasospasm or rebleeding.

Between 15 and 22 percent of people die as a result of the first episode of intracerebral bleeding from a ruptured aneurysm. Many of these people never reach a hospital alive. Others arrive at a treatment center in a stuporous or comatose state. Of those who survive the initial episode of bleeding, rebleeding can occur in 30 to 50 percent of patients during the first year following the initial hemorrhage. The first two weeks after hemorrhage onset carry the greatest risk of rebleed. The mortality associated with rebleeding is high and has been estimated to range from 42 to 80 percent.

Thought Question

What are the similarities and differences between an AVM and an aneurysm in terms of cause, location, and risk of mortality?

Arteriovenous Malformations

Arteriovenous malformations (AVMs) consist of a tangle of dilated blood vessels that form an abnormal communication between the arterial and venous systems. AVMs can occur in any part of the brain, brainstem, or spinal cord. They are only one-tenth as common as saccular aneurysms. There are three distinct components of AVMs (Figure 24-16 ■): (1) arteries that feed into the AVM; (2) the core, or nidus, composed of a snakelike, vascular tangle of abnormally thin-walled blood vessels; and (3) the draining veins from which the core shunts blood directly from the feeding arteries.

The tangled blood vessels of the core may proliferate and enlarge with time. This explains why AVMs most often produce their symptoms in people over the age of 30. Most AVMs are asymptomatic and found incidentally when neuroimaging is done for other reasons. Typically, they do not have to be treated—they are small, and the risk of bleeding or causing neurological symptoms is also low. Repeat imaging every few years indicates if and how the AVM is progressing. AVMs vary in size from a few millimeters in diameter to large masses that may occupy most of the lobe of a cerebral hemisphere. Most large AVMs occur in a cerebral hemisphere at the junction points of the major cerebral arteries. If large AVMs grow, they may produce slowly progressive neurologic deficits

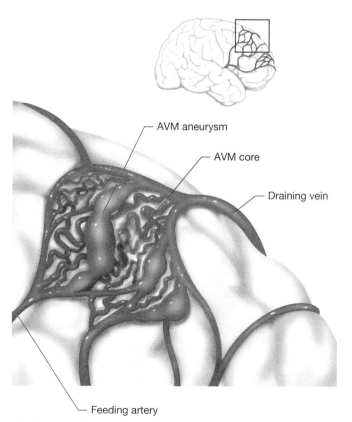

AVM aneurysm

AVM core

Draining vein

Feeding artery

FIGURE 24-16 Arteriovenous malformation (AVM) with dilation of the core. This AVM is illustrated on the surface of the cerebral cortex. However, most large AMVs occur in the central part of a cerebral hemisphere.

Neuropathology Box 24-8: Cerebral Amyloid Angiopathy

The incidence of small intracerebral hemorrhages in elderly individuals is often correlated with amyloid disease in the microcirculation of the brain. The risk increases with age, with the current association of intracerebral hemorrhages occurring in 12 percent of patients over the age of 85. Incidental evidence of microhemorrhages noted on MRI is almost 25 percent. The amyloid appears to be similar to the amyloid present in the senile plaques of Alzheimer's disease. The location of these hemorrhages is lobular, especially in the posterior brain. This is to be distinguished from the location of primary intracerebral hemorrhages that tend to be in the deeper structures, supplied by the penetrating intracranial circulation. There is a high correlation of this pathology in patients who express the APOE e4 gene, further linking the likely pathological process to Alzheimer's disease.

because of compression of neighboring structures by the enlarging mass of vessels.

There are three common presenting characteristics of AVMs: hemorrhage, seizure, and headache. When AVMs leak, they produce intermittent, various-sized hemorrhages that are partly intracerebral and may extend into the subarachnoid space. The intracerebral hemorrhage may cause focal neurological deficits such as a hemiparesis or hemiplegia. While hemorrhage is the most common and dangerous presentation of AVMs, the risk of major neurologic deficits (30 percent) and mortality (15 percent) is lower than with rupture of a saccular aneurysm. In about 30 percent of patients, a focal seizure may be the only manifestation. In another 20 percent of patients, a headache is the only symptom. Often, the headache is mistaken for migraine, but many AVMs do not cause any symptoms.

A number of diagnostic and imaging studies may be done to identify and characterize the AVM. Cerebral angiography will demonstrate AVMs larger than 5 mm in diameter and will reveal all three anatomical components of the AVM. Computerized tomography scans will show AVMs in about 95 percent of patients. MRA is particularly sensitive to small AVMS and is more valuable than cerebral angiography in disclosing the relationship of the AVM to

adjacent brain tissue—especially brain tissue that is neurologically indispensable.

CLINICAL CONNECTIONS

Although the causes and prognosis from ischemic and hemorrhagic strokes are quite different, the clinical consequences can be similar. Hence, similar examination strategies are used in both cases. It is important to recognize, however, that in hemorrhagic stroke, it may not be possible to predict the symptoms that will occur based on the vessel involved. This is because consequences of the hemorrhage can extend well beyond the territory of that vessel. The clinician can, however, draw inferences regarding locations of the affected structures based on examination findings. With regard to intervention, the rehabilitation professional draws on the same types of strategies as are used for people with ischemic stroke.

> **Thought Question**
>
> In what ways would rehabilitation for a person with a hemorrhagic stroke be similar to, and in what ways different from, rehabilitation for a person with an ischemic stroke?

Summary

This chapter began with an overview of stroke and its causes. The identification and modification of risk factors is of extreme importance because tissue damage has almost always occurred before the individual receives medical attention. A variety of factors exist that can modify the severity of a stroke in a given person. Thus, a one-to-one relationship does not exist between an arterial occlusion and the state of the brain tissue nourished by an occluded vessel such that occlusion of the same vessel in different people can result in a markedly different array of clinical signs.

Two major causes of stroke were identified: ischemic and hemorrhagic. One cause of ischemic stroke is an embolism, in which a fragment, usually of a thrombus, breaks off and travels in the brain circulation until it lodges in a vessel too small to permit its further passage. A second cause is a thrombosis, in which a blood clot develops in an atherosclerotic vessel. Infarctions from an embolus or thrombus usually can be differentiated from one another by their onset and clinical course.

Identifiable syndromes result from ischemia in the three major cerebral arteries because of the unique, functionally specific, cortical and subcortical areas supplied by each. Occlusion of the internal carotid artery may also result in the unique carotid border-zone syndrome, which cogently illustrates the hydrodynamics of cerebral perfusion. Lacunar syndromes are distinct in that they result from multiple small infarctions in the territories of the small-diameter arteries that penetrate into the substance of structures such as the thalamus, internal capsule, or brainstem.

Hemorrhagic strokes are due to blood escaping from a damaged vessel and may result from a primary intracerebral hemorrhage, a ruptured cerebral aneurysm, or an arteriovenous malformation. Differences were discussed between hemorrhagic and ischemic strokes with respect to onset and prognosis.

Clinical consequences were discussed for both ischemic and hemorrhagic strokes. Prognosis of each was considered. The importance of understanding the location and type of lesion was illustrated with respect to examination strategies and intervention approaches for people with ischemic strokes. Intervention approaches were analyzed with respect to remediation, compensation, and preventive strategies. Similar considerations apply to people with hemorrhagic strokes.

Applications

1. Jason McDowd is 63 years old with a history of atrial fibrillation, hypertension, and diabetes mellitus. His body mass index (BMI) is high; in fact, he has battled obesity most of his adult life. He has smoked for more than 40 years. One week ago, he experienced a period of confusion accompanied by right arm and leg numbness that lasted about 10 minutes. Since it resolved on its own, he did not seek medical advice or care. However, when he awoke this morning, he could not move his right arm or leg. He appeared confused and was unable to communicate verbally. His wife drove him to the hospital, where he was diagnosed with a stroke.

   a. Identify his risk factors for stroke.
   b. What is the term used to describe the initial symptoms that he experienced one week ago?
   c. What type of stroke do you think he had, ischemic or hemorrhagic? Justify your response.
   d. Which vessel do you think was involved?
   e. Comment on general factors affecting his prognosis.

2. Ha Dho is a 15-year-old girl with a history of migraine headaches. These headaches caused

throbbing pain, and she often had visual complaints. Specifically, she described being unable to see objects in her lower right visual field. Today, her headache was severe and she fell to the ground with a seizure due to hemorrhage. She was rushed to the emergency department.

   a. What could have caused this hemorrhagic event?
   b. What types of imaging procedures may be used to properly identify her problem?
   c. What hemisphere do you think will have an identifiable problem? Justify your response.

3. For the examples of the infarcts of three major vessels, depicted in Figure 24-12:

   a. Make a list of key anatomical structures that are affected at each level represented in the cross sections of Figure 24-12. Differentiate cortical from subcortical structures.
   b. To understand the consequences of these infarcts, relate the affected regions to the deficits identified in Tables 24-1, 24-2, and 24-3. Consider laterality (right versus left).
   c. Compare what would happen if the infarct is due to stenosis of the proximal vessel (stem), penetrating vessels, or distal vessels (cortical).

References

Barnett, H. J. M., Mohr, J. P., Stein, B. M., and Yalsu, F. M., eds. *Stroke: Pathophysiology, Diagnosis, Management*, 2nd ed. Churchill Livingston, New York, 1992.

Bowman, J. P., and Giddings, F. D. *Strokes: An Illustrated Guide to Brain Structure, Blood Supply, and Clinical Signs*. Prentice Hall, Upper Saddle River, NJ, 2003.

Brodal, A. *Neurological Anatomy in Relation to Clinical Medicine*, 3rd ed. Oxford University Press, New York, 1981.

Brott, T. Thrombolysis for stroke. *Arch Neurol* 53:1305, 1996.

Duvernoy, H. M. *The Human Brainstem and Cerebellum: Surface, Structure, Vascularization and Three-dimensional Sectional Anatomy with MRI.* SpringerWein, New York, 1995.

Duvernoy, H. M. *The Human Brain: Surface, Blood Supply, and Three-dimensional Sectional Anatomy*, 2nd ed. SpringerWein, New York, 1999.

Giaquinto S., Buzzelli S., Di Francesco L., Lottarini A., Montenero P., Tonin P., and Nolfe, G. On the prognosis of outcome after stroke. *Acta Neurol Scand* 100;202–208, 1999.

Greenberg, S. M, Rapalino, O., and Frosch, M. P. Case records of the Massachusetts General Hospital. Case 22-2010. An 87-year-old woman with dementia and a seizure. *N Eng J Med* 363:373, 2010.

Grundy, S. M., ed. *Atlas of Atherosclerosis: Risk Factors and Treatment*, 4th ed. Current Medicine, Philadelphia. 2005.

Guthkelch, A. N., and Misulis, K. E., eds. *The Scientific Foundations of Neurology*. Blackwell Science, Cambridge, UK, 1996.

Kelly, P. J., Furie, K. L., Shafqat, S., Rallis, N., Chang, Y., and Stein, J. Functional recovery following rehabilitation after ischemic stroke. *Arch Phys Med Rehabil* 84:968–972, 2003.

Mohr, J. P. and Gautier, J. C., eds. *Guide to Clinical Neurology*. Churchill Livingston, New York, 1995.

The National Institute of Neurological Disorders and Stroke rt-PA Stroke Study Group. Tissue plasminogen activator for acute ischemic stroke. *N Eng J Med* 333:1581; 1995.

Ng, Y. S., Stein, J., Ning, M. M., and Black-Schaffer, R. M. Comparison of clinical characteristics and functional outcomes of ischemic stroke in different vascular territories. *Stroke*. 38:2309–2314, 2007.

Ropper, A. H., and Brown, R. H. Ch. 34. Cerebrovascular diseases. In: *Adams and Victor's Principles of Neurology*, 8th ed. McGraw-Hill, New York, 2005.

Ross, R. W., ed. *Vascular Diseases of the Central Nervous System*, 2nd ed. Churchill Livingston, New York, 1983.

Tatu, L., Moulin, T., Bogousslavsky, J., and Duvernoy, H. Arterial territories of human brain: Brainstem and cerebellum. *Neurology*, 47:1125, 1996.

Toole, J. F. *Cerebrovascular Disorders*, 4th ed.: Raven Press, New York, 1990.

Vinken, P. J., Bruyn, G. W., and Klawans, H. L., eds. *Handbook of Clinical Neurology*, vol. 53, Vascular diseases. Elsevier, Amsterdam, 1988.

PEARSON
myhealthprofessionskit™

Use this address to access the Companion Website created for this textbook. Simply select "Physical Therapy" from the choice of disciplines. Find this book and log in using your username and password to access self-assessment questions, a glossary, and more.

The Brain's Environment and Brain Injury

LEARNING OUTCOMES

This chapter prepares the reader to:

1. Discuss the structure and function of the layers of the meninges and the space separating them.

2. Discuss the potential long-term consequences of viral, fungal, and bacterial meningitis and implications for the rehabilitation professional.

3. Explain the sequence of events that could lead to brain herniation.

4. Discuss the production, location, and purpose of cerebrospinal fluid.

5. Discuss disorders associated with CSF and mechanisms for testing for these disorders.

6. Explain the importance and limitations of the blood–brain barrier and discuss the mechanism that determines whether or not substances cross the blood–brain barrier.

7. Compare and contrast the blood–brain, blood–nerve, blood–cerebrospinal, and blood–retinal barriers in terms of structure and function.

8. Contrast the following conditions and their consequences: concussion, cerebral concussion, contusion, and laceration.

9. Explain why coup–contrecoup occurs with TBI.

10. Contrast epidural and subdural hematomas with respect to cause, location, and consequences.

11. Describe the cascade of events that can occur following TBI and explain the consequences of each in terms of symptoms and eventual outcome.

12. Compare and contrast the damage and consequences of TBI with consequences of lesions to specific blood vessels as occurs with stroke.

13. Discuss the consequences of repeated concussion.

14. Compare and contrast decerebrate and decorticate posturing following TBI and relate these two conditions to neuroanatomical location of injury.

15. Discuss causes of traumatic brain injuries, consequences, classification, and prognosis.

16. Compare and contrast the Glasgow Coma Scale with the Ranchos Los Amigos Scale.

17. Discuss concepts used in rehabilitation for examination and intervention for people who have sustained a TBI.

18. Compare and contrast the approach to examination and intervention strategies when working in rehabilitation with people who have sustained strokes and TBIs.

ACRONYMS

AIDS Acquired immunodeficiency syndrome

CT Computerized tomography

CNS Central nervous system

CSF Cerebrospinal fluid

CVO Circumventricular organs

HIV Human immunodeficiency virus

HRP Horse radish peroxidase

ICP Intracranial pressure

L-Dopa Levadopa

MAO Monoamine oxidase

MRI Magnetic resonance imaging

MS Multiple sclerosis

NPH Normal pressure hydrocephalus

PD Parkinson's disease

PNS Peripheral nervous system

RPE Retinal pigment epithelial

TBI Traumatic brain injury

Introduction

The semisolid structures making up the CNS are easily damaged and therefore require support and protection. Three types of structures fulfill the supportive and protective functions: bony, membranous, and liquid. As noted in Chapter 1, the CNS is encased in a bony vault with the spinal cord being located in the vertebral column and the brain in the cranium. The CNS is invested by three connective tissue membranes (the meninges) and floats in a clear, watery medium (the cerebrospinal fluid).

While all three of these structural systems clearly fulfill a supportive and protective function, they paradoxically represent important components that, under adverse circumstances, can contribute to the location and distribution of brain pathology. Although they themselves typically are not the primary cause of a particular pathology, they contribute significantly to the location and distribution of damage. The cause of the pathology can be a microorganism (a bacterium or virus) that causes meningitis, a tumor or hemorrhage that occupies space within the cranial vault, or edema due to a blow to the head or a stroke.

These three structural systems provide protective support for gross brain structure. There is, in addition, a vital system—the blood–brain barrier—that isolates the brain from the general systemic circulation and regulates the transfer of nutrients and metabolites between the blood and nervous tissue. The microenvironment within which neurons reside must be closely regulated to ensure normal neuronal function and survival, and the blood–brain barrier fulfills this function by regulating the chemical composition of the extracellular fluid within which neurons and neuroglia are bathed. The blood–brain barrier is commonly regarded as being protective, but in some circumstances the barrier can be broken, permitting the passage of microorganisms, inflammatory blood cells, and chemical substances that are harmful, sometimes even fatal, to neurons.

The first three sections of this chapter present structural and functional roles of the meninges (the first section), the cerebrospinal fluid (second section), and the blood–brain barrier (third section). Finally, in the fourth section we consider traumatic brain injury (TBI). TBI is one of the most common causes of neurologic damage and permanent functional disability. TBI is a physical injury to the brain caused by an external force and is a major focus of this chapter. The incidence of TBI in the United States is estimated to be between 1.5 and 2 million new cases each year. This makes TBI at least twice as common as stroke.

MENINGES AND VENOUS DRAINAGE OF THE BRAIN

Clinical Preview · · · · · · · · · · · · · · · ·

Karen Lowry is 10 years old. She recently recovered from a case of viral meningitis. Jason Brown is 12. He too had meningitis, but his was a bacterial form of the disease. As you read through this chapter, consider the following:

- What symptoms should you be aware of if one of these children seeks your care in your outpatient clinic?
- What determines whether meningitis is likely to result in permanent deficits?
- Under what circumstances would these two children likely require rehabilitation?
- What aspects of rehabilitation might be important?

Meninges

The three connective tissue meninges (the dura mater, arachnoid mater, and pia mater) investing the CNS were introduced in Chapter 1 (see Figure 1-6) and those of the spinal cord were detailed in Chapter 5 (see Figure 5-1). Because the arachnoid and pia mater are similar histologically and are interconnected, they often are referred to as the pia-arachnoid. Two actual spaces and one potential space are associated with the three meninges: an epidural space external to the dura that is normally present only in the spinal meninges, a potential subdural space between the dura and arachnoid that may become an actual space under certain pathological conditions, and a normally present subarachnoid space between the arachnoid and pia that is present in both cranial and spinal meninges. The subarachnoid space is filled with cerebrospinal fluid.

Dura Mater

The most external of the meninges, the dura, is thick, tough, and poorly extensible. The dura of the spinal cord and brain differ in their relationship to surrounding bone due to the fact that, unlike the vertebral canal, the inner surface of the cranium lacks its own periosteum. Cranial dura thus consists of two layers: an outer periosteal layer that serves as cranial periosteum and an inner meningeal layer representing the true dura. The periosteal layer is adherent to the inner surface of the calvaria, somewhat loosely in most places but firmly in the regions of skull sutures, the transverse sinus, and base of the skull. Thus, there is normally no cranial epidural space; the two dural layers are fused. (Recall, however, that in contrast, there is an epidural space in the spinal cord). There is no sharp histological boundary, except in the regions occupied by the large venous channels draining blood from the brain,

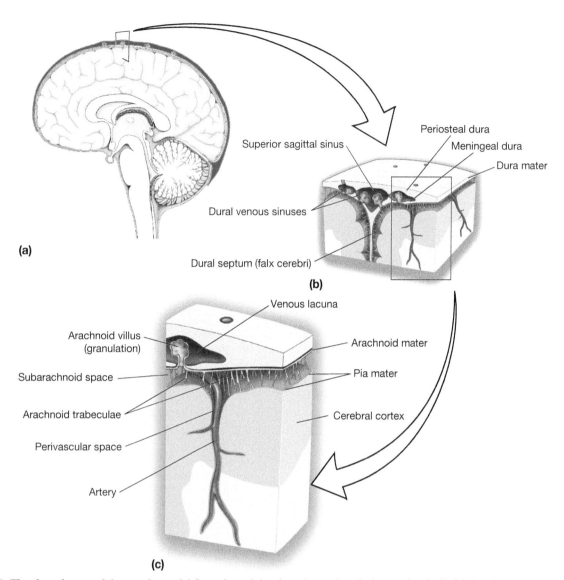

(a)

(b)

(c)

FIGURE 25-1 The three layers of the meninges. (a) Location of the three layers in relation to the skull. (b) Two layers of the dura mater: the periosteal and meningeal layers; also shown is their relationship to the dural septum. (c) The arachnoid mater and pia mater, as well as the subarachnoid space and the arachnoid villi.

the **dural venous sinuses**. Here, the layers separate to form the walls of the sinuses (Figure 25-1 ■). The major venous sinuses are somewhat triangular in cross section, the most superficial wall being made up of the periosteal layer; the other two walls are formed by the meningeal layer.

The meningeal layer is reflected from the periosteal layer to form several **dural septa** or reflections that partition the cranial vault into three compartments (Figure 25-2 ■). Most prominent of these septa is the sickle-shaped **falx cerebri**, a vertical midline partition located in the longitudinal fissure between the cerebral hemispheres. Its free, inferior border is dorsal to the corpus callosum and roughly follows the latter's conformation. The **tentorium cerebelli** is a transversely oriented partition separating the superior surface of the cerebellum from the inferior surface of the occipital lobes. It forms the roof of the posterior fossa. The tentorium is tent shaped; at its elevated midline region, the tentorium and falx cerebri fuse with one another. The free anterior border of the

tentorium is in the shape of a deep notch and is called the **tentorial incisure** or **tentorial notch**, within which the midbrain is situated. The **falx cerebelli** is a small midsagittal septum situated ventral to the tentorium. It partially separates the cerebellar hemispheres. The **diaphragma sellae** is a small dural sheet forming the fibrous roof of the hypophyseal (pituitary) fossa. It is perforated by the infundibulum that joins the hypothalamus with the pituitary gland.

The tentorium and falx cerebri divide the cranial vault into paired lateral compartments housing the cerebral hemispheres and a single posterior compartment for the cerebellum, pons, and medulla. A common clinical usage is to refer to the former as the *supratentorial* compartment and the latter as the *infratentorial* compartment. In addition to supporting soft neural tissue, the compartments constrain fore-aft and side-to-side movement of the brain during head motion, minimizing the potential for brain trauma.

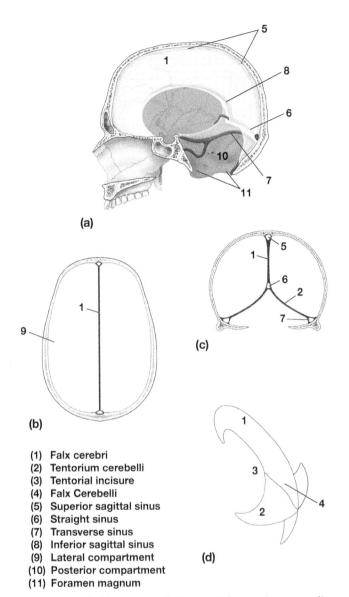

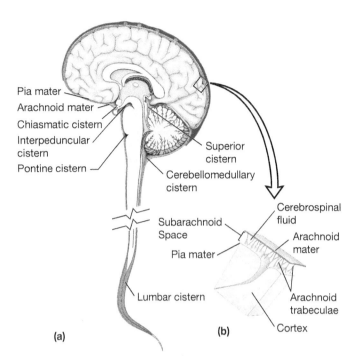

FIGURE 25-3 The subarachnoid cisterns, which contain large amounts of cerebrospinal fluid. (a) Mid-sagittal section. (b) Section from the cortex illustrating the relationship to the arachnoid and pia mater of the subarachnoid space traversed by the arachnoid trabeculae.

(1) Falx cerebri
(2) Tentorium cerebelli
(3) Tentorial incisure
(4) Falx Cerebelli
(5) Superior sagittal sinus
(6) Straight sinus
(7) Transverse sinus
(8) Inferior sagittal sinus
(9) Lateral compartment
(10) Posterior compartment
(11) Foramen magnum

FIGURE 25-2 The septa and sinuses of the cranium, as well as the two lateral and one posterior compartments. (a) Mid-sagittal view. (b) Horizontal view. (c) Coronal view. (d) Major septa.

Thought Question

Consider the implications of the bony and dural structures of the cranial vault with respect to brain injury following trauma. What sites do you think might be particularly vulnerable to injury?

Arachnoid Mater

The thin *avascular* arachnoid mater is the middle meningeal layer between the dura mater and the innermost layer, the pia mater. It is closely applied to the inner surface of the dura, and thus the subdural space in life is really only a potential space. The CSF-containing subarachnoid space is located between the arachnoid and pia. It is traversed by numerous **arachnoid trabeculae**, delicate fibrous threads given off from the inner surface of the arachnoid and

attaching the latter to the pia (Figure 25-3 ■). This gives the arachnoid the appearance of a cobweb, hence, its name (Gr., *arachne*, web).

Cells of the arachnoid are joined together by tight junctions that serve to isolate the general extracellular fluid of the body from the extracellular fluid of the brain. The latter includes the cerebrospinal fluid occupying the subarachnoid space. The arachnoid is an important component of the blood–brain barrier (discussed later) because cerebrospinal fluid cannot penetrate the arachnoid.

The arachnoid conforms only to general brain shape and thus bridges over sulci, fissures, and other irregular contours of the brain surface. As a result, the size of the subarachnoid space varies considerably at different brain locations. At the base of the brain, where pia and arachnoid become widely separated, focal enlargements of the space are present, and because they contain relatively large amounts of CSF, they are called **subarachnoid cisterns**. The largest of these is the cerebellomedullary cistern, or cisterna magna, which is located between the inferior cerebellar and dorsal medullary surfaces (Figure 25-3).

The arachnoid contains areas of specialization for the passage of CSF from the subarachnoid space into the venous system, specifically into the dural venous sinuses. These are the *arachnoid villi*. Arachnoid villi are most numerous along the walls of the superior sagittal sinus and in outpocketings from the sinus, called venous lacunae. Arachnoid villi are small evaginations of the arachnoid

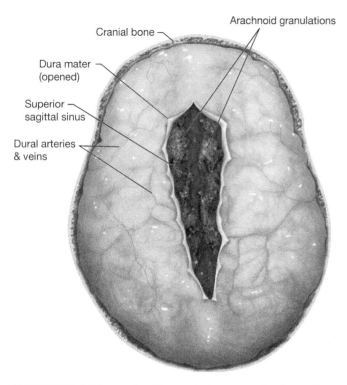

Cranial bone

Arachnoid granulations

Dura mater
(opened)

Superior
sagittal sinus

Dural arteries
& veins

FIGURE 25-4 The arachnoid granulations are collections of arachnoid villi that allow for passage of cerebrospinal fluid from the subarachnoid space into the venous system. The superior sagittal sinus, which extends along the superiorly attached border of the falx cerebri, is overlaid by the dura mater.

extending through the dural wall of a sinus. At such sites, the connective tissue of the dura is absent so that CSF and venous blood are separated only by a layer of arachnoidal cells and the layer of endothelial cells lining the sinus. Collections of villi are termed **arachnoid granulations** (Figure 25-4 ■).

> **Thought Question**
>
> Traumatic injury can result in both subdural and subarachnoid hemorrhage. Compare and contrast the anatomical locations.

Pia Mater

The pia mater is a delicate connective tissue layer that is the innermost of the meninges. It firmly adheres to the surface of the brain such that it follows all brain contours and dips into all sulci (see Figure 25-1). Astrocytes of the CNS have fine processes that terminate as end feet in the pia, serving to anchor it to neural tissue (see Figure 3-9). Like dura, the pia consists of two layers: a superficial epipial layer and a deeper layer, the intima pia. However, the epipia of the cerebrum is not well developed. The cerebral blood vessels lie on the surface of the intima pia, within the subarachnoid space. At sites where blood vessels penetrate neural tissue, the intima pia is invaginated to form the

outer wall of the perivascular space that persists until the vessel becomes a capillary (see Figure 25-1). Perivascular spaces are important anatomical landmarks in the diagnosis of neurological diseases such as multiple sclerosis.

Venous Drainage

The cerebral venous system exhibits greater variability than does the cerebral arterial system discussed in Chapter 7. Vessels of the two systems do not run together. After emerging from brain parenchyma, cerebral veins run in the subarachnoid space, penetrate the arachnoid, run for a short distance between the dura and arachnoid, and empty into dural venous sinuses.

Sinuses of the Dura Mater

Dural sinuses are located between the outer, periosteal and the inner, meningeal dural layers. Because their walls are composed of dense fibrous connective tissue and because of their firm attachment to the inner surface of the cranium, dural sinuses do not collapse. Thus, dural sinuses are capable of sustaining a negative pressure in the upright position, which is important to the absorption of cerebrospinal fluid (discussed later). The intracranial sinuses are devoid of valves. In addition to receiving blood from the brain, dural sinuses communicate with veins superficial to the skull (including the nasal cavity) via a system of emissary veins that perforate the cranium. Emissary veins may act as pressure valves under conditions of elevated intracranial pressure, in which case the direction of blood flow in them reverses. They can also allow the hematogenous spread of infection from the nasal cavity or scalp into the cranial vault and cause meningitis.

The **superior sagittal sinus** extends along the superiorly attached border of the falx cerebri, increasing in size as it progresses posteriorly (see Figure 25-4). It contains, especially along its middle portion, a number of lateral outpocketings—the venous lacunae—into which arachnoid villi extend. The paired **transverse sinuses** run along the posterior, attached border of the tentorium cerebelli, while the **straight sinus (sinus rectus)** runs posteriorly and inferiorly in the line of attachment of the falx cerebri and tentorium. The paired transverse, straight, and superior sagittal sinuses meet in variable combinations at the **confluence of sinuses**, located at the internal occipital protuberance. The ascending **occipital sinus** joins the confluence. In most individuals, the confluence is asymmetrical, with the superior sagittal sinus turning to the right to become continuous with the right transverse sinus and the straight sinus turning to the left to join the left transverse sinus (Figure 25-5 ■). The **sigmoid sinus** is a continuation of the transverse sinus at the occipitopetrosal junction, where the transverse sinus leaves the tentorium. Each sigmoid sinus pursues an S-shaped course toward the jugular foramen to empty into the internal jugular vein.

The small, **inferior sagittal sinus** runs posteriorly in the free, inferior border of the falx cerebri. It empties into

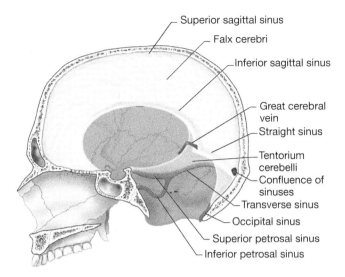

FIGURE 25-5 Dural sinuses of the cranium.

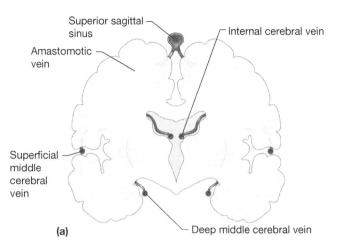

(a)

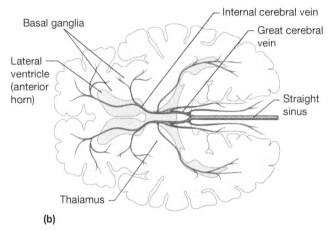

(b)

FIGURE 25-6 Relationship of veins to sinuses. (a) Coronal view. (b) Horizontal view.

the straight sinus. The **cavernous sinus** is a paired network of interconnecting channels situated on either side of the sella turcica; the two sides are connected by anastomotic venous channels passing in front of and behind the hypophysis. Posteriorly, the cavernous sinus is drained by the **superior** and **inferior petrosal sinuses**, the former joining the transverse sinus, the latter the internal jugular vein.

Cerebral Veins and Typical Drainage Pattern

Cerebral veins are divided into superficial and deep groups. Vessels within and between each group are interconnected by anastomoses (Figure 25-6a ■). Such intra- and extra-cerebral anastomoses are numerous and effective, thereby providing alternative routes of drainage in the event a cerebral vein becomes clogged.

Superficial veins drain the cerebral cortex and subjacent white matter. Those on the upper lateral and medial hemispheral surfaces drain into the superior sagittal sinus that, in turn, drain toward the confluence of sinuses. Most of the venous drainage of the cerebral cortex subsequently ends up in the right transverse and sigmoid sinuses and right internal jugular vein. Superficial veins draining other hemispheral surfaces empty into the cavernous, petrosal, and transverse sinuses (the so-called basal sinuses).

Deep cerebral veins (Figure 25-6b) drain more deeply situated cerebral structures, including deep white matter, basal ganglia, and choroid plexus, as well as portions of the diencephalon. Veins from these regions eventually empty into the internal and great cerebral veins. The paired internal cerebral veins run caudally in the roof of the third ventricle (dorsal to the thalamus); they join in the region of the pineal gland to form the short, unpaired great cerebral vein (of Galen) that, in turn, empties into the straight sinus. Blood from these areas flows sequentially into the left transverse and sigmoid sinuses and left internal jugular vein. The rest of the venous systems of the cranium are otherwise variable in location, similar to the rest of the body.

CLINICAL CONNECTIONS

Meningitis

A number of pathological processes involve the meninges either directly or secondarily. **Meningitis** is an inflammation of the pia-arachnoid and the fluid in the resulting enclosed space. The infection can be both cerebral and spinal because the subarachnoid space is continuous so that an infective agent gaining access to one part rapidly accesses all other parts of the CNS. The responsible agent may be bacterial, viral, fungal, or even protozoan. Fungal and protozoan infections are more common in immunologically compromised people. In most cases of meningitis, the responsible organism gets into the cranium by way of a hematogenous spread, often from the original infection of the lungs or gut. The other pathway is through a local spreading from scalp or sinus infections.

Typically, the consequences of bacterial, fungal, and protozoan meningitis tend to be severe. These forms of meningitis often result in abscesses, with resulting tissue damage and long-term consequences for movement, cognition, and other brain functions. Viral meningitis, in contrast, tends to be self-limiting and without significant complications. However, certain viruses (e.g., herpes simplex, West Nile) can cause encephalitis that can then potentially lead to permanent damage, including seizures and cognitive problems.

In general, as long as the infection is restricted to the meninges, it will not have long-term consequences. However, an infection that involves both the meninges and the brain—referred to as a **meningoencephalitis**—is serious and likely to cause localized clinical symptoms, compromise of consciousness, disability, or even death.

The first clinical signs of meningitis usually include fever and headache, associated with a stiff and painful neck (nuchal rigidity). Pain may also occur in the lumbar area or the posterior aspects of the thigh. Because meningitis is a form of infection, inflammation occurs. As the inflammation progresses, if left untreated, it can result in edema in the brain with a wide variety of possible symptoms that result from the increased intracranial pressure (discussed later), causing vomiting, papilledema, and even seizures. In addition, meningoencephalitis can cause focal neurologic signs such as cranial nerve palsies, sensory loss, cognitive and language loss, or motor loss. In severe cases, the person may be left with paralysis, dementia, stupor, or even persistent coma. If left untreated, bacterial meningitis can be fatal.

Thought Question

Contrast the clinical consequences of viral meningitis, bacterial meningitis, meningiomas, and herniations.

Meningioma

A **meningioma** is a primary extrinsic tumor of the CNS arising most commonly from arachnoidal cells, especially those of the arachnoid villi. Venous sinuses are thus favored locations of these tumors. In general, meningiomas are slow growing and benign. Meningiomas smaller than 2 cm in diameter often are found upon autopsy in older persons who had no observable symptoms during life (clinically silent). However, malignant meningiomas occur in 1 to 10 percent of cases. Meningiomas may displace, compress, and invaginate the brain, but they do not actually infiltrate neural tissue. Those involving, in particular, meninges of the lateral and superior hemispheral surfaces are amenable to surgical removal because the neoplasm is always sharply demarcated from neural tissue. Until they cause symptoms from seizures or compression of brain tissue, it is not usually necessary to treat a meningioma by surgery. Specific symptoms depend on on tumor location, with seizures being the most common symptom associated with skull-based lesions.

Herniations

Herniation results from elevated intracranial pressure. To understand the causes of herniation, it is important to recall that the cranial vault of the adult is a rigid, nonexpansible chamber with a restricted volume. It contains blood, CSF, and neural tissue—all of which are relatively incompressible substances within the confines of the vault. Because the total volume of these components remains constant, any space-occupying lesion (such as a tumor, edema, increased volume of CSF, intracranial hematomas, or hemorrhage) taxes intracranial space and results in elevated intracranial pressure. Brain herniation is a possible consequence of a severe rise in intracranial pressure because of the compartmentalization of the cranial vault by the relatively rigid falx cerebri and tentorium cerebelli. Pressure from a space-occupying lesion in one compartment will not be distributed evenly to the other compartments. Soft neural tissue thus shifts (i.e., *herniates*) from one compartment, where the pressure is higher, to another compartment, where it is lower. A major cause of herniation is traumatic brain injury (TBI). Following trauma to the skull, the meninges may trap blood in the epidural space or in the subarachnoid space. This is discussed in the detail in the section on TBI.

Three herniations are common: the *subfalcial, temporal lobe-tentorial* (or *uncal*), and *cerebellar-foramen magnum* (Figure 25-7 ■). In subfalcial herniation, the adjacent cingulate gyrus is pushed under the falx cerebri. The clinical consequence is usually alteration of consciousness without any focal neurological findings. In temporal lobe-tentorial herniation, the medial part of one temporal lobe is forced into the tentorial incisure. The herniated tissue displaces the third cranial nerve, leading to pupil and eye movement changes. If the midbrain is compressed or displaced, the herniation may have severe consequences, leading to motor function alterations, respiratory changes, and coma. If the increased pressure is due to a generalized increase of intracranial pressure, a cerebellar-foramen magnum herniation may occur. Here, tissue of the inferior and medial portions of the cerebellum are displaced into the foramen magnum, compressing the caudal brainstem and upper cervical cord.

Thought Question

Edema can cause the brain to press on bony and other poorly extensible structures. Thinking ahead—and drawing on your current knowledge of the anatomy of the skull and its related tissues, crevices, and foramina—which structures might pose the greatest threat to integrity of the brain under these circumstances?

Clinically important cerebrovascular problems can occur with herniation because the anterior cerebral and posterior cerebral arteries can be compressed by the herniated tissue against the dural invaginations, causing a stroke in their distribution. Involvement of the venous system is relatively infrequent because of the hydrodynamics and

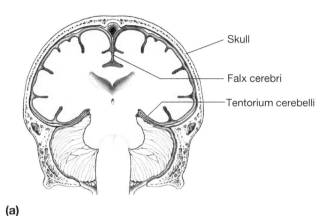

(a)

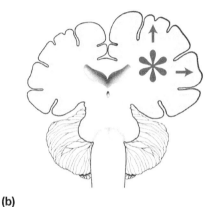

(b)

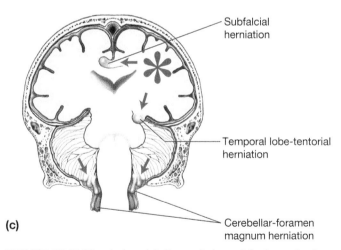

(c)

FIGURE 25-7 Herniation. (a) Coronal view of the intact brain. (b) In the absence of the skull, a space-occupying lesion would cause expansion of the cortical areas. (c) Because the brain is contained by the skull, pressures cause herniation of the neural tissue to other compartments. The three most common types of herniation are the subfalcial, temporal lobe-tentorial (uncal herniation), and cerebellar-foramen magnum.

anatomy of the system. For example, because of the extensive and effective anastomoses within and between superficial and deep cerebral veins, one group of veins may, when the necessity arises, drain areas ordinarily drained by members of the other group. Thus, a slowly developing

occlusion may be compensated for by a shifting of blood to another region, thereby equalizing the local pressure increases attending the occlusion. As a result, only slight transitory clinical effects occur—or none at all may appear. A rapidly developing occlusion or pressure increase, on the other hand, may produce a marked passive hyperemia (the presence of an increased amount of blood) and possible hemorrhage from rupture of the vessel wall.

Intracranial thrombophlebitis is a central venous inflammation resulting in the formation of a thrombus. This process typically involves the major dural sinuses (cavernous, transverse, and superior sagittal) with potential spread to the veins emptying into them. Most commonly, the thrombophlebitis is due to hematogenous spread from a primary focus of infection in the middle ear; paranasal sinuses; or skin around the eyes, nose, or upper lip. Other causes include dehydration, birth control medications, pregnancy, and the postpartum period. Symptoms vary depending on the sinus involved. Thrombophlebitis of the superior sagittal sinus may result in increased intracranial pressure, seizures, and cortical motor and sensory problems. The disease often is associated with other types of intracranial suppuration—for example, bacterial meningitis. Treatment consists of large doses of antibiotics and possible surgical decompression.

> **Thought Question**
>
> Drawing on information presented in Chapters 13, 14, and 15, explain why herniation leading to compression of the midbrain can result in coma or death.

CEREBROSPINAL FLUID

Clinical Preview ·················

Marilyn Leskovitz experienced severe and unrelenting headaches over a four-day period. Initially, her primary care physician was unable to determine the cause of the headaches and suggested that the headaches might be migraines. Imaging with a CT scan was normal. Eventually, however, he decided to perform a lumbar puncture to assess her cerebrospinal fluid. The lumbar puncture revealed viral meningitis.

As you read through this section, consider the following:

- What is the purpose of the lumbar puncture?

- What conditions other than migraine could cause unrelenting headaches?

- What could be the consequence of waiting too long to treat Marilyn's condition?

Cerebrospinal fluid (CSF) is a clear, colorless fluid present within the ventricular system, subarachnoid space, and central canal of the spinal cord. Recall from Chapter 2 that the ventricular system consists of the paired lateral ventricles (one within each cerebral hemisphere), a midline third ventricle in the diencephalon, and a fourth ventricle overlying the pons and medulla. The ventricles are in communication with one another: the lateral ventricles with the third ventricle via the interventricular foramina (of Monro) and the third with the fourth ventricle via the cerebral aqueduct in the midbrain. The fourth ventricle communicates with the subarachnoid space via two lateral apertures (the foramina of Luschka) and a single midline aperture (the foramen of Magendie). The central canal of the spinal cord may not be patent in the adult. Its small size lends itself to occlusion from normal cellular debris. This is of no apparent clinical significance. The CSF functions to protect, support, and nourish the parenchyma of brain and spinal cord.

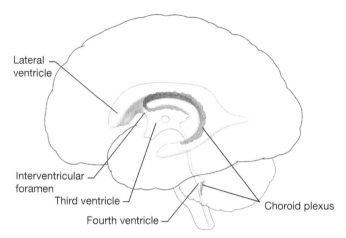

FIGURE 25-8 Cerebrospinal fluid is produced by the choroid plexus within the ventricles.

> **Thought Question**
>
> CSF does not remain static, but rather circulates constantly. What is the underlying mechanism, and why is this important?

Production

CSF is produced primarily by the **choroid plexus** of the ventricular system. CSF is essentially an ultrafiltrate of blood serum, with few proteins and cells. It is similar to extracellular fluid in the brain and spinal cord, allowing free exchange of extracellular fluid and CSF.

During development, the pia—accompanied by its arterioles, venules, and capillaries—invaginates a ventricular cavity and pushes ependyma ahead of it. Overlying ependymal cells then specialize to form choroid epithelium. The complex of capillaries, pia, and choroid epithelium form choroid plexus.

Choroid plexus is present in all four of the brain's ventricles (Figure 25-8 ■). Most is present as a long, continuous band in each of the lateral ventricles, where it extends from the tip of the inferior horn through the body of the ventricle until it reaches the interventricular foramen through which it often protrudes. Each interventricular foramen leads into the unpaired third ventricle. Thus, there are two strands of choroid plexus that occupy the roof of the midline third ventricle. These two continuous strips of choroid plexus end in the posterior third ventricle and do not extend into the cerebral aqueduct of the midbrain. Within the fourth ventricle, two adjacent strands of choroid plexus occupy the roof of the caudal half of the ventricle. On each side, a strand extends laterally into the lateral recess of the ventricle and protrudes through the foramen of Luschka into the subarachnoid space of the cerebellomedullary cistern (cisterna magna). Thus, choroid plexus of the fourth ventricle is T-shaped, with a tuft in the cisterna magna of each side.

Several structures other than choroid plexus contribute to the formation of CSF. These other structures, estimated to produce around 30 percent of total CSF volume, include ependymal cells, neural tissue, and the capillary bed of the brain.

Adult choroid plexus is a highly tufted structure. So extensive are the infoldings of its free ventricular surface (think of cauliflower), that choroid plexus is estimated to amount to approximately two-thirds of the total ventricular surface area. Choroid plexus is composed of a single layer of cuboidal epithelial cells enclosing a dense capillary network that is embedded in a connective tissue stroma (Figure 25-9 ■). Unlike capillaries elsewhere in the brain (with a number of specific exceptions relating to the circumventricular organs), those of the choroid plexus are fenestrated, thereby allowing solutes to filter from blood plasma into the loose, extra-capillary connective tissue network. However, most solutes cannot pass into ventricular CSF. This is because the apical regions of adjacent choroid epithelial cells are surrounded and connected by tight junctions. Such junctions comprise the so-called **blood–CSF barrier** that functions to regulate the composition of CSF: substances that enter CSF must be transported across the choroid epithelium. The blood–CSF barrier is part of the overall blood–brain barrier.

Although details of the process by which CSF is produced have not been resolved entirely, CSF is considered to be an actively secreted fluid. This is consistent with the shape of choroid epithelial cells, as well as with their complement of organelles and enzymes—all of which are characteristic of metabolically active secretory cells. Additionally, metabolic inhibitors depress the formation of new CSF. Interestingly, transcellular transport may be bidirectional, even though the primary direction is from choroidal blood vessels to ventricular CSF.

CSF is produced continuously, the production amounting to approximately 500 to 700 ml CSF/day. The

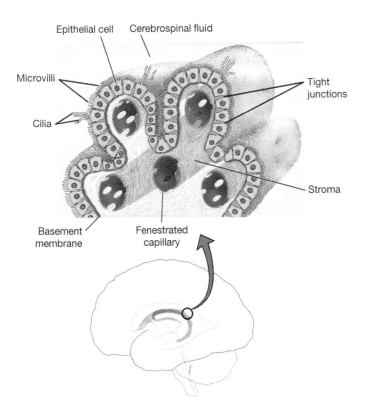

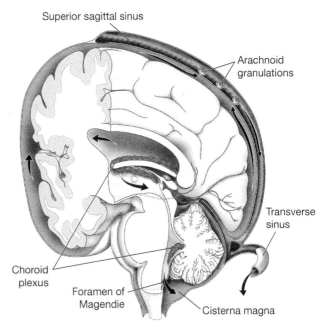

FIGURE 25-10 Production, circulation, and reabsorption of cerebrospinal fluid.

FIGURE 25-9 An expanded view of the choroid plexus illustrating its infolded structure and tight junctions.

total volume of CSF in the ventricles and subarachnoid space is about 140 ml, only 20 to 25 ml of which is in the ventricles. Thus, the total volume of CSF is renewed approximately three times per day. The rate of CSF production is fairly constant and largely independent of intraventricular pressure. Because increasing intracranial pressure from a space-occupying lesion does not elicit a compensatory drop in production, the lesion and CSF have an augmentative effect in taxing intracranial volume and increasing intracranial pressure. Osmotic diuretics (such as mannitol) are sometimes administered to reduce the volume of CSF. By elevating plasma osmolality, the excessive intravascular fluid is excreted, and the overall vascular volume is decreased, thereby decreasing the amount of CSF produced.

Circulation and Absorption

The bulk of CSF is produced by choroid plexus of the lateral ventricles. It then flows sequentially through the interventricular foramina, third ventricle, cerebral aqueduct, and fourth ventricle, being augmented in both ventricles by CSF from their own choroid plexuses (Figure 25-10 ■). It then passes through the foraminae of Luschka and Magendie into the subarachnoid space (the cerebello-medullary and pontine cisterns). Once within the subarachnoid space, the major circulatory route is directed superiorly over the convexities of the hemispheres. A less dynamic circulation occurs caudally through the subarachnoid space of the spinal cord into the lumbar cistern.

As noted in earlier, CSF is reabsorbed into venous blood of the dural sinuses through arachnoid villi (granulations) and nasal lymphatics. The villi have been depicted as functioning like one-way flow valves: they permit the one-way hydrostatic bulk flow of CSF from the subarachnoid space into the dural venous sinuses. The majority of CSF flows into the superior sagittal sinus and its associated lacunae. Because the composition and anatomical bindings of the dural sinuses prevent their collapsing, they are capable of sustaining a pressure less than that of subarachnoidal CSF. When CSF pressure is greater than venous pressure, the valves open and CSF moves into the dural sinus. When venous pressure exceeds that of CSF (as in lifting a heavy load or coughing), the valves close, thus preventing the backflow of venous blood into the CSF. Although dependent on a pressure gradient, the actual absorptive mechanism has not been defined. The villi may contain continuously open tubules that communicate directly with venous blood, or CSF may be transported across the villi by the formation of giant vacuoles.

Several mechanisms maintain the continuous circulation of CSF through the ventricular system and subarachnoid space. First, and likely most important, is the combination of secretory pressure and absorptive suction at opposite ends of the system. CSF is produced at a hydrostatic pressure of 15 ml of H_2O, and this is sufficient to push it through the ventricular system and into the subarachnoid space. Second, arterial pulsations of the highly vascular choroid plexus likely contribute to interventricular CSF circulation. These pulses can be readily seen with intracranial pressure measuring devices and, when they become muted, indicate a pathological increase of intracranial pressure.

Function

CSF is supportive to neural tissue in both physical and metabolic capacities. The most obvious and frequently cited function of CSF is as a water cushion, protecting brain parenchyma from traumatic injury. Although only a thin layer of fluid surrounds much of the brain, the buoyancy of CSF is high. In the laboratory, a brain with a mass of 1,500 grams in air weighs only 50 grams when immersed in CSF.

The constant turnover of CSF indicates it has other functions as well. Among the metabolic functions suggested for CSF are the transport of nutrients to neurons and the removal of waste products of neuronal metabolism and other compounds from the intracranial tissues. CSF also contributes to the regulation of the composition of the extracellular fluid bathing neurons. Because CSF is in free communication with the extracellular fluid of the brain, substances secreted by the choroid plexus have ready access to the extracellular compartment. There is no effective CSF–brain barrier. Another important role for CSF is in the transport of hormones, or hormone-releasing factors, locally within the ventricular system. And, finally, alterations in the pH, calcium, magnesium, and potassium ion concentrations of CSF affect neurons of the brain, thereby modifying heart rate, respiration, blood pressure, muscle tone, and emotional state. Additionally, the choroid plexus itself actively removes certain drugs and neurotransmitters from the CSF.

> **Thought Question**
>
> Contrast the location, role, and composition of CSF to that of blood with respect to brain function.

CLINICAL CONNECTIONS

The cranio-vertebral cavity with its dural lining is a tightly closed compartment. Nerves and blood vessels having access to the compartment are sealed to meninges and bone. Because the contents of the cavity (CSF, blood, and neural tissue) are incompressible, any local space-occupying process will transmit hydrostatic pressure to all parts of the cavity, even remote recesses. Thus, an intracranial tumor or edema will register in the lumbar cistern of the spinal cord as elevated CSF pressure (Figure 25-11 ■). When possible, imaging of the brain should be performed before there is any attempt to examine the spinal fluid because if there is a mass with increased intracranial pressure, the spinal tap can cause the brain to herniate. Disease processes, especially those with space-occupying properties, frequently alter the shape and communicative status of the CSF containing spaces of the brain and spinal cord. These changes can be visualized by imaging technologies such as CT scanning and MRI.

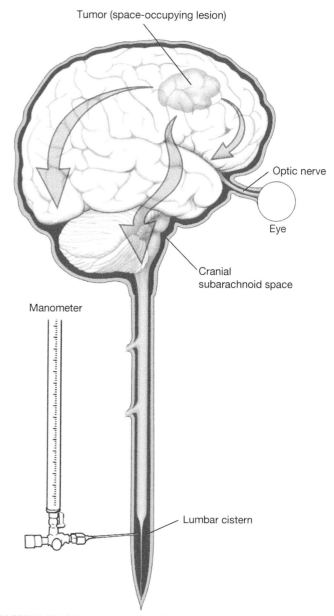

FIGURE 25-11 A space-occupying structure causes increased hydrostatic pressure throughout the cranial vertebral cavity that can be measured in the lumbar cistern.

Papilledema

Clinically, an increase of intracranial pressure may be detected by examining the optic disc through an ophthalmoscope to determine whether it is swollen. Because the optic nerve is ensheathed in a continuation of the meninges and subarachnoid space, it too will be compressed by any rise in intracranial pressure (see Figure 25-11). Such compression has a twofold effect: (1) the pressure on optic nerve axons as they exit the eyeball to enter the subarachnoid space behind the eye interferes with axoplasmic transport, causing the axons in the optic disc to swell, and (2) because blood vessels, especially the veins, draining the retina run with the nerve, they too will be compressed with a consequent venous engorgement. Conjointly, these factors lead to what is called a *choked disc*, or **papilledema**.

Lumbar (Spinal) Tap

An important diagnostic test is the spinal tap, or lumbar puncture; it is performed by inserting a needle into the lumbar subarachnoid space (cistern). This test is performed either when the patient is lying on his or her side with the knees flexed in a fetal position or when the patient is sitting and flexing the spine. Flexion of the vertebral column spreads the spinal processes of the vertebra apart and makes insertion of the needle easier. Under aseptic conditions and with the skin covering the lower lumbar vertebrae anesthetized, a long needle is inserted in the midline between the spines of L3 and L4 vertebrae, or L4 and L5. There is no risk of injuring the spinal cord because it terminates above these levels. Because the nerve roots of the cauda equina are floating in CSF, they are usually deflected aside by the needle and thus not injured. (Figure 25-12 ■).

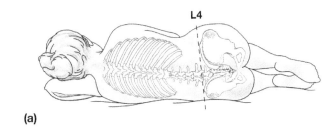

(a)

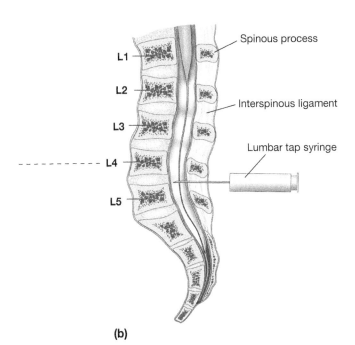

L1 — Spinous process
L2
L3 — Interspinous ligament
L4
L5 — Lumbar tap syringe

(b)

FIGURE 25-12 (a) Side-lying position for the lumbar tap, with L4 at the level of the iliac crest. (b) Spinal tap into the lumbar cistern.

CSF pressure is measured by a manometer attached to a needle inserted in the lumbar cistern (subarachnoid space). A CSF sample may also be withdrawn for analysis of alterations in its physical, chemical, cellular, and immunological characteristics, as well as for the presence of bacteria—all of which may be reflective of disease processes affecting the meninges or brain parenchyma. Given the importance of evaluating CSF to the diagnosis of a variety of CNS disorders, the retrieval of CSF from the lumbar cistern is an important clinical tool.

A lumbar puncture is a risky procedure and should not be performed when intracranial pressure may be elevated. With elevated intracranial pressure, removal of CSF from the lumbar cistern would lower pressure below the cranial vault and could result in herniation of brain tissue into the vertebral canal, which could potentially be fatal.

One of the important diagnostic uses of the lumbar puncture is to examine for possible subarachnoid hemorrhage. Normally, CSF is clear and colorless, like water. However, with subarachnoid hemorrhage, gross blood may be present in the CSF sample. Within a few hours of a subarachnoid hemorrhage, red blood cells begin to hemolyze, and the CSF undergoes a predictable sequence of color changes over time. Within two to three days, for example, bilirubin appears and may remain in the CSF for several weeks, imparting to the CSF a yellow color referred to as xanthochromia. Bleeding into the brain ventricles, for example, in primary intracerebral hemorrhage, may produce the same results as subarachnoid hemorrhage.

In bacterial meningitis, CSF may be under increased pressure and cloudy with increased numbers of white blood cells, especially polymorphic leukocytes. Normally, CSF contains very few red or white blood cells with one to five cells per microliter of lymphocytes considered to be normal. In bacterial meningitis, however, the white blood cell count may be markedly elevated. The presence of polymorphic leukocytes in the spinal fluid indicates a pathological problem. CSF may be cultured and stained to identify the responsible bacterial organism. CSF can be assayed for antigens and antibodies associated with various viral infections.

Hydrocephalus

A delicate balance normally exists between the rate of formation and the rate of absorption of CSF. Disruption of this balance, most typically by direct or indirect interference with circulation and/or absorption, results in

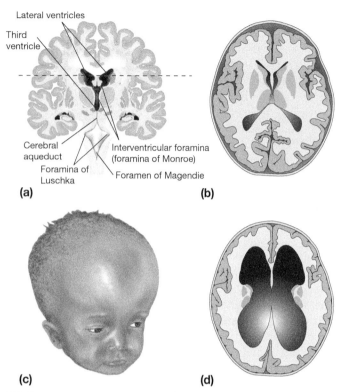

FIGURE 25-13 Hydrocephalus. (a) Coronal section of the brain and brainstem illustrating the level of a transverse section in relationship to the ventricles. (b) The transverse section of an intact brain. (c) Infant with overt hydrocephalus, resulting in an enlarged head. (d) Enlarged ventricles of the infant.

hydrocephalus (Figure 25-13 ■). Hydrocephalus is an abnormal accumulation of CSF within the ventricles that, when sufficiently pronounced, can lead to significant enlargement of the skull in infants. In an adult, it can lead to increased intracranial pressure, with clinical symptoms of headache, nausea, vomiting, and papilledema; it may even lead to herniation.

Hydrocephalus has a wide variety of etiologies. Although rare, there may be a congenital absence or malformation of the cerebral aqueduct, fourth ventricle foramina, or arachnoid villi. Recall from Chapter 1 that hydrocephalus often accompanies neural tube defects such as spina bifida with myelomeningocele. Tumors may cause hydrocephalus by direct compression of the cerebral aqueduct or foramina or by compressing the superior sagittal sinus, causing an increase in venous pressure and upsetting the absorption pressure gradient. Subdural hematomas, by virtue of their space-occupying properties, may have similar effects. Infectious etiologies include meningitis and ependymitis, the latter causing stenosis of the cerebral aqueduct. Meningitis may affect the arachnoid villi or foramina of Luschka and Magendie, or its purulent exudate may occlude the subarachnoid space or CSF exit sites at the nerve root sheaths, interfering with the flow of CSF. Normal aging and fibrosis of the arachnoid villi can result in hydrocephalus in the older person.

Two major syndromes of hydrocephalus are distinguished clinically: one in which the head enlarges (*overt hydrocephalus*), the other in which head size remains normal (*occult hydrocephalus*). The distinction is based on the age of onset. In infants, the fontanels have not fused. (Fusion occurs by the end of the second year of age.) Hence, overt hydrocephalus typically occurs within the first few months of life. However, skull sutures may separate in a child up to about 5 years of age in the event of a particularly rapidly evolving increase in intracranial pressure. The difference between the fused and unfused skull has implications for symptoms resulting from hydrocephalus. For a child whose fontanels are not closed, head enlargement can occur. In contrast, in older children whose fontanels have fused and in adults, the brain is in a closed vault; hence, swelling can result in symptoms such as headaches, nausea and vomiting, irritability, and visual symptoms because of pressure on cranial nerves, but it will not result in an enlarged head.

At one time, a *communicating hydrocephalus* was distinguished from a *noncommunicating hydrocephalus*. The differentiation was based on whether communication existed between CSF of the ventricular system and that of the subarachnoid space. In communicating (or external) hydrocephalus, the blockage was held to be outside the ventricular system, whereas in noncommunicating (internal or obstructive) hydrocephalus, the blockage was considered to be within the ventricular system. In actual fact, the dynamics of hydrocephalus is not that simple. Complete obstruction of, for example, the cerebral aqueduct in the midbrain is incompatible with survival for more than a few days.

Because CSF production is largely independent of blood and intraventricular pressure, interference with absorption does not elicit a compensatory drop in production. The resultant increase in CSF volume and attendant rise in intracranial pressure cause a dilation of one or more ventricles. Ventricular expansion compresses brain parenchyma against the walls of the cranium: brain tissue becomes thinner, convolutions widen, and in the infant, sutures of the skull ultimately begin to separate. With marked cerebral compression, the arterial supply is compromised, and tissues become ischemic; they may eventually undergo infarction and necrosis.

The symptoms of hydrocephalus, although multiple and varied, are for the most part referable to cerebral compression. Neurologic signs may entail changes in the personality and level of consciousness of the person, as well as cortical sensory and/or motor deficits.

Thought Question

Some children with developmental disabilities with whom rehabilitation professionals work have hydrocephalus. What is this condition, why is it of concern, and how is it treated?

Normal Pressure Hydrocephalus

Normal pressure hydrocephalus (NPH) is a condition that can develop in elderly individuals or individuals who have had an intracranial hemorrhage or infection. The process is so insidious that the ventricles can dilate without an increase of intracranial pressure. Although the exact cause is unknown, the problem seems to be a diminished absorption of the spinal fluid by the arachnoid villae. The theory is that with the increases of ventricular area, there is an increase in the force exerted on the neighboring brain tissue. Especially vulnerable are the long fiber tracts responsible for bladder and leg control as well as the hippocampus. The consequences of NPH typically include three symptoms: urinary incontinence, difficulties with gait, and cognitive decline. The person with NPH may initially have impairments similar to those seen in people with early Parkinson's disease (PD): gait is shuffling, balance declines, the person has difficulty rising from a chair, and he or she may have a stooped, flexed posture. However, urinary incontinence and memory deficits in combination with other findings are indicative of NPH but not of early PD. Intervention for these individuals includes, first and foremost, the use of a ventricular shunt to reduce the pressure from CSF. In some cases, use of the shunt reverses the deficits, although in other people, deficits may persist. In addition to the use of the shunt, physical intervention strategies are important. Because of the similarity in presentation with PD, similar intervention approaches are used, although there is little evidence in the literature regarding the efficacy of such approaches.

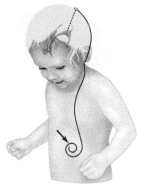 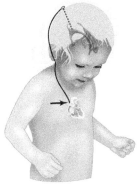

Ventriculoperitoneal shunt   Ventriculoatrial shunt

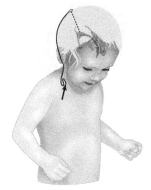 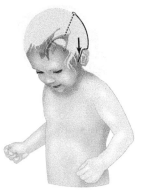

Ventriculoatrial shunt   Shunt to subarachnoid space
to internal jugular vein

FIGURE 25-14 Various shunts provide alternate routes for cerebrospinal fluid.

> **Thought Question**
>
> The findings associated with NPH are similar to those associated with PD. What are the commonalities and what are the major differences between the two conditions? How might rehabilitation of these two types of individuals be similar or different?

> **Thought Question**
>
> You have just begun working for the first time in an intensive care unit that specializes in treating patients who sustained traumatic brain injury. You notice that several of the patients have something referred to as a *shunt*. Explain the purpose of this device and the likely causes that led to the need for the device.

Use of Shunts in Treatment of Hydrocephalus

Current therapeutic efforts to treat hydrocephalus in both children and adults involve the implantation of various shunts to provide alternate routes for CSF to escape (Figure 25-14 ■). Tubes equipped with small, pressure-sensitive valves are implanted to bypass the obstruction and may run from a ventricle to the subarachnoid space, superior sagittal sinus, internal jugular vein, right cardiac atrium (ventriculoatrial), or peritoneal (ventriculoperitoneal) cavity. Treatment is highly successful for most people with developmental hydrocephalus but may have varying success for adults. Even without shunts, many individuals develop alternative pathways for CSF circulation that reach a steady state accommodating the increased fluid volume.

BLOOD–BRAIN BARRIER

In order for neurons and glia to survive and function normally, the composition of the extracellular fluid within which they are bathed must be stable and maintained within rigid limits. Given that communication between neurons is so dependent on the composition of the extracellular environment in which they reside, it is to be expected that the nervous system possesses elaborate mechanisms by which to regulate that environment. This is accomplished by a series of regulatory barriers, comprised of lipids, surrounding and within both the CNS and PNS. In the brain and spinal cord, these barriers are collectively called the **blood–brain barrier**, while in the peripheral nervous system the same barriers are referred to as the **blood–nerve**

barrier or *blood–nerve interface*. Even in the retina, there is a barrier separating the systemic circulation from the extracelluar fluid of the retinal neurons (the **blood–retinal barrier**). The idea that substances dissolved in the blood have a restricted passage into the brain arose from the observations of Paul Erlich in 1885. Although Erlich did not actually develop the concept of a blood–brain barrier, he found that vital dyes, such as trypan blue, when injected into the blood of a mature animal, stained practically all body tissues except the brain.

It should be noted that this blood–brain barrier mechanism is predominantly regulatory, not protective. Hence, the term *barrier* is somewhat misleading from the standpoint that it should not be assumed that the barrier is present for the specific purpose of protecting the brain from potentially harmful organic substances. The ability of a chemical or biologic agent to cross the blood–brain barrier depends on on lipid solubility or various transport systems such as those that transport immunoglobulins and interleukins across the barrier. The barrier often defeats medical management. For example, the barrier restricts transport of dopamine into the brain for the treatment of Parkinson's disease and blocks the access of many antibiotics, used to treat infections, into the intracranial structures.

A substance present in the blood can gain access to the extracellular fluid compartment either by crossing the membranes of capillary endothelial cells or by a more circuitous route (Figure 25-15 ■). The latter involves the substance (1) passing through the fenestrated capillaries of the choroid plexus, (2) crossing the membranes of choroid epithelial cells to enter the CSF compartment, and (3) passing between the spaces separating the ependymal cells lining the ventricles. An additional route involves a substance leaving an extracerebral fenestrated capillary and moving through cells of the arachnoid membrane. Capillary endothelial cells of the brain and spinal cord, choroid epithelial cells, and cells of the arachnoid membrane are all joined together by tight junctions, and this feature represents the structural basis of the blood–brain barrier. Thus, in order for a substance to gain access to neurons, axons, and glia, it must actually pass through the membranes of these barrier cells—unless there is a physical breech of the blood–brain barrier, such as would occur with a trauma (e.g., a cranial fracture, gunshot wound).

Compared to the capillaries of peripheral organs (i.e., systemic capillaries), those of the brain possess a number of unique morphological and functional features. In the peripheral organs, the endothelial cells have clefts between cells and specialized cytoplasmic fenestrations. In contrast, in the brain, the capillary endothelial cells are joined together by complex arrays of tight junctions that block diffusion across the vessel wall. Additionally, brain endothelial cells contain vastly increased numbers of mitochondria that are necessary to support energy-dependent transport mechanisms. Finally, more than 95 percent of the abluminal surface of a brain capillary is covered by the end feet of astrocytes. (It was originally

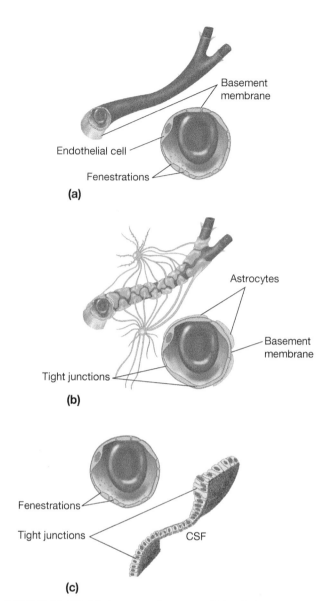

FIGURE 25-15 (a) Access to the extracellular fluid by way of fenestrated capillaries in the systemic system. (b) In the blood–brain barrier, capillaries are covered by end feet of astrocytes. (c) In the blood–brain barrier, tight junctions block diffusion across the vessel wall.

thought that this astroglial sheath was the site of the blood–brain barrier.)

Given these unique features of brain capillaries, what determines whether a substance crosses the vessel wall? First are the biochemical and biophysical characteristics of the solute present in blood plasma. Most important is the lipid solubility of the solute. Because the blood–brain barrier is comprised of lipids, lipid-soluble gasses such as O_2 and CO_2 cross the vessel wall easily, the exchange being limited only by the surface area of the vessel wall and cerebral blood flow. The extent to which a solute binds to plasma proteins is also important because the binding may result in a molecule too large to readily penetrate the barrier. Certain molecules needed for brain metabolism, however, cross the barrier more readily than their lipid solubility alone would predict. Such observations suggest the existence of specific carrier-mediated transport systems for these molecules. These transport systems represent the second major factor in determining what crosses the barrier.

In the adult, neurons rely exclusively on glucose as a source of energy. However, glucose has a low lipid solubility. The carrier-mediated transport system for glucose operates at the luminal membrane of an endothelial cell to transport glucose from the blood into the cell and at the abluminal membrane to transport glucose out of the endothelial cell and into the extracellular fluid of the brain. The glucose transporter is not energy dependent, and therefore, it cannot move glucose against a concentration gradient. It is a facilitative transporter that moves glucose from its relatively higher concentration in plasma into the brain for use by neurons and glia.

Three distinct carrier systems are involved in transporting amino acids across the barrier. A facilitative transporter drives large neutral amino acids, such as phenylalanine, leucine, and valine, down their concentration gradients from blood into the brain. This carrier system also transports systemically administered L-Dopa (the precursor to the neurotransmitter dopamine), the primary drug treatment for people with Parkinson's disease (see Chapter 19). Two energy-dependent carriers transport small neutral amino acids across the barrier. However, these transporters are located only at the abluminal surface of the endothelial cell. Thus, small neutral amino acids are transported out of the brain against a concentration gradient. In the spinal cord, one of these carriers may limit the accumulation of the inhibitory neurotransmitter glycine; in the brain, it may limit the accumulation of the excitatory neurotransmitter glutamate.

The transport of substances across the blood–brain barrier may be regulated to some extent according to metabolic need. During suckling, for example, fat derived from the mother's milk helps fuel the infant's brain metabolism. Associated with this shift to fat metabolism, there is

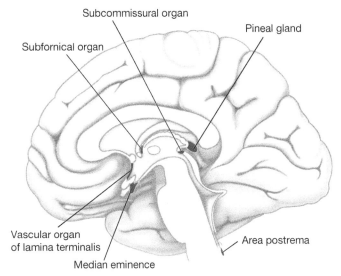

FIGURE 25-16 Circumventricular organs.

an increase in the transport of beta-hydroxybutyrate, the form in which fat enters the brain. During starvation, the brain no longer relies exclusively on the metabolism of glucose for energy, and products of fat metabolism (monocarboxylic acids) appear in the plasma in high concentrations. Normally, they are transported poorly across the blood–brain barrier. However, within a few days of fasting, an increase in transport occurs, indicating that an induction of transport mechanisms has taken place.

Other Related Barriers

Blood–Nerve Barrier

Like cells of the CNS, peripheral nerve fibers and their associated glial cells function within a specialized extracellular fluid compartment, called the *endoneurial space*. Functional equivalents of the arachnoid barrier and blood–brain barrier continue in the PNS as the **blood–nerve barrier**.

An entire peripheral nerve is surrounded by the **epineurium**, a connective tissue sheath that represents

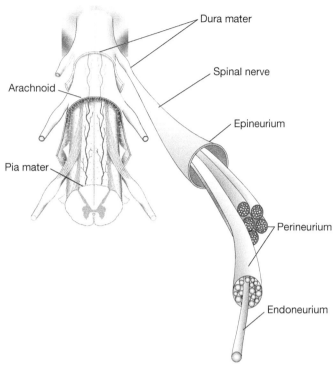

FIGURE 25-17 Peripheral nerve, surrounded by the connective tissue sheath.

the direct continuation of the dura mater in the CNS (Figure 25-17 ■). In all but the smallest of peripheral nerves, axons are arranged in bundles called fascicles. Each fascicle is enclosed by a second connective tissue sheath called the **perineurium**. Finally, individual nerve fibers have a delicate connective tissue covering, the **endoneurium**.

The perineurium forms the boundary of the endoneurial space. It is analogous to the arachnoid membrane in the CNS. The perineurium consists of a layer of thin, concentrically arranged cells that are connected to one another by tight junctions. The tight junctions isolate the endoneurial space around peripheral nerve fibers from the general extracellular fluid of the body. Like brain capillaries, the endothelial cells of capillaries within the perineurium are joined by tight junctions. Therefore, access to the extracellular fluid bathing peripheral nerve axons and glia is limited and controlled, just as in the CNS. However, at the terminals of some peripheral nerve fibers, such as at the neuromuscular junction, the perineurium is open ended. This permits the endoneurial microenvironment to communicate with the general extracellular fluid of the body. Such sites provide certain toxins and viruses with a means of access to the nervous system. The herpes simplex, herpes zoster, and rabies viruses utilize this peripheral nerve pathway to invade and infect cells of the peripheral and central nervous systems. They are actively transported into the CNS axoplasmically along the outside of peripheral nerves.

Blood–Cerebrospinal Fluid Barrier

As noted earlier, the connective tissue stroma of a choroid plexus contains capillaries that are fenestrated. Thus, protein tracers, or horse radish peroxidase (HRP), when injected intravascularly will pass through the pores of choroidal capillaries to fill the connective tissue stroma, but they will not enter the CSF because of the tight junctions that surround the apical regions of choroid epithelial cells. Like the blood–brain barrier, the blood–CSF barrier is responsible for carrier-mediated active transport. Micronutrients like vitamin C are transported into the epithelial cells by an energy-dependent active transporter on the basal membrane and released into CSF by facilitated diffusion (requiring no energy) at the apical surface of the cell. Essential ions also are exchanged between CSF and blood plasma.

Thought Question

Contrast the mechanism by which the following substances are transported across the blood–brain barrier: glucose, alcohol, amino acids, herpes simplex, rabies, HIV, pharmacological agents, and micronutrients.

CLINICAL CONNECTIONS

The Blood–Brain Barrier and Brain Pathology

A variety of pathological conditions affect the function of the blood–brain barrier. This barrier breaks down in the blood vessels of malignant primary brain tumors, such as glioblastomas or anaplastic astrocytomas, or systemic cancers that have metastasized to the brain. This may be due to chemical factors secreted by the tumor cells or to a lack of normal interaction between astrocytes and tumor endothelial cells. The breakdown is limited to the lesion site, which is clinically significant. Albumin labeled with radioactive iodine can be used as a tracer to locate a tumor because the protein enters only the lesion site, not normal brain tissue where the barrier is still intact. The tumor thus stands out as an island of radioactivity in computer-generated images of the brain.

A number of pathologic processes result in increased permeability of brain capillary endothelial cells and a significant increase in the volume of extracellular fluid, a condition called vasogenic brain edema. The edema may be local (e.g., in areas surrounding a tumor, infarct, or contusion), or it may be general (e.g., in head injury and meningitis). The general breakdown of the barrier in meningitis may be exploited clinically. The antibiotic penicillin does not normally penetrate the barrier to reach the brain in significant amounts because of its large size and poor lipid solubility. With the general breakdown of the barrier in meningitis, however, penicillin enters the brain in quantities sufficient to be therapeutically effective.

Several systemic diseases alter the permeability of the blood–retinal barrier. For example, diabetes and arterial hypertension increase the permeability of the barrier. Likewise, trauma may increase barrier permeability. Finally, magnetic resonance imaging has shown that the initial event in multiple sclerosis (MS) is a focal breakdown of the blood–brain barrier. Early MS lesions are, invariably, immediately adjacent to cerebral veins, thus indicating a characteristic breakdown of the barrier in MS.

The Blood–Brain Barrier and Pharmacological Interventions

The blood–brain barrier can pose problems for introducing pharmacological interventions into the nervous system. Psychoactive drugs such as nicotine, heroin, and diazepam (Valium) penetrate the barrier easily because of their high lipid solubility. Uptake of anticonvulsant medications such as phenobarbital and phenytoin, on the other hand, is lower than would be predicted from their lipid solubility because they bind to plasma proteins (mainly albumin). The large molecular size of the resultant complex reduces passage across the barrier.

The problem of medication for people with Parkinson's disease (PD) was addressed in Chapter 19. Recall that one of the greatest challenges to effective management of this condition is that of replacing dopamine through exogenous mechanisms. The role of the blood–brain barrier in keeping substances out of the nervous system explains this problem. In addition to transport systems that regulate the composition of the extracellular fluid, capillary endothelial cells contain enzymes that provide a barrier to some neurotransmitters and their precursors.

As discussed in Chapter 19, Parkinson's disease is a disorder characterized by a degeneration of dopamine-producing neurons in the brain, resulting in a dramatic reduction in the brain's content of the neurotransmitter dopamine. Dopamine will not cross the blood–brain barrier, but its immediate precursor, L-Dopa, does via the facilitative transporter discussed earlier. Thus, the mainstay in the treatment of Parkinson's disease is systemically administered L-Dopa. However, capillary endothelia contain relatively high amounts of monoamine oxidase (MAO) and dopa decarboxylase. Dopa decarboxylase converts the precursor L-Dopa into the neurotransmitter dopamine, and MAO metabolizes dopamine while still in the endothelial cell. These actions reduce the entry of L-Dopa into the brain. This efficient mechanism illustrates why the simultaneous administration of a decarboxylase inhibitor (carbidopa) is standard protocol in L-Dopa treatment of people with Parkinson's disease. Significantly, the carrier-mediated diffusion system that transports L-Dopa across the blood–brain barrier is saturable. This explains why a dose of L-Dopa is less effective following a high-protein meal: other dietary amino acids are competing for the transport carrier.

Thought Question

What are the implications of the blood–brain and related barriers with respect to pharmacological interventions?

TRAUMATIC BRAIN INJURY

Clinical Preview

Chris Chang is an 18-year-old young man who was drinking with his friends, drove his car while inebriated, and ran off the road into a tree. He sustained a head injury and was initially in a coma. By the third day, he was categorized as Glasgow coma scale 10. As you read through this section, consider the following:

- What is meant by a Glasgow coma score, and how well does this score predict Chris's future deficits?

- What types of lasting deficits (impairments and limitations in functional activities) could this young man have?

- In what ways might his deficits be similar to those of people who have had a stroke, and in what ways might they be different?

- What does this suggest regarding rehabilitation strategies?

One of the most frequent neurological problems requiring medical care and rehabilitation is generalized brain injury, which can result from trauma or anoxia (e.g., from near drowning, exposure to gas, or attempted suicide). The biochemistry of anoxia is the same for stroke (see Chapter 24); however, the consequences are more generalized. Here, we focus on **traumatic brain injury (TBI)**, recognizing that brain injury caused by anoxia can result in similar clinical consequences.

Traumatic brain injury results from a blow to the head: either a rapidly moving object striking the stationary head or the rapidly moving head being flung against a hard, immobile surface. Among the most common causes of TBI are accidents (e.g., automobile, falls, sports related), violence, and abuse. Males are more likely to sustain a TBI than are females. Among young adults, common causes of TBI include car accidents, sports injuries, and violence, while falls (resulting in subdural hematomas) are a common cause of TBI among elderly individuals. Child abuse is the most common cause of TBI in infants. Suicide attempts are among the common causes of violent injuries. The cause of the injury is of importance when considering rehabilitation because of the implications with respect to the premorbid social and emotional context.

Some head injuries produce scalp lacerations or skull fractures. Although rigid, the skull possesses sufficient flexibility to yield to a blow severe enough to injure the brain without causing skull fracture. Thus, significant neurological symptoms may be present without such external evidence of head trauma. This is referred to as a **closed head injury**. Note that the term **concussion** refers to any injury resulting from impact with an object and is to be distinguished from the term **cerebral concussion**, which is a specific clinical syndrome (defined later).

Concussive effects may be associated with multiple types of brain pathology involving the gross brain, including neurons and glia and microvascular structures and nerves, depending on the severity of head trauma. Thus, the brain may be bruised, swollen (edematous), and/or lacerated; there may be intracerebral or meningeal hemorrhages; or there may be areas of localized white matter necroses or diffuse axonal injury (as well as herniations of brain tissue discussed earlier). A *cerebral contusion* represents a local area of swelling and capillary hemorrhage resembling a bruise. The extravasated blood remains beneath the pia-arachnoid that is not ruptured. *Cerebral lacerations* involve actual tears in neural tissue. Both types of injury tend to occur at favored sites of the cortical surface, and a brief discussion of their mechanism of production follows.

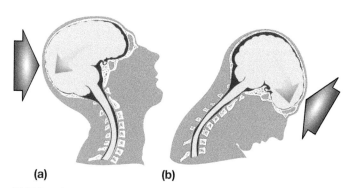

FIGURE 25-18 Coup–contrecoup forces.

> ### Thought Question
>
> Describe the sequence of events that can occur during traumatic brain injury, beginning with the initial injury and continuing with the cascade of subsequent events. What is the relative importance of this sequence of events in determining ultimate impairments and functional consequences of TBI?

Mechanisms Involved in Concussion

When the head is struck, the inertia of the soft and suspended brain causes it to be flung against the side of the skull that was struck. Simultaneously, the brain is pulled away from the opposite side and then rebounds back against bony prominences. This explains why there are some contusions and lacerations beneath the point of impact (**coup injury**), often with even more extensive damage on the opposite side of the brain (**contrecoup injury**). The mechanism of coup–contrecoup contusions is illustrated in Figure 25-18 ■.

Additionally, the brain is subjected to rotational forces that can result in injury to areas of the central nervous system quite removed from the site of impact. The first location wherein these forces can cause problems is the brainstem. The cerebrum is tethered to the brainstem at a high midbrain–subthalamic level. Trauma-induced head motion usually occurs in an arc, owing to the head's attachment to the neck. The brain is thus subjected to shearing stresses primarily in the sagittal plane that are focused at its point of tethering in the region of the upper brainstem reticular formation.

Second, rotational forces cause soft cerebral tissue to be impelled against bony prominences on the inner surface of the skull. Such bony protrusions are especially pronounced in the portion of the middle cranial fossa housing the undersurface of the anterior temporal lobe and temporal pole, as well as in the portion of the anterior cranial fossa housing the undersurface of the anterior frontal lobe and frontal pole. This explains the preferential occurrence of contusions and lacerations at the anterior poles and undersurfaces of the temporal and frontal lobes (Figure 25-19 ■). Lack of occipital lobe damage is explained by the smooth, inner surfaces of the occipital bones and the tentorium cerebelli. Additionally, the corpus callosum is also prone to injury because it can be flung against the falx cerebri.

Head trauma leads to variable degrees of vasogenic brain edema. In *vasogenic edema*, there is a breakdown in the blood–brain barrier such that there is increased permeability of capillary endothelial cells—either because of a defect in their tight junctions or because of increased vesicular transport across the cells. In either case, plasma proteins enter

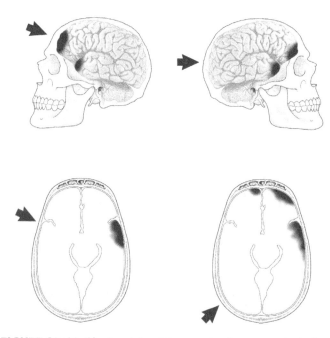

FIGURE 25-19 The frontal and temporal poles are particularly vulnerable to rotational forces.

the extracellular space, and this draws excess water into the space. For some unexplained reason, white matter is especially vulnerable to vasogenic edema. Cerebral edema may be massive and catastrophic, especially in children, and may lead to secondary brainstem compression and/or herniation with potentially dire consequences due to a compromise of respiration, heart rate, and blood pressure. In addition to vasogenic cerebral edema, *cytotoxic edema* can occur. Cytotoxic edema occurs when increased intracranial pressure decreases blood flow, causing neuronal and glial ischemia. The cells cannot maintain metabolic balance and water seeps into the cells, resulting in intracellular edema. Steroids are more effective in treating vasogenic edema because of patching the tight junctions of the capillaries, but they have little effect on cytotoxic edema. With cytotoxic edema, mannitol is used to try to reduce the total fluids of the body. If that intervention is not successful, it may be necessary to decompress the brain by removing a part of the skull to reduce pressure.

> ## Thought Question
>
> What are the typical locations for damage with concussive forces? Refer back to Chapters 21, 22, and 24, and contrast the specific impairments that would occur with damage at these different sites.

Traumatic Brain Injury and the Meninges

Two types of hematoma can occur as a result of head injury, with very different consequences: epidural and subdural hematomas. **Epidural hematomas** occur when a fracture results in a torn meningeal artery. Blood then escapes into the extradural space (between the dura and cranium). Most commonly, this results from a skull fracture of the temporal bone that extends across the grooves containing branches of the middle meningeal artery, thereby tearing the artery (Figure 25-20 ■). The arteries that can be affected are those that lie between the dural membranes (osseous and membranous). These membranes are held very tightly together. When the fracture occurs, there are often no clinical findings (referred to as a "lucid interval") because the membrane sequesters the bleeding. However, once the bleeding reaches a sufficient pressure to dissect the membranes, there can be an abrupt deterioration in the person's condition, sometimes leading to death. The key factor here is that the bleed is associated with an artery with the blood under considerable pressure.

Subdural hematomas, in contrast, are associated with venous drainage and are, therefore, under lower pressure, so the damage can occur more slowly. It is possible for a person to have a subdural hematoma with no clinical consequences, whereas others may have immediate acute symptoms, and some may become chronic. When deterioration of the person's condition occurs, the time course may not be as abrupt (such as occurs in the epidural hematomas), and the results are not typically fatal.

In *acute subdural hematomas*, these rapidly evolving subdural hematomas are due to the tearing of superficial cerebral veins as they cross from the cortical surface to the venous sinuses that are formed from the dura matter. Acute subdural hematomas are particularly problematic in elderly individuals and individuals who are alcoholics because shrinkage of the brain has occurred and results in

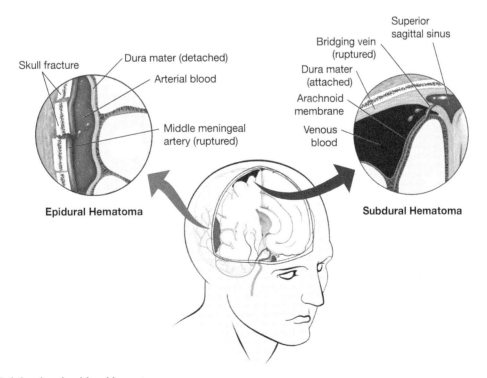

FIGURE 25-20 Subdural and epidural hematomas.

veins that are more taut. This type of injury is particularly common in infants as well.

In *chronic subdural hematoma*, the individual may not have any symptoms, or the symptoms may progress very slowly and be more nonspecific such as giddiness, headaches, slowness in thinking, confusion, drowsiness, apathy, and occasionally seizures. The changes in thinking and consciousness may fluctuate over time. In some instances, the hematoma will have resolved and a hygroma (space with fluid or proteinacious liquid) will be found serendipitously.

Fractures of the Skull

Fractures of the skull are illustrated in Figure 25-21 ■. Skull fractures may provide a vent for excessive intracranial pressure, but they are important for a number of other reasons as well. First, the presence of a fracture provides an indication of the site and potential severity of brain damage. Second, if the fracture crosses a location where a cranial vessel is located, an epidural hematoma may occur. Third, basal skull fractures are a major cause of cranial nerve deficits, referred to as cranial nerve palsies. Fourth, if accompanied by scalp laceration, fractures provide pathways for microbes or air to enter the cranial vault, with resultant meningitis and abscess formation. If the underlying meninges are also torn, fractures provide a route of egress for cerebrospinal fluid; the fluid may present as a watery discharge from the nose (*CSF rhinorrhea*) or external ear canal (*CSF otorrhea*).

The existence of a fracture involving the base of the skull is commonly indicated by signs of cranial nerve damage. When basilar fractures extend across a foramen housing a cranial nerve, the nerve may be either torn or compressed, producing signs appropriate to the function of the particular

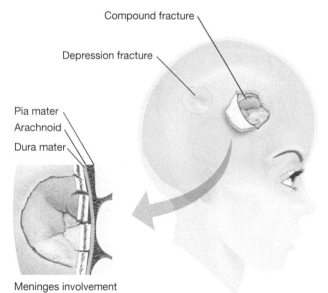

Compound fracture

Depression fracture

Pia mater
Arachnoid
Dura mater

Meninges involvement

FIGURE 25-21 Compound fractures with meningeal involvement and depression fractures are two common fractures of the skull. When the meninges are disrupted, these fractures provide a route by which cerebrospinal fluid can leave the cranium, reducing intracranial pressure. However, if the scalp is lacerated, they also provide a route by which bacteria and viruses can enter the cranium.

nerve (see Chapter 13). Pupil reaction and eye movement can be tested in the comatose patient and are important clinical markers for the patient's prognosis. A comatose patient with pupil dilation and loss of caloric responses after two days has a very poor prognosis (i.e., if the person even survives, he or she will have very poor functional outcome).

Concussion and Coma

Concussion

One of the consequences of mild or severe head trauma is cerebral concussion. This is a clinical entity defined as an immediate, reversible, trauma-induced impairment of neurologic function lasting seconds, minutes, hours, or days. If the patient is comatose, the duration of unconsciousness is the most reliable indicator of the severity of the concussive injury. Additional symptoms include headache, dizziness, confusion, disorientation, amnesia, and visual disturbances. CT and MRI scans do not show any obvious fracture or hematoma. Given the immediacy of onset and often complete reversibility of symptoms, the causative factor is believed to be transient neuronal dysfunction rather than cell death.

No satisfactory explanation can be given of the pathophysiology of concussion in humans. However, evidence from experiments with animal models provides considerable insight that helps to explain the consequences of concussion and has also led to new interventions for concussion. These experiments indicate that biomechanical injury to the brain immediately sets into motion a cascade of neurometabolic changes, some of which are described here. There is an abrupt neuronal depolarization and indiscriminate release of excitatory neurotransmitters (e.g., glutamate), leading to further depolarization and a massive efflux of K^+ and influx of Ca^{2+}. These ionic shifts can lead to more chronic changes in cellular physiology. For example, excessive intraneuronal Ca^{2+} activates a self-destructive cellular cascade involving multiple calcium-dependent enzymes, such as phosphatases, proteases, and lipases. Lipid peroxidation results in the production of free radicals that can lead to cell death. Intraneuronal accumulation of excessive Ca^{2+} also may lead to the activation of *death genes* involved in programmed cell death (apoptosis). Excessive intracellular Ca^{2+} accumulation in mitochondria results in impaired oxidative metabolism with eventual energy failure.

> ### Thought Question
>
> Two high school students recently sought your assistance for musculoskeletal injuries following a football injury. The first had neck pain and stiffness; the second had low back pain. In taking their histories, you learned that each of these young men was also having difficulty concentrating and with memory since the incidents. Why would these two students have both musculoskeletal and cognitive impairments?

Although a person may have a single concussion and get better, repeated concussions have been shown to have cumulative and potentially deleterious effects, as seen in athletes with repetitive minor injuries. Over time, these repeated concussions may lead to mild or profound cognitive deficits. Not only can there be chronic cognitive problems, but evidence is accumulating that repeated head trauma can lead to amyotrophic lateral sclerosis (ALS, or Lou Gehrig's disease) and Alzheimer's type pathology. Another possible consequence of concussion is **axonal shearing** or **diffuse axonal injury**. This occurs because of the shear stresses in the white matter of the cerebrum and brainstem during rotational acceleration or deceleration of the head, resulting in a stretching of nerve fibers without tearing them. Diffusion tensor imaging, a new radiological technique, has been used to demonstrate axonal damage even in people who have sustained only a mild TBI; furthermore, this technique has demonstrated an association between such damage and persistent neurological problems, including deficits of executive function. Postmortem examination of patients who have survived has also shown axonal injury.

Thought Question

Recently, considerable attention has been paid to the long-term consequences of repeated concussion associated with sports. What could be the potential neurological consequences of such injuries for youth who participate in school sports? How are these similar to or different from elite athletes such as boxers and football players who are in professional leagues?

Coma

Coma represents a profound state of unconsciousness from which the patient cannot be aroused by external stimuli or inner need. Thus, the patient, whether with eyes open or closed, cannot be brought to a state even of partial alertness or function. Prolonged coma following head injury represents the accumulation of several processes affecting the brainstem and thalamic reticular activating systems. These processes could include the direct tearing and laceration of the tissue, the consequences of herniation, infarctions and hemorrhages, the biochemical cascades triggered by flooding the brain with excitatory neurotransmitters, and axonal damage.

Cranial trauma is one of the three major causes of coma (the other two causes are cardiac arrest and stroke). Given the immediate loss of consciousness with severe head injury causing coma, coma from head trauma always evolves from a substrate of concussion. However, there is accompanying evidence of gross brain pathology. For example, cerebral contusions, lacerations, scattered intracerebral hemorrhages, subdural hematomas, displacement of the thalamus and midbrain, and sometimes transtentorial herniation can be visualized on CT scans.

Abnormal posturing may occur in comatose patients. Although there are numerous exceptions, such posturing may assume one of two forms, referred to as decerebrate and decorticate, after their initial descriptions in animals following transection of the brainstem at different levels resulting in **decerebrate rigidity** or **decorticate rigidity**.

In decerebrate posturing, associated with decerebrate rigidity, there is a clenching of the jaws and stiff extension of the extremities with internal rotation of the arms and plantar flexion of the feet (Figure 25-22 ■). Generally, such extensor posturing is not a fixed steady state but is intermittent. Decerebrate rigidity occurs with lesions at or below the level of the red nucleus. The classical explanation for decerebrate (extensor) posturing is that there is a loss of extensor inhibition normally exerted on the brainstem reticular formation by the cerebral cortex. Specifically, inhibition is lost to the

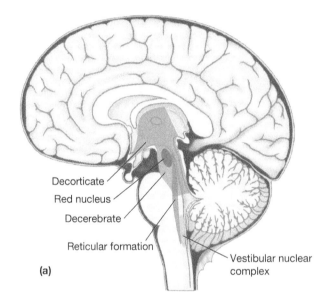

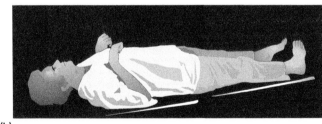

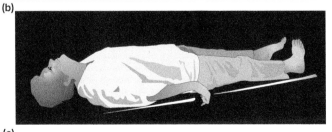

FIGURE 25-22 Decorticate and decerebrate posturing.
(a) Lesions resulting in the two types of abnormal posturing.
(b) Decorticate (upper extremity flexor) posture.
(c) Decerebrate (extensor) posture.

reticulospinal and vestibulospinal tracts. Consequently, spinal extensor motor neurons are driven by reticulospinal neurons originating in the extensor facilitatory parts of the reticular formation.

Thought Question

Consider what you know about decorticate and decerebrate posturing and the anatomical location thought to underlie each condition. Based on this information, how would you interpret the likely damage sustained by individuals with head injury who display these postures? Furthermore, based on the neuroanatomy, what does this posturing suggest about other impairments that could likely occur?

Decorticate rigidity occurs when the lesion is above the level of the red nucleus. In decorticate posturing, associated with decorticate rigidity, the arms are flexed and adducted and the legs extended. Such flexor posturing is thought to result from lesions at a higher level of the neuraxis in the thalamus, internal capsule, or cerebral white matter. Posturing of the upper extremities in flexion results from the intact rubrospinal tract that has been rendered free from inhibitory influences from higher centers. (The intact rubrospinal tract serves to facilitate lower motor neurons that activate upper extremity flexor muscles.)

CLINICAL CONNECTIONS

Thought Question

Contrast the cause of ischemic stroke, hemorrhagic stroke, and TBI. Relate the cause of the disorder to the expected deficits. Summarize the ways in which the impairments associated with these three types of injury might be similar and the ways in which they might be different. Now stretch your mind and think about the possible implications for rehabilitation strategies.

Traumatic injuries to the brain can result in a spectrum of consequences—from those that are mild to those that are very severe. Traumatic brain injuries result in multifocal and diffuse impairments both because the initial impact can affect diverse areas of the brain and because of the additional pathology that occurs, such as diffuse axonal injury and diffuse excitatory neurotransmitter release. Damage to the anterior temporal lobes is common with traumatic brain injuries (with implications for cognitive function), and damage to the frontal lobes frequently occurs, resulting in deficits of executive function. Furthermore, because the pathology associated with TBI often is extensive, massive edema and herniation can occur. Finally, the individual who sustains a TBI is also at risk of injury to the brainstem, which can affect vital centers associated with respiration and cardiac function and can, therefore, lead to death.

When an individual survives a TBI, the motor and sensory consequences are, in many ways, similar to the consequences from stroke. However, an individual who sustains a TBI is likely to have impairments affecting diverse combinations of impairments. For a particular individual, these consequences may or may not include motor, sensory, cognitive, emotional, and memory impairments.

Classification of Coma

The **Glasgow Coma Scale** (Table 25-1 ■) is used routinely to classify patients based on the degree of severity of the injury. It is relatively simple and is used across the spectrum of health care providers, including emergency medical technicians, neurologists and neurosurgeons, and rehabilitation professionals. Individuals with a score of 15 are fully alert and interactive. Individuals with scores of 13 to 15 are considered to have a mild injury. Individuals with a score of less than 5 are considered to have severe head injury.

Mild injury refers to people with a Glasgow Coma Scale score of 13, 14, or 15. People with mild TBI may remain conscious and only feel dazed, or "not quite themselves." Typically, they do not have motor deficits; however, they may complain of headache, confusion, amnesia, ringing in

---

Neuropathology Box 25-2: Decerebrate and Decorticate Posturing

The terms *decerebrate* and *decorticate rigidity* are misleading in as much as both conditions actually are consistent with the definition of spasticity presented in Chapter 11. It should be noted that these two conditions were described early in the 20th century. Indeed, Sir Charles Sherrington, the "father of modern neurophysiology," was the first to describe decerebrate ridigity. These terms have been in common usage long before the 1970s, when a group of neurophysiologists and clinicians arrived at the definition of spasticity that we have used in this text. It is important for the rehabilitation professional to understand the difference in mechanisms underlying spasticity (typically associated with upper motor neuron disorders) and rigidity (typically associated with basal ganglia disorders). Technically, neither rigidity nor spasticity should be equated to fixed postures, given that both are identified in response to passive movement of the limb or body part. As such, the terms *decerebrate posturing* and *decorticate posturing* are more accurate from a neurophysiological perspective.

Table 25-1 The Glasgow Coma Scale

The eye opening part of the Glasgow Coma Scale has four scores:

    4 Patient can open eyes spontaneously.

    3 Patient can open eyes on verbal command.

    2 Patient opens eyes only in response to painful stimuli.

    1 Patient does not open eyes in response to any stimulus.

The best verbal response part of the test has five scores:

    5 Patient is oriented and can speak coherently.

    4 Patient is disoriented but can speak coherently.

    3 Patient uses inappropriate words or incoherent language.

    2 Patient makes incomprehensible sounds.

    1 Patient gives no verbal response at all.

The best motor response test has six scores:

    6 Patient can move arms and legs in response to verbal commands.

    5–2 Patient shows movement in response to a variety of stimuli, including pain.

    1 Patient shows no movement in response to stimuli.

their ears, dizziness, "seeing stars," fatigue, loss of appetite or a "bad taste." Even when an injury may appear to be mild, some people subsequently develop a postconcussion syndrome, including headache, dizziness, neuropsychiatric symptoms, and cognitive impairment. These individuals may have problems with attention and concentration, memory, and learning. Postconcussion symptoms typically develop in the first days after mild traumatic brain injury. Generally, they resolve within a few weeks to a few months, although, in rare cases, they may persist.

Recently, there has been considerable attention to the *second impact syndrome*, especially as it relates to athletes. This term is used when diffuse cerebral swelling occurs after a second concussion and while an athlete is still symptomatic from an earlier concussion. Second impact syndrome in children can cause massive edema, which can be devastating or even fatal. The reason for the massive edema, compared with the initial impact, is unknown. Although there is controversy regarding this syndrome, current guidelines are that athletes should not return to play while signs or symptoms of concussion are present. Furthermore, guidelines are under development, determining whether an athlete can resume participation in sports who has experienced any loss of consciousness other symptoms of concussion, or post-traumatic amnesia.

Moderate injury refers to people with a Glasgow Coma Score of 9 to 12. These individuals may have a combination of deficits. They may have difficulties in any or all

of the following functions: motor, sensory, and/or cognitive. People who have had moderate TBI may have an unrelenting and worsening headache, nausea and vomiting, excessive sleepiness, inability to be aroused from sleep, confusion, restlessness, and agitation. There may be loss of coordination and weakness and numbness of the limbs. Small children who have had moderate to severe TBI may have persistent crying and may not nurse or eat. Anyone with signs of moderate TBI should receive medical attention as soon as possible.

Severe injury refers to people with a Glasgow Coma Score of 8 or less. These individuals have persistent motor and sensory findings in addition to the cognitive/personality changes. Such injuries are not easily localized to specific brain areas, as is the case in stroke, because brain trauma results in multifocal and diffuse injury. The process of diffuse axonal injury is dynamic, with symptoms evolving over a period of time because of the cascading nature of the injury. Patients with the most severe TBI often have midline diencephalic herniation and a constellation of clinical findings. Decerebrate or decorticate posturing can occur, depending on the location of damage, along with disturbances of pupil reactions, eye movement and changes in breathing and in consciousness.

The long-term consequences of TBI may include any combination of impairments, including motor, sensory, cognitive, emotional, memory, and behavioral. For example, if the brainstem is involved, there may be disruption of critical functions of arousal and awakeness. Right-sided hemispheric lesions can cause problems of visual-spatial processing, while left-sided lesions could cause deficits in verbal processing. If the amygdala is damaged, there may be heightened arousal, which enhances sensory information processing and is linked to heightened emotional responses. If the hippocampus is injured (as is the case with temporal lobe tentorial herniation), memory processing can be altered. Therefore, in addition to use of the Glasgow Coma Scale or other measures to classify injury, the rehabilitation professional applies tests and measures similar to those used with people who have sustained strokes (see Chapter 24), as well as specific tests of cognitive function (especially executive function), memory, and perception (see Chapters 21 and 22).

Prognosis

Among the great challenges to the rehabilitation professional is the difficulty in predicting the outcome from a TBI. This can be particularly disconcerting to patients and their families. Some broad indicators are helpful. Included are the depth of impaired responsiveness, duration of altered consciousness, and the duration of post-traumatic amnesia. Loss of pupillary light reflexes is suggestive of a poorer prognosis because this indicates brainstem damage. The degree of hypoxemia and hypotension early after injury can also have an effect on prognosis. However, even with good prognostication, the outcome is predicted incorrectly in about 10 to 20 percent of patients.

People who have had even a so-called mild injury may experience impairments of memory, emotion, executive function, and other cognitive functions long after recovery otherwise appears to be complete. Among other issues that have the greatest impact on daily function are difficulties with divided attention and a reduction in information-processing capacity, speed, or the amount of information that can be processed. Such deficits may be related to the more diffuse white matter lesions that occur with TBI. These deficits can have profound implications for return to school, work, or home responsibilities, even in cases where all motor function has returned. Deficits of cognition, memory, and executive function are also problematic (e.g., difficulty with work performance following injury) and for older adults who may already be at risk for cognitive decline.

Further compounding the prognosis for people who have sustained a TBI is that they may also have musculoskeletal injuries associated with the trauma. These injuries can significantly complicate the rehabilitation and outcomes, especially when the individual has behavioral, emotional, and cognitive dysfunction, as well as chronic pain.

Thought Question

What are the factors to consider in estimating the prognosis for a person who has sustained a TBI?

Examination

The examination strategy includes determination of the level of coma; the time course of recovery from coma; the extent of impairments related to cognition, emotion, and memory; and the degree to which sensory and motor functions are impaired. Function is examined, not just in relation to motor performance, but also with regard to the person's judgment and safety. Interventions are then developed to improve function that address each of the underlying deficits. The examination strategy used with the person who has a TBI is similar to the strategy used for the person who has had a stroke (see Chapter 24). However, a few issues are of particular importance and should be emphasized.

First, it is necessary to establish the overall effects of the TBI, as well as the specific cognitive ramifications. The Glasgow Coma Scale (discussed earlier) is helpful in establishing the overall status with respect to injury. The Rancho Los Amigos Hospital Scale of Cognitive Function provides a more detailed categorization of overall cognitive status and identifies specific issues of particular importance in determining the rehabilitation strategy. Some of the key issues assessed in the Rancho Los Amigos scale are summarized in Table 25-2 ■. Two scoring systems have been devised to address the amount of injury sustained in sports injuries. These are the Standardized Assessment of Concussion (SAC) and the Rivermead Post-Concussion Symptom Questionnaire.

Table 25-2 The Ranchos Los Amigos Hospital Scale of Cognitive Function

LEVEL	RESPONSE	AMOUNT OF ASSISTANCE	DESCRIPTION
I	No response	Total	No response to any stimuli
II	General response	Total	Generalized response to painful stimuli
III	Localized response	Total	Responds directly to stimuli Responds inconsistently to simple commands
IV	Confused, agitated	Maximal	Brief and nonpurposeful attention, unable to cooperate with treatment efforts
V	Confused, inappropriate Nonagitated	Maximal	Inconsistently responds to simple commands May become agitated in response to external simulation
VI	Confused, appropriate	Moderate	Consistently follows simple directions
VII	Automatic appropriate	Minimal	Unaware of own limitations; oppositional/uncooperative
VIII	Purposeful, appropriate	Stand-by	Consistently oriented; independently attends to and completes familiar task; aware of own limitations; may be depressed, irritable

What are the strengths and weaknesses of the Glasgow Coma Scale and the Ranchos Los Amigos Scale? When would it be most appropriate to use each when examining a person who sustained a TBI?

Second, many individuals who have sustained a TBI are young adults or teenagers. Of critical importance is an understanding of the individual's premorbid life situation, including the activities preferred, performance in school, sociability level, and home situation. It is important to weigh this individual's current intellectual, social, and emotional status against his or her prior status. For people who sustained a brain injury following an attempted suicide, clearly a psychological evaluation is paramount. And for infants with abuse-related injuries, consultation is required with the proper authorities. With such infants, there are ramifications regarding the caregivers with whom the clinician will interact.

Third, because emotional, cognitive, and memory deficits typically occur with TBI, these areas require extensive assessment, using both qualitative assessment and standardized tests. A number of relevant tests were discussed in Chapters 21 and 22.

Fourth is the necessity to assess functional ability, including tasks related to balance, gait, upper extremity function, and self-care. The tests and measures are similar to those used for people who have sustained a stroke (Chapter 24).

Finally, specific tests also are used to assess the motor, somatosensory, language, and perceptual systems, as well as tests of working memory, speed of response, and judgment. When localized injury has been identified, the predicted impairments assist the clinician to identify tests and measures that should be applied. For example, if there is brainstem or cerebellar involvement, tests should be implemented of the vestibular system and related reflexes (Chapter 17). If a lesion is localized to the left hemisphere, language, motor planning, and praxis can be affected and should be considered; and if the lesion involves the right temporo-parieto-occipital region, perception should be assessed (Chapter 18). In situations where diffuse injury has occurred, the clinician makes judgments regarding what to measure and how to focus the intervention based on overall impressions and findings.

Given what you know so far about TBI and stroke, what are the likely similarities and differences in the examination and intervention strategies used by the rehabilitation professional?

Intervention Strategies

Medical Management

The medical management of a person with head trauma severe enough to cause coma is basically to provide support. Basic intensive care procedures include maintaining adequate oxygenation, blood pressure, and nutrition and preventing thrombophlebitis and skin breakdown. Edema can be managed by using high doses of methylprednisolone (steroids). Mannitol may be used to reduce fluid, thereby reducing intracranial pressure. In some cases, a coma is induced to decrease the metabolic demand on the cerebral tissue. It is customary to insert a device to measure the intracranial pressure. Common techniques include use of a pressure manometer device in the epidural space or a catheter inserted into the ventricles. In some cases, a drain is used to reduce the intracranial pressure. When a patient has an intracranial monitoring device or a drain, the position of the head of bed is determined by the neurosurgeon. In some instances, it is crucial to keep the head elevated (e.g., 30 to 45 degrees) to maintain constant intracranial pressure.

Rehabilitation

Physical management should be initiated as soon as possible to prevent secondary sequelae. Included are impairments of range of motion and postural alignment, cardiovascular and musculoskeletal deconditioning, skin breakdown, and other general consequences of immobility.

Many of the rehabilitation strategies used when working with people who have sustained a TBI are similar to those used with people following a CVA (see Chapter 24). However, as with examination strategies, some specific issues are of particular importance following a TBI. First is the critical role of the team approach. Because many of the patient's deficits are likely to involve multiple domains (psychological, physical, and behavioral), it is of paramount importance that various members of the team work closely together. This applies to working with individuals in the ICU (where the medical condition can change hour to hour or even minute to minute) to working in acute and chronic rehabilitation (where cognitive/emotional issues can affect every aspect of the intervention) to the home setting (where safety and judgment can affect ability to be independent). Strategies directed at improving function must be specifically tailored to the individual. Recovery of functional skills and return to community can be particularly challenging for this population. Given that the cognitive, emotional, and behavioral impairments can be pervasive, they must be addressed both in and of themselves and also when deciding how best to structure interventions focused on restoration of physical function (e.g., walking, eating, and self-care).

Summary

This chapter began with a consideration of the meningeal and cerebrospinal fluid environments within which the CNS is embedded. We also discussed the nature of clinical conditions related to these structures.. For example, the meninges can trap blood between their layers in the event of traumatic brain injury or a cerebral hemorrhage. CSF serves as a "water cushion" for the brain and spinal cord, serving to minimize or prevent damage in the event of mechanical trauma. Additionally, CSF provides a vehicle for the transport of nutrients to and the removal of waste products from brain tissue. Its composition is routinely analyzed because its cellular, chemical, and microbial makeup can reveal many pathological conditions that affect the CNS such as encephalitis, meningitis, and intracranial hemorrhage. Hence, the spinal tap is one of the procedures discussed in the chapter.

The second major section focused on the blood–brain and related barriers. This regulatory barrier ensures that appropriate nutrients reach neurons to fuel their high metabolism and that appropriate molecular substrates such as amino acids are able to access neurons, allowing them to synthesize the vast array of proteins they need to function properly. However, because of the factors that regulate the passage of substances across the barrier, certain toxic agents can breach the barrier, causing damage to cells of the central nervous system with resulting impairment of function.

The third major section considered traumatic brain injury. The mechanical factors that cause concussive TBI resulting in coup and contrecoup contusions and lacerations were discussed, as were the factors causing vasogenic and cytotoxic edema. Trauma-induced tearing of arteries and veins may result in extravasated blood becoming trapped in the epidural or in the subdural spaces of the meninges. The cellular pathophysiology of concussion was addressed, including the cascade of cellular events that follow trauma. We then considered the ramifications of this cascade of events and the diffuse nature of injury from TBI compared with stroke. We ended this chapter with a discussion of the implications for rehabilitation. With respect to examination, we included specialized scales for coma, as well as issues that should be considered specific to people with TBI. With respect to intervention, we discussed similarities as well as differences in strategies as compared with people who sustained a stroke.

Applications

1. Jamie Singleton is a 6-year-old boy who fell while riding his bike. He was not wearing a helmet. His parents report that he may have lost consciousness for a very short period. They had him rest and he seemed fine that evening. Days later, however, he still had a headache and told his parents that he couldn't see well. His parents interpreted his description to indicate that he may have blurry vision. Jamie's parents took him to his pediatrician who completed a physical examination and ordered an MRI—all of which were normal. The physician told the parents that he had had a minor concussion.

   a. What does a diagnosis of concussion mean?
   b. Comment about the usefulness of the Glasgow and Rancho Los Amigos scales in assessing Jamie's injury.
   c. What was the purpose of the imaging? Given that the MRI was normal, what was the physiological basis for Jamie's symptoms?
   d. Comment about the impact of sustaining a single concussion versus repeated concussions.
   e. What would have been the likely impact of Jamie's fall had he been wearing a helmet?

2. Mark Andrews is 54 years old with a long-standing history of chronic alcoholism. He drank sufficiently to have a blackout, during which he fell and hit his head. His wife called 911, and he was transported by ambulance to the Emergency Department (ED) of his local hospital. On admission, Mr. Andrews was unresponsive and had a Glasgow Coma Score of 3. A CT scan revealed a subarachnoid hemorrhage in his right cerebral hemisphere.

   a. What other tests might have been used to diagnose the subarachnoid hemorrhage?
   b. What does the Glasgow score of 3 indicate about the severity of his head injury? Given this score, what might be his score on the Ranchos Los Amigos Scale?
   c. What types of impairments could be associated with a right subarchnoid hemorrhage?
   d. Given that Mr. Andrews has a long-standing problem with alcoholism, what might be the implications for his recovery from the current brain injury?

References

Meninges

Bo-Abbas, Y., and Bolton, C. F. Roller-coaster headache. *New Engl J Med* 332:1585, 1995.

Davson, H., Hollingsworth, G., and Segal, M. B. The mechanism of drainage of the cerebrospinal fluid. *Brain* 93:665, 1970.

Fox, R. J., et al. Anatomic details of intradural channels in the parasagittal dura: A possible pathway for flow of cerebrospinal fluid. *Neurosurg* 39:84, 1996.

Laine, F. J., et al. Acquired intracranial herniations: MR imaging findings. *Am J Roentgenol* 165:967, 1995.

Penfield, W., and McNaughton, F. Dural headache and innervation of the dura mater. *Arch Neurol Psychiatr* 44:43, 1940.

Upton, M. L. and Weller, R. O. The morphology of cerebrospinal fluid drainage pathways in human aerachnoid granulations. *J Neurosurg* 63:867, 1985.

Zhang, E. T., Inman, C. B. E., and Weller, R. O. Interrelationships of the pia mater and the perivascular (Virchow-Robin) spaces in the human cerebrum. *J Anat* 170:111, 1990.

Venous Drainage

Duvernoy, H. M. *The Human Brain: Surface, Three-Dimensional Sectional Anatomy with MRI, and Blood Supply*, 2nd ed. Springer-Verlag, Vienna, 1999.

Schaller, B. Physiology of cerebral venous blood flow: From experimental data in animals to normal function in humans. *Brain Res Rev* 46:243–260, 2004.

Cerebrospinal Fluid

Brightman, M. W., and Reese, T. S. Junctions between intimately apposed cell membranes in the vertebrate brain. *J Cell Biology* 40:648, 1969.

Bull, J. W. D. The volume of the cerebral ventricles. *Neurol* 11:1, 1961.

Cutler, R. W. P., et al. Formation and absorption of cerebrospinal fluid in man. *Brain* 91:707, 1968.

DiChiro, G. Observations on the circulation of the cerebrospinal fluid. *Acta Radiol (Diagn)* 5:988, 1966.

Dohrmann, G. J., and Bucy, P. C. Human choroid plexus: A light and electron microscopic study. *J Neurosurg* 33:506, 1970.

Gutierrez, Y., Friede, R. L., and Kaliney, W. J. Agenesis of arachnoid granulations and its relationship to communicating hydrocephalus. *J Neurosurg* 43:553, 1975.

Kier, E. L. The cerebral ventricles: A phylogenetic and ontogenetic study. In: Newton, T. H., and Potts, D. G.,eds. *Radiology of the Skull and Brain*, vol 3, Anatomy and pathology. Mosby, St. Louis, 1977.

Lenfeldt, N., Koskinen, L.-O. D., Bergenheim, A. T., et al. CSF pressure assessed by lumbar puncture agrees with intracranial pressure. *Neurology* 68:155–158, 2007.

McConnell, H., and Bianchine, J., eds. *Cerebrospinal Fluid in Neurology and Psychiatry*, Chapman and Hall, London, 1994.

Nicholson, C. Signals that go with the flow. *Trends Neurosci* 22:143, 1999.

Nilsson, C., Lindvall-Axelsson, M., and Owman, C. Neuroendocrine regulatory mechanisms in the choroid plexus-cerebrospinal fluid system. *Brain Res Rev* 17:109, 1992.

Schurr, P. H., and Polkey, C. E., eds. *Hydrocephalus*. Oxford University Press, New York, 1993.

Silverberg, G. D. Normal pressure hydrocephalus (NPH): Ischemia, CSF stagnation or both. *Brain* 127:947–948, 2004.

Strazielle, N., and Ghersi-Egea, J.-F. Choroid plexus in the central nervous system: Biology and physiopathology. *J Neuropath Exp Neurol* 59:561, 2000.

Blood–Brain Barrier

Bradbury, M. W. B. *The Concept of a Blood–Brain Barrier*. John Wiley & Sons, New York, 1979.

Bradbury, M. W. B. The structure and function of the blood–brain barrier. *Fed Proc* 43:186-190, 1984.

de Vries, H. E., Kuiper, J., de Boer, A. G., et al. The blood–brain barrier in neuroinflammatory diseases. *Pharmacol Rev* 49:143–155, 1997.

Floris, S., Blezer, E. L. A., Schreibelt, G., et al. Blood–brain barrier permeability and monocyte infiltration in experimental allergic encephalomyelitis. *Brain* 127:616–627, 2004.

Ford, D. H. Blood–brain barrier: A regulatory mechanism. *Ann Rev Neurosci* 2:1–42, 1976.

Goldstein, C. W., and Betz, A. L. The blood–brain barrier. *Sci Am* 255:74–93, 1986.

Hart, Jr., W. M. *Adler's Physiology of the Eye, Clinical Application*, 9th ed. Mosby Year Book, St Louis, 1992.

Hickey, W. F. Migration of hematogenous cells through the blood–brain barrier and the initiation of CNS inflammation. *Brain Pathol* 1:97–105, 1991.

Huber, J. D., Egleton, R. D., and Davis, T. P. Molecular physiology and pathophysiology of tight junctions in the blood–brain barrier. *Trends Neurosci* 24:719–725, 2001.

Johanson, C. E. Ontogeny and phylogeny of the blood–brain barrier. In: E. Neuwelt, ed. *Implications of the Blood–Brain Barrier and Its Manipulation*, Vol. 1, Basic science aspects. Plenum Press, New York, 1989.

Laterra, J., and Goldstein, G. W. Ventricular organization of cerebrospinal fluid: Blood–brain barrier, brain edema, and hydrocephalus. In: Kandel, E. R., Schwartz, J. H., and Jessell, T. M., eds. *Principles of Neural Science*, 4th ed. McGraw-Hill, New York, 2000.

Latour, L. L., Kang, D.-W., Ezzeddine, M. A., et al. Early blood–brain barrier disruption in human focal brain ischemia. *Ann Neurol* 56:468–477, 2004.

Lipton, M. L., Gulko, E., Zimmerman, M. E., et al. Diffusion-sensor imaging implicates prefrontal axonal injury in executive function impairment following very mild traumatic brain injury. *Radiology* 252:816–824, 2009.

Nolte, J. *The Human Brain: An Introduction to Its Functional Anatomy*. Mosby Elsevier, Philadelphia, 2009.

Prat, A., Biernacki, Wosik, K., and Antel, J. P. Glial cell influence on the human blood–brain barrier. *Glia* 36:145–155, 2001.

Rapoport, S. I. *Blood–Brain Barrier in Physiology and Medicine*. New York: Raven Press, 1976.

Ropper, A. H., and Brown, R. H. *Adams and Victor's*

Principles of Neurology, 8th ed. McGraw-Hill, New York, 2005.

Tarnai, I., and Tsuji, A. Transporter-mediated permeation of drugs across the blood-brain barrier. *J Pharm Sci* 89:1371–1388, 2000.

Traumatic Brain Injury

Adair, J. Damage control for traumatic brain injury. *Neurology*. 67:748–755, 2006.

Adriano, C., Gianmartino, B., Dossena, M., Mutani, R., and Mora, G. Severely increased risk of amyotrophic lateral sclerosis among Italian professional football players. *Brain* 128:472–476, 2005

Giza, C. C. and Hovda, D. A. The neurometabolic cascade of concussion. *J Athletic Training* 36(3):228–235, 2001.

King, N. S., Crawford, S., Wenden, E. J., Moss, N. E. G., and Wade, D. T. The Rivermead Post-Concussion Symptoms Questionnaire: A measure of symptoms commonly experienced after head injury and its reliability. *J Neurol* 242:587–592, 1995.

McCrea, M., Kelly, J. P., and Randolph, C. *Standardized Assessment of Concussion (SAC): Manual for Administration, Scoring and Interpretation*, 3rd ed. Comprehensive Neuropsychological Services, Waukesha, WI, 2000.

NIH Consensus Development Panel of Rehabilitation of Persons with Traumatic Brain Injury. Rehabilitation of persons with traumatic brain injury. *JAMA* 282:974–983, 1998.

Povlishock, J. T., and Katz, D. I. Update of neuropathology and neurological recovery after traumatic brain injury. *J Head Trauma Rehabil* 20:76–94, 2005.

Ropper, A, H., and Brown, R. H. Ch. 35. Craniocerebral trauma. *Adams and Victor's Principles of Neurology*, 8th ed. McGraw-Hill, New York, 2005.

Moore, K. L., and Dalley, A. F. Ch. 7. Head. *Clinically Oriented Anatomy*, 4th ed. Lippincott Williams & Wilkins, Philadelphia, 1999.

Brain Plasticity: Injury, Recovery, and Rehabilitation

LEARNING OUTCOMES

This chapter prepares the reader to:

1. Discuss the role of long-term potentiation and long-term depression in plasticity.

2. Explain how neural recovery differs from neural compensation and discuss the importance of this distinction.

3. Explain why change at the level of the gene is of importance in plasticity.

4. Discuss the role of plasticity in the development of ocular dominance columns and in the development of language.

5. Discuss animal experiments that implicate plasticity in the expression of cortical maps.

6. Describe adaptive and maladaptive responses that result in adaptations to cortical maps among humans.

7. Contrast adaptive and maladaptive plasticity and provide examples of each.

8. Discuss critical periods of development and provide examples of their impact on development in both animal models and humans.

9. Discuss evidence related to neural plasticity with regard to recovery from stroke.

10. Discuss the relationship of diaschisis and plasticity to recovery following stroke.

11. Discuss the evidence related to ipsilesional and contralesional consequences of stroke and their implications for recovery.

12. Analyze the relevance and importance of experiments conducted in animal models and their implications for rehabilitation of people who have sustained brain injury.

13. Identify 10 principles related to recovery of function following brain injury.

14. Relate the same 10 principles to implications for rehabilitation.

ACRONYMS

AMPA Alpha-amino-3-hydroxyl-5-methyl-4-isoxazolepropionate

BDNF Brain-derived neurotrophic factors

CIMT Constraint-induced movement therapy

CNS Central nervous system

CVA Cerebrovascular accident

EEG Electroencephalography

EPSP Excitatory postsynaptic potential

fMRI Functional magnetic resonance imaging

GABA Gamma-amino butyric acid

LGB Lateral geniculate body

LTD Long-term depression

LTP Long-term potentiation

M1 Primary motor area

MEG Magneto-encephalography

MEP Motor-evoked potential

mRNA Messenger ribonucleic acid

NMDA N-methyl-D-aspartic acid

PD Parkinson's disease

PET Positron emission tomography

SCI Spinal cord injury

SMA Supplementary motor area

TMS Transcranial magnetic stimulation

Introduction

Plasticity is the brain's capacity to be shaped by experience. Chapter 4 addressed plasticity at the cellular level of the synapse and in the behavioral context of learning and memory. In this chapter, we draw on that information but extend these concepts to the entire organism, drawing from work with animal models (both rodents and primates) and from humans.

The first major section of this chapter provides a basis for considering plasticity by summarizing and expanding on information that was presented in Chapter 4. To this end, we discuss changes in cell structure, long-term potentiation, and long-term depression (LTP and LTD), as well as the relevant mediators.

Our focus in the second major section of this chapter is on plastic changes that can be observed in the organization of the central nervous system (CNS) during development and following specialized training or damage to the adult nervous system. First, we consider cortical columns and the critical periods of development related to the visual system. Then we consider the research on plasticity that is concerned with what is called map plasticity. As we saw in Chapter 7, the body's receptive surface is mapped onto the primary somatosensory cortex in exquisite detail. Map plasticity refers to changes in the extent of representation of body parts, in particular within the cerebral cortex, under a variety of circumstances. In this section, we also discuss two conditions that occur because of maladaptive plasticity: phantom limb pain and fibromyalgia.

The third major section of this chapter focuses on plasticity that occurs following damage to the nervous system in primates, including humans. Here, we consider emerging evidence from animal models related to cortical reorganization following ischemic injury and people with a variety of neurological disorders.

In the final major section, we address some of the salient issues surrounding application of current models and information to rehabilitation of individuals who have sustained cortical damage.

NEURAL PLASTICITY REVISITED

Plasticity can be observed as a change in structure or function of individual neurons or can be inferred from measures taken across populations of neurons. Thus (as discussed in Chapter 4), plasticity can be observed as changes in the number of synapses or the strength of those synapses. These changes can be manifested at the systems level as alterations in neural networks and reorganization of representational maps, as discussed later in this chapter. For plasticity to be of functional relevance, it is necessary that these changes also result in behavioral changes (e.g., sensory, motor, cognitive). Although changes in sensory, motor, or cognitive performance may result from plasticity, measures of these behaviors are not themselves direct measures of plasticity nor can changes in these measures be interpreted in isolation as evidence of plasticity. Yet, these are the measures that are most easily applied in humans. And indeed, many of the techniques used to study plasticity in animal models are invasive and, as such, cannot be applied to studying plasticity in humans. While much can be learned from studies at the cellular level and from animal models, it is challenging to make direct links from cellular mechanism to neural rearrangement and then to functional changes. Tantalizing information is available and inferences can be drawn, but much is yet to be learned about the mechanisms of plasticity in humans.

One of the challenges in the quest to elucidate mechanisms of neuroplasticity is to differentiate changes that represent true neural recovery from those that represent changes due to compensations. Neural recovery depends on restoration of brain function in neural tissues that were initially lost as a result of injury or disease. Recovery can also refer to the ability to perform tasks and overall behaviors at the same level as was possible prior to the injury or disease, referred to as *functional recovery*. The term *compensation*, on the other hand, refers to residual neural tissue taking over functions of damaged or lost tissue, potentially resulting in differences in motor and task performance from that which was observed prior to injury or disease.

Neural Plasticity from Cells to Organisms

Brain plasticity can be described at several different levels of the central nervous system, from individual cells to networks of neurons to behavior. A central aspect of plasticity is the increase (or decrease) in synapses, because it is through synapses that cells communicate and, hence, through synapses that changes in communication can occur between neurons. Structural manifestations of plasticity at the level of individual cells include increases in dendritic arborization, spine density, numbers of synapses, and receptor density through increased dendritic spine formation, pruning, remodeling, and addition of new synapses. These structural changes at the level of the cell lead to structural changes within groups of cells (e.g., cortical columns, cortical maps), which in turn can result in changes in thickness of the structure, gray matter cell density, or patterns of activity within neural networks. These changes, in turn, can lead to changes in behavior as evidenced by motor actions and sensory perceptions, possibly resulting in changes in overall task performance. Considerable evidence now demonstrates the role of training in mediating such structural changes.

Measurement of Neural Plasticity

Thought Question

In preparation for this chapter, it is important to review information in Chapter 4 about neuronal signaling. What are the mechanisms underlying LTP and LTD?

Four different categories of neural plasticity can be considered, each of which has been applied in different experimental studies. The first two categories of neural plasticity relate to individual neurons and are differentiated into structural and functional changes. Structural changes in individual neurons include changes in dendritic arborization, spine density, synapse size and number, axonal arborization, and receptor density. Functional changes in individual neurons include excitatory postsynaptic potentials (EPSPs), neural activity, and intrinsic excitability.

Recall from Chapter 4 that changes to neuronal signaling can result in long-term potentiation (LTP) and/or long-term depression (LTD). LTP and LTD in some synapses depend on an interaction between the two types of glutamate receptors, N-methyl-D-aspartic acid (NMDA) receptors and alpha-amino-3-hydroxyl-5-methyl-4-isoxazolepropionate (AMPA) receptors. Both LTP and LTD begin with the same signal—namely, the entrance of Ca^{2+} through the NMDA receptor. Thus, important molecules involved in plasticity include Ca^{2+}, NMDA receptors, and AMPA receptor trafficking. Brain-derived neurotropic factor (BDNF) also influences neural plasticity. BDNF affects neural plasticity directly through modulation of cellular processes and indirectly through modulation of other factors that influence plasticity (e.g., can rapidly depolarize postsynaptic neurons and elicit short-term, post-synaptic effects on ion channels and NMDA). Hence, the presence of circulating BDNF is sometimes used as a measure indicating plastic changes.

It should not be surprising that changes in gene expression (i.e., the process by which information from the gene is used to synthesize related products such as amino acids and hormones) also are central to long-term changes in the nervous system. After all, plasticity involves memory and learning (whether at the level of cells or of the person). Learning, in turn, implies a long-term change, manifested by changes in distribution or density of postsynaptic AMPA receptors (among others). Hence, long-term change requires a change in the gene expression itself, which is mediated by changes of messenger ribonucleic acid (mRNA) and related proteins. Such changes in gene expression and protein synthesis have been linked to plasticity in, for example, the mammalian hippocampal formation.

Just as individual neurons can demonstrate plastic changes, so too can populations of neurons. Likewise, these changes can be differentiated into structural and functional changes. Structural changes in populations of neurons can be measured by such variables as thickness of particular structures and gray matter density. Functional changes can be measured structurally by quantifying changes to sensory and motor maps.

Techniques used to measure structural and functional changes include electroencephalography (EEG), which measures brain activity generally; positron emission tomography (PET), used to image neural activity within the cerebral cortex; functional magnetic resonance imaging (fMRI), used to measure changes in blood flow as an indirect measure of synaptic activity during specific tasks; and magneto-encephalography (MEG), a technique used to map brain activity by recording magnetic fields produced naturally in the brain. In addition, transcranial magnetic stimulation (TMS) is used extracranially to either stimulate or inhibit underlying cortex and has been combined with other imaging techniques to investigate neural changes. These responses can be measured with motor-evoked potentials (MEPs), which are recorded from muscles following direct stimulation of the exposed cortex.

Techniques to observe changes following training with or without neural damage or injury have substantial limitations. Many of the techniques to observe changes at the level of the individual neuron cannot be applied in studies of humans, relying rather on animal models. Although intracellular and extracellular electrophysiological recording can identify changes and indicate whether these changes are inhibitory or excitatory, they are limited in terms of the number of networks that can be examined at one time. In contrast, imaging techniques used to examine changes in populations of neurons can easily be applied in studies of humans and can provide information about localized neural activity, but these techniques cannot determine if the activity is inhibitory or excitatory at the neuronal level.

Thought Question

What are the relationships among memory, learning, genes, and plasticity?

Behavioral Consequences of Neural Plasticity

Animal experiments illustrating the behavioral consequences of neuronal plasticity demonstrate how changes in neuronal response can change motor behavior. This is demonstrated well by a condition that is analogous to epilepsy. Specifically, a stimulating neuron is implanted in the amygdala and weakly stimulated on a daily basis. At first, there is no response to the stimulation, but with daily repeated stimulation, the stimulation results in full-blown seizure activity. This process is referred to as *kindling* because it is likened to kindling a fire. Once the full-blown seizure occurs, it can be initiated even a year later by a single weak stimulation.

To date, much of the study of plasticity has revolved around two behavioral changes: motor skill acquisition and memory. Given the role of the basal ganglia, motor cortex, and cerebellum in motor skill acquisition and performance

(Chapter 20), it is not surprising that studies related to these functions have centered on changes in these areas, associated with motor performance, motor learning, or re-learning following injury. Similarly, because of the role of the hippocampus and amygdala in memory (Chapter 21), studies related to memory and cognition have centered around these latter structures.

PLASTICITY OF CORTICAL STRUCTURES

Clinical Preview

You are a rehabilitation professional, working in an early intervention clinic. Your spouse also is a rehabilitation professional and works in an adult neurological rehabilitation clinic. As you read through this section, consider the following:

*   What are the implications of critical periods for the likely response to neurological injury of neonates compared with adults?

*   What might be the similarities and differences in alteration of cortical columns in neonates compared with adults who have brain injury?

*   What might findings about critical periods and cortical columns imply regarding the likelihood that neonates with neurological injury could develop typical motor and sensory abilities?

Plasticity during Development

Ocular Dominance Columns

Thought Question

In preparation for this section, review ocular dominance columns discussed in Chapter 18.

The visual system provides a well-studied example of developmental neuronal plasticity. An orderly sequence of events occurs in the primary visual cortex during development that underlies the establishment of normal binocular vision and depth perception (**stereoscopic vision**, or **stereopsis**). An early event is the development of **ocular dominance columns** (actually stripes or bands) in layer IVC of the visual cortex. As noted in Chapter 18, these are sets of contiguous neurons arranged in stripes, with each stripe occupying a cortical width of approximately 0.5 mm. Neurons within a given ocular dominance column respond to **lateral geniculate body (LGB)** input from just one eye. On each side of the brain, the columns alternate with one another: one receiving input from the right eye, its neighbor input

from the left eye, its neighbor from the right eye, and so on (see Figure 18-13). This segregation of input from the LGB neurons serving each eye occurs before birth in monkeys and is apparently due to LGB axons following molecular guidance signals. The columns are then defined sharply by the thousands of left eye and right eye terminal arbors of afferents from the lateral geniculate body disentangling their overlapping terminals from one another. Discrete ocular dominance columns are generated by the remodeling of these terminal arbors.

An important postnatal event is the development of cortical neurons that respond to input from both eyes—that is, binocular neurons. Binocular responsive neurons develop in the cortical layers above and below layer IVC, specifically in layers II, III, V, and VI. Their development depends on at least two factors: (1) a convergence onto the same layer III neuron of input from adjacent right and left eye ocular dominance columns in layer IVC (Figure 26-1 ■) and (2) a temporally coincident arrival of input from neurons of right and left eye ocular dominance columns subserving corresponding points on the two retinas. A critical question here is what occurs when pathology impairs fulfillment of these criteria.

The question is important because two clinical conditions exist in human infants that affect this normal development sequence. The first is congenital **cataract**, in which the opacity of the lens of the eye impairs normal light input. As a consequence, the perception of patterned input and form also are altered. The second clinical condition is **strabismus**, commonly referred to as *lazy eye*. Strabismus affects the temporal correlation of input to

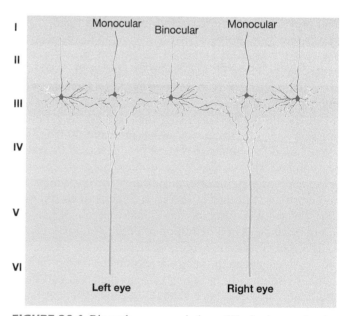

FIGURE 26-1 Binocular neurons in layer III of primary visual cortex receive input from neurons in layer IVC. The neurons in layer IV receive input either from the left or from the right eye. The neurons in layer III receive inputs from neurons in layer IV, some of which received inputs from the right and some from the left eye. Thus, the mixing of information from the two eyes occurs in layer III.

binocular neurons. Normally, both eyes are directed to exactly the same point on a visual target because the activity of a given muscle in one eye is precisely balanced by reciprocal activity in the opposite eye. The result is that corresponding points on the two retinas image the same location in visual space at the same time. So what happens to ocular dominance columns and binocular neurons in the visual cortex in these two clinical conditions?

Animal experiments in both monkeys and cats have addressed these questions and, in so doing, revealed that the wiring of cells in the primary visual cortex has a remarkable, although temporally limited, degree of plasticity. It is to be emphasized that the cat and monkey visual systems are more developed at birth than is the human visual system. Although ocular dominance columns develop prenatally in these animals, their organization can be influenced postnatally by altering the balance of visual input. This is accomplished by suturing one eyelid closed. This procedure eliminates all patterned vision in the sutured eye but does not otherwise injure the eye.

Monocular visual deprivation produces a dramatic alteration in the ocular dominance columns in primary visual cortex. When a radioactive tracer is injected into the open eye, the columns are found to have expanded (Figure 26-2 ■). Significantly, the overall configuration and periodicity of the columns is unaffected. In contrast, when a radioactive tracer is injected into the sutured eye, the columns (stripes) of the closed eye are found to have severely narrowed compared with the unsutured eye.

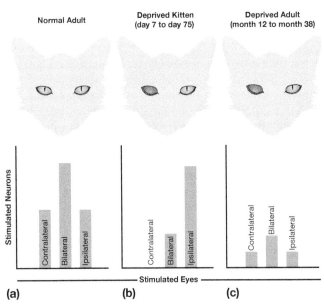

FIGURE 26-3 Monocular deprivation affects development of the ocular dominance columns in the primary visual cortex. (a) The ocular dominance columns in the normal animal. (b) Ocular dominance columns in the adult animal deprived of vision *during* the critical period, demonstrating that ocular dominance columns respond only to the non-sutured eye. (c) Ocular dominance columns in the adult animal deprived of vision *after* the critical period, demonstrating that the ocular dominance columns respond to both eyes, although they may be attenuated.

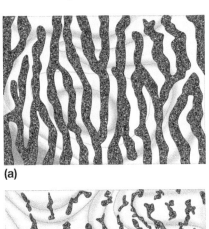

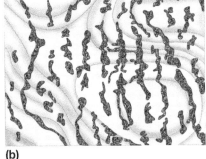

FIGURE 26-2 Monocular deprivation affects development of the ocular dominance columns in the primary visual cortex. Layer IV cells are segregated into a series of alternating stripes, with one set related to the left eye and the other to the right eye. (a) Stripes in an animal without visual deprivation. (b) Stripes in an animal with monocular deprivation.

The mechanism is as follows (Figure 26-3 ■). The two eyes compete for synaptic contacts upon stellate cells in layer IVC. The absence of light onto the retina of the sutured eye imposes a severe handicap on the closed eye in this contest. This leads to excessive pruning of the terminal arbors of geniculate cells driven by the deprived eye so that the deprived eye loses many of the connections already established at birth. The ocular dominance columns of the deprived eye thus shrink. The open eye profits in this contest by sprouting geniculate terminals beyond their usual boundary to occupy territory relinquished by terminals of the deprived eye. Thus, the columns of the open eye expand.

The functional correlate of this abnormality in the size of ocular dominance columns in monocularly deprived animals is that most neurons in the visual cortex respond exclusively to stimulation through the normal (unsutured) eye. In normal animals, most neurons in the visual cortex are binocular, although most respond more vigorously to stimulation of one eye than the other (Figure 26-3a).

This animal experimentation led to the development of the concept of a critical period. The critical period is the time during which the wiring of visual cortex neurons remains malleable and thus vulnerable to the effects of visual deprivation. For example, when one eye is sutured closed in a kitten 7 to 38 days following birth, the ocular dominance column never develops a response to the sutured eye. Thus, in the adult animal, only the nonsutured eye develops an ocular column (Figure 26-3b). In contrast, when the eye is sutured after the critical period, no alteration results in the morphology of ocular dominance columns (Figure 26-3c). This is the case even when the animal is subjected to years of monocular deprivation. Correspondingly, electrode recordings from neurons in the visual cortex of animals visually deprived as adults reveal a normal distribution of binocular neurons.

Monocular closure in animals at different ages shows that kittens and macaque monkeys are vulnerable to the deleterious effects of eyelid suture only for a few months after birth. During this critical period, the deleterious effects of monocular eyelid closure can be corrected by "reverse" eyelid suture (i.e., by opening the sutured eye). The formerly shrunken deprived eye columns reexpand, but only if the reverse suture is carried out during the critical period.

Language Acquisition

Critical periods found in language acquisition are a related example, analogous to critical periods in development of vision. A considerable body of research has evolved related to the acquisition of a second language in the developing child. If the child is exposed to a second language by the age of 3, he or she will be able to acquire that second language as a native speaker. If the child is not exposed to the second language by age 7, the child will be fluent but will not have the innuendos of a native speaker. A child who is not exposed to the second language until puberty will have limitations on the number of words and, more importantly, the sense of grammar of the second language.

> **Thought Question**
>
> This is a good time to synthesize information. How are ocular dominance columns established, what is the critical period in this process, and what happens when the animal does not experience the necessary stimulus?

Map Plasticity in the Adult Nervous System

Normal (Adaptive) Map Plasticity

> **Thought Question**
>
> In preparation for this section, it is important to review information in Chapter 7 related to cortical maps. How does experience influence cortical maps?

Recall from Chapter 7 that the detail of resolution in the cortical maps of different body parts is dictated by somatosensory innervation density. For the body, innervation density is greatest in the digits (along with the tongue) such that the cortical somatosensory map for the body has its greatest extent and detail for the digits. The representational map in the postcentral gyrus has been studied extensively

in terms of its plasticity. Importantly, in any single individual (barring catastrophic events such as limb amputation or massive peripheral deafferentation), there is an intrinsic and lifelong stability in the sequential order of the representation of body parts along the postcentral gyrus. Maps may differ across individuals in terms of the proportion of cortex allotted to different body parts, depending on experience, but the topographic sequence remains stable.

MAP PLASTICITY AMONG MUSICIANS That anatomical markers of exceptional skills should exist in the brain seems intuitively obvious. This led to the study of map plasticity in the brains of professional musicians compared to nonmusicians. Long-term intensive practice in keyboard players results in increases in the volume of gray matter in those structures that participate in mediating keyboard playing. These changes are extensive enough to be detected on a macroanatomical level using specialized magnetic resonance imaging techniques. Extensive practice induces expansions not only in motor representations, but also in sensory representations. Thus, on the motor side, the volume of gray matter in the finger–hand representation in the cerebellum and in the left precentral gyrus is increased in practiced musicians relative to nonmusicians or amateur musicians. On the sensory side, changes occur in the right parietal lobe as would be anticipated given its role in processing visuospatial information and guiding skilled motor function (i.e., sight-reading musical notation, and transforming into motor plans). The right postcentral gyrus and posterior parietal lobe have greater gray matter volumes in practiced musicians. Additionally, Heschl's gyrus in the left temporal lobe also is expanded, this being a neocortical region of obvious importance in auditorily monitoring the accuracy of keyboard finger placements.

Not only does training induce an increase in gray matter volume, but plasticity also occurs in the white matter. It has been a common finding across such skill acquisition studies that there is a use-dependent functional enlargement in the CNS structures that mediate the particular skill. The term *functional* is used here because the structural reorganization of the brain has not yet been identified with the current state of neuroimaging technology.

> **Thought Question**
>
> Changes in cortical maps can be either adaptive or maladaptive. Thinking ahead, what might be the consequences of these two responses?

Map Plasticity in Response to Injury

Because innervation density is so great in the digits, and because the cortical somatosensory map has such detail of the digits, there have been numerous investigations into the question of what happens to cortical maps of the body surface when the innervation to those maps is altered. For example, what happens to the map when a finger is amputated? Does the representation of that digit atrophy and disappear? What happens to the map when a finger is stimulated more than is normal? Does it expand? The answers to these questions have obvious importance for the recovery of function following amputations of body parts or peripheral nerve injuries. These questions were initially addressed in the 1980s in experiments on monkeys, who possess an elaborate cortical representation of the digits.

When a digit is removed from the hand of a monkey, the somatosensory cortical representation of the missing finger does, indeed, seem to disappear. However, the former representation is taken over by expansions of the representations of neighboring digits. Thus, when digit 3 is amputated, the representations of digits 2 and 4 take over the area formerly represented by digit 3 (Figure 26-4 ■). Of course, in monkeys it is not possible to determine the perceptual consequences to sensory experience of this cortical reinnervation. Conversely, when the cortical input from specific digits is increased by training a monkey to use them for a rewarded task repeated thousands of times, the cortical representation of those active digits expands at the expense of other less used digits. Significantly, the *receptive fields* of neurons in the expanded cortical regions are correspondingly smaller than those of the fingers of the untrained hand, thereby providing a more detailed cortical representation of the trained fingers. Thus, the receptive field becomes smaller with training (i.e., greater synaptic density for more precise localization) while, concomitantly, the overall size of the map becomes larger (i.e., more cortex is devoted to this function).

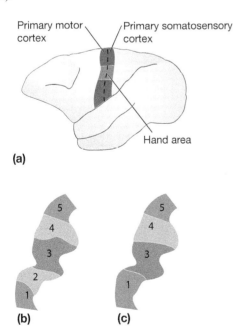

FIGURE 26-4 Cortical maps change in the area for the hand of an animal when a digit is removed. The numbers indicate the digit. (a) Somatosensory and motor cortices for the hand area. (b) Distribution of digit representations within the somatosensory and motor cortices when all five digits are present. (c) Redistribution of the digit representations when digit 2 is removed.

Maladaptive Plasticity
Phantom Limb Pain

A particularly compelling example of map plasticity concerns the *phantom limb phenomenon* that occurs in humans who have sustained amputations. People with amputated extremities often continue to experience vivid sensations from the missing limb—sensing not only its continued existence, but its movement and, sometimes, excruciating pain related, for example, to a perception that the limb is locked in an awkward and painful posture. The appearance of phantom limb sensations indicates that the cortical representation of the extremity in the postcentral gyrus remains, despite the amputation. Further, the perceptual illusion results from the projection of postcentral activation into the perceptual operations of the somatic sensory system. The phantom limb is usually perceived as an integral part of the body image. Leg and arm phantoms are frequently foreshortened, terminating at their distal ends in a normally sized foot or hand. Thus, the general representation of the body form in the postcentral gyrus has been preserved, although it has been modified by the magnification factors for different body parts.

What occurs in some of these individuals who experience phantom limb pain is a reorganization of sensory input to the primary somatosensory cortex. This reorganization is explained by a mechanism consistent with that underlying the reorganization seen following amputation of a digit in monkeys. Namely, body part representations adjacent to the missing extremity invade the deafferented cortex.

To understand what happens in people who have amputated extremities, several factors must be understood. First, recall that the representation of the hand is located in the contralateral cortex adjacent to the representation of the face (see Figure 7-7). Thus, representation of the hand is between the arm and the face. When an extremity is amputated, afferents from the face invade the cortex formerly innervated by afferents from the missing hand. The map of the hand remains as a complete and very detailed map; the topography of all the digits is faithfully represented, despite the fact that the hand is no longer there and the innervation originates elsewhere. At least over the short term, the hand representation within the area of cortex now invaded by the face or arm is still interpreted by the brain as occurring in the missing hand. As a consequence, stimulation of the face evokes not only the expected experience of facial stimulation, but also sensation referred to the phantom hand (Figure 26-5 ■).

Thought Question

Here's a question to stretch your mind. Given that phantom limb pain occurs because of maladaptive plasticity, what might be the prognosis for rehabilitation?

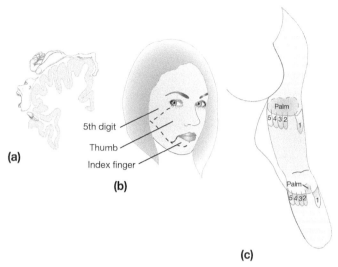

FIGURE 26-5 Phantom hand sensation evoked by stimulation of the face or arm. (a) Somatosensory homunculus illustrating the relationship of the normal hand to the arm and face. (b) In the patient with perception of a phantom limb, stimulation of facial areas produces phantom sensations of the missing hand. (c) Likewise, in the patient with perception of a phantom limb, stimulation of the forearm and brachium produces phantom sensations of the entire missing hand, including all digits.

At one time, it was thought such cortical reorganization might be an adaptive process after amputation that protects the person from developing phantom limb pain. However, there is a high positive correlation between the magnitude of phantom limb pain and the extent of cortical reorganization in the representational map. Although the cause of phantom limb pain remains speculative, this cortical reorganization occurs in all persons experiencing phantom limb pain. However, it has been noted that this cortical reorganization also occurs among people who have amputations with nonpainful phantoms. Thus, an adapted and changed postcentral representational map appears to be a necessary, but not sufficient, condition for the development of a painful phantom. In some cases, this cortical reorganization seems to be maintained dynamically by continuing peripheral input. When anesthetization of the amputation stump by blockade of the brachial plexus leads to an elimination of pain during the period of arm anesthesia, there is a reversal to normal of the postcentral maps. But this is not seen in all people with amputations who

have painful phantoms. So what are potential explanations for the cortical reorganization?

Changes in the dynamics of network operation in existing neuronal assemblies is one possibility; activation of silent synapses is probably involved as well (see Chapter 4). This is likely involved in changes that appear almost instantaneously. But this also appears to be a factor in the maintenance of longer-term changes, as mentioned earlier with anesthetization of an amputated stump. Structural changes may be operative in long-term changes. One possibility is the capture of denervated neurons by collateral sprouting in surviving innervations. Sprouting could occur at every level of the somatic afferent system after peripheral denervation. Therefore, sprouting even in the dorsal entry zone of the spinal cord could account for the large areas of change found in the postcentral cortical map. This mechanism may account for the significant changes in postcentral representational maps, where large-scale shifts on the order of 12 to 20 mm seem too large to be accounted for by changes in the dynamics of local circuit operation.

The paradoxical activation of the hand representation by stimulation of the face or shoulder is a maladaptive plastic change of no functional utility to somatic sensory perception. Nonetheless, these findings on the phantom limb phenomenon demonstrate that intact sensory systems have the capacity to gain access to CNS structures they do not normally serve. What this means for rehabilitation is not clear at this time, but the principle that an intact neural system can be exploited to activate a dormant one is certainly exciting.

Fibromyalgia

Another important clinical example of aberrant plasticity of the nervous system is fibromyalgia. There is increasing evidence that some, if not a major, contribution to this syndrome of diffuse musculoskeletal pain is due to central nervous system sensitization. It is not clear which came first, the muscular pain syndrome or the central nervous system changes. In any event, there appears to be a genetic predisposition to this chronic pain syndrome. Polymorphism of the catecholamine methyltransferase gene (COMT) implicates a possible genetic aberrant capability of serotonin and catecholamine metabolism. This may be only a substrate for the changes that eventually take place in the

Neuropathology Box 26-1: Mirror Therapy and Phantom Limb Pain

In 2007, researchers at the Walter Reed Army Medical Center reported using mirror therapy for treating phantom limb pain. They used three types of visualization. One group of individuals was trained in mental visualization, one group viewed a covered mirror, and the third group observed a

reflected image in a mirror. The group of individuals who viewed the intact limb in the mirror had significant reduction of the phantom pain. This concept builds on the approach of Ramachadran, who introduced this approach to retraining the brain to decrease phantom experiences in 1996.

brain of the individual with this syndrome. In many individuals with fibromyalgia, triggering events can be identified that may vary from actual muscle injury to viral or bacterial infections. Once the symptoms are established, functional neuroimaging demonstrates decreased dopaminergic activity throughout the brain and increased activation in the insula, anterior cingulate, and somatosensory cortex. In addition, spinal fluid markers of neurogenesis are altered, with increased brain-derived neurotrophic factor (BDNF) and abnormal levels of substance P. These factors are especially active in many plastic behaviors. However, the concurrent symptoms of sleep disorders and depression present in many of these people tend to cloud a more definitive explanation for this chronic problem.

CLINICAL CONNECTIONS
Cataracts and Strabismus in Infants

Amblyopia refers to decreased visual acuity in one eye without detectable organic disease of the other eye. *Amblyopia ex anopsia* is a severe form of amblyopia attributable to nonuse and cortical suppression of vision. It develops when the retina is deprived of patterned visual stimulation, but vision may be partially or totally recoverable. Animal experimentation has provided important guidelines to the treatment of infants with cataracts and severe strabismus.

In children, amblyopia ex anopsia is caused by any dense opacity of the ocular media, most commonly due to dense unilateral cataract or severe ptosis. Reverse suture experiments in kittens and monkeys provide a strong rationale for early intervention in such children. Effective therapy depends on the early surgical removal of the offending cataract and vigorous patching of the normal eye, along with appropriate refractive correction. Indeed, the newborn infant suffering from dense, bilateral lens opacities must be treated soon after birth to avoid permanent visual loss from bilateral amblyopia. Cataract extraction performed after the critical period has elapsed prevents the child from having the possibility of enjoying normal vision.

By documenting the visual outcome in children after surgical removal of congenital cataracts performed at different ages, it has been established that the critical period in humans extends for at least several years after birth. This finding agrees with the fact that the visual system of humans is less well developed at birth than that of the macaque. Likewise, patching the dominant eye to improve vision in a person with amblyopia seems fruitless if instigated beyond the end of the critical period. However, after the critical period has ended, the visual system is impervious to the deleterious effects of sensory deprivation. Thus, in adults, a lack of patterned visual input induced by slowly advancing cataracts does not permanently impair visual function. Removal of the cataracts, even decades after their development, fully restores visual function.

Thought Question

Compare and contrast the recovery of vision in infants with severe congenital cataracts, kittens in which the eye is sewn shut, and adults with cataracts.

Several important caveats must be attached to extrapolating these experimental findings to clinical practice. First, comparing a cataract in infancy to the suturing of an eyelid closed seems questionable. Are cataracts ever dense enough to exclude the amount of light eliminated by the latter experimental procedure? Second, the idea that depth perception never develops unless severe strabismus is surgically corrected during infancy is not uniformly the case.

The perception of depth depends largely on the presence of neurons in the visual cortex that respond to input from both eyes and that are capable of detecting the exceptionally small retinal disparities that result from the space separating the two eyes (the interocular separation). To some extent, children compensate spontaneously for strabismus-induced diplopia. Either viewing an object at very close range (2 inches or so) or tilting the head such that the affected eye is aligned with the normal eye (refer to Chapter 18) would result in at least some retinal disparity detecting cells being activated. Thus, the total elimination of any binocular experience whatsoever during the critical period cannot always be assumed. If even a few binocular neurons survive, the essential substrate for stereopsis may exist in a person who alternately fixates with the two eyes. Appropriate and rigorous vision therapy to regain binocular fixation (fusion) may then restore stereopsis, even after decades of alternate ocular fixation.

Adults with Visual Loss

Among adults who are blind, there is evidence for changes to polymodal association areas. Similarly, in experiments in which juvenile mammals (rats, monkeys, or cats) are deprived of vision, the number of neurons that respond to somatosensory and auditory information increases in multimodal areas such as the superior colliculus, the anterior ectosylvian region (cats), and the parietal cortex (primates). Furthermore, experiments have demonstrated that areas that typically respond to visual stimuli in animals with sight begin to respond to other stimuli in animals deprived of sight. As examples, the anterior ectosylvian cortex becomes predominantly auditory or somatosensory in those animals that are deprived of sight; Brodmann's area 19 (which is visual cortex in monkeys) responds to tactile stimulation in monkeys without sight.

Use of behavioral, electrophysiological, and neuroimaging techniques has demonstrated similar changes in people who lose sight (and also in those who lose hearing). As an example, fMRI studies have demonstrated increased recruitment of the auditory areas in the inferior parietal lobe (Brodmann's area 40) when individuals who are blind process stimuli from other modalities. Taking this a step further, there is evidence that the primary cortex for a modality that is lost (e.g., loss of vision) might be able to process other modalities; in addition, the association cortices associated with that modality might become responsive to other modalities. In humans, then, studies with MEG and PET, and with combined fMRI and TMS, have demonstrated that the posterior visual areas are activated during somatosensory processing in people who are blind, whereas the auditory areas are activated during visual and somatosensory processing in people who are deaf. Mechanisms underlying cross-modal plasticity are under investigation.

PLASTICITY IN HUMANS DURING RECOVERY FROM BRAIN DAMAGE

Clinical Preview ·················

Melissa Arndt was just admitted, following a brain injury, to the acute rehabilitation unit where you work. You are committed to utilizing the most up-to-date information in determining the appropriate intervention strategy for her. Some of your colleagues have suggested that you should begin with compensatory strategies to allow her to improve function as quickly as possible. Others suggest that you should never use compensatory strategies. As you read through this section, consider the following:

- What is known about motor recovery following brain injury in adults?

- Does sufficient evidence exist to guide you in your decision regarding use of compensatory strategies?

In both animals and humans, the nature of cortical reorganization that follows damage to the CNS varies depending on age, the extent and location of brain injury, the specific brain pathology, and the implementation of appropriate rehabilitative training. Additionally, individual variation in anatomy, development, and function plays an as-yet-undefined role. Thus, it should not be surprising that the study of patient populations has yielded a bewildering variety of plastic brain changes following injury.

The patterns of reorganization thus far described do seem to follow a logical rule when considered at a systems level: that is, the reorganization is within system. In Alzheimer's disease, for example, neuroimaging reveals that functional compensation occurs within the memory system: surviving hippocampal neurons may be more active than normal (i.e., doing the same with less), or information processing may be shifted to different modes within the linked memory system (e.g., to the prefrontal cortex for working memory). Similarly, in motor recovery following stroke, reorganization occurs in other components of the motor system.

Recovery from Stroke

Animal models have been used in experimental exploration of the changes that might occur following stroke and other neurological injuries. Findings from rodents that are subjected to experimental lesions demonstrate increased synaptogenesis and alterations in the number and shape of dendrites. These changes all demonstrate that the brain responds to the lesion, whether or not specific rehabilitation strategies are implemented. Furthermore, in animal models of stroke, it has been shown that synaptogenesis and dendritic remodeling are associated with increases in neurological activity of *motor maps* in both ipsilesional and contralesional cerebral cortex. With training, there is an upregulation (or increased synthesis) of BDNF, which is known to be important in neurogenesis and in learning.

Neuroimaging data in humans using a variety of brain activation tasks suggest that functional recovery after stroke is mediated primarily by an evolving reorganization of cortical activity within the perilesional cortex and structures connected to the lesion site within the damaged hemisphere—and not by a shifting of function exclusively to the contralateral undamaged hemisphere, although this may occur. Structural and metabolic brain imaging and electrophysiological recording document reorganization of neuronal activity in both ipsilesional and contralesional primary motor cortices and the dorsal premotor cortex.

Neuroimaging studies are beginning to shed light on how to predict which individuals are likely to recover motor function following stroke. For example, individuals with low contralesional primary motor cortex activity and evidence of motor evoked potentials (MEPs) in response to transcranial magnetic stimulation (TMS) are more likely to recover from stroke-associated motor deficits than are individuals who do not exhibit such responses. Additionally, some individuals have measurable MEPs following stimulation with TMS, whereas others do not. Those with measurable MEPs appear to have a better prognosis. Individuals who lack the MEP response can be further divided through use of diffusion tensor imaging, which allows for assessment of the white matter tracts in the brain. Diffusion tensor imaging is an MRI technique dependent on structural characteristics of water diffusion that can specifically image white matter connections between brain regions. People with significantly lower white matter tract integrity on the ipsilesional side were unlikely to have meaningful recovery. Preliminary examination of corticospinal tracts suggests that integrity of these tracts may be the most important factor with respect to recovery during the acute stage following a stroke, whereas changes on local motor cortex circuitry might be most important at three months poststroke. Nervous system stimulation using techniques such as TMS is also under investigation. Almost all of the studies to date have demonstrated increased excitability in response to such stimulation of the ipsilesional motor cortex (M1). However, these trials had small sample sizes and confirmatory studies are needed.

Recovery from stroke appears to be mediated by mechanisms that are unique to this mode of brain damage and does not occur following, for example, traumatic brain injury—at least insofar as this has been revealed by the study of animal models. In traumatic brain injury, perilesional cortex (lying outside of a rim of glial scar tissue) generates a favorable microenvironment that facilitates two cellular events: (1) axonal sprouting such that new connections can be formed within the injured hemisphere and (2) a migration of immature neurons into perilesional cortex from periventricular stem cells.

> ### Thought Question
>
> What are the possible cortical changes that underlie recovery of hand function and language following a cortical stroke?

Impact of Pharmacological Interventions

A number of pharmacological interventions have received considerable attention as potential mediators of neuroplasticity following stroke. Here, the concept is to use pharmacological agents that can upregulate the endogenous intracellular signaling pathways that drive synaptic plasticity. For example, amphetamine has been implicated in neuroplasticity through its role in modulation of cortical excitability. Preclinical studies have been carried out with rodent and cat models to test whether amphetamine treatment in combination with activity can enhance recovery.

Amphetamines are of interest because they are known to increase presynaptic release of dopamine and norepinephrine while inhibiting neurotransmitter uptake. Another approach is to use drugs that enhance the activity of the cholinergic system. This system is of interest because it is known to modulate neural activity throughout the cortex and has been demonstrated to enhance memory and executive function in people who have Alzheimer's disease. While the findings are enticing, it should be noted from the outset that the data from a number of studies remain contradictory. One possible explanation for the differences in findings among studies is that other factors, such as motivation, may play an important modulating role that needs to be accounted for.

Emerging Principles Related to Recovery from Stroke

It appears that a common theme in plasticity research is that plasticity is distributed functional and/or structural changes that occur in multiple, not single, areas. Nowhere is this more clearly illustrated than in the spinal cord. With localized traumatic spinal cord injury and intensive postinjury treadmill training, virtually the entire spinal cord undergoes a plastic redistribution of activity such that locomotor kinematics re-approximate those of normal subjects. However, the patterns of muscle activity associated with both supralesional and infralesional segments are different from those of normal subjects, indicating that novel muscle synergies underlie the recovery. Such distributed plasticity is likely subserved by mechanisms at both spinal and cortical levels.

Based on evidence available to date, some general principles are emerging with regard to plasticity and recovery following damage to the brain. First, it should be recalled that after injury or disease, **diaschisis** occurs, meaning that there is dysfunction within structurally intact brain structures. This can be conceptualized as *disfacilitation* following loss of excitatory input. Diaschisis results from changes in metabolism, blood flow, inflammation, edema, and neuronal excitability; the net result can be a temporary loss of function. Functional improvement following the injury can occur as these issues resolve. However, the functional loss can be compounded if the individual develops compensatory behavioral strategies that avoid the use of compromised areas in function. With compensatory strategies, motor circuits that could have functioned normally are neglected, thus further compounding the person's loss. Restoration of function may then require regaining control of existing, but unused, pathways. For these reasons, functional improvement should not be confused with neuroplasticity per se. Within the realm of plasticity, it is not entirely clear yet to what extent the cerebral cortex adapts to existing functions and to what extent it takes on new functions and circuits.

In this regard, Nudo and colleagues conducted a series of experiments in monkeys in which they first carefully mapped the motor cortical map for hand representation. They then created a very small cortical infarction stroke in an area representing hand and wrist motion. This resulted in the monkey having difficulty producing skilled movements of the wrist and digit and concomitant loss of the wrist and hand representation in motor cortex. Of importance, the cortical loss extended beyond the wrist and hand area of the initial lesion. With task training that required wrist and digit use, the monkeys' functional use of the extremity improved, and the representations of the motor map likewise were partially restored. These experimental findings were interpreted to mean that neural connectivity was reestablished with those areas. This experiment may illustrate diaschisis with resulting loss of connectivity due to disuse and recovery of function with reactivation of still-existing pathways through training.

> ### Thought Question
>
> Contrast neural plasticity with other potential causes of decline or improvement in function in people who have had a stroke.

What does seem clear is that recovery following brain damage involves learning; hence, a comprehensive understanding of the neurobiology of learning is important in determining appropriate rehabilitation strategies. Failure to drive specific brain functions can lead to functional degradation, as is illustrated by the experiments following amputation of digits that result in changes to cortical maps. In this context, it is important to realize that there is remodeling even in the absence of rehabilitation. Thus, three critical questions should be answered:

1. What can drive remodeling in an optimum direction?
2. How can we optimize the extent of remodeling?
3. To what extent can brain structure and function remodeling occur in days, months, and even years postinjury?

Finally, it should be recognized that age is likely to play an important role in determining the extent to which plasticity can occur. Neuroplastic capability is altered in the aged brain. Widespread neuronal synaptic atrophy occurs with reduction in experience-dependent synaptic potentiation, synaptogenesis, and cortical map reorganization.

Thought Question

Using what you learned in previous chapters plus information about critical periods and cortical columns and neurophysiological alterations with cortical injury, answer the following: How is an adult who sustains brain injury similar or different to a neonate with respect to redeveloping typical motor and sensory abilities?

Recovery of Hand Function

Recovery of hand function following a stroke that damages the primary motor cortex may occur by shifting activity to alternative cortical areas in the damaged hemisphere that have direct access to lower motor neurons in the spinal cord via the pyramidal system (see Chapters 11 and 20). These would include the premotor cortex, the supplemental motor area (SMA), and cingulate motor cortex—all of which are somatotopically organized and may exhibit increased activity in motor tasks involving the recovered hand. Additionally, the laterality of activity may change. For example, in normal subjects, low-rate finger movement is accompanied by exclusively contralateral activation of the primary motor and premotor cortices irrespective of which hand is used. In contrast, in people who have recovered hand function following stroke, use of the affected hand in the same low-rate finger movement is accomplished by a *bilateral* activation of the primary motor and premotor cortices.

The mechanisms underlying the foregoing neocortical plastic shifts in neural activity remain speculative for humans. But the potential makes intuitive sense. For one thing, localized body part representations are maintained by laterally directed intracortical inhibitory interneurons that release the transmitter gamma-amino butyric acid (GABA). When such inhibitory intracortical neurons are damaged,

body part representations could expand by unmasking preexisting but ineffective neural connections. Other potential mechanisms include dendritic growth and the proliferation of additional spines, axonal sprouting with new synapse formation, changes in synaptic efficacy like LTP and LTD, and rehabilitative training protocols.

Recovery of Language

The recovery of language function following stroke involves shifts in activity that occur within the language system. The study of chronic stroke patients with aphasia indicates that recovery of language is mediated by an increase in activity of undamaged, perilesional tissue in the affected left hemisphere, as well as by a recruitment of homologous "language areas" in the right hemisphere (which is, apparently, of lesser importance). However, this is not an entirely transparent revelation of recovery mechanisms. For example, hemispheric shifts in activity may depend on the phase of recovery and thus vary in a patient population over time.

In this regard, the impact of music with lyrics on the rehabilitation of people who have undergone strokes has been examined. Exposure to music enhances brain plasticity by increasing neurogenesis in the hippocampus; modifying the expression of glutamate receptor GluR2 in the auditory cortex and in the anterior cingulate; increasing brain-derived neurotrophic factor (BDNF) levels in the hippocampus and in the hypothalamus; and increasing the levels of tyrosine kinase receptor B (TrkB), a BDNF receptor, in the cerebral cortex.

Thought Question

Here's another question to stretch your mind. What might the findings on the impact of music on recovery from stroke suggest regarding the broader context of the impact of emotion and well-being on recovery?

EXERCISE AND PLASTICITY

Clinical Preview ·················

Let's return to Melissa Arndt, who you met in the last section. You are now treating her in an outpatient rehabilitation center. Some of your colleagues have suggested that it is critical to focus only on skill-based interventions. Others suggest that aerobic conditioning is of greater importance for her recovery of brain function. As you read through this section, and drawing on information presented earlier in this chapter, consider the following:

• What is known about mechanisms of changes within the nervous system following injury?

- What is known about the role of skill-based interventions and aerobic exercise with respect to neural changes and/or motor recovery following brain injury in adults?

- Does sufficient evidence exist to guide you in your decision regarding whether to use one or both of these strategies?

- Based on the available evidence, what key issues should you consider in developing an intervention program for Mrs. Arndt in the hope of facilitating neural plasticity and recovery?

- Is it possible that changes in function represent behavioral changes but do not represent neural plasticity?

Animal Models

Because map plasticity has been shown to occur in the adult human cerebral cortex as a result of training, plasticity carries with it the great hope of developing and implementing novel therapies to improve the successful rehabilitation of people who have sustained strokes or other forms of nervous system injury. Work in this area is in its infancy, but preliminary results are promising.

Thought Question

Evidence is beginning to emerge regarding various physiological changes that might relate to plasticity. As you read the remainder of this chapter, make a list of all possible factors. Consider which might be mediated by learning (e.g., of skill-related activities) and which might be mediated by aerobic activities.

Exercise-induced increases have been demonstrated in rodents for BDNF, messenger ribonucleic acid (mRNA), and protein. Such changes have been demonstrated in the cerebral cortex, cerebellum, and spinal cord—sometimes in as little as 30 minutes.

In animal models (rodents and primates) of Parkinson's disease (PD), various forms of exercise, including endurance training, can lead to symptomatic changes in the disease as well as central changes within the basal ganglia and its corticostriatal connections. Specifically, animal studies have shown that exercise may reduce the degree of dopaminergic neuronal cell loss, facilitate dopamine release and synaptic occupancy, increase dopamine D2 receptor type expression, elevate neurotrophic factor function, normalize glutamatergic neurotransmission at corticostriatal synapses, reverse dendritic spine loss within the medium spiny neurons of the striatum, and enhance blood flow to the striatum with angiogenesis.

In animal models of stroke, focal ischemic lesions to the motor cortex of rodents and primates lead to loss of ability to elicit movements in adjacent regions of the cortex. This loss is prevented such that structural and functional reorganization is promoted by rehabilitative training using reaching tasks (Figure 26-6 ■). Cumulative training with restraint of the noninvolved extremity promotes movement-associated activation in the remaining motor cortex of the damaged hemisphere. Synaptogensis and increased synaptic responses occur in monkeys and rats trained in specific tasks postinjury (e.g., see the earlier discussion of digit representation within primary motor cortex). For example, in experiments with squirrel monkeys, initial motor impairment occurs following an ischemic lesion, accompanied by loss of hand representation in the motor map. After several weeks of training using tasks requiring wrist flexion and extension, both the motor maps and function improved.

So, at what point in time should intensive exercise begin? Findings to date provide conflicting insight. In some studies using animal models of stroke, intense exercise too early after injury led to exaggerated tissue loss with worse functional outcomes. However, in other situations, this seems not to be the case. For example, use of the

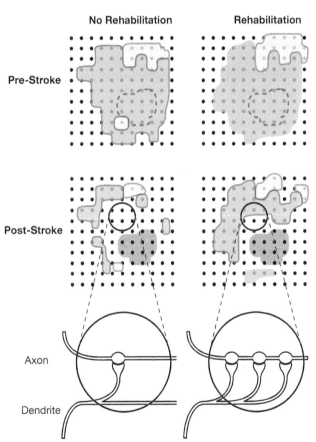

FIGURE 26-6 Cortical reorganization with exercise (motor rehabilitation) following stroke in an animal model. Following stroke, the motor map greatly diminishes in size, and synapses are reduced following stroke. Motor rehabilitation restores part of the cortical map and number of synapses.

neurotoxin 6-hydroxy dopamine to damage dopamine-producing neurons (and, therefore, produce an animal model of PD) suggest that exercise needs to start early to maximally promote recovery of function.

It should be noted that a growing body of evidence suggests that endurance exercise such as that provided by aerobic conditioning may also result in neuroplastic changes. Possibly, endurance and skill approaches to exercise work through different mechanisms.

CLINICAL CONNECTIONS

Findings are beginning to emerge from studies exploring the effects of intense exercise on structures of the brain as well as behavioral changes. One of best studies demonstrating both structural and functional changes associated with exercise relates to cognitive changes in older adults. A one-year aerobic exercise program led to increased size of the hippocampus, whereas people who were in a stretching program had an expected degree of decline in the size of the hippocampus over the year. In addition, the people who exercised vigorously had improvements on tasks that required spatial memory (thus demonstrating both anatomical and behavioral improvements). Furthermore, changes in circulating BDNF level was associated with increased hippocampal volume.

Intervention Strategies

Several strategies have been developed to assist with motor recovery that might be explained based on animal experiments of plasticity-related changes. Constraint-induced movement therapy (CIMT) is one such strategy that has been investigated in people post-CVA. In CIMT, the limb ipsilateral to the lesion is constrained for many hours during the day, such that the upper extremity with impaired function must function in an active manner. There are criteria for the degree of function required in order to use this approach, including (among others) a minimal degree of active wrist and hand movement of the affected upper extremity.

CIMT has been shown to improve motor ability of the paretic arm, as well as functional use of the extremity. The forced-use movements during CIMT presumably elicit remodeling of cortical structures subserving the improvements in motor function. A related approach is that of body weight–supported treadmill training, which has been used with people who have a variety of conditions, including spinal cord injury (SCI), cerebrovascular accident (CVA) or stroke, and developmental disabilities (such as Down syndrome), among others. In this approach, the individual exercises on a treadmill, with part of his or her body weight supported by a harness such that he or she is able to walk despite deficits of balance and motor control. The treadmill is set at a relatively vigorous speed. One possible explanation of the benefits of this approach is that, like the constraint-induced movement therapy, it could potentially drive central nervous system remodeling through the repetition of the walking movement that the patient would otherwise be too weak to perform without partial unloading of body weight.

Intervention Principles

Drawing from the available animal work, as well as recent evidence in humans, Kleim and Jones recently suggested 10 principles of experience-dependent neural plasticity and their translation to the damaged brain. Their principles are summarized as follows:

Principle 1: Use it or lose it. If a person doesn't exercise following brain damage, it is likely that degradation of pathways and further degradation of function will occur.

Principle 2: Use it and improve it. Here, the converse is considered. Training that drives a specific brain function can lead to an enhancement of that function.

Principle 3: Specificity of training matters. In this regard, evidence indicates that it is necessary to train for skill acquisition, not just for use. For example, rats with unilateral lesions in the motor cortex that were required to make skilled reaching movements showed increases in related cortical areas, whereas those rats that made unskilled movements did not. Similarly, humans trained to make skilled ankle movements showed corticospinal excitability, whereas participants who were trained on repeated nonskilled ankle movements did not.

Principle 4: Repetition matters. The number of repetitions required to produce detectable changes in the brain are much greater than the number of repetitions to produce behavioral changes. This has been demonstrated in experiments with rats in which behavioral changes occurred early in training, but several days of exercise were required for the strength and number of synapses to change.

Principle 5: Intensity matters. In addition to repetition, the intensity of the stimulus is important. Indeed, low-intensity stimulation can actually result in a weakening of synaptic responses (LTD), whereas high-intensity stimulation can strengthen the responses (LTP). There is, however, a caveat: there must be a balance between sufficient intensity to result in neuroplasticity without using intensity sufficient to result in further damage to the nervous system.

Principle 6: Timing matters. Several issues are of importance here. First, it is important to recall that brain injury is a process, not a single event. Recall from Chapter 25 that a whole series of events occur from the molecular to the cellular to structural changes. Just as there are critical periods during development, it appears that there may be critical periods during restoration of function following brain injury. If intense activity occurs too early, it may be destructive rather than constructive. And if it occurs too late, the critical period may have passed.

Principle 7: Salience matters. It is important for interventions to have meaning in order to make changes to the nervous system. It has long been known that emotion modulates the strength of memory consolidation. Similarly, experiments with animal models demonstrate that motivation and attention are necessary for rehabilitative strategies to effect changes.

Principle 8: Age matters. It is clear that the younger brain is more plastic than the older brain.

Principle 9: Transference. Transference refers to the ability of one set of neuronal circuits to promote concurrent or subsequent plasticity. For example, it is known that training on a fine-digit movement task can lead to increased corticospinal excitability with expansion of the cortical areas representing hand muscles. It has been shown that the use of repeated TMS over the motor cortex at the same time as a task is being practiced can enhance acquisition of the skill. This concept has been applied to motor retraining after stroke and is also being explored in treatment of depression.

Principle 10: Interference. Interference refers to the concept that plasticity within a given neural circuitry can interfere with or prevent expression of new plasticity within the same circuitry. In this regard, rehabilitation that benefits one skill may, in fact, be detrimental to another skill. For example, rodents trained in a spatial learning task have demonstrated that saturation of synaptic potentiation within the hippocampus impairs subsequent learning. Also, rats that are trained to use the ipsilateral extremity following a unilateral cortical lesion were found to have decreased use for the impaired forearm. This is of particular relevance in determining when and to what extent it is appropriate to retrain patients to compensate for the effects of a stroke.

While these findings are tantalizing, much is yet to be learned before we will know the most effective intervention strategies to drive both nervous system and behavioral changes in motor function following nervous system damage. For example, it is necessary to identify the patients for whom such strategies should be applied. Further, it is important to determine the time at which the intervention should occur and the most appropriate strategies, based on nature and degree of injury. Finally, much is yet to be learned about the relationship between behavioral and cortical changes that underlie changes in function.

Summary

This chapter on neuroplasticity explores long-held observations and emerging theories and constructs related to this critical area of neuroscience. We began by discussing neuroplasticity from cells to organisms, contrasting neural recovery with neural compensation. Next, we considered evidence for cortical plasticity including critical periods during development, drawing from classic experiments related to ocular dominance columns, as well as language development. We next turned our attention to map plasticity, including both appropriate adaptive plasticity and maladaptive plasticity, as evidenced by phantom limb pain.

Drawing on the principles presented in the first portion of this chapter, we then turned our attention to more recent experiments related to recovery from brain damage, with an emphasis on recovery from stroke. And finally, we dipped into some of the recent and tantalizing investigations into the role of exercise in facilitating plastic changes in the nervous system. Here, we drew from experiments in both animal models and humans. This area of investigation is just beginning to blossom; over the next decade, it has the potential to radically alter approaches to physical intervention.

Applications

1. Kenzo Kobyashi is a 15-year-old boy who sustained an incomplete thoracic cord injury with accompanying traumatic brain injury. Immediately after the injury, he was in spinal shock and had an initial Glasgow Coma Score of 14. He has now recovered sufficiently to be transferred to the rehabilitation facility where you work. You are using body weight–supported treadmill training as one part of your intervention strategy.

   a. Revisit spinal shock (Chapter 11), and explain what this condition implies in terms of Kenzo's initial condition.

   b. Now consider diaschisis (Chapter 25), and explain its role in his initial condition.

   c. Given the initial spinal shock and diaschisis, explain why you are using body weight–supported treadmill training with Kenzo.

   d. What mechanisms underlie the possibility that body weight–supported treadmill training might lead to neural recovery?

   e. What principles of neuroplasticity and recovery will guide your use of body weight–supported treadmill training and other intervention strategies?

2. Charles Young sustained a stroke resulting in a relatively mild left hemisphere lesion. He has some movement of his right hand (which is his dominant hand) but does not have sufficient control to use the hand functionally. He has slight aphasia.

   a. What are the probable neurophysiological events that will occur following brain injury, whether or not he receives rehabilitation therapy?
   b. Discuss how the ipsilateral and contralateral hemisphere regions are involved in the recovery of hand and language functions.
   c. Would you expect Mr. Young to benefit from constraint-induced movement therapy (CIMT)? Why or why not?
   d. What is the relationship of CIMT to neuroplasticity?
   e. Would you expect CIMT to be beneficial in a patient who sustained a severe stroke and who has no movement of the forearm and hand?

References

Bavelier, D., and Neville, H. J. Cross-modal plasticity: Where and how? *Nature Rev* 3:443–452, 2002.

Beck, H., Goussakov, I. V., Lie, A., et al. Synaptic plasticity in the human dentate gyrus. *J Neurosci* 20:7080–7086, 2000.

Behrman, A. L., Bowden, M. G., and Nair, P. M. Neuroplasticity after spinal cord injury and training: An emerging paradigm shift in rehabilitation and walking recovery. *Phys Ther* 86:1406–1425, 2006.

Bengtsson, S. L., Nagy, Z., Skare, S., et al. Extensive piano practicing has regionally specific effects on white matter development. *Nature Neurosci* 8:1148–1150, 2005.

Birbaumer, N., Lutzenberger, W., Montoya, P., et al. Effects of regional anesthesia on phantom limb pain are mirrored in changes in cortical reorganization. *J Neurosci* 17:5503–5508, 1997.

Bronshtein, A. I., and Petrova, E. P. The auditory analyzer in young infants. In: Brackbill, Y. and Thompson, G., eds. *Behavior in Infancy and Early Childhood*. Free Press, New York, 1967.

Buccino, G., Solodkin, A., and Small, S. L. Functions of the mirror neuron system: Implications for neurorehabilitation. *Cog Behav Neurol* 19:55–63, 2006.

Butefisch, C. M., Kleiser, R., Korber, B., et al. Recruitment of contralesional motor cortex in stroke patients with recovery of hand function. *Neurology* 64:1067–1069, 2005.

Carmichael, S. T. Cellular and molecular mechanisms of neural repair after stroke: Making waves. *Ann Neurol* 59:735–742, 2006.

Chen, R., Cohen, L. G., and Hallet, M. Nervous system reorganization following injury. *Neuroscience* 111: 761–773, 2002.

Cooke, S. F., and Bliss, T. V. P. Plasticity in the human central nervous system. *Brain* 129:1659–1673, 2006.

Dimyan, M. A., and Cohen, L. G. Neuroplasticity in the context of motor rehabilitation after stroke. *Nat Rev Neurol* 7:76–85, 2011.

Dimyan, M. A., and Cohen, L. G. Contribution of transcranial magnetic stimulation to the understanding of mechanisms of functional recovery after stroke. *Neurorehabil Neural Repair* 24:125–135, 2011.

Dipietro, L., Krebs, H. I., Fasoli, S. E., et al. Changing motor synergies in chronic stroke. *J Neurophysiol* 98: 757–768, 2007.

Erickson, K. I., Voss, M. W., Prakash, R. S., et al. Exercise training increases size of hippocampus and improves memory. *Proc Nat Acad Sci* 108:3017–3022, 2011.

Finan, P. H., Zautra, A. J., Davis, M. C., et al. Genetic influences on the dynamics of pain and affect in fibromyalgia. *Health Psychol* 29:134, 2010.

Flor, H. Phantom-limb pain: Characteristic, causes, and treatment. *Lancet Neurol* 1:182–289, 2002.

Flor, H., Elbert, T., Knecht, S., et al. Phantom-limb pain as a perceptual correlate of cortical reorganization following arm amputation. *Nature* 375:482–484, 1995.

Gaser, C., and Schlaug, G. Brain structures differ between musicians and non-musicians. *J Neurosci* 23: 9240–9245, 2003.

Grafton, S. T. Doing more with less: The plight of the failing hippocampus. *Ann Neurol* 56:7–9, 2004.

Grasso, R., Ivanenko, Y. P., Zago, M., et al. Distributed plasticity of locomotor pattern generators in spinal cord injured patients. *Brain* 127:1019–1024, 2004.

Hlustik, P., and Mayer, M. Paretic hand in stroke: From motor cortical plasticity research to rehabilitation. *Cog Behav Neurol* 19:34–40, 2006.

Hubel, D. H., and Weisel, T. N. Receptive fields and functional architecture of monkey striate cortex. *J Physiol (Lond)* 195:215, 1968.

Hubel, D. H., and Weisel, T. N. Laminar and columnar distribution of geniculocortical fibers in the macaque monkey. *J Comp Neurol* 146:421, 1972.

Hubel, D. H., and Wiesel, T. N. Functional architecture of macaque monkey visual cortex. *Proc R Soc Lond B* 198:1–59, 1977.

Hubel, D. H., Wiesel, T. N., and LeVay, S. Plasticity of ocular dominance columns in monkey striate cortex. *Phil Trans R Soc Lond B* 278:377, 1977.

Jenkins, W. M., Merzenich, M. M., Ochs, M. T., and Guic-Robles, E. Functional reorganization of primary somatosensory cortex in adult owl monkeys after behaviorally controlled tactile stimulation. *J Neurophysiol* 63:82–104, 1990.

Karni, A., Meyer, G., Jezzard, P., et al. Functional MRI evidence for adult motor cortex plasticity during motor skill learning. *Nature* 377:155–158, 1995.

Kleim, J. A., and Jones, T. A. Principles of experience-dependent neural plasticity: Implications for rehabilitation after brain damage. *J Speech, Lang, Hear Res* 51:S225–S239, 2008.

LeVay, S., Connolly, M., Houde, H., et al. The complete pattern of ocular dominance stripes in the striate cortex and visual field of the macaque monkey. *J Neurosci* 5:486, 1985.

LeVay, S., Wiesel, T. N., and Hubel, D. H. The development of ocular dominance columns in normal and visually deprived monkeys. *J Comp Neurol* 191:1, 1980.

Merzenich, M. M., Nelson, R. J., Stryker, M. P., Cynader, M. S., and Schoppman, A. Somatosensory cortical map changes following digit amputation in adult monkeys. *J Comp Neurol* 224:591–605, 1984.

Nudo, R. J., and Milliken, G. W. Reorganization of movement representations in primary motor cortex following focal ischemic infarcts in adult squirrel monkeys. *J Neurophysiol* 75:2144–2149, 1996.

O'Dell, S. J., Gross, N. B., Fricks, A. N., Casiano, B. D., Nguyen, T. B., and Marshall, J. F. Running wheel exercise enhances recovery from nigrostriatal dopamine injury without inducing neuroprotection. *Neuroscience* 144:1141–1151, 2007.

Pearson-Fuhrhop, K. M., and Cramer, S. C. Genetic influences on neural plasticity. *PMR* 2:S227–S240, 2010.

Petzinger, G. M., Fisher, B. E., Van Leeuwen, J. E., et al. Enhancing neuroplasticity in the basal ganglia: The role of exercise in Parkinson's disease. *Mov Disord.* 25(Suppl 1):S141–5, 2010.

Pothokos, K., Kurz, M. J., and Lau, Y. S. Restorative effect of endurance exercise in the chronic mouse model of Parkinson's disease with severe neurodegeneration. *EMC Neuroscience* 10:6, 2009.

Ramachandran, V. S. Behavioral and magnetoencephalographic correlates of plasticity in the adult human brain. *Proc Natl Acad Sci USA* 90:10413–10420, 1993.

Ramachandran, V. S., and Rogers-Ramachandran, D. Synaesthesia in phantom limbs induced with mirrors. *Proc Biol Sci* 263:377–386, 1996.

Rhyu, I. J., Bytheway, J. A., Kohler, S. J., et al. Effects of aerobic exercise training on cognitive function and cortical vascularity in monkeys. *Neuroscience* 167(4):1239–1248, 2010.

Sacks, O. A neurologist's notebook: Stereo Sue. *The New Yorker*, June 19, 2006, pp. 64–73.

Särkämö, T., Tervaniemi, M., Laitinen, S., et al. Music listening enhances cognitive recovery and mood after middle cerebral artery stroke. *Brain* 131:866–876, 2008.

Saur, D., Lange, R., Baumgaertner, A., et al. Dynamics of language reorganization after stroke. *Brain* 129:1371–1384, 2006.

Small, S. L. Therapeutics in cognitive and behavioral neurology. *Ann Neurol* 56:5–7, 2004.

Sutoo, D., and Akiyama, K. Regulation of brain function by exercise. *Neurobiol Dis* 13(1):1–14, 2003.

Tillerson, J. L., Caudic, W. M., Reveon, M. E., and Miller, G. W. Exercise induces behavioral recovery and attenuates neurochemical deficits in rodent models of Parkinson's disease. *Neuroscience* 119:899–911, 2003.

Tsao, J. W., et al. Mirror therapy for phantom limb pain. *N Engl J Med* 357:2206–2207, 2007.

Warraich, Z., and Kleim, J. A. Neural plasticity: The biological substrate for neurorehabilitation. *PMR* 2:S208–S219, 2010.

Weisel, T. N., and Hubel, D. H. Comparison of the effects of unilateral and bilateral eye closure in cortical unit responses in kittens. *J Neurophysiol.* 28:1029–1040, 1965.

Wolf, S. L., Winstein, C. J., Miller, J. P., et al. Effect of constraint-induced movement therapy on upper extremity function 3 to 9 months after stroke. The EXCITE randomized clinical trial. *JAMA* 296;2095–2104, 2006.

Wolpaw, J. R. Treadmill training after spinal cord injury. *Neurology* 66:466–467, 2006.

Yunnus, M. B. Fibromyalgia and overlapping disorders: The unifying concept of central sensitivity syndromes. *Semin Arthritis Rheum* 36:339, 2007.

Zacks, J. M., Michelon, P., Vettel, J. M., and Ojemann, J. G. Functional reorganization of spatial transformations after a parietal lesion. *Neurology* 63:287–292, 2004.

Zigmond, M., and Smeyne, R. J. Foreword: Exercise and the brain. *Brain Res* 1341:1–2, 2010.

PEARSON
myhealthprofessionskit™

Use this address to access the Companion Website created for this textbook. Simply select "Physical Therapy" from the choice of disciplines. Find this book and log in using your username and password to access self-assessment questions, a glossary, and more.

APPENDIX Responses to Applications

CHAPTER 1

1. Refer to Figure 1-18 to identify the sulcus limitans, alar plate, basal plate, and neural crest cells.

2. Refer to Figure 1-22 to diagram the cross-sectional representation of the embryonic spinal cord during the sixth week of development.

3. Refer to Figure 1-22. With respect to the relationship of sensory and motor information, in the adult spinal cord sensory nuclei and roots are located in the dorsal portion of the spinal cord, and motor nuclei and roots are located in the ventral portion.

4. Refer to Figure 1-23 to diagram the cross-sectional representation of the adult medulla. Note that in the adult medulla, sensory cranial nerve nuclei are located lateral to the sulcus limitans, and motor cranial nerve nuclei are located medial to the sulcus limitans.

CHAPTER 2

1. Students will need to bring or have access to the following: Figure 2-6 and Table 2-1 from the chapter, reflex hammers, cotton swabs, and safety pins.

2. The insula lies buried in the depths of the lateral fissure, hidden from view by portions of the frontal, parietal, and temporal lobes and the limbic system.

3. The circle of Willis is an arterial polygon that may be able to provide effective collateral circulation when there is occlusion of one internal carotid artery (located in the neck). It is formed by the bilateral anterior cerebral arteries, posterior communicating arteries, internal carotid arteries, posterior cerebral arteries, and the single anterior communicating artery. If one vessel is occluded, the circle of Willis may allow for collateral circulation, preventing neurological damage. See Figure 2-29.

CHAPTER 3

1. Oligodendrocytes and Schwann cells are both glial cells that form and maintain the myelin sheaths of axons. The myelinated sheaths are interrupted by periodic gaps, where ion channels are concentrated and action potentials are propagated. These gaps, called nodes of Ranvier, increase the speed of conduction. Oligodendrocytes are found in the CNS, while Schwann cells are found in the PNS. A single oligodendrocyte myelinates 7 to 70 CNS neurons. In contrast, a single Schwann cell makes up one segment of myelin in the PNS; hence, many Schwann cells are needed to myelinate a single axon. Demyelination decreases the speed of conduction because demyelination means that the insulation is lost. Multiple sclerosis is an example of a demyelinating disease of the CNS, and acute inflammatory demyelinating polyradiculoneuropathy (also known as Guillian Barré syndrome) is an example of a demyelinating disease of the PNS.

2. Glial cells function as support cells for neurons. Many of the functions of glial cells require increased numbers of glial cells. For example, in response to injury of the nervous system, astrocytes (a type of glial cell) increase both in size and in number. They can be replaced when or if destroyed. However, their ability to divide and proliferate also makes them the primary source of intrinsic tumors of the CNS.

3. The herpes simplex virus is thought to invade the peripheral nervous system via the trigeminal nerve and to be transported to the sensory ganglion of the nerve via the retrograde axoplasmic transport system. Once it gains access to the nervous system, the herpes simplex virus then resides latent in the sensory ganglion of the trigeminal nerve. Upon reactivation, the virus spreads along trigeminal axons into the brain. Trigeminal axons innervate the pia mater and arachnoid mater of the meninges in the anterior and middle fossae of the cranium (see Chapter 13). This innervation explains the characteristic distribution pattern of hemorrhagic necrotic lesions in the inferior and medial temporal lobes and orbitomedial parts of the frontal lobes. Note that acute encephalitis is discussed in greater detail in Chapter 25.

CHAPTER 4

1. Discovered in the 1800s, clostridium botulinum was known as the "sausage poison" because it was linked to improper handling of meat products. Botulinus toxin, causing botulism or food poisoning, blocks the release of acetylcholine at the neuromuscular junction. An early use was in treatment of strabismus. Current medical uses include treatment for dystonia and spasticity. Known commercially as "Botox," the clostridium toxin is also used for cosmetic purposes to temporarily diminish wrinkles.

2. See Figures 4-21, 4-22, 4-23, and 4-24. Chemical synaptic transmission is broken down into five distinct steps: synthesis, storage, release, interaction with a receptor, and inactivation. Chlordiazepoxide, prescribed for anxiety, alters transmitter–receptor interaction by increasing the frequency of opening of GABA-gated Cl^- channels. Phenelzine sulfate is a monoamine oxidase (MAO) inhibitor that prevents inactivation of MAO, thereby increasing the availability of the neurotransmitter. MAOs may be prescribed for depression. Sertraline hydrochloride, also prescribed for depression, selectively blocks the re-uptake of serotonin, thus interfering with inactivation.

3. a. The myelin sheath of axons in the central nervous system is one of the primary neuroanatomical sites of dysfunction in multiple sclerosis. With destruction of the myelin sheath, the axonal conduction is slower than in a healthy neuron. Note that the axon can also be damaged and neuronal cell death can occur. Finally, it should be noted that multiple sclerosis also affects gray matter.

   b. Elevated temperature is an aggravating factor in patients with multiple sclerosis because the reliability of conduction in the demyelinated fibers is already reduced. As temperature is raised, the ion channels in the axon membrane open and close faster. This means that the action potential occurs faster so that less current is generated in any given region of the axon. The reduction in available current reduces the safety factor. When this temperature-dependent reduction is added to the already present disease-related reduction, the conduction of action potentials may fail altogether. Because of the already compromised myelin sheath, the rise in temperature from the shower slowed conduction sufficiently to cause a change in her vision.

CHAPTER 5

1. a. The weakness of his left gastrocnemius and hamstring muscles, loss of the Achilles reflexes, and the distribution of the sensory losses, along with diagnosis of a herniated intervertebral disc, together suggest damage to the left L5-S1 nerve root.

    b. Given that the nerve roots exit below the vertebra in this region of the spinal cord, the likely herniation is located between L4 and L5. Note this is a frequent location for disc herniation.

2. a. Damage to the corticospinal tract, if complete, produces a loss of the capacity for voluntary movement. This is referred to as a paralysis. Destruction of the lower motor neurons supplying a muscle also produces paralysis.

    b. The spinothalamic tract is concerned with the conscious appreciation of pain and temperature, whereas the dorsal columns are concerned with discriminative touch and position sense. Given her symptoms, it appears that the spinothalamic tract was damaged, but the dorsal columns were spared.

    c. The ventral portion of the spinal cord was damaged bilaterally at T12. Bilateral damage to the ascending spinothalamic tracts explains Maria's bilateral diminished responses to pain and temperature. Damage to the descending corticospinal tracts explains her bilateral motor losses. These tracts are located in the ventral spinal cord. Ventral portions of the lower thoracic and lumbosacral spinal cord are vascularized by branches of the abdominal aorta. This loss of pain and temperature sensibility and of motor function corresponds to involvement of the branches of the abdominal aorta. In contrast, the posterior spinal arteries vascularize the posterior spinal cord. Maria had normal and accurate responses to light touch and position sense. This suggests that the posterior spinal arteries appear to have been spared at T12, thus preserving the dorsal columns.

CHAPTER 6

1. a. Damage to the ascending spinothalamic tract or its projections could result in a loss and/or change in the perception of pain and temperature. This includes damage to the primary afferents, the long ascending tracts of the spinal cord and brainstem, the thalamic relay nuclei, the cortical projections, or the somatosensory cortex of the parietal lobe.

    b. Mrs. Jeffries' problems are characteristic of the thalamic pain syndrome because of the description of unrelenting pain in combination with dysthesias and ataxia. This syndrome is typically caused by a vascular lesions. Small, penetrating branches of the posterior cerebral arteries nourish most of the thalamus. Occlusion of these arteries can result in the thalamic syndrome.

    c. The lesions is on the left, contralateral to her symptoms.

2. a. An astrocytoma is a tumor that develops from astrocytes. (Recall from Chapter 3 that glial cells maintain their mitotic capacity and therefore can proliferate inappropriately.)

    b. Astrocytomas are a common form of brain tumors in children. Prognosis depends on the type, location, timeliness, and success of treatment.

    c. The vestibulocerebellum is involved in the regulation of balance and eye movements. Jacquelyn's difficulty focusing, the presence of gaze nystagmus, and her problems with balance are, therefore, attributable to damages of the vestibulocerebellum. The spinocerebellum receives input from the spinal cord. Jacquelyn's wide base of support and staggering gait are symptomatic of damage of the spinocerebellum. The cerebrocerebellum is involved with skilled movement and cognition. Jacquelyn's difficulty carrying objects while walking suggests difficulty with motor planning, which can be attributed to damage of the cerebrocerebellum.

CHAPTER 7

1. a. Mr. Brown was having trouble both speaking and understanding language. Trouble speaking (decreased fluency) indicates motor aphasia; difficulty with comprehension indicates sensory aphasia. Thus, Mr. Brown had a combination of motor and sensory aphasia. Note that this is referred to as global aphasia, which will be discussed in depth in Chapters 22 and 24.

    b. Mr. Brown's motor and sensory losses were right-sided, indicating damage to the left hemisphere. In addition, he had language deficits. Language faculties for the vast majority of humans are mediated by the left cerebral hemisphere. Thus, we can be confident that Mr. Brown's lesions was in the left hemisphere. The motor loss and motor aphasia indicate the lesions involves the frontal lobe, whereas the somatosensory loss and sensory aphasia indicate that the lesions involves the parietal lobe. Thus, Mr. Brown appears to have sustained a large lesions that includes the left frontal and parietal lobes. Specifically, Mr. Brown appears to have sustained damage to Brodmann's areas 3, 1, 2, 39, 40, 4, 44, and 45.

2. a. Ms. Andrews had full comprehension of language, but difficulty producing the right words. Her problem was with fluency. Trouble speaking (decreased fluency) is termed Broca's aphasia or motor aphasia.

    b. Ms. Andrews's language deficits localize her lesions to Broca's area, which is Brodmann's areas 44 and 45 in the dominant hemisphere (see Table 7-2). Additionally, she had right arm weakness. Broca's area and the motor representation for the arm are both located laterally in the frontal lobe. Ms. Andrews's lesions is of the motor areas of the left lateral frontal lobe.

3. Mr. Brown has several risk factors for stroke, including his age, hypertension, diabetes mellitus, and hypercholesterolemia. Ms. Andrews, although she had no co-morbid issues, has social and lifestyle risk factors of smoking, use of alcohol, and stress. Both Mr. Brown and Ms. Andrews have risk factors that are modifiable by lifestyle changes, diet, and exercise.

CHAPTER 8

1. If damage occurs *rostral* to the decussation, motor function will be affected contralateral to the lesions. If damage occurs *caudal* to the decussation, motor function will be affected ipsilateral to the lesions.

2. a. The loss of kinesthesia and vibration sensibility in Chris's right leg and trunk indicates that the right dorsal column was damaged. His loss of pain and temperature sensibility of the left leg and trunk indicates damage to the right spinothalamic tract.

   b. We can assume that the injury was at spinal cord levels C8-T1 because Chris has atrophy of the intrinsic muscles of the right hand, indicating lower motor neuron damage, which can occur when there is damage either to the cell body or the nerve itself. As we will see in response to the other questions, we can rule out damage to the peripheral nerve because of other co-occurring symptoms. Additionally, Chris has loss of all cutaneous sensibility over a strip along the ulnar side of the right arm. This also indicates damage at C8-T1.

   c. The right half of Chris's spinal cord was damaged. At the level of the lesions, Chris has atrophy of the intrinsic muscles of the *right hand.* Atrophy is a lower motor neuron sign. The lower motor neurons exit the spinal cord to innervate muscles on the ipsilateral side; therefore, the right-sided atrophy indicates that the lesions is on the right side. There was a loss of all cutaneous sensibility over a strip along the ulnar side of the right arm, again indicating that the damage is on the right side. Below the lesions, he has spastic paresis on the right with exaggerated knee-jerk reflexes. Spastic paresis on the right indicates damage to the descending tract on the right. Any lesions that happens caudal to the pyramidal decussation (in the medulla) results in ipsilateral symptoms. Thus, the right-sided spastic paresis also indicates that the lesions is on the right. He had loss of kinesthesia and vibration sensibility on the right and loss of pain and temperature sensibility below C8-T1 (the level of the lesions) on the left. Loss of kinesthesia and vibration sensibility indicates damage to the dorsal columns. The dorsal columns ascend in the ipsilateral side of the spinal cord until they decussate at the level of the medulla. Hence, damage in the dorsal columns of the spinal cord also results in symptoms ipsilateral to the lesions. Finally, there was a loss of pain and temperature sensibility over the entire left half of the body at the level of the third rib. Pain and temperature sensibility is carried by the spinothalamic tract (STT). Recall that the STT decussates in the spinal cord, near the level at which the sensory neurons enter the cord. Therefore, the STT ascends the *contralateral cord;* hence, damage to the ascending tract results in symptoms contralateral to the lesions. The symptoms affect transmission of pain and temperature that entered the cord caudal to the lesions (i.e., the lower extremities and trunk).

   d. The spinal nerves that innervate the leg arise from cell bodies located in the ventral gray of the lumbar spinal cord. Therefore, injury to these structures would result in lower motor neuron symptoms in the leg, with the specific symptoms depending on the level of the injury. Chris has spastic paresis of muscles of the lower extremity, an upper motor neuron sign, which indicates damage to the descending spinal tract. He does not have lower motor neuron signs for the lower extremity. Recall, however, that he does have lower motor neuron signs for the upper extremity at the level of the lesions.

CHAPTER 9

1. a. The spinothalamic tract (STT) carries pain and temperature information.

   b. Small-diameter, lightly myelinated primary afferent fibers enter the dorsal fasciculus, where they may ascend or descend as many as three segments. They then synapse upon cell bodies in the dorsal horn of the spinal cord within Rexed's lamina I/II. The axons of the second-order neurons decussate in the anterior white commissure and then ascend the spinal cord in the contralateral anterolateral fasciculus. The second-order neurons project to the ventral posterior nucleus (VPL) of the thalamus, where they synapse on the third-order neurons. Third-order neurons project from the VPL to the postcentral gyrus of the parietal lobe. Because of the decussation, the fibers that convey the sensation of pain and temperature synapse in the VPL and postcentral gyrus *contralateral* to the extremity in which the experience of pain and temperature arose.

   c. The single lesions that could cause these symptoms is at the point at which spinothalamic tracts from both the right and left side decussate. This is in the anterior white commissure in lower cervical levels of the spinal cord, specifically including C4/5 to C8/T1. Damage to this area of the spinal cord could be the result of a condition referred to as syringomyelia, which would be confirmed by MRI.

   d. Figure 11-20 provides a depiction that illustrates a lesions similar to that of Jason's lesions.

2. a. Damage to the dorsal column–medial lemniscal system (DC-ML) results in deficits of kinesthesia, stereognosis, graphesthesia, direction of tactile stimulus, and vibration. Damage to the STT results in deficits of fast pain, temperature, light touch, and some discriminative touch.

   b. i. Loss of DC-ML and STT sensibility in the distribution of the right radial nerve.

   ii. Loss of DC-ML and STT sensibility in the right C6 dermatome.

   iii. Loss of DC-ML sensibility on the right at and below C5 dermatome.

   iv. Loss of STT sensibility on the left below C5 dermatome.

   v. Loss of STT sensibility bilaterally below C5 dermatome.

   vi. Loss of DC-ML and STT sensibility of the left side of the body.

   vii. Loss of DC-ML and STT sensibility of the left side of the body and head.

CHAPTER 10

1. a. Poliomyelitis is an acute infection that attacks ventral horn cells of the spinal cord.

   b. The ventral gray is comprised of the cell bodies of the alpha lower motor neurons. Lesions of the ventral horn will result in lower motor neuron symptoms. Such lesions will not result in upper motor neuron signs, which are associated with lesions of the descending motor tracts connecting the descending tracts to the alpha lower motor neuron.

   c. Poliomyelitis is classified as a neurogenic motor neuron disease because it affects the cell bodies of lower motor neurons. Myopathic disorders, in contrast, affect the muscle itself.

   d. No set pattern occurs with respect to which alpha lower motor neurons will be affected by the polio virus. Overall, the severity of the infection, along with the number of anterior horn cells infected, will predict the variability and severity of muscle involvement.

   e. An ounce of prevention is the best treatment. The poliomyelitis vaccine, developed in the mid-1950s, has nearly eradicated polio in the United States. Poliomyelitis is an enterovirus spreading primarily through a fecal–oral route.

Therefore, proper hand washing is also recommended to prevent spread from infected persons. During acute infection, treatment is provided to make the individual safe and comfortable. If the nerves associated with muscles of respiration are affected, mechanical ventilation may be required. For comfort, treatments may include analgesics for pain, fluids, and bed rest. After the infection has run its course, physical therapy is indicated for restoration of muscle strength and improvement of function, despite the remaining weakness.

f. Collateral sprouting is the process by which unaffected lower motor neurons form collateral branches to muscles that lost their original innervations. Such sprouting is induced by the denervation caused by the infection. The resulting collateral branches innervate muscles that had previously been innervated by the lower motor neurons that were affected by polio. Collateral sprouting does not typically result in complete reinnervation of the affected muscles. This also contributes to the variable pattern of restoration of muscle strength in people who have had polio.

g. Postpolio syndrome occurs 20 to 30 or more years after the acute paralytic disease. It is characterized by a worsening of weakness, which in turn may cause a further loss of function. Postpolio syndrome is not yet entirely understood. However, it is attributed in part to loss of lower motor neurons that occurs with aging. With aging, the lower motor neurons that formed collateral branches are taxed metabolically and may no longer function as effectively. Furthermore, muscles that were reinnervated by collateral branches do not have as robust a pattern of innervations as would normally occur. Thus, if neurons that provided collateral innervations die off through aging, the muscles affected in the process of polio may no longer be sufficiently innervated to function effectively.

2. a. Larry had both UMN and LMN signs. Hyperreflexia is a UMN sign; the fasciculations are an LMN sign. Weakness and mild atrophy could be either a UMN or LMN sign.

b. Amyotrophic lateral sclerosis (ALS) is a disorder in which both UMN and LMN symptoms are present.

c. Treatments for ALS are designed to manage symptoms and improve quality of life. Rilozule is believed to decrease damage to motor neurons by decreasing the release of glutamate, although no treatments have been found to stop the progression of the disorder. In the early stages, physical intervention is important to assist the individual to maintain joint range of motion and to preserve strength to the extent possible. As the disorder progresses, rehabilitation is important to maximize function despite the disorder and to prevent problems associated with immobility and complications (e.g., from falls). As ALS progresses, respiratory involvement is common, at which time ventilator support may be indicated.

d. ALS is a fast-progressing degenerative neurological disease that decreases life expectancy. Larry is expected to live about 5 years after diagnosis.

e. Early in the disorder, rehabilitation professionals may have a role in providing Larry with adaptive equipment to increase mobility, assisting him to learn energy-conservation techniques to decrease fatigue, and providing an exercise program designed to maintain muscle strength and range of motion and alleviate pain and stiffness. The rehabilitation professional may also work with the individual in the home and work environments to improve independence

and safety. Throughout the disorder, rehabilitation professionals would have a role in educating Larry and his family about ALS.

3. a. Myasthenia gravis is an autoimmune disease in which antibodies bind to and destroy the acetylcholine (ACh) receptors of the neuromuscular junction. In this disorder, the lower motor neuron generates the nerve impulse, which releases ACh at the neuromuscular junction. ACh crosses the neuromuscular junction, but there are fewer receptors with which it can bind (because antibody has bound to and destroyed receptors). As a consequence, muscle contractions are compromised.

b. Treatments may include a combination of medications, immunotherapy, and plasmapheresis. Anticholinesterase treatments are prescribed to increase the amount of acetylcholine present at the neuromuscular junction, immunotherapy is prescribed to alter immune response, and plasmapheresis is used to remove the circulating antibodies.

c. Physical rehabilitation cannot reverse myasthenia gravis. However, a rehabilitation professional can have an important role in treating an individual with myasthenia gravis. Examples of the focus of treatment include education about energy-conservation techniques, modification of the home and work environment, and development of compensatory strategies for safety and function.

CHAPTER 11

1. The monosynaptic reflex occurs in response to tapping the tendon of a muscle with a reflex hammer. The receptor for this reflex is the muscle spindle, which is the primary ending of the Ia afferent neuron. The Ia afferent synapses directly on the alpha motor neuron in the central nervous system (e.g., the anterior horn of the spinal cord). An example is the knee-jerk reflex. Figure 11-5 depicts this reflex.

2. The inverse myotatic reflex is an example of a polysynaptic reflex (see Figure 11-6). The receptor for this reflex is the Golgi tendon organ. Unlike the monosynaptic reflex, the Ib afferent fiber synapses on *interneurons*, which then synapse on the alpha motor neuron.

3. a. Most likely, you will have a sudden and very brisk withdrawal reaction in which you quickly lift your right foot. At the same time, you will likely have a strong extension reaction of your left lower extremity. This is referred to as the *flexor withdrawal and crossed extension* reflex.

b. This response to painful stimuli begins with excitation of nociceptors. The primary afferents involved in this response include lightly myelinated A-delta fibers that synapse with multiple interneurons. These interneurons synapse with alpha motor neurons within the anterior horn of the spinal cord. See Figures 11-7 and 11-9 for examples.

4. a. Peripheral neuropathy affects the primary afferent neurons for all sensory pathways, including the DC-ML and STT.

b. This will depend on the severity of the peripheral neuropathy. If the neuropathy is mild, she may have a delayed or diminished response. However, if the neuropathy is severe, such that most of the somatosensory neurons are destroyed, she will not have a response.

c. An individual with peripheral neuropathy may not feel sensory stimuli. This can be problematic because many such stimuli provide a warning of potential tissue damage.

She should wear properly fitting shoes to avoid tissue damage (e.g., blisters). She should inspect her feet regularly to ensure that the skin is intact. Because she may not have good proprioceptive awareness (which is important for balance control), she may require an assistive device for balance and should be cautious when walking on unpredictable terrain. (Note that proprioceptive input is one of the key components of balance.) Furthermore, she may need to rely on vision to compensate for proprioceptive and tactile loss.

CHAPTER 12

1. a. Spinal shock occurs as a result of sudden compression of the spinal cord. It is characterized by loss of all sensation, motor, and reflex activity below the level of the lesions. Spinal shock is a temporary condition, which may be followed by spastic paresis below the level of the lesions.

   b. Spastic paresis is an upper motor neuron sign. It is the result of interruption of the descending corticospinal tract, but preservation of some of the local inteneuronal connections such that, below the level of the lesions, hyperreflexive responses may occur in the absence of volitional movement.

   c. Autonomic dysreflexia is an overreaction of the sympathetic nervous system. In people with spinal cord injury above the sixth thoracic level, the normal balance of the sympathetic and parasympathetic control over blood pressure and heart rate is disrupted because the descending parasympathetic signals cannot be transmitted below the level of the injury. In Patrick's case, these signals cannot be transmitted below C8. Thus, Patrick's blood pressure was elevated and his heart rate slowed, with potentially life-threatening consequences. Common triggers of autonomic dysreflexia include bladder infections and bowel impactions.

   d. Both conditions occur because the normal modulating influence is disrupted. In the case of hyperreflexia, the corticospinal tract is disrupted such that it is not possible to control movements volitionally, yet the local interneuronal connections are still present, initiating muscle responses. In the case of autonomic dysreflexia, the parasympathetic control is lost such that the sympathetic system works locally without modulation.

   e. Symptoms of autonomic dysreflexia include pounding headachc, sudden increase in blood pressure, bradycardia, skin-flushing, and profuse sweating above the level of injury. The individual may also report blurred vision. Because autonomic dysreflexia is potentially life-threatening, it is critical to respond urgently. Initially, it is treated by sitting the individual up immediately, thus lowering blood pressure. This is followed by obtaining vital signs and then identifying and alleviating the cause.

2. a. Horner's syndrome consists of a combination of miosis (meaning a constricted pupil), ptosis (meaning drooping of the eyelid), and apparent enophthalmos (the eyeball appears to be recessed).

   b. Lesions of the central nervous system that damage the cervical spinal cord (or the lateral portions of the brainstem) may result in Horner's syndrome. Lesions of the peripheral nervous system resulting in Horner's syndrome involve preganglionic sympathetic fibers that emerge from T1 and T2, postganglionic sympathetic neurons (at any point along their course) that emerge from the superior cervical ganglion, or the superior cervical ganglion itself.

   c. The symptoms of Horner's syndrome are ipsilateral to the lesions.

   d. Tumors of the cervical spinal cord can also result in Horner's syndrome. Syringomyelia in the upper thoracic or cervical cord could likewise result in the findings of Horner's syndrome.

CHAPTER 13

1. a. • Hearing loss left ear (VIII).
   • Left facial droop (VII).
   • Talkative, but with dysarthric speech (VII).
   • Difficulty eating (VII).
   • Drooling from left side of mouth (VII).
   • Complained of dizziness and feeling "off balance" (VIII, vestibular nuclei).
   • Difficulty going sit to stand (VIII, vestibular nuclei, inferior cerebellar peduncle).
   • Wide-based, slow and uncoordinated gait (VIII, vestibular nuclei).
   • Normal discriminative touch, proprioception, and pain and temperature sensibility in the face and body (medial lemniscus and spinothalamic tracts unaffected).
   • Norrmal strength of her arms and legs (corticospinal tracts unaffected).

   b. The lesions is located at the pontomedullary junction, where all the affected structures are in close proximity.

   c. The predicted results of the corneal reflex exam are as follows: because cranial nerve VII is impaired on the left, Maria will demonstrate impaired corneal blink on the left when the reflex is elicited from either eye. Conversely, her right eye would blink normally with stimulation of either eye. Because of this, Maria may be at risk for left eye injury. An eye patch or protective eyewear is recommended.

   d. Practice testing cranial nerves VII and VIII.

   e. Maria presents with impairments of hearing, dizziness, and balance. Her functional limitations include difficulty with talking, eating, and slow gait speed and difficulty with sit to stand. She may need more time at home to complete tasks and may need help from her family. Maria may have concerns about participating in activities with her peer group—for example, eating and socializing with friends at school. She may have limitations in the classroom due to hearing loss.

2. a. Cranial nerve V (trigeminal nerve) has three peripheral branches providing somatosensory innervations to the face and motor innervation to the muscles of mastication. The motor branch travels with the mandibular sensory branch. The trigeminal nerve enters and exits the brainstem at the ventrolateral pons.

   b. Central damage to cranial nerve V can present as somatosensory loss in the distribution of its three branches, and if descending motor fibers are affected, a brisk jaw reflex may be present. Peripheral damage may present as sensory loss and weakness of the muscles of mastication.

   This cranial nerve conveys somatosensory information from the face and parts of the head (e.g., jaw) and motor function as relates to muscles of mastication. Cranial nerve V also serves as the afferent limb for the corneal reflex. Somatosensory function of cranial nerve V is tested by assessing the individual's response to light touch and the ability to discriminate between sharp and dull stimuli. Motor function of this cranial nerve is tested by having an individual clench his or her teeth and resist jaw opening and deviation. The examiner may also palpate the masseter muscles for contraction. The corneal reflex and jaw-jerk reflex also provide information about the integrity of cranial nerve V.

CHAPTER 14

1. a. Trigeminal neuralgia (also referred to as tic douloureux) is a condition in which the individual experiences neuropathic pain in the distribution of the trigeminal nerve that can be severe and disabling. The condition may be caused by compression of the trigeminal nerve from blood vessels or local tumors. Alternatively, this condition may occur in people who have multiple sclerosis, wherein demyelination of the trigeminal nerve occurs as it enters the brainstem. The condition is somewhat more common in men and may run in families.

   b. Treatments may include anticonvulsant medications, tricyclic antidepressants, decompression surgeries, and rhizotomies.

   c. Trigeminal neuralgia is a nonfatal disorder characterized by recurrences and remissions. The successive recurrences may incapacitate the patient. Because the pain is so intense, some people with this disorder may become incapacitated just from fear of an impending attack. Some people find support groups for help in understanding and coping with the condition and its recurrences.

2. Franco's presentation is remarkable for dysarthria and emotional incontinence, both of which are consistent with progressive and pseudobulbar palsy. The presence of lower motor neuron signs would indicate progressive bulbar palsy. Specifically, atrophy and fasciculations of the tongue would be expected. Therefore, it would be important to ask Franco to stick out his tongue and to observe whether he has atrophy of the tongue or fasciculations. The absence of these lower motor neuron signs would suggest pseudobulbar palsy. The presence of upper motor neuron signs would indicate pseudobulbar palsy. Therefore, it would be important to test for upper motor signs such as a hyperactive jaw-jerk reflex.

CHAPTER 15

1. Refer to images in Chapter 1 illustrating motor nuclei medial to the sulcus limitans and sensory nuclei located laterally.

2. See the descriptions and images of the syndromes provided in Chapter 15; specifically, refer to Figures 15-13 through 15-17. In addition, it would be beneficial to review cross-sectional representations from a variety of sources. Pay particular attention to the following: (a) The medial lemniscus moves from a more medial position in the caudal medulla to a more posterolateral position in the midbrain. (b) The spinothalamic tract is located in a lateral position throughout the brainstem. (c) The corticospinal tract is located in the ventral brainstem.

3. The organizing principles of the through tracts outlined in the beginning of the chapter can be applied to understand how these long tracts are positioned as they traverse the brainstem. Note how the somatosensory tracts approximate each other as they ascend the brainstem. Specifically,

observe how the dorsal column–medial lemniscus moves from its posterior position in the spinal cord to a more medial position in the rostral medulla and, finally, to a more lateral position in the midbrain such that this tract approximates the lateral spinothalamic tract. Both of these tracts then project to the VPL of the thalamus. Discuss how the pontine nuclei and fibers break up the appearance of the ventral pons. In contrast to the sensory tracts, the descending corticospinal tracts remain in the ventral brainstem throughout their descent to the spinal cord.

CHAPTER 16

1. a. Samuel was diagnosed with complex regional pain syndrome. This type of pain, by definition, is neuropathic in nature. Neuropathic pain is due to nervous system pathology in the absence of peripheral nociceptor activation. Neuropathic pain results most commonly from injury or inflammation of peripheral nerves and far less often from pathological involvement of neurons of the CNS. Nociceptive pain, in contrast, is due to the activation of peripheral nociceptors in the skin in response to tissue injury and inflammation. As such, nociceptive pain would be expected during the acute event, but should not persist three months later.

   b. Dorsal horn neurons on which both nociceptive and low-threshold touch afferents converge are called wide, dynamic-range neurons (WDRs). Wide, dynamic-range neurons may monitor the precise location of a noxious stimulus on the body surface. Following localized injury, allodynia spreads into cutaneous areas, where there is no apparent inflammation such that an ordinarily painless tactile stimulus is experienced as being painful. This occurs as a result of central sensitization. Central sensitization is both triggered and maintained by the abnormal noxious input resulting from peripheral sensitization. Central sensitization results from an altered processing by dorsal horn WDR neurons of impulses entering the spinal cord over A-beta touch afferents. This alteration is caused by a sensitization of dorsal horn neurons, whereby A-beta afferents acquire the capacity to drive WDR neurons that they previously did not drive.

   c. Injury to afferent peripheral axons can result in hyperalgesia. The axon, after injury, can undergo segmental demyelination. At these areas of demyelination, there is a remodeling of the cells membrane marked by excessive Na^+ channels. This renders the axon hyperexcitable. Samuel was experiencing severe pain and allodynia, a consequence of hyperexcitablity and ectopic discharge.

   d. No. Ectopic discharge and the alterations of WDR neurons are examples of nonproductive plasticity of the nervous system.

   e. Samuel's right lower limb was red, swollen, and warm to the touch months after the original injury and surgery. This is related to autonomic system dysfunction.

2. Modalities that rely on heat and cold decrease the activation of nociceptors in the periphery; hence, they are used to treat the injury at peripheral sites. Cold agents work by decreasing local blood flow and nerve conduction velocities. Even a modest reduction in temperature (less than 5°C) can have a substantial impact on both blood flow and nerve conduction velocity. Thus, the use of cold can affect pain through reduction of inflammation (via reduced

blood flow) and by slowing conduction of nerve impulses. Heat is used to increase local circulation and remove the mechanical irritants from the nervous system, thereby reducing nociceptive input to the CNS. Electrophysiological approaches such as ultrasound and short-wave diathermy can provide significant heating of deeper tissues via energy absorption mechanisms. In contrast to heat and cold, transcutaneous electrical nerve stimulation (TENS) acts at the afferent fibers. *High-frequency, low-intensity TENS* is used to stimulate large-diameter afferents, which in turn inhibit the responses in the dorsal horn evoked by nociceptive inputs; *low-frequency, high-intensity TENS* activates smaller C fibers in addition to the larger-diameter fibers. Furthermore, low-frequency, high-intensity TENS activates descending brainstem pathways, thereby activating the descending inhibitory systems involved in reduction of hyperalgesia. These supraspinal mechanisms provide longer-lasting pain control.

CHAPTER 17

1. The Rinne test compares hearing by bone conduction and air conduction. It is performed by placing the end of a vibrating tuning fork firmly against the mastoid process. This examines hearing by bone conduction. The subject reports when vibration is no longer heard. The U of the tuning fork is then placed beside the external auditory meatus (without touching it), and the patient again indicates when the vibration is no longer heard. This examines hearing by air conduction. Normally, the tuning fork is heard about twice as long by air conduction than by bone conduction because normally air conduction is greater than bone conduction. The Weber test is a test for lateralization. It is performed by placing the end of a vibrating tuning fork firmly against the vertex of the skull. The subject is asked to indicate where he or she hears the sound. Normally, the sound will be heard equally in both ears. If heard louder in one ear, the sound is said to be lateralized to that side.

2. a. Bacterial meningitis is an infection that spreads through the cerebrospinal fluid. This results in inflammation of the pia and arachnoid maters of the spinal cord and brain.

   b. Gentamicin is an aminoglycoside antibiotic. It has a known side effect of ototoxicity and can damage hair cells of the auditory and vestibular systems. Damage of the hair cells results in impairments of equilibrium and hearing.

   c. Ototoxicity is largely irreversible. The prognosis for these structures to heal is poor.

   d. Yes. Balance is the integration of vestibular, visual, and proprioceptive systems. Kaitlin could benefit from physical therapy to compensate for her vestibular impairments and prevent falls. She has the potential for functional improvements. Note also that bacterial meningitis could have primary effects on the vestibular system. If this occurs, the prognosis will be quite different than if the only effects on the vestibular system are a result of the gentamicin.

CHAPTER 18

1. a. Papilledema is swelling of the optic disk due to an increase in intracranial pressure. Increases in intracranial pressure can be caused by brain tumors, traumatic brain injuries, infections of the brain or meninges, and bleeding within the brain.

   b. Homonymous hemianopsia is the loss of vision from the same visual field from both eyes. This can occur with lesions posterior to the optic chiasm—specifically, unilateral lesions of the optic tract or of the visual cortex.

   c. Lower facial weakness indicates upper motor neuron damage to the corticobulbar fibers of CN VII. Injury to the facial motor nuclei or to the peripheral nerve would produce weakness of both the upper and lower facial muscles.

   d. Left arm weakness and hyperreflexia could occur with damage to the right frontal lobe motor cortex, internal capsule, or descending corticospinal tract.

   e. Damage to motor areas of the right motor cortex could explain the presence of hyperreflexia.

   f. The sensory losses described by Jennifer could occur with damage to the fasciculus cuneatus, thalamus, or right parietal lobe somatosensory cortex.

   g. Jennifer's symptoms could be explained by the presence of a tumor located in the frontal and parietal lobe affecting Brodmann's areas 4, 3, 1, 2 and the optic radiations.

2. a. Diplopia is the technical term for double vision. It signifies a disruption of binocular vision. It is caused by defective function of the extraocular muscles or of the cranial nerves that innervate them (CN III, IV, VI).

   b. For this woman, cranial nerves I, II and III are affected.

   c. The loss of vision is of the superior temporal field of each eye. The loss is homonymous. The nasal retinal portion decussates in the optic chiasm. The fields are inverted. Therefore, the inferior portion of the nerve in the optic chiasm is affected.

   d. i. Head pain suggests a space-occupying lesions. This is consistent with her gradual progression of symptoms.

      ii. Amenorrhea suggests a hormone balance, related to pituitary dysfunction.

   e. A pituitary tumor near the optic chiasm explains all of the findings.

CHAPTER 19

1. a. Nausea, vomiting, ataxia, dysmetria, intention tremor, and dysdiochokinesia are all symptoms related to cerebellar dysfunction. Her symptoms are on the right side, so this indicates a right cerebellar lesions because unilateral lesions produce ipsilateral deficits.

   b. Mrs. Patel has multiple risk factors for stroke: advanced age, hypertension, atrial fibrillation, and migraine history. An abrupt onset is also suggestive of stroke. The most likely location of the infarct is the right cerebellar hemisphere and vermis. The cerebellar peduncles could also be involved. These areas are vascularized by the vertebrobasilar system.

2. a. Yes, his work history is significant. There have been considerable efforts to understand the etiology of many neuromuscular diseases, including Parkinson's disease (PD). Environmental theory has identified several risk factors. Mining and exposure to heavy metals could be a risk factor.

   b. His lack of facial expression is characteristic of masked facies as seen in people with PD. His difficulty with swallowing is likely due to bradykinesia and rigidity, producing a slow, less efficient swallow.

   c. Mr. Bartlett is demonstrating signs and symptoms consistent with PD. He has cardinal signs of resting tremor, bradykinesia, rigidity, and postural instability.

CHAPTER 20

1. a. Rhythmic auditory stimulation (RAS) utilizes pathways from the auditory cortex to the premotor cortex, bypassing the cortico-basal ganglia-thalamo-cortico circuit.

   b. People with PD have difficulty initiating movement through the cortico-basal ganglia-thalamo-cortico circuit because of loss of dopamine in the substantia nigra of the midbrain and the resulting loss of disinhibition of the thalamus. By initiating movement via auditory stimuli, this deficit can be bypassed.

   c. As with RAS, the visual stimuli allows for initiation and continuation of movement, bypassing the cortico-basal ganglia-thalamo-cortico circuit.

2. a. Ms. Balenscu is demonstrating signs of ideomotor apraxia. She is unable to demonstrate the movements in a clinical setting but is able to perform the movements in a functional setting.

   b. Ideomotor apraxia may result from a lesions to the left hemisphere, specifically of the supramarginal gyrus and superior parietal lobule.

CHAPTER 21

1. a. The cortical regions affected by the stroke likely involve the right frontal and parietal lobes. Specifically, damage to the motor cortex accounts for her motor loss, and damage to the primary somatosensory cortex accounts for her somatosensory loss. Damage to the posterior association cortex accounts for her neglect.

   b. The presence of neglect is predictive of functional disability and poor outcomes for people with stroke. The reason for the poor prognosis is that it is very difficult for a person to compensate for a deficit if he or she is unaware that there is a deficit. This lack of awareness is due to a fundamental inability of the brain itself to attend to and interpret certain information (e.g., visual, proprioceptive). Neglect can improve with nervous system recovery. However, in instances where improvement does not occur, rehabilitation strategies are not typically effective in engaging the brain mechanisms for attention.

   c. Neglect may be detected by asking her to draw a clock face with time set at 9:20 or to bisect a line. Observing her behavior may also give clues to the presence of neglect. For example, does she bathe and groom both sides of her body? Does she eat from both sides of the plate?

   d. Her unawareness of her deficits (a cognitive negation) could be called anosoagnosia or asomatoagnosia.

2. a. Motor symptoms of PD include the following: resting tremor, bradykinesia, rigidity, and postural instability. Nonmotor symptoms include the following: cognitive decline, motivational apathy, dementia, sleepiness, hallucinations, and autonomic dysfunction.

   b. Tremor may be identified by observing the person at rest and during purposeful movement. A resting tremor will be more apparent at rest. Bradykinesia can be identified through observation of finger tapping, foot tapping, and fist opening and closing. Rigidity may be identified during passive movements of the limbs, torso and neck. Postural instability may be identified by assessing the person's ability to recover balance in response to external perturbations, such as a brisk displacement to the posterior from the pelvis or shoulders. Nonmotor signs may be identified by the individual as well as by family report. For example, the individual may report having difficulty remembering familiar names and places, taking medications on time or managing her finances. Individuals or family members may report that the spouse is now more likely to be in charge of important decisions. Clinical tests such as the WCST may also identify cognitive deficits in people with PD. Note that the person and/or family member may also describe other nonmotor symptoms such as sleepiness, fatigue, and depression. Standardized tests can also be used to quantify these difficulties.

CHAPTER 22

1. a. Positive symptoms are an exaggeration of normal function. Examples related to seizure activity include aura, illusions, hallucinations, disturbances of sensation, and convulsions.

   b. Negative symptoms reflect the loss of particular functions. Examples related to seizure activity include amnesia, loss of sensation, and impairment of mental functioning.

   c. Seizures result from sudden and excessive discharge of neurons. These events occur with discharge in the temporal, parietal, and frontal lobes and within structures of the limbic system. The symptoms associated with the seizures correspond to the location of neurons affected. For example, a person with seizure of the temporal and limbic cortex may experience anterograde amnesia because this area is responsible for storing short-term memory. In contrast, discharge of neurons in the motor cortex can result in posturing and movements associated with clonic activity or convulsions. Discharge of neurons in the somatosensory cortex results in somatosensory manifestations such as paresthesias or tingling.

   d. Other examples of positive signs, not associated with seizure, include hyperreflexia (associated with upper motor neuron disorders), tremor and rigidity (associated with Parkinson's disease), and fasciculations and fibrillations (associated with damage to the lower motor neuron). Other negative signs that we have discussed previously include hyporeflexia and hypotonia. Anopsia (or loss of vision) is another negative sign that likewise can occur with either central or peripheral damage to the visual system.

2. a. Global aphasia is a language deficit of both fluency and comprehension. The lesions includes Broca's territory anteriorly and Wernicke's territory posteriorly, as well the neocortex between them. As a result, all aspects of language are severely impaired. That is, the person with global aphasia can neither express him- or herself using propositional language (Broca's area) nor understand and interpret spoken words (Wernicke's area).

   b. Alphonso, having global aphasia, will have great difficulty with verbal communication because he will have problems both generating and comprehending language. Furthermore, if the global aphasia persists, he will not be able to read or write. However, over time, he may learn to communicate more through emotional language such as gesture, tone, and facial expression. Such emotional language—expressing responses to immediate environmental circumstances—does not exclusively depend on structures of the dominant cerebral hemisphere (as does propositional language) and most likely involves processing via the nondominant hemispheres.

   c. It is likely that in addition to global aphasia, Alphonso will also have weakness of his right arm, trunk, and leg (due to damage in the left frontal motor areas) and somatosensory losses of his right arm, trunk, and leg (due to damage of the left somatosensory areas of the parietal lobe).

CHAPTER 23

1. a. The somatosensory system contributes to balance and gait, particularly through the DC-ML, providing information about the sense of position and kinesthesia relayed from the lower extremities. The vestibular system mediates both conscious and unconscious orientation of head position and coordination of vision and head position for voluntary movement, as well mediating reflex adjustments of the motor system for posture, balance, and gait. The visual system contributes by interpreting the external environment. The motor system is the effector system through which balance and postural control mechanisms act. This system contributes both to volitional and automatic components of movement, with peripheral contributions made by muscle and LMNs and central contributions of UMNs and planning by way of the basal ganglia and thalamus. Additionally, cortical contributions are made by association areas for spatial processing, problem solving, executive functioning, and memory. In summary, Antonio could have deficits in balance related to changes in the somatosensory and/or special sensory systems, in the motor system (either cortically or peripherally), and in higher cortical processing. Individual small changes in several of these systems can be asymptomatic, while cumulative effects of small changes in many systems (as occurs with aging) can manifest in difficulties with balance and gait.

    b. Normal aging can alter each of the systems. Reaction times are known to increase with normal aging. Decreased muscle output and decreased visual acuity are also associated with normal aging. In addition, older individuals who would be considered generally healthy may typically have a number of disorders such as diabetes mellitus, hypertension, cataracts, and arthritis that can affect these various systems.

2. a. Alec is having problems with memory (i.e., word-finding, misplacing items, asking the same question throughout the day). This is characteristic of consequences of medial temporal lobe damage known to occur with AD—and to the hippocampal gyrus in particular. He is also having difficulty with emotion as evidenced by outbursts, crying, and yelling. This, too, can be associated with temporal lobe damage. His difficulties with posture, balance, and gait could be associated with neuronal losses in a variety of areas, including the motor and sensory cortices, as well as diffuse cortical and subcortical structures (e.g., generalized cerebral atrophy, basal ganglia).

    b. Although Alec and Antonio are both 77-year-old males with problems related to balance and gait, Alec has a poorer prognosis given his diagnosis of AD. AD is a progressive disorder that can lead to profound impairment and death within 5 to 10 years. Further, his emotional issues and lack of memory may decrease his safety awareness and judgment, which could in turn impair balance and gait. In contrast, Antonio's difficulties may progress slowly or not at all.

CHAPTER 24

1. a. His risk factors include HTN, atrial fibrillation, diabetes, smoking history, and obesity.

    b. Jason's symptoms lasted only 10 minutes, which is characteristic of a transient ischemic attack (TIA). Recall that a TIA is a warning sign for stroke and warrants medical attention.

    c. His symptoms are consistent with an ischemic stroke, given that the event occurred during the night and given that

TIAs are typically associated with ischemic strokes. Finally, the combination of risk factors is most closely associated with ischemic stroke. Note that both hypertension and atrial fibrillation put him at risk for developing a thrombus and throwing emboli. This is consistent with his earlier TIA and the eventual ischemic stroke.

    d. The symptoms are consistent with involvement of the left MCA and possibly the stem, given that he has impairments of the sensory, motor, and language systems. Note that it is not always possible to determine where in the blood distribution the stroke occurred during the first few hours to days after the incident.

    e. MCA strokes have a relatively poor prognosis compared with some other vessels. Larger strokes also have a poorer prognosis. At this time, it appears that his stroke may involve the stem on the left, in which case his prognosis is not as good as if the stroke occurred in a more distal branch of the artery. (Recall that when the stem is involved, the distributions of both the penetrating and distal vessels are affected.) Because the stroke is on the left, he should not have perceptual deficits, which would have further complicated his prognosis. However, he could have persistent language deficits, which can be emotionally distressing. Further, his other health issues should be considered with respect to overall prognosis.

2. a. Hemorrhagic events can result from primary intracerebral hemorrhage (i.e., direct leakage from a vessel), rupture of an aneurysm, or the rupture of an arteriovenous malformation (AVM).

    b. Types of imaging that can be used include cerebral angiography, computerized tomography scanning (CT), magnetic resonance imaging (MRI), and magnetic resonance arteriogram (MRA).

    c. The hemorrhage occurred in the left hemisphere, given that she has visual deficits on the right.

3. a. *MCA*—The infarct to the MCA, depicted in this example, affected both cortical and subcortical structures as outlined here.

    Level a: Highest level shown: only cortical areas are affected. Most of the affected territory is in the lateral hemisphere, including both frontal and parietal lobes.

    Level b: The lateral hemisphere is affected (frontal and parietal lobes) along with the anterior limb of the internal capsule.

    Level c: The same areas are affected as in Level b; in addition, subcortical areas are affected (i.e., parts of the basal ganglia).

    Level d: Inferior frontal and parietal lobe are affected and possibly the most anterior portion of the temporal lobe. All of these areas are cortical.

    This example of an infarct did not affect the temporal lobe, cerebellum, or brainstem depicted in Levels e and f.

    ACA—The infarct to the ACA, depicted in this example, affected both cortical and subcortical structures as outlined here.

    Level a: Medial surfaces of the frontal and parietal lobe (cortical areas) are affected.

    Level b: The same areas are affected as in part a; in addition, the infarct begins to encroach into the head of the caudate (subcortical area), as well as the anterior limb of the internal capsule.

    Level c: The same areas are affected as in part b; in addition, more of the basal ganglia (subcortical), more of the internal capsule, and the anterior thalamus (subcortical) are affected.

Level d: Anterior inferior frontal lobe (cortical) is affected.

This example of an infarct did not affect the temporal lobe, cerebellum, or brainstem depicted in Levels e and f.

PCA—The infarct to the PCA, depicted in this example, affected both cortical and subcortical structures as outlined here.

Level a: Medial surface of the occipital parietal lobes (cortical) is affected.

Level b: The same areas are affected as in part a; in addition, the infarct encroaches into the posterior limb of the internal capsule.

Level c: Inferior medial occipital lobe and the tail of the caudate nucleus (subcortical) are affected.

Levels d, e, f: A small portion of the inferior medial temporal lobe is affected.

b. The difference between infarcts on the right versus left is important in relation to language versus somatosensory perception and visual-spatial perception.

c. The emphasis here is on (1) the size of the lesions and the resulting deficits when the stem is infracted, as opposed to an infarct of the more distal distribution of the major arteries, and (2) the affects of lesions in the penetrating branches that affect subcortical but not cortical structures. Trace the specific areas of the cross sections that would be most likely affected with infarcts of the distal and penetrating vessels. [For example, with infarcts of the penetrating vessels, the lesions would not extend into levels (1) and (2).]

CHAPTER 25

1. a. A concussion indicates a traumatic event has affected the nervous system. Clinically, these events are considered reversible, although as was discussed, even a so-called mild concussion can result in long-term problems with higher cortical function.

b. These two scales are used to assess patients who have sustained a coma but are not appropriate for a person with an apparently mild concussion, such as that sustained by Jamie.

c. Imaging is used to determine whether a hemorrhage occurred during the injury. The fact that the imaging was normal is consistent with a mild concussion. Despite the fact that Jamie did not have any intracranial bleed, he may still have deficits as a result of biochemical and metabolic changes associated with mild axonal injury.

d. While a person can recover completely from a single concussion, he or she may have profound and permanent cognitive deficits with repeated concussions. This issue has been highlighted recently by the profound deficits experienced by some elite athletes who sustained repetitive injuries. Furthermore, second-impact concussion can lead to death because of massive edema that sometimes accompanies the second injury. This issue is equally important for school and recreational athletes. Indeed, some school systems are developing stringent guidelines regarding when a student athlete can resume play and when he or she must first recover from injury. The American Association of Neurology has developed guidelines for on-the-field examination to guide these decisions.

e. Use the literature to find current and relevant information. The use of helmets has been shown to substantially decrease the incidence and consequences of TBI.

2. a. An MRI or CTA would be used to determine whether Mark's symptoms are due to an anuerism. An angiogram would reveal whether there was an aneurismal subarachnoid hemorrhage.

b. A Glasgow coma score of 3 is one of the very lowest scores. It indicates that he has no motor response, no eye opening, and no response to verbal stimuli. He has the lowest score for each category on the Glasgow scale, indicating that he doesn't even respond to painful stimuli. This score indicates that he has sustained a severe injury. These findings correspond to a I on the Rancho Los Amigos Scale, indicating that he has no response to stimuli.

c. Because Mr. Andrews sustained a right subarachnoid hemorrhage, we would expect deficits on the left side (e.g., motor and somatosensory), along with sensory perceptual and visual perceptual deficits such as neglect, as well as generalized attentional deficits.

d. Chronic alcoholism can result in generalized cerebral atrophy and cerebellar dysfunction. Because of the atrophy, these individuals are at greater risk for a hematoma. Sensory and motor deficits due to a right hemisphere hemorrhage are, therefore, compounded by the degree to which the brain has already sustained either overt or covert generalized damage. Furthermore, should Mr. Andrews begin to recover responsiveness, the premorbid psychosocial complications of chronic alcoholism may make it difficult for him to cooperate fully and appropriately with rehabilitation, thus further impeding recovery.

CHAPTER 26

1. a. Spinal shock is the temporary and transient condition that occurs following injury to the spinal cord. It is characterized by loss of sensation, loss of voluntary movement, and loss of reflexes. The cause of this loss is thought to be the sudden interruption of facilitatory suprasegmental descending fibers that keep spinal motor neurons in a state of response readiness. The condition resolves spontaneously. Once the condition passes, the individual may recover motor and sensory function (depending on whether the injury is complete or incomplete). In addition, hyperreflexia (including spasticity) typically develops over time.

b. Diaschisis refers to dysfunction within structurally intact brain structures and results from changes in metabolism, blood flow, inflammation, edema, and neuronal excitability. The net result can be a temporary loss of function. Diaschisis, like spinal shock, is a temporary condition that can resolve on its own or may require intervention to restore activity within the suppressed pathways. Kenzo likely experienced both spinal shock and brain diaschisis from his injury.

c. Once the spinal shock and diaschisis resolve, the patient's underlying impairments and capabilities are revealed. In this example, Kenzo, who had a relatively mild TBI and an incomplete SCI, is able to begin to walk with body weight support. It is also possible that some of the recovery represents reactivation of existing pathways that were affected by diaschisis.

d. Evidence suggests that both intensity and repetition might facilitate changes in association with neural plasticity, including increased synaptogenesis, alterations in the number and shape of dendrites, and increased neurological activity in the motor map in the ipsilesional and contralesional cerebral cortex.

e. The first issue is to determine that Kenzo has sufficient movement capability to begin to walk with support of some of his body weight. If he is able to do so, it is important to begin walking, based on the principle that if he does not exercise following damage, further degradation can occur, whereas if he does exercise, it is possible that neural connections will be enhanced. Additionally, specificity matters. Because walking is of functional critical importance, he needs to practice walking to relearn walking. Finally, the treadmill allows for repetition and the body weight support facilitates intensity with safety.

2. a. Diaschisis is the first event that will likely occur following injury. With disachisis, changes occur with metabolism, blood flow, inflammation, and edema. With recovery, functional improvement may occur. In addition, neuroplasticity could occur, including the following events that have been identified during recovery from brain injury: increased synaptogenesis, alterations in the number and shape of dendrites, and increased neurological activity in the motor maps of the ipsilesional and contralesional cerebral cortex.

b. Recovery of hand function following a stroke may occur by shifting neural activity to alternative cortical areas in the damaged hemisphere and/or by change in the laterality of the activity. Similarly, the recovery of language function following stroke can be accomplished by increased activity in the perilesional tissue or by recruitment of homologous contralateral hemisphere.

c. Constraint-induced movement therapy (CIMT) has been shown to improve function for people who have had a stroke. One of the important criteria is availability of some wrist and hand movement. Given that Charles has some ability to move his hand, he may be a candidate to benefit from CIMT (assuming he meets the other basic criteria).

d. Possibly, CIMT is effective because it drives neural reorganization. CIMT may also alter function through behavioral changes without neurological reorganization. Insufficient data are available at present to determine the underlying mechanism.

e. Such an individual would not meet the criteria for use of CIMT and, therefore, would not be an appropriate candidate for this strategy.

INDEX